Savita Pahwa

Fourth International Congress of Immunology

IMMUNOLOGY 80

Progress in Immunology IV

Participants' edition in one volume

Fourth International Congress of Immunology

IMMUNOLOGY 80

Progress in Immunology IV

edited by

M.Fougereau and J.Dausset

1980

ACADEMIC PRESS

A Subsidiary of Harcourt Brace Jovanovich, Publishers

London New York Toronto Sydney San Francisco

ACADEMIC PRESS INC. (LONDON) LTD.
24/28 Oval Road, London NW1 7DX

United States Edition published by
ACADEMIC PRESS INC.
111 Fifth Avenue, New York, New York 1003

International Congress of Immunology,
4th, Paris, 1980
Immunology 80.
1. Immunology–Congresses
I. Title II. Fougereau, M
III. Dausset, J
574.2′9 QR180.3 80–49682

ISBN 0–12–262940–X

Filmset by Northumberland Press Ltd, Gateshead, Tyne and Wear
Printed in Great Britain by Fletcher and Son Ltd, Norwich

Contributors

The following is a list of all authors who contributed to this publication

ALLISON, A. C., D.Phil., B.M., F.R.C.Path.

Director, International Laboratory for Research on Animal Disease, P.O. Box 30709, Nairobi, Kenya

ALPER, A. C., M.D.

Professor of Pediatrics, Harvard Medical School; Director, Center for Blood Research, Boston, Massachusetts 02115, USA

ASKENASE, P. W., M.D.

Associate Professor of Medicine, Yale University School of Medicine, New Haven, Connecticut 06510, USA

AUSTEN, K. F., M.D.

Theodore Bevier Bayles Professor of Medicine, Harvard Medical School; Chairman, Department of Rheumatology and Immunology, Brigham and Women's Hospital, Boston, Massachusetts, USA

BACH, J.-F., M.D., D.Sc.

Professeur Agrégé d'Immunologie Clinique, Hôpital Necker, 75730 Paris Cedex 15, France

BEER, A. E., M.D.

Professor and Chairman, Department of Obstetrics and Gynecology, University of Michigan Medical Center, Ann Arbor, Michigan 48109, USA

BENACERRAF, B., M.D.

Department of Pathology, Harvard Medical School, Boston, Massachusetts, USA

BINZ, H., M.D.

Senior Lecturer, Institute of Immunology and Virology, University of Zürich, P.O.B. CH-8028 Zürich, Switzerland

BIOZZI, G., M.D.

Directeur du Groupe de Recherches genetiques de l'INSERM; Directeur de Recherche au CNRS; Chef du Service d'Immunogenetique de l'Institut Curie, Section de Biologie, 75231 Paris Cedex 05, France

BLAKE, J. T.

Research Fellow, Department of Immunology, Merck Sharp & Dohme Research Laboratories, Rahway, New Jersey, USA

BODMER, W. F., Ph.D., F.R.S.

Director of Research, Imperial Cancer Research Fund, P.O. Box 123, Lincoln's Inn Fields, London WC2A 3PX, UK

BOEHMER, H. von, M.D., Ph.D.

Member of the Basel Institute for Immunology, Postfach 4005, Basel 5, Switzerland

BONNARD, G. D., M.D., Swiss Specialty Title (FMH) Ped.

Senior Investigator, Laboratory of Immunodiagnosis, National Cancer Institute, National Institutes of Health, Bethesda, Maryland 20205, USA

CANCRO, M. P., Ph.D.

Assistant Professor, Department of Pathology, University of Pennsylvania, Philadelphia, Pennsylvania 19104, USA

CANTOR, H., M.D.

Professor of Pathology, Harvard Medical School; Chief, Laboratory of Immunopathology, Farber Cancer Institute, Boston, Massachusetts 02115, USA

CAPRA, J. D., M.D.

Professor of Microbiology and Internal Medicine, Department of Microbiology, The University of Texas Health Science Center at Dallas, Dallas, Texas, USA

CAPRON, A. R. G., M.D.

Professor of Immunology, Faculty of Medicine, Lille; Director, Centre d'Immunologie et de Biologie Parasitaire, Institut Pasteur, Lille, France

CAPRON, M., Ph.D.

Lecturer, Faculty of Medicine, Lille; Senior Research Assistant, Centre d'Immunologie et de Biologie Parasitaire, Institut Pasteur, Lille, France

CAZENAVE, P. A.

Professor, University of Paris VII; Head, Unit of Analytical Immunochemistry, Institut Pasteur, 75724 Paris Cedex 15, France

CEROTTINI, J.-C.

Director and Member, Unit of Human Cancer Immunology, Ludwig Institute for Cancer Research, Lausanne; Professor of Immunology, Faculty of Medicine, University of Lausanne, Lausanne, Switzerland

CLARK, M. R., B.Sc.

Research Student, MRC Laboratory of Molecular Biology, The Medical School, Cambridge CB2 2QH, UK

CLOSS, O., M.D., Ph.D.

Senior lecturer, Department of Immunology, University of Oslo, Norway

COHEN, SIDNEY, C.B.E., M.D., Ph.D., F.R.C.Path., F.R.S.

Professor of Chemical Pathology, Guy's Hospital Medical School; Consultant Chemical Pathologist, Guy's Hospital, London SE1, UK

COHEN, STANLEY, M.D.

Professor of Pathology, University of Connecticut Health Center, Farmington, Connecticut 06032, USA

COHN, M., Ph.D.

Fellow, The Salk Institute, P.O. Box 85800, San Diego, California 92138, USA

COOPER, M.D., M.D.

Professor, Departments of Pediatrics and Microbiology; Director, Cellular Immunobiology Unit of the Tumor Institute, University of Alabama in Birmingham, Birmingham, Alabama 35294, USA

CUELLO, A.C., M.D.

University Lecturer, Departments of Pharmacology and Human Anatomy, University of Oxford, Oxford, UK

DAUSSET, J., M.D.

Professeur au College de France; Member de l'Institut; Directeur, Unite de Recherches sur l'Immuno-genetique de la Transplantation Humaine (INSERM U.93); Institut de Recherches sur les Maladies du Sang, Hôpital Saint Louis, Paris X, France

DAVIES, A. J. S., Ph.D., D.Sc., F.I.Biol.

Head, Division of Biology, Institute of Cancer Research, Chester Beatty Research Institute, London SW3 6JB, UK

DESSAINT, J. P., M.D.

Lecturer, Faculty of Medicine, Lille; Senior Research Assistant, Centre d'Immunologie et de Biologie Parasitaire, Institut Pasteur, Lille, France

DIERICH, M. P., M.D.

Professor, Institut für Medizinische Mikrobiologie, Johannes Gutenberg-Universität, Mainz, West Germany

DIXON, F. J., M.D.

Director, Research Institute of Scripps Clinic, La Jolla, California 92037, USA

DOHERTY, P. C., M.V.Sc, Ph.D.

Professor, The Wistar Institute, Philadelphia, Pennsylvania 19104, USA

DONALDSON, V. H., M.D.

Professor of Pediatrics, Children's Hospital, Cincinnati, Ohio 45229, USA

EPPLEN, J. Th., M.D.

Deutsches Forschungsgemeinschaft Postdoctorate Fellow (University of Göttingen), City of Hope Research Institute, Duarte, California 91010, USA

ESTESS, P.

Research Fellow, Department of Microbiology, The University of Texas Health Science Center at Dallas, Dallas, Texas, USA

FAUCI, A. S., M.D.

Head, Clinical Physiology Section, Laboratory of Clinical Investigation; Deputy Clinical Director, National Institute of Allergy and Infectious Diseases, National Institutes of Health, Bethesda, Maryland, USA

FAULK, W. PAGE, M.D., B.Sc., M.R.C. Path.

Honorary Consultant, Queen Victoria Hospital, East Grinstead; Professor, Royal College of Surgeons of England, London; Director, Blond McIndoe Centre for Transplantation Biology, East Grinstead, Sussex RH19 3DZ, UK

FAUVE, R. M., M.D.

Unité d'Immunophysiologie Cellulaire, Institut Pasteur, 75015 Paris, France

FERREIRA, V. C. A., Ph.D.

Bolsista do Conselho Nacional de Desenvolvimento Cientifico e Tecnologico, Instituto Biologico, Sao Paulo, Brazil

FRANKLIN, E. C., M.D.

Professor of Medicine; Chairman, Rheumatic Diseases Study Group; Director, Irvington House Institute; New York University Medical Center, New York, New York 10016, USA

FRANSSEN, J. D.

Research Scientist, Laboratory of Animal Physiology, University of Brussels, Belgium

FUJINAMI, R. S., Ph.D.

Research Associate, Department of Immunopathology, Scripps Clinic and Research Foundation, La Jolla, California, USA; Postgraduate Research Immunopathologist, University of California, San Diego, USA

FUKS, Z., M.D.

Professor and Chairman, Department of Radiation and Clinical Oncology, Hadassah University Hospital School of Medicine, p.o.b. 12000, il-91120 Jerusalem, Israel

GALFRE, G., M.Sc., Ph.D.

Scientific Staff, MRC Laboratory of Molecular Biology, The Medical School, Cambridge CB2 2QH, UK

GECKELER, W., Ph.D.

The Salk Institute, P.O. Box 85800, San Diego, California 92138, USA

GERSHON, R. K.

Director, Laboratory of Cellular Immunology, The Howard Hughes Medical Institute; Professor of Pathology and Biology, Department of Technology, Yale University School of Medicine, New Haven, Connecticut 06510, USA

GOOD, R. A., Ph.D., M.D.

President and Director, Sloan-Kettering Institute, New York; Director of Research, Memorial Hospital, New York, New York 10021, USA

GORELIK, E., M.D., PH.D.

Visiting Scientist, National Cancer Institute, National Institutes of Health, Bethesda, Maryland 20205, USA

GOREVIC, P. D., M.D.

Assistant Professor of Medicine, State University of New York at Stony Brook, Stony Brook, New York 11794, USA

GOTTLIEB, P. D., Ph.D.

Professor of Microbiology, Department of Microbiology, University of Texas at Austin, Austin, Texas 78712, USA

GREENE, M. I., M.D., Ph.D.

Associate Professor of Pathology, Harvard Medical School, Boston, Massachusetts 02115, USA

GRESSER, I., M.D.

Institut de Recherches Scientifiques sur le Cancer, 94800 Villejuif, France

GUPTA, S. K., M.Sc.

Senior Scholar (Lady Tata Memorial Trust), All-India Institute of Medical Sciences, Ansari Nagar, New Delhi 110029, India

HARBOE, M., M.D., Ph.D.

Professor of Medicine, Department of Immunology, University of Oslo, Norway

HAYAKAWA, K., M.D., D.M.S.

Research Associate, Department of Immunology, Faculty of Medicine, University of Tokyo, Bunkyo-ku, Tokyo, Japan

HAYNES, B. F., M.D.

Senior Investigator, Clinical Physiology Section, Laboratory of Clinical Investigation, National Institute of Allergy and Infectious Diseases, National Institutes of Health, Bethesda, Maryland, USA

HERBERMAN, R. B., M.D.

Chief, Laboratory of Immunodiagnosis, National Cancer Institute, National Institutes of Health, Bethesda, Maryland 20205, USA

HOLGATE, S. T., M.D.

Research Fellow in Medicine, Harvard Medical School; Research Fellow, Department of Rheumatology and Immunology, Brigham and Women's Hospital, Boston, Massachusetts, USA

HOM, J. T.

Graduate Student in Immunology, University of California, San Francisco, California, USA

HOZUMI, T., Ph.D.

Postdoctorate Fellow (Wakunaga Pharmaceutical Co. Central Institute, Kodachi, Japan), City of Hope Research Institute, Duarte, California 91010, USA

HÜBNER, L., Ph.D.

Research Associate, Institute of Virology and Immunobiology, University of Würzburg, 8700 Würzburg, West Germany

IBANEZ, O. M., Ph.D.

Bolsista do Conselho Nacional de Desenvolvimento Cientifico e Tecnologico, Instituto Biologico, Sao Paulo, Brazil

IRVINE, W. J., D.Sc., M.B.Ch. B., F.R.C.P.Ed., F.R.C.Path., F.R.S.Ed.

Consultant Physician, Endocrine Unit/Immunology Laboratories (Medicine) and General Medicine, Royal Infirmary, Edinburgh; Reader, University Department of Medicine, Edinburgh, UK

ISHIZAKA, K., M.D.

O'Neill Professor of Medicine and Microbiology, School of Medicine, Johns Hopkins University, Baltimore, Maryland, USA

ITO, Y., M.D., Ph.D.

Recombinant DNA Research Unit, National Institute of Allergy and Infectious Diseases, National Institutes of Health, Bethesda, Maryland 20205, USA

IZUI, S., M.D.

Assistant Member, Department of Immunopathology, Research Institute of Scripps Clinic, La Jolla, California 92037, USA

JANEWAY, C. A., Jr., M.D.

Lecturer, Yale University; Investigator, Howard Hughes Medical Institute at Yale University; Assistant Professor of Pathology, Yale University School of Medicine, New Haven, Connecticut 06510, USA

JOTEREAU, F. V.

Licenciée ès Sciences Naturelles; Docteur d'Etat; Maître-Assistante à L'Université de Nantes, Faculté des Sciences, 44072 Nantes, France

KAPLAN, H. S.

Maureen D'Ambrogio Lyles Professor of Radiology; Director, Cancer Biology Research Laboratory, Stanford University School of Medicine, Stanford University Medical Center, Stanford, California 94305, USA

KAPOOR, N., M.D.

Research Associate, Sloan-Kettering Institute, New York; Assistant Attending Pediatrician, Memorial Hospital, New York, New York 10021, USA

KATZ, D. H., M.D.

Member and Chairman, Department of Cellular and Developmental Immunology, Scripps Clinic and Research Foundation, La Jolla, California 92037, USA

KAZATCHKINE, M. D., M.D.

First Chief Resident, Medical Clinic, Hôpital Broussais, Paris, France

KINLEN, L. J., D.Phil., M.R.C.P.

Gibb Fellow, Cancer Research Campaign, University of Oxford, Radcliffe Infirmary, Oxford, UK

KLEBANOFF, S. J., M.D., Ph.D.

Professor of Medicine and Chief, Division of Allergy and Infectious Disease, Department of Medicine, University of Washington, Seattle, Washington 98195, USA

KLEIN, J., Ph. D.

Director, Max-Planck-Institut für Biologie, Abteilung Immunogenetik, Tübingen; Honorary Professor, Eberhard-Karls-Universtät, Tübingen, West Germany

KLEIN, G., M.D., D.Sc.

Professor and Head, Department of Tumour Biology, Karolinska Institute, S-104 01 Stockholm 60, Sweden

KLINMAN, N. R., M.D., Ph.D.

Member, Department of Cellular and Developmental Immunology, Scripps Clinic and Research Foundation, La Jolla, California 92037, USA

KOPROWSKI, H., M.D.

Wistar Professor of Research Medicine, University of Pennsylvania; Director and Institute Professor, The Wistar Institute of Anatomy and Biology, Philadelphia, Pennsylvania 19104, USA

LANGMAN, R., Ph.D.

Assistant Professor, The Salk Institute, P.O. Box 85800, San Diego, California 92138, USA

LAMBERT, P. H., M.D.

Head, WHO Immunology Research & Training Center, University Hospital, Geneva, Switzerland

LEDER, P.

Chief, Laboratory of Molecular Genetics, National Institute of Child Health and Human Development, N.I.H., Bethesda, Maryland 20014, USA

LEDERER, E., D. Phil., D. Sc.

Professor Emeritus, Université Paris-Sud, Centre d'Orsay, 91405 Orsay, France; Director Emeritus, Institut de Chimie des Substances naturelles, CNRS, 91190 Gif sur Yvette, France

LE DOUARIN, N. M.

Agrégée ès Sciences Naturelles; Docteur d'Etat, Paris; Professeur d'Université; Directeur de Recherche au C.N.R.S.; Directeur de l'Institut d'Embryologie du C.N.R.S. et du Collège de France, 94130 Nogent-sur-Marne, France

LENNOX, E. S., Ph. D.

Medical Research Council, Laboratory of Molecular Biology, University Postgraduate Medical School, Cambridge CB2 2QH, UK

LEO, O.

Research Scientist (Belgian FNRS), Laboratory of Animal Physiology, University of Brussels, Belgium

LEWIS, R. A., M.D.

Assistant Professor of Medicine, Harvard Medical School; Assistant Physician, Department of Rheumatology and Immunology, Brigham and Women's Hospital, Boston, Massachusetts, USA

MANHAR, S. K., B.Sc.

All-India Institute of Medical Sciences, Ansari Nagar, New Delhi 110029, India

MARIAMÉ, B. Ph.D.

Research Scientist, Laboratory of Animal Physiology, University of Brussels, Belgium

MATSUNAGA, T., Ph.D.

Junior Research Scientist, Division of Biology, City of Hope Research Institute, Duarte, California 91010, USA

MAX, E. E.

Laboratory of Molecular Genetics, National Institute of Child Health and Human Development, N.I.H., Bethesda, Maryland 20014, USA

McCONAHEY, P. J., B.S

Assistant Member, Department of Immunopathology, Research Institute of Scripps Clinic, La Jolla, California 92037, USA

McCUMBER, L. J., Ph.D.

Assistant Professor, Department of Microbiology and Immunology, The University of South Carolina, School of Medicine, Columbia, South Carolina, USA

McDEVITT, H. O., M. D.

Professor of Medicine and Medical Microbiology, Division of Immunology, Stanford University School of Medicine, Stanford, California 94305, USA

MELCHERS, F.

Basel Institute of Immunology, Postfach CH-4005, Basel 5, Switzerland

MILLER, J. F. A. P., M.D., F.A.A., F.R.S.

Head, Experimental Pathology Unit, The Walter and Eliza Hall Institute of Medical Research, Post Office, Royal Melbourne Hospital, Victoria 3050, Australia

MILSTEIN, C., D.Q., Ph.D., F.R.S.

Head of Subdivision, Medical Research Council Scientific Staff, MRC Laboratory of Molecular Biology, The Medical School, Cambridge CB2 2QH, UK

MINGARI, M. C., Ph.D.

Assistant Member, Ludwig Institute for Cancer Research, Epalinges sur Lausanne, Switzerland; on leave of absence from Istituto di Microbiologia, University of Genoa, Italy

MITCHELL, G. F., R.D.A., B.V.Sc., Ph.D.

Laboratory Head, The Walter and Eliza Hall Institute of Medical Research, Victoria 3050, Australia

MITCHISON, N. A., M.A.

Hon. Director, Imperial Cancer Research Fund Tumour Immunology Unit; Professor of Zoology and Comparative Anatomy, Department of Zoology, University College London, London WC1E 6BT, UK

MIYASAKA, N., M.D.

Postdoctoral Fellow, Veterans Administration Medical Center, San Francisco, California 94121, USA

MÖLLER, E. B. I., M.D.

Acting Chairman, Department of Immunology, Karolinska Institute Medical School, S-104 05 Stockholm 50, Sweden; Consultant in Transplantation Immunology, Department of Clinical Immunology, Karolinska Institute, Huddinge Hospital, Huddinge, Sweden

MÖLLER, G., M. D., Ph.D.

Professor of Immunobiology and Chairman, Department of Immunobiology, Karolinska Institute, 104 05 Stockholm 50, Sweden

MORETTA, A., M.D.

Postdoctoral Fellow, Ludwig Institute for Cancer Research, Epalinges sur Lausanne, Switzerland

MORETTA, L., M.D.

Associate Member, Ludwig Institute for Cancer Research, Epalinges sur Lausanne, Switzerland; on leave of absence from Istituto di Microbiologia, University of Genoa, Italy

MORLING, N., M.D.

Research Assistant, Tissue-Typing Laboratory of the Blood Grouping Department, State University Hospital of Copenhagen, K-2100 Copenhagen, Denmark

MOUTON, D., Ph.D.

Chargé de Recherche à l'INSERM, Institut Curie, Section de Biologie, Paris, France

MÜLLER-EBERHARD, H. J., M.D.

Chairman, Department of Molecular Immunology; Associate Director, Science Research Institute of Scripps Clinic, La Jolla; Adjunct Professor, Department of Pathology, University of California, San Diego, La Jolla, California 92037, USA

NELSON, D. S., Ph.D., D.Sc., M.B., B.S., B.Sc.(Med.), F.R.C.P.A., F.R.A.C.P.

Director, Kolling Institute of Medical Research, Royal North Shore Hospital of Sydney, St. Leonards, New South Wales 2065, Australia

NISONOFF, A., Ph.D.

Professor of Biology, Rosenstiel Research Center, Brandeis University, Waltham, Massachusetts 02257, USA

NOBUYUKI, M., M.D.

Postdoctoral Fellow, Veterans Administration Medical Center, San Francisco, California, USA

NOSSAL, G. J. V., M.B., B.S., Ph.D.

Professor of Medical Biology, University of Melbourne; Director, The Walter and Eliza Hall Institute of Medical Research, Post Office, Royal Melbourne Hospital, Victoria 3050, Australia

NUSSENZWEIG, V., M.D.

Professor of Pathology, New York University Medical Center, New York, New York 10016, USA

NYDEGGER, U. E., M.D.

Head, Medical Service, Central Laboratory of the Swiss Red Cross, Blood Transfusion Service, 3000 Berne 22, Switzerland

OHNO, S., D.V.M., Ph.D., D.Sc.

Chairman, Division of Biology, City of Hope Research Institute, Duarte, California 91010, USA

OLDSTONE, M. B. A., M. D.

Department of Immunopathology, Research Institute, Scripps Clinic and Research Foundation, La Jolla, California 92037, USA

O'REILLY, R. J., M.D.

Associate, Sloan-Kettering Institute; Director, Bone Marrow Transplantation Program, Memorial Hospital, New York, New York 10021, USA

ORTALDO, J. R., B.S., M.S., Ph.D.

Senior Investigator-Laboratory of Immunodiagnosis, National Cancer Institute, National Institutes of Health, Bethesda, Maryland 20205, USA

OUTZEN, H. C., Ph.D.

Staff Scientist and Assistant Director (Training), The Jackson Laboratory, Bar Harbor, Maine 04609, USA

OWEN, J. J. T., M.A. B.Sc. M.D.

Sands Cox Professor and Head of the Department of Anatomy, Medical School, University of Birmingham, UK

PACIFICO, A., M.D.

Research Fellow, Department of Microbiology, The University of Texas Health Science Center at Dallas, Dallas, Texas, USA

PAHWA, R. N., M.D.

Associate, Sloan-Kettering Institute; Assistant Attending Pediatrician, Memorial Hospital, New York, New York 10021, USA

PIKE, B. L., M.Sc. (Melb.), F.A.I.M.L.S.

Cellular Immunology Unit, Walter and Eliza Hall Institute of Medical Research, Post Office, Royal Melbourne Hospital, Victoria 3050, Australia

PLATZ, P., M.D.

Research Assistant, Tissue-Typing Laboratory of the Blood Grouping Department, State University Hospital of Copenhagen, DK-2100 Copenhagen, Denmark

PREHN, R. T., M.D.

Senior Scientist, The Jackson Laboratory, Bar Harbor, Maine 04609, USA

RAMAKRISHNAN, S., M.Sc., Ph.D.

Research Officer, All-India Institute of Medical Sciences, Ansari Nagar, New Delhi 110029, India

RAUM, D. Ph.D.

Center for Blood Research, Boston, Massachusetts 02115, USA

ROSEN, F. S., M.D.

James L. Gamble Professor of Pediatrics, Harvard Medical School; Chief, Division of Immunology, Children's Hospital Medical Center, Boston, Massachusetts 02115, USA

ROSENTHAL, A. S., M.D.

Executive Director, Department of Immunology, Merck Sharp & Dohme Research Laboratories, Rahway, New Jersey, USA

ROUBINIAN, J. R., M.D.

Assistant Professor of Medicine, University of California, San Francisco, California; Clinical Investigator, Veterans Administration Medical Center, San Francisco, California, USA

RÜMKE, P., M.D.

Internist, The Netherlands Cancer Institute, 1066 CX Amsterdam, The Netherlands

RYDER, L. P., M.Sc.

Senior Biochemist, Tissue-Typing Laboratory of the Blood Grouping Department, State University Hospital of Copenhagen, D-2100 Copenhagen, Denmark

SACHS, D. H., M.D.

Chief, Transplantation Biology Section, Immunology Branch, National Cancer Institute, National Institutes of Health, Bethesda, Maryland 20205, USA

SCHIMPL, A., Ph.D., M.Sc.

Professor of Immunobiology, University of Würzburg, 8700 Würzburg, West Germany

SCHROER, J., Ph.D.

Laboratory of Immunogenetics, National Institute of Allergy & Infectious Diseases, National Institutes of Health, Bethesda, Maryland, USA

SEIDMAN, J. G.

Laboratory of Molecular Genetics, National Institute of Child Health and Human Development, N.I.H., Bethesda, Maryland 20014, USA

SELA, M., Ph.D.

Professor of Immunology, Department of Chemical Immunology, and President, The Weizmann Institute of Science, Rehovot, Israel

SHARON, N., Ph.D.

Head, Department of Biophysics, The Weizmann Institute of Science, Rehovot, Israel

SHEAR, H., Ph.D.

Assistant Professor of Medicine, Department of Medicine, New York University Medical Center, New York, New York 10016, USA

SIEGELMAN, M.

Research Fellow, Department of Microbiology, The University of Texas Health Science Center at Dallas, Dallas, Texas, USA

SIQUEIRA, M., Ph.D.

Chief, Laboratory of Immunology, Instituto Biologico, Sao Paulo, Brazil

SISSONS, J. G. P., M.D., M.R.C.P.

Assistant Member I, Department of Immunopathology, Scripps Clinic and Research Foundation, La Jolla, California, USA; Senior Lecturer in Medicine, Royal Post-graduate Medical School, London, UK

SLAVIN, S., M.D.

Senior Lecturer, Immunobiology Research Laboratory, Department of Medicine A, Hadassah University Hospital School of Medicine, p.o.b. 12 000, il-91 120 Jerusalem, Israel

STIFFEL, C., Ph.D.

Maître de Recherche au CNRS, Institut Curie, Section de Biologie, Paris, France

STROBER, S., M.D.

Associate Professor of Medicine; Chief, Division of Immunology, Department of Medicine, Stanford University Medical Center, Stanford, California 94305, USA

STROMINGER, J. L., M.D., Sc.D. (honorary)

Professor of Biochemistry, Harvard University, Cambridge, Massachusetts 02138, USA

STROSBERG, A. D., D.Sc.

Professor of Biochemical Pathology, School of Medicine, Free University of Brussels, Belgium; Professor of Biochemistry and Immunology, Faculty of Sciences, University of Paris VII, 75221 Paris cedex 05, France

SVEJGAARD, A., M.D., Ph.D.

Lecturer in Immunology, University of Copenhagen; Director of the Tissue-Typing Laboratory of the Blood-Grouping Department, State University Hospital of Copenhagen, DK-2100 Copenhagen, Denmark

TADA, T., M.D., D.M.S.

Professor and Chairman, Department of Immunology, Faculty of Medicine, University of Tokyo, Bunkyo-ku, Tokyo, Japan

TALAL, N., M.D.

Professor of Medicine, University of California, San Francisco, California; VA Medical Investigator and Chief, Immunology/Arthritis Section, Veterans Administration Medical Center, San Francisco, California, USA

TALWAR, G. P., Docteur es Sciences, F.A.M.S., F.A.Sc., F.N.A.

Jawahar Lal Nehru Fellow; Head, ICMR-WHO Research and Training Centre in Immunology; Professor and Head, Department of Biochemistry, All-India Institute of Medical Sciences, Ansari Nagar, New Delhi-110 029, India

TANDON, A., M.Sc.

Tutor, All-India Institute of Medical Sciences, Ansari Nagar, New Delhi 110029, India

THEOFILOPOULOS, A. N., M.D.

Associate Member, Department of Immunopathology, Research Institute of Scripps Clinic, La Jolla, California 92037, USA

THOMAS, J. W., M.D.

Postdoctoral Fellow, The Jewish Hospital of St. Louis, Washington University Medical Center, St. Louis, Missouri 63110, USA

THOMSEN, M., M.D.

Medical Assistant, Tissue-Typing Laboratory of the Blood Grouping Department, State University Hospital of Copenhagen, DK-2100 Copenhagen, Denmark

TIMONEN, T. T., B.M., M.D., Ph.D.

Visiting Scientist, National Cancer Institute, National Institutes of Health, Bethesda, Maryland 20205, USA

URBAIN, J.

Professeur à l'Université Libre de Bruxelles; Directeur, Laboratoire de Physiologie Animale, Rhode-St-Genese, Belgium

WALDSCHMIDT, T.

Research Fellow, Department of Microbiology, The University of Texas Health Science Center at Dallas, Dallas, Texas, USA

WECK, A. L. de, M.D.

Professor of Immunology, University of Bern; Director, Institute of Clinical Immunology, Inselspital, 3010 Bern, Switzerland

WECKER, E., M.D.

Director of the Institute of Virology and Immunobiology; Member of the Senate, Deutsche Forschungsgemeinschaft; Professor of Virology and Experimental Immunobiology, University of Würzburg, 8700 Würzburg, West Germany

WEIGERT, M.

Institute for Cancer Research, University of Pennsylvania, Philadelphia, Philadelphia 19111, USA

WEST, A., M.A.

Editor, Sloan-Kettering Institute, New York, New York, USA

WIGZELL, H.

Department of Immunology, Box 582, Biomedical Centre, Uppsala University, 75123 Uppsala, Sweden

WIKLER, M., Ph.D.

Research Scientist, Laboratory of Animal Physiology, University of Brussels Belgium

WINCHESTER, R. J., M.D.

Director, Department of Rheumatic Diseases, Hospital for Joint Diseases, Orthopaedic Institute; Professor of Medicine, Mt. Sinai School of Medicine; Adjunct Professor, The Rockefeller University, New York, New York 10003, USA

WONG, C. A., B.Sc.

Fellow of the DAAD, Institute of Virology and Immunobiology, University of Würzburg, 8700 Würzburg, West Germany

WYLIE, D. E., Ph.D.

Fellow, Department of Cellular and Developmental Immunology, Scripps Clinic and Research Foundation, La Jolla, California 92037, USA

YATZIV, S., M.D.

Associate Professor, Department of Pediatrics, Hadassah University Hospital School of Medicine, p.o. 6. 12000, il-91120 Jerusalem, Israel

ZAN BAR, I., Ph.D.

Senior Scientist, Department of Cell Biology, The Weizmann Institute of Science, Rehovot, Israel

ZINKERNAGEL, R. M., M.D., Ph.D.

Associate Professor, Division of Experimental Pathology, Universitaetsspital, 8091 Zurich, Switzerland

Preface

The fourth International Congress of Immunology was held in Paris in July 1980. On this occasion, we realized that Immunology was doing very well for a centenarian, although—and probably because—it is still raising more questions than providing answers. The spectacular achievements in the molecular approach to immunoglobulin gene organization bringing nearer elucidation of the origin of antibody diversity, the revolution provided by the explosion of hybridomas and monoclonal antibodies, the rapid progress concerning the genetics, biology and biochemistry of the major histocompatibility complex in man and mouse, the increasing interest in medical aspects of immunology and the development of new areas such as immunology of reproduction undoubtedly witness the vitality of the discipline.

Needless to say, it is impossible to write exhaustive Proceedings of such a Congress. We decided rather to prepare a book that would reflect its character and polymorphism. Outstanding specialists who were invited to deliver a symposium lecture were therefore asked to write, on this occasion, a "position paper", giving a comprehensive review of their subject, including both their own work and a synthesis of the topic. These reviews have been grouped according to the 18 themes of the Congress. As these manuscripts were prepared before the Congress, they could not therefore, include the up-to-date developments that were presented and discussed in the various workshops. For each theme, an eminent personality in the field was asked to under take the almost impossible task of writing a synthesis including the latest results and ideas which were presented up to the very last minute of the Congress.

The conjunction of the position papers and of the synthesis written "on the spot" will—we hope—constitute a real up-to-date review of Immunology in 1980.

We would like to take this opportunity to thank all the authors for their hard work in preparing and presenting their manuscripts; their contribution is inestimable. Gratitude is also due to those who worked on theme syntheses throughout the Congress, faced with the extremely difficult task of assimilating large amounts of new information and preparing a manuscript in a very few days.

The understanding and co-operation of the authors has enabled us to produce this book so soon after the Congress. We hope that it will thus provide a useful and efficient tool for immunologists throughout the world.

October, 1980

M. Fougereau, D.Sc., D.V.M
*Centre d'Immunologie
de Marseille-Luminy,
Marseille, France*

J. Dausset, M.D.
*Institut de Recherches sur
les Maladies du Sang,
Hôpital Saint Louis,
Paris, France*

Contents

The order of Themes in this publication has been changed from that of the original Congress. References given in the Theme Summaries to Theme Workshop numbers use the original numbers as listed in the book of Abstracts: Abstracts IVth International Congress of Immunology, Paris, 1980

Theme 3

Expression of Antigen Receptors in Lymphocytes and Cellular Activation Mechanisms

Presidents: K. RAJEWSKY and S. AVRAMEAS
Symposium chairman: B. ASKONAS

Theme 4

Nonantigen-specific Receptors

Presidents: N. L. WARNER and J. L. PREUD'HOMME
Symposium chairman: H. J. KUNKEL

Theme 5

Ontogeny and Differentiation of T and B Lymphocytes

Presidents: J. T. T. OWEN and J. F. BACH
Symposium chairman: M. FELDMAN

Theme 6

Cellular Co-operation

Presidents: J. F. A. P. MILLER and W. H. FRIDMAN
Symposium chairman: D. W. TALMAGE

Theme 7

Genetic Regulation of Immune Responsiveness

Presidents: B. BENACERRAF and G. BIOZZI
Symposium chairman: M. SELA

Theme 8

The MHC and its Role in the Immune Defence

Presidents: A. SVEJGAARD and L. DEGOS
Symposium chairman: W. F. BODMER

Theme 9

Viral Immunity—T Killer Cells (including Alloreactivity)

Presidents: R. M. ZINKERNAGEL and J. P. LEVY
Symposium chairman: K. T. BRUNNER

Theme 10

Tumour Immunology

Presidents: G. KLEIN and J. C. SALOMON
Symposium chairman: G. MATHÉ

Theme 11

Natural Immunity and Macrophages (including Immunity against Bacteria)

Presidents: B. R. BLOOM, G. CUDKOWICZ and P. H. LAGRANGE
Symposium chairman: D. S. NELSON

Theme 12

Effector and Escape Mechanisms in Host–Parasite Relationships

Presidents: B. H. WAKSMAN and A. CAPRON
Symposium chairman: K. S. WARREN

Theme 13

Immediate and Delayed-type Hypersensitivity

Presidents: K. F. AUSTEN and A. DE WECK
Symposium chairman: C. STEFFEN

Theme 14

Mechanisms of Autoimmune Phenomena and Immune Deficiencies

Presidents: M. D. COOPER, N. TALAL and J. P. REVILLARD
Symposium chairman: P. GRABAR

Theme 15

Complement and Immune Complexes

Theme 16

Immunology of Reproduction and Embryonic Development

Theme 17

Manipulation of the Immune System

Presidents: I. M. ROITT and P. GALANAUD
Symposium chairman: S. KOTANI

Theme 18

Human and Experimental Immunopathology

Presidents: F. ROSEN and M. SELIGMANN
Symposium chairman: J. HUMPHREY

Theme 1

Immunoglobulin Structure and Molecular Organization of Immunoglobulin Genes

Presidents:
J. D. CAPRA
M. FOUGEREAU

Symposium chairman
E. A. KABAT

1

The Arsonate System of A/J Mice: Structural and Serologic Studies on the Induced Serum Antibodies and the Products of B and T Cell Hybridomas

PILA ESTESS, LARRY McCUMBER, MARK SIEGELMAN, THOMAS WALDSCHMIDT, ANTONIO PACIFICO and J. DONALD CAPRA

Department of Microbiology, The University of Texas Health Science Center at Dallas, Texas, USA

Introduction

Homogeneous antibody populations from a variety of sources have proved extraordinarily useful in deducing the structure of immunoglobulin molecules. Serological studies of myeloma proteins, in particular, have been invaluable

Supported by grants from the National Science Foundation (PCM 79–23480) and the National Institutes of Health (AI12127).

in delineating many aspects of normal immunoglobulin structure, and both myeloma proteins and induced antibody populations in a variety of species have been used extensively in defining and localizing individual antigenic specificities or idiotypes (Slater *et al.*, 1955; Oudin and Michel, 1963; Brient and Nisonoff, 1970; Kindt, 1975). Subsequently, Williams *et al.* (1968) and Kunkel *et al.* (1974), demonstrated shared cross-idiotypic specificities among cold agglutinin and anti-γ-globulin antibody populations isolated from genetically unrelated individuals, thus suggesting a relationship between idiotype and antibody specificity.

Amino acid sequence analysis of homogeneous antibodies has also provided investigators with a much clearer understanding of antibody molecules, particularly with regard to structure–function relationships. For example, the domain hypothesis of antibody structure was only formulated when complete primary structures could be compared (Edelman and Gall, 1969). Compilation of sequence data from several laboratories yielded the concept of subgroups (Milstein, 1967; Niall and Edman, 1967; Köhler *et al.*, 1970), and hypervariable regions (Wu and Kabat, 1970; Capra, 1971; Capra and Kehoe, 1975). Affinity-labelling studies of purified antibodies have subsequently demonstrated that the hypervariable regions are those portions of the molecule that make contact with an antigenic determinant and are responsible for antigenic specificity (Goetzl and Metzger, 1970; Ray and Cebra, 1972).

Efforts in our laboratory over the past 10 years have been devoted to the serological and structural dissection of an induced antibody system in an attempt to understand its molecular and genetic implications. All A/J mice when immunized with the hapten *p*-azophenylarsonate (Ar) coupled to keyhole limpet haemocyanin (KLH), make a restricted anti-Ar response, 20–70% of which bear a cross-reactive idiotype (CRI) detected by an appropriately absorbed rabbit antiserum (Kuettner *et al.*, 1972). The CRI is linked to the immunoglobulin heavy-chain locus (Pawlak *et al.*, 1973) and has been one of the variable (V)-region markers used to demonstrate linkage of variable and constant regions of immunoglobulin heavy chains in mice. Recently, linkage of the CRI to the κ-chain locus has been demonstrated as well (Laskin *et al.*, 1977; Brown *et al.*, 1980).

All structural analyses done to date indicate that the serum anti-Ar response is extremely restricted. Thus, IgG_1 CRI-positive heavy chains isolated from conventional anti-Ar antibodies exhibit a homogeneous sequence that includes their hypervariable regions (Capra *et al.*, 1975a, b; Friedenson *et al.*, 1975; Capra and Nisonoff, 1979). CRI-negative heavy chains are homogeneous and identical to the CRI-positive chains with the exception of their hypervariable regions, which are quite heterogeneous. CRI-positive light chains appear to be drawn from at least three different V_k-subgroups, but also have homogeneous and identical hypervariable region sequences (Capra *et al.*, 1975a, b, 1976, 1977). The CRI-negative light chains were too heterogeneous to sequence.

These results suggested that the CRI-positive anti-Ar response is under strict genetic control and that the cross-idiotypic specificity measured serologically is comprised of amino acids in the hypervariable regions.

To explore further the relationships between the CRI-positive and CRI-negative molecules and to verify the presumed homogeneity of the serum anti-Ar response, we undertook the generation of monoclonal anti-Ar antibodies by somatic cell fusion. Serologic analysis of the hybridoma antibodies indicates heterogeneity in their ability to react with a conventional anti-idiotypic reagent raised against serum anti-Ar, and suggests that each hybridoma product may possess in addition to the cross-reactive idiotypic determinant(s), unique antigenic specificities (Brown *et al.*, 1980; Gill-Pazaris *et al.*, 1979; Estess *et al.*, 1979; Estess and Capra, 1980).

Several laboratories have recently studied the role of T cells and their products in the arsonate system. Suppressor T cells have been shown to bear idiotypic determinants similar to those found on B cells and/or their antibody products. Furthermore, arsonate specific suppressor factors have been characterized as proteins of a molecular weight between 33 000 and 68 000 bearing determinants encoded within the major histocompatibility complex (Lewis and Goodman, 1978; Bach *et al.*, 1979a, b; Green *et al.*, 1979). However, a serious limitation of these studies has been the lack of single clonal products—especially those that could be propagated indefinitely.

The ability to make T cell hybrids has led several investigators to use this technique to study T cell functions, T cell surface markers and T cell products (Taniguchi *et al.*, 1976; Hammerling, 1977; Goldsby *et al.*, 1977; Taniguchi and Tokuhisa, 1980; Taniguchi *et al.*, 1980). The present study was undertaken with the aim of identifying such antigenic specific, "nonimmunoglobulin" T cell products in the A/J arsonate system. Our long range goal is to understand the molecular relationships between such T cell products and the products of B cell hybridomas with similar idiotypic characteristics.

B cell hybridomas

Production and characterization of anti-Ar producing hybridomas

The 8 monoclonal anti-Ar antibodies subjected to amino acid sequence analysis were generated in 2 separate fusion experiments. In the first experiment, 21/54 hybrids were positive for anti-Ar activity. Since the frequency of positive wells was high, hybridoma products (HPs) 93G7, 91A3, 92D5 and 94B10 were cloned by limiting dilution to insure their monoclonality. In the second experiment, only 39 out of 268 potentially positive hybrids exhibited anti-Ar activity. Since the Poisson distribution predicts that when no greater than 66% of the items under study are positive for a given parameter each positive represents the result of a single event and since the frequency of anti-Ar positive hybridomas in this experiment was only 15%, the cells were not cloned and four of the hybrids, HPs 121D7, 123E6, 124E1 and 123E4 were chosen for further study. Sequence analyses indicate that in terms of the anti-Ar producing population of cells, the hybrids are monoclonal.

Supernatants from the 8 cell lines, as well as purified anti-Ar antibody from (Balb/c × A/J)F_1 ascites, were tested for their ability to inhibit the binding of radiolabelled, purified, CRI-positive antibodies from A/J mice to the rabbit anti-CRI reagent. As indicated in Table I, 4 of the hybridoma products

TABLE I

Displacement of labelled A/J anti-Ar from its rabbit anti-idiotypic antibodies by unlabelled A/J anti-Ar antibodies or hybridoma products with anti-Ar activity[a]

Unlabelled inhibitor	*Amount required for 50% inhibition (ng)*	*Per cent inhibition by 2 μg*
Serum anti-Ar	11	97
HP93G7	12	90
HP121D7	300	71
HP123E6	1900	51
HP124E1	2900	47
HP91A3	±	4
HP123E4	±	2
HP94B10	±	0
HP92D5	±	4

[a] Each assay used 10 ng of ^{125}I-labelled, specifically purified A/J anti-Ar antibodies and slightly less than an equivalent amount of anti-idiotype.
±50% inhibition never achieved.

effectively inhibit the binding of the ^{125}I-labelled CRI-positive antibodies by 50%, although marked quantitative differences in their ability to do so are evident. One hybridoma product, HP93G7, appears almost as effective as serum anti-Ar as an inhibitor of the CRI/anti-CRI reaction. The remaining 4 anti-Ar antibodies are unable to inhibit the reaction at all, even in very large amounts. By Ouchterlony analysis, all 8 hybridoma products are of the IgG1 subclass.

Amino terminal amino acid sequence analysis

Eight monoclonal anti-Ar antibodies have been selected for complete amino acid sequence analysis. Four of these molecules bear the A/J anti-Ar CRI as defined by their ability to inhibit by at least 50% the reaction between serum or ascites CRI-positive molecules and a rabbit anti-CRI reagent. The other 4 molecules are negative for the idiotype. Isolated heavy and light chains from each of the 8 molecules were subjected to automated sequence analysis. Each PTH amino acid was subjected to 3 analytical procedures and unambiguous assignments could be made at every position. The results are shown in Figs 1 and 2, where the first framework segments are compared to the

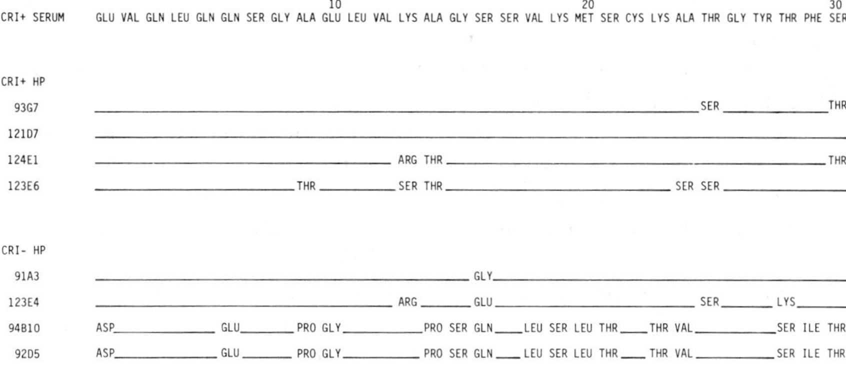

FIG. 1. *Comparison of the amino acid sequences of the CRI-positive and CRI-negative hybridoma heavy chain variable regions with the sequence of CRI-positive heavy chains found in serum. Identical residues are indicated by a line and only differences are noted.*

previously reported structures of anti-Ar heavy and light chains isolated from hyperimmunized A/J mice.

While antibodies from hyperimmune A/J serum consistently gave a nearly homogeneous sequence, clear differences from this sequence exist in the heavy chains of the hybridoma antibodies. With the exception of the Lys-Ser interchange at position 13 in HP123E6, all of the CRI-positive heavy chain substitutions could have arisen from a single base change in the DNA encoding the major (serum) sequence.

The 4 CRI-negative heavy chains can be divided into 2 groups according to their amino-terminal framework sequences (see Fig. 1). Two of the molecules, HP91A3 and HP123E4, are clearly as related to the serum heavy chain sequence as they are the CRI-positive hybridoma heavy chains; that

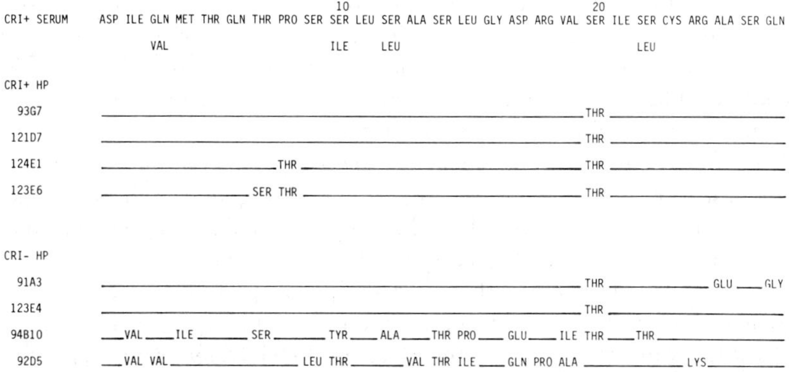

FIG. 2. *Comparison of the amino acid sequences of the CRI-positive and CRI-negative hybridoma light chains with the sequence of CRI-positive light chains found in serum. Identical residues are indicated by a line and only differences are noted. The major framework sequence of pooled antibody is listed on top with the minor sequence noted below for positions 3, 10, 12 and 22.*

is, they belong to the V_{HII} subgroup of mouse immunoglobulin in heavy chains. Again, however, definite differences from the serum sequence are noted in each of the chains. As with the CRI-positive chains, substitutions are found at several different positions.

The sequences of both CRI-positive and CRI-negative anti-Ar hybridoma light chains are illustrated in Fig. 2, along with the sequences found in serum A/J anti-Ar antibodies positive for the cross-reactive idiotype. Several striking features are apparent. First with respect to V_k-subgroup, the hybridoma molecules are *more* restricted than the CRI-positive molecules in A/J serum. Although only one heavy chain V-region subgroup is present in the serum CRI-positive molecules, it is found in association with at least 3 different light chain V-region subgroups. Six of the 8 hybridoma light chains (4 with the CRI and 2 without) clearly belong to the same V_k-subgroup as the major population of serum anti-Ar light chains, while none belong to the 2 other subgroups.

Preliminary structural analysis of V_H and V_L domains of CRI-positive hybridoma products

Figures 3 and 4 present preliminary data indicating our progress in completion of the variable domain structures of these molecules. Light chain sequences were largely derived from completely reduced and alkylated light chains treated with trypsin or chymotrypsin. Peptides were separated by molecular sieve chromatography followed by paper chromatography. Certain peptides were isolated from tryptic digests which were subjected to high pressure liquid chromatography. In some instances, CNBr digestion of intact molecules (done to isolate heavy chain V-region structures) resulted in the isolation of certain light chain V-region peptides as well. Heavy chain sequences were derived from CNBr digestion of the intact, unreduced hybridoma product. Common structural features of these molecules include the methionine residues at positions 20 and 83 which allow the single step isolation of virtually the entire V-region following CNBr digestion and chromatography on ACA-34 in 5 M guanidine. This large V-region fragment was subsequently digested with trypsin and the resultant peptides isolated as above.

The tentative amino acid sequence of the heavy chain of the CRI-positive hybridoma, 93G7, is shown in Fig. 3 where it is compared to the serum pool sequence and some fragments of the 123E6 heavy chain (also derived from a CRI-positive hybridoma). Structurally, the 2 hybridomas seem to be more related to each other than either is to the serum pool sequence. However, there are positions in which one of the two hybridoma heavy chains contains the "serum sequence" while the other does not (in 93G7, for example, positions 9, 13, 14, 24, 31, 58). While both 93G7 and 123E6 were derived from molecules which bore the cross-reactive idiotype, their capacity to inhibit in the standard idiotype assay differs markedly (see Table I). The completion of these V-domain structures should help in the definition of the region(s) of the molecule

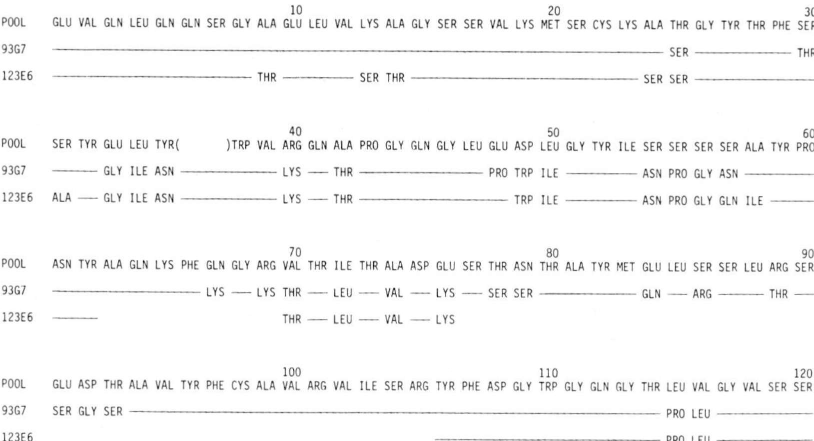

10 20 30
POOL GLU VAL GLN LEU GLN GLN SER GLY ALA GLU LEU VAL LYS ALA GLY SER SER VAL LYS MET SER CYS LYS ALA THR GLY TYR THR PHE SER
93G7 —— SER —— THR
123E6 —— THR —— SER THR —— SER SER ——
40 50 60
POOL SER TYR GLU LEU TYR( )TRP VAL ARG GLN ALA PRO GLY GLN GLY LEU GLU ASP LEU GLY TYR ILE SER SER SER SER ALA TYR PRO
93G7 —— GLY ILE ASN —— LYS —— THR —— PRO TRP ILE —— ASN PRO GLY ASN ——
123E6 ALA —— GLY ILE ASN —— LYS —— THR —— TRP ILE —— ASN PRO GLY GLN ILE ——
70 80 90
POOL ASN TYR ALA GLN LYS PHE GLN GLY ARG VAL THR ILE THR ALA ASP GLU SER THR ASN THR ALA TYR MET GLU LEU SER SER LEU ARG SER
93G7 —— LYS —— LYS THR —— LEU —— VAL —— LYS —— SER SER —— GLN —— ARG —— THR ——
123E6 —— THR —— LEU —— VAL —— LYS
100 110 120
POOL GLU ASP THR ALA VAL TYR PHE CYS ALA VAL ARG VAL ILE SER ARG TYR PHE ASP GLY TRP GLY GLN GLY THR LEU VAL GLY VAL SER SER
93G7 SER GLY SER —— PRO LEU ——
123E6 —— PRO LEU ——

FIG. 3. *Tentative partial sequence analysis of the heavy chains derived from CRI-positive hybridomas compared to the pooled serum CRI-positive sequence.*

10 20
SERUM POOL ASP ILE GLN MET THR GLN THR PRO SER SER LEU SER ALA SER LEU GLY ASP ARG VAL SER ILE SER CYS ARG ALA SER GLN
(VAL) (ILE) (LEU) (LEU)
93G7 —— THR —— GLU
124E1 —— THR —— THR ——
123E6 —— SER THR —— THR ——

30 40 50
SERUM POOL ASP LEU SER GLN TYR LEU PHE TRP TYR GLN GLN LYS PRO GLY GLN PRO PRO LYS LEU LEU ILE TYR ARG VAL SER ARG LEU
(PHE) (GLU) (ALA)
93G7 —— ILE —— ASN —— ASN —— LYS —— ASP GLY THR VAL ——
124E1 —— ILE ASN ASN —— ASN ——
123E6

60 70 80
SERUM POOL THR ASN GLY VAL PRO ASP ARG PHE SER GLY SER GLY SER GLY THR ASP PHE THR LEU THR ILE ASP PRO MET GLU GLU ASP
(THR) (ARG) (SER SER VAL) (ALA)
93G7 ILE —— ALA —— TYR —— ASN ——
124E1 —— TYR —— GLU ILE ASN —— GLN GLU
123E6

90 100 108
SERUM POOL ASP THR ALA THR TYR PHE CYS GLN GLN SER ARG LEU ILE PRO ARG THR PHE GLY GLY GLY THR LYS LEU GLU ILE LYS ARG
(ASP) (GLN) (ARG)
93G7 MET ——
124E1 —— ILE —— ——
123E6 MET ——

FIG. 4. *Tentative partial sequence analysis of the light chains derived from CRI-positive hybridomas compared to the pooled serum CRI-positive sequence. Alternate residues, which were identified in the serum sequence, are noted below the major sequence in parenthesis.*

likely to be responsible for the CRI determinant(s). Note that the third hypervariable region and the "J" segment of the heavy chain of 93G7 and the "J" segment of 123E6 bear a striking similarity to the serum pool, more so than in any other contiguous stretch.

The presently available light chain variable region sequences are shown in Fig. 4. Again, in many respects, the hybridoma light chains resemble each other more than they do the serum pool (see, for example, positions 20, 29, 31, 34, 71, 77, 93). *Note that all three hybridoma light chains and the serum pool have identical sequences in the "J" segments.*

Collectively, these data might be explained by a large number of "V" genes (1–96, for example, in the light chain) associated with a single "J" segment. While this would reduce the "germ line load", the diversity noted in the amino terminal 27 residues (every hybridoma sequence was different) suggests that if this explanation is correct, the A/J repertoire for the hapten *p*-azophenylarsonate must be enormous. How such a diverse group of molecules could all share a cross-reacting idiotype remains obscure, unless the J segment represents the inherited genetic element which gives rise to the cross-reacting idiotype.

T cell hybrids

Construction of T cell hybrids

Mice were immunized intravenously with Ar-coupled spleen cells and tested for suppression by footpad swelling induced by Ar-coupled spleen cells. Those mice which clearly demonstrated specific suppression of the DTH reaction were killed by cervical dislocation and their spleens removed for hybridization with the AKR thymoma, BW5147.

Three separate fusions were performed and cell growth was observed in 324 of 1080 wells. A radioinhibition assay was performed on the 238 hybrids which survived passage to larger wells. A sample of the initial screening of 48 of these 238 wells tested for inhibition of the binding of a hybridoma product to BSA-Ar coated polyvinyl plates is shown in Fig. 5. Wells 5, 36 and 41 showed considerable inhibition of binding and the cells in these wells were selected for further study.

The hybrids in wells 5, 36 and 41 were cloned by limiting dilution and for this study, the hybrid clone which was originally derived from well 5 is referred to as T34G6 and the clone derived from well 36 T33D5. This latter clone was subsequently subcloned.

Characterization of the T cell hybrids

The hybrid nature of each clone was confirmed by growth in HAT medium. A subclone of T33D5 was tested for Thy 1 antigens and over 95% of the cells expressed both Thy 1·1 and Thy 1·2 on their surface by indirect immunofluorescence. In order to test for the presence of the H–2 complex of the A/J

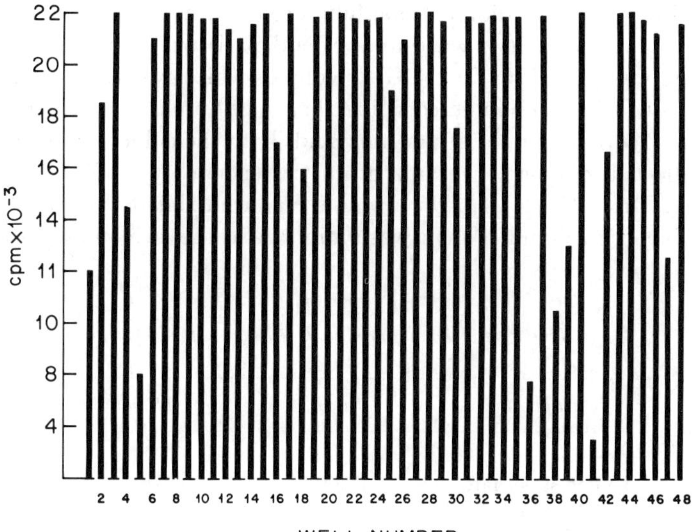

FIG. 5. *An example of the screening assay for nonimmunoglobulin arsonate specific T cell products. This illustrates tests on 48 of the 238 growth positive wells. No inhibition was observed in over two-thirds of the wells. Of the approximately one-third which did inhibit the reaction, some (for example, wells 5, 36 and 41) inhibited markedly and were chosen for further study.*

parent in the hybrids, the T33D5 subclone was tested by indirect immunofluorescence with B10.BR anti-B10.D2 which had been previously absorbed with the BW (AKR) parent line. A weak, but clearly positive reaction was evident.

On the basis of biosynthetically incorporated leucine, arginine and lysine, we estimate that from 0·1 to 0·2% of the material in culture supernatants is the arsonate specific product. Whether this is actively secreted, shed from living cells, or released after cell death and lysis has not been investigated. The amount of material that can be isolated has remained reasonably constant over the 6 months these clones have been extensively studied and, in addition, the Ar specific product appears stable as no proteolytic breakdown has been observed in stored culture fluids.

Isolation of arsonate specific T cell hybrid products

Antigen specific T cell products were isolated from 3 of the cloned T cell hybrids by biosynthetic labelling with a mixture of ^{3}H-leucine, ^{3}H-arginine and ^{3}H-lysine. Other biosynthetic studies involved ^{14}C amino acids as outlined below. In addition, unlabelled T cell hybrid products were isolated from one clone (T33D5).

Table II illustrates one experiment with the T33D5 clone biosynthetically labelled with ^{3}H-leucine. One ml of culture supernate was collected and a portion tested in the radioimmunoinhibition assay; in this particular experiment about 31% inhibition was found. After dialysis, one ml of this radioactive supernate was placed on an HGG-Ar column which was then exhaustively washed with phosphate buffered saline. The T cell product was then isolated by hapten elution with 0·1 M arsanilic acid. Both the effluent and the eluate were collected, dialysed, lyophilized and resuspended in 250 μl of PBS. As shown in Table II, the T33D5 arsonate eluate inhibited the reaction over 90%, while the column effluent was inhibitory at the level of only 16%.

TABLE II
Inhibition of binding by T cell hybridoma products

Inhibitor	*Ct/min*	*Per cent inhibition*
PBS	15 000	0
T33D5 supernate	10 300	31·4
T33D5 Ar eluate	1 400	90·7
T33D5 effluent	12 600	16·0
BW51 supernate	14 600	2·7
T33B3 supernate	14 600	2·7

Ar-BSA coated plates plus HP93G7 anti-Ar + ^{125}I-rabbit antimouse Ig.

When the arsonate specific eluate was applied to an HGG column with no hapten coupled, all radioactivity appeared in the effluent. In addition, after elution of an active T cell supernate with the arsonate hapten, further stripping of the column with 5 M guanidine resulted in the recovery of relatively few counts.

Serologic characterization arsonate specific T cell hybrid products

Since with the techniques employed, one is able to isolate relatively large amounts of biosynthetically labelled T cell hybridoma products with antigen specificity, experiments could be done on the purified material, rather than on whole culture supernates. In typical experiments, 3000 ct/min of leucine, arginine and lysine labelled Ar eluates were placed in serial tubes and specific and facilitating antisera added. After overnight incubation, the pellets were counted. This is a substantially different system than employed by other investigators studying T cell products and is one of the significant advantages of isolating hapten specific material. As can be seen in Table III of all the antisera tested, only rabbit anti-CRI and A.TH anti-A.TL resulted in specific precipitation of the T33D5 T cell hybridoma product. These studies demonstrate that the T33D5 hybrid produces a product which has determinants which are recognized by a rabbit anti-CRI, as well as containing determinants which are recognized by antisera directed against the whole *I* region of the murine major histocompatibility complex.

TABLE III
Serological characterization of T33D5 arsonate specific T cell product

Antiserum	*Ct/min precipitated*
Rabbit anti-CRI	2857 ± 275
A.TH anti-A.TL	2981 ± 127
A.TL anti-A.TH	405 ± 37
Anti-H-2K^k	330 ± 44
Anti-H-2D^d	487 ± 56
Anti-Slp	550 ± 65
Rabbit antihuman C4	604 ± 93
Rabbit antimouse Ig	783 ± 83
Mouse antihuman IgGK	468 ± 50
Goat antimouse Ig	403 ± 47
Goat antirabbit Ig	409 ± 56

Each reaction system included 3000 ct/min of ^{3}H L, R, K biosynthetically labelled Ar eluate and 50 μl of appropriate antisera.

Chemical characterization of arsonate specific T cell hybrid products

The arsonate eluates from all 3 products were run both on SDS polyacrylamide gel slab as well as tube gels with appropriate molecular weight markers, and the apparent molecular weight of each is 62 000. Figure 6 illustrates an SDS

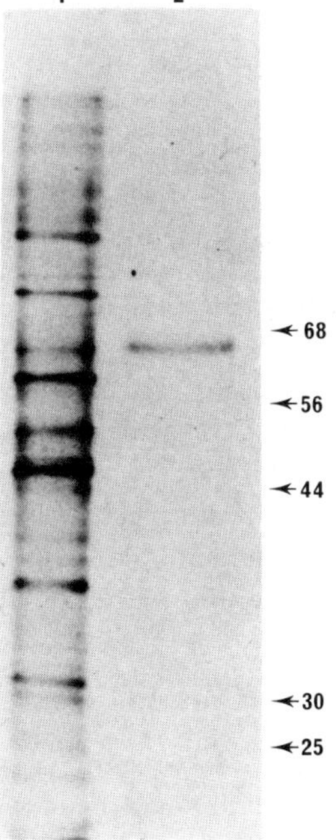

FIG. 6. *Fluorographic analysis of biosynthetically labelled T35D5 supernate (Lane 1), and the Ar eluate (Lane 2). Molecular weight markers are indicated on the right.*

slab gell of whole biosynthetically labelled T cell supernatant (Lane 1) as well as the arsonate eluate from an HGG-Ar column (Lane 2). As can be seen, the Ar eluate is a single band of 62 000 daltons. A band of comparable molecular weight is clearly evident in the whole cell supernatant.

Complete reduction and alkylation of the Ar eluate did not appreciably change its apparent molecular weight. Thus, the T cell product appears to be either a single 62 000 dalton molecule, or multiple 62 000 dalton subunits noncovalently associated.

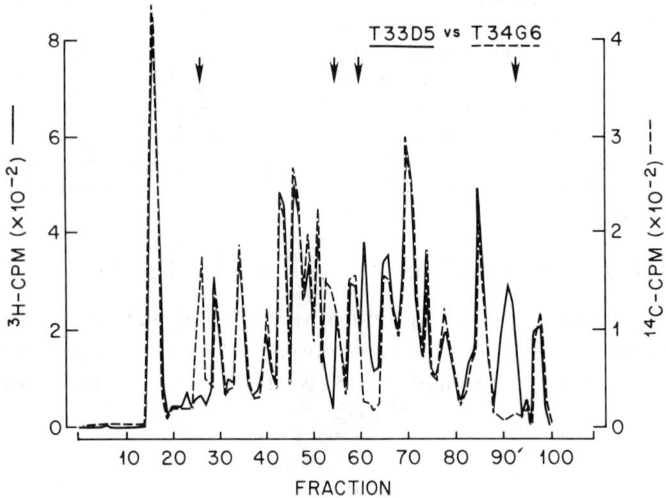

FIG. 7. *High pressure liquid chromatographic analysis of tryptic digests of the T35D5 and T34G6 specifically purified T cell products.* ^{3}*H-labelled* (——) *T33D5 is compared with* ^{14}*C-labelled* (– – –) *T34G6. The 4 peptides which are clearly distinct between the two T cell products are indicated by arrows. All other peptides appear identical by this analysis. This particular analysis was performed on a radial compression module with an acetic acid-acetonitrile gradient.*

Figure 7 shows the results of an HPLC analysis of the tryptic peptides of two of the T cell products, both of which react with the anti-CRI. Twenty peptides were clearly resolved by HPLC and the vast majority of the peptides were shared by both T cell products. However, from 2 to 4 peptides were clearly distinct. These results indicate that while these two T cell products are remarkably similar, they have unique features as well.

Conclusions

Barring unexpected serologic cross-reactivity, the data presented strongly suggest that a single polypeptide chain bears antigenic determinants which are thought to be encoded on *different* chromosomes. Thus, the antigen binding function and the CRI are encoded on chromosomes 6 and 12 (light and heavy chain loci) while *I*-region structures are encoded on chromosome 17. Four possibilities should be considered for this unprecedented finding: (1) the V-region loci have been duplicated and they, or structures related to them, are encoded on chromosome 17; (2) the *I*-region loci have been duplicated and exist on chromosomes 6, and/or 12 as well as chromosome 17; (3) protein or RNA ligases exist which splice either nucleic acids or proteins from different chromosomes; or (4) the *I*-region loci (possibly *I–J* since previous results seem to rule out *I–A* or *I–E/C*) do not encode the structural genes for the polypeptide chains in question, but rather encode modifying enzymes which actually dictate the serologic specificities.

The relationship of these T cell products to molecules described by other investigators is speculative at present since we have not determined any functional activity for these arsonate specific products. Our approach has been to search for a specific molecule and with this homogeneous product available, design experiments to test potential function. Nonetheless, the relationships of these antigen specific, idiotype positive, *I*-region containing structures to suppressor, helper or allogeneic effector factors and to the T cell receptor problem itself are now approachable.

References

Bach, B., Greene, M., Benacerraf, B. and Nisonoff, A. (1979a). *J. Exp. Med.* **149**, 1084.

Bach, B. A., Sherman, L., Benacerraf, B. and Greene, M. I. (1979b). *J. Immunol.* **121**, 1460.

Brient, B. W. and Nisonoff, A. (1970). *J. Exp. Med.* **132**, 951.

Brown, A. R., Estess, P., Lamoyi, E., Gill-Pazaris, L., Gottlieb, P. D., Capra, J. D. and Nisonoff, A. (1980). *In* "Membranes, Receptors and the Immune Response" (E. P. Cohen and H. Köhler, eds) p. 231. Alan R. Liss, New York.

Capra, J. D. (1971). *Nature (Lond.)* **230**, 61.

Capra, J. D. and Kehoe, J. M. (1975). *Adv. Immunol.* **20**, 1.

Capra, J. D., Klapper, D. G., Tung, A. S. and Nisonoff, A. (1976). *Cold Spring Harbor Symp. Quant. Biol.* **41**, 847.

Capra, J. D. and Nisonoff, A. (1979). *J. Immunol.* **123**, 279.

Capra, J. D., Tung, A. S. and Nisonoff, A. (1975a). *J. Immunol.* **114**, 1548.

Capra, J. D., Tung, A. S. and Nisonoff, A. (1975b). *J. Immunol.* **115**, 414.

Capra, J. D., Tung, A. S. and Nisonoff, A. (1977). *J. Immunol.* **119**, 993.

Edelman, G. M. and Gall, W. E. (1969). *Ann. Rev. Biochem.* **38**, 415.

Estess, P. and Capra, J. D. (1980). *In* "Membranes, Receptors, and the Immune Response" (E. P. Cohen and H. Köhler, eds) p. 249. Alan R. Liss, New York.

Estess, P., Nisonoff, A. and Capra, J. D. (1979). *Molecular Immunol.* **16**, 1111.

Friedenson, B., Tung, A. S. and Nisonoff, A. (1975). *Proc. Natn. Acad. Sci. U.S.A.* **72**, 3676.

Goetzl, E. J. and Metzger, H. (1970). *Biochemistry* **9**, 1267.

Goldsby, C. A., Osborne, B. A., Simpson, E. and Herzenberg, L. A. (1977). *Nature (Lond.)* **267**, 707.

Gill-Pazaris, L. A., Brown, A. R. and Nisonoff, A. (1979). *Ann. Immunol. (Paris)* **130**, 199.

Green, M. I., Bach, B. and Benacerraf, B. (1979). *J. Exp. Med.* **149**, 1069.

Hammerling, G. J. (1977). *Eur. J. Immunol.* **7**, 743.

Kindt, H. G. (1975). *Adv. Immunol.* **21**, 35.

Köhler, H., Shimizu, A., Paul, C., Moore, V. and Putnam, F. W. (1978). *Nature (Lond.)* **227**, 1318.
Kuettner, M. G., Wang, A.-L. and Nisonoff, A. (1972). *J. Exp. Med.* **135**, 579.
Kunkel, H. G., Winchester, R. J., Joslin, F. G. and Capra, J. D. (1974). *J. Exp. Med.* **139**, 128.
Laskin, J. A., Gray, A., Nisonoff, A., Klinman, N. R. and Gottlieb, P. D. (1977). *Proc. Natn. Acad. Sci. U.S.A.* **74**, 4600.
Lewis, G. K. and Goodman, J. W. (1978). *J. Exp. Med.* **148**, 915.
Milstein, C. (1967). *Nature (Lond.)* **216**, 330.
Niall, H. D. and Edman, P. (1967). *Nature (Lond.)* **216**, 262.
Oudin, J. and Michel, M. (1963). *C. R. Hebd. Seances Acad. Sci.* **257**, 805.
Pawlak, L., Mushinski, E. B., Nisonoff, A. and Potter, M. (1973). *J. Exp. Med.* **137**, 22.
Ray, A. and Cebra, J. J. (1972). *Biochemistry* **11**, 3647.
Slater, R. J., Ward, S. M. and Kunkel, H. G. (1955). *J. Exp. Med.* **101**, 85.
Taniguchi, M., Hayakawa, K. and Tada, T. (1976). *J. Immunol.* **116**, 542.
Taniguchi, M., Takei, I. and Tada, T. (1980). *Nature* **283**, 227.
Taniguchi, M. and Tokuhisa, T. (1980). *J. Exp. Med.* **151**, 517.
Williams, R. C., Kunkel, H. G. and Capra, J. D. (1968). *Science (Wash. D.C.)* **161**, 379.
Wu, T. T. and Kabat, E. A. (1970). *J. Exp. Med.* **132**, 211.

2

Monoclonal Antibodies from Hybrid Myelomas

C. MILSTEIN, M. R. CLARK, G. GALFRE and A. C. CUELLO*

*Medical Research Council Laboratory of Molecular Biology, Cambridge, England and *Departments of Pharmacology and Human Anatomy, University of Oxford, England*

Introduction

The introduction of hybrid myelomas for the continuous supply of monoclonal antibodies (McAb), was the result of basic advances in immunology and in cell biology. Burnet's clonal selection theory established that the enormous heterogeneity of antibodies was due to the existence of an equally complex population of clones of cells, each one synthesizing a single antibody. Myelomas and similar lymphoproliferative disorders could then be considered as tumours of such "antibody" producing cells. The immunoglobulins produced by such

The immunocytochemical studies on 5HT and substance P were done in collaboration with J. V. Priestley and B. Wright. The help of J. M. Jarvis and B. Wright is gratefully acknowledged.

tumours had a single chemical structure, since they arose from the clonal expansion of a single cell. M. Potter at NIH induced such tumours in the BALB/c strain of mice but the efforts to induce myelomas synthesizing specific antibodies were unsuccessful. These mouse tumours became the subject of intensive research and eventually were adapted to grow permanently in culture. Lines of plasmacytomas actively secreting immunoglobulin became available for further work from Horibata and Harris (1970). From them we received the cell lines P1 and P3 and derived mutants suitable for cell hybridization studies. Around this time the spontaneous tumours of the Lou strain of rats were characterized and shown to secrete large amounts of immunoglobulin (Bazin *et al.*, 1972). One of these tumours (S210) was adapted to grow in tissue culture and provided a second type of cell from which suitable mutants could be isolated in preparation for the first fusion between two myeloma cell lines.

Somatic cell hybrids (see Ringerts and Savage, 1976) formed by spontaneous fusion of two different cells in culture were discovered in 1960. This was a very rare event, and hybrid cells became a tool for basic research when methods for their production and selection were developed in 1964 and 1965. One was the introduction of inactivated Sendai virus to increase the efficiency of hybrid formation. The other was the use of mutant cells and selective media for the isolation of hybrid cells. Up to 1976, somatic cell hybrids were used for two purposes. For gene mapping purposes, interspecific hybrids were produced between cells of different organisms. The chromosome segregation was then correlated with the segregation of species specific biochemical markers, like enzymes with characteristic electrophoretic mobilities. For studies of gene expression, intraspecific hybrids obtained by fusing two different cell types from the same species were prepared. This was followed by a study of the retention as well as complementation of biochemical, immunological, and other phenotypic properties. The fusion of two myeloma type cells, a critical step in the origin of the "hybridoma" technology, belongs to this category.

Hybrids between two antibody producing cells did not obey the rules of isotype, allotype, and idiotype exclusion (i.e. one cell one antibody species)—a subject finally settled in the Cold Spring Harbor Symposium of 1967. In hybrids, there was codominant expression of the heavy and light chains of both parental cells. This gave rise to the production of hybrid immunoglobulin molecules made by random association of the heavy and light polypeptide chains of both parents (Cotton and Milstein, 1973; Köhler and Milstein, 1975; Margulis *et al.*, 1976).

Immortalization of differentiated functions by cell fusion

The production of hybrids between a mouse myeloma cell and a normal antibody producing cell from the same species, for the continuous production of monoclonal antibodies, introduced a new concept. This involved the use of normal and transformed cells, genetically and phenotypically as closely related as possible, for the immortalization of specific differentiated functions (Köhler and Milstein, 1975).

The essential features of the derivation of hybrid myelomas secreting a specific antibody are as follows. The myeloma parent contributes to the hybrid the malignant phenotype and its ability to grow permanently in tissue culture. Being a mutant defective in the enzyme hypoxanthine guanine phosphoribosyl transferase, it cannot grow under conditions where incorporation of hypoxanthine is essential to cell growth (HAT medium). The spleen parental cell provides the enzyme and permits the hybrid cells to grow under those conditions. In addition it contributes with the rearranged *V* and *C* genes for both heavy and light chains which code a specific antibody.

The myeloma parental line also provides the phenotype for high production and secretion to hybrids with cells which may not have such properties. In other words, the nonsecreted immunoglobulin of a cell can be effectively secreted in a hybrid with a myeloma partner (Raschke *et al.*, 1979).

TABLE I

Selective fixation of differentiated functions in established hybrids (taken from Milstein et al., *1979)*

Parental and hybrid lines	*Cell phenotype*			
	Ig secreted		*Thy-1 surface antigen*	
	Parental myeloma	*Other Ig*	*Thy-1, 1*	*Thy-1, 2*
X63 (myeloma)	>95%	0	0	0
(X63 × spleen) hybrids	> 90%	~65%	0	0
Spleen	0	~5%	0	~40%
(BW × spleen) hybrids	0	0	>90%	~70%
BW (T lymphoma)	0	0	>95%	0

The surviving hybrids do not represent a random immortalization of the phenotypic properties of the donor spleen cells. This is illustrated in Table I. When the same population of spleen cells is used to fuse with either a myeloma or a T cell lymphoma the result is quite different. When the fusion parent is the myeloma, the growing hybrids express preferentially the antibody secreting phenotype acquired from the parental spleen. On the contrary, when the fusion parent is a T cell lymphoma, the growing hybrids preferentially express T cell characteristics acquired from the parental spleen cells. The "T cell hybridomas" have been the subject of intensive study, but I will not have time to discuss them. The main message of these experiments is that T cell lymphomas immortalize T cell properties. Myelomas immortalize the antibody production and confer secretion phenotype when this is lacking.

The selective effect of the myeloma, described in Table I, is even more pronounced when the rat cell line Y3 is used (Galfre *et al.*, 1979). More recently these results have been confirmed in a much more elaborate series of experiments. In these experiments several myeloma lines from both mouse and rat origin were fused to spleen cells from mice and rats in all four combinations (mouse × mouse; rat × rat; rat × mouse and mouse × rat). The fusion mixtures were fractionated into about 50 cultures and allowed to grow. Cultures vigorously growing were then analysed as soon as they had sufficient cells. The analysis of the products secreted by them was done by incorporation of radioactive amino acids and analysis of secreted heavy chains by SDS-gel electrophoresis. A statistical treatment was then applied to estimate the number of clones present in each culture (the details of the method will be the subject of a separate communication). In this way the number of successful hybrids prepared with the different myelomas which fail to express the spleen immunoglobulin heavy chains can be compared. Table II shows that while the mouse myeloma parents produce a minimum of 20%–50% of negative hybrids, the

TABLE II

The expression of the spleen parental immunoglobulin is better in hybrids prepared with rat myelomas than with mouse myelomas

		Negative hybrid clones as % of growing clones		
Fusion	*Parental cells*	*Minimum value* (%)	*Maximum value* (%)	*Best estimate* (%)
Mouse × mouse				
NN1	NSI/1.Ag.4.1 × B10.D2 spleen	18	85	<44
NN2	NSI/1.Ag.4.1 × C3H spleen	35	99	<60
NOA1	NSI/1.Ag.4.1/0 × BALB/c spleen	41	89	60
XOA1	X63 Ag.8.653 × BALB/c spleen	50	75	50
Rat × rat				
YS4/5	Y3 Ag.1.2.3 × DA spleen	0	37	7
YA5	Y3 Ag.1.2.3 × DA spleen	0	50	<30
YA5	Y3 Ag.1.2.3 × DA spleen	0	50	<30
YOL1	YB2/3.0.Ag × Lou spleen	10	51	<35
Mouse × rat				
NR5/6	NSI/1.Ag.4.1 × Lew spleen	50	99	<96
Rat × mouse				
YN5/6	Y3 Ag.1.2.3 × C3H spleen	3	54	<36

The results were obtained 3–4 weeks after fusion by analysis of the immunoglobulin secreted by all successfully growing hybrids followed by a statistical calculation of the number of growing clones (details to be published elsewhere).

equivalent value with the rat myelomas is 0%–10%. Whether this is due to more selectivity on the part of the rat line, better stability of the hybrids, or a combination of both, remains to be seen.

Derivation and uses of hybrid myelomas

The protocol for the derivation of hybrid myeloma cell lines secreting a monoclonal antibody of predefined specificity has remained essentially the same as when first published (Köhler and Milstein, 1975, 1976). The most important changes have been the use of polyethylene glycol as fusing agent instead of Sendai virus, the introduction of a battery of assay methods to detect the presence of antibody in the supernatants of cultured hybrid cells, and the development of a wider spectrum of myeloma cell lines to be used as parental cells.

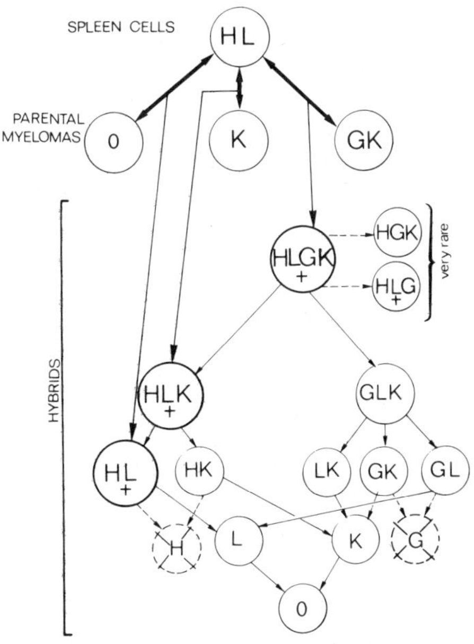

FIG. 1. *Ig chains made by hybrid clones and segregants. H and L represent the heavy and light chains originating from the spleen parental cell, G and K the equivalent chains from the myeloma parent. Myelomas with defective Ig expression synthesize only κ chains or no chains at all (see also Table III). The loss of heavy chains precedes the loss of light chains (see text). Synthesis of multiple chains produces hybrid Ig molecules. However, probably because of structural restrictions, hybrids between μ and γ chains have not been demonstrated to become associated to form mixed class molecules. Mixed subclasses of γ chains have been demonstrated in several instances (Secher and Herzenberg, quoted in Herzenberg* et al.*, 1978; Köhler* et al.*, 1978) including mouse × rat hybrid combinations (Howard* et al.*, 1979).*

Immunoglobulin structure in hybrids and segregation of chains

Hybrid cells derived from fusion to each of those different lines secrete immunoglobulin molecules made up by combination of the heavy and light chains of both parental cells. From them it is easy to derive segregants, particularly soon after fusion, in which some of the chains are no longer expressed. The pattern of loss of expression is schematically shown in Fig. 1. A remarkable feature of the diagram is that the segregants do not develop in a random fashion. The loss of heavy chains precedes the loss of light chains (Margulis *et al.*, 1976; Köhler *et al.*, 1978). This has been interpreted as owing to the toxic effect of free heavy chains. This conclusion has been supported by the pattern of losses of chains of triple hybrids (Köhler, 1980). The importance of the insolubility of the free heavy chains is supported in studies on heavy chain deletion mutants and the hybrids derived from them (Wilde and Milstein, 1980).

The loss of immunoglobulin chains in segregants is rather fast during the early period of proliferation of the hybrids. At the same time, segregants with

TABLE III

Screening of variants for reversion to specific antibody production by SRBC plaque assays and to Ig production by reverse plaque assays. Inclusion of SP3/HL or Sp3/HK cells was used as a control, showing that Ig secreting cells can be detected from among the large excess of inactive cells

Number of cells plated		*SRBC*	*Number of cells plated*		*Anti-P3-Ox RBC*
Sp2/L(K)	*Sp3/HL*	*plaques*	*Sp2/L(K)*	*Sp3/HK*	*plaques*
10^7	400	212	10^7	10^3	432
10^7	40	26	10^7	100	55
10^7	—	0	10^7	—	0
10^7	—	0	10^7	—	0
$2{\cdot}5 \times 10^7$	—	0	10^7	—	0

Numbers of cells screened for revertants. This table summarizes the data given for Sp2/L(K) above together with those for other variant lines which were similarly investigated

Cell line	*Reversion to anti-SRBC antibody production*	*Reversion to Ig production*	*Total cells screened*
Sp1/L(K)	$1{\cdot}5 \times 10^7$	$1{\cdot}5 \times 10^7$	3×10^7
Sp2/O-Ag	$3{\cdot}5 \times 10^7$	$4{\cdot}2 \times 10^7$	$7{\cdot}7 \times 10^7$
Sp2/L-Ag	$4{\cdot}5 \times 10^7$	4×10^7	$8{\cdot}5 \times 10^7$
Sp2/L(K)	$4{\cdot}5 \times 10^7$	4×10^7	$8{\cdot}5 \times 10^7$
Sp3/O	$1{\cdot}5 \times 10^7$	$1{\cdot}5 \times 10^7$	3×10^7
Sp3/L	$1{\cdot}8 \times 10^7$	$1{\cdot}8 \times 10^7$	$3{\cdot}6 \times 10^7$
Sp3/L(K)	3×10^7	$4{\cdot}2 \times 10^7$	$7{\cdot}2 \times 10^7$
Sp3/(K)	3×10^7	5×10^7	8×10^7

Data from Wilde and Milstein (1980)

lower chromosome content and better growth characteristics arise. Clonal competition and chain loss play overlapping roles often leading to loss of antibody activity of uncloned hybrids. This process is faster in the early stages of hybrid growth and gradually slows down as chromosomes are being lost. Successful growth characteristics and secretion of specific antibody do not seem to be correlated in either a positive or negative way. In practice this means that when searching for McAb, very successful fusions can be allowed to "mature", i.e. to allow clonal competition to choose the best growing hybrids which retain the expression of the antibody.

Loss of immunoglobulin chains appears to be an irreversible process (see Table III) and is thought to be generally due to chromosome losses. Correlation of loss of specific chromosomes and loss of immunoglobulin chains has been used as a way to assign the location of the respective genes. In this way it has been suggested, for instance, that the mouse κ and heavy chain genes are in chromosomes 6 and 12 respectively (Hengartner *et al.*, 1978), the human heavy chain in chromosome 14 (Croce *et al.*, 1979; but see also Smith and Hirschorn, 1978), and the rat heavy chain in chromosome 14 (Schröder *et al.*, 1980).

Monospecific antibodies from impure antigens

From the beginning it was clear that the preparation of McAb by the hybrid myeloma method had one overwhelming advantage over conventional antisera. When an animal is immunized with an antigenic preparation, the animal responds to many antigenic determinants in a very complex way (Fig. 2). Minor impurities may be antigenically dominant and antibodies to specific components are mixed with antibodies to all the components. Multiple antibodies are likely to be produced against a single antigen and even against a single determinant. Sometimes partial purifications are possible by specific absorptions but the process, as we all know, is painfully complex. Each antibody species is made by different immunocytes, and therefore by different hybrid myelomas. The purification of the antibody is therefore confined to the purification, by the simple device of cloning, of one clone producing it. This very simple basic principle is what makes the hybrid myeloma approach such a powerful tool in a wide range of basic and applied problems.

From the point of view of basic immunology, in principle one should be able to isolate and describe all the antibody variants which an animal can theoretically produce. This is the ultimate goal in describing the extent of antibody diversity.

Monoclonal antibodies in medicine

Antibodies prepared by the hybrid myeloma method have very definite practical advantages over the conventional antisera obtained from immunized animals. Traditional antisera consist of mixtures of antibody species, which

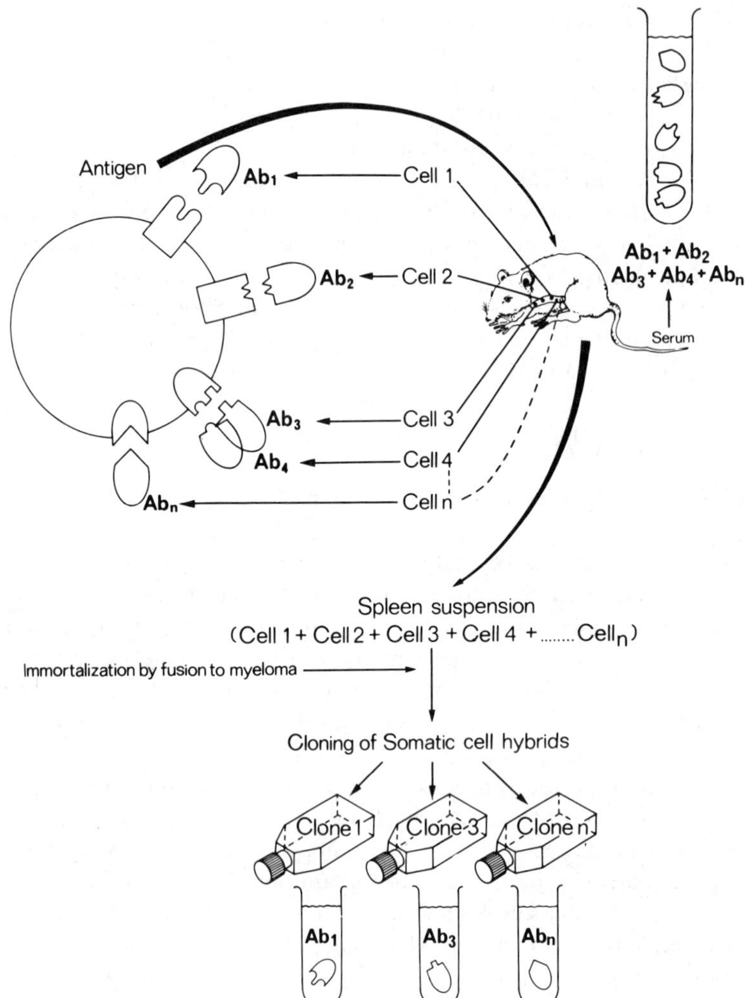

FIG. 2. *The hybrid myelomas permit the dissection of the immune response. The response of an animal to an antigen is very complex. But each antibody is synthesized by individual cells. These can be immortalized by cell fusion to provide an inexhaustible supply of monoclonal antibody. Taken from Milstein* et al. *(1979).*

vary from animal to animal and even with different bleedings of the same animal. Lack of reproducibility has been a major drawback in the use of antisera as biochemical reagents. In contrast, hybrid myeloma lines can be kept indefinitely: the first line derived, Sp1, is today better than it was when first obtained in 1974. The antibodies produced by hybrid myelomas are defined molecular species and not unknown mixtures. For this reason, monoclonal antibodies and defined blends are likely to substitute conventional antisera as standard reagents in laboratory practice. There are several instances where monoclonal antibodies to viral antigens and to peptide hormones are being introduced for radioimmunoassays.

As laboratory reagents, monoclonal antibodies need not only recognize specifically the desired antigen, but in addition have certain desired properties. For instance, they may be required to be cytotoxic, haemagglutinating of high avidity for radioimmunoassays, etc. All this must be taken into consideration when developing hybrid lines suitable for use in defined laboratory tests. For instance, in radioimmunoassays, the avidity of the antibody is essential. Therefore, it is advantageous in screening the activity of the supernatants of hybrids to use tests designed to select reagents displaying the desired property. Only high avidity antibodies were detectable by the screening method (a radioimmunoassay) used to isolate clone NCI/34 producing a McAb to the neurotransmitter substance P. In a radioimmunoassay, it was capable of detecting down to about 10 fmol of substance P (Cuello *et al.*, 1980).

The blood grouping reagents, on the other hand, have completely different requirements. They are used in haemagglutination tests and must be able to give fast and accurate results under both routine and emergency situations. The antiblood group A should be highly specific but capable of recognizing the weak A cells of A_2B and some cord bloods. The preparation of ABO typing reagents in the UK uses 1200 litres of human serum annually from 6000 blood donations. There are in addition powerful economic reasons for an alternative source of antiblood group reagents apart from the variation in the individual serum donations which require large numbers of tests on each of them. From among a variety of hybrid myeloma clones we have chosen one (MH2/6D4) which displays the necessary qualities as a provider of a standard anti-A reagent (Voak *et al.*, 1980). The McAb was used with 1421 samples in manual tests, including 169 cord samples. They all gave satisfactory reaction and no false reactions were detected. In automatic tests, using the Auto Grouper 16C machine, 1911 random samples including many A_1B and A_2B gave satisfactory results. The reagent was prepared as the spent medium of stationary phase MH2/6D4 cells. Potency increases by concentrating the spent medium, to provide a reagent with an avidity time of 12–15 s, which is generally regarded as sufficient. With further adaptation of the cells, the concentration of antibody in the spent medium has already doubled or even trebled over the earlier values. We are confident that the required potency can be achieved without the need of concentrating it. We have concluded that mass culture production of this monoclonal anti-A provides a cost-effective model for the use of monoclonal antibodies as a new generation of better standardized potent reagents for routine blood typing. The reagent is at present being tested in the UK on a national scale.

I have described an example which is now at a reasonably advanced stage of generalized usage. At present, I would not dare to list others related to tissue typing, haematology, clinical virology or endocrinology.

Monoclonal antibodies and cell subpopulations

Since its introduction (Williams *et al.*, 1977) the hybrid myeloma strategy has been very successful in providing a host of new (and reproducible !) reagents to define markers of cell subpopulations in rat, mouse and humans.* In principle, the method allows the preparation of antibodies to any of the many antigenic structures of the cell surface. In practice the ease with which each specificity can be produced depends to a large extent on the relative antigenicity of the particular marker. Immunization schedules and specific assays are essential considerations.

But as more reagents are accumulated, the likelihood of repeats increases. This can be avoided and a frontal attack on the characterization of all the components of a complex mixture of antigens should be possible by using the McAb cascade purification approach (Milstein and Lennox, 1980). An antigenic mixture (for instance, a solubilized cell membrane preparation) is injected into an animal and a random collection of monoclonal antibodies prepared by fusion. These are then used to prepare immunoadsorbant columns which can be used to remove the relevant antigens from the total cell membrane preparation. The eluate containing all the components not retained by the immunoadsorbants, can be used as antigens to generate a new set of monoclonal antibodies. These allow the preparation of new immunoadsorbant columns to further remove antigens and repeat the immunizations. As the purification proceeds, new McAb can be generated which are directed against the more elusive antigenic components.

The monoclonal antibodies prepared so far have provided a variety of new reagents which are very valuable as markers of cell subpopulations. The list is now much too long to be summarized here. Indeed, the flood of information is presenting us with a serious cataloguing problem. And yet each new reagent is of great potential value because they are necessary for the correct definition of the surface antigens of a cell. As we have pointed out before (Milstein and Lennox, 1980), more than by the expression of individual antigens, cell subpopulations and cell lineages are best characterized by the ensemble of the antigenic markers.

* A number of reviews are now available in "Monoclonal Antibodies" (1980). (Kennett, McKearn and Bechtol, eds). Plenum, New York; *Immunological Reviews* **47** and "Current Topics of Developmental Biology", Vol. 14, ((1980) M. Friedlander, ed.) Academic Press, New York and London.

Monoclonal antibodies to human lymphocytes are now being used not only to define the human lymphoid subpopulations but also as a means to study leukaemias. Furthermore, their possible use in therapy is being seriously considered. For instance, the monoclonal antibody YD1/23 is very weakly expressed on bone marrow precursors (such as CFUc and TdT^+ cells) and on blast cells in the common form of ALL. But reacts frequently with almost all blast cells in thymic ALL as well as thymocytes and mature lymphocytes. Reagents of this type can be tested for their capacity to remove residual thymic ALL cells from the bone marrow of patients prior to autologous marrow transplantation, or for the elimination of bone marrow T lymphocytes (responsible for graft versus host disease) prior to allogeneic marrow transplantation (Janossy *et al.*, 1980).

The characterization of differentiation antigens by monoclonal antibodies has revealed a persistent involvement of carbohydrates (lipopolysaccharides and glycoproteins) and the frequent recognition of antigenic determinants which are common to subpopulations of cells belonging to different differentiation pathways. We refer to them as "jumping" specificities. One such specificity is H9/25. It is an alloantigenic marker and its strain distribution shows very close genetic linkage with previously defined markers like Ala-1 and Ly-6 (Takei *et al.*, 1980a, b). But H9/25 is expressed on different functional subsets (Table IV). It is most likely, therefore, that these surface markers

TABLE IV
Expression of Ly-2, Ly-6, Ala-1 and H9/25 Ag on lymphocyte subsets

Lymphocyte subset	*Ly-6*	*Ala-1*	*Ly-2*	*H9/25*
Allokiller T	+	+	+	+
Precursor of allokiller T	−	−	+	+
Helper T	+	+	−	−
Suppressor T	+	+?	+	+?
PFC	+	+	−	+
Virgin B	−	−	−	−
B memory	?	?	−	−

Taken from Takei *et al.* (1980b)

originate from a genetic region controlling the expression of a variety of differentiation antigens. Once again, the temptation to suggest the involvement of carbohydrates (more precisely the enzymes responsible for their synthesis) is difficult to resist. But this is a subject in which speculation may be unnecessary. The same monoclonal antibodies which define the markers hopefully will allow the isolation of the antigenic molecules and their subsequent chemical characterization.

Monoclonal antibodies as immunoadsorbants

The hybrid myeloma strategy allows the preparation of an antibody capable of recognizing specifically a minor component of a mixture. The antibody is then the means of purifying the antigen. This approach had been used previously with cell surface components but its most dramatic development has been with interferon (Secher and Burke, 1980). The starting material was an interferon preparation—less than 1% pure—to immunize animals. The difficulties were great because the biological assay for interferon was tedious and not really suited for screening methods. In spite of that, a hybrid clone (NK2) was isolated and with it McAb to interferon were prepared. In pilot experiments the antibody proved to be very useful in interferon purification. Crude interferon could be purified over 5000-fold in a single step using an immunoadsorbant made with the monoclonal antibody, prepared in large quantities from tumour bearing mice. The material after a single passage over the immunoadsorbant column is already over 50% pure, and better than 90% when subjected to a second treatment.

Now that purified interferon can be prepared with no difficulty, the preparation of other McAb to it becomes a simpler problem. And it is made even simpler by the use of the present McAb for interferon assay. In our laboratory, D. S. Secher has developed such an assay which has proved to be of excellent sensitivity and great simplicity. This will be invaluable in the control of interferon production as well as in clinical trials and screenings (D. S. Secher, pers. comm.).

Monoclonal antibodies in immunocytochemistry and pharmacology

For its capacity to reveal unknown components in complex biological systems, the hybrid myeloma strategy is likely to have an important impact in many other areas. I would like to single out the characterization and visualization of neurotransmitter substances, their receptors, their biosynthetic enzymes and of the subsets of cells in the nervous system. The potential widespread availability of relevant McAb is an important step to mapping of neurotransmitter and/or candidate substances in the central nervous system. This will also minimize discrepancies between results from different laboratories.

In the case of receptors, a good start has been made by the recent derivation of McAb to the nicotinic acetylcholine receptor (Moshly-Rosen *et al.*, 1980; Gomez *et al.*, 1980). A variety of McAb have been prepared reacting with different functional parts of the receptor. The reagents provide a new powerful tool in functional studies, structural analysis and mapping of the receptor. They could help to understand the role of antibodies in *Myasthenia gravis.*

Antibodies to neurotransmitters are not easy to prepare, because they are usually very poor antigens, even when conjugated to carrier proteins. This has been a serious limitation in the use of immunological methods. The hybrid myeloma approach does not solve the problems created by the poor immunogenicity, but it ensures that such problems need only be solved once to ensure an unlimited supply of "rare" or "difficult" antibodies. The first example was provided by the preparation and use of the antisubstance P monoclonal antibody NCI/34 (Cuello *et al.*, 1979). The reagent was shown to be excellent when used in immunocytochemistry for tissue preparation. Staining by either immunofluorescence or immunoenzyme procedures yielded remarkably clean patterns. The monoclonal antibody is essentially free of contaminating immunoglobulins from the same species eliminating a major source of background.

More recently we have developed a rat hybrid line (YC5/45.HLK) secreting McAb to serotonin (5HT). When tested by standard methods of fluorescent immunocytochemistry, it specifically detected the 5HT cell bodies and terminals in all brain regions as previously reported by other methods. However, in specificity studies the reagent cross-reacted with almost equal avidity with the related amines 5-methoxytryptamine and dopamine. This provides an example of antibody cross-reactivity resulting from the multirecognition of different antigenic structure by a *single antibody* combining site. This cross-reactivity should not be confused with the one resulting from the *heterogeneity* of conventional (polyclonal) antisera. The interesting point is that in spite of the cross-reaction, when the McAb preparation was tested in tissue preparations, it completely failed to reveal dopamine sites in areas of the brain where the presence of the amine is well documented (e.g. *zona compacta* of the *substantia nigra*). What we find exciting about these contradictory observations is our ability to exclude artifacts due to the antibody heterogeneity. More important, the problem can be investigated without the fear of running out of a preparation which displays such properties. In fact, our present hypothesis is that the specificity of the histochemical reaction is introduced by the procedure used for the fixation of the tissue. Staining specificity should be regarded as the combination of the specificity of the combining site of the antibodies themselves and the "method specificity" due to the conditions of incubation, preparation of tissue, differential penetration by different antibody classes or fragments, etc.

Another advantage of the hybrid myeloma methods comes from the ability of cells in culture to produce internally radiolabelled monoclonal antibody using radioactive amino acid precursors in the tissue culture medium. The application of internally labelled antibodies offers unique possibilities in immunocytochemistry. The internally labelled antibodies offer substantial advantages over coupling of ^{125}I to purified antibody from conventional antisera which require purification of specific antibody by affinity columns. Internal labelling is superior to ^{125}I coupling to monoclonal antibodies in several respects: (i) several labels can be used (^{14}C, ^{35}S, ^{3}H) which have a much longer half-life than ^{125}I; (ii) external labelling methods involve chemical modifications and partial or severe inactivation of the antibody with consequent increase in background; (iii) the use of internally labelled amino acids is a procedure which does not require the handling precautions and restriction of ^{125}I. Radioactive contamination of laboratory workers, a common event with ^{125}I, is easily avoided.

The preparation of internally labelled monoclonal antibody is quite simple. Cells are grown under chosen conditions in the presence of ^{3}H-lysine, for example. The supernatant fluid is radiochemically about 60% pure, after removal of small molecular weight components. The radioactive reagents we have prepared have a radioactivity of about 300–2000 Ci/mmol. It has been successfully used for both light and electron microscopy (Cuello *et al.*, 1980). The most commonly used peroxidase (or ferritin) labelling methods sacrifice preservation of cell structure to allow the penetration of large complexes of antibody-enzyme molecules. Internally labelled antibody allows minimal disruption hence more detailed analysis of immunoreactive structures. Perhaps more exciting is the potential of combining immunoenzyme and radioimmunocytochemical methods for the simultaneous staining of a single preparation. This is an approach we are investigating with our antisubstance P and anti-5HT antibodies.

Uncharacteristic and unexpected serological properties of monoclonal antibodies

Monoclonal antibodies display certain features which would be uncharacteristic of conventional antisera. Unless the antigen contains multiple subunits, monoclonal antibodies are unlikely to give precipitating reactions as no three-dimensional lattices will be produced. In unpublished studies we have shown that several monoclonal antihuman IgG antibodies directed against the γ chain or the light (κ) chain did not precipitate human IgG. But the combination of pairs of them did so in double diffusion analysis (Fig. 3) or in Mancini plates. On the other hand, three different McAb directed against different sites of human C3 complement failed to give precipitin reactions under several conditions, including low concentrations of polyethylene glycol (Lachmann *et al.*, 1980). We are confronted here with a well defined example of non-precipitating antibodies. Such antibodies are an old serological puzzle not yet fully explained.

Cytotoxic reactions are affected not only by the class of the McAb, but also by the local distribution of the determinants on the cell surface. Local concentrations can be increased by multiple antibodies recognizing neighbouring determinants of the same antigen. This situation arises when using conventional (polyclonal) antisera. The importance of such synergistic effects has been clearly demonstrated using monoclonal antibodies to rat histocompatibility antigens (Howard *et al.*, 1979). A series of monoclonal antibodies seemed to recognize two independent sites of the same histocompatibility antigens. These were called P and S sites. Individual monoclonal antibodies were poorly cytotoxic or not cytotoxic. On the contrary, when McAb were

A

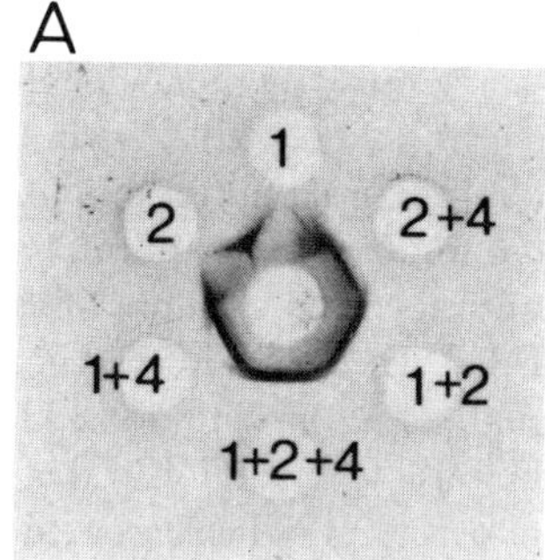

B

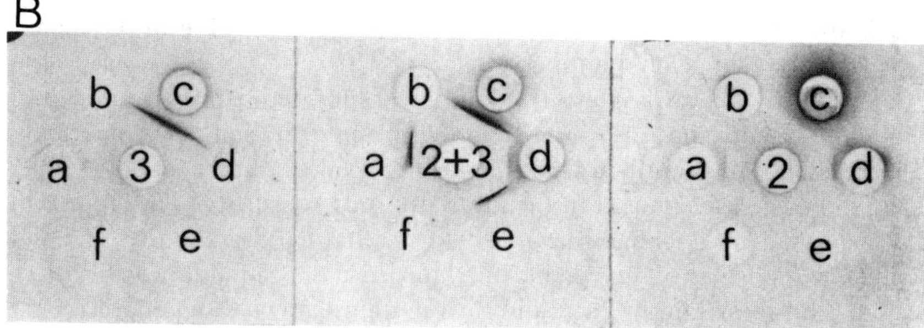

FIG. 3. *Double diffusion analysis with monclonal antibodies. A. The centre well contains human serum (diluted 1:3); the outer wells ascites fluid from mice bearing the following hybrid myeloma clones (derived in collaboration with M. Spitz and H. Waldmann) secreting antihuman IgG antibodies: 1: NH2/17 (anti-γ); 2: NH3/130 (anti-γ); 3: NH3/41 (anti-κ); 4: NH3/75 (anti-γ). Notice that a single McAb does not give a precipitin line. However, between two neighbouring wells containing different McAb (1 and 2) a precipitation zone occurs where the two McAb mix. B. The centre well contains NH3/41 (anti-κ on the left), NH3/130 (anti-γ on the right) and a mixture of the two in the centre. The outer wells contain myeloma proteins of the following sub-classes and types: [a] IgG1 (κ); [b] IgG2 (λ); [c] IgG3 (κ) (probably an aggregated preparation); [d] IgG4 (λ); [e] IgG4 (κ) Bence-Jones protein (κ). The fact that IgG3 (κ) is precipitated by NH3/41 alone is interpreted as due to multivalency of the antigen due to aggregation. The failure of the anti-γ to precipitate the aggregates could be due to steric hindrance. Note the shortening of the precipitin line in [e] and [a] due to competition by the fast diffusing Bence-Jones protein in [f].*

mixed, the blend was strongly cytotoxic. The synergistic effect was observed with McAb to P and S sites but not with different McAb directed to the same site (Howard *et al.*, 1979). This type of phenomenon explains the difficulty in detecting certain types of antibody secreting cells by cytotoxic methods and shows the way to solve the problem. Rat red cells are pretreated with one (nonlytic) monoclonal antibody. They then become excellent targets to reveal the presence of antihistocompatible antibody forming cells (by ordinary Jerne plaque assay) in appropriately immunized animals (Howard and Corvalan, 1979). Each antibody forming cell produces an antibody which is itself monoclonal and probably not lytic. But it can act synergistically with the (different) monoclonal antibody used to pretreat the red cells to produce a plaque.

Co-operative effects are also likely to be one of the reasons why monoclonal antibodies are sometimes poorer agglutinators of red cells (and coated red cells) than conventional antisera (Lachmann *et al.*, 1980), but there are other complications. A rat monoclonal antimouse Ig was tested for its ability to agglutinate sheep red cells coated with mouse antibody. The antisheep red cells used for coating were two monoclonal antibodies, Sp2 and Sp3. In the SRBC (sheep red blood cells) there are about 20 times more available binding sites for Sp2 than for Sp3. The addition of ^{3}H YA2/40 (a rat antimouse IgG) demonstrated binding in both cases. But agglutination was only observed to red cells coated with the *low* density binder Sp3 (Galfre *et al.*, 1979). The precise reasons for such effects may involve structural features and/or ratios of molecular species which are difficult to achieve and which are very critical due to the homogeneity of the monoclonal antibodies.

Unusual behaviour of monoclonal antibodies to soluble proteins in coprecipitation reaction has also been reported. Coprecipitation of an internally labelled monoclonal antibody mixed with a polyvalent antiserum is a method likely to be extensively used in the future to study specificity. This approach has been used by Lachmann *et al.* (1980) to characterize McAb to human complement. It was observed that the labelled monoclonal antibodies were able to bind to precipitin lines, and then to diffuse further and coprecipitate in a second precipitin line. This is contrary to the normal rules where precipitin lines act as diffusion barriers. It seems that an antibody to a single antigenic determinant hence (nonprecipitating by itself) present at a relatively high concentration can saturate the precipitin line (produced by the polyvalent carrier) without dissolving it. The excess McAb can then diffuse through and is available to coprecipitate with other precipitin lines which contain the relevant antigenic determinant.

References

Bazin, H., Deckers, C., Beckers, A. and Heremans, J. F. (1972). *Intern. J. Cancer* **10**, 568.

Cotton, R. G. H. and Milstein, C. (1973). *Nature* **244**, 42.

Croce, C. M., Shander, M., Martinis, J., Cicurel, L., D'Ancona, G. G., Dolby, R. W. and Koprowski, H. (1979). *Proc. Natn. Acad. Sci. U.S.A.* **76**, 3416.

Cuello, A. C., Galfre, G. and Milstein, C. (1979). *Proc. Natn. Acad. Sci. U.S.A.* **76**, 3532.

Cuello, A. C., Galfre, G. and Milstein, C. (1980). *In* "Receptors for Neurotransmitters and Peptide Hormones" (Pepeu, Kuhar and Enna, eds), pp. 349. Raven Press, New York.

Galfre, G., Milstein, C. and Wright, B. (1979). *Nature* **277**, 131.

Gomez, C. M., Richman, D. P., Berman, P. W., Burres, S. A., Arnason, B. G. W. and Fitch, F. W. (1980). (Submitted for publication).

Hengartner, H., Meo, T. and Müller, E. (1978). *Proc. Natn. Acad. Sci. U.S.A.* **75**, 4494.

Herzenberg, L. A., Herzenberg, L. A. and Milstein, C. (1978). *In* "Handbook of Experimental Immunology" (D. M. Weir, ed.), pp. 25.1. Blackwell Scientific Publications, Oxford.

Horibata, K. and Harris, A. W. (1970). *Exp. Cell Res.* **60**, 61.
Howard, J. C. and Corvalan, J. R. F. (1979). *Nature* **278**, 449.
Howard, J. C., Butcher, G. W., Galfre, G. and Milstein, C. (1979). *Immunol. Rev.* **47**, 139.
Janossy, G., Tidman, N., Crawford, D., Papageorgiou, E. S., Francis, G., Bradstock, K. F., McConnell, I., Secher, D. S. and Milstein, C. (1980). *Protides Biol. Fluids* **28** (in press).
Köhler, G. (1980). *Proc. Natn. Acad. Sci. U.S.A.* **77**, 2197.
Köhler, G. and Milstein, C. (1975). *Nature* **256**, 495.
Köhler, G. and Milstein, C. (1976). *Eur. J. Immunol.* **6**, 511.
Köhler, G., Hengartner, H. and Milstein, C. (1978). *Protides Biol. Fluids* **25**, 545.
Lachmann, P., Oldroyd, R. G., Milstein, C. and Wright, B. W. (1980). *Immunology* (in press).
Margulis, D. H., Kuehl, W. M. and Scharff, M. D. (1976). *Cell* **8**, 405.
Milstein, C. and Lennox, E. S. (1980). *In* "Current Topics in Developmental Biology", Vol. 14 (M. Friedlander, ed.). Academic Press, New York and London.
Milstein, C., Galfre, G., Secher, D. S. and Springer, T. (1979). CIBA Foundation Symposium No. 66, pp. 251. Excerpta Medica, Amsterdam.
Moshly-Rosen, D., Fuchs, S. and Eskhar, Z. (1980). (Submitted for publication.)
Raschke, W. C., Mather, E. L. and Koshland, M. E. (1979). *Proc. Natn. Acad. Sci. U.S.A.* **76**, 3469.
Ringerts, N. R. and Savage, R. E. (1976). *In* "Cell Hybrids", (N. R. Ringerts and R. E. Savage, eds). Academic Press, New York and London.
Secher, D. S. and Burke, D. C. (1980). *Nature* **285**, 446.
Schröder, J., Autio, J., Jarvis, J. M. and Milstein, C. (1980). *Immunogenetics* **10**, 125.
Smith, M. and Hirschorn, K. (1978). *Proc. Natn. Acad. Sci. U.S.A.* **75**, 3367.
Takei, F., Galfre, G., Alderson, T., Lennox, E. S. and Milstein, C. (1980). *Eur. J. Immunol.* **10**, 241.
Takei, F., Waldmann, H., Lennox, E. S. and Milstein, C. (1980). *Eur. J. Immunol.* (in press).
Voak, D., Sacks, S., Alderson, T., Takei, F., Lennox, E. S., Jarvis, J., Milstein, C. and Darnborough, J. (1980). *Vox sanguinis* (in press).
Wilde, C. D. and Milstein, C. (1980). *Eur. J. Immunol.* **10**, 462.
Williams, A. F., Galfre, G. and Milstein, C. (1977). *Cell* **12**, 663.

3

The Organization of Immunoglobulin Genes and the Origin of Their Diversity

P. LEDER, E. E. MAX and J. G. SEIDMAN

Laboratory of Molecular Genetics,
National Institute of Child Health and Human Development,
National Institutes of Health,
Bethesda, Maryland, USA

Introduction

Our insight into the nature of the immunoglobulin genes is growing so rapidly that one is tempted to wait a few months in order to allow the results of experiments in progress to form a complete picture. Indeed, with only a few (albeit important) gaps left, our image of how immunoglobulin light chain genes are assembled and how they generate diversity is nearly complete and many important aspects of heavy chain gene structure and assembly are being revealed from work proceeding in almost a dozen laboratories. Given this

We are grateful to Marion Nau and Barbara Norman for their expert help in this work. We are also grateful to Terri Broderick for expert assistance.

situation, it still seems useful to consider in detail now the mechanisms used to generate diversity in light chain genes while treating some of the newer and emerging features of heavy chain assembly in broader outline.

The problem and the Dreyer-Bennett solution

The problem that confronts those of us who have been concerned with the nature of antibody diversity became clear almost two decades ago from the early studies of immunoglobulin structure. The unique fact that antibody subunits constituted classes of polypeptides that were identical in their carboxy-terminal amino acid sequences, but variable in their amino-terminal portions, required a genetic explanation. The additional fact that this variation in the amino-terminal portion of light and heavy chains provided the antigen-binding specificity of each antibody molecule lent additional physiological relevance and interest to the problem (see review and references in Leder *et al.*, 1974).

During the sixties and early seventies a profusion of general and detailed models, many of them experimentally useful, were advanced to account for the unusual structure of antibodies and to relate their structure to the generation of antibody diversity. The most simple model had great appeal, namely that antibody genes were encoded in the germline colinearly with the structure of each immunoglobulin subunit; i.e. a thousand heavy and light chain genes encoded with variable and constant regions adjacent to one another. This argument required no unprecedented biochemical events to generate a large antibody gene repertoire. Gene duplication, amplification and the general mechanisms that accomplish divergence among other genes would allow evolution alone to provide the diverse variable region repertoire.

While this germline argument was attractive in its simplicity, it had a flaw that was quickly recognized by Dreyer and Bennett (1965). They were troubled by the necessity of postulating a thousand discrete segments of DNA somehow divided so that the initial portion of each could vary during evolution while the terminal portion was held absolutely constant. Selection alone provided an unsatisfactory mechanism for maintaining the unaltered sequence of the constant region, because it was clear that the constant regions of both light and heavy chains could tolerate amino acid substitutions (e.g. the difference between κ and λ chains). Faced with this paradox, they made a radical proposal that would neatly solve the problem. They suggested that variable and constant regions were separately encoded and, moreover, that there were many variable region genes but only one copy of the constant region sequence. Such an arrangement would automatically provide for a single constant region sequence in all immunoglobulin subunits of a given class. One had only then to assume (as Dreyer and Bennett did) that this single constant region gene was capable of being joined to any one of the many variable region genes. As we shall see below, their model, proposed in 1965, has been proved to be substantially correct.

Molecular biology enters

A light chain locus

The development of techniques for protein purification and amino acid sequencing provided the facts from which our initial picture of antibody structure and diversity emerged. A generation of immunologists had developed the critical molecular details as well as the intellectual framework for the problem, but a new technology whose roots were in molecular genetics and the chemistry and enzymology of DNA provided the final answers and often confirmed theoretical proposals made years before.

The earliest efforts of molecular biologists to reconcile the diversity parodox were directed towards testing a strong prediction of the Dreyer-Bennett hypothesis. The germline models required many (a thousand or more) copies of constant region genes, whereas the Dreyer-Bennett model required only one. Technical developments in the field had advanced to the stage that an immunoglobulin light chain mRNA could be translated, purified and converted into a highly labelled DNA sequence (cDNA) using the then newly discovered viral enzyme, reverse transcriptase. This cDNA, which could be manipulated to correspond only to the constant region coding portion of the mRNA, was used as a hybridization probe in several laboratories to show that there were, at the most, very few copies of the light chain constant region genome (see review in Leder *et al.*, 1974). This result, of course, was entirely consistent with the Dreyer-Bennett proposal and, given that the many known variable region amino acid sequences strongly suggested the presence of many germline variable region genes, it inevitably strengthened the notion that these genes were separately encoded.

A precise picture of the κ light chain gene

The discovery of the restriction endonucleases and their application to the mapping of gene sequences on DNA allowed Hozumi and Tonegawa (1976) to do an elegant experiment which tested this notion in a more direct fashion. They cleaved DNA from embryonic and plasma cells (the latter derived from an immunoglobulin-producing plasmacytoma) with a restriction endonuclease, then separated the cleaved fragments according to size by electrophoresis and assayed for variable (V) and constant (C) region genes using appropriate cDNA probes. Their results indicated that constant and variable region genes resided on different fragments in DNA derived from embryonic tissue, whereas these genes resided on the same fragment in DNA derived from immunoglobulin-producing cells. Obviously, the Dreyer-Bennett prediction was correct and it was also evident that V/C assembly took place at the level of DNA.

That these conclusions were correct could be demonstrated in a very direct way by making use of the tools of recombinant DNA technology (Seidman *et al.*, 1978a; Tonegawa *et al.*, 1978; Brack *et al.*, 1978; Seidman and Leder, 1978b). Indeed, the cloned genes are easily visualized electronmicroscopically and the fact that they are in different configurations in antibody-producing cells as compared to other cells was made obvious by visualizing the clones (Fig. 1) (Seidman *et al.*, 1979). Apart from directly demonstrating the fact that V and C regions are separately encoded and undergo somatic recombination to form an active κ gene, detailed sequencing studies revealed further interesting and unexpected features of their structure. The germline V region gene (Fig. 1A) only encoded amino acids through position 95, though the V region conventionally had been associated with positions 1 to 108 (Seidman *et al.*, 1978; Tonegawa *et al.*, 1978). Furthermore, electronmicroscopic and sequence analysis showed that the remaining 13 codons of the V region were separately encoded about 3·7 kb to the 5′ side of the C region gene (Fig. 1B) (Brack *et al.*, 1978; Bernard *et al.*, 1978; Seidman and Leder, 1978; Sakano *et al.*, 1979). This segment (the J segment) encoded the remaining codons of the V region, but also specified the site at which the V region joined close to the C region to form the active gene (Fig. 1C). Since additional studies involving *in situ* hybridization indicated that there were several hundred separately encoded V region genes in the germline (Seidman *et al.*, 1978; Valbuena *et al.*, 1978), this somatic recombination mechanism could theoretically utilize any germline V region by joining it at the J site near the single constant region gene. Genes for the κ, λ and heavy chains appear to be similar in this regard (see below).

Diversity is amplified by the availability of multiple J regions

The additional feature of the structure of these genes that is a powerful element in generating their diversity is that there is not just 1 J coding segment near the κ constant region gene, as is the case with the mouse λ genes (Bernard *et al.*, 1979; Sakano *et al.*, 1979). Moreover, 4 of these appear to be active in that they correspond to amino acid sequences that appear in sequenced mouse light chains. The central J fragment, J3, encodes a sequence that has never been found in a light chain and we have suggested that a single nucleotide change at its 3′ border inactivates a signal necessary for RNA splicing (Max *et al.*, 1979). Thus its mRNA precursor should not be assembled coherently.

It is immediately clear that the combinational power of joining one of several hundred V regions with 1 of 4 J segments can generate over a thousand different light chain sequences. An analogous situation seems to exist for the mouse heavy chain, except that an additional segment seems to be separately encoded (the D segment; see below) between V and J and therefore must be involved in somatic recombination (Early *et al.*, 1980). While the existence of such D segments has only been inferred, this would obviously require an additional DNA joining event to form an active V/D/J segment. This reaction would further amplify the diversity available in the heavy chain.

In its final structure, an active light chain gene is composed of 3 discrete coding segments. These are shown diagrammatically in Fig. 2. The initial segment encodes a hydrophobic leader sequence (usually codons -19 to -4) that is separated from the somatically joined V/J segment (codons -3 to 108) by a small (100–200 bp) intervening sequence. These 2 V segments are

EMBRYONIC

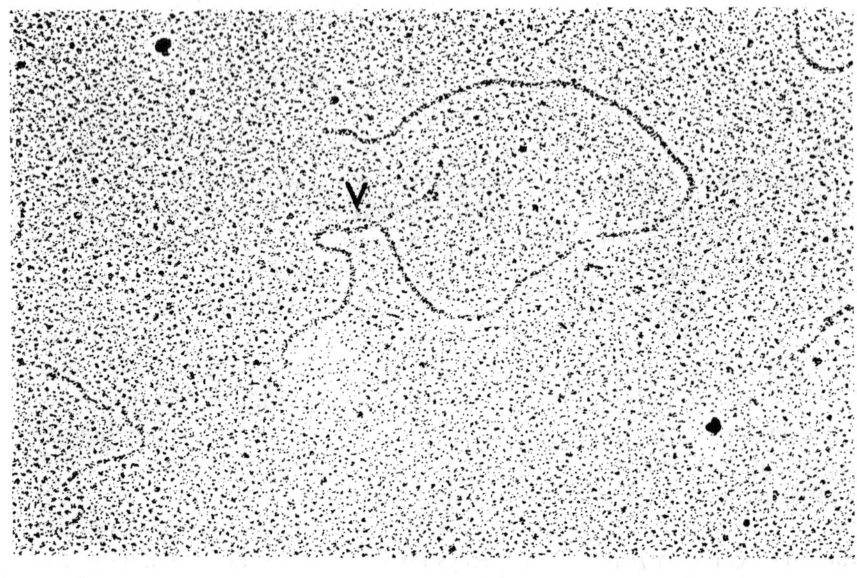

(A)

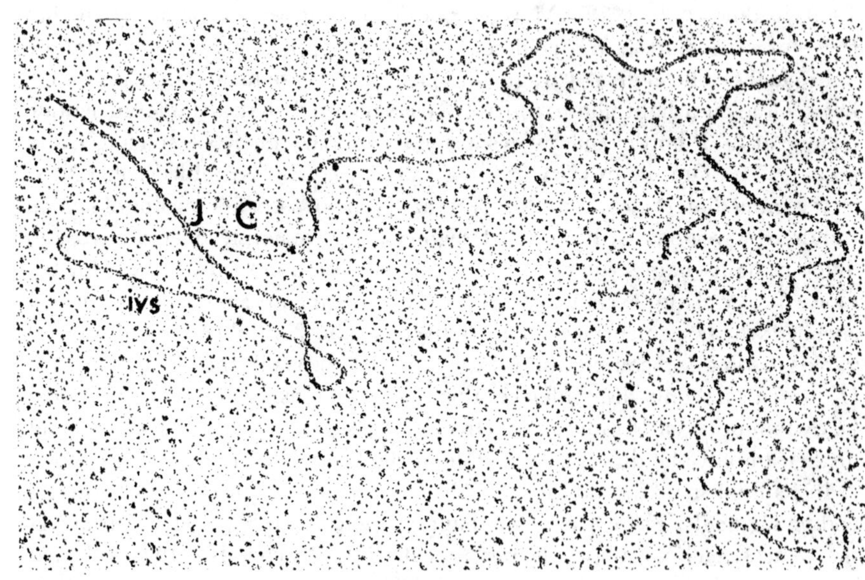

(B)

RECOMBINANT

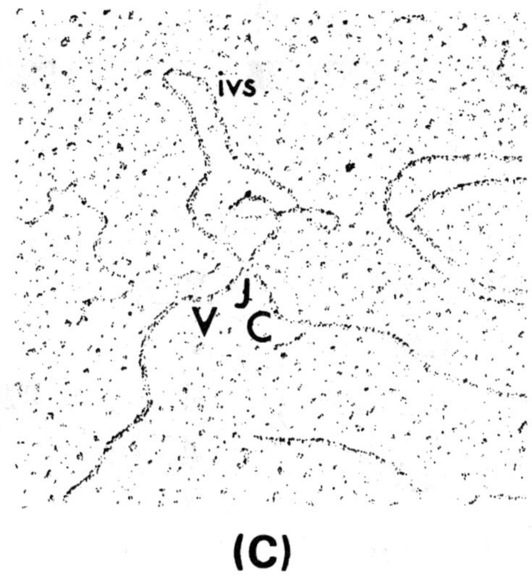

(C)

FIG. 1. *Electronmicroscopic visualization of mouse chain genes in their germline and somatically rearranged configurations. The electronmicrographs represent (A) germline variable (V), (B) germline constant (C), and (C) somatically rearranged, active κ light chain genes. The cloned fragments of "germline" DNA were derived from 12-day-old mouse embryos; the cloned fragment of the active light chain gene was derived from the κ chain producing plasmacytoma MOPC-41. The segments of DNA corresponding to the mRNA are visualized by annealing mRNA to each fragment under special conditions, displacing the strand of DNA that is identical to the mRNA. This region appears as a bubble (R-loop) in the electronmicrograph. Occasionally, mRNA sequences not present on a fragment can be visualized as an unannealed tail. In addition, it can be seen in the germline C R-loop that the fragment crosses itself at the edge of C R-loop. This is because a coding segment, the J (or joining) region, is encoded 3·7 kb away from the main body of the C region and the mRNA has annealed to it (see diagram in Fig 2). The germline V region is joined to this J segment in the active gene (C), leaving the gene interrupted by 3.7 kb intervening sequence. The gene is interrupted by one other small intervening sequence that separates a hydrophobic leader sequence from the body of the V region gene. This interruption is too small (~100 bases) to be visualized in the electronmicrograph. The structure of these genes in germline and active configuration is indicated diagrammatically in Fig. 2. (Reprinted with permission from Seidman* et al., *1979.)*

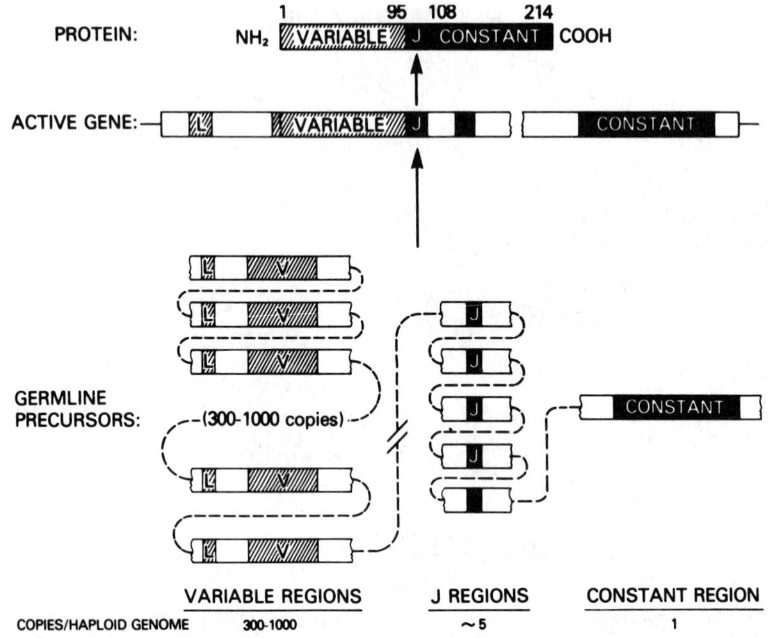

FIG. 2. *Diagrammatic representation of the germline and active κ chain gene configurations. The bottom diagram represents the germline configuration of the V, J and C region genes. The middle diagram represents the structure of an active κ gene formed by somatic recombination between one of the germline Vs and Js. The uppermost diagram represents the structure of the mature light chain. The hatched areas marked L and V are the leader (codons −19 to −4) and body (codons −3 to +95) of the V region respectively. The solid areas marked J and Constant represent those regions respectively. The numbers above the uppermost figure refer to amino acid positions.*

separated by a much larger intervening sequence (3·7–2·4 kb) from the C segment. Depending upon which J region has been used for somatic recombination, a number of unused J segments are "trapped" within the intervening sequence. Obviously the active J region must provide some sort of signal for DNA recombination (see below) on one of the faces (5′) while it also provides a signal for RNA splicing on the other (3′). The final immunoglobulin mRNA is assembled by splicing the coding segments from a larger RNA precursor (Gilmore-Hebert *et al.*, 1978; Rabbits, 1978; Perry *et al.*, 1979). Evidently the inactive Js are not used as splice signals (Perry *et al.*, 1979), an observation that suggests that they are activated by V/J recombination.

The flexible nature of V/J recombination: an additional source of diversity

From the standpoint of the molecular geneticist, the V/J joining reaction is an extraordinarily interesting one. Not only is it a means of generating diversity and of creating an active gene, it must be a carefully controlled reaction, playing, as it does, a cardinal role in the development of the lymphocyte. While V and C regions are thought to be located on the same germline

```
                                    <--*--> TrpThrPheGlyGlyGlyThrLysLeuGluIleLysArg
GGAGGGTTTTTGTACAGCCAGACAGTGGAGTACTACCACTGTGGTGGACGTTCGGTGGAGGCACCAAGCTGGAAATCAAACGTAAGTAG      J5
-------------

                                             *
                                    <--*--> TyrThrPheGlyGlyGlyThrLysLeuGluIleLysArg
GCTCAGTTTTTGTATGGGGGTTGAGTTAAGGGACACCAGTGTG TACACGTTCGGAGGGGGGACXAAGCTGGAAATAAAACGTAAGTAG      J4
-------------                             TG
                                             *        *  *                       *
                                    <--*--> IleThrPheSerAspGlyThrArgLeuGluIleLysPro
GGAGGG TTTTGT  GGAGGTAAAGTTAAAATAAATCACTGTAAATCACATTCAGTGATGGGACCAGACTGGAAATAAAACCTAAGTAC      J3
------ ------
                                             *           *
                                    <--*--> PheThrPheGlySerGlyThrLysLeuGluIleLysArg
GGCAGGTTTTTGTAAAGGGGGCGCAGTGATATGAATCACTG GATTCACGTTCGGCTCGGGGACAAAGTTGGAAATAAAACGTAAGTAG      J2
-------------
                                             *           *                 *
                                    <--*--> LeuThrPheGlyAlaGlyThrLysLeuGluLeuLysArg
GGCAGGTTTTTGTAGAGAGGGGCATGTCATAGTCCTCACTGTGGCTCACGTTCGGTGCTGGGACCAAGCTGGAGCTGAAACGTAAGTAC      J1
-------------

                                    <--*-->
                                    CACXGTG
```

FIG. 3. *The nucleotide sequences of the J gene recombination site. The nucleotide sequences of the 5 J regions are shown. Above each sequence are the translated 13 amino acids that comprise each J region. An asterisk appears above each amino acid that differs from the J 5 sequence. A double headed arrow marks each heptanucleotide palindrome and the consensus palindrome is shown at the bottom of the figure. A T region about 20–23 nucleotides to the 5′ side of the palindrome is also underlined in each sequence. Both these regions are complementary to sequences identified on the 3′ of the V region joining sites and can be drawn as the stem structure shown in Fig. 4. The data are from Max* et al., *1979.*

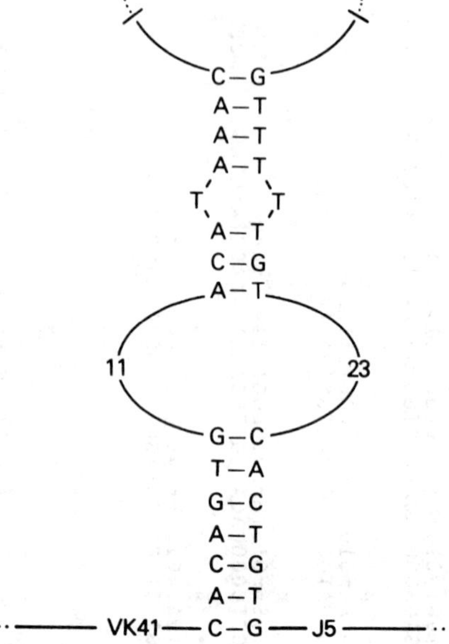

FIG. 4. *Complementary sequences at the germline V/J junction. The diagram represents the V and J regions as if they were encoded in a 5′ to 3′ order. A complementary stem is drawn between the conserved sequences shown in Fig. 3 and complementary sequences from the germline K41 V region gene. The nucleotide sequence at the V/J junction that forms the mouse K41 gene is shown (Seidman)* et al., *1979*).

chromosome, their precise location and orientation are not known. Nevertheless several experimental facts provide some insight into V/J recombination reaction.

There is a small, self-complementary, palindromic heptanucleotide sequence recognizable just to the 5′ side of all J regions thus far sequenced (Fig. 3). This sequence (CACTGTG), in addition to a T rich sequence about 20 bases 3′ to the palindrome, can be shown as a stem-like structure (Fig. 4) drawing a V and J region together across its base. If such a structure were relevant to recombination, joining of the V and J region segments should be accompanied by the deletion of intervening V and J region segments. *In situ* hybridization experiments clearly indicate that such deletions occur (Sakano *et al.*, 1979; Seidman *et al.*, 1980).

A further interesting point about the recombination reaction follows from the observation that all the mouse BALB/c κ chains sequenced through the J region correspond to 1 of the 4 germline J region amino acid sequences at every position except position 96. For example, an ARG or PRO can be substituted for the TRP position in germline J5 sequence. More importantly, position 96 seems to be involved in the formation of the antibody–antigen combining site and its variation should contribute greatly to physiological diversity by altering antibody specificity (Padlan *et al.*, 1976).

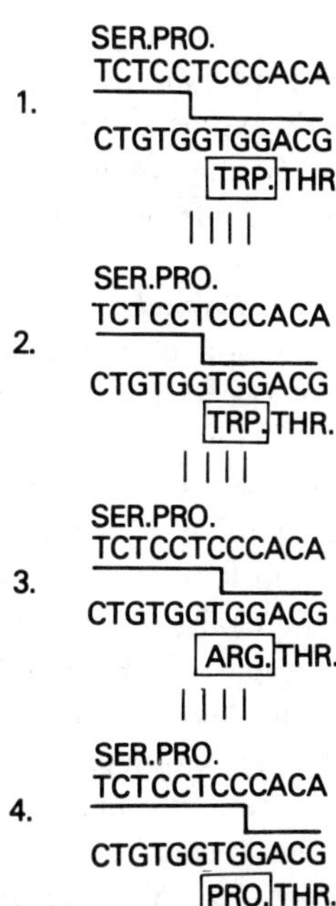

FIG. 5. *Altering the frame of somatic recombination accounts for diversity at amino acid codon 96. The sample nucleotide sequences of germline V and J regions are aligned at the V/J recombination site. The examples are VK41 (top) and J5 (bottom). The cross-over point of recombination is indicated by the line under/over each sequence. The translation of the product of 4 cross-overs is shown. The boxed amino acid is at the cross-over point.*

This discrepancy at this critical position could easily be accounted for by making a simple assumption about the nature of the V/J recombination event itself; namely, that it could vary in the cross-over point of recombination. The consequences of such variation are shown in Fig. 5 where the sequence of the V/J junction of the germline V region gene (VK41) and a germline J region (J5) are used as examples. In cross-over 3 and 4 in that figure, the codons for ARG and PRO are easily generated by using a recombinational cross-over point that differs from that shown in cross-over 1 and 2 which retain the germline amino acid sequence. Thus, such a mechanism would vastly amplify the diversity available through the V/J recombination reaction by altering the amino acids at and around position 96.

We have been able to confirm that variation in the cross-over point of recombination actually occurs by determining the nucleotide sequences of several myeloma recombinants. These are shown diagrammatically in Fig. 6. The recombination event that formed the MOPC 41 (Seidman *et al.*, 1979) and MOPC 321 (Sakano *et al.*, 1979) genes preserved the germline sequence. The recombination event that formed the MOPC 173B sequence deleted a single base forming a cryptic gene with a nonsense J sequence (Max *et al.*, 1980), while the recombination event that formed the S107B sequences deleted 2 codons to form an in-phase, but foreshortened J region (S.-P. Kwan, E. E.

Max, J. G. Seidman, M. Scharff, and P. Leder, unpub. results). It is clear from these analyses that V/J recombination can occur using various cross-over points *and* that it does not always occur in proper phase. The lack of a mechanism to assure in-phase (with coding sequences) recombination must be responsible for the exclusion of one of the pair of immunoglobulin alleles from antibody production (see below).

Point mutations remote from the V/J recombination site

One aspect of the somatic variation of V region sequences remains to be explained. Extensive studies of the amino acid sequences of closely related BALB/c mouse λ light chains had revealed single amino acid alterations that clustered in the hypervariable regions that form the antigen-antibody combining site (Cohn *et al.*, 1974). Similar restricted alterations were found in κ chains in NZB mice (Weigert and Riblet, 1977). The nucleotide sequences of the genes of one of these light chains further revealed discrete nucleotide changes that differed from the apparent germline V region sequence and that accounted for the amino acid alterations (Bernard *et al.*, 1978). The molecular basis for these solitary base changes is obscure, although the elegant proposal that they are the result of assembling smaller mini-genes (Kabat *et al.*, 1978) appears to be ruled out by the known structure of V region sequences in non-lymphocyte (Seidman *et al.*, 1978b; Tonegawa *et al.*, 1978) and sperm (Early *et al.*, 1980a) DNA.

Perhaps one clue to the origin of these changes comes from a more careful consideration of sequence changes that accompany V/J and non-V/J recombination. In particular, we have noted a single base change in the third hypervariable that accompanies the V/J recombination event that forms the MOPC173B gene (Max *et al.*, 1980). Further, we have noted a "spray" of several nucleotide changes that occur within the intervening sequence of a MOPC149 non-V/J recombinant (Max, Seidman and Leder, unpublished). In short, it seems that these recombination events may be accompanied by faulty DNA repair processes that scatter nucleotide changes at a considerable distance from the recombination site. While such an error-prone repair system seems attractive, it does not account for the apparent specificity that the clustered amino acid alterations suggest. In this regard, it will be interesting to see whether this clustered relationship persists in the growing numbers of sequenced V regions.

The molecular basis of allelic exclusion

Most lymphocytes produce only heavy and light chains that correspond to one of their two chromosomal alleles. This phenomenon is called allelic exclusion and much of what we have learned about the organization of immunoglobulin genes in plasmacytoma is relevant to its molecular basis. Obviously, if one of the two light (or heavy) chain alleles remains in the germline configuration it will not be expressed. Such a situation is not uncommon (Seidman and Leder, 1978; Joho and Weissmann, 1980). On the other hand, we have just seen that V/J recombination can occur out-of-phase, creating a nonsense J. If the other gene were properly formed, this cell would

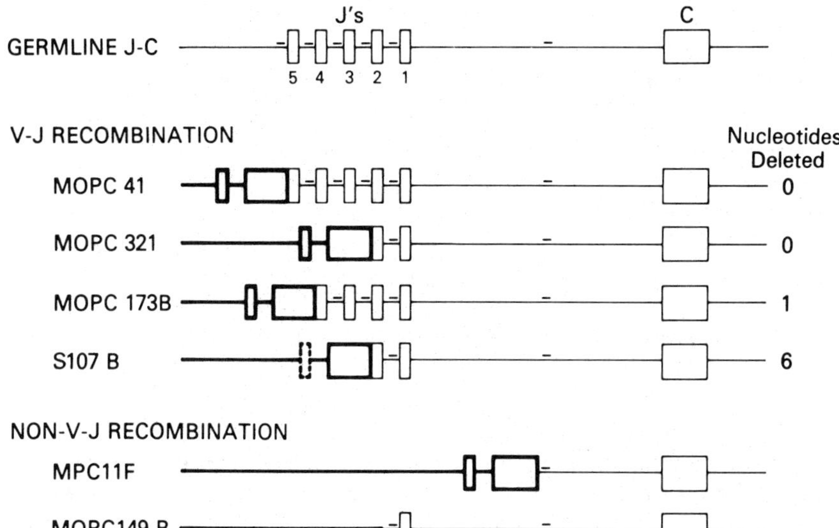

FIG. 6. *Diagrammatic representation of the structure of several normally and aberrantly recombined κ light chain genes. The fine line represents the germline J/C region sequences; the heavy line represents V regions. The small palindrome referred to in the text is represented as a short dash. Each recombinant is discussed in the text where relevant references are indicated.*

phenotypically express only one light chain allele. In addition, it is clear that some of the recombinational activity that affects light chain genes is unrelated to V/J joining and creates "null" recombinants, that is, recombinants that cannot form an active light chain (see MOPC-149 in Fig. 6).

Interestingly, there is one special, but possibly common, type of null recombinant that produces a mutant fragment of a κ light chain (Kuehl and Scharff, 1974). The gene in this plasmacytoma (MPC-11, see Fig. 6) has recombined at a site *between* J and C sequences, exactly at the only non-J CACAGTG palindrome within 5 kb of the 5′ side of the C region (Seidman and Leder, 1980). Since there is RNA splice signal at the 3′ end of the V region this gene directs the synthesis of a light chain fragment consistent of a leader sequence and a C region. A survey of mRNAs produced by a bank of plasmacytomas suggests that null recombinants of this type are quite common (Perry *et al.*, 1980). In any event, it seems clear that while these recombinational mechanisms serve to generate enormous diversity, they accomplish it at considerable cost to the organism in terms of generating null recombinants.

The heavy chain locus

While the structure and rearrangement of heavy and light chain genes are similar in many important ways, there are a number of differences that add interesting complexities to the heavy chain system. Lymphocyte differentiation involves the initial appearance of a μ chain in the cytoplasm of a pre-B cell (Raff, 1976; Cooper *et al.*, 1976) followed by the appearance of surface IgM

(Lala *et al.*, 1979; Kearney *et al.*, 1977) and, often, IgD (Goding and Layton, 1976; Vittetta and Uhr, 1977). The specificity and idiotype of IgM and IgD molecules expressed on the same cell are identical, which suggests that their V regions are also identical (Abney and Parkhouse, 1974; Fu *et al.*, 1975; Coffman and Cohn, 1977). In addition, further maturation of the lymphocyte results in the loss of IgD production with the continued production of membrane bound IgM and, often simultaneously, a new immunoglobulin heavy chain class. Continued development may result in eventual loss of IgM production and a switch to the exclusive production of one or another of the mature heavy chain classes IgM (secreted), IgG, IgA or IgE. The process that allows a change in the heavy chain constant region component while maintaining the expression of the same V region is called the heavy chain class switch. Much of what has been learned about the organization of immunoglobulin heavy chains over the last 2 years has shed light on these switching mechanisms as well as upon the mechanism that generates diversity in the variable region of the heavy chain. While this information is accumulating rapidly and uncertainties remain, a reasonably reliable map of the mouse heavy chain locus can be constructed by putting together data from a number of laboratories. Such a map is shown diagrammatically in Fig. 7.

Three elements form the heavy chain V region

While formation of a complete heavy chain region involves the joining of germline V and J regions, it appears to involve a third element as well. Early *et al.* (1980a) and Sakano *et al.* (1980) were able to show that the sequences present in germline V and J region genes did not include the amino acids that appeared between codon positions 95 and 102 (using the numbering system of Kabat *et al*, 1977) in cloned, active heavy chain genes. They suggested that these amino acids, including almost the entire third hypervariable region, were separately encoded in what is now called a D segment, and that formation of the V_H sequence involved 2 joining events that form the V/D/J sequence. V/D/J recombination is thought to involve the same signals that may play a role in light chain V/J joining (see above). The consequences of such a putative recombination event are shown diagrammatically in Fig. 7. At present, there is no direct evidence supporting the existence of a discrete D region segment.

Simultaneous μ/δ chain production

The simultaneous production of IgM and IgD might be accounted for without invoking DNA rearrangements. Recent cloning studies (Liu *et al.*, 1980) have established the relative map position of μ and δ heavy chain genes which lie, respectively, in a 5′/3′ orientation approximately 2·5 kb from one another in the mouse genome (see Fig. 7). The proximity of these genes, their orientation, the fact that both μ and δ are heavy chains that are simultaneously associated with the same V region, and the fact that alternative RNA splice or termination choices appear to account for the simultaneous expression of membrane and secreted μ chains (see below), prompted these authors to suggest that μ and δ chains arise from the differential processing of an RNA precursor. Such precursors would be processed so as to include or exclude the μ or γ sequence. The model is plausible and, above all, experimentally testable.

The μ/γ-α switch

Lymphocyte maturation often involves a shift from IgM production to the synthesis of either IgG or IgA. The possibility that the heavy chain class switch could be brought about by a recombination event involving the deletion of the active μ chain and the joining of an active V_H region gene to one of an array of γ or α heavy chain sequences was first tested experimentally by Honjo and Kataoka (1978) using hybridization kinetic analyses to determine the copy number of γ genes in IgA producing myeloma cells. Their conclusions regarding the deletion of genes to the 5′ side of expressed heavy chain and of the order of the heavy chains in the germline chromosome have subsequently been confirmed in a series of detailed and more precise studies (Cory and Adams, 1980; Rabbits *et al.*, 1980; Coleclough *et al.*, 1980; Cory *et al.*, 1980; Yaoita and Honjo, 1980a, b). Although the order of the γ and α genes has not been established directly (the internal order of the 4 γ genes has been directly established by gene cloning (Honjo *et al.*, 1980)), the deletion data are consistent with the arrangement shown in Fig. 7. Germline configurations and sequences of numbers of γ (Miyata *et al.*, 1980; Sakano *et al.*, 1980) and α (Davis *et al.*, 1980a, b) have also been determined.

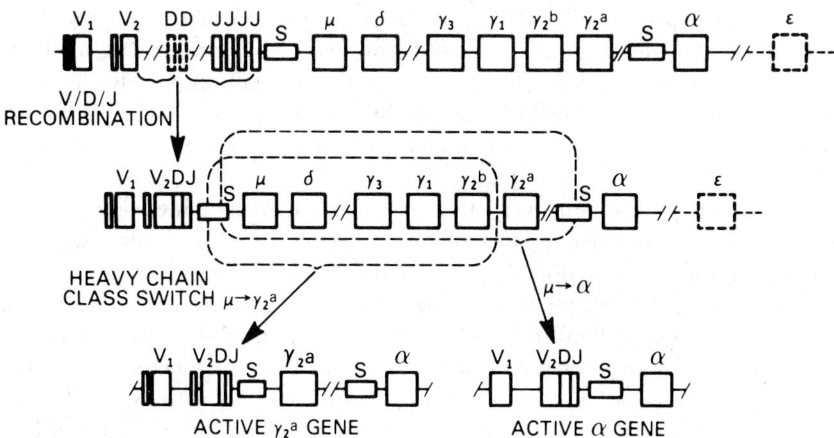

FIG. 7. *Diagrammatic representation of the heavy chain gene locus in germline and recombined configuration. The map is not to scale and does not represent the detailed structure of the constant region domains. Broken lines represent gene orders that are likely, though not established. Dashed lines represent sequences not yet cloned and the boxed S represents putative switch regions. The uppermost map represents the germline configuration; the middle map represents a rearranged, active μ gene; and the lower 2 maps represent "switched" γ and α genes as indicated. The brackets enclose segments deleted by the recombination events that lead to V/D/J joining or the 2 indicated switches. References relevant to the derivation of this map are given in the text.*

In contrast to the relatively precise nature of the V/J recombination event the heavy chain class switch seems to occur at a variety of recombination sites included within the intervening sequences of the μ, γ or α germline sequence (Davis *et al.*, 1980a; Kataoka *et al.*, 1980; Maki *et al.*, 1980; Takahashi *et al.*, 1980). Thus, as indicated in Fig. 7, an active γ or α gene will be assembled from an active V/D/J sequence and its adjacent μ intervening sequence which is joined to the 5′ flanking sequence of a germline γ or α gene. The precise signals that are responsible for the various heavy chain class switches are not known, but the occurrence of runs of repeated sequences around the switching site in μ, γ and α chains offer an attractive basis for speculation (Davis *et al.*, 1980b; Dunnick *et al.*, 1980; Takahashi *et al.*, 1980; Rabbits *et al.*, 1980; Tyler and Adams, 1980; Sakano *et al.*, 1980). Indeed, recent comparisons of these switch regions that have been conserved between mouse and human μ and α genes suggest that the μ/α switch may depend upon extensive homology in the switch region (Ravetch *et al.*, 1980). The fact that such an extensive homology is lacking between μ and γ genes further suggests that the two different class switches may depend upon somewhat different mechanisms. The extreme variability in the switch site and the lack of characteristic V/J complementing sequences in the switching region (Sakano *et al.*, 1980) at least suggest that these different recombination steps depend upon different systems of enzymes.

RNA processing determines μ chain secretion

We considered earlier the possibility that simultaneous μ and δ chain production might depend upon differential processing of an mRNA precursor containing sequences encoding both structures. Strong precedent for such a mechanism is provided by what has recently been learned about the gene responsible for the membrane bound and secreted forms of the μ chain (Melchers and Uhr, 1973). These two forms of μ chain appear to differ by virtue of a lengthened, possibly hydrophobic, peptide present at the C terminal portion of the membrane bound μ chain (M. Kehry, cited in Rogers *et al.*, 1980).

Both polypeptide chains turn out to be encoded by the same μ gene (Early *et al.*, 1980b). The C terminal portion of the μ gene consists of a coding segment corresponding to the C_μ domain, separated by a 1·85 kb intervening sequence from 2 small coding segments that together constitute a 26 amino acid long hybrophobic peptide flanked by charged amino acid residues. Two alternative RNA splicing patterns or poly A addition sites determine whether or not the membrane (M) peptide coding segment becomes a part of the μ RNA (Rogers *et al.*, 1980; Alt *et al.*, 1980). If a splice occurs between a site within the $C\mu4$ domain and M domain, a termination codon is eliminated and a longer membrane bound domain is produced. If this splicing event fails to occur or the transcript does not reach the M coding segment, the membrane anchor peptide is not synthesized and secreted form of the μ chain is produced instead. Thus the immune system not only uses various sequence combinations at the DNA level to produce antibody diversity, but employs the same principles to expand genetic possibilities at the RNA level as well.

Summary

The major sources of diversity for the light chain arise from a somatic recombination events that join one of several hundred V region sequences to one of a short series of J region segments. In addition to various combinations inherent in this process, the cross-over point of recombination can itself vary and thereby generate additional diversity, particularly at the amino acid codons formed at the critical V/J recombination site. Heavy chain diversity is similarly generated but appears to involve the incorporation of a third segment (D) between V and J sequences. Heavy chain class switching among μ, γ and α chains appears to occur by recombination between large sites that lie within the flanking sequences 5′ to each of these germline genes and that shifts active V region sequences close to the appropriate heavy chain coding segment. Alternative RNA splicing patterns also play a role in altering constant regions, particularly in determining whether a μ chain will contain a membrane anchor peptide or not. Such mechanisms may also be involved in simultaneous association of a given V region with both μ and γ heavy chains.

References

Abney, E. and Parkhouse, R. M. E. (1974). *Nature (Lond.)* **252**, 600.

Alt, F. W., Bothwell, A. L. M., Knapp, M., Siden, E., Mather, E., Koshland, M. and Baltimore, D. (1980). *Cell* **20**, 293–301.

Bernard, O., Hozumi, N. and Tonegawa, S. (1978). *Cell* **15**, 1133–1144.

Brack, C., Hirama, M., Lenhard-Schuller, R. and Tonegawa, S. (1978). *Cell* **15**, 1–14.

Cohn, M., Blomberg, B., Geckeler, W., Raschke, W., Riblet, R. and Weigert, M. (1974). *In* "The Immune System: Genes, Receptors, Signals" (E. Sercarz *et al.*, ed.), p. 89. Academic Press, New York and London.

Coleclough, C., Cooper, D. and Perry, R. P. (1980). *Proc. Natn. Acad. Sci. U.S.A.* **77**, 1422–1426.

Cooper, M. D., Kearney, J. F., Lydyard, P. M., Grossi, C. E. and Lawton, A. R. (1976). *Cold Spring Harbor Symp. Quant. Biol.* **41**, 139.

Cory, S. and Adams, J. (1980). *Cell* **19**, 37–51.

Cory, S., Jackson, J. and Adams, J. M. (1980). *Nature (Lond.)* **285**, 450–455.

Davis, M. M., Calame, K., Early, P. W., Livant, D. L., Joho, R., Weissmann, I. L. and Hood, L. (1980a). *Nature (Lond.)* **283**, 733–739.

Davis, M. M., Kim, S. K. and Hood, L. E. (1980b). *Science* **209**, 1360–1365.

Dreyer W. and Bennett, J. C. (1965). *Proc. natn. Acad. Sci U.S.A.* **54**, 864–868.

Dunnick, W., Rabbits, T. H. and Milstein, C. (1980). *Nature (Lond.)* **286**, 669–675.

Early, P., Huang, H., Davis, M., Calame, K. and Hood, L. (1980a). *Cell* **19**, 981–992.

Early, P., Rogers, J., Davis, M., Calame, K., Bond, M., Wall, R. and Hood L. (1980b). *Cell* **20**, 313–319.

Gilmore-Hebert, M., Hercules, K., Komaromy, M. and Wall, R. (1978). *Proc. Natn Acad. Sci. U.S.A.* **75**, 6044–6048.

Goding, J. W. and Layton, J. E. (1976). *J. Exp. Med.* **144**, 852.

Honjo, T. and Kataoka, T. (1978). *Proc. Natn. Acad. Sci. U.S.A.* **75**, 2140.

Honjo, T., Kataoka, T., Yaoita, Y., Shimizu, A., Nikaido, T., Nakai, S., Obata, M., Kawakami, T. and Nishida, Y. (1980). *Cold Spring Harbor Symp. Quant. Biol.* (in press).

Hozumi, N. and Tonegawa, S. (1976). *Proc. Natn. Acad. Sci. U.S.A.* **73**, 3628–3632.

Joho, R. and Weissmann, C. (1980). *Nature* (*Lond.*) **284**, 179–181.
Kabat, E. A., Wu, T. T. and Bilofsky, H. (1978). *Proc. Natn. Acad. Sci. U.S.A.* **75**, 2429–2433.
Kataoka, T., Kawakami, T., Takahashi, N. and Honjo, T. (1980). *Proc. Natn. Acad. Sci. U.S.A.* **77**, 919–923.
Kearney, J. F., Cooper, M. D., Klein, J., Abney, E. R., Parkhouse, M. E. and Lawton, A. R. (1977). *J. Exp. Med.* **146**, 297.
Kuehl, W. M. and Scharff, M. (1974). *J. Mol. Biol.* **89**, 409–421.
Lala, P. K., Layton, J. E. and Nossal, G. J. V. (1979). *Eur. J. Immunol.* **9**, 39.
Leder, P., Honjo, T., Packman, S., Swan, D., Nau, M. and Norman, B. (1974). *Proc. Natn. Acad. Sci. U.S.A.* **71**, 3659–3663, 1974.
Liu, C.-P., Tucker, P. W., Mushinski, J. F. and Blattner, F. R. (1980). *Science* **209**, 1348–1353.
Max, E. E., Seidman, J. G., Miller, H. I. and Leder, P. (1980). *Cell* (in press).
Melchers, U. and Uhr, J. W. (1973). *J. Exp. Med.* **138**, 1282–1287.
Miyata, T., Yasunaga, T., Yamawaki-Kataoka, Y., Obata, M. and Honjo, T. (1980). *Proc. Natn. Acad. Sci. U.S.A.* **77**, 2143–2147.
Nathans, D. (1979). *Science* **206**, 903–909.
Padlan, E. A., Davies, D. R., Pecht, I., Givol, D. and Wright, C. (1976). *Cold Spring Harbor Symp. Quant. Biol.* **41**, 627–637.
Pernis, B., Forni, L. and Luzzatti, A. L. (1976). *Cold Spring Harbor Symp. Quant. Biol.* **41**, 175.
Perry, R. P., Kelley, D. E. and Schibler, U. (1979). *Proc. Natn. Acad. Sci. U.S.A.* **76**, 3678–3682.
Perry, R. P., Kelley, D. E., Coleclough, C., Seidman, J. G., Leder, P., Tonegawa, S., Matthyssens, G. and Weigert, M. (1980). *Proc. Natn. Acad. Sci. U.S.A.* **77**, 1937–1941.
Rabbits, T. H. (1978). *Nature* (*Lond.*) **275**, 291–296.
Rabbits, T. H., Forster, A., Dunnick, W. and Bentley, D. L. (1980). *Nature* (*Lond.*) **283**, 351–356.
Raff, M. C. (1976). *Cold Spring Harbor Symp. Quant. Biol.* **41**, 159.
Ravetch, J., Kirsch, I. R. and Leder, P. (1980). *Proc. Natn. Acad. Sci. U.S.A.* (in press).
Rogers, J., Early, P., Carter, C., Calame, K., Bond, M., Hood, L. and Wall, R. (1980). *Cell* **20**, 303–312.
Sakano, H., Huppi, K., Heinrich, G. and Tonegawa, S. (1979). *Nature* (*Lond.*) **280**, 288–294.
Seidman, J. G. and Leder, P. (1978). *Nature* (*Lond.*) **276**, 790–795.
Seidman, J. G., Leder, A., Edgell, M. H., Polsky, F., Tilghman, S., Tiemeier, D. C. and Leder, P. (1978a). *Proc. Natn. Acad. Sci. U.S.A.* **75**, 3881–3885.
Seidman, J. G., Leder, A., Nau, M., Norman, B. and Leder, P. (1978b). *Science* **202,** 11–17.
Seidman, J. G., Max, E. E. and Leder, P. (1979). *Nature* (*Lond.*) **280**, 370–375.
Seidman, J. G., Nau, M., Norman, B., S.-P. Kwan, Scharff, M. and Leder, P. (1980). *Proc. Natn. Acad. Sci. U.S.A.* (in press).
Takahashi, N., Kataoka, T. and Honjo, T. (1980). *Gene* (in press).
Tonegawa, S., Maxam, A. M., Tizard, R., Bernard, O. and Gilbert, W. (1978). *Proc. Natn. Acad. Sci. U.S.A.* **75**, 1485–1489.
Tyler, B. M. and Adams, J. M. (1980) (in press).
Valbuena, O., Marcu, K. B., Weigert, M. and Perry, R. P. (1978). *Nature* (*Lond.*) **276**, 780–784.
Vitetta, E. S. and Uhr, J. W. (1977). *Immunol. Rev.* **37**, 506.
Yaoita, Y. and Honjo, T. (1980a). *Biomedical Res.* **1**, 164–175.
Yaoita, Y. and Honjo, T. (1980b). *Nature* (*Lond.*) **286**, 852–853.

Theme 1: Summary

Immunoglobulin Structure and Molecular Organization of Immunoglobulin Genes

M. WEIGERT

University of Pennsylvania, Philadelphia, USA

A "standard model" for the organization and expression of antibody genes can be advanced. This model (Fig. 1) is in fact equivalent to the organization, before and after, the expression of the mouse λ locus described by Tonegawa and coworkers in 1978 (*Cell*, **15**). Even though the mouse λ locus is the simplest known, other loci in mouse and other species differ only in detail; the mouse κ locus including more *V* genes and *J* genes, the heavy chain locus including more *V* genes, *J* genes, *C* region domain genes and possibly additional *V* gene segments called *D*. Inherent in the standard model are signal sequences or substrates for enzymes that mediate expression of an antibody gene. Such signals are involved in the initial events of expression, *V-J* or *V-D-J* joining, and other kinds of signals are used for the heavy chain class switch.

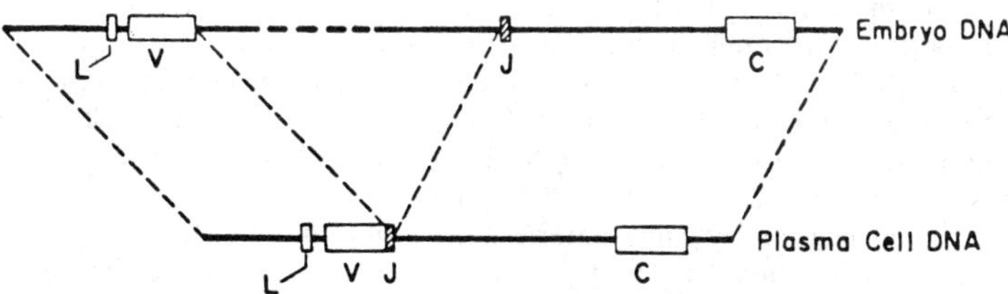

FIG. 1. *The organization of an antibody gene in embryo and plasma cell DNAs. Adapted from Brack, C., Hirama, M., Lenhard-Schuller, R. and Tonegawa, S. (1978).* Cell ***15**, 1.*

The standard model seems to have survived the IVth International Congress. New findings presented here have shown the universality of the model and indicate important consequences of this kind of gene organization. In addition, it appears that new elements may have to be added to the model and possible exceptions may need to be considered.

This Congress signals an important new trend in molecular immunology. Our understanding of antibody genes, the standard model, is derived from the analysis of the mouse genome. This of course reflects the dependence of this research on Michael Potter's mouse myeloma system. Exploiting the structural gene homology between man and mouse, investigators have used mouse antibody probes to find and clone human genes thus paving the way for a complete molecular analysis of human antibody loci. These recent studies of Leder, Rabbits, and their coworkers have already yielded important new results and conclusions. Remarkable homolgies have been detected between these species, particularly in regions that determine antibody gene expression.

Rabbits, Mathiessens and Bently find regions of intervening sequence homology at points associated with V region genes that are probably involved in the joining mechanisms. This applies both to V_H and V_κ, and the DNA sequence 3′ of human V_κ has the same features and organization as mouse V_κ that complement sequences next to the J_κ genes (i.e., 7 and 10 complementing nucleotides separated by 11 nucleotides). Leder (Chapter 3) finds that the human κ locus is organized in a manner similar to the mouse κ locus with respect to the number of J_κ gene segments to each other and to the C_κ gene. Similarly, homologies between man and mouse are found at regions associated with different H-chain constant region genes (α and μ so far). These regions encompass what in the mouse is thought to include the signals for the H-chain switching. These homologies at the signal sequences are underscored by studies of Dunnick and Rabbits who have shown homologies for the switch sites of the different heavy chain classes of the mouse and by studies of Hozumi who has shown exact identity of the J_κ regions of different strains of mice.

One consequence of the organization of antibody genes is the opportunity for diversification by combinatorial association offered by multiple V and J genes in one locus. Such a diversification mechanism could be inferred from the nature of the mouse κ locus as described by Leder, Tonegawa and their coworkers and that it actually operates is clear from V_κ amino acid sequences. In addition, as reiterated by Leder, another effect of V-J joining could be to generate new codons at the junction site due to alternate modes of cutting and joining. Such joining alternatives could lead to amino acid substitutions as well as insertions and deletions at the V-J junction. The kinds of amino acid substitutions would be dictated by the signal sequences in or near V and J, and Leder's thesis is generally borne out by a comparison of the amino acid sequences to the known DNA sequences of the relevant regions. Rudikoff has extended the potential of this mechanism by discovering a new amino acid substitution (isoleucine) at the $V_\kappa J_\kappa$ junction of galactan antibodies; neither are accounted for by germ line J_κ genes nor can be generated by known V_κ region signal sequences. He proposes that different V_κ genes may have different signal sequences that will have the effect of broadening the range of amino acid residues that can be generated by joining. The obvious liability of this mechanism is the chance of generating frameshift mutations leading to prematurely terminated L or H chains, and Leder and colleagues have indeed found such an example. Hence antibody loci appear to be willing (or even anxious, see below) to sacrifice integrity for diversity.

Somatic diversification by combinatorial association and V-J joining clearly occur but do they lead to functional diversity, i.e., by creating new specificities. Two important studies argue that they do: Davies and coworkers report further refinements of the structure of the combining site of antibody M603 including residue 96 of V_κ. They conclude that this site, in addition to playing a role in V_H interaction, has a profound influence on combining shape. Pecht and Zidovertzki (1.5.09, 1.5.10*) have extended their analysis of ligand induced conformational change to galactan binding antibodies of known sequence. Again they point out that the mechanics of the observed conformational transition is inherent in the structural domains, but emphasize that the parameters of the transition are modulated by the amino acid sequence in J and/or D.

It may be important to add what now appears to be an essential element to the standard model. As noted by the Leder and Tonegawa groups, the mouse κ locus includes a nonfunctional J gene segment or pseudogene. In addition, both groups have observed pseudo-joining signals in the κ locus that also cause nonproductive rearrangements. These types of elements have now been discovered in both the mouse heavy chain and κ chain loci. Bernard and coworkers have found a pseudo-J_κ and a pseudo-J_H

* Reference numbers indicate Abstract numbers in: Abstracts 4th International Congress of Immunology, Paris, 1980.

gene segment. A pseudo-joining signal may occur in the heavy chain locus. Johnson, Meo, and Tonegawa have developed an ingenious system for analysing heavy gene rearrangements; namely somatic cell hybrids carrying structurally distinguishable homologies of chromosome 12 and different heavy chain alleles that allow the necessary chromosome bookkeeping. They show that the heavy chain locus on both chromosomes is changed in context but on the unexpressed chromosome a rearrangement has occurred to a site that may be analogous to pseudo-joining sites in the κ locus described by Leder and Tonegawa.

The impulse, when only single pseudo-elements were known, was to regard these as relics of previously functional genes. By the homology of these pseudo-elements to functional elements they clearly have evolved from a common gene, but the recent finding that pseudo-elements are present in all loci suggests they may be maintained in the genome for a purpose. One possible role for such elements may be to provide a form of allelic exclusion. Though one form of allelic exclusion is manifested by having one rearranged and one unrearranged (hence unexpressed) allele, another form (as observed in plasmacytomas by several groups) is manifested by one productively and one non-productively rearranged allele. The latter is a result of joining to a pseudo-J or pseudo-joining signal. Thus these elements may play a key role in ensuring allelic and perhaps isotypic (κ versus λ) exclusion.

Certain exceptions or apparent exceptions to the standard model now need to be considered. One consequence of this organization of antibody genes is that joining events delete DNA between structural genes. For example, as originally shown by Honjo and coworkers, the heavy chain class switch must result from DNA deletions upstream of the gene expressed. Lymphocytes that simultaneously express two heavy chain classes, μ and δ, would seem to require a different mechanism for δ expression since, as shown by Blattner and colleagues, the δ gene is located downstream from the μ gene. Expression of both μ and δ could, however, be explained if both chromosomes were active, but this alternative is now excluded by recent experiments of Wabl and coworkers. They have isolated somatic cell hybrids expressing both μ and δ and that have only one chromosome 12 which includes the heavy chain locus as shown by Swan and coworkers. Therefore, it is possible that expression of certain heavy chain classes such as δ may be determined at another level such as RNA processing.

An apparent exception to the standard model may have been raised by Leder's direct demonstration that there are multiple C_λ genes in man, as had previously been inferred from amino acid sequence data. It is known that V_λ genes can be joined to any C_λ isotype, but Leder's data does not seem to allow for independent clusters of V_λ genes affiliated with the different C_λ genes. This raises the question, how do V_λs arrive at different C_λs. This may be achieved by affiliating J_λ genes with the separate C_λ genes as suggested by the analysis of Deutsch which shows that certain J_λ amino acid sequences may be unique to certain C_λ isotypes. Hence these new discoveries on C_λ isotypes in man do not require new mechanisms of DNA joining. λ isotypes in mouse are probably not organized in this manner. Azuma, Steiner and Eisen have now shown that there are at least 2 λ isotypes (λ_1 λ_2) and from $V\lambda_2$ amino acid sequences would argue that the λ_1 and λ_2 isotypes are discrete *V-J-C* loci.

So far V regions appear to be coded by single genes that for V_λ, V_κ and V_H include most or a part of the third complementarity determining region. That this may not be a standard organization has already been suggested by the finding that V_H genes and J_H genes alone do not code for a number of V_H region amino acid sequences. Hood and coworkers have proposed a new set of gene segments called D to account for this discrepancy. Kabat argues from recent comparisons of rabbit V_L regions that further gene segmentation may occur. Although this is not indicated from the mouse *V* gene sequences yet, further *V* gene analysis in the mouse or in other species may reveal additional segmentation or mini-genes. Hence there may not be a standard organization of *V* region genes.

Will the standard model extend to all antibody genes? Close homologies of joining signals have been observed between different loci in mouse and between different species. These signals were probably a feature of ancestral antibody genes and possibly the same signals for rearrangement and expression are used by other kinds of antibodies such as the T cell receptor. Though the structural genes for different antibodies (κ, λ, IgT) may have diverged considerably, the signals and proteins (enzymes) that mediate antibody expression may be common to all loci and all lymphocytes. Kemp and coworkers consider this possibility in light of their important new findings on μ-RNA and μ gene rearrangement in thymocytes and T cell lymphomas. They find that μ transcription and rearrangements may not have a functional relevance *per se* since these μ-RNAs are qualitatively different from μ-RNA in plasma cells in size, do not code for variable regions and are not translated. It is difficult to consider a functional role for these transcripts. By the same token the occasional rearrangements in the J_H gene region observed in T cell lymphomas appear to be abortive and may indeed be due to joining at the pseudo-J_H described by Bernard. Though these features may have no functional relevance for the T cell, they may reflect the presence of a common enzymology and in turn a similar organization for conventional antibody genes and T cell antibody genes.

Theme 2

Idiotypy, Allotypy and Network Regulation

Presidents:
J. URBAIN
P. CAZENAUE

Symposium chairman
J. OUDIN

4

Regulation through Idiotypic Determinants of the Immune Response to the *p*-Azophenylarsonate Hapten in Strain A Mice

ALFRED NISONOFF and MARK I. GREENE

Rosenstiel Research Center and Department of Biology, Brandeis University, Massachusetts and Department of Pathology, Harvard Medical School, Boston, Massachusetts

Introduction

In this paper we will summarize recent investigations in our laboratories relating to regulation of the immune response. Many of the mechanisms to be discussed involve regulation at the level of idiotype. The idiotypic system we have worked with is that associated with anti-*p*-azophenylarsonate (anti-Ar) antibodies of A/J mice (Kuettner *et al.*, 1972; Nisonoff *et al.*, 1977). On the average, about half of the antibodies produced in response to the Ar-derivative of keyhole limpet haemocyanin (KLH) bear a cross-reactive idiotype (CRI). Recent studies of CRI^+ hybridoma products indicate that the antibodies expressing this idiotype actually constitute a family of closely related but nonidentical molecules (Estess *et al.*, 1979, 1980; Lamoyi *et al.*, 1980a; Marshak-Rothstein *et al.*, 1980; Alkan *et al.*, 1980). Serological data indicate that at least one of these idiotypic determinants is highly conserved within the family, although "private" idiotypic determinants can readily be identified on individual monoclonal antibodies (Lamoyi *et al.*, 1980a, b). Inheritance of the idiotype is linked to the *Igh* locus (Pawlak *et al.*, 1973b) and also to the *VK-1* locus associated with light chain biosynthesis (Laskin *et al.*, 1977; Gottlieb *et al.*, 1979). The latter genetic locus is in turn tightly linked to the *Lyt-3* locus which controls a thymocyte surface alloantigen (Gottlieb, 1974). Most strains of mice, with the exception of a few strains demonstrated by P. D. Gottlieb to differ from the others at the *VK-1* locus, are capable of synthesizing light chains that can complement the appropriate heavy chains for the production of CRI^+ anti-Ar antibodies (Laskin *et al.*, 1977; Gottlieb *et al.*, 1979; A. R. Brown, P. D. Gottlieb and A. Nisonoff, unpublished data). Linkage of CRI synthesis to the *Igh* locus has been demonstrated by backcross studies (Laskin *et al.*, 1977) and also by the observation that C.AL-20 congenic mice, which have the heavy chain allotype of the AL/N strain on a BALB/c background, produce CRI^+ anti-Ar antibodies (Pawlak *et al.*, 1973b). C.AL-20 and BALB/c mice were used in several of the studies to be discussed below, to demonstrate genetic linkage of the inheritance of certain phenotypes to the *Igh* locus.

We will first briefly review earlier work on the suppression of the anti-Ar

Abbreviations
anti-id: anti-idiotype or anti-idiotypic; Ar: *p*-azophenylarsonate; BSA: bovine serum albumin; CRI: cross-reactive idiotype; DTH: delayed-type hypersensitivity; IBC: idiotype-binding capacity; i.v.: intravenous; KLH: keyhole limpet haemocyanin; NMG: normal mouse globulin; PC: phosphoryl-choline; s.e.: standard error of the mean; TNP: trinitrophenyl; Ts_1: suppressor T cell with CRI^+ receptors; Ts_2: suppressor T cells with anti-idiotypic receptors; TsF_1: T cell-derived suppressor factor with CRI^+ receptors; TsF_2: T cell-derived suppressor factor with anti-idiotypic receptors.

CRI and the induction of idiotype-suppressor T cells. Studies on idiotypic and anti-idiotypic T cell suppressor factors (TsF) will then be described. We will also discuss our recent studies, comprising a series of experiments that have analysed two identifiable sets of interactions. The first set occurs when ligand, associated with self-components, interacts with receptors on antigen-reactive T or B cells. This interaction will be discussed in terms of ligand-receptor events. Consequent to the activation of clones of antigen-reactive cells, idiotypic determinants on the receptors of such cells appear to induce a second series of events leading to the stimulation of anti-idiotypic suppressor cells. This phenomenon will be discussed in terms of receptor–antireceptor (idiotype–anti-idiotype) interactions. Finally, we will focus on the mechanism whereby anti-idiotypic cells ultimately interact with idiotype-bearing cells and lead to regulation of clonal expression. The data will be considered in the context of their historical documentation. Our collaborators on the more recent investigations are Drs Bruce Bach, Baruj Benacerraf, Alan R. Brown, Yoshitane Dohi, Ronald Germain, Paul D. Gottlieb, Yoshikatsu Hirai and Man-Sun Sy.

Suppression of the idiotypic component of the anti-Ar response by anti-id antibodies

Once it had been observed that a substantial portion of the anti-Ar antibodies of A/J mice express a common idiotype, it was feasible to attempt to suppress the idiotype by administration of anti-id antibodies (Hart *et al.*, 1972; Pawlak *et al.*, 1973a). Inoculation of rabbit anti-id antibodies caused virtually complete suppression of the CRI in A/J mice with very little effect on total anti-Ar synthesis. Suppression could be achieved in adult as well as neonatal mice. In these experiments roughly 5 μg of anti-id antibodies were used for suppression. Fab and $F(ab')_2$ fragments of anti-id were found to be ineffective. Suppression was maintained for 6 weeks in all of the mice and for the 5-month duration of the experiment in almost half of the mice. The anti-id antibody was far less effective when administered after, rather than several days before the antigen (KLH-Ar).

Other early examples of the suppression of major idiotypes were the experiments of Cosenza and Köhler (1972) on the *in vitro* synthesis of an idiotype associated with antiphosphorylcholine antibodies in BALB/c mice; the suppression of the same idiotype in neonatal BALB/c mice (Strayer *et al.*, 1974); and the studies of Eichmann (1974) on suppression of the idiotype associated with antibodies to Group A streptococci in the A strain. Eichmann made the interesting observation that guinea-pig IgG_2, but not IgG_1, anti-id antibodies were effective in causing suppression, and demonstrated the induction of idiotype-specific suppressor T cells by anti-id (discussed below). Bordenave (1975) was able to demonstrate idiotype-suppression in an adult rabbit by preparing homologous anti-id against antibodies isolated after a primary response and using these anti-id antibodies to suppress the reappearance of the idiotype in the same rabbit in a late response.

Suppression of delayed-type hypersensitivity (DTH) by anti-id antibody

It was found that inoculation of rabbit anti-CRI antibodies greatly suppresses the DTH response to the Ar hapten group in A/J mice (Sy *et al.*, 1979b). The anti-id antiserum was administered on 5 successive days after subcutaneous immunization with 3×10^7 Ar-coupled syngeneic leukocytes. The mice were challenged in the footpad on day 5 with the diazonium salt of *p*-arsanilic acid. As shown in Table I, as little as 1 μg of idiotype-binding capacity (IBC) of anti-id caused significant suppression of DTH and suppression with 10 μg was virtually complete. Inoculation of anti-id had no effect on DTH to an unrelated hapten, trinitrochlorobenzene, as measured by ear swelling. In contrast with these results, 10 μg IBC of $F(ab')_2$ fragments of anti-id antibodies had no significant effect on DTH to the Ar hapten. As discussed above, $F(ab')_2$ is similarly ineffective in suppressing the idiotypic component of the humoral A/J anti-Ar response.

Inoculation of anti-id also brought about suppression of DTH in C.AL-20 mice, but was ineffective in BALB/c. (Mice of the C.AL-20, but not the BALB/c strain produce anti-Ar antibodies with the major CRI.) Thus, the same genetic restrictions apply to humoral antibody production and to DTH, which is mediated by a subset of T cells; i.e., the inheritance of the capacity to undergo anti-idiotypic suppression of DTH and the production of the CRI

TABLE I

Inhibition of DTH in A/J mice by rabbit anti-CRI antibodies (Sy et al., *1979b)*

Total amount of anti-CRI	*Footpad swelling*[a]	P
μg IBC[b]	mm × 10^2 (s.e.)	
0	38 (2·7)	
0·1	35 (2·6)	N.S.[c]
1	23 (1·8)	<0·001
10	10·5 (1·3)	<0·001
Challenge only	5·6 (2·0)	

[a] Normal A/J mice were injected subcutaneously with 3×10^7 Ar-coupled syngeneic spleen cells. They were injected i.v. on 5 successive days with 0·2 ml of rabbit anti-CRI antiserum. On day 5 they were challenged in the footpad with the diazonium salt of *p*-arsanilic acid and footpad swelling was measured 1 day later.
[b] Idiotype-binding capacity.
[c] No significant difference from control.

are both linked to the *Igh* locus. The results are also consistent with the widely accepted view that T and B cell receptors utilize similar V_H regions (Binz and Wigzell, 1977; Rajewsky and Eichmann, 1977; Ramseier *et al.*, 1977). The failure of anti-id to suppress DTH in BALB/c mice is consistent with the absence of a suitable target cell, having receptors that are CRI^+ and specific for the Ar hapten.

In the same study (Sy *et al.*, 1979b) it was found that suppression of DTH by anti-id is mediated by suppressor T cells; this will be considered further below.

Induction of suppressor T cells by anti-id antibodies

Humoral responses

Eichmann (1975) demonstrated that administration of low doses (0·1 μg idiotype-binding capacity) of guinea-pig IgG_2 anti-id suppressed the appearance of CRI associated with antibodies to the carbohydrate of Group A streptococci in A/J mice. Suppression by this low dose of anti-id was maintained for several months and the treatment was found to stimulate suppressor T cells, as shown by adoptive transfer experiments.

In the A/J anti-Ar system, Owen *et al.* (1977a, b) showed that idiotype-suppressor T cells are present in mice that have been suppressed with anti-id and hyperimmunized with KLH-Ar. Most of the suppressor cells present after a rest period of 8–12 weeks have anti-idiotypic receptors, as shown by their capacity to form rosettes with A/J red blood cells coated with CRI^+ Fab fragments. Removal of the rosettes eliminated the suppressor activity and the rosettes themselves were highly suppressive. The suppressor cells had little or no effect, however, on an ongoing immune response; i.e., they did not cause suppression of idiotype when transferred into KLH-Ar-primed mice (Owen and Nisonoff, 1978).

DTH responses

We have already considered the suppression of DTH responses to the Ar hapten caused by inoculation of anti-CRI antibodies into strain A or C.AL-20 mice. The results in Table II show that this is accompanied by the formation of suppressor cells that can adoptively transfer the suppressed state to naïve recipients (Sy *et al.*, 1979b). Transfer of 5×10^7 leukocytes from the spleen, lymph node or thymus of idiotypically suppressed mice resulted in the suppression of the DTH response upon subsequent immunization with Ar-coupled cells and challenge of the recipients. Treatment of the transferred cells with anti-Thy-1.2 antiserum and complement destroyed the suppressor activity, indicating that the suppressors are T cells.

Although these experiments demonstrate that suppressor cells are induced by the anti-id antibodies, they do not prove that the suppressor cells are solely responsible for suppression in those mice that have received anti-id; the anti-id antibodies themselves might play a direct role in suppression. This question was approached by treating mice with cyclophosphamide (50 mg/kg) 2 days before administration of anti-id antibodies. Such treatment was found to abrogate completely the suppression by anti-id, indicating that the suppression takes place principally or solely through the induction of suppressor T cells (Sy *et al.*, 1979b).

TABLE II

Induction of suppressor cells in A/J mice with anti-CRI antibodies (Sy et al., *1979b)*[a]

Treatment of donors	*Number of cells transferred*	*Footpad swelling mm × 10^2 (s.e.)*	P
—	None	27 (2·8)	
Normal rabbit serum	5 × 10^7 spleen	26 (1·5)	N.S.
Anti-CRI	5 × 10^7 lymph node	15·6 (2·0)	0·01
Anti-CRI	5 × 10^7 thymocytes	12·5 (2·1)	0·004
Anti-CRI	5 × 10^7 spleen	10·6 (2·3)	0·002
Challenge only		5·6 (0·9)	

[a] Normal A/J mice were injected i.v. with 2 μg IBC of anti-CRI daily for 5 days. On day 6 they were sacrificed and 50 × 10^6 viable leukocytes were transferred to naïve recipients, which were then immunized subcutaneously and challenged in the footpad 5 days later; after 24 h swelling was measured.

The virtually complete suppression of DTH by anti-id contrasts with the results obtained in the humoral response; there is little effect of anti-id on the total anti-Ar response, although the major idiotypic component is generally undetectable (Pawlak *et al.*, 1973a). Two possible explanations are that the T cell compartment makes greater use of the major idiotype or that idiotype-mediated suppression of DTH also generates nonspecific, or antigen-specific cells or soluble factors that suppress nonidiotypic components as well. This question is currently being investigated.

Similar results were reported by Yamamoto *et al.* (1979) who showed that DTH against the phosphorylcholine hapten group in BALB/c mice can be suppressed by inoculations of anti-id antibodies raised in A/J mice, and that this treatment results in the induction of idiotype-suppressor T cells. They also demonstrated that the anti-id antibodies inhibited the induction of DTH responsiveness but were not suppressive at the effector phase of the response.

Suppression of idiotypic humoral responses and of DTH responses to the Ar hapten group by inoculation of CRI$^+$ antibodies coupled to leukocytes

Humoral responses

Until recently the selective suppression of the expression of an idiotype had always involved the use of anti-idiotypic antibody. After the identification of idiotype-suppressor T cells with anti-id receptors (Owen *et al.*, 1977a, b), it seemed reasonable to attempt to achieve idiotype suppression and the induction of suppressor cells by inoculating CRI$^+$ molecules, or such molecules conjugated to syngeneic leukocytes. Rowley *et al.* (1976) had shown that the response to phosphorylcholine (PC) was greatly decreased in BALB/c mice after inoculation of the PC-binding myeloma protein, T15. It was impractical in that system to look for selective idiotype suppression, since a very large

TABLE III

Suppression of synthesis of idiotype by inoculation of idiotype-conjugated thymocytes (Dohi and Nisonoff, 1979)[a]

No. of mice	*Preinoculations*	*Antibody response, day 38* — *Anti-Ar titre µg/ml*	*Anti-Ar antibody required for 50% inhibition, ng*
7	None	930, 1600, 980, 1800 1800, 400, 850	17, 36, 14, 28, 39, 7, 18
5	A/J thymocytes	200, 2000, 550, 4800, 5800	18, 7, 13, 12, 76
8	Conjugate,A/J thymocytes-anti-Ar	180, 3600, 180, 1800, 4300, 6000, 4900, 8100	>4600, >89 000 >4600 >46 000, >110 000, >150 000, >120 000, 190 000
4	Conjugate,A/J thymocytes-normal mouse IgG	200, 7900, 200, 15 000	25, 8, 10, 10
6	Anti-Ar antibody, 100 µg twice	580, 2400, 420, 790, 740, 3200	8, >59 000, 52, 34, 51, 8
7	Mixture A/J thymocytes + anti-Ar[b]	9, 46, 1600, 380, 1500, 7500, 4300	25, 60, 70, 8300, 14, >190 000, 5300
6	Conjugate, BALB/c thymocytes-anti-Ar	1900, 240, 2100, 1800, 1000, 7800	500, 80, 1100, 300, 650, 1500

[a] Preinoculations were given on days -42 and -21. When thymocytes were injected, 25×10^6 were used. Conjugated thymocytes contained 12 ± 2 µg purified A/J anti-Ar antibody/25×10^6 cells. All recipients received 0·25 mg KLH-Ar i.p. in CFA on days 0 and 28.

[b] 25×10^6 cells + 12 µg Ab/injection (not conjugated).

fraction of the anti-PC response involves a major idiotype. Evidence on suppressor cell formation was not reported.

The data in Table III (Dohi and Nisonoff, 1979) indicate that selective suppression of the CRI can be achieved in A/J mice by preinoculation of CRI^+ molecules conjugated to A/J thymocytes. Suppression also occurred after inoculation of the mixture (unconjugated) of thymocytes and CRI^+ antibody, but the suppression did not take effect in all of the mice.

Other observations in this study included the following. The carrier of the CRI^+ antibody is not H-2 restricted; C57BL/10 and BALB/c thymocytes were equally as effective as A/J thymocytes. Selective suppression of CRI expression also occurred, after inoculation of cell-coupled CRI^+ antibody, in C.AL-20 or (A/J × BALB/c)F_1 mice. In the latter two strains unconjugated CRI^+ antibody was quite ineffective in inducing a state of idiotype suppression.

It was also found that A/J mice treated with CRI-coupled cells developed suppressor cells, shown to be T cells, that adoptively transfer the suppressed state into mildly irradiated (200 R) A/J recipients. Although many of the suppressed mice produced undetectable amounts of the CRI, no pronounced decrease in anti-Ar titre after immunization with KLH-Ar was observed in the recipients.

Inoculation of CRI-coupled cells had no significant effect on mice that had already received antigen; i.e., a secondary response was not affected. The failure of idiotype-suppressor cells to influence the secondary response had been noted earlier (Owen and Nisonoff, 1978).

These experiments demonstrated the feasibility of selectively suppressing a cross-reactive idiotype, and generating suppressor T cells, without the use of anti-id antibodies or antigen.

Suppression of DTH with idiotype-coupled cells

It was found that DTH to the Ar hapten group could be suppressed by preinoculation of idiotype-coupled spleen cells (Sy *et al.*, 1979a). In this experimental system it is difficult to ascertain whether an idiotypic component of the response or the entire response is being affected, and, indeed, there is as yet no proof that the effector T cells in the DTH response carry idiotypic or anti-idiotypic receptors. In any event a profound effect was noted on DTH to the Ar hapten when A/J mice were inoculated with CRI-coupled splenic leukocytes before immunization and challenge. Some of the data obtained in this study are shown in Table IV. Inoculation of CRI-coupled syngeneic spleen cells caused suppression of DTH in A/J and C.AL-20 mice but not in the CRI^- BALB/c strain. Thus, inheritance of the capacity to undergo inhibition of DTH is linked to the *Igh* locus. The carrier used for the CRI^+ antibodies is not critical since CRI^+ molecules conjugated to either BALB/c or A/J cells were suppressive in A/J mice. Other results showed that cells coupled with CRI^- anti-Ar antibody, obtained from idiotypically suppressed

TABLE IV
Inhibition of Ar-specific DTH by inoculation of CRI-coupled syngeneic spleen cells; linkage to the Igh *locus* (*Sy* et al., *1979a*)[a]

Strain	*Tolerogen*	*Immunization (hapten-cells)*	*Footpad swelling mm × 10² (s.e.)*	P
A/J	None	Ar-A/J	29 (1·6)	
A/J	NMG-A/J[b]	Ar-A/J	27 (2·4)	N.S.
A/J	CRI-A/J	Ar-A/J	12 (1·2)	<0·001
BALB/c	None	Ar-BALB/c	41 (1·7)	
BALB/c	NMG-BALB/c[b]	Ar-BALB/c	39 (2·1)	N.S.
BALB/c	CRI-BALB/c	Ar-BALB/c	41 (2·1)	N.S.
C.AL-20	None	Ar-C.AL-20	44 (2·9)	
C.AL-20	NMG-C.AL-20	Ar-C.AL-20	42 (2·7)	N.S.
C.AL-20	CRI-C.AL-20	Ar-C.AL-20	18 (2·0)	<0·001
A/J	None	Ar-A/J	30 (2·2)	
A/J	CRI-BALB/c	Ar-A/J	10 (1·3)	<0·001

[a] Mice were inoculated i.v. with 5×10^7 conjugated splenic leukocytes. They were immunized 7 days later with Ar-coupled cells and were challenged after 5 more days by footpad inoculation.
[b] NMG, normal mouse globulin conjugated to leukocytes of the strain specified.

A/J mice, were not capable of inducing unresponsiveness to DTH in the A/J strain.

It was found, in addition, that inoculation of CRI-coupled cells generated suppressor T cells, present in the thymus or spleen, that could adoptively transfer unresponsiveness to syngeneic recipients (Sy *et al.*, 1979a).

Production of suppressor T cells with anti-id receptors in the CRI⁻ BALB/c strain

As indicated in the previous section, injection of CRI-coupled cells into BALB/c mice, which are CRI^-, failed to induce DTH unresponsiveness to the Ar hapten. The possibility was considered that anti-id suppressor T cells might none the less have been induced, but that these failed to affect DTH because of the absence of an appropriate (CRI^+) target cell. To test this hypothesis BALB/c mice were treated with CRI-coupled syngeneic cells (Sy *et al.*, 1980b). The data in Table V indicate that such mice develop suppressor cells that can induce DTH unresponsiveness to the Ar hapten group in C.AL-20 mice, which produce humoral antibodies that are CRI^+, but not in BALB/c or B10.D2 mice, whose anti-Ar antibodies are CRI^-. (Both the BALB/c and B10.D2 strains, as well as C.AL-20 are $H\text{-}2^d$.) Other experiments indicated that the suppression of DTH is antigen-specific, since there was no effect on the DTH response to dinitrofluorobenzene, and that it is mediated by T cells.

TABLE V

BALB/c anti-id suppressor cells (Ts_2) are active in C.AL-20 (CRI^+) mice but not in BALB/c or B10.D2 (CRI^-) (Sy et al., *1980b)*

Tolerogen	*Donors (5 × 10⁷ cells)*	*Recipients*	*Footpad swelling mm × 10² (s.e.)*	P
Control (BALB/c)	None	—	24 ± 1·8	
Id-coupled cells	BALB/c	BALB/c	23 ± 1·5	N.S.[a]
Control (C.AL-20)	—	—	19 ± 1·8	
Id-coupled cells	BALB/c	C.AL-20	9·5 ± 0·8	0·003
Control (B10.D2)	None	—	20 ± 1·4	
Id-coupled cells	BALB/c	B10.D2	20 ± 1·2	N.S.

[a] Not significant.

Finally, it was shown that the suppressor T cells induced by id-coupled cells in BALB/c mice have anti-idiotypic determinants (Table VI). T cells that were adherent to CRI-coated polystyrene plates caused suppression when $1{\cdot}4 \times 10^6$ cells were transferred, whereas 19×10^6 nonadherent cells had no significant effect.

TABLE VI

Ts induced in BALB/c mice by id-coupled cells have anti-idiotypic receptors (Sy et al., *1980b)*[a]. *Recipients of cells are C.AL-20 mice*

Cell enrichment	*Number of cells transferred*	*Units of footpad swelling mm × 10² ± s.e.*	P
Control C.AL-20	None	25 ± 0·9	—
T cells	19 × 10⁶	14 ± 0·9	<0·001
T cells nonadherent[b] to CRI	19 × 10⁶	21·7 ± 3·1	0·3
T cells adherent[c] to CRI	1·4 × 10⁶	6·5 ± 1·7	<0·001

[a] BALB/c mice were challenged with 3×10^7 CRI-coupled BALB/c splenic leukocytes. T cells were prepared from spleen and adoptively transferred into C.AL-20 recipients which were then immunized and challenged in the footpad.
[b] Nonadherent to polystyrene dishes coated with CRI^+ anti-Ar.
[c] Adherent to, and recovered from CRI-coated plates by temperature shift and mechanical pressure.

Thus, while there are allotype-linked restrictions on the capacity to undergo suppression by idiotype-coupled cells or by anti-id, the inoculation of idiotype-coupled cells can induce anti-id suppressors even in a CRI^- strain. It seems likely that the repertoire of receptors on suppressor T cells is very extensive and is not limited by the repertoire of major idiotypes within the strain.

On the basis of the network theory of Jerne (1974), one might predict that there are T cells in BALB/c mice with receptors that are complementary to anti-CRI (i.e., are CRI^+) but that they may not possess anti-Ar specificity in the BALB/c strain.

Induction of unresponsiveness to DTH by inoculation of Ar-coupled cells; generation of Ts with idiotypic receptors

The subcutaneous inoculation of Ar-coupled spleen cells immunizes A/J mice so that a subsequent footpad challenge with Ar-coupled cells, or with the diazonium salt of *p*-arsanilic acid, causes the swelling characteristic of DTH. In contrast, intravenous inoculation of Ar-coupled spleen cells results in unresponsiveness to a subsequent subcutaneous injection and footpad challenge (Bach *et al.*, 1978). Similar effects on tolerance induction have been observed with other antigens (Battisto and Bloom, 1966; Baumgarten and Geczy, 1970; Claman and Miller, 1976; Scott and Long, 1976; Greene *et al.*, 1978). In addition to inducing unresponsiveness, Ar-coupled cells injected intravenously stimulate suppressor T cells (Ts) which can adoptively transfer the state of unresponsiveness to syngeneic recipients (Bach *et al.*, 1978).

In this section we will discuss two types of result which manifest a role for idiotypy in this process. First, the Ts induced by Ar-coupled cells in A/J mice have anti-Ar receptors and can be killed by treatment with anti-CRI antibodies and complement; thus, these Ts have CRI^+ receptors (Dietz *et al.*, 1980). Second, the same cells elaborate a soluble factor (TsF) which can also adoptively transfer the state of suppression (Bach *et al.*, 1979). This TsF has an anti-Ar binding site, and a large fraction of the soluble suppressor activity is removed by passage through a column containing immobilized anti-CRI antibodies. Other properties of the factor will be described. Finally, inoculation of the CRI^+ TsF into A/J mice induces another set of suppressor cells which have anti-idiotypic rather than idiotypic receptors (Sy *et al.*, 1980a).

The data in Table VII demonstrate that Ts induced by inoculation of Ar-coupled cells have CRI^+ receptors, since the activity of the cells is abrogated by treatment with anti-id and complement. Specificity is shown by the failure of the anti-id treatment to affect spleen cells which can adoptively transfer suppression of DTH to the TNP group. It was also found that BALB/c splenic suppressor cells, induced by inoculation of Ar-coupled BALB/c cells, are not affected by treatment with anti-CRI prepared against A/J anti-Ar antibodies; this is consistent with the absence of the CRI in BALB/c humoral antibodies and confirms the similarity of T and B cell receptors with respect to V_H repertoire. We will refer to suppressor T cells having CRI^+ receptors as Ts_1; suppressor cells with anti-id receptors are designated Ts_2.

Other experiments, carried out with enriched T cells, demonstrated that Ts_1 adhere to Ar-BSA-coated polystyrene plates but not to TNP-BSA-coated plates (Dietz *et al.*, 1980); very little suppressor activity remained in the cell population that was nonadherent to Ar-BSA and the adherent cells, when recovered, were much more potent on a numerical basis as suppressors than the unfractionated T cell population. All of the data are consistent in indicating that Ts induced initially by the i.v. inoculation of ligand-coupled cells have hapten-binding receptors that are CRI$^+$.

TABLE VII

Ts induced by Ar-coupled syngeneic leukocytes have receptors that are CRI$^+$ (Dietz et al., *1980)*

Tolerogen[a]	*Number of spleen cells transferred*[b]	*Treatment of cells*	*Units of footpad swelling mm × 10^2 ± s.e.*	P
None (control)	—	—	19 ± 1·4	—
Ar-coupled spleen cells	5 × 10^7	Normal rabbit serum + C	9·4 ± 1·0	<0·01
Ar-coupled spleen cells	5 × 10^7	Anti-CRI + C	20 ± 1·5	N.S.
None (control)[c] (TNP system)	—	—	20·8 ± 1·4[c]	—
TNP-coupled spleen cells	5 × 10^7	Normal rabbit serum + C	9·6 ± 0·9[c]	<0·01
TNP-coupled spleen cells	5 × 10^7	Anti-CRI + C	8·9 ± 1·0[c]	<0·01

[a] 3 × 10^7 cells administered i.v. into A/J mice.
[b] Into naive A/J recipients.
[c] Mice immunized and challenged with TNP-coupled cells.

Properties of a T cell-derived suppressor factor (TsF) obtained from suppressor cells stimulated by inoculation of Ar-coupled cells

It was found that TsF can be obtained from splenic or thymic cells present in A/J mice 7 days after i.v. inoculation of Ar-coupled spleen cells (Bach *et al.*, 1979). The soluble factor can be prepared by freeze-thaw or sonication of cells which are sensitive to anti-Thy-1.2 and complement. It is also present in culture supernatants of the cells. TsF is assayed by measuring its capacity to prevent subsequent development of DTH to the Ar hapten when inoculated into normal A/J mice. Typically, TsF from 3 × 10^7 spleen cells from a tolerized mouse is used to suppress another A/J mouse. The data in Table VIII show that much of the suppressor activity of the soluble factor is retained on a column containing insolubilized F(ab′)$_2$ fragments of rabbit anti-CRI antibodies and can be recovered by elution at pH 2·8. Some of the activity, however, is always recovered in the initial filtrate, indicating the presence of TsF that does not express the major CRI. A control column, containing bound nonspecific rabbit F(ab′)$_2$ fragments, failed to retain the suppressor factor.

Since, as shown above, suppressor T cells present 7 days after i.v. inoculation of Ar-coupled cells have CRI$^+$ TsF, (TsF_1) must be derived from the T cells (Ts_1) with CRI$^+$ receptors. The possibility has not been ruled out that TsF is the T cell receptor itself. Arguing against this possibility is the failure of Rajewsky's group to identify H-2 determinants on the T cell receptors that they isolate on derivatized nylon (Krawinkel *et al.*, 1977). Taussig and Holliman (1979) report that the TsF they isolated, which is specific for sheep red blood cells, carries H-2-encoded determinants and the antigen-binding site on separate polypeptide chains. However, Dr J. D. Capra (pers. comm.) has

TABLE VIII

Absorption and elution of suppressor factor from anti-idiotypic immunoadsorbent (*Bach* et al., *1979a*)

Material injected[a]	*Immunoadsorbent column specificity*	*Footpad swelling*[b] *mm* × *10*² ± *s.e.*	P
—	—	20·3 ± 1·8	—
Filtrate	Rabbit anti-CRI[c]	12·2 ± 2·1	<0·01
Acid eluate	Rabbit anti-CRI	4·8 ± 2·1	<0·005
Unfractionated TsF	—	4·0 ± 1·4	<0·005
Filtrate	Normal rabbit Ig[c]	3·8 ± 1·8	<0·005
Acid eluate	Normal rabbit Ig	20·5 ± 1·6	N.S.[d]

[a] Material obtained from columns was adjusted to 2×10^7 cell eq/0·2 ml per mouse and administered daily for 5 days into A/J mice.

[b] Mice were immunized i.p. with 3×10^7 Ar-coupled spleen cells and challenged in the footpad with 25 μl of 10 mM diazonium salt of *p*-arsanilic acid.

[c] $F(ab')_2$ fraction.

[d] Not significant.

found the antigen-binding site and H-2-encoded determinants on a single polypeptide chain in molecules secreted by a T cell hybridoma. Additional work is needed to reconcile these reports and in particular to ascertain whether various groups are working with the same material.

Other properties of the TsF just described will be summarized briefly (Bach *et al.*, 1979). The factor is bound to immobilized Ar hapten groups as well as to anti-id antibody. It has a molecular weight by gel filtration of 30 000–60 000 daltons and possesses antigenic determinants controlled by the *I–J* subregion of the *H–2* MHC (Sy *et al.*, 1980a). The H-2 determinants, idiotypic determinants, and hapten-binding site are all on the same molecular complex, as shown by successive filtration through pairs of columns containing bound hapten, bound anti-id, or bound anti-H-2 antibodies. The factor does not possess antigenic determinants recognized by conventional anti-Ig reagents.

TsF obtained from A/J or C.AL-20 mice was bound to an immobilized anti-CRI column and could be eluted at low pH, whereas TsF from B10.A or BALB/c mice was not retained (Bach *et al.*, 1979; Greene and Benacerraf, 1980). Thus, inheritance of the capacity to produce CRI$^+$ TsF is linked to the *Igh* locus but not to the *H-2* MHC. It seems probable that the TsF has V_H regions similar to those in CRI^+ anti-Ar antibodies.

Our data do not establish whether or not the products of the MHC and V_H genes are on the same polypeptide chain. As indicated above, Dr Capra's results would indicate that this is the case. If so, this would suggest the presence on a single polypeptide chain of segments encoded by chromosomes XII (*Igh*) and XVII (*H-2*). In any case the V_H gene product is undoubtedly responsible for the antigen-binding specificity; the MHC-controlled portion of the molecule may be directly involved in a cell-signalling function, which might include a direct interaction with cellular receptors.

Existence of TsF with idiotypic (TsF_1) and anti-idiotypic (TsF_2) receptors

The experiments to be described next were carried out by using the humoral response as the method for assaying activity of TsF. Activity was demonstrated by suppression of the major idiotypic component of the response to the Ar hapten in strain A mice. In contrast to the DTH response, we have not observed a major effect of TsF on total anti-Ar production (Hirai and Nisonoff, 1980).

The TsF used in these experiments was obtained from supernatants of cultured splenic leukocytes of mice that had been suppressed by inoculation of rabbit anti-id antiserum and then immunized with KLH-Ar. Only those mice were used as a source of TsF that had produced high titres of anti-Ar antibodies with undetectable CRI. After hyperimmunization, mice were allowed to rest for 3 weeks before sacrifice. Active TsF could be prepared

TABLE IX
Time-course of appearance of TsF in culture supernatants[a]
(*Hirai and Nisonoff, 1980*)

Duration of culture h	Serum titres, day 30: Anti-Ar μg/ml	Serum titres, day 30: Anti-Ar Ab required for 50% inhibition ng
0	510, 600, 660, 780, 780	14, 66, 30, 64, 92
6	340, 660, 900, 1050, 1400	8600, 16 000, 20, 15, 82
12	600, 780, 960, 1350, 1590	6000, 66, 4800, >33 000, 8000
24	840, 840, 1200, 1300, 1400	>21 000, >21 000, >30 000, >34 000, >34 000

[a] The spleen cells cultured were from mice that had been idiotypically suppressed, hyperimmunized and allowed to rest for 3 weeks. Each irradiated (560 rad) recipient was given 5×10^7 spleen cells that had been incubated with culture supernatant from 5×10^7 cultured cells.

from culture supernates of erythrocyte-free splenic T cells as well as whole spleen cell preparations; either source was equally effective. Typically, a cell suspension containing 2×10^7 cells/ml was cultured for 24 h at 37°C; the supernate was recovered by centrifugation and incubated with normal A/J spleen cells for 4 h. Fifty $\times 10^6$ cells were transferred to irradiated (560 rad) A/J recipients, which were then immunized with KLH-Ar. Sera were tested by quantitative radioimmune assays for anti-Ar and CRI content.

The data in Table IX demonstrate the suppressor activity of TsF and show the time course of its appearance in a culture supernatant (Hirai and Nisonoff, 1980). It is evident that cells incubated with cell-free culture supernates from spleen cells of hyperimmunized suppressed mice can produce high titres of anti-Ar antibodies after adoptive transfer; however, these antibodies are devoid of CRI. On the basis of the data in Table IX, cells were cultured for 24 h for subsequent preparations of TsF.

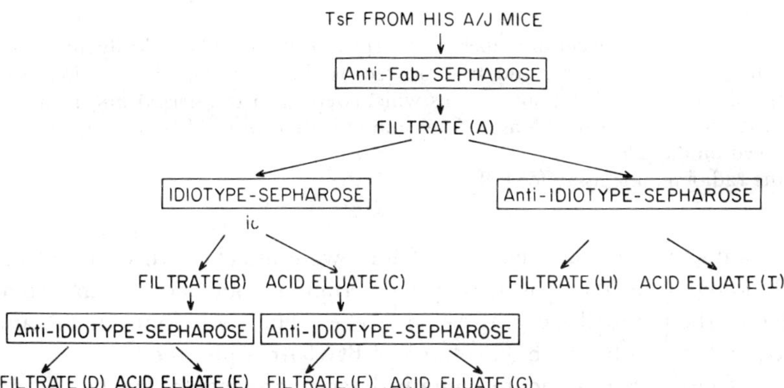

FIG. 1. *Fractionation procedure used for TsF from 2×10^9 spleen cells of hyperimmunized suppressed mice. Acid elution was done with glycine (0·1 M)-HCl buffer, pH 2·8.*

Some of the evidence indicating the existence of two types of TsF, with idiotypic or anti-idiotypic receptors, is shown in Fig. 1 and Table X. Each recipient mouse was given 5×10^7 normal spleen cells incubated with a volume of TsF solution that would have contained 5×10^7 cell equivalents if all of the TsF applied had been recovered in that fraction (filtrate or eluate). The filtrate from anti-Fab-Sepharose (Fraction A) possessed suppressor activity. The activity was not completely retained on either an idiotype-Sepharose or anti-idiotype-Sepharose column; i.e., Fractions B and H both had suppressor activity. However, successive passages over idiotype-Sepharose followed by anti-idiotype Sepharose completely removed the suppressor activity (Fraction D). In addition, the acid eluates from both id-Sepharose and anti-id-Sepharose (Fractions C and I) were both active. In other experiments (not shown) it was found that the anti-idiotypic TsF, eluted from id-Sepharose was bound, as expected, to another CRI^+ column but was not bound by Sepharose to

TABLE X

Evidence for the existence of TsF with idiotypic or anti-idiotypic receptors[a] *(Hirai and Nisonoff, 1980)*

Fraction (*see Fig. 1*)	*Anti-Ar titre* $\mu g/ml$	*Anti-Ar Ab required for 50% inhibition*[b] *ng*
A	200–320	2500, >4200, >5200, 4100
B	42–450	>1000, 3700, 30, >6400, >10 800, 45
C	230–560	>5620, >6700, 9, 11 000, >14 000
D	60–660	8, 19, 39, 41, 18, 16
E	32–300	>800, 210, 750, 18, 23, >7500
F	58–430	>1500, 3000, 1500, >4100, 24, 11 000
G	44–330	11, 1400, 45, 13, 11
H	180–990	4500, 450, 960, 2100, 4200, 5000
I	150–360	750, 180, 2700, >5300, >5300, 720
Control (culture medium)	150–640	27, 52, 110, 150, 19

[a] TsF was obtained from culture supernates of spleen cells from idiotypically suppressed, hyperimmunized A/J mice, and fractionated as shown in Fig. 1. Fractions were incubated with normal A/J spleen cells which were then transferred into irradiated recipients (5×10^7 cells per mouse). After immunization with KLH-Ar recipient mice were bled on day 25.

[b] In the radioimmune assay for CRI.

which anti-Ar antibodies that were CRI^- were attached; this showed that the binding is mediated by idiotypic determinants and not by an antigen bridge to the immobilized anti-Ar antibodies. The CRI^+ but not the anti-idiotypic TsF was bound by a column of BGG-Ar-Sepharose.

Both factors were found to contain determinants controlled by the *H-2* MHC; more recent experiments have localized these to the *I–J* subregion. The molecular weight of either factor, as estimated by gel filtration, is 50 000–100 000 and each factor is inactivated by pronase and not by DNase or RNase. Cells that elaborated either factor were killed with treatment with anti-Thy-1.2 and complement (Hirai and Nisonoff, 1980).

Demonstration of anti-idiotypic TsF (TsF_2) in the DTH system

We have already discussed data which establish the existence of a suppressor factor (TsF_1) with CRI^+ receptors, which suppresses DTH to the Ar hapten through the induction of anti-idiotypic suppressor T cells (Ts_2). More recently (manuscript in preparation) we have shown that these Ts_2 elaborate a suppressor factor which cannot be bound by immobilized hapten or by nonspecific A/J Ig but which is bound by CRI^+ anti-Ar antibodies. Thus the existence of idiotypic and anti-idiotypic TsF can be demonstrated by suppression of DTH as well as by selective suppression of the major idiotypic component of the humoral response. In other recent experiments we have shown that differences in the mechanism of action of TsF_1 and TsF_2 can be demonstrated by kinetic experiments. Thus, TsF_1 (idiotypic) was effective when administered on days 0–4 after immunization with Ar-coupled syngeneic cells but was inactive when given on days 3 and 4. (Footpad challenge was on day 4.) In contrast TsF_2 was inactive when given on days 3 and 4 (as well as days 0–4). The data suggest that TsF_2 but not TsF_1 works at the effector limb of the DTH response and that TsF_1 acts at the afferent limb.

We have already discussed data indicating that TsF_1 induces anti-idiotypic suppressor T cells (Ts_2). Other experiments suggest that the suppressor function of TsF_1 is mediated only through its capacity to induce Ts_2. Thus TsF_1 suppresses DTH in C.AL-20 mice but does not do so in BALB/c mice; however, it does induce anti-idiotypic Ts_2 in BALB/c mice, which can suppress DTH when adoptively transferred into C.Al-20 recipients.

Genetic control of the structural composition of TsF

As mentioned in the Introduction, the CRI present on humoral A/J anti-Ar antibodies is under control of both the *Igh* and *VK-1* loci. Thus, several strains of mice which are Lyt-3·1 do not produce the L chains necessary for the expression of CRI^+ antibody molecules. Using appropriate F_3 offspring of A/J and PL/J mice we examined the genetic control of idiotypic determinants on TsF. The results are shown in Table XI. TsF obtained from mice that have *Igh-1*^{e} genes, characteristic of strain A mice, are retained on an anti-CRI

TABLE XI

Influence of Igh and Lyt genes on the expression of the A/J CRI in TsF (*Sy* et al., *in prep.*)

Donors of suppressor factor Igh-1	Lyt-3	Fractionation on anti-CRI column	Footpad swelling in recipients mm × 10^2 ± s.e.	P
Control A/J (no factor injected)			20·2 ± 0·4	
e	3·1	Unfractionated	11·3 ± 1·8	<0·01
		Filtrate	20 ± 1·8	N.S.
		Acid eluate	10 ± 1·7	<0·01
e	3·2	Unfractionated	9·2 ± 0·9	<0·01
		Filtrate	20·2 ± 1·7	N.S.
		Acid eluate	8·1 ± 0·7	<0·01
a	3·1	Unfractionated	8·6 ± 0·8	<0·01
		Filtrate	9·5 ± 0·9	<0·01
		Acid eluate	20·5 ± 1·9	N.S.
a	3·2	Unfractionated	10·1 ± 1·0	<0·01
		Filtrate	10·9 ± 1·8	<0·01
		Acid eluate	21 ± 1·2	N.S.

[a]The mice used for breeding were A/J (Igh-1^e, Lyt-3·3) and PL/J (Igh-1^a, Lyt-3·1).

column irrespective of the *Lyt-3* genes present (*Lyt-3·1* or *3·2*). These results contrast with those obtained with humoral antibodies, for which *Lyt-3·2* genes are needed for the expression of CRI^+ antibodies, and are consistent with the possibility that TsF_1 does not contain a light chain corresponding to that in CRI^+ A/J anti-Ar antibodies (Sy *et al.*, 1980b).

Discussion

The regulation of the immune response to *p*-azophenylarsonate involves a complex series of cellular interactions, some of which can be mediated by defined molecular entities (TsF). We do not as yet know the relative importance of Ts and TsF *in vivo*; i.e., whether some or all Ts activity is mediated through TsF. Another unsettled question is whether TsF is a cell receptor. In the reactions of T cells and B cells to the Ar hapten, both idiotypic and anti-idiotypic elements are essential for co-ordinated regulation. Experimentally, we have studied regulation by the inoculation of anti-id antibody, of ligand coupled to cells or by CRI^+ molecules coupled to cells.

Intravenous inoculation of ligand(AR)-coupled cells leads to expansion of regulatory cell populations capable of dampening idiotype-bearing T cell (DTH) responses, an effect described by Battisto and Bloom (1966), by Claman and Miller (1976) and by Scott and Long (1976). We showed that the inhibitory effect is attributable to a population of suppressor T cells capable upon adoptive transfer of limiting DTH to the Ar hapten. More recently we have found that such treatment also suppresses cytotoxic and proliferative responses, both of which are mediated by T cells (manuscript in preparation). The data discussed in this paper relate to the effects on T cell-mediated DTH. A detailed analysis of the functional and phenotypic character of ligand-induced first order suppressor T cells (Ts_1) has revealed the following.

Ts_1 are idiotype-bearing and are bound to Ar-coated polystyrene plates, but not to idiotype-coated plates. Their Ly phenotype has not yet been defined but in terms of their similarity to other inducer cells in regulatory systems may be Lyt-1 or Lyt-1,2,3 (Cantor *et al.*, 1978). Such Ts_1 cells must be given on or shortly after the day of immunization in order to cause suppression. Moreover, such Ts_1 are allotype-restricted; ligand-induced BALB/c Ts_1 will cause suppression upon adoptive transfer into BALB/c but not into C.AL-20 recipients, and vice versa. This restriction with respect to allotype indicates that the mechanism by which Ts_1 causes suppression cannot relate solely to antigen specificity. The process may involve the release, production or expression of an idiotype-bearing $I\text{-}J^+$ molecule (TsF_1) which can stimulate the clonal expansion of secondary suppressor cells (Ts_2) with complementary anti-idiotypic receptors.

General structural characteristics of TsF_1 have been studied in some detail. They can be obtained from Ts_1 cells by physical disruption or from supernatants obtained after culturing Ts_1 *in vitro*. TsF_1 capable of causing suppression of either the CRI-component of the anti-Ar antibody response or of the Ar-specific, T-dependent DTH reaction have a number of comparable features, and may indeed be the same molecule. The molecular weights estimated for the two TsF preparations by gel filtration are 33 000–68 000 in the case of the DTH-active molecule and 50 000–100 000 for TsF_1 active in the humoral response. Both preparations have antigenic determinants encoded by the H-2 region of the MHC and, in the case of the TsF active in DTH, the determinants have been shown to be encoded by the I-J subregion. Both TsF_1 preparations are specifically bound to immobilized Ar hapten groups or anti-idiotype. TsF_1 preparations can be inactivated by treatment with pronase but not by DNase or RNase. The molecular properties of TsF_2 are so far indistinguishable from those of TsF_1 except for binding activity. (TsF_2 is bound specifically by idiotype rather than by hapten or anti-idiotype.)

In the case of TsF_1 induced by ligand-coupled cells we have also analysed the contribution of the *VK-1* locus, using DTH as the measure of activity. Actually, assays were carried out for Lyt-3 antigens; as shown by P. D. Gottlieb, the *Lyt-3* locus is very tightly linked to the *VK-1* locus. We bred mice which possessed *Igh-1^e^* genes but which varied at the *Lyt-3* locus. The mice were tested for the capacity to make CRI^+ TsF. It had been shown earlier that the production of CRI^+ anti-Ar antibody required the presence of *Lyt-3·2* genes, associated with the A strain (Laskin *et al.*, 1977). In contrast, expression of CRI^+ TsF_1 was independent of the genes present at the *VK-1* locus, but did require the presence of *Igh-1^e^* genes. Thus, the genes controlling light chains which are needed for CRI^+ antibody biosynthesis are apparently not necessary for the synthesis of TsF_1 that is CRI^+. Other experiments suggest that the anti-id antibodies that are responsible for binding the TsF are directed to the V_H region of the molecule and not to the binding site (Sy *et al.*, in prep.).

The presence of I-J-coded determinants as well as CRI^+ structures on TsF indicate that at a minimum two separate genes must control TsF. One is present in chromosome XII and encodes the $Igh\text{-}1^e$ complex, and the other is in chromosome XVII.

The mechanism of action of TsF_1 was investigated in considerable detail and was found to include the generation of a second set of suppressor T cells (Ts_2) in naive recipients. The induction of Ts_2 by TsF with undefined idiotypic properties was reported by Waltenbaugh *et al.* (1977) and by Tada (1977). Examination of genetic restrictions on this interaction revealed that TsF_1 induced Ts_2 in each strain of mouse tested, but that such Ts_2 could only be detected when transferred into the strains whose humoral antibodies (and presumably T cells) are CRI^+. Thus, TsF_1 from A/J mice induced Ts_2 in either C.AL-20 or BALB/c mice. The BALB/c mice were not directly suppressed (although C.AL-20 were), presumably because the CRI is not expressed in the BALB/c strain. However, Ts_2 activity could be demonstrated in such BALB/c mice by adoptive transfer of their cells into C.AL-20 recipients. The T cells responsible were shown to have anti-idiotypic receptors; they were bound to CRI-coated, but not to Ar-coated polystyrene plates. These experiments have been done by using both DTH (Sy *et al.*, 1980b) and the humoral idiotypic response (Hirai *et al.*, in prep.) as the assays.

C.AL-20 mice are directly suppressed by CRI^+ TsF_1 and the activity of Ts_2 present can be demonstrated by adoptive transfer into C.AL-20 but not into BALB/c mice. The allotype restriction of both Ts_1 and TsF_1 suggest that they may function exclusively through the induction of Ts_2.

Anti-idiotypic Ts_2 have several structural and functional properties which clearly distinguish them from Ts_1. Ts_1 bind to ligand-coated plates but not to idiotype-coated plates, whereas the opposite is true of Ts_2. Ts_1 were suppressive of DTH only when given early in the immune response (days 0 or 1). Ts_2 was functionally suppressive when administered either early or late (days 3 and 4), a property consistent with effector-level suppression. The early action of Ts_1 (afferent-suppression) is of course consistent with the inducing-function of this subset. Similar functional studies have been performed in the NP (nitrophenylacetyl) system in C57BL mice by Weinberger *et al.* (1979, 1980).

More recently (unpublished results), we have found that Ts_2 (as well as Ts_1) releases a soluble factor that suppresses DTH. This TsF_2 is anti-idiotypic, bears H-2 encoded structures, and suppresses immune T cells that are matched with respect to both allotype and H-2. As discussed in the text anti-idiotypic TsF_2 have also been demonstrated by using the humoral response as an assay, in mice that were suppressed by inoculation of anti-idiotypic antibodies followed by hyperimmunization; the specificity of the T cells secreting this TsF_2 has not yet been established but by analogy with the DTH studies the cells are probably Ts_2. Also by analogy with the findings on DTH (efferent suppression by Ts_2) it seems likely that these anti-id TsF may interact directly with idiotypic structures on B or T cells to cause suppression. It should be noted that such idiotype-bearing target cells have not been proven to be the actual effectors.

Thus we can envision that ligand-induced suppressor T cells function by virtue of a defined molecular mediator (TsF_1) which is $I\text{-}J^+$ and CRI^+. Such TsF_1 can induce Ts_2 in other strains, without H-2 or Igh restrictions. However, if these strains are directly examined only those which are CRI^+ (with respect to humoral antibody production) are suppressed by the Ts_2. The presence of Ts_2 can be demonstrated, however, by adoptive transfer into an H-2 identical, CRI^+ strain.

We will now consider humoral antibody production and DTH, in which mice were treated with idiotypic antibody conjugated to cell surfaces. Such idiotype-coupled cells, administered by a tolerogenic route, readily induced anti-idiotypic Ts_2 cells in each of the recipient strains tested; thus Ts_2 can be induced by TsF_1 or by idiotype-coupled cells. Ts_2 cells induced by id-coupled cells are active in H-2 matched recipients which are CRI^+. Such Ts_2 can be produced in a CRI^- strain, and its activity demonstrated by adoptive transfer to an H-2 matched CRI^+ strain. The Ts_2 can cause suppression of DTH or the idiotypic component of the humoral anti-Ar response. Thus there is a requirement for matching of the inductive signal (CRI^+ structure) and the target (which must be CRI^+) in order for suppression to be observed. CRI^- mice treated with idiotype-coupled cells exhibited no suppression of DTH although they did produce anti-idiotypic suppressor cells, as shown by adoptive transfer into an appropriate strain.

This series of experiments helps to define the restrictions observed in certain systems involving suppressor T cells. Gershon and his colleagues have, for example, identified V_H restrictions between inducer subsets in the regulation of the immune response to sheep erythrocytes (Eardley *et al.*, 1979). However, in these studies inducer and target cells were not matched. Hence the failure to observe suppression does not exclude the possibility that anti-idiotypic Ts were generated across an allotype barrier but did not cause suppression because of the absence of a suitable target.

The experiments described here have defined similar effects for either T cell or B cell responses to the Ar hapten and suggest a generalized scheme necessary for ordered regulation of immunity. We envision that after ligand has activated clones of antigen-reactive T or B cells, their idiotypic receptors (analogous to idiotype-coupled cells) activate anti-idiotypic Ts which can cause inhibition by interacting with T or B cells expressing the relevant idiotype. The data reported are consistent with the hypothesis of Jerne (1974) concerning the existence of idiotype-anti-idiotype networks. The data reported so far suggest that anti-idiotypic T cells may play a more significant role in regulation than auto-anti-idiotypic antibodies.

In the case of the humoral response, the existence of a network is indicated by the demonstration of TsF with idiotypic and anti-idiotypic receptors. Also, treatment with anti-idiotypic antibody followed by immunization with antigen results in the appearance of Ts_2 with anti-idiotypic receptors. Since the initial target of either anti-idiotype or antigen would be expected to be an idiotype-bearing cell, it seems quite likely that the anti-idiotypic suppressors are stimulated by cells (or factors) with idiotypic receptors (Owen *et al.*, 1977a, b). In the DTH system the induction of Ts_2 by TsF_1 was demonstrated directly.

A related recent finding is the induction of idiotype-bearing T effector cells by the administration of anti-idiotype, either subcutaneously to untreated mice or i.v. to cyclophosphamide-pretreated mice. Again it seems probable that anti-id initially induces idiotype-bearing elements.

In summary, regulation of the response to a hapten has been evaluated for both T and B cell reactivities. A variety of symmetrical features of the network have been defined in which two gene complexes, the *Igh* locus and the *H-2* MHC, provide structural elements which are important in regulation. Although these studies have focused on reactions to a hapten group, many of the principles may be applicable to other types of antigens, including proteins and particulate antigens, and to tumour immunity. Recent experiments have demonstrated that anti-idiotypic $I\text{-}J^+$ Ts can limit the secretion of idiotypic antibodies by a myeloma tumour. Such studies on regulation of a tumour may eventually have therapeutic implications.

Diagrams outlining some of our conclusions are shown in Figs 2 and 3.

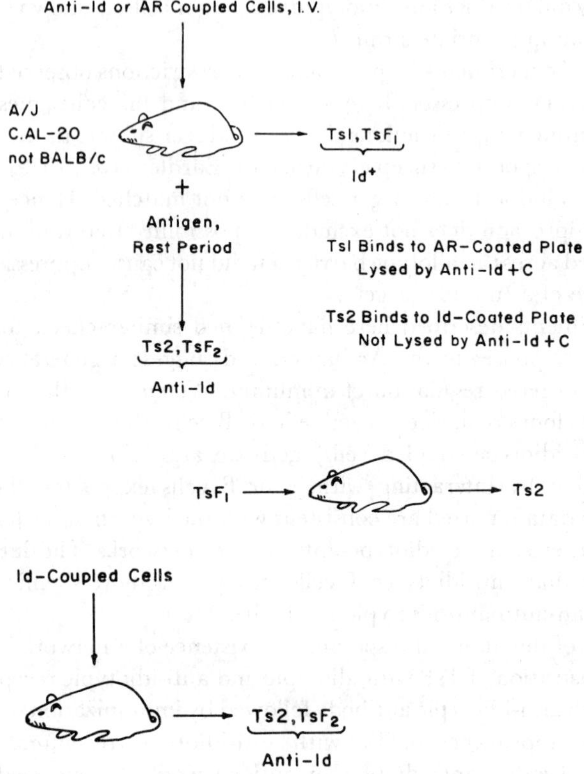

Ts2 Can Be Produced in BALB/c Mice (That Do Not Express the Idiotype)

Such Ts2 are Active in the CRI$^+$ C.AL-20 Strain, Not BALB/c.

Conclusion: C.AL-20 Express Suitable CRI$^+$ Targets; BALB/c Do Not.

FIGS 2 and 3. *Proposed mechanisms in the regulation of the anti-Ar response mediated by idiotypic determinants.*

References

Alkan, S. S., Knecht, R. and Braun, D. G. (1980). *Hoppe-Seyler's Z. Physiol. Chim.* **361**, 191.

Bach, B. A., Sherman, L., Benacerraf, B. and Greene, M. I. (1978). *J. Immunol.* **121**, 1460.

Bach, B. A., Greene, M., Benacerraf, B. and Nisonoff, A. (1979). *J. Exp. Med.* **149**, 1084.

Battisto, J. R. and Bloom, B. R. (1966). *Nature* **212**, 156.

Baumgarten, A. and Geczy, A. F. (1970). *Immunology* **19**, 205.

Binz, H. and Wigzell, H. (1977). *Contemp. Topics Immunobiol.* **7**, 113.
Bordenave, G. R. (1975). *Immunology* **28**, 635.
Brown, A. R., Estess, P., Lamoyi, E., Gill-Pazaris, L., Gottlieb, P. D., Capra, J. D. and Nisonoff, A. (1980). *Prog. Clin. Biol. Research* **42**, 231.
Cantor, H., Hugenberger, J., McVay-Boudreau, L., Eardley, D. D., Kēmp, J., Shen, F. W. and Gershon, R. K. (1978). *J. Exp. Med.* **148**, 871.
Claman, H. N. and Miller, S. D. (1976). *J. Immunol.* **117**, 480.
Cosenza, H. and Kohler, H. (1972). *Science* **176**, 207.
Dietz, M. H., Sy, M-S., Greene, M. I., Nisonoff, A., Benacerraf, B. and Germain, R. N. (1980). Submitted for publication.
Dohi, Y. and Nisonoff, A. (1979). *J. Exp. Med.* **909**, 150.
Eardley, D. D., Shen, F. W., Cantor, H. and Gershon, R. K. (1979). *J. Exp. Med.* **150**, 44.
Eichmann, K. (1974). *Eur. J. Immunol.* **4**, 296.
Eichmann, K. (1975). *Eur. J. Immunol.* **5**, 511.
Estess, P., Nisonoff, A. and Capra, J. D. (1979). *Mol. Immunol.* **16**, 1111.
Estess, P., Lamoyi, E., Nisonoff, A. and Capra, J. D. (1980). *J. Exp. Med.* **151**, 863.
Germain, R. N., Ju, S-T., Kipps, T. J., Benacerraf, B. and Dorf, M. E. (1979). *J. Exp. Med.* **149**, 613.
Gottlieb, P. D. (1974). *J. Exp. Med.* **140**, 1432.
Gottlieb, P. D., Wan, H., Brown, A. R. and Nisonoff, A. (1979). *In* "Cell Biology and Immunology of Leukocyte Function", Proc. 12th Leukocyte Culture Conf., p. 317. Academic Press, New York and London.
Greene, M. I., Sugimoto, M. and Benacerraf, B. (1978). *J. Immunol.* **120**, 1605.
Greene, M. I. and Benacerraf, B. (1980). *Immunol. Rev.* **50**, 163.
Hart, D. A., Wang, A. C., Pawlak, L. L. and Nisonoff, A. (1972). *J. Exp. Med.* **135**, 1293.
Hirai, Y. and Nisonoff, A. (1980). *J. Exp. Med.* **151**, 1213.
Jerne, N. K. (1974). *Ann. Immunol.* (Paris) **125c**, 373.
Krawinkel, U., Cramer, M., Imanishi-Kari, T., Jack, R. S., Rajewsky, K. and Makela, O. (1977). *Eur. J. Immunol.* **7**, 566.
Kuettner, M. G., Wang, A. and Nisonoff, A. (1972). *J. Exp. Med.* **135**, 579.
Lamoyi, E., Estess, P., Capra, J. D. and Nisonoff, A. (1980a). *J. Immunol.* **124**, 2834.
Lamoyi, E., Estess, P., Capra, J. D. and Nisonoff, A. (1980b). *J. Exp. Med.* (in press).
Laskin, J. A., Gray, A., Nisonoff, A., Klinman, N. R. and Gottlieb, P. G. (1977). *Proc. Natn. Acad. Sci. U.S.A.* **74**, 4600.
Marshak-Rothstein, A., Siekevitz, M., Margolies, M. N., Mudgett-Hunter, M. and Gefter, M. (1980). *Proc. Natn. Acad. Sci. U.S.A.* **77**, 1120.
Nisonoff, A., Ju, S-T. and Owen, F. L. (1977). *Immunol. Rev.* **34**, 189.
Owen, F. L. and Nisonoff, A. (1978). *J. Exp. Med.* **148**, 182.
Owen, F. L., Ju, S-T. and Nisonoff, A. (1977a). *J. Exp. Med.* **137**, 1559.
Owen, F. L., Ju, S-T. and Nisonoff, A. (1977b). *Proc. Natn. Acad. Sci. U.S.A.* **74**, 2084.
Pawlak, L. L., Hart, D. A. and Nisonoff, A. (1973a). *J. Exp. Med.* **137**, 1442.
Pawlak, L. L., Mushinski, E. B., Nisonoff, A. and Potter, M. (1973b). *J. Exp. Med.* **137**, 22.
Rajewsky, K. and Eichmann, K. (1977). *Contemp. Topics Immunobiol.* **7**, 67.
Ramseier, H., Aguet, M. and Lindenmann, T. (1977). *Immunol. Rev.* **34**, 50.
Rowley, D. A., Kohler, H., Schreiber, H., Kaye, S. T. and Lorbach, I. (1976). *J. Exp. Med.* **144**, 946.
Scott, D. W. and Long, C. A. (1976). *J. Exp. Med.* **144**, 1369.
Strayer, D. S., Consenza, H., Lee, W. M. F., Rowley, D. A. and Kohler, H. (1974). *Science* **186**, 640.
Sy, M-S., Bach, B. A., Brown, A. R., Nisonoff, A., Benacerraf, B. and Greene, M. I. (1979a). *J. Exp. Med.* **1229**, 150.

Sy, M-S., Bach, B. A., Dohi, Y., Nisonoff, A., Benacerraf, B. and Greene, M. I. (1979b). *J. Exp. Med.* **1216**, 150.

Sy, M-S., Dietz, M. H., Germain, R. N., Benacerraf, B. and Greene, M. I. (1980a). *J. Exp. Med.* **151**, 1183.

Sy, M-S., Dietz, M. H., Nisonoff, A., Germain, R. N., Benacerraf, B. and Greene M. I. (1980b). Submitted for publication.

Tada, T. (1977). *In* "The Immune System: Genetics and Regulation". (E. Sercarz, L. A. Herzenberg and C. G. Fox, eds), p. 345. Academic Press, New York and London.

Taussig, M. J. and Holliman, A. (1979). *Nature* **277**, 308.

Waltenbaugh, C., Theze, J., Kapp, J. A. and Benacerraf, B. (1977). *J. Exp. Med.* **146**, 970.

Weinberger, J. Z., Germain, R. N., Ju, S-T., Greene, M. I., Benacerraf, B. and Dorf, M. E. (1979). *J. Exp. Med.* **150**, 761.

Weinberger, J. Z., Benaceraff, B. and Dorf, M. E. (1980). *J. Exp. Med.* **151**, 1413.

Yamamoto, H., Nonaka, M. and Katz, D. H. (1979). *J. Exp. Med.* **150**, 818.

5

Idiotypic Induction and Immune Networks

J. URBAIN, P. A. CAZENAVE, M. WIKLER, J. D. FRANSSEN, B. MARIAMÉ and O. LEO

Laboratory of Animal Physiology, Université de Bruxelles, Belgium

Introduction

The astonishing diversity of the immunological repertoire is best illustrated by the phenomenon of idiotypy (or individual antigenic specificity) (Oudin and Michel, 1969a, b; Kunkel, 1963; Kelus and Gell, 1968). When different animals from one species are confronted with the same antigen, they respond by the synthesis of antibodies displaying different idiotypic specificities. Exceptions to this rule, which have been called cross-reactive, major, public or recurrent idiotypes, have been extensively studied, but it should be stressed that the number of idiotypes defined "à la Oudin" exceeds by far the number of recurrent idiotypes (for review, see Eichmann, 1979).

The somatic mutation theory was the most obvious explanation to account for idiotypy. Since, in this theory, the repertoire is built *de novo* in each individual from a few germ line genes, different immunological repertoires will arise in different individuals and there will be no Mendelian inheritance of idiotypic expression. However, another explanation would be to assume that complex mechanisms of activation and suppression involving idiotypes lead to the expression of different idiotypes in different individuals. In this hypothesis, we have to distinguish between the potential immunological repertoire and the repertoire available to an antigen.

Since one immunoglobulin can be an antibody recognizing an external antigen and also can behave as an antigen by inducing the appearance of anti-idiotypic antibodies, we are faced with an amazing paradox. At first sight, there seem to be two sets of antibodies. The first set contains conventional antibodies raised against external antigens; the second set contains all antibodies against antibodies (anti-idiotypic antibodies). Since each animal can make anti-idiotypic antibodies against any idiotype and anti-idiotypic antibodies can themselves induce anti-(anti)-idiotypic antibodies and so on, it seems that the two sets are largely overlapping, if not identical (Jerne, 1974, 1976; Lindenmann, 1973). Now if the two sets are really one set, several interesting things can be deduced. First, there should be coexistence of complementary idiotypes and autoanti-idiotypes within the immune repertoire of one individual (formal network). This has now been proved beyond doubt (for review see Rodkey, 1980). Therefore, this could be the basis for a new way of communications between lymphocytes, based on self recognition (functional idiotypic network).

Since the universe of paratopes is complete and since the number of idiotypes is as high as the number of paratopes, the immune system should contain imperfect internal images of external antigens. In appropriate conditions, such internal images could substitute for antigen (see below).

We suggested that the immune system could be a functional idiotypic network on the basis of quite different premises (Urbain, 1974; Urbain, 1978).

The crux and the burden of germ line theories has always been the selection problem. How could a species keep genes apparently useless during the lifetime of one individual since many of these genes would code for antibodies directed against unforeseen antigenic stimuli? How could a system evolve in anticipation of future needs? If the external selection pressure due to antigens is clearly insufficient, there could be an internal selective pressure allowing to conserve a large number of genes. This internal selective pressure should be as diversified as the world of antigens. Therefore, if any immunoglobulin is in fact an anti-idiotype of another immunoglobulin and if these idiotypic interactions are physiologically relevant, or, in other words, if the immune system is a functional idiotypic network, the burden of germ line theories can be removed. The recent DNA data show that the number of germ line genes is indeed very large (Seidman *et al.*, 1980).

Many data which have accumulated during the last decade allow us to paint a new picture of the immune system. If we compare with the concepts of clonal selection theory, a fair description of the immune system 15 years ago, two main things have emerged:

(a) The immune system can no longer be considered as a library of small independent immune systems (clones), awaiting activation by antigen. This reductionist approach has to be replaced by network concepts. Each lymphocyte speaks to some others and the language of communication forms the basis of immunoregulatory circuits. This conclusion stems from the fact that (i) antigen can bridge T and B lymphocytes from different immunological specificities (Mitchison, 1971), and (ii) T lymphocytes can be subdivided into subsets or compartments performing different functions (help, suppression etc.). More precisely, Lyt-1 lymphocytes in addition to inducing B cells to secrete antibody, induce resting Lyt-23 T cells to exert feedback suppressive activity. Activation of suppressors leads to a reduction in helper activity which in turn leads to decreased antibody production and therefore decreased suppressor cell induction (see Cantor, 1979).

(b) The immune system is indeed a functional idiotypic network in the sense that idiotypes are involved in clonal interactions. T lymphocytes use a dual recognition system. They "see" one epitope, only when this epitope is associated with the "correct" membrane environment (for review, see Zinkernagel, 1978). These last two findings imply that self recognition is a key feature within the immune system.

As pointed out by Vaz and Varela (1978), "the acknowledgement that the immune responses are actually loop in a complex web of intercellular events is important but it adds little to our understanding of how the system operates". We have to define precise rules of the immunological game. We have to understand the relationships between the cellular network, the idiotypic network and the restrictive recognition association with T lymphocytes.

Before facing these questions, we shall discuss data which strongly suggest that the immune system is a functional idiotypic network. We will restrict ourselves here to those experiments concerning the induction of specific idiotypes. A more detailed review can be found elsewhere (Urbain *et al.*, 1980; Bona and Hiernaux, 1980).

Induction of specific idiotypes

Induction by internal images

As stated above, network concepts led to the view that an immune system already contains within it imperfect images or homobodies of antigens.

During a study of the specificity of idiotypic reactions in the tobacco mosaic virus system we found that one anti-idiotypic serum contained antibodies with strange properties (O. Leo, B. Mariamé, M. Slaoui and J. Urbain, in prep.).

(a) These "anti-idiotypic antibodies" were recognizing not only the idiotypic anti-TMV antibodies used for immunization (as is to be expected), but were also reacting with part of anti-TMV antibodies from all rabbits immunized against TMV. No linkage with allotypes of the a group was apparent since anti-TMV antibodies from a1/a1, a2/a2, a3/a3 rabbits are recognized. These special Ab-2 never react with antibodies from rabbits immunized against other antigens. They are therefore exquisitely specific for antibodies specific for TMV.

(b) The epitopes which are recognized by these "peculiar" anti-idiotypic antibodies are not species specific since a similar reactivity was discovered with anti-TMV antibodies from all mice, horses, goats, chickens etc. tested. In other words, these antiantibodies react with any anti-TMV serum.

(c) These same anti-idiotypic antibodies, when injected into mice in the total absence of TMV, induce the appearance of anti-TMV antibodies.

In summary, these special Ab-2 behave like the antigen: they react with anti-TMV antibodies and they are also able to promote the synthesis of anti-TMV antibodies. They are therefore good candidates for being considered as the internal image of tobacco mosaic virus. These results also strongly support the assertion that the immune system is a functional idiotypic network, since the immune system can be triggered by elements of the system itself, without intervention of external antigens.

Induction of recurrent idiotypes

Eichmann and Rajewsky (1975) showed that minute amounts of guinea-pig anti-idiotypic antibodies belonging to the IgG_1 class were able to sensitize B cells and T helper cells positive for the A5A idiotype (a recurrent idiotype which appears when A/J mice are immunized with *Streptococcus* of the A group). Similar results were obtained for the T15 idiotype by Julius *et al.* (1977).

Recently, similar kinds of experiments have been performed by Kelsoe *et al.* (1980) using well defined monoclonal anti-idiotype antibodies directed against NP antibodies. Primary anti-NP antibodies represent a family of idiotypically cross-reactive antibodies. Several groups of mice were injected with graded amounts of anti-idiotope antibodies from 10 ng to 10 μg. Mice were subsequently immunized with the hapten NP coupled to chicken immunoglobulins 1–8 weeks after anti-idiotope antibodies injection. Doses of 10 and 100 ng lead to a striking enhancement of idiotype expression, but this effect was only seen if antigen is given at least 4 weeks after anti-idiotopes treatment. Higher doses promoted suppression of idiotype expression.

As these authors point out, several aspects are worth emphasizing. The system seems to be well programmed since similar dose effects are found in individual mice. Regulatory effects are observable only after a long time delay. From this, the authors conclude that "quite in the sense of the original network concept, the anti-idiotope disturbs the idiotypic balance of the system and a new equilibrium is reached by a complex series of reactions which proceed over many weeks, and in which a large number of idiotypes and anti-idiotypic molecules and cells are involved". Although we do not negate this interpretation, we propose that such time delays are necessary because regulatory effects are exerted mainly on cells which are in an early stage of differentiation. The effects, at the level of humoral synthesis of idiotype, are only seen after complete differentiation of those early cells influenced by anti-idiotope treatments. It is of utmost importance that minute amounts of anti-idiotypic antibodies, which are in the range of natural antibodies, can result in such profound changes of idiotope expression.

Binz *et al.* (1979) have succeeded in demonstrating a functional mimicry between anti-idiotypic antibodies specific for antiallo-MHC reactive T cell receptors and the corresponding allo-MHC antigen. Normal T lymphocytes from relevant individuals were incubated with anti-idiotypic antibodies in the absence of complement for various times *in vitro*. Prolonged incubation periods were necessary to observe a generation of highly specific killer T cells.

Antiarsonate antibodies induced in A/J mice display a recurrent idiotype (Nisonoff and Bangasser, 1975). Anti-idiotypic antibodies injected intravenously usually induce specific suppressor T cells. However, the same antibodies passively administrated, under appropriate conditions, induce T cell mediated immunity. Interestingly, pretreatment of mice with low doses of cyclophosphamide before i.v. injection of anti-CRI antibodies induces a significance-specific DTH reaction (Sy *et al.*, 1980). Moreover, injection of $(Fab)'_2$ fragments of an anti-CRI antibodies also induced DTH, instead of suppressing it. Subcutaneous injections of anti-CRI promote DTH.

It is therefore clear that the same antibodies can have opposite physiological effects depending on the route of administration, the status of the host (absence or presence of the suppressor compartment and so on). From all the results described above, it can be concluded that helper or suppressor T cells are not essentially linked with idiotypic or anti-idiotypic specificities. Idiotypes are involved in clonal interactions, but the nature of the ongoing interactions is not dictated by the idiotypic–anti-idiotypic interactions but by the compartments to which the interacting cells belong.

Induction of idiotypes "à la Oudin"

All the findings described above and others show clearly that it is possible to promote the induction of recurrent idiotypes by the use of anti-idiotypic antibodies in appropriate conditions. In some way, anti-idiotypic antibodies can mimic and replace antigens. However, in those cases, we know that animals are already programmed to make the desired idiotypes, because antigen alone always triggers the appearance of the idiotype. We would now like to consider the following questions: what happens with idiotypes *sensu stricto*, idiotypes "à la Oudin" which are specific for one antigen and one individual? Do these idiotypes correspond to the occurrence of different somatic mutations in different individuals, or do they represent *differential expression* of a basic germ line immunological repertoire? It could be that, starting with the same total repertoire, different repertoires available to antigen will emerge in different individuals, which will experience different *antigenic histories*. In their two famous papers of 1969, Oudin and Michel suggested that "things seem to happen as if the idiotypic specificities of one given individual were lot-drawn among a set of a very large number of possibilities which are common to all individuals of the same genotype (in terms of immunoglobulin allotypy)".

The following data strongly suggest that Oudin's proposal is fundamentally correct and gives precision to the meaning of lot-drawn. One of the first indications came from studies of irradiated rabbits repopulated with a mixture of bone marrow, lymph node and spleen cells taken from rabbits hyperimmunized with tobacco mosaic virus. Donor and recipient rabbits were displaying different allotypic specificities of V_H (donors were a1/a1 and recipients were a3/a3) (Van Acker *et al.*, 1979; Urbain-Vansanten *et al.*, 1979).

The results indicated that recipient rabbits, after being grafted with allogeneic immune cells and immunized with the same antigen, were immediately synthesizing high affinity antibodies, but the antibodies were bearing recipient allotypic specificities. In contrast, recipients from nonimmune donors synthesized antibodies of a much lower affinity. These results suggested that antibodies were produced by host cells which differentiated during radiation recovery and that the repertoire expressed by host cells had been strongly influenced by the presence of donor cells (which are rejected within 2 weeks). The most striking finding was a high level of idiotypic cross-reactivity between donor and recipient antibodies.

An interpretation of the results was proposed in the light of network concepts. A rabbit confronted with an antigen would be capable of producing a wide range of different antibodies bearing different idiotypic specificities. The antibody which is actually produced is the one which escaped suppression by the regulatory idiotypic network. Suppression is likely to be due to autoanti-idiotype. Irradiated rabbits are grafted with donor cells bearing receptors characterized by given idiotypic specificities (id 1). As new host B cells are emerging during radiation recovery, some will display receptors idiotypically cross-reactive (id 1′). This set would be in equilibrium with a corresponding inhibitory set (anti-idiotypic set). The presence of donor cells during the first weeks after irradiation and transfer could lead to the inactivation of the inhibitory set. Such a blocking would allow escape from suppression of the set id 1′, cross-reactive with the donor set. Also, these results suggested that the repertoire available to antigen is not only due to antigenic selection but also to the idiotypic history of the animal. However, these results were obtained using a rather sophisticated model and it was desirable to obtain more precise data using another experimental scheme (Urbain *et al.*, 1977; Cazenave, 1977; Wikler *et al.*, 1979; Urbain *et al.*, 1980).

Normally rabbit, say, I and rabbit, say, X produce different idiotypes when confronted with the same antigen. If we suppose that the immune repertoire of rabbit X contains some silent lymphocytes, endowed with the capacity to produce immunoglobulins displaying idiotypic specificities normally found in rabbit I after antigen immunization, it should be possible in principle to relieve these silent lymphocytes from suppression by raising immunity against the suppressors. The receptors of suppressors should be specific for the silent idiotype.

The following experimental scheme was therefore tried. A first antibody is isolated (call it Ab-1). Conventional anti-idiotypic antibodies (Ab-2) were raised in allotype-matched rabbits. These Ab-2 antibodies were isolated and used as immunogen in a third series of rabbits to elicit the production of anti-(anti)-idiotypic antibodies (Ab-3). Antigen was therefore given for the first time in this third series of rabbits which synthesized specific antibodies (call it Ab-1′).

This protocol has been successfully used in rabbits, now using 4 different antigens (carbohydrate from *Micrococcus*, peptidoglycan from *Micrococcus*, tobacco mosaic virus and ribonuclease).

The main results can be summarized as follows:

(a) in most cases (27 out of 28), Ab-1′ antibodies are idiotypically cross-reactive with Ab-1. In some cases, Ab-1 and Ab-1′ can be idiotypically identical using radioimmunoassay methods.

(b) in most cases, Ab-3 antibodies (antianti-idiotypic antibodies) do not react with antigen. However, there is a sharing of idiotypic specificities between Ab-1 and Ab-3 since Ab-4 antibodies (which are anti-idiotypic against Ab-3 or anti-(antianti)-idiotypic antibodies do recognize specifically Ab-1 and Ab-1′ antibodies belonging to the same chain of immunization.

In the case of *Micrococcus*, 60 unrelated rabbits hyperimmunized were used as controls. Only in one case was a clear idiotypic cross-reaction obtained. Interestingly, Ab-4 sera do not react with the 60 sera, with the exception of the one recognized by Ab-2.

Therefore, a strange mathematic begins to appear: idiotypically Ab-3 looks like Ab-1 and Ab-4 looks like Ab-2. Diversity is not increasing along the immunization chain (Ab-4 is as specific as Ab-2) and therefore the rules which are valid at the first step (different idiotypes are expressed in different individuals immunized with the same antigen) are no longer valid when one enters inside the networks. These results clearly suggest that the network is not open-ended but is in some way circular.

A large proportion of rabbits possess closely related idiotypic repertoires, even though these rabbits express different idiotypes when confronted with the same antigen. A randomly chosen animal can be reprogrammed and can learn to make the idiotype of another individual, familially unrelated. Several points can be mentioned Ab-1′ and Ab-3 antibodies are idiotypically cross-reactive, but Ab-3, unlike Ab-1′, do not recognize antigen significantly. Ab-1′ and Ab-3 antibodies which are synthesized in the same rabbits could be the equivalent of the so-called “nonspecific” immunoglobulins and antibodies which are simultaneously induced by antigen and which are sharing idiotypic specificities (Oudin and Cazenave, 1971).

In many instances, Ab-1 and Ab-1′ antibodies are not identical but constitute a large family of idiotypically interrelated molecules. This is after all not surprising since:

(a) even the so-called “public idiotypes” which were believed to be the products of a few germ line genes appear now as a collection of idiotypically related molecules (Brown *et al.*, 1980).

(b) in normally immunized animals, heterogeneous antibodies are not just a random collection of immunoglobulins which happen to fit with antigen, but are made up of idiotypically cross-reactive subpopulations (for review, see Urbain *et al.*, 1980).

A working hypothesis to explain the data described above is the presence in rabbits synthesizing Ab-3 and Ab-1′ antibodies of T helper cells whose immunological receptors are idiotypically cross-reactive with Ab-1 and Ab-3 (and/or T helper whose receptors are autoanti-idiotypic). These T helper cells would counteract suppressors which normally block the expression of silent idiotypes.

Idiotypic manipulations have also been achieved in mice (Bona and Paul, 1979; Cazenave and Le Guern, 1979). The expression of MOPC 460 idiotype has been studied in different strains of mice, using a BALB/c antiserum raised against the myeloma protein MOPC 460 and a monoclonal anti-idiotypic antibody (F6-51) obtained by the hybridoma tool. This idiotype is a recurrent one in the BALB/c strain (10–20% of antibodies in BALB/c mice immunized with TNP-Ficoll or DNP-ovalbumin react with the anti-idiotypic antibodies) but is normally never expressed in DBA/2, NZB strains. All strains synthesize Ab-3 antibodies when immunized with either one of the Ab-2 antisera. Following immunization with TNP-Ficoll or DNP-OVA, an enhanced expression of the MOPC 460 idiotype is observed in BALB/c mice. In complete agreement with the rabbit data, DBA/2 mice and NZB mice, which normally do not express the MOPC 460 idiotype, after preimmunization with Ab-2 antibodies, synthesize anti-DNP antibodies, some of which are M460 idiotype positive.

The cellular basis for the enhancement of the M460 idiotype in BALB/c mice has been studied (Bona and Paul, 1979; for review, see Bona and Hiernaux, 1980).

BALB/c spleen cells depleted of T lymphocytes and immunized *in vitro* with TNP-Nocardia (Nocardia is a polyclonal B cell activator) exhibit an increased synthesis of the M460 idiotype positive component of the anti-TNP response. Subsequent experiments revealed that suppressor T cells which limit the expression of the M460 idiotype display the Ly-2, Qa-1 phenotype.

Moreover, plate binding experiments showed that these suppressor T lymphoctes can be specifically removed by Petri dishes coated with the MOPC 460 protein (Bona *et al.*, 1979). Such suppressor T lymphocytes could not be detected in mice synthesizing Ab-3 antibodies. Furthermore, passive injection of Ab-3 antibodies can lead to the same effects as immunization with Ab-2. All these findings suggest that anti-M460 idiotype suppressor T cells are inactivated by Ab-3 antibodies. Furthermore, the immunological receptors of suppressor T cells and the anti-idiotypic antibodies seem to be idiotypically cross-reactive.

Several important questions remain to be answered. One of the most important is perhaps this. Silent idiotypes are under active suppressive mechanisms. The removal of suppressor T cells is necessary to obtain induction of these idiotypes. Is this removal necessary and sufficient? This question cannot be answered since, in the experiments of Bona and Paul, after specific removal of T_S specific for the M460 idiotype, spleen cells were immunized with TNP coupled to a polyclonal B cell activator which obviates the need for specific T helper cells.

Since our previous experiments have revealed that it was indeed possible to inhibit the activity of *intrinsic suppressors* (suppressors not intentionally induced which keep many idiotypes silent), we decided to investigate whether it was also possible to block the activity of *induced suppressors*.

In some tumour systems, it has been shown that cytotoxic T cells induced by the cancerous cells are very soon inhibited by suppressor T lymphocytes. After grafting of a syngeneic T2 sarcoma into C57BL/6 mice, two waves of cytotoxic activity are found at 1 week and 4 weeks. No cytotoxic activity can be found at 2 weeks and, moreover, lymph node cells taken at that time are able to suppress the cytotoxic activity. Suppressor cells can be highly enriched by sedimentation velocity (Schaaf-Lafontaine, 1978). Suppressor cells were purified from a pool of 10 mice and injected with adjuvant in C57BL mice in order to elicit immunity against suppressors. The effects of blast iso-immunization were evaluated by measuring the weight of sarcoma grafted 1 week after the last immunization. A considerable reduction of sarcoma T2 growth was evident in mice previously immunized against blast suppressor cells. Even in a few cases (20% of cases), no growth at all is found (A. F. Tilkin, N. Schaaf-Lafontaine, A. Van Acker, M. Boccadoro and J. Urbain, in prep.).

Induction of idiotypes by polyclonal activators

The results described above show that it is possible to transform one idiotype into a recurrent one. It was therefore interesting to confirm these findings by the use of polyclonal B cell activators, which bypass the normal regulatory mechanisms and which force the differentiation of B lymphocytes (D. Juy, D. Primi and P. A. Cazenave, in prep.). The silent part of the repertoire should be revealed by polyclonal activators, just as antiself antibodies can be demonstrated by such tools.

Expression of the MOPC 460 idiotype was therefore studied *in vitro*, using spleen cells from BALB/c or DBA/2 mice depleted in T cells. B cells were activated by LPS and the expression of the MOPC 460 idiotype was measured at different times. At day 3 in culture of BALB/c spleen cells, the addition of syngeneic anti-M460 antibodies inhibited 40% of the anti-TNP plaques. No such effect could be detected with DBA/2 spleen cells. However, at day 6 the situation was completely reversed: DBA/2 spleen cells gave anti-TNP PFC which were M460 idiotype positive. At the same time, the expression of the M460 idiotype has disappeared in BALB/c mice. By day 10, the response of

DBA/2 mice also waned. This decline could be due to activation of clones with anti-M460 specificity. This is strongly suggested by the fact that addition of anti-anti-M460 (Ab-3 antibodies) reverses the decrease in the expression of the M460 idiotype. A likely interpretation of these results is that, in the absence of regulatory T cells, B cells are able to modify clone size by idiotypic–anti-idiotypic interactions.

Immunoregulatory role of maternal idiotype: ontogeny of immune networks

Suppression is dominant in the functioning of the immune system since the potential idiotypic repertoire of one individual is far greater than the repertoire expressed after antigen immunization.

This again raises the question: why do different animals synthesize different idiotypes when injected with the same antigens? One possible answer to this comes from studies of the immunoregulatory role of maternal idiotypes (Wikler *et al.*, 1980; Cazenave and Voetglé, in prep.). By the Ab-1-Ab-2-Ab-3 tool, one animal can learn to make idiotypes normally silent. Female rabbits were injected with anti-idiotypic antibodies (Ab-2) to elicit the synthesis of anti-(anti)-idiotypic antibodies (Ab-3). Let us recall that Ab-3 antibodies are sharing some idiotypic specificities with Ab-1 but do not react with antigen. These female rabbits producing Ab-3 antibodies were then crossed with naïve males. From 5 female rabbits, we obtained 32 surviving siblings. Three months after birth, both the mothers and the offsprings were given antigen (*Micrococcus*) for the first time. All mothers, and around 40% of the offsprings, produced antibodies idiotypically cross-reactive with the starting idiotype. It is therefore obvious that maternal immunoglobulin of Ab-3 type have strongly influenced the emergence of the available idiotypic repertoire.

Analogies have been drawn between the immune system and the nervous system. It is known in the nervous system that the initial network is genetically programmed and that the connectance is greater than in the adult nervous system. The final structure of the nervous network depends on the selective stabilization of some pathways functioning during an early critical period. An imprint of the environment is built in the initial nervous system (Changeux and Danchin, 1966).

In the case of the immune system, there is also an early critical period. Only negative signals can be given by antigen or anti-idiotypic antibodies to immature B lymphocytes. If different individuals start with the same basic idiotypic repertoire, the presence of different self antigens in an outbred species, the presence of different maternal immunoglobulins and the unpredictable arrival of external antigens will drive the initial network into different functional states in different individuals. Different pathways of response will be chosen in different individuals.

Some fragmentary conclusions

If we put together all the findings discussed above and others, a new picture of the immune system seems to emerge.

(a) Despite the fact that different individuals use different available repertoires when confronted with the same antigen, the total idiotypic repertoire of all individuals of a given species is more or less the same. Suppression is dominant in the functioning of the immune system and silent clones are not insignificant minorities, but are kept under active suppressive mechanisms. In agreement with DNA data, this suggests that the germ line repertoire is largely diversified.

(b) The immune system is a functional idiotypic network in the sense that idiotypes are involved in clonal interactions and in the regulatory circuitry of the immune system. Taken together with the H-2 restriction phenomenon, we are led to the idea that *self recognition is one of the key features of the immune system.*

(c) There is no convincing evidence, in our opinion, that physiological signals are delivered via idiotypic anti-idiotypic interactions. Idiotypic interactions allow the meeting of complementary partners and signals are given by the compartment to which interacting cells belong. For example, a T helper bearing autoanti-idiotypic receptors will promote the differentiation of B cells bearing the complementary idiotypes, while T suppressors bearing autoanti-idiotypic receptors have the opposite effect.

The physiological signal could be delivered either by the constant part of the T cell receptors or via another surface molecule. We make no distinction between interactions of an anti-idiotype with an idiotope located within or outside the paratope, since, when antigen is absent, the receptor does not know where the paratope is located.

The real meaning of H-2 restriction could be the identification of the nature of the interacting partner, since different lymphocyte compartments display different restricting elements.

(d) The idiotypic network is probably not open-ended but rather it turns back onto itself. This is strongly suggested by the fact that, idiotypically, Ab-3 looks like Ab-1 and Ab-4 looks like Ab-2 and different Ab-2 synthesized by different individuals against the same Ab-1 share idiotypic specificities.

(e) The presence of idiotypes (or anti-idiotypes) during an early stage of the differentiation of the immune system have tremendous effects on the locking of the idiotypic network in a given equilibrium state. This is not unlike the nervous system in which the adult connectance is determined both by the genetic envelope and by the selective stabilization and degenerescence of some pathways (see above).

(f) The existence of a functional idiotypic network could be a solution to the problem of selection and conservation of a large germ line repertoire and, therefore, of genes apparently useless during the lifetime of one individual. How can a rabbit make antibodies against unforeseen antigens? How can the immune system evolve in anticipation of future needs? As stated by Ohno: "While a shelved *V* gene is ignored by natural selection there is nothing to prevent it from undergoing random changes. A shelved *V* gene is likely to become a derelict before the need for it arises" (Ohno, 1978). Yet even if selection of somatic mutations offers a partial solution to the selection dilemma, the problem remains because many clones are present but silent. The solution to the dilemma may be the functional idiotypic network. If idiotypic interactions are physiologically relevant (and this seems to be the case), there may be an internal selective pressure which promotes for conservation of otherwise apparently useless genes. Rabbits can make antibodies against koala albumin because these antibodies are in fact anti-idiotypes towards other immunoglobulins in a functional idiotypic network (Urbain *et al.*, 1980).

References

Binz, H., Frischknecht, H. and Wigzell, H. (1979). *Ann. Immunol.* (*Inst. Pasteur*) **130C**, 273.

Bona, C. and Hiernaux, J. (1980). *In* "Critical Reviews in Immunology" (in press).

Bona, C. and Paul, W. E. (1979). *J. Exp. Med.* **149**, 592.

Bona, C., Hooghe, R., Cazenave, P. A., Le Guern, C. and Paul, W. E. (1979). *J. Exp. Med.* **149**, 815.

Brown, A., Esten, P., Lamoyi, E., Gill-Pazaris, L., Gottlieb, P. D., Capra, J. D. and Nisonoff, A. (1980). *In* "Membrane Receptors and the Immune Response". La Rabida, University of Chicago Institute (in press).

Cantor, H. (1979). *Ann. Rev. Med.* **30**, 269.

Cazenave, P. A. (1977). *Proc. Natn. Acad. Sci. U.S.A.* **74**, 5122.

Cazenave, P. A. and Le Guern, C. (1979). *In* "Cells of Immunoglobulin Synthesis", p. 343. Academic Press, London and New York.

Changeux, J. P. and Danchin, A. (1976). *Nature* **264**, 705.

Eichmann, K. (1979). *Adv. Immunol.* **25**, 195.

Eichmann, K. and Rajewsky, K. (1975). *Eur. J. Immunol.* **5**, 661.

Fernandez, C., Hammarström, L., Möller, G., Primi, D. and Smith, C. (1979). *Immunol. Rev.* **43**, 1.

Frischknecht, H., Binz, H. and Wigzell, H. (1978). *J. Exp. Med.* **147**, 500.

Jerne, N. K. (1974). *Ann. Immunol.* (*Inst. Pasteur*) **125C**, 373.

Jerne, N. K. (1976). *Harvey Lectures* **70**, 93.

Julius, M. H., Augustin, A. and Cosenza, H. (1977). *In* "Regulatory Genetics of the Immune System" (E. E. Sercarz, L. A. Herzenberg and C. F. Fox, eds), Vol. 6, p. 179. Academic Press, New York and London.

Kelsoe, G., Reth, M. and Rajewsky, K. (1980). *Immunol. Rev.* (in press).

Kelus, A. S. and Gell, P. G. (1968). *J. Exp. Med.* **127**, 215.

Kunkel, H. G. (1963–1964). *Harvey Lectures* **59**.

Lindenmann, J. (1974). *Ann. Immunol.* (*Inst. Pasteur*) **125C**, 171.

Mitchison, N. A. (1971). *Eur. J. Immunol.* **1**, 18.

Nisonoff, A. and Bangasser, S. (1975). *Transplant. Rev.* **27**, 100.

Ohno, S. (1978). *In* "Comprehensive Immunology" 5 (B. G. Litman and R. A. Good, eds), Vol. 5, p. 197. Plenum Medical Book Company, New York.
Oudin, J. and Cazenave, P. A. (1971). *Proc. Natn. Acad. Sci. U.S.A.* **68**, 2616.
Oudin, J. and Michel, M. (1969a). *J. Exp. Med.* **130**, 595.
Oudin, J. and Michel, M. (1969b). *J. Exp. Med.* **130**, 619.
Rodkey, L. S. (1980). *In* "The Handbook of Cancer Immunology" (Watern Garland, ed.), Vol. 9. STPM Press (in press).
Schaaf-Lafontaine, N. (1978). *Int. J. Cancer* **21**, 329.
Seidman, J. G., Max, E. and Leder, P. (1980). *Nature* **280**, 370.
Sy, M. S., Brown, A. R., Benaceraff, B. and Greene, M. I. (1980). *J. Exp. Med.* **151**, 896.
Urbain, J. (1974). *Arch. Biol.* **85**, 139.
Urbain, J. (1978). *In* "Immunology" (J. Gergely, G. A. Medgyesi and S. R. Hollan, eds), p. 47. Akademiaï Kiado, Budapest.
Urbain, J., Wikler, M., Franssen, J. D. and Collignon, C. (1977). *Proc. Natn. Acad. Sci. U.S.A.* **74**, 5126.
Urbain, J., Collignon, C., Franssen, J. D., Mariamé, B., Leo, O., Urbain-Vansanten, G., Van de Walle, P., Wikler, M. and Wuilmart, C. (1979). *Ann. Immunol. (Inst. Pasteur)* **130C**, 397.
Urbain, J., Wuilmart, C. and Cazenave, P. A. (1980). *Contemp. Topics Mol. Immunol.* **8** (in press).
Urbain, Vansanten, G., Van Acker, A., Mariamé, B., Tasiaux, N., De Vos-Cloetens, C. and Urbain, J. (1979). *Ann. Immunol. (Inst. Pasteur)* **130C**, 397.
Van Acker, A., Urbain-Vansanten, G., De Vos-Cloetens, C., Tasiaux, N. and Urbain, J. (1979). *Ann. Immunol. (Inst. Pasteur)* **130C**, 385.
Vaz, N. and Varela, F. J. (1978). *Med. Hypotheses* **4**, 231.
Weigert, M. and Riblet, R. (1978). *Springer Sem. Immunopathol.* **1**, 133.
Wikler, M., Franssen, J. D., Collignon, C., Leo, O., Mariamé, B., Van de Walle, P., De Groote, D. and Urbain, J. (1979). *J. Exp. Med.* **150**, 184.
Wikler, M., Demeur, C., Dewasme, G. and Urbain, J. (1980). *J. Exp. Med.* (in press).
Zinkernagel, R. (1978). *Immunol. Rev.* **42**, 24.

6

Lymphocyte Receptors

HANS WIGZELL and HANS BINZ

Department of Immunology, Uppsala University, Uppsala, Sweden and Institute of Medical Microbiology, University of Zürich, Zürich, Switzerland

Introduction

Few terms are as widely abused in cellular immunology as receptors. Frequently when some structure or particle can be shown to display a somewhat select binding ability to a subset of lymphoid cells, this is claimed to display the existence of a receptor for that substance. In the present discussion on antigen-binding receptors on lymphocytes, we have tried whenever possible to link structure with function. It is clear, however, that this is particularly difficult when one comes to deal with thymus-dependent T lymphocytes. It is thus possible that some of the molecules we will discuss have no true receptor function.

Antigen-specific receptors on B lymphocytes

It has been known for quite some time that the clonally distributed, antigen-binding receptors on B lymphocytes carry all the hallmarks of being Ig molecules very similar to the serum immunoglobulin molecules. This was shown with regard to fine antigen-binding specificity using various fractionation procedures (Wigzell and Andersson, 1971). Direct biochemical analysis of membrane-bound Ig molecules have now shown minor differences allowing the separation of humoral versus cellbound Ig molecules of the same Ig class even at the level of the messenger RNA (Rogers *et al.*, 1980).

The Ig molecules on a B lymphocyte would all seem to have the very same antigen-binding specificity and idiotypes. A switch in Ig class would not result in a change in antigen-binding sites of the newly synthesized molecules. In fact, stability of the area of the antigen-combining region of Ig molecules produced by the immunocompetent B cell is probably well paralleled by the stable idiotypic pattern of B cell malignancies.

The number of Ig molecules present on a B cell surface would seem to be in the order of 10^5 for small, as well as activated, B blasts. These molecules are able to express significant binding to the correct epitopes, as is shown by a multitude of physical fractionation experiments involving the separation of specific, antigen-reactive B cells with antigen. Still, it would seem clear that the Ig molecules on a B cell do only play a partial role in the induction of antibody synthesis and that they normally require the parallel collaboration with other surface components in order to constitute a functional receptor unit.

Part of this knowledge has come from the analysis of the functional requirements for T independent antigens (Coutinho and Möller, 1974) where the antigen-specific membrane Ig molecules would seem to act as a mere focusing device for B cell mitogens. Actual triggering of antibody synthesis would here occur via interaction with mitogen receptors physically distinct from the Ig molecules. Likewise, the activation of Ig production by T dependent antigens would also seem to act in an intricate manner involving membrane-bound Ig molecules, as well as Ia molecules and hypothetical receptors for mitogenic factors.

It is thus clear that the Ig molecules on B cell surfaces fail to fulfil our requirements for a receptor capable of delivering a complete, triggering signal leading to the activation of Ig synthesis. It is, however, suggested by several independent studies that interaction with Ig molecules on the cell surface may have consequences as to B cell proliferation or select change in Ig turnover. It would accordingly be premature to regard the Ig molecules as a mere concentrating device for immunogenic molecules, which then in a secondary manner will induce the further necessary triggering signals.

Figure 1 describes in a summary form the B cell surface structures collaborating in the induction of high rate Ig production by T independent and dependent antigens. Further analysis of the exact molecular and cellular requirements would here require clones of B cells studied at defined stages of activation, as this can be shown to have significant impacts on the specificity requirements for activation (Andersson *et al.*, 1980).

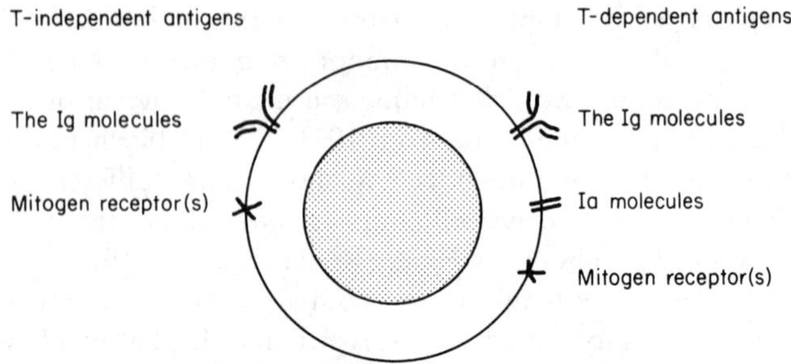

FIG. 1 *The receptor for antigen on B lymphocytes*

T cell receptors for antigen

Intense research activities have been focused on these structures over the last decade and the rest of this paper is devoted to this topic. Although considered quite "elusive" by several investigators, it has been possible during the last few years to accumulate significant information concerning features and functions of these molecules.

Successful approaches to T cell receptors

Initial attempts to prove in any conclusive way the physical presence of antigen-binding receptors on T lymphocytes that could be linked to function all ended in frustration. The first successful method allowing the demonstration of relevant receptors was introduced by Brondz (1968), who used monolayers of allogeneic cells to selectively remove T cells. We now understand that his success was due to the fact that early methods used in attempts to study antigen-binding T cells in other systems failed to include major histocompatibility antigens on antigen-presenting cells as alternative immunosorbants. Using the Brondz-technique it was subsequently possible to prove the actual clonal distribution of receptors for alloantigens on T lymphocytes (Golstein *et al.*, 1971).

As soluble antigens in most systems would fail to interact in an avid manner with helper or killer T cells (due to their true specificity involving MHC antigens in collaboration with antigen), an alternative highly successful approach involved the use of antireceptor antibodies as initially suggested by Ramseier and Lindenmann (1972). Applying this concept, it was thus possible (Binz and Wigzell, 1975a) to prove the actual presence on the outer surface of idiotypic, antigen-binding receptors on T lymphocytes. These T receptors could be shown to share idiotypic determinants with B cell receptors directed against the same antigens. Anti-idiotypic analysis has subsequently been found fruitful in a variety of idiotypic studies of T cell receptors and antigen-specific factors as reviewed by Eichmann (1978). The reason for this success would seem to be energy of interaction where the anti-idiotypic reagents can be shown to display high avidity interactions with the proper T cell receptors, which allow the actual physical separation of idiotypic T lymphocytes (Binz and Wigzell, 1975c).

Finally, as suppressor T lymphocytes were defined as a distinct set of cells, it became clear that, in contrast to most helper and killer cells, suppressor T cells frequently react with soluble antigen in a manner similar to B lymphocytes. This allowed the actual development of techniques using antigen-coated solid surfaces to enrich for specific suppressor cells (Okumura *et al.*, 1977). In a few cases, fusions of suppressor T cells with T lymphomas have subsequently been shown to result in a T suppressor hybrid lymphoma with useful producing abilities of antigen-specific factors (for example, see Taniguchi *et al.*, 1980).

The genetic basis of T cell receptors

Three successful approaches have been adopted in the analysis of the underlying genetics coding for T cell receptors for antigen. As our understanding of the biochemistry of these molecules is still far from complete (see under Biochemistry), it should be understood that there is still uncertainty at several levels regarding the finer details of this genetic information.

The inheritance pattern of idiotypes can in many systems be shown to be under control by a single locus, mostly the V_H gene clusters linked to the *Ig* heavy chain genes. With the realization that T cells may express idiotypic receptors, it then became possible to study the linkage patterns of idiotypes presented on T cells. Both in mice (Krawinkel *et al.*, 1977) and rats (Binz and Wigzell, 1977), a clearcut correlation between the expression of a particular T cell idiotype and the inheritance of *IgG* or *IgA* allotypic genes could be shown. Failure to find any linkages to the inheritance pattern of light chain *Ig* genes has been reported in several systems. In one system a possible direct contribution of MHC genes to the structure of T cell idiotypes has been indicated (Krammer and Eichmann, 1977), but as the actual target antigen for these receptors was an MHC alloantigen, other reasons for this finding are obvious.

A second approach yielding, in essence, similar results has been obtained by the use of anti-V_H framework specific antisera (Neriah *et al.*, 1980), which in several murine T cell systems have been shown to interfere selectively with T cell function, or react with antigen-specific factors derived from T cells. Similar attempts using anti-V_L antisera have to our mind failed to yield convincing results as to presence of reactive antigenic determinants on T cell receptors.

The third approach where repeated success has been reported by some workers has been in the use of particular anti-Ia sera (notably anti-I-J specific), where convincing results demonstrating the association of Ia determinants to certain antigen-specific factors from T cells have been obtained (for review see Tada and Okumura, 1979). The implications of these findings will be discussed later in this paper (see Biochemistry).

In conclusion, the genetic analysis of inheritance pattern and serological display of determinants of T cell receptors has, in every system so far studied in detail, shown contributions of V_H genes for the build-up of these molecules. Contribution of structures coded for by MHC-associated genes would seem to be relevant for the biological activity of some antigen-specific molecules, but may not participate in all T lymphocyte receptor systems.

Specificity of T cell receptors

Analysis of the fine antigen-binding activity of T cell receptors has been slow in most systems. This is due to the low amount of receptor material available and the fact that in several systems the "true" antigen may involve a composite unit of MHC structures and extraneous antigen. Many studies exist which yield results on this topic in secondary manner, i.e. they link the induction of a particular specific T cell function to the specificity of the T receptors in a relatively direct manner. In all, however, there now exists, within these limitations, considerable information concerning the selective binding abilities of T cell-derived, antigen-specific molecules.

The most straightforward system used has been that of Krawinkel *et al.* (1979). They have been using solid support matrices coated, for example, with a hapten, and have allowed the attachment of antigen-binding lymphocytes and their release of membrane structures onto these antigen-coated surfaces. The recovered material, which has conclusively been shown to be derived from T cells, has also been shown to exhibit select, comparatively high avidity binding to the hapten. The binding specificity using cross-reacting haptens could be shown at the level of the T receptor to express a unique V_H-linked profile also found in conventional Ig antibodies with the same specificity. Other systems using soluble factors, mostly involved in the generation of suppressor T cells (Tada and Okumura, 1979), have shown significant avid binding to antigen-coated columns in a selective manner, which, in some systems, would nicely match the selective behaviour of the T lymphocytes themselves. In all, these results prove beyond doubt that certain T cells, at least, notably suppressor cells, can express binding to antigen in a way which is almost indistinguishable from conventional Ig antibodies against the same epitopes.

A very large proportion of T lymphocytes would seem to have clonally distributed receptors for MHC antigens (self or allo), as shown in several sets of experimental systems. Likewise, T cells with specificity for Ig-coded determinants (class, allotype or idiotype specific) have also been found in a variety of systems to contribute in a significant manner to the immune response and its deviations. The limited number of studies that have been performed in such specificity systems using soluble T cell receptor molecules have, in principle, yielded results of a similar nature to those in the above reported systems (Binz *et al.*, 1979b). In short, these latter results showed that rat T cell receptors purified over anti-idiotypic immunosorbants so as to enrich for molecules carrying idiotypic determinants. This indicates a particular anti-allo-MHC reactivity which would also display strong selective binding to such purified MHC antigens. An additional point of interest found in these experiments was the fact that such strong allo-MHC (here = anti-Ia) reactive T cell receptors would also react in a weak, but measurable, manner with "self-Ia" but not with third party Ia molecules. This suggested that the specificity of the allo-MHC reactive molecules may indeed represent a heteroclitic reactivity pattern where the "true" selective force for this receptor-carrying cell may have been the self-Ia reactivity (as suggested initially by Jerne, 1971). In a recent set of experiments (Binz and Wigzell, in prep.), further proof for such an opportune behaviour of alloreactive T cell receptors with regard to "self" was observed. Here it was found that, using the same anti-idiotypic immunosorbant, it was possible to purify T cell receptors from two congenic rat strains (differing at MHC only) with the "same" idiotypes signifying potential strong binding to MHC antigens of a third strain. Analysis of the binding properties of these two batches of T cell receptors showed that both reacted strongly to the corresponding allo-Ia molecules. However, each batch could be shown to bind in a weak (as to forces involved) manner with "self" Ia only and not with the Ia of the other congenic strain. Thus, T cell receptors with the same (similar) idiotypes linked to strong alloreactivity of MHC type will behave in an opportune manner with regard to binding to self Ia structures, which must be explained on the basis of a positive selective

TABLE I

T cell receptors with "Lewis-anti-DA" idiotypes display strong binding to DA MHC chains and select but weak binding to "self" Ia chains

Origin of T receptors[a]	*Binding of MHC polypeptide chains*[b]								
	DA			*BN*			*Lewis*		
	44K	*34K*	*27K*	*44K*	*34K*	*27K*	*44K*	*34K*	*27K*
Lewis	+ + + +	+ + + +	+ + +	−	−	−	−	+	−
L.BN	+ + + +	+ + + +	+ + + +	−	+	+	−	−	−

[a] Isolated using the same anti-idiotypic immunosorbant from large volumes of normal serum and further isolated using chromatography (Binz and Wigzell, 1979b). Lewis and L.BN rats are congenic differing only at MHC (L.BN has the BN MHC).

[b] Binding of isotope labelled isolated MHC chains in low concentrations of detergent to immunosorbants made of T receptor material. + + + or + + + + denotes retention of more than 50% of applied material whereas + denotes retardation of more than 50% of applied material.

force in the generation of peripheral normal T lymphocytes. These results would thus strongly suggest that alloreactive T lymphocytes may, in their interactions with allo-MHC, use the same receptors that could also be used for recognition of self-MHC in the context of extraneous antigen. In short, this would mean that the reason for the immune system to have such an unusually high frequency of allo-MHC reactive T cells is indeed that the true reactivity in the biological context of these cells is for self-Ia plus additional antigen. Table I presents this set of results in a summary form. It should be clear, however, that these results do not allow any final conclusions as to "altered self" versus "dual recognition" concepts of T cell recognition. In order to solve this it would be necessary to show that *all* antigen-binding T receptors from a cloned T cell line would behave in the very same manner. The results would, however, suggest that association of MHC-coded structures with antigen-binding T receptor molecules may occur in the physiological non-immune situation using a variable region interaction with specificity for "self-MHC" of unusual avidity.

Idiotypic determinants on T cell receptors

Idiotypic determinants can be shown to exist on T cell receptors, as has already been discussed, and auto-anti-idiotypic reactions against such receptors can be shown to have drastic consequences in some systems for the respective idiotype positive cell. One system to which we have devoted much analysis is the auto-anti-idiotypic regulation of anti-allo-MHC immune reactions (Aguet *et al.*, 1978). As the reactions here can serve as principal examples of auto-anti-idiotype regulations of T cell functions in general, a summary of these findings will be made. The idiotypic determinants on T cell receptors can be found to be represented on single heavy chains, but not light chains derived from IgG antibodies carrying similar idiotypes to the T receptors (Binz and Wigzell, 1977). Idiotypic T cell receptors or single heavy chains derived from idiotypic IgG antibodies would seem to be the best immunogens to induce and auto-anti-idiotype immune reaction in syngeneic animals, whereas the use of intact Ig molecules will frequently result in anti-idiotypic reactions involving predominantly B cell receptors. Note here that experiments in the mouse have so far indicated the existence of unique B cell idiotypes (V_H-V_L determined) whereas no unique T cell idiotypes have yet been shown to exist (Eichmann, 1978).

The display of idiotypes as to frequency distribution would seem to vary greatly according to T cell subset. It could thus be shown that in anti-allo-MHC systems in the mouse, T blasts generated across an entire H-2 barrier will display different idiotypes depending on their function and Lyt-phenotype (Binz *et al.*, 1979c). This would be in agreement with the concept that the major phenotype (Lyt-1^+2^-) of the anti-Ia reactive cells would be distinct from that of the anti-H-2 K/D reactive killer cells (Lyt-1^-2^+). Whether a similar disproportion as to idiotypic spectra will exist on T lymphocyte groups recognizing the same soluble antigen is unknown.

Elimination or triggering of idiotype-positive T cells could be shown to be possible using auto-anti-idiotypic reactions in the murine or rat system. Elimination could be carried out using anti-idiotypic killer T cells or anti-idiotypic antibodies in the presence of complement. Confrontations between idiotypic normal T cells and anti-idiotypic factors *in vitro* (factors = antibodies, or possibly also T derived molecules) in the absence of complement could be shown to cause a highly efficient induction of proliferating or cytolytic T cells with the correct allo-MHC specificity (Frischknecht *et al.*, 1978). This efficiency was in fact greater than when using allogeneic spleen cells as a stimulating agent and may allow the bypass of the normal requirement of helper T cells for efficient generation of killer T cells.

In conclusion, idiotypic (or anti-idiotypic) receptors on T cells can be shown to function as important target structures in idiotypic regulation. The strength of the reactions between idiotypic and anti-idiotypic receptors may be similar to allo-MHC reactions with regard to T cell activation, that is, quite efficient.

Biochemistry of T cell receptors

A general agreement amongst immunologists trying to study T cell receptors for antigen that these receptors would seem to display V_H-coded idiotypic determinants, significant controversy and confusion does exist as to the biochemical build-up of these molecules. Strikingly opposite results have been presented from different laboratories and here we will only try to give the general picture and important points in this area of research. It may well be that this analysis will show streaks of personal bias in emphasizing certain but not other data.

One important problem yet to be solved is the principal build-up of the T cell receptor as to polypeptide chains. Researchers working with soluble antigen-specific factors derived from T cells, and with the ability to effect certain select functions in the presence of antigen, have produced significant results indicating a two chain structure in at least some of these systems (see Tada and Okumura, 1979 for review). This conclusion is based in part on the use of various immunosorbant columns (antigen specific, anti-I-J specific or anti-idiotype specific) showing, in most of these systems, a simultaneous expression of V_H-idiotypes, antigen-binding specificity and the presence of Ia-associated determinants on the active "factors". Using T suppressor hybridomas, two groups (Taussig *et al.*, 1978; Taniguchi *et al.*, 1980) have been able to demonstrate the physical existence of two distinct chains with distinguishing markers (antigen-binding versus I-J positivity). Likewise, when the antigen-binding system of Krawinkel *et al.* (1979) has been used where the effector function of the molecules is unknown (receptor? pharmacological activity?), results have been obtained over the years which indicate a molecular composition superficially quite similar to IgG molecules. However, the heavy chain would here be of a new Ig class unique for T cells and the light chain has no antigenic features in common with conventional light chain Ig molecules. This receptor material has, however, consistently been found to be Ia negative. It is also still not certain that the smaller chains by necessity represent distinct molecules on their own and not breakdown products of the larger chain. These molecules can actively inactivate haptenated bacteriophages, and bivalent interactions are required for such inactivation to occur. To our minds, however, it is not as yet clear whether this inactivation could not occur, considering that monovalent units attached to membrane pieces contain more than one such hypothetical unit. Results of a more preliminary nature have also been obtained by other groups suggesting additional variation and two chain structures. It is possible that all the studies indicating two chain units are derived from T cells involved in the suppressor circuits.

In the allo-MHC system of the rat we have ourselves consistently failed to find convincing evidence for more than one chain participating in the build-up of idiotypic, antigen-binding receptors (Binz and Wigzell, 1976; Binz *et al.*, 1979a). The chain size is close to 70 000 (70K) and it may occur as a dimer or in fragments obtained during "spontaneous" proteolysis resulting in predominant fragments around 50K and 35K. The chain would seem to be quite susceptible to proteolysis and, unless precautions as to stop proteolysis are used, loss of activity via extensive fragmentation will frequently occur. This single chain would seem to be devoid of Ia or other MHC-associated serological epitopes and does not react with conventional anti-Ig antisera. So far we have failed to find evidence for significant amounts of carbohydrate on the chain. It is possible to produce heteroantisera against this structure in rabbits and such hetero-antisera can be shown not only to precipitate the rat allo-MHC T receptors in a selective manner, but it will also react with suppressor T cell factors in the mouse. It is, however, not clear whether this reactivity is directed against constant or variable region determinants. One confusing aspect is that such suppressor factors may also appear to be present as single chains in some systems (R. K. Gershon, pers. comm.) with no display of Ia associated determinants. Other workers studying human reactivity (Lea *et al.*, 1979; Preudhomme *et al.*, 1977) have obtained biochemical results on T cell receptors (here with binding ability to soluble antigens) strongly suggesting a single chain as the unit building stone for T cell receptors. Additional groups having antigen specific suppressor and killer T cell lines have also found evidence for a single chain nature of such receptors. It must be deemed clear that antigen-binding factors derived from T lymphocytes can exist in several forms and the same is probably true for membrane-bound "receptors". How many of the differences present are due to differences in handling and assessing the various molecules is yet to be established. It is clear, however, that receptor material from cloned T cells would be required to solve finally several of the remaining questions as to T cell receptors for antigen.

Conclusions

This paper aims to inform immunologists interested, but not working in this area of cellular immunology as to our past and present understanding of antigen-binding receptors on lymphoid cells. The facts presented have been selected according to the limited space available and our personal feelings as to which parts of receptor studies should be emphasized. It seems clear that there is still a long way to go before these receptors will be fully characterized as to features and functions.

References

Aguet, M., Andersson, L. C., Andersson, R., Wight, E., Binz, H. and Wigzell, H. (1978). *J. Exp. Med.* **145**, 51.
Andersson, J., Schreier, M. and Melchers, F. (1980). *Proc. Natn. Acad. Sci., U.S.A.* **77**, 1612.
Binz, H. and Wigzell, H. (1975a). *J. Exp. Med.* **142**, 197.
Binz, H. and Wigzell, H. (1975b). *J. Exp. Med.* **142**, 1218.
Binz, H. and Wigzell, H. (1975c). *J. Exp. Med.* **142**, 1231.
Binz, H. and Wigzell, H. (1976). *Scand. J. Immunol.* **5**, 559.
Binz, H. and Wigzell, H. (1977). *Progr. Allerg.* **23**, 154.
Binz, H., Frischknecht, H., Mercolli, C., Dunst, S. and Wigzell, H. (1979a). "Proc. Internat. Congr. Regulation by T cells" (D. G. Kilburn, J. G. Levy and H. S. Teh, eds).
Binz, H., Frischknecht, H., Mercolli, C., Dunst, S. and Wigzell, H. (1979b). *J. Exp. Med.* **150**, 1084.
Binz, H., Frischknecht, H., Shen, F. W. and Wigzell, H. (1979c). *J. Exp. Med.* **147**, 500.
Brondz, D. B. (1968). *Fol. Biol., Prague* **14**, 115.
Coutinho, A. and Möller, G. (1974). *Scand. J. Immunol.* **3**, 133.
Eichmann, K. (1978). *Adv. Immunol.* **26**, 195.
Frischknecht, H., Binz, H. and Wigzell, H. (1978). *J. Exp. Med.* **147**, 500.
Golstein, P., Svedmyr, E. A. J. and Wigzell, H. (1971). *J. Exp. Med.* **134**, 1385.
Jerne, N. K. (1971). *Eur. J. Immunol.* **1**, 1.
Krammer, P. and Eichmann, K. (1977). *Nature* **270**, 733.
Krawinkel, U., Crammer, M., Berek, C., Hämmerling, G., Black, S. J., Rajewsky, K. and Eichmann, K. (1977). *Cold Spring Harbor Symp. Quant. Biol.* **41**, 285.
Krawinkel, U., Crammer, M., Kindred, B. and Rajewsky, K. (1979). *Eur. J. Immunol.* **9**, 815.
Lea, T., Förre, Ö., Michaelsen, T. E. and Natvig, J. (1979). *J. Immunol.* **122**, 2413.
Neviah, Y. B., Givol, D., Lonai, P., Simon, M. and Eichmann, K. (1980). *Nature* **285**, 287.
Okumura, K., Takemori, T., Tokuhisa, T. and Tada, T. (1977). *J. Exp. Med.* **146**, 1234.
Preud-homme, J. L., Klein, M., Labaume, S. and Seligmann, M. (1977). *Eur. J. Immunol.* **7**, 840.
Ramseier, H. R. and Lindenmann, J. (1972). *Transplant. Rev.* **10**, 57.
Rogers, J., Early, P., Carter, C., Calame, C., Bond, M., Hood, L. and Wall, R. (1980). *Cell* (in press).
Tada, T. and Okumura, K. (1979). *Adv. Immunol.* **28**, 1.

Taniguchi, T., Takei, I. and Tada, T. (1980). *Nature* **283**, 227.
Taussig, M. J., Corvalan, J. R. F., Binns, R. M. and Holliman, A. R. (1978). *Nature* **277**, 305.
Wigzell, H. and Andersson, B. (1971). *Ann. Rev. Microbiol.* **25**, 291.

Theme 2: Summary

Idiotypy, Allotypy and Network Regulation

A. D. STROSBERG

Institut de Recherche en Biologie Moléculaire, Université de Paris, Paris VII, France

How an organism controls the extent and the diversity of an immune response is still not clear. Humoral responses are known at times to be extremely diverse and abundant and at others to be quite restricted. The extent of proliferation of lymphocytes and their plasmocyte offspring also varies from antigen to antigen, and obvious rules governing immune responses have been difficult to define.

A number of regulatory mechanisms have been proposed to explain both this variety of reactions and their limitation in time. These mechanisms generally involve all the active elements of the immune system; antigens, antibodies, B and T lymphocytes and a whole array of soluble factors. Antigenic determinants on both variable and constant regions of the immunoglobulins have also been suggested to act as recognition signals in control mechanisms. The multiple interactions between these numerous elements are now usually said to be enmeshed in "networks".

Network concepts rest on the positive (inductive) and negative (suppressive) interactions between multiple components which may either be cells, chemical messengers or both. They suppose necessarily a great diversity of elements in line with the many functions taken care of.

In earlier days it was generally assumed that the immune response was essentially based on "positive" interactions involving for instance a foreign antigen and antigen-receptor bearing lymphocytes. Cells recognizing self-antigens would be remorsely and continuously eliminated thus avoiding autoimmune reactions. More recently however it has been suggested that this "negative" type of interaction which would involve a kind of "autocensure" may only explain partially the apparent tolerance towards self-antigens. In fact it is now felt quite strongly that the immune system continuously generates autoimmune reactions which involve the production of anti-idiotypic antibodies in response to synthesis of antibodies specific for a given antigen. This humoral type of regulatory network has its cellular counterpart which puts on stage T suppressor and helper cells, cytotoxic cells, idiotype or anti-idiotype bearing cells.

We will here summarize some aspects of regulatory networks involving idiotypic and allotypic epitopes both in solution and at the surface of immunocompetent cells.

The major points discussed during the symposium concerned successively the regulatory role in the immune response of suppression and induction and serological and the biochemical identification of the molecules which in solution or at the surface of lymphocytes participate in the regulatory networks. Rather than trying to summarize the numerous data which were presented, I will attempt briefly to evoke some of the questions which were raised.

An early observation pointed out that an immune response can be either enhanced, modified or even suppressed by anti-idiotypic antibodies or by T cells able to recognize the idiotype or the anti-idiotype. Al Nisonoff described suppression studies both of the humoral response and of the delayed hypersensitivity to arsonate. In the first case,

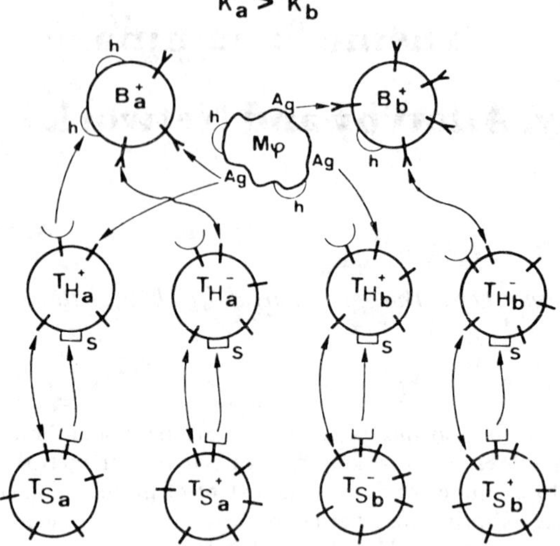

suppression is restricted to the antiarsonate antibodies which bear the major idiotype. In delayed hypersensitivity, one gets an almost complete suppression of the response.

Suppression can be induced by anti-idiotypic antibodies, by the ligand coupled on syngeneic leukocytes and by the idiotype conjugated on cells. Suppression is always transferable by T cells and can be transferred by B cells after suppression and hyperimmunization.

SUPPRESSION OF DTH BY IDIOTYPE-CONJUGATED CELLS,
OTHER OBSERVATIONS

ANTIGEN-SPECIFIC

INOCULATION OF IDIOTYPE-NEGATIVE ANTI-Ar CONJUGATED TO SPLEEN CELLS DOES NOT SUPPRESS DTH.

INOCULATION OF IDIOTYPE-CONJUGATED CELLS STIMULATES FORMATION OF SUPPRESSOR T CELLS (AS SHOWN BY ADOPTIVE TRANSFER).

THESE SUPPRESSORS CANNOT BE KILLED BY ANTI-id + C (IN CONTRAST TO SUPPRESSORS STIMULATED BY Ar-COUPLED CELLS I.V.).

AS SHOWN BY DATA FOR C.AL-20 AND BALB/c, CAPACITY FOR SUPPRESSION OF DTH BY IDIOTYPE-CONJUGATED CELLS IS LINKED TO Igh LOCUS.

The T suppressor cells seem to secrete a T suppressor factor which possesses ligand-binding specificity, is devoid of immunoglobulin determinants, binds to anti-idiotype antibody and may possess Ia antigenic determinants.

An interesting point concerns the nature of the idiotypic determinants to be found on T cells. How well do these compare and overlap with those of the B cell products, the antibodies? Many investigators have concluded in the presence of V_H determinants on T cell, but few will support the presence of V_L. Since the idiotypic determinants often depend on the interaction of both regions, one must at least suppose that the idiotype determinants on the T cell represent necessarily only a part of the B cell product idiotype repertoire.

Jacques Urbain developed the concept that the production of antibodies induces the subsequent production of anti-antibodies which will serve as regulators both in terms of quantity but also quality of the immune response. The coexistence at any moment in the lifetime of an organism of both idiotype bearing immunoglobulins and autoantibodies directed against these idiotypes forms the basis of a regulatory network. A parallel situation could describe relationships between B cells and T suppressor cells.

The antigen and the anti-idiotype each have a particular relationship with the idiotype-bearing molecule: in fact, the anti-idiotype antibody could constitute a certain "internal image" of an immunogen which may be a molecule never seen by the individual or even the species.

The logical extension of the concept of internal image is that the anti-idiotype antibody may by itself also stimulate an immune response, thereby inducing antibodies able to react with antigen.

A number of situations have now been described in which both antibodies and anti-antibodies have been shown to coexist during an immune response and to influence its evolution. Conditions for stimulating the production of the anti-idiotype antibodies may involve maternal immunoglobulin, polyclonal activation of idiotype-bearing molecules and again "internal image"-like molecules. The extensiveness of the anti-idiotype repertoire prior to antigen introduction, the existence of B cells which display idiotypic determinants without binding antigen, the possibility to suppress in nude mice and finally the physiological significance of the idiotype network remain at the present time open questions: it will require some sophisticated experimentation to outline the *in vivo* role of auto-anti-idiotype antibodies.

The presentation of Hans Wigzell and most of the workshop discussions concerned the serological and the biochemical description of the various markers (allotypes, idiotypes and T cell suppressor factors) involved in the network interactions.

The first workshop concerned itself mostly with analyses of the public and private idiotypic specificities in normal immune responses: public idiotypes are in fact families of closely related, but nonidentical clonotypes whose heterogeneity has now been studied by isoelectric focusing, amino acid sequencing and most recently by monoclonal anti-idiotypic antibodies. The heterogeneity within an intraspecies public idiotype may include minor allelic differences associated with the haplotype of the individual: such an allelic variation was described for the T15 idiotype.

It was also reported that the monoclonal anti-idiotype antibodies appeared to be more restricted in their specificity than in their ability to suppress.

What became especially evident at the meeting is the strong impact of the hybridoma technology on the study of idiotypes, allotypes and immunological receptors. I will specifically mention two examples. The only mouse homogeneous proteins available for sequence studies used to be myeloma proteins which happened to bind ligands such as phosphorylcholine or DNP and at the same time were recognized by anti-idiotypic antibodies. Now, however, homogeneous monoclonal antibodies can be produced at will by fusing vector cells with antibody-producing lymphocytes: these functional hybridoma proteins have been shown to display many of the idiotypic determinants previously identified on antiarsonate or antiphosphorylcholine antibodies from sera of hyperimmunized animals. Although it is not clear yet whether the lymphocytes involved in the somatic fusion events belong to specific categories of cells, or whether they are picked purely at random, the immunoglobulins produced by the hybridoma certainly appear to be representative of every subgroup, class, and subclass present in the serum. They may even have escaped a severe selection process which, during an immune response, may eliminate less performing antibodies, minor idiotypes and so on.

Intense efforts by several groups have permitted the first sequence comparisons between idiotype-bearing hybridoma antibodies and should, in the near future, allow a precise molecular mapping of the idiotypic determinants, both in the sequence and in the tridimensional structure of immunoglobulins.

The second example concerns the use of somatic cell fusion as a means to perpetuate a given cell in view of studying the product of a single clone: I will develop that type of experiment as my conclusion.

The spectrum of identified allotypic markers in the rabbit and in the mouse continues to widen thanks mainly to studies performed on wild animals. These new allotypes are located both in the variable and constant region of the mouse and rabbit immunoglobulin chains. Reagents have now also been described which recognize similar antigenic structures on immunoglobulins of different species. The structural correlates of various allotypes are actively studied as well.

Whereas Oudin's early definition of allotypy and idiotypy clearly precluded any confusion between the two concepts, a large number of intriguing observations have lately established that the control of expression of idiotypes may actually serve as an example to how some allotype's expression may be regulated.

Two workshops addressed themselves to the problem of allotype's expression. In the first, still more examples were presented in man, mouse and rabbit on the appearance of latent allotypes, expressed in patients or in animals which genetically were not thought to contain these markers. It was established that the latent allotypes cannot be distinguished serologically nor structurally from their nominal counterparts. When found on cells, the latent allotypes always accompany nominal markers.

The induction in isolated cells of latent allotypes by antiallotype antisera was described in studies which sounded quite familiar to those who have used similar methods in the study of idiotypes. The existence of T suppressor cells for allotypes was postulated quite a while ago in the mouse: the *in vitro* studies on rabbit will certainly appreciably contribute to clarify this issue. Little doubt remain after this meeting that latent allotypes are but one more piece of evidence for the existence of functional networks of interactions in the immune system.

Another workshop addressed itself to the phenomenon of suppression. The mechanism by which administration or induction of antiallotype antibodies may effectively suppress the target allotype was again abundantly discussed during the present meeting. The role of auto-antiallotype antibodies, in maintaining a prolonged state of suppression in rabbits was compared to that of a particular set of B cells which seem responsible for allotype suppression in the chicken. The manner by which the pecking order in isotype expression is maintained can clearly be viewed within the context of self-regulation at work in autorecognition systems controlling B cell differentiation.

In nude mice, generally thought to be devoid of T cells, the relative expression of the different isotypes mimicks the recently proposed order of constant region genes mapping to the right of V region. Reconstitution of nude mice with syngeneic T cells confirmed T cell regulation of B cell differentiation.

Several groups have now isolated from T cell lysates or supernatants antigen-specific T cell products on affinity columns containing antigen anti-idiotype or antivariable region (V_H) antibody. Despite the diversity of systems that are used, the general molecular properties of the isolated T cell products bear striking resemblances. A large component was repeatedly found with a molecular weight between 62 000 and 68 000 daltons. This T cell product, referred to as the "T cell receptor" carries V_H determinants as shown by the binding of specific anti-idiotype antibodies and of antibodies directed against V_H framework determinants. In addition several groups have indicated that Ia determinants, coded for by *I-J* genes are also found on the 62 000 to 68 000 daltons T cell product. In contrast, no known immunoglobulin heavy chain constant region or light chain antigenic determinant could be detected on the T cell receptor. The T cell product, whether isolated from spleen, form cloned cells or from T cell hybridoma may effectively display suppressor activity. A number of investigators have shown that the 62 000 to 68 000 component could be resolved into 40 000–45 000 and 25 000 components either by simple reduction of disulphide bonds, mild acid cleavage, spontaneous or provoked proteolytic digestion. The larger component bears the V_H determinants, the smaller the Ia antigenic markers. Rather than trying to imagine a new type of genetic control which would explain how both immunoglobulin and Ia determinants could be expressed on a single polypeptide chain, some investigators suggest that the native T cell receptor is in fact a two-chain molecule. Others propose that the active antigen binding receptor is a dimer of the 62 000–68 000 daltons component. This could explain the reconstitution of functional idiotypic determinants generally not encountered on isolated immunoglobulin V_H regions nor on heavy chains.

The latest and most promising development concerns the study of T cell hybridoma products. In Chapter 1 Capra described the purification of a 68 000 daltons arsonate-specific T cell product. Although functional studies were not initiated yet, this molecule had all the binding properties of a bona fide receptor. Comparative peptide maps of products from several different T hybridomas revealed structural variability in about 25% of the T cell receptor.

In this field, as in the other subjects discussed during the symposium on idiotypy, allotypy and network regulation, the availability of somatic cell fusion and cloning has opened important new avenues for research and has created renewed enthusiasm for solving the question of how the immune response is regulated.

METHOD OF SUPPRESSION	EFFECT ON RESPONSE	
	Humoral AB	DTH to the Ar hapten
Anti-Id	Suppresses cri only	suppression
Ligand (Ar)-coupled cell	Partial tolerance	suppression
Idiotype-coupled cells	Suppresses cri only	suppression

Suppression is always transferable with T cells.

After suppression and hyperimmunization humoral cri suppression is transferable with B cells.

Theme 3

Expression of Antigen Receptors in Lymphocytes and Cellular Activation Mechanisms

Presidents:

K. RAJEWSKY

S. AURAMEAS

Symposium Chairman

B. ASKONAS

7

Expression of Receptor Diversity in T Lymphocytes

HARALD VON BOEHMER

Basel Institute for Immunology, Basel, Switzerland

The available receptor repertoire of B lymphocytes can be studied by analysis of antibodies. Its size has been estimated to exceed several millions of different antibodies in mammals (Jerne, 1971; Köhler, 1976). Estimates of the number of different antibodies fitting a single epitope range from 10^2 to 10^3 (Köhler, 1976; Fazekas de St Groth, 1980). The antibody repertoire is considered to be complete and degenerate.

The number of germ line genes underlying antibody diversity is not known. Phenotypic diversity is increased by rearrangement of Ig-coding DNA segments in somatic cells (Sakano *et al.*, 1979), as well as by mutations within

Abbreviations
CTL: Cytotoxic T lymphocyte; D^d: *D* region of the MHC in mice expressing the *d* haplotype; H-2: MHC of mice; Ia: *I* region coded antigens; Ig: Immunoglobulin; Ir: Immune response; J: J—or joining—DNA segment; *K*, *D*: *K* or *D* region of MHC; MHC: Major histocompatibility complex; TCGF: T cell growth factor; V_H: Variable part of immunoglobulin heavy chain.

these genes (Bernard *et al.*, 1978). The mechanism by which the available repertoire is selected from the potential repertoire is yet to be defined.

As the molecular composition and fine specificity of antibodies can be relatively easily analysed, the diversity of B cell Ig receptors is also well known.

T cells do not secrete antibodies. Rather, their effector function is induced and exerted through interaction with other cells. The available T cell repertoire must therefore be analysed by a study of these complex cell interactions. T cells fall into several subclasses, known as T helper cells, cytolytic T cells and T suppressor cells. Even members of different subclasses interact; for instance, T killer cells are completely dependent on T helper cells. It is necessary, therefore, to consider the steps of T cell activation when trying to reach some conclusions about the repertoire of T cells.

The steps leading to activation and clonal expansion of T helper and killer cells are relatively well understood, partly because clones of both cell types are now available. Activation and effector functions of suppressor cells are more obscure (at least to the author) and will therefore be neglected in this article. (Suppressor cells are treated extensively in other chapters of this volume.) My aim here is to link some facts known about activation of T helper and killer cells with observations made on the available repertoire of these cell types.

T helper cells

Activation, growth and effector function of T helper cells

The available experimental evidence indicates that binding of their specific antigen is not sufficient to induce T helper cells to clonal expansion, but they require interaction with other, nonlymphoid accessory cells which "present" antigen on their surface. For instance, cloned T helper cells, specific for sheep red blood cells (SRC), cannot be induced to grow by SRC unless accessory cells are added (Schreier *et al.*, 1980a). It is not understood how macrophages bind and "present" antigen; it is conceivable that antibody is involved in the uptake.

The mere presence of macrophages is not sufficient: T helper cells are not induced unless they interact with Ia antigens of the accessory cells. This follows from the fact that accessory cells expressing the "wrong" Ia antigens do *not* induce T helper cells. The Ia restriction of macrophage–T cell interaction was first noted by Rosenthal and Shevach (1973). Steps following the interaction of helper and accessory cells are still conjectural; it may be that on binding between T cell receptors and Ia antigen the accessory cells produce substances inducing growth in the T helper cells. Extensive clonal expansion is only observed in those helpers which have engaged with the accessory cell. Thus, accessory cells do not seem to produce polyclonal T cell activators.

The induced helper cells can activate resting, small B cells to proliferation and antibody secretion (a step once again Ia-restricted (Andersson *et al.*, 1980; Katz *et al.*, 1973a; Sprent, 1978)). They also produce soluble factors inducing *antibody secretion without proliferation* in *small, resting B cells* or *antibody secretion with proliferation* in *large B cell blasts*, irrespective of their Ia type (Schreier *et al.*, 1980b).

Properties of cloned T helper cells

Several T helper cell clones have been described (Schreier *et al.*, 1980; Watson and Mochizuki, 1980; von Boehmer *et al.*, 1980). They all are Ia-restricted and of the Lyt-1$^+$, 2$^-$ phenotype. Some of these clones can be grown in media containing factors from concanavalin A (Con A) stimulated spleen cells (Schreier *et al.*, 1980a, b; Watson *et al.*, 1980) in the absence of accessory cells, while the growth of others is absolutely dependent on accessory cells (von Boehmer *et al.*, 1980). It might be that clones independent of accessory cells represent variants with less stringent growth requirements during prolonged culture (Haas *et al.*, 1980). All clones, apart from inducing antibody secretion in B cells, produce T cell growth factors (Smith, 1980). T cell growth factors induce growth only in those T cells—including T killer cells—which have interacted with antigen or lectin (Paetkau *et al.*, 1980; Larsson and Coutinho, 1980; Schreier *et al.*, 1980a, b). These findings allow the conclusion that T cells providing help for B cells and T killer cells belong to the same T cell subclass (Glasebrook and Fitch, 1979).

It has been observed several years ago (von Boehmer, 1974) that after interaction with H-2 antigens on other cells, T cells produce factors mitogenic for B as well as T cells. The recent facts are that only T helper cells can produce these factors, and that resting, small T as well as B cells are not induced by growth factors without previous receptor–ligand interaction by their antigen receptors. It appears then that T helper cells represent the lymphocyte subclass capable of responding to antigen assembled in immunogenic form on the surface of macrophages.

The repertoire of T helper cells

The available repertoire of Lyt-1$^+$, 2$^-$ cells is heavily biased towards recognition of Ia antigens. Up to several percent of Lyt-1$^+$, 2$^-$ cells can be induced by allogeneic cells expressing Ia antigen coded by a single haplotype (MacDonald *et al.*, 1980). It is not known whether allospecific T cells recognize allo-Ia antigens on their own or allo-Ia antigen plus some other cell surface antigens. In the latter case they could be regarded as allo-Ia restricted T helper cells. It is clear, however, that the phenotype of H-2 restriction is not determined by the H-2 genotype of T helper cells: T helper cells restricted to allogeneic Ia antigens can be obtained in chimaeric mice (von Boehmer *et al.*, 1975; Waldmann and Munro, 1975).

Ia antigens cannot be substituted for by *K* or *D* region antigens: for instance, looking at male-specific responses in various mouse strains, the only Lyt-1$^+$, 2$^-$ T cells capable of being induced by male cells are Ia-restricted. Thus, Ia antigens, whether syngeneic or allogeneic, are mostly involved in T helper cell activation. Since it is difficult to imagine how a T cell repertoire specific for various Ia antigens only could be selected, we are led to the view that recognition of Ia antigens is in most cases a prerequisite for T helper cell induction. This might also be the first step in the production of lymphocyte activating factors by accessory cells.

Finally, the repertoire of T helper cells is influenced by so-called *Ir* genes, located in the *I* region of the H-2 complex (McDevitt and Chinitz, 1969). To return to the example of male-specific helper cells, we found that such cells could easily be induced in mice expressing I-A^b antigens but not in I-A^k mice (von Boehmer *et al.*, 1980). Initially, this type of finding was interpreted to indicate that *H-2* genes encode T cell receptors (Benacerraf, 1974). In the meantime, however, it has become apparent that the "Ir phenotype" is independent of the "Ir genotype" of T cells (von Boehmer *et al.*, 1978; Kappler and Marrack, 1978). Thus, T cells of high responder genotype, when restricted to low responder I-A antigens, display the low responder phenotype and vice versa (Katz *et al.*, 1973a, b; von Boehmer *et al.*, 1978; Kappler and Marrack, 1978). In other words, there is a strict correlation of the "H-2 restriction phenotype" and the "Ir phenotype".

T cell receptor serology

Using anti-idiotype sera, it was found that antigen-specific T helper cells share idiotypic determinants with antibodies directed against the same antigens. Thus, Binz and Wigzell (1977) found that roughly 6% of T cells expressed receptors to alloantigens of a foreign haplotype and their idiotypes were shared by less than 1% of B cells. There were "extra" idiotypes on antibodies not shared by T cells, but not the other way around. Linkage studies suggested that expression of idiotypes was linked to the Ig heavy chain locus.

Idiotypes shared by antibodies and T helper cells specific for various antigens were reported also by Hämmerling *et al.* (1977).

The data suggest that either V_H genes encode part of the T cell receptor (structural genes) or indirectly regulate expression of idiotypes on T cells (regulatory genes). The decision between these two possibilities can best be made by looking at the DNA of T helper cells. An answer to the question whether T helper cells express V_H genes still does not explain the bias of the T helper repertoire towards Ia antigens and the *Ir* gene control of T helper cell responses.

Cytolytic T cells

Activation of cytolytic T cells

Isolated cytolytic T cells (CTL) of the Lyt-2$^+$ phenotype (in some assays Lyt-1 is detected) cannot be induced to clonal expansion by antigen alone. Whenever cloned CTL were studied, they could be induced to grow only when Lyt-1$^+$, 2$^-$ T helper cells were supplied or TCGF added to the culture medium (for review, see Möller, 1980). TCGF itself stimulates the growth of CTL only when their receptors had bound antigen (MacDonald *et al.*, 1980). This indicates that clonal expansion of primed (and probably also of unprimed) CTL is absolutely helper-cell dependent.

Clones of cytolytic T cells

Most CTL clones express Lyt-2 antigens. Their killing can be inhibited with anti-Lyt-2 sera (Nabholz *et al.*, 1980). Some of these clones can be grown over long periods of time in TCGF-supplemented media without losing their specificity. They are likely to represent variants particularly well adapted to growth of TCGF (Hass *et al.*, 1980), since not all CTL will grow well in such media in the absence of accessory cells (Glasebrook and Fitch, 1979).

The repertoire of cytolytic T cells

Up to several percent of CTL precursors can be activated by foreign antigens coded by genes of a *single* H-2 haplotype (Miller *et al.*, 1977). *K* and *D*, but also Ia (Wagner *et al.*, 1975) and other antigens coded by genes of the mouse chromosome 17, are recognized (Fischer-Lindahl and Hausmann, 1980). Fifty different clonotypes specific for a single foreign K molecule could be analysed by testing clones obtained by limiting dilution on a panel of mutant targets (Sherman, 1980). While this could be interpreted as a K molecule consisting of 50 epitopes, it is equally consistent with the view that a few epitopes are recognized by CTL receptors of differing affinity. Again, it is not known whether CTL are *restricted* by allo K, D antigens or recognize allo K, D antigen *per se*.

CTL specific for non-MHC antigens are H-2 restricted by K and D antigens. Apparently, CTL restricted by *I* region antigens do not exist: for instance, we failed to obtain male-specific CTL restricted to I-A^b in B10.A(5R) mice where no male-specific CTL restricted to either K or D can be induced, yet male-specific helpers restricted to I-A^b were readily demonstrated (von Boehmer *et al.*, 1980). Thus, while allogeneic Ia antigens can induce CTL which are not restricted by K and D (Wagner *et al.*, 1975), self Ia-restricted CTL are not inducible.

The phenotype of H-2 restriction of CTL is independent of the H-2 genotype, i.e. under appropriate conditions CTL restricted to allogeneic K or D antigens can be demonstrated (for review, see Möller, 1978). Experiments have been performed which show that self-H-2 restricted CTL can kill allogeneic target cells (Bevan, 1977; Lemonnier *et al.*, 1977; von Boehmer *et al.*, 1978): some male-specific CTL clones restricted to D^b lyse female targets expressing D^d. The extent of the overlap between the H-2-restricted and allo-H-2-specific repertoire is at present unknown.

The repertoire of CTL is controlled by *Ir* genes located in the *K* or *D* region of the H-2 complex. Several investigators have consistently failed to generate male-specific CTL restricted to K^b or D^d and the B10.A(5R) strain expressing these antigens is a nonresponder strain, despite the fact that I-A^b-restricted, male-specific helper cells are found. In other mice the defect is not in the induction of killer cells, but at the induction of helper cells: we were unable to find male-specific helper cells restricted to I-A^k, and H-2^k mice are therefore low responders, even though K^k- or D^k-restricted CTL can be obtained in mice expressing I-A^b (Simpson and Gordon, 1977). Before we knew about the requirement of helper cells for CTL expansion, the experiments would have suggested that *Ir* genes located in the *I* region controlled the repertoire of CTL.

As with helper cells the "Ir genotype" of CTL has no influence on the "Ir phenotype". CTL from low responder strains raised under appropriate conditions express the high responder phenotype and vice versa. Again, as with helper cells, there is a strict correlation of "H-2 restriction phenotype" and "Ir phenotype".

The close analogy of *Ir* gene control in helper and killer cells indicates that selection and expression of their repertoire is governed by the same principles, the only difference being the orientation of helper cells towards Ia and of killer cells towards *K*, *D*.

Analysis of receptors of CTL

CTL receptors have been studied by serological methods, but no analysis of linkage has been reported. Inhibition of killing by anti-Lyt-2 sera is an interesting observation, but has to be further exploited. Studies on gene rearrangements in killer cell clones are presently performed by Tonegawa and collaborators: they indicate that V_H–J joining, as present in antibody-producing B cells, is not an obligatory step for expression of antigen specificity in CTL.

Conclusion

Studies on activation of T helper and killer cells indicate that T helper cells represent the class which initiates immune responses on activation by antigen-presenting accessory cells. Ia antigens are crucially involved in the activation process and may function as special signal transmitters both on accessory cells and on small, resting B cells. K, D, Ia and other proteins coded by mouse chromosome 17, may be involved in the activation of primary CTL, and certainly have a specialized function transmitting effector signals of CTL (Langmann, 1978). The interaction of CTL precursors with such antigens alone is not sufficient to clonally expand CTL: clonal expansion requires growth factors provided by T helper cells.

The available repertoire of T helper or cytolytic T cells is heavily biased towards recognition of Ia or K and D antigens, respectively. This is evident by the high proportion of helper or killer cells which can be induced by cells expressing H-2 antigens coded by a single foreign haplotype.

The available T cell repertoire of individuals, but *not* of the species, seems incomplete. The repertoire is controlled by *Ir* genes, which map in the *I* region for helpers and in the *K* or *D* region for killers.

Bias—in terms of frequency—towards H-2 antigens, as well as gaps in the repertoire, have not been detected in B cells. It should be remembered, however, that there is a fundamental difference in the activation and effector function of T and B cells and hence in the way we probe the repertoire. In general (some exceptions are known), T cells have to bind to H-2 antigens on other cells to be activated and exert their effector function. In that sense, B cells are passive. They bind antigen with their Ig receptors and T cells "see" the antigen in the context of the B cell's Ia antigens. The equivalent of the B cell receptor is subsequently secreted and can be assayed. Thus, we may assess the repertoire of B cells by the antibodies they secrete, but the T cell repertoire must be probed through cell interactions.

Only if we assume that T cell specificity is reflected in measurable binding affinity of their solubilized receptors (some evidence points in that direction (Binz and Wigzell, 1977; Krawinkel *et al.*, 1977)), can we say that receptors on T and B cells must be different. The bias of T cells towards H-2 may be introduced by gene products partly or totally different from those expressed in B cells. Alternatively, T cells may only use a subset of *V* genes coding for immunoglobulin, which would lead to an "H-2 oriented repertoire". Finally, it could be argued that the available T cell repertoire is simply the outcome of a selection process different from that selecting the B cell repertoire. The latter assumption gains some support by the fact that H-2 antigens, as expressed on an X-irradiated thymus, can have a profound influence on the available T cell repertoire (Zinkernagel *et al.*, 1978; Bevan and Fink, 1978).

MHC "linked" *Ir* genes or, better, *MHC* genes control the available repertoire of MHC-restricted T cells specific for non-MHC antigens. MHC polymorphism is therefore associated with distinct T cell repertoires (incomplete repertoires) in individual members of the species. We wonder whether this phenomenon is a chance correlate of or is causally related to MHC polymorphism.

We cannot yet tell how genes exert their influence on the T cell repertoire, except to note that we find a strict correlation of "MHC restriction phenotype" and "*Ir* gene phenotype". Both are independent of the MHC genotype of T cells and thus the proposition that *H-2* genes are structural genes for T cell receptors fails to explain MHC *Ir* gene control of the T cell repertoire. This fact was predicted by Jerne (1971). It follows from his theory on the "somatic generation of immune recognition", but in itself cannot prove the correctness of the theory. Other hypotheses explaining the bias of the T cell repertoire towards MHC and *Ir* gene control have been proposed (for review, see Möller, 1980). It is a difficult task to disprove any of the hypotheses as long as the T cell receptor remains hidden in the T cell membrane and T cell receptor genes are not identified.

References

Andersson, J., Schreier, M. H. and Melchers, F. (1980). *Proc. Natn. Acad. Sci. U.S.A.* **77**, 1612.
Benacerraf, B. (1974). *Ann. Immunol. (Inst. Pasteur)* **125C**, 143.
Bernard, O., Hozumi, N. and Tonegawa, S. (1978). *Cell* **15**, 1113.
Bevan, M. J. (1977). *Proc. Natn. Acad. Sci. U.S.A.* **74**, 2094.
Bevan, M. J. and Fink, P. J. (1978). *Immunol. Rev.* **42**, 3.
Binz, H. and Wigzell, H. (1977). *Cold Spring Harbor Symp. Quant. Biol.* **41**, 275.
von Boehmer, H. (1974). *J. Immunol.* **112**, 70.
von Boehmer, H., Hudson, L. and Sprent, J. (1975). *J. Exp. Med.* **142**, 989.
von Boehmer, H., Haas, W. and Jerne, N. K. (1978). *Proc. Natn. Acad. Sci. U.S.A.* **75**, 2439.
von Boehmer, H., Hengartner, H., Nabholz, M., Lernhardt, W., Schreier, M. H. and Haas, W. (1979). *Eur. J. Immunol.* **9**, 592.
von Boehmer, H., Haas, W. and Melchers, F. (1980). *Immunol. Rev.* (in press).
Cosenza, H., Augustin, A. A. and Julius, M. H. (1977). *Cold Spring Harbor Symp. Quant. Biol.* **41**, 709.
Fazekas de St Groth, S. (1980). *In* "XXVIIth Annual Colloquium on Proteids of the Biological Fluids". Brussels.
Fischer-Lindahl, K. and Hausmann, B. (1980). *Eur. J. Immunol.* **10**, 289.
Glasebrook, A. L. and Fitch, F. W. (1979). *Nature* **278**, 171.
Haas, W., Mathur-Rochat, J., Pohlit, H., Nabholz, M. and von Boehmer, H. (1980). *Eur. J. Immunol.* (in press).
Hämmerling, G. J., Black, S. J., Berek, C., Eichmann, K. and Rajewsky, K. (1977). *J. Exp. Med.* **143**, 861.
Jerne, N. K. (1971). *Eur. J. Immunol.* **1**, 1.
Jerne, N. K. (1972). *In* "Ontogeny of Acquired Immunity", pp. 1–15. CIBA Foundation Symposium, Associated Scientific Publications, Amsterdam.
Kappler, J. W. and Marrack, P. (1978). *J. Exp. Med.* **148**, 1510.
Katz, D. H., Hamaoka, T. and Benacerraf, B. (1973a). *J. Exp. Med.* **137**, 1405.
Katz, D. H., Hamaoka, T., Dorf, M. E., Maurer, P. H. and Benacerraf, B. (1973b). *J. Exp. Med.* **138**, 734.
Köhler, G. (1976). *Eur. J. Immunol.* **6**, 340.
Krawinkel, V., Cramer, M., Berek, C., Hämmerling, G., Black, S. J., Rajewsky, K. and Eichmann, K. (1977). *Cold Spring Harbor Symp. Quant. Biol.* **41**, 285.
Langmann, R. E. (1978). *Rev. Phys. Biochem. Pharm.* **81**, 1.
Larsson, E-L. and Coutinho, A. (1980). *Immunol. Rev.* **51**, 61.

Lemonnier, F., Burakoff, S. J., Germain, R. N. and Benacerraf, B. (1977). *Proc. Natn. Acad. Sci. U.S.A.* **74**, 1229.

MacDonald, H. R., Cerottini, J. C., Ryser, J. E., Maryanski, J. L., Taswell, C., Widmer, M.B. and Brunner, K. T. (1980). *Immunol. Rev.* **51**, 93.

McDevitt, H. O. and Chinitz, A. (1969). *Science* **163**, 1202.

Miller, R. G., Teh, H. S., Harley, E. and Phillips, R. A. (1977). *Immunol. Rev.* **35**, 38.

Möller, G. (ed.) (1978). *Immunol. Rev.* **42**.

Möller, G. (ed.) (1980). *Immunol. Rev.* **51**.

Nabholz, M., Conzelmann, A., Acuto, O., North, M., Haas, W., Pohlit, H., von Boehmer, H., Hengartner, H., Mach, J. P., Engers, H. and Johnson, J. (1980). *Immunol. Rev.* **51**, 125.

Paetkau, V., Shaw, J., Mills, G. and Caplan, B. (1980). *Immunol. Rev.* **51**, 157.

Rosenthal, A. S. and Shevach, E. M. (1973). *J. Exp. Med.* **138**, 1194.

Sakano, H., Hüppi, K., Heinrich, G. and Tonegawa, S. (1979). *Nature* **280**, 288.

Schreier, M. H., Andersson, J., Lernhardt, W. and Melchers, F. (1980a). *J. Exp. Med. 151*, 194.

Schreier, M. H., Iscove, N. N., Tees, R., Aarden, L. and von Boehmer, H. (1980b). *Immunol. Rev.* **51**, 315.

Sherman, L. (1980). *J. Exp. Med.* **151**, 1386.

Simpson, E. and Gordon, R. D. (1977). *Immunol. Rev.* **35**, 79.

Smith, K. A. (1980). *Immunol. Rev.* **51**, 337.

Sprent, J. (1978). *Immunol. Rev.* **42**, 108.

Wagner, H., Götze, D., Ptschelinezew, L. and Röllinghoff, M. (1975). *J. Exp. Med.* **142**, 1477.

Waldmann, H. H. A. and Munro, A. J. (1975). *Nature, London* **258**, 728.

Watson, J. and Mochizuki, D. (1980). *Immunol. Rev.* **51**, 257.

Zinkernagel, R. M. (1978). *Immunol. Rev.* **42**, 224.

8

Mechanisms that Govern Repertoire Expression

NORMAN R. KLINMAN, DWANE E. WYLIE and MICHAEL P. CANCRO*

*Department of Cellular and Developmental Immunology, Scripps Clinic and Research Foundation, La Jolla, California, USA and *Department of Pathology, University of Pennsylvania, Philadelphia, Pennsylvania, USA*

Introduction

Because a comprehensive understanding of repertoire diversity is crucial to any consideration of immune responsiveness, a considerable amount of investigation has centred on an effort to define the antibody repertoire, particularly that of inbred murine strains where the genetic component of repertoire expression can be controlled. The availability of myeloma proteins, monoclonal responses, and techniques such as isoelectric focusing and idiotypic analyses, have provided a growing body of knowledge concerning the processes responsible for repertoire expression and the general constitution of the antibody repertoire. From these studies it was perceived that the adult murine B cell repertoire is extraordinarily diverse, containing more than 10^7 distinct specificities or clonotypes (reviewed by Sigal and Klinman, 1978). In addition, it was clear that various clonotypes are disproportionately represented within the repertoire, some being expressed by a much higher proportion of B cells than others (Blomberg *et al.*, 1972; Eichmann, 1972; Pawlak and Nisonoff, 1973; Lieberman *et al.*, 1974; Gearheart *et al.*, 1975; Makela and Karjalainan, 1977). In most cases the disproportionately high representation of certain clonotypes is genetically inherited as a Mendelian codominant trait linked to either the heavy chain allotype locus or both the heavy and light chain loci (Makela and Imanishi, 1975; Laskin *et al.*, 1977).

Recently, our perception of repertoire expression and our experimental approach to its delineation have been greatly affected by the advent of new experimental models, particularly the availability of hybridoma antibodies and gene cloning technology. Furthermore, there has been a growing recognition that repertoire expression is as much a product of the interaction of developing B cells with antigens and other cells in their milieu as it is of the structural genes responsible for the immunoglobulin products themselves. The dissection of repertoire itself has been greatly facilitated by a new awareness of the capabilities of panel analyses for delineating antibody specificities (Cancro *et al.*, 1978a), as well as an abundance of new anti-idiotypic reagents provided by the availability of hybridomas (Reth *et al.*, 1978; Ju *et al.*, 1980; Marshak-Rothstein *et al.*, 1980). Comparative repertoire analysis has also been pursued with neonates as well as adults (Klinman and Press, 1975a; Sigal *et al.*, 1976; Cancro *et al.*, 1979) and recent advances in T cell technology that have enabled similar clonotype analyses of the T cell repertoire (Sherman, 1980). Finally, a greater understanding of the parameters of tolerance induction (Cambier *et al.*, 1976; Metcalf and Klinman, 1976; Stocker, 1977; Teale *et al.*, 1979), and an increased awareness of the potential effects of immunoregulatory phenomena, particularly with respect to idiotype recognition, on repertoire expression (Jerne, 1974; Rodkey, 1974; Nisonoff *et al.*, 1977; Pierce and Klinman, 1977; Kohler *et al.*, 1979) has changed the emphasis of our overall approach towards a greater understanding of the factors that control what is ultimately expressed from among the vast array of potential clonotypes.

Immunoglobulin gene structure and repertoire expression

The current status of the experimental probing of immunoglobulin gene structure has been presented in great detail in another symposium in this volume. Several of the findings relevant to consideration of immunoglobulin repertoire expression are depicted in Fig. 1. It is now clear that the major amino terminal portions of both heavy and light chain variable regions are inherited as a multiplicity of gene sets (Brack *et al.*, 1978; Seidman *et al.*, 1978; Schilling *et al.*, 1980). Individual members of these sets are combined by splicing mechanisms to at least one and maybe two second gene sets that account for the carboxy terminal end of these variable region genes. If one assumes that a major proportion of these genes can be utilized, then combi-

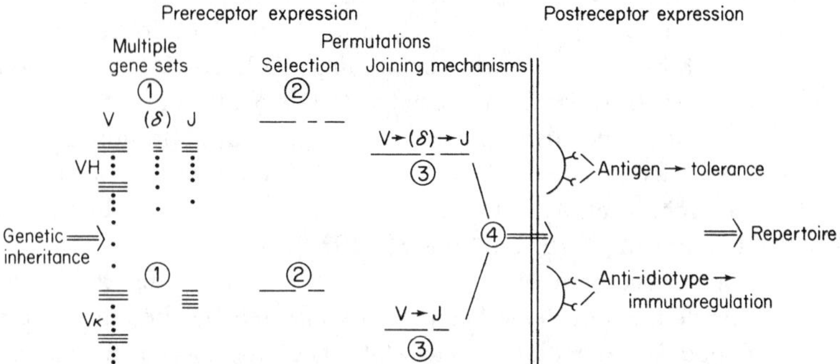

FIG. 1. *Mechanisms that govern repertoire expression.* (*1*) *Inheritance of multiple gene sets;* (*2*) *determination of appropriate combinations of V,* (δ) *and J;* (*3*) *variability at joining regions;* (*4*) *determination of appropriate combinations of VH and VL.*

natorial association among the component parts of any given variable region could account for a considerable amount of diversity (Seidman and Leder, 1978; Weigert *et al.*, 1980). Additionally, there appears to be considerable diversity created by the joining process itself. Thus, particularly for murine κ light chains and heavy chains, many thousands of protein sequences seem possible even in the absence of additional somatic mutational events at the DNA level. Since the combinatorial association of heavy and light chains is essential for the formation of antibody combining sites, it is apparent that many millions of distinct antibody clonotypes could be generated by combinatorial processes alone. Mutation at the DNA level may additionally magnify repertoire diversity.

As studies at the molecular level progress, it can be anticipated that additional modes of diversification may be revealed. Of direct concern to the genetic analysis of repertoire expression *per se* will also be information pertaining to the extent of polymorphism of the inherited genes themselves among the various murine strains. This would enable a clearer understanding of the basis for the apparent polymorphisms in antibody structure among strains. Finally, it may be hoped that we will also obtain greater insights into the mechanisms that determine which of the members of the gene sets are expressed and the mechanisms that control the joining processes themselves. Of particular interest may be the questions of whether these mechanisms are themselves polymorphic; the location of the genes which control these processes; and whether such processes can act in a *trans* fashion. As will be presented below, disparities in the repertoire of parental and F_1 strains may ultimately be accounted for at the level of the control of gene expression, rather than at the level of structural genes themselves. Nonetheless, knowledge gained at the molecular level indicating that the potential for inherited diversity may be far greater than even the highest estimates of expressed repertoire, and that the synthesis of the polypeptide chains themselves may be subject to control at several levels, has had a profound impact on all considerations of repertoire expression and its control.

Control of repertoire expression postreceptor acquisition

As our knowledge of the immune mechanism increases, it is increasingly apparent that the ultimate expression of the mature repertoire is the product of not only the molecular mechanisms responsible for generating a vast array of clonotypes, but also the environment in which the B cells expressing this repertoire develop. Although many elements of the environment may influence the developmental fate of B cells prior to receptor acquisition, with respect to repertoire expression, *per se*, it is convenient to divide the factors that govern repertoire expression, as depicted in Fig. 1, into those which obtain prior to receptor acquisition and those which influence the repertoire of B cells which bear antigen receptors. Events prior to receptor expression would primarily involve the inheritance and expression of immunoglobulin structural genes. Events that occur postreceptor expression would include all of those mechanisms which specifically select, from among the repertoire, clonotypes which will ultimately constitute the mature B cell population as opposed to those to be eliminated prior to maturation. Two mechanisms that could potentially eliminate developing clones have been recently defined; tolerance induction and idiotype specific suppression.

The fact that individuals rarely respond to their own antigenic determinants has led investigators to believe that a specific mechanism exists for the elimination of antiself reactivities. Over the years, a considerable amount of evidence has accumulated demonstrating that the elimination of such reactivities is possible from both B and T cell repertoires and that the specificities that might have existed do not normally exist in the mature individual (Triplett, 1962). Recently, several laboratories have demonstrated that both *in vivo* and *in vitro* developing B cell clones are exquisitely susceptible to a tolerance mechanism (Metcalf and Klinman, 1976; Cambier *et al.*, 1976; Teale *et al.*, 1979; Etlinger and Chiller, 1979; Kay *et al.*, 1980). The reactivity of such cells is eliminated by antigen concentrations which are several orders of magnitude lower than that found necessary for diminishing the reactivity of mature B cells. Furthermore, such tolerance can be induced by antigenic molecules that are incapable of rendering mature cells tolerant. Thus hapten, polyvalently substituted on essentially any carrier moiety, is capable of tolerizing responsive immature B cells at determinant concentrations as low as 10^{-9} M. Furthermore, this tolerance induction is exquisitely specific, discriminating between even closely related moieties such as 2,4-dinitrophenyl (DNP) and 2,4,6-trinitrophenyl (TNP) (Metcalf and Klinman, 1976). Given the availability of such a mechanism and the apparent need for elimination of certain clonotypes, in particular those that are specific for self immunogens that are polymorphic within the species, it is highly likely that this mechanism plays a central role in shaping the expressed mature B cell repertoire.

The second mechanism which presumably plays an important role in shaping the mature repertoire is the elimination of developing clones via their recognition by other cells in the immune system. Such "network" recognition is most likely accomplished via recognition of the idiotypic determinants of a developing B cell's antigen receptor. Since a determinant concentration of 10^{-9} M is necessary for tolerance induction it is unlikely that cells bearing receptors recognizing idiotypic determinants would themselves be eliminated via a tolerance mechanism (i.e., any given idiotype is not likely to be present on more than a few B cells, and thus would be very dilute in the system as a whole). Several experimental systems have demonstrated that such anti-idiotypic recognition can be generated even as a consequence of antigenic stimulation (Rodkey, 1974; Nisonoff *et al.*, 1977; Pierce and Klinman, 1977; Kohler *et al.*, 1979). In one system such anti-idiotypic reactivity has been shown to eliminate idiotype bearing cells from the mature repertoire (Accolla *et al.*, 1977; Kohler *et al.*, 1979). Thus neonatal induction of suppression to the TEPC 15 idiotype is capable of eliminating TEPC 15 bearing phosphorylcholine (PC) responsive cells from the mature repertoire. Furthermore, recent studies have indicated that individuals normally accumulate a considerable amount of such immunoregulatory phenomena during the course of their lifetime (Klinman, 1980). These studies have demonstrated that aged individuals can suppress the responses of B cells bearing their own homologous idiotypes, but do not suppress B cells of strains that are allogeneic in the allotype, and thus much of the idiotype locus.

The impact of regulation by mechanisms that occur postreceptor expression has not yet been evaluated. It should be noted, however, that several anomalies in repertoire expression may be the result of such mechanisms. In several systems the expression and predominance of clonotypes appears to be under multigenic control (Cancro *et al.*, 1978b; Stein *et al.*, 1980). It is likely that some of the involved genes participate only after receptor expression. Furthermore, much of repertoire polymorphism is apparent only subsequent to antigenic stimulation (Cancro *et al.*, 1978b; Stashenko and Klinman, 1980). The extent to which environmental antigens and immunoregulatory phenomena dictate repertoire expression will not be fully evaluated until an accurate analysis of the prereceptor B cell repertoire has been carried out. The first stages of such an analysis are presented later in this chapter.

The adult B cell repertoire

The majority of studies of the mature adult B cell repertoire have involved analyses of responses that are dominated by a single readily definable set of clonotypes. Whereas initially many of these responses were thought to involve a single clonotype, with one exception they all appear to represent large sets of clonotypes that behave as a single unit both genetically and subsequent to antigenic stimulation. At the present time, only the response to PC in mice of the Igh^a haplotype appears to have a single predominant clonotype (Cosenza and Kohler, 1972; Lieberman *et al.*, 1974). This clone, which is identical to the TEPC 15 myeloma protein, is represented by approximately 1 in 40 000 BALB/c B cells (Gearhart *et al.*, 1975; Sigal *et al.*, 1975). However, it is now clear that even the BALB/c response to PC is highly heterogeneous (Sigal *et al.*, 1977). Indeed, several other clonotypes share in part, the TEPC 15 idiotype (Gearhart *et al.*, 1977). All other "predominant" responses now appear to represent highly heterogeneous clonotype sets. It has long been known that the response in BALB/c mice to the α-1,3 dextran determinant is dominated by a set of closely related clonotypes which share a common idiotypic determinant and which bear the λ light chain (Blomberg *et al.*, 1972; Cohn *et al.*, 1974). Recent sequence analyses using hybridoma antibodies have indicated not only the location and sequence of the cross-reactive idiotypic determinant but also the enormous diversity of clonotypes which share these characteristics (Schilling *et al.*, 1980). Recent findings also indicate a considerable degree of heterogeneity in the family of clonotypes responsive to the (4-hydroxy-3-nitrophenyl) acetyl (NP) determinant which dominate the response in mice of the Igh^b haplotype. These clonotypes are characteristically heteroclitic in their binding for heterologous determinants such as (4-hydroxy-

TABLE I

Fine specificity of primary anti-NP specific clones

Fine specificity		*Number of clones (%)*	
		BALB/c	*B10.D2*
Homoclitic	Total	24 (45·3)	7 (14·0)
	κ	23	6
	λ	1	1
	RPs	6	4
Heteroclitic	Total	29 (54·7)	43 (86·0)
	κ	14	15
	λ	15	28
	RPs	10	7

5-iodo-3-nitrophenyl) acetyl (NIP), bear the λ light chain, and share a cross-reactive idiotypic determinant (Karjalainen and Makela, 1978). Table I presents a summary of an analysis of monoclonal responses to NP in B10.D2 mice (Igh^b) and BALB/c mice (Igh^a) (Stashenko and Klinman, 1980). This analysis demonstrates that the heteroclitic clonotypes are heterogeneous and that the considerable differences between these strains observed in late serum antibodies is not as apparent at the precursor cell level. Another clonotype set which had initially been thought to involve a single clonotype, the response to the *p*-azophenyl arsonate (ARS) determinant in Igh^e mice (Nisonoff and

Bangasser, 1975), has also recently been shown to include an extremely diverse array of clonotypes (Marshak-Rothstein *et al.*, 1980). Similarly, diverse clonotype sets appear to dominate responses in various strains to sheep erythrocytes (McCarthy and Dutton, 1975), levan (Bona *et al.*, 1979) and amino acid copolymers (Ju *et al.*, 1980). *In toto*, these findings indicate that immune responses to certain antigenic determinants can be dominated by a closely related set of clonotypes which are inherited as a single or tightly linked set of genetic loci. Inheritance of these expressions is linked primarily to the heavy chain allotype locus, but is also dependent in some instances on an appropriate light chain locus (Laskin *et al.*, 1977) and other genetic loci as well.

Both the genetic mechanisms responsible for predominant clonotype expression and the control mechanisms which account for the predominance of these clonotype sets in the various responses are as yet unknown. It should be noted, that while many examples of such dominance have been identified, these types of responses remain relatively rare when compared to overall B cell responsiveness, and thus, may reflect the effects of special mechanisms which may be responsible for both the genetic fidelity of their expression and the mechanisms that enable their dominance in the responsive cell pools. Nonetheless, given the frequency of B cells of these clonotype sets in the B cell repertoire (Stashenko and Klinman, 1980) and the enormous diversity within these sets, any given clonotype (with the exception of TEPC 15) is likely to be represented by fewer than 1 in 10^6–10^7 B cells. If, indeed, all potential clonotypes of each of these sets are expressed in all of the individuals of an inbred strain, these findings would constitute strong evidence for genetic control of repertoire expression, even to the level of 10^6–10^7 total expressed clonotypes. Recent studies by Marshak-Rothstein *et al.* (1980) imply that this may indeed be the case. Using anti-idiotypic antibodies that recognize only one of the set of anti-ARS clonotypes, they were able to show that the immune serum from all tested A/He individuals contained this idiotype to the level of 0·1 to 1% of their total anti-ARS antibody.

The total extent of diversity of the entire murine B cell repertoire has been analysed using more general approaches to evaluate the array clonotypes responsive to nonrestrictive antigenic determinants. These studies have involved the responsive B cells of inbred murine strains to haptenic determinants such as DNP and NIP, which are capable of stimulating a high proportion of B cells, as well as complex antigens such as β-galactosidase and influenza which present multiple antigenic determinants to the immune system. In general, the clonotypes responsive to such determinants are delineated using either isoelectric focusing or reactivity pattern analysis. Thus, several years ago, Kreth and Williamson (1973) were able to demonstrate that the response of CBA/H mice to the NIP determinant included 3×10^3 to 25×10^3 distinct clonotypes. Similarly, Pink and Askonas (1974) were able to determine that the BALB/c response to DNP included at least 10^3 to 3×10^3 clonotypes. By the use of isoelectric focusing and substrate binding properties, Kohler (1976) was able to demonstrate several hundred clonotypes in the

BALB/c response to β-galactosidase. By using reactivity pattern analysis, Cancro *et al.* (1978a) were able to demonstrate that hundreds of clonotypes are available in adult BALB/c mice which recognize determinants on the PR8 influenza haemagglutinin molecule (PR8-HA). Given the overall frequency of B cells responsive to each of these antigens and the number of clonotypes involved in the particular response, in essentially every instance it can be calculated that fewer than 1 in 10^7 B cells bears the clonotype in question. In addition, in none of these studies was a predominant clonotype identified. If all B cells are reactive to at least one antigenic determinant, then it is clear that the B cell repertoire contains more than 10^7 distinct specificities.

It should be noted that all of these studies are likely to underestimate the size of the repertoire since calculations are based on the frequency of repeats of a single clonotype within a given analysis. Since neither isoelectric focusing nor reactivity panel analysis is totally discriminatory, it is likely that many clonotypes judged to be identical are not truly identical. Furthermore, even among these "minor" clonotypes, it is likely that disparities exist in the frequency with which they are represented in the B cell pool. Repeats may most often occur among the more highly represented of these clonotypes and thus falsely lower repertoire estimates. The fact that these clonotypes are so rare has made any meaningful comparison among individuals or among strains impossible. Thus it has not been possible to use the analyses of "minor" clonotypes to help resolve issues such as the degree of polymorphism among strains in repertoire expression, or the effects of various regulatory factors on repertoire expression *per se*.

The developing repertoire

As mentioned above, the extraordinary diversity of the adult murine B cell repertoire has precluded meaningful repertoire comparisons either between individuals or between strains. Several strategies have been adopted in an attempt to analyse a more restricted repertoire in which all clonotypes present would be represented by a greater proportion of the total B cell pool. Recently, du Pasquier and Wabl (1978) carried out an intensive investigation of the antibody repertoire of genetically identical frogs. These studies revealed that, at certain times of development, frogs display a relatively limited repertoire and genetically identical individuals display considerable repertoire overlap. Similar findings have been obtained from the studies of Huang and Dreyer (1978) who used experimental bursectomy to truncate the B cell repertoire of genetically identical chickens. Again, relatively restricted repertoires were observed with a considerable degree of repertoire overlap between similarly treated chickens.

Since neonatal mice contain far fewer B cells than adults, it may be assumed that their repertoire should also be considerably more restricted. This, plus the obvious relevance of the developing repertoire to questions of repertoire acquisition provided the rationale for an intensive analysis of the B cell repertoire in neonatal and developing inbred mice. Studies of the late foetal and early neonatal repertoire provided considerable evidence for repertoire restriction both in individuals and in the strain as a whole (Klinman and Press, 1975a; Sigal *et al.*, 1976; Sigal, 1977; Cancro *et al.*, 1979). In BALB/c neonates during the first few days after birth, the responses to DNP, TNP, ARS and dansyl, were shown to be dominated by a very small set of clonotypes. Each of these clonotypes was apparently representative of approximately 1 in 10 000 B cells. B cells responsive to a variety of other antigenic determinants such as fluorescein, PC, and PR8-HA were either absent or very rare representing *in toto* less than any one of the aforementioned dominant clonotypes. Importantly, many of these frequencies are totally disproportionate to the ultimate adult representation of the relevant specificities. Because of this, and the extraordinary reproducibility of the appearance of the dominant clonotypes among early BALB/c neonates, we concluded that the early murine B cell repertoire is highly restricted and genetically determined. Among the most striking findings was the reproducible occurrence of cells responsive to PC between the 5th and 7th days after birth (Sigal *et al.*, 1976). These responses included both the TEPC 15 clonotype and non-TEPC 15 clonotypes specific for the PC determinant. This finding provided the first indication that a defined clonotype might appear relatively late in development in a totally reproducible and genetically determined fashion, implying a patterned acquisition of the repertoire throughout early development. Recent studies by other laboratories (Fung and Kohler, 1980) have confirmed the late and reproducible expression of the PC responsive B cells in the splenic population. These studies also imply that these clonotypes may occur at an earlier time in the liver. This may indicate that the patterned acquisition of the repertoire may differ in different organs and possibly different B cell subpopulations. These findings, plus those of other laboratories implying the reproducible late occurrence of various clonotypes responsive to the levan (Bona *et al.*, 1979) and α,1,6 dextran (Fernandez and Möller, 1978) imply that the repertoire might be relatively restricted even quite late in postnatal development.

In order to evaluate the fidelity of repertoire expression after a considerable amount of diversification and assess the affects of environment on repertoire expression itself, we initiated a detailed study of the PR8-HA specific repertoire in 2-week-old mice. This analysis has been greatly facilitated by the availability of a large panel of closely related antigens. As mentioned above, the repertoire of adult BALB/c and B10.D2 mice to this antigen is extremely diverse, including apparently hundreds of distinct clonotypes (Cancro *et al.*, 1978; Cancro and Klinman, 1980). The anti-PR8-HA specific repertoire of 12 to 14-day-old BALB/c neonates was found to be extraordinarily restricted (Cancro *et al.*, 1979). Only 9 RPs have been identified in an analysis of 78 monoclonal antibodies derived from 28 individual mice. A detailed statistical analysis of this data indicates not only that the neonatal repertoire is far more restricted than that of adults, but also that there is a significant degree of repertoire sharing among genetically identical individuals at a similar stage in development. Since the average representation of each clonotype at this stage is approximately 1 in 10^6 B cells, it is apparent that considerable diversification has occurred between birth and 12–14 days of age; yet, repertoire acquisition continues to be highly patterned and genetically predetermined (Klinman *et al.*, 1977). Importantly, although a considerable amount of diversification has occurred, the techniques available for analysis of the PR8-HA specific repertoire are capable of totally defining the murine repertoire at 12–14 days of age. A similar analysis has now been carried out of the repertoire of neonatal B10.D2 mice (Cancro and Klinman, 1980). Again, the neonatal repertoire was found to be significantly more restricted than that of the adult displaying only 8 RPs in an analysis of 70 monoclonal antibodies from 32 individuals. A comparison was carried out between the PR8-HA specific repertoires of 12 to 14-day-old B10.D2 and BALB/c mice. While some overlap was noted, the majority of the repertoire was clearly distinct in these 2 strains. Thus, similar to findings with predominant adult clonotypes mentioned above, there appears to be strain-associated differences in the expression of the neonatal B cell repertoire.

The finding that 2 murine strains differ significantly in their expressed repertoire at 12–14 days and the demonstration that analytical techniques are adequate to define fully repertoire at this stage provides a unique opportunity for analysis of genetic and environmental control of repertoire expression. Our first approach to this analysis has been to conduct a comprehensive analysis of the repertoire of the F_1 progeny of BALB/c and B10.D2 mice (Cancro and Klinman, 1980). At days 12–14 after birth F_1 neonates display an extremely restricted PR8-HA specific repertoire displaying only 8 reactivity patterns in an analysis of 98 monoclonal antibodies from 41 individuals. Reproducibility of this repertoire expression among F_1 neonates is equally as great as that of both parental strains. A comparison of the repertoire of F_1 neonates with that of both parents was carried out. While a small amount of repertoire overlap was present between the F_1 repertoire and that of both parental strains, the major portion of the repertoire of F_1 individuals was completely distinct from that expressed by either parent. Thus, although the inherited genetic information of F_1 individuals must be assumed to be the sum of the genetic information of the inbred parental lines, the temporal acquisition of definable clonotypes is quite distinct from that displayed by either of the two parental strains.

Since findings with predominant adult clonotypes clearly demonstrate the codominant behaviour of at least some specificities, it may be assumed that the repertoire expressed by F_1 individuals may ultimately more closely reflect the sum of the two parental repertoires. However, differences in both the temporal acquisition of repertoire and the ultimate composition of repertoire between F_1 and parental individuals could readily be explained at several levels in the process of repertoire generation and expression. As shown in Fig. 1, prior to receptor expression, if *trans* effects can take place at the level of control of any of the multiple complex processes which lead to a viable heavy and light chain, then the temporal sequence and ultimate repertoire expression of F_1 individuals may differ considerably from that of the parental strain. Post-receptor expression, it may be anticipated that the F_1 environment would select differently on the expressed repertoire than either of the parental environments alone. Such selection could affect either the expressed repertoire *in toto* or its temporal acquisition. Given the ability to dissect the developing repertoire and the wide array of available recombinant murine strains, it should now be possible to carefully delineate those factors which may contribute to such disparities in repertoire expression.

The adult prereceptor B cell repertoire

As implied in Fig. 1, the most direct approach to evaluating the relative contributions of prereceptor and postreceptor mechanisms to repertoire expression would be to compare the repertoire in adults of developing B cells prior to their expression of surface immunoglobulin with that of mature B cells. Findings from this and other laboratories using the splenic focus technique have indicated that, in the presence of optimal T cell help, very immature B cells may be given the opportunity to develop and be stimulated to monoclonal antibody production *in vitro* (Klinman and Press, 1975b; Teale *et al.*, 1979; Fung and Kohler, 1980). A series of experiments has now been initiated to evaluate the efficacy of a comprehensive analysis of the repertoire of B cells from adult bone marrow prior to their acquisition of receptors. It is assumed that such B cells would be truly naive and display repertoire exclusive of tolerogenic and other environmental mechanisms which require interaction with the expressed surface receptor. In order to remove immunoglobulin-bearing cells, bone marrow cells were subjected to anti-IgM panning procedures (Wysocki and Sato, 1978). The characteristics of the unbound cell population are presented in Table II. It can be seen that by fluorescence microscopy and fluorescence activated cell sorter analysis, these cells bear no detectable surface immunoglobulin. These cells represent approximately 25% of clonal precursor cells in the bone marrow, give rise to IgM but not IgG producing clones, and, consistent with previous findings with bone marrow B cells, are exquisitely susceptible to *in vitro* tolerance induction (Metcalf and Klinman, 1977). Most important for the present analysis is the fact that these cells show no evidence of having interacted with environmental influences. One month after tolerance induction with 2 mg of DNP_{56} DGL, the copolymer of D-glutamic acid and D-lysine (Katz *et al.*, 1971), when the frequency of responsive immunoglobulin-bearing cells in the spleen and marrow has been reduced by greater than 80%, very little reduction in the DNP responsive prereceptor B cells is apparent (Klinman, N. R. and Katz, D. H., unpublished observations). Thus, in spite of the presence of tolerogen in the environment, the prereceptor B cell popula-

TABLE II
Characteristics of prereceptor B cells

	Prereceptor[a] *B cells*	*Postreceptor B cells*
Surface Ig	−	+
Frequency of DNP responsive cells (per 10^6 injected cells)	0·7	2·2
Tolerance susceptibility	>80%	<5%
IgG production	<5%	>60%
Environmental influence		
Presence during tolerance	>80%	<20%

[a] Adult bone marrow cells not removed by anti-IgM panning.

tion remains essentially intact throughout the course of the tolerance regimen.

An analysis is now being carried out to evaluate the characteristics of the PR8-HA specific repertoire in these prereceptor B cells. Initial findings indicate that the repertoire as expressed in these cells is diverse and not reflective of the early neonatal restricted repertoire (Wylie and Klinman, 1980). This implies that a considerable degree of repertoire diversification occurs prior to receptor acquisition. Thus, contact with environmental antigens or receptor specific immunoregulatory mechanisms are not necessary for diversification *per se*. Second, individuals displaying a given clonotype in their prereceptor B cell repertoire display multiple precursors of that clonotype. Thus, it would appear that considerable clonal expansion occurs prior to receptor acquisition. This finding is in agreement with previous reports by Osmond (1980) indicating that the major division potential of bone marrow B cells occurs prior to surface expression of immunoglobulin.

While all of these investigations with prereceptor B cells are in a preliminary stage, they give considerable promise for enabling a clear delineation between the relative contributions of prereceptor and postreceptor mechanisms in the ultimate determination of the repertoire. Furthermore, they may provide the basis for a better understanding of the mode of action of postreceptor mechanisms in general. Several laboratories are currently engaged in isolating and defining B cell populations at very early stages of their development. Given new probes for repertoire delineation, the availability of hybridomas and the comparative and molecular analyses they provide, it may soon be possible to place each of the elements involved in repertoire diversification and expression into an appropriate molecular and developmental perspective.

References

Accolla, R. S., Gearhart, P. J., Sigal, N. H., Cancro, M. P. and Klinman, N. R. (1977). *Eur. J. Immunol.* **7**, 876.

Blomberg, G., Geckeler, W. and Weigert, M. (1972). *Science (Wash. D.C.)* **177**, 178.

Bona, C., Mond, J. J., Stein, K. E., House, S., Lieberman, R. and Paul, W. E. (1979). *J. Immunol.* **123**, 1484.

Brack, C., Hiromon, M., Lenhard-Schuller, R. and Tonegawa, S. (1978). *Cell.* **15**, 1.

Cambier, J. C., Kettman, J. R., Vitetta, E. S. and Uhr, J. W. (1976). *J. Exp. Med.* **144**, 293.

Cancro, M. P. and Klinman, N. R. (1980) (submitted).

Cancro, M. P., Gerhard, W. and Klinman, N. R. (1978a). *J. Exp. Med.* **147**, 776.

Cancro, M. P., Sigal, N. H. and Klinman, N. R. (1978b). *J. Exp. Med.* **147**, 1.

Cancro, M. P., Wylie, D. E., Gerhard, W. and Klinman, N. R. (1979). *Proc. Natn. Acad. Sci. U.S.A.* **76**, 6577.

Cohn, M., Blomberg, B., Geckeler, W., Rashke, W., Riblet, R. and Weigert, M. (1974). *In* "The Immune System: Genes, Receptors, Signals" (E. E. Sercarz, A. R. Williamson and C. F. Fox, eds) p. 89. Academic Press, New York.

Cosenza, H. and Kohler, H. (1972). *Science* **176**, 1027.

du Pasquier, L. and Wabl, M. R. (1978). *Eur. J. Immunol.* **8**, 128.

Eichmann, K. (1972). *J. Exp. Med.* **137**, 603.

Etlinger, H. M. and Chiller, J. M. (1979). *J. Immunol.* **122**, 2558.

Fernandez, C. and Möller, G. (1978). *J. Exp. Med.* **147**, 645.

Fung, S. J. and Kohler, H. (1980). *J. Immunol.* (in press).

Gearhart, P. J., Sigal, N. H. and Klinman, N. R. (1975). *J. Exp. Med.* **141**, 56.

Gearhart, P. J., Sigal, N. H. and Klinman, N. R. (1977). *J. Exp. Med.* **145**, 876.

Huang, H. V. and Dreyer, W. J. (1978). *J. Immunol.* **121**, 1738.

Jerne, N. K. (1974). *Ann. Immunol.* (*Inst. Pasteur*). **125**, 373.

Ju, S-T., Benacerraf, B. and Dorf, M. E. (1980). *J. Immunol.* **124**, 2870.

Karjalainen, K. and Makela, O. (1978). *Eur. J. Immunol.* **8**, 105.

Katz, D. H., Davie, J. M., Paul, W. E. and Benacerraf, B. (1971). *J. Exp. Med.* **134**, 201.

Kay, T. W., Pike, B. L. and Nossal, G. J. V. (1980). *J. Immunol.* **124**, 1579.

Klinman, N. R. (1980). Abstracts 4th International Congress of Immunology, Paris 1980.

Klinman, N. R. and Press, J. L. (1975a). *J. Exp. Med.* **141**, 1133.

Klinman, N. R. and Press, J. L. (1975b). *Transplant. Rev.* **24**, 41.

Klinman, N. R., Sigal, N. H., Metcalf, E. S., Pierce, S. K. and Gerhart, P. J. (1977). *Cold Spring Harbor Symp. Quant. Biol.* **41**, 165.

Kohler, G. (1976). *Eur. J. Immunol.* **6**, 340.

Kohler, H., Kaplan, D., Kaplan, R., Fung, J. and Quintans, J. (1979). *In* "Cells of Immunoglobulin Synthesis" (B. Pernis and H. J. Vogel, eds) p. 357. Academic Press, New York.

Kreth, H. W. and Williamson, A. R. (1973). *Eur. J. Immunol.* **3**, 141.

Laskin, J. A., Gray, A., Nisonoff, A., Klinman, N. and Gottlieb, P. D. (1977). *Proc. Natn. Acad. Sci. U.S.A.* **74**, 4600.

Lieberman, R., Potter, M., Mushinski, E. B., Humphrey, Jr, W. and Rudikoff, S. (1974). *J. Exp. Med.* **139**, 983.

McCarthy, M. M. and Dutton, R. W. (1975). *J. Immunol.* **115**, 1327.

Makela, O. and Imanishi, T. (1975). *J. Exp. Med.* **141**, 840.

Makela, O. and Karjalainen, K. (1977). *Immunol. Rev.* **34**, 119.

Marshak-Rothstein, A., Beneditto, J. D. and Gefter, M. L. (1980). *J. Immunol.* (in press).

Metcalf, E. S. and Klinman, N. R. (1976). *J. Exp. Med.* **143**, 1327.

Metcalf, E. S. and Klinman, N. R. (1977). *J. Immunol.* **118**, 2111.

Nisonoff, A. and Bangasser, S. A. (1975). *Transplant. Rev.* **27**, 100.

Nisonoff, A., Ju, S.-T. and Owen, F. L. (1977). *Transplant. Rev.* **34**, 89.

Osmond, D. (1980). *In* "Immunoglobulin Genes and B Cell Differentiation" (J. R. Battista and K. L. Knight, eds). Elsevier/North-Holland, New York (in press).

Pawlak, L. L. and Nisonoff, A. (1973). *J. Exp. Med.* **137**, 855.
Pierce, S. K. and Klinman, N. R. (1977). *J. Exp. Med.* **146**, 509.
Pink, J. R. L. and Askonas, B. (1974). *Eur. J. Immunol.* **4**, 426.
Reth, M., Hammerling, G. J. and Rajewsky, K. (1978). *Eur. J. Immunol.* **8**, 393.
Rodkey, L. S. (1974). *J. Exp. Med.* **139**, 712.
Schilling, J., Clevinger, B., Davie, J. M. and Hood, L. (1980). *Nature* **283**, 35.
Seidman, J. G. and Leder, P. (1978). *Nature* **276**, 790.
Seidman, J. G., Leder, A., Edgell, M. H., Polsky, F., Tilghman, S., Tiemeir, D. C. and Leder, P. (1978). *Proc. Natn. Acad. Sci. U.S.A.* **75**, 3881.
Sherman, L. A. (1980). *J. Exp. Med.* **151**, 1386.
Sigal, N. H. (1977). *J. Immunol.* **119**, 1129.
Sigal, N. H. and Klinman, N. R. (1978). "Advances in Immunology", Vol. 26, p. 255. Academic Press, London and New York.
Sigal, N. H., Gearhart, P. J. and Klinman, N. R. (1975). *J. Immunol.* **68**, 1354.
Sigal, N. H., Gearhart, P. J., Press, J. L. and Klinman, N. R. (1976). *Nature* (*Lond.*) **259**, 51.
Sigal, N. H., Cancro, M. P. and Klinman, N. R. (1977). *In* "ICN-UCLA Symposia on Molecular and Cellular Biology, Col. VI. Immune System: Genetics and Regulations" (E. E. Sercarz, L. A. Herzenberg and C. F. Fox, eds) p. 217. Academic Press, New York.
Stashenko, P. and Klinman, N. R. (1980). *J. Immunol.* (in press).
Stein, K., Bona, C., Lieberman, R., Chien, C. and Paul, W. E. (1980). *J. Exp. Med.* **151**, 1088.
Stocker, J. W. (1977). *Immunology* **32**, 282.
Teale, J. M., Layton, J. E. and Nossal, G. J. V. (1979). *J. Exp. Med.* **150**, 205.
Triplett, E. L. (1962). *J. Immunol.* **89**, 505.
Weigert, M., Perry, R., Kelly, D., Hunkapillar, T., Schilling, J. and Hood, L. (1980). *Nature* **281**, 497.
Wylie, D. E. and Klinman, N. R. (1980). In prep.
Wysocki, L. J. and Sato, V. L. (1978). *Proc. Natn. Acad. Sci. U.S.A.* **75**, 2844.

9

Antibody Receptor Diversity and Diversity of Signals

G. J. V. NOSSAL and BEVERLEY L. PIKE

The Walter and Eliza Hall Institute of Medical Research Post Office, Royal Melbourne Hospital, Victoria, Australia

Our sincere thanks are due to Kim Bamford and Helen Bathard for excellent technical assistance. This work was supported by the National Health and Medical Research Council, Canberra, Australia; and by Grant Number AI-03958 from the National Institute for Allergy and Infectious Diseases, US Public Health Service.

Introduction

Academic immunology is concerned principally with two spectra of questions, namely the mechanisms by which lymphocytes become somatically diversified and committed to the expression of a single immunological specificity; and the nature, source and regulation of the intermolecular and intercellular signals, both inductive and suppressive, that govern the cellular repertoire's response to the entry of antigen. The other authors in this symposium address principally the former question. The focus of our presentation will be on the latter, and especially on mechanisms of negative signalling, constituting the group of phenomena embraced by the term immunological tolerance. Nevertheless, the validation of the concept of a specificity repertoire enshrined in a population of monospecific lymphocytes confined to the expression of one element of the repertoire is so crucial to all arguments concerning signalling that we wish briefly to address this issue.

Validation of the clonal selection approach

Though the clonal selection theory (Burnet, 1957) is generally accepted as the framework for thinking about antibody formation, formal proof has been provided only recently (Nossal and Pike, 1978a; Nossal *et al.*, 1978a). The proof demands that lymphocytes from an unimmunized animal be fractionated on the basis of the antigen-binding specificity of their surface immunoglobulin (Ig) receptor (postulated to constitute a single specificity), and then be able to be triggered by that antigen (but by no other) to secrete the corresponding unique antibody. This demands two separate technologies, namely antigen affinity fractionation methods for B lymphocytes, and ways of challenging single B cells to develop into antibody-forming clones. As regards the former, we have found it necessary to adopt two-cycle fractionation procedures to obtain really satisfactory results. The initial step involves an affinity-adherence procedure based on attachment of lymphocytes to a thin layer of a hapten coupled to gelatin (Haas and Layton, 1975). The second step is either the selection of a high avidity subset of these hapten-binding cells by use of the fluorescence-activated cell sorter (FACS), or a rosetting procedure involving haptenated erythrocytes. The latter approach has also been used successfully by Diener's group (Shiozawa *et al.*, 1980). The *in vitro* cloning of single B lymphocytes has been achieved by a microculture system involving inclusion of anti-Ia and complement-treated thymus cells as "fillers", and triggering of the B cells by a T cell-independent antigen, namely hapten-polymerized flagellin (Nossal and Pike, 1976).

With these techniques, we have been able to show that B cells fractionated for reactivity against a given hapten such as NIP or fluorescein (FLU) can develop into the relevant hapten-specific antibody-forming cell clones with a cloning efficiency of 1 in 3 to 1 in 10. They fail to form antibody against unrelated haptens. The question may then be posed: why does not every cell respond? This can be answered by reference to the work of Andersson *et al.* (1979). Using techniques similar to our own, they asked what proportion of B cells can be fired off into clonal proliferation and IgM synthesis by a T cell-independent mitogen, *E. coli* lipopolysaccharide (LPS). The answer they obtained was 1 in 3 to 1 in 10. The technique was unable to differentiate whether the nontriggerable cells belonged to a different B cell subset, or whether it was simply a matter of cloning efficiency, bearing in mind the fragility of lymphocytes in tissue culture, but this does not affect the argument. The absolute identity of the effective cloning efficiencies is striking, and proves that our nontriggered cells were not silent because they possessed some unsuspected specificity. The logical chain for clonal selection, at least as far as the B lymphocyte is concerned, now appears to be complete.

The situation with respect to the T lymphocyte is much less clear-cut. Clonal diversity is apparent at the level of the effector cell, but studies on the equivalent of the "virgin" B cell, namely the T cell that is the antigen-activatable precursor of cytotoxic, helper, suppressor or delayed hypersensitivity T effector cells, are hampered by the apparently poor or limited display of antigen receptors, which militate against robust and reproducible antigen-affinity fractionation techniques. Methods involving the cloning of cytotoxic T lymphocyte precursors (Skinner and Marbrook, 1976) suggest clonal precommitment to a unique specificity, and there are no cogent reasons to believe that clonal selection is not the operative principle for the T lymphocyte as well. However, until our knowledge of the T lymphocyte's receptor for antigen, and of its recognition mechanisms for "self" major histocompatibility components (MHC), improves considerably, the precision of experiments designed to test this proposition will continue to leave much to be desired.

Framework for addressing diversity of signals

Activation of B lymphocytes

It is possible to decompose the activation of a B lymphocyte into at least four sets of events which, though linked, may nevertheless be subject to separate controls. The first is the conversion of a noncycling, small membrane immunoglobulin (m-Ig) positive B lymphocyte into a larger, more active cell. The second is the initiation and maintenance of a series of mitotic divisions creating a clone of B cells with the given specificity. The third is the development of a specialized protein synthesizing and secreting mechanism changing the cell from one simply displaying m-Ig to one actively secreting Ig. The fourth is a switch in isotype secreted from IgM to one or more of the other Ig classes by cells of the same clone. Though these four sets of events usually proceed in parallel, there are many examples of a partial or complete dissociation. Thus, T cell helper factors acting alone and without specific antigen, may activate steps 1 and 4 alone, causing small lymphocytes to differentiate into antibody-forming cells without intervening cell division (Fu *et al.*, 1979; Andersson *et al.*, 1980). The combined action of agar mitogens and macrophage-derived factors can activate steps 1 and 2 alone, causing B cells to divide exponentially and form large colonies without developing into typical antibody-forming cells (Metcalf *et al.*, 1975); macrophage-derived factors produced in a typical *in vivo* immune response can cause certain B cells to transform into rapidly dividing nonantibody—secreting blasts in an antigen—nonspecific manner (Shortman *et al.*, 1978); this activation of the "pre-progenitor" subset being an example of steps 1 and 2 alone. However, there is also recent evidence that accessory cell-derived factors can specifically force step 3—the conversion from dividing blast to antibody-forming cell (Shiozawa *et al.*, 1980), the target cells in this case being "direct progenitors" of antibody-forming cells. While it is generally believed that step 4, isotype switching, is consequent on specific T lymphocyte-mediated effects, a limited degree of switching can be noted in microcultures driven by T-independent antigens (Nossal and Pike, 1976). These are but a few of the complexities surrounding the cell biology of lymphocyte triggering. We have discussed elsewhere (Schrader and Nossal, 1980) the strategy of more incisive experimental approaches to the various roles of accessory cells in this process.

It is therefore premature to attempt to put forward a detailed model of B cell activation. The initial events involve binding of antigen and receipt of signals (? factors) from macrophages and specific helper T cells. The T cell requirement, but probably not the macrophage requirement, can be bypassed through the use of "T-independent" antigens. The subsequent clonal expansion and differentiation depends on the further action of antigen (Pike and Nossal, 1976) and factors from macrophages and T cells which may or may not be the same as those needed for activation.

Negative signalling of B lymphocytes

Bretscher and Cohn (1970) were initially responsible for the theory that lymphocyte activation depended on two classes of signals, Signal 1 being delivered via the m-Ig receptor binding its antigen, and Signal 2 representing the helper T lymphocyte input. They put forward the idea that Signal 1 acting alone might negatively signal the cell, causing immunological tolerance; whereas Signal 1 and Signal 2 acting together would constitute the positive signal. Over the past several years, we have been taking this hypothesis as a broad frame of reference for addressing B lymphocyte tolerance, with the caveat that certain T-independent antigens may themselves possess "Signal 2" properties, either because they directly stimulate the B cell (Möller, 1975) or because they cause macrophage activation and thus Signal 2 generation (Schrader, 1974). We have measured the strength of the negative signal by exposing various B cell subsets to antigen alone, or to anti-immunoglobulin mimicking antigen, for various periods. Following this the B cells were activated in one of a variety of B lymphocyte cloning assays. Before summarizing the results of this research, a brief review of the possible cellular mechanisms of immunological tolerance is presented.

Theories of tolerance induction

B lymphocytes

The first category of possible cellular mechanisms of B lymphocyte tolerance induction are suppressor mechanisms, as shown in Fig. 1. On this view, B

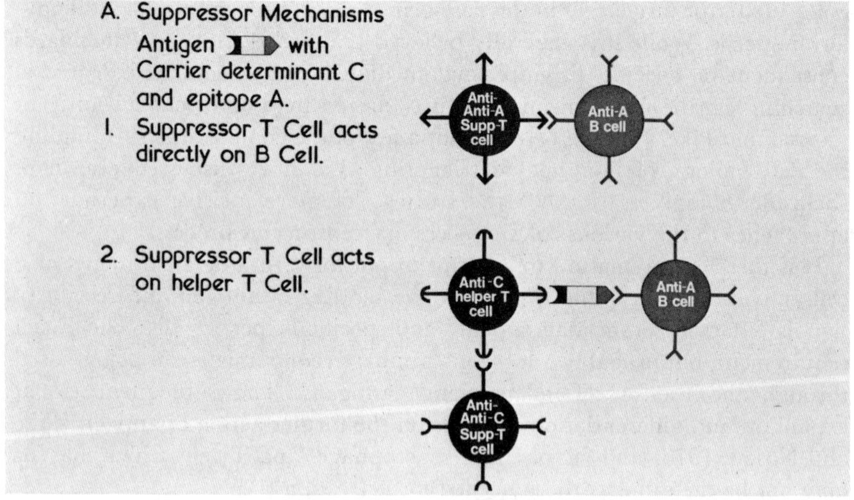

FIG. 1. *Suppressor mechanisms of B lymphocyte tolerance.*

cells with receptors for a given epitope A are held in check, unable to be activated to antigen A, by the existence of suppressor T cells. Two variants of this theme can be envisaged, namely a suppressor T cell acting directly on the B cell, possibly because of possession of anti-idiotypic receptors directed against the B cell's anti-A receptors (Fig. 1, A1); or a suppressor T cell acting to antagonize the action of a helper T lymphocyte. Figure 1, A2, considers the case of an animal rendered tolerant to the antigen AC. The anti-A B cell requires the help of an anti-C helper T cell to respond, but this is prevented through a suppressor cell acting on the helper cell, perhaps via an anti-idiotypic determinant anti-C.

Even though this is contrary to current dogma, one can envisage the possibility that, under some circumstances, suppressor T cells could possess

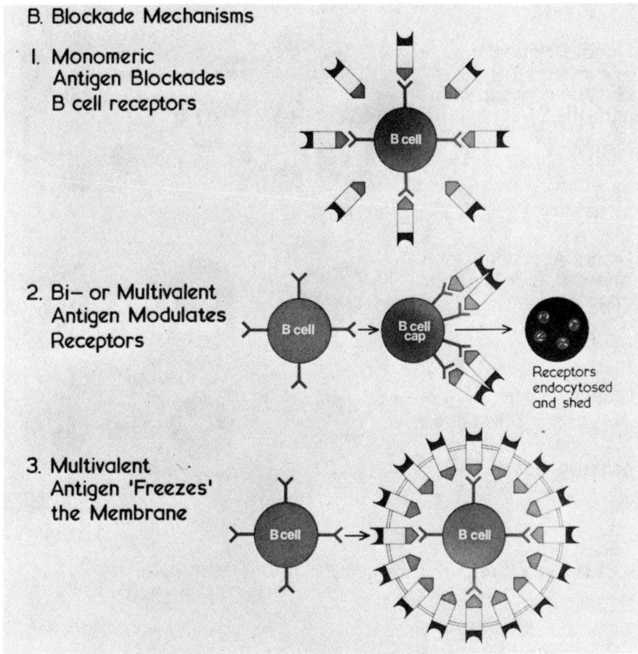

FIG. 2. *Blockade mechanisms of B lymphocyte tolerance.*

cytotoxic properties. In that case, mechanism A1 would resemble B cell clonal deletion, as would A2 in respect of anti-C T cells.

The second category of possibilities are various types of blockade mechanisms, as shown in Fig. 2. Monomeric antigens could be seen as incapable of signalling the B cell while in monomeric form, though this remains a postulate rather than a proven fact. In that case, at high molarity, they could occupy the B cell's m-Ig receptors to such an extent as to prevent macrophage-associated or other immunogenic forms of antigen from gaining access to the B cell. Bivalent or multivalent antigens, including antigen-antibody complexes in the zone of antigen excess, could deprive the cell of its m-Ig receptors through the patching–capping–endocytosis cycle, a process that has been termed modulation. There is evidence that immature B cells may be unduly susceptible to irreversible modulation, thus providing a link between this mechanism and that shown in Fig. 3, C2. It has been reported that high concentrations of certain multivalent antigens can immobilize m-Ig receptors, thus "freezing" the membrane, at least in respect of m-Ig (Diener and Paetkau, 1972). Given the efficacy of the modulation cycle, this is unlikely to be a general mechanism.

The third category of possible cellular mechanisms consists of a purging or a functional silencing of elements of the B cell repertoire. Variants on this

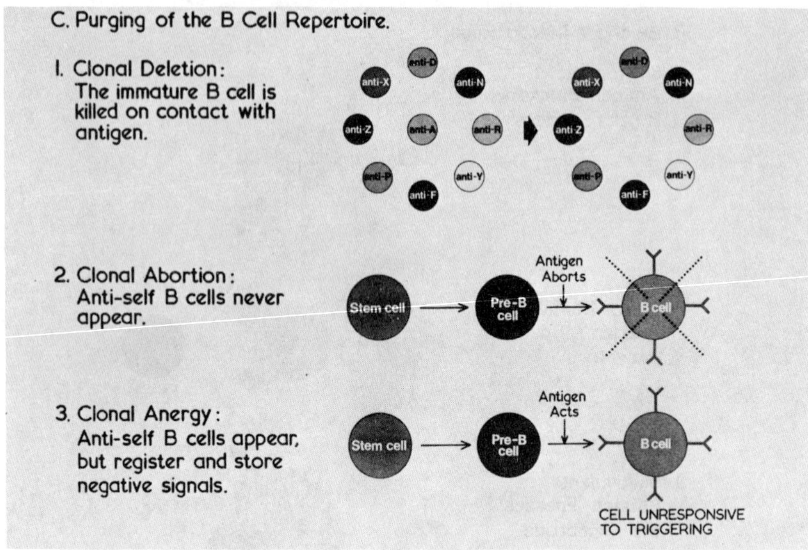

FIG. 3. *Repertoire purging mechanisms of B lymphocyte tolerance.*

theme are shown in Fig. 3. One could imagine, as Burnet (1957) originally postulated, a deletion of immature B cells that meet antigen. A refinement of that idea is the notion of clonal abortion (Nossal and Pike, 1975b), where it is visualized that antiself B cells never appear in competent form because early contact with antigen prevents the proper sequence of maturation. Mechanism C3 of Fig. 3 allows the appearance of m-Ig receptors, but in a cell that has been functionally silenced through premature contact with antigen.

T lymphocytes

Fundamentally, the possible mechanisms for T lymphocyte tolerance are no different. Taking the cytotoxic T lymphocyte precursor (CTL-P) as an example, the possibilities are schematized in Fig. 4. The chief reason for drawing attention to the T lymphocyte here is to flag the point (canvassed in more detail in the section: Basis of T lymphocyte tolerance) that limiting dilution techniques essentially analogous to those that have been worked out for B cells should prove most useful in an analysis of mechanisms of T lymphocyte tolerance.

It is not suggested that the mechanisms listed on Figs 1 to 4 be regarded as mutually exclusive. Indeed, it seems certain that different models of the tolerant state result from different mechanisms, and a diversity of mechanisms may even be operative in a given model. As "self" antigens occur in such diverse forms and concentrations, it seems likely that the same is true for physiological self-tolerance.

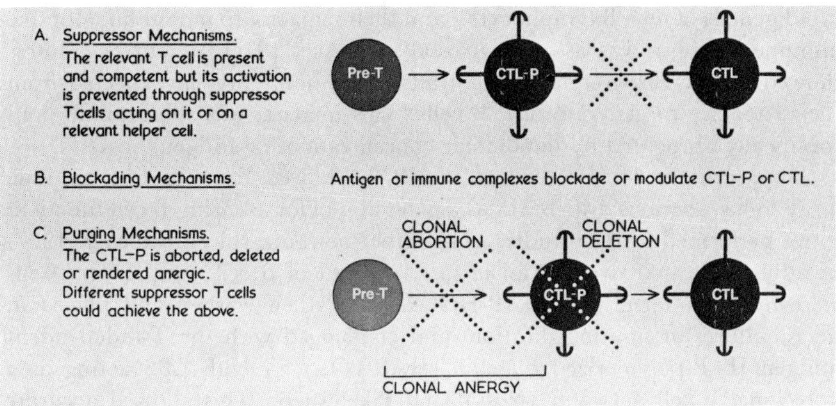

A. Suppressor Mechanisms.
The relevant T cell is present and competent but its activation is prevented through suppressor T cells acting on it or on a relevant helper cell.
Pre-T
CTL-P
CTL
B. Blockading Mechanisms.
Antigen or immune complexes blockade or modulate CTL-P or CTL.
C. Purging Mechanisms.
The CTL-P is aborted, deleted or rendered anergic. Different suppressor T cells could achieve the above.
CLONAL ABORTION
CLONAL DELETION
Pre-T
CTL-P
CTL
CLONAL ANERGY

FIG. 4. *Possible mechanisms of T lymphocyte tolerance.*

Results favouring clone silencing or purging mechanisms of B lymphocyte tolerance

We shall list below the chain of reasoning and experimentation that has convinced us that B lymphocyte tolerance is intimately tied to B cell differentiation and to the ontogeny of the lymphoid system. The initial attraction of the "clonal abortion" notion was its intrinsic elegance. What better way to silence an unwanted antiself reactivity than to programme in an early phase of differentiation where the cell was exquisitely sensitive to negative signalling by encounters with its antigen? In the presence of such a mechanism, the threat of autoimmunity would be neutralized. In some ways, having silenced the cell, it would make little sense to preserve it. Before we could address the question of whether the silenced cell would be destroyed in some way, the first necessity was to demonstrate that cells differentiating from precursor cells into competent B cells indeed passed through a phase of great sensitivity to tolerance induction.

The first model system we chose (Nossal and Pike, 1975a) allowed the emergence of B cells from foetal liver stem cells in lethally irradiated, syngeneic mice. An analogous system was later (independently) described by Elson (1977). In this situation, new B cells first appear 8 days after irradiation and restoration, and reach normal numbers 2 weeks after that. Antigens acting as putative tolerogens were injected during the regeneration phase. A variety of antigens could be shown to be highly effective tolerogens in this situation.

This experimental design, of an entirely *in vivo* nature, was next supplemented by one where the tolerance was induced *in vitro*. Hapten-human γ globulin (HAP-HGG) was added to cultures of adult bone marrow, a site of rapid genesis of new B lymphocytes, and their capacity to mount an adoptive immune response was assessed (Nossal and Pike, 1975b). Control cultures showed an increased capacity for transferring immunity, as expected from their capacity to generate new B cells. This increase was substantially and specifically abrogated by nanomolar concentrations of antigen.

Subsequent work (Howard *et al.*, 1979) showed the adoptive immune assay to have serious drawbacks as a general tool for assessing B cell function, so we performed further studies using either newborn spleen (Stocker, 1977) or adult bone marrow and an *in vitro* read-out of B cell competence. Cells were first incubated with HAP-HGG *in vitro*; then washed and placed in microcultures at limiting dilution, and challenged with the T-independent antigen HAP-polymerized flagellin (HAP-POL), or with LPS acting as a polyclonal B cell activator (Nossal and Pike, 1976). This allowed accurate quantitation of the degree of tolerance induced, namely an exact enumeration of the number of anti-HAP B cells in the control population versus the putatively tolerized one. This work confirmed that immature B cell sources were far more susceptible to negative signalling than mature splenic B cells. A particularly telling experiment was the direct comparison of newborn and adult splenic B lympyhocytes that had been fractionated on HAP-gelatin dishes (Nossal and Pike, 1978b). These two cell populations were shown to have virtually identical spectra of antigen-binding avidities, yet displayed a 1000-fold difference in their capacity to be rendered tolerant.

Following the work of Metcalf and Klinman (1976), who showed a great sensitivity to tolerance induction amongst immature B cells using a T-dependent splenic microfocus B cell cloning system, we introduced this elegant tool into our laboratory. We were able to show that m-Ig negative cells, whether derived from foetal, newborn or adult sources, maturing to immunocompetence *in vitro*, passed through a phase of tolerance sensitivity as judged by this different assay as well (Teale *et al.*, 1978).

Having developed a great deal of confidence in B cell cloning assays as accurate and reproducible tools for the quantitation of B lymphocyte tolerance, we returned to a consideration of *in vivo* tolerance induction (Kay *et al.*, 1980). We injected adult or newborn mice with various doses of HAP-HGG, established serum antigen levels by trace labelling techniques, and killed mice at various intervals. Spleen cells were then tested for the numbers of anti-HAP B cells competent to react in the T-independent limiting dilution microculture cloning system. We showed that newborn animals were rendered tolerant by these criteria with 230-fold lower antigen concentrations than were adult animals.

In subsequent experiments, as yet unpublished, we followed in the steps of Waters *et al.* (1980) who introduced antigen into the foetal circulation via the placenta by intravenous injection of pregnant mice. Again using our clone frequency enumeration technology, we showed that the threshold for tolerance induction was 200 to 1000-fold lower than for the newborn when HAP-HGG was introduced 2 days prior to the first appearance of any B cells in the foetus, and thus 5000 to 23 000-fold lower than for adults. This was strong evidence that the pre-B to B transition period displayed still greater sensitivity to negative signalling than that phase when the B cell was already m-Ig positive but still immature. Of course, in the physiological situation, a potential "anti-self" B cell would first "see" antigen when m-Ig receptors were emerging during the pre-B to B transition, and not at the latter, somewhat less tolerance-sensitive phase. The molarity thresholds observed in our various model situations are summarized in Table I.

TABLE I
Molarity thresholds for tolerance induction using FLU_5-HGG[a]

	Initial serum conc.[b] c. *1 week* in vivo	*Culture conc.* *1 day* in vitro
Pre-B to B transition[c]	5×10^{-13} M	N.T.
Immature B cell[d]	5×10^{-10} M	$3{\cdot}6 \times 10^{-9}$ M
Mature B cell[e]	2×10^{-7} M	$1{\cdot}9 \times 10^{-7}$ M

[a] The hapten fluorescein coupled to human γ globulin at a ratio of 5 mol hapten to one of protein.
[b] As judged by trace labelling techniques.
[c] Mice injected at 14·5 days gestation, killed 3 days after birth and spleen cells challenged *in vitro* with FLU-polymerized flagellin.
[d] Newborn mice injected *in vivo* and tested 7 days later; or cultured for 1 day with tolerogen and challenged *in vitro*.
[e] Adult mice. Spleen cells tested.

The special sensitivity of immature cells of the B lineage has also been shown in numerous other systems (Metcalf and Klinman, 1976; Cambier *et al.*, 1977; Szewczuk and Siskind, 1977; Elson, 1977; McKearn and Quintans, 1980). Some aspects of this work have been reviewed elsewhere (Nossal *et al.*, 1978b). While an effect has thus been established with great clarity, it is necessary to refer now to some of the constraints limiting the generality of the phenomenon.

Constraints relating to clonal silencing of immature B cells

The valency constraint

Hapten valency has a major effect on the experimental results obtained when immature cells of the B lineage are exposed to tolerogens. In our early work, satisfactory results were obtained with HAP_1-HGG, but conjugates displaying this mean hapten frequency per mole would have contained many molecules with 2 or more haptens per protein molecule. Both Klinman's (Metcalf and Klinman, 1976) and Siskind's (Szewczuk and Siskind, 1977) groups have alluded to the need for multivalency in causing tolerance amongst immature B cells. Accordingly, we have tested fluorescein (FLU)-HGG at a mean substitution rate of 0·3 haptens per protein in the transplacental transfer system, a conjugate presumably poor in bi- or multivalent molecules. We have found this to be ineffective (unpublished results). We have also studied a great variety of multivalent conjugates for their capacity to silence B cells from newborn mouse spleen *in vitro* during 24 h incubation. The results (upper panel of Table II) show that tolerogenicity increased markedly with increased

TABLE II

Approximate protein concentrations of FLU-conjugates required to produce 50% reduction in clonable anti-FLU B lymphocytes in vitro[a]

Conjugate	*Concentration of conjugate (μg/ml)* *Newborn spleen*	*Adult spleen*	*Factorial difference*[b]
FLU_2HGG	16	98	6
FLU_5HGG	0·60	32	53
FLU_8HGG	0·19	4·5	24
$FLU_{12}HGG$	0·04	0·28	7
FLU_5FAB[c]	12	230	19
FLU_8FAB	0·80	4·8	6
$FLU_{12}FAB$	0·11	1·3	12
FLU_5BSA	10	60	6
$FLU_{12}BSA$	2·7	18	7

[a] Spleen cells were incubated for 24 h with various concentrations of the different conjugates and were then challenged with FLU-POL. The assay was for the development of FLU-specific PFC clones.
[b] Factor by which newborn cells were more sensitive than adult cells.
[c] Fluorescein conjugated to the $F(ab)'_2$ fragment of HGG.

hapten valency, not only for the more sensitive newborn cells, but even for mature adult splenic B cells.

This raises important questions about physiological mechanisms of self-tolerance. It suggests that receptor cross-linking is involved in signal generation, and that many autologous proteins, present in serum and extracellular fluids in monovalent form, may not cause self-tolerance by this mechanism unless they become associated with some cell membrane, thereby gaining an operational multivalency. Of course, many key "self" antigens are predominantly presented to the developing lymphoid system in multivalent form, such as the major histocompatibility complex determinants, which exist as cell membrane macromolecules.

The role of the carrier

The early work of Havas (1969) already showed that the nature of the protein carrier for a hapten could profoundly influence the capacity of hapten-protein conjugates to cause hapten-specific B cell tolerance. This line of work was extended by Golan and Borel (1971), who showed that certain Ig classes were especially favourable carriers. The question has been thoughtfully pursued by Diener's group, who have shown that apparently minor chemical changes can convert a tolerogenic carrier into a completely ineffective one (Diner and Diener, 1979). Recent work from this group is of special concern (Waters *et al.*, 1980). Using the transplacental route to introduce protein tolerogens, they found that while HGG worked well, many other proteins appeared to be entirely nontolerogenic, even at quite high dose, and even though transplacental transfer was proven.

We have investigated the role of the carrier to a limited extent in our *in vitro* tolerance induction model (Table II, lower two panels). At relatively low hapten density, e.g. 5 FLU residues per mol of protein, HGG is more effective than its $F(ab)'_2$ fragment or albumin. This lack of an Fc piece can be partially compensated for by increasing hapten valency. Interestingly, at high hapten valency, albumin is not nearly as effective as the $F(ab)'_2$ fragment, for reasons that are presently not clear.

In view of these constraints, it is certainly not possible to assert that clonal silencing of immature B cells is the major mechanism of self-tolerance within the B cell compartment. Furthermore, it has become eminently clear that no "all-or-none" difference exists between an immature, tolerance-susceptible cell and a mature, immunizable one. Rather, there is a gradation of sensitivities, with the pre-B to B transition at one extreme and the mature B cell at the other. Just how the carrier exerts such a profound role is obscure at present. We do not even know whether this reflects secondary events at the B cell surface after the hapten epitope has bound to the Ig receptor; or whether it is due to differential binding of carriers to some other cell, which then acts to present tolerogen to the B cell. When HGG acting as a carrier can bind via the Fc receptor as well as the Ig receptor, this obviously augments the tolerogenic signal. However, this cannot be a dominant effect, given the efficacy of FLU_{12}-FAB as a tolerogen. The availability of populations of fractionated hapten-specific B cells should allow at least some of these issues to be addressed experimentally.

Does tolerance induction involve deletion of the B cell?

The question of whether animals tolerant of a given antigen actually exhibit a lack or diminution of B cells with specificity for that antigen has been posed in a variety of models. We thought the availability of the FACS provided a more objective approach to the question than enumeration of (rare) antigen-binding cells by radioautographic or immunofluorescence methods. Accordingly, we induced nonreactivity by injections of FLU_5-HGG into foetal, newborn or adult mice, ensuring coverage of a wide range of dosages so that we always knew on which portion of the dose : response curve we were working. Unfortunately, one-step analysis of the situation by searching in the FACS for cells capable of binding various FLU-proteins proved unrewarding. Despite our attempts to introduce specificity by prelabelling cells with non-haptenated carrier; and though we varied the nature of the labelling conjugate, its concentration, and the parameters of the sorting procedure (including light-scattering characteristics) within wide limits, it proved impossible to validate the specificity of the sorted cells as FLU-reactive B cells by clonal analysis. Their capacity to yield anti-FLU PFC clones proved to be several times lower than that of cells pre-sorted by the HAP-gelatin procedure and then re-fractionated in the FACS to the same fluorescence intensity threshold. This discrepancy is due in part to the inclusion of nonlymphoid cells including eosinophils and monocytes in the one-step procedure; and to the influence of noncellular particulate matter and other machine artifacts when the sorter is asked to identify very rare cells. Accordingly, we adopted a two-cycle strategy for the enumeration and analysis of FLU-binding B cells. The number of hapten-binding cells was first established by counting the numbers of cells adhering specifically to FLU-gelatin dishes, and then their FLU-binding avidity profiles were measured in the FACS. This approach rapidly yielded clear-cut and reproducible results (Nossal and Pike, 1980).

When the mice were rendered tolerant with amounts of FLU-HGG greater than those required to produce maximal tolerance, there was a modest (30 to 50%) and transient reduction in anti-FLU B cell numbers, without any selective loss of high avidity cells. More importantly, when low concentrations of tolerogen were used, sufficient to induce substantial partial tolerance, there was no reduction whatever in FLU-binding B cells. In either situation, FLU-specific cells could be harvested from FLU-gelatin dishes, and shown to be incapable of responding to FLU-POL or to LPS. In other words, the immature B cells had received and stored some negative signal without having been eliminated, or without their receptors having been stripped from the cell. Furthermore, when cells were "caught" by tolerogen in the transition phase from pre-B cell to immature B cell, as in the transplacental induction experiments, the negative signal could be effectively registered without detriment to the emergence of the cell's m-Ig receptor coat.

Given that antigen-binding B cells incapable of reacting to antigen or mitogen can exist in an animal in a functionally silenced state, even when the antigen had been introduced into the foetus before any B cells had emerged, the process whereby such tolerance is induced is more accurately termed "clonal anergy" than "clonal abortion".

Basis of T lymphocyte tolerance

Four categories of T cells need to be considered in any analysis of T lymphocyte tolerance, namely those responsible for cell-mediated lympholysis, helper effects, suppressor effects and delayed hypersensitivity. Little is known about degrees of overlap amongst these populations, or about subsets within any one category. There is no doubt of the importance of suppressor cells in some models of tolerance, as has been amply demonstrated in other chapters of this volume. We were anxious to explore whether immature T cells, like immature B cells, were unduly sensitive to negative signalling by antigen. In adopting a conceptual approach similar to that for B cells, we were handicapped by two considerations. First, while a good deal is known about the effector cells of the above phenomena, much less is known about the "virgin" T lymphocytes that act as the antigen-activatable precursors of effector cells. Secondly, with the exception of cytotoxic T lymphocytes (CTL), functional cloning systems for accurate quantitation of the effects of various tolerogens are not yet available.

Accordingly, we have begun by studying tolerance to MHC antigens induced by injection of semi-allogeneic cells into newborn mice. We have been stimulated by the suggestion of Gorczynski and MacRae (1979) that, in this classical tolerance system, two sorts of T suppressor cells make their appearance, one responsible for preventing the conversion of bone marrow cells into competent, allogeneically reactive CTL precursors (CTL-P); and the other suppressing the conversion of CTL-P into CTL. It has occurred to us that detailed analysis of this suggestion can be performed at limiting dilution. If the phenotype of a T lymphocyte population is suppressor, those suppressor cells have to be removed in some way before the population can be examined for its content of CTL-P. We do not yet know enough about the cell surface phenotypes of the various populations of T cells to be confident about achieving this with isoantisera and complement, so one good way of approaching the problem is to ensure that the suppressor cells are so diluted out that they cannot exert any action on the CTL-P, if present.

Our experiments on limiting dilution analysis of CTL-P from tolerant mice are based on the prior work of Skinner and Marbrook (1976) and Lindahl and Wilson (1977). Newborn CBA mice were injected with 5×10^7 CBA $\times$ BALB/c F_1 adult spleen cells (or with CBA $\times$ C57Bl F_1 spleen cells as a control). The mice were killed 1–8 weeks later and small numbers of thymus or spleen cells were cultured in 96-well microculture trays with 4×10^5 3000 rad-irradiated BALB/c spleen cells in the presence of T cell growth factor derived from the supernatant of concanavalin A-stimulated spleen cells. After 7 days, the cultures were harvested and individually assayed for their capacity to lyse ^{51}Cr-labelled P 815 mastocytoma cells. The CTL-P frequency was calculated by Poisson analysis.

TABLE III

Cytotoxic lymphocyte precursors in organs of tolerant mice[a]

	CTL-P per 10^6 *cells reactive against P815 (H2-d)*		
	$(CBA \times C_{57})F_1$ *injected-Control*	$(CBA \times BALB/c)F_1$ *injected-Tolerant*	
2-week thymus	53·9	4·68	(8·7%)
2-week spleen	277	193	(69·7%)
6-week thymus	324	32·8	(10·1%)
6-week spleen	1470	115	(7·8%)

[a] Newborn CBA mice were injected with 5×10^7 semi-allogeneic spleen cells, and later their spleens and thymuses were examined by limiting dilution analysis for CTL-P reactive against H2-d MHC antigens. Cultures were supported by T cell growth factor. ^{51}Cr release of P815 cells was measured.

Some typical results are given in Table III. It is evident that, as well as any suppression that may have been induced, there was a marked diminution in activatable anti-BALB/c CTL-P in both thymus and spleen at 6 weeks, and in the thymus at 2 weeks. Whether this represented their destruction through early contact with antigen; their functional silencing through a mechanism akin to B cell clonal anergy; the *in vivo* action of a suppressor cell preventing their creation; or some mixture of these phenomena, remains to be determined. The CTL-P purging or silencing is manifest very early, preliminary results (not shown) suggesting a defect in clonable CTL-P already at one week in the thymus. This may speak for a mechanism directly mediated by antigen rather than one dependent on the prior *in vivo* creation of suppressor cells interfering with correct CTL-P ontogeny. The point is certainly moot, however, and deserving of critical study.

As a next phase of this work, we intend to use HAP-HGG as a tolerogen for HAP-specific CTL-P, using the generation of clones of anti-HAP CTL as the assay system. This would allow a more direct comparison of relative tolerizability of T versus B lymphocytes than has been possible before.

Summary

Now that the phenotypic diversity of lymphocytes has been clearly established, an understanding of the regulation of the immune response must centre around the diversity of signals to which lymphocytes respond. These include signals received from antigens, from other lymphocytes, from accessory cells, and from serum factors including antibodies and immune complexes. This paper has concentrated on negative signals engendered by antigens acting on immature lymphocytes. It has shown that certain antigens acting on immature cells can markedly depress the capacity of corresponding B lymphocytes to be triggered by antigen or mitogen. This functional silencing is not accompanied by destruction of the cell, or by blockade or modulation of its m-Ig receptors. Instead, it appears that such early contact with antigen can induce a profound clonal anergy. The most sensitive phase of the B cell's life history appears to be the pre-B cell to B cell transition, when m-Ig receptors are first appearing. Anergy can be induced without impairing the appearance of a normal m-Ig receptor coat.

Less is known about the effects of antigenic signalling on immature T lymphocytes, but preliminary results are consistent with the view that the precursors of cytotoxic lymphocytes can also be rendered anergic (or eliminated) through early contact with antigen.

References

Andersson, J., Coutinho, A. and Melchers, F. (1979). *J. Exp. Med.* **149**, 553.
Andersson, J., Schreier, M. H. and Melchers, F. (1980). *Proc. Natn. Acad. Sci. U.S.A.* **77**, 1612.
Bretscher, P. and Cohn, M. (1970). *Science* **169**, 1042.
Burnet, F. M. (1957). *Austral. J. Sci.* **20**, 67.
Cambier, J. C., Vitetta, E. S., Uhr, J. W. and Kettman, J. R. (1977). *J. Exp. Med.* **145**, 778.
Diener, E. and Paetkau, V. H. (1972). *Proc. Natn. Acad. Sci. U.S.A.* **69**, 2364.
Diner, U. and Diener, E. (1979). *J. Immunol.* **122**, 1886.
Elson, C. J. (1977). *Eur. J. Immunol.* **7**, 6.
Fu, S. M., Chiorazzi, N., Hurley, J. N., Halper, J. P. and Kunkel, H. G. (1979). *In* "Cells of Immunoglobulin Synthesis" (B. Pernis and H. J. Vogel, eds) pp. 127–139. Academic Press, New York.
Golan, D. T. and Borel, Y. (1971). *J. Exp. Med.* **136**, 1046.
Gorczynski, R. M. and MacRae, S. (1979). *J. Immunol.* **122**, 747.
Haas, W. and Layton, J. E. (1975). *J. Exp. Med.* **141**, 1004.
Havas, H. F. (1969). *Immunology* **17**, 819.
Howard, M. C., Fidler, J. M., Baker, J. and Shortman, K. (1979). *J. Immunol.* **122**, 309.
Kay, T. W., Pike, B. L. and Nossal, G. J. V. (1980). *J. Immunol.* **124**, 1579.
Lindahl, K. F. and Wilson, D. B. (1977). *J. Exp. Med.* **145**, 508.
McKearn, J. P. and Quintans, J. (1980). *J. Immunol.* **124**, 77.
Metcalf, D., Nossal, G. J. V., Warner, N. L., Miller, J. F. A. P., Mandel, T. E., Layton, J. E. and Gutman, G. A. (1975). *J. Exp. Med.* **142**, 1534.
Metcalf, E. S. and Klinman, N. R. (1976). *J. Exp. Med.* **143**, 1327.
Möller, G. (1975). *Transplant. Rev.* **23**, 126.
Nossal, G. J. V. and Pike, B. L. (1975a). *In* "Immunological Aspects of Neoplasia" (E. M. Hersch and M. Schlamowitz, eds) pp. 87–101. Williams and Wilkins, Baltimore.
Nossal, G. J. V. and Pike, B. L. (1975b). *J. Exp. Med.* **141**, 904.
Nossal, G. J. V. and Pike, B. L. (1976). *Immunology* **30**, 189.
Nossal, G. J. V. and Pike, B. L. (1978a). *J. Immunol.* **120**, 145.
Nossal, G. J. V. and Pike, B. L. (1978b). *J. Exp. Med.* **148**, 1161.
Nossal, G. J. V. and Pike, B. L. (1980). *Proc. Natn. Acad. Sci. U.S.A.* **77**, 1602.
Nossal, G. J. V., Pike, B. L. and Battye, F. L. (1978a). *Eur. J. Immunol.* **8**, 151.

Nossal, G. J. V., Pike, B. L., Teale, J. M., Layton, J. E., Kay, T. W. and Battye, F. L. (1978b). *Immunol. Rev.* **43**, 185.
Pike, B. L. and Nossal, G. J. V. (1976). *J. Exp. Med.* **144**, 568.
Schrader, J. W. (1974). *Eur. J. Immunol.* **4**, 20.
Schrader, J. W. and Nossal, G. J. V. (1980). *Immunol. Rev.* (in press).
Shiozawa, C., Longenecker, M. B. and Diener, E. (1980). *J. Immunol.* **125**, 68.
Shortman, K., Howard, M. C. and Baker, J. A. (1978). *J. Immunol.* **121**, 2060.
Skinner, M. A. and Marbrook, J. (1976). *J. Exp. Med.* **143**, 1562.
Stocker, J. W. (1977). *Immunology* **32**, 283.
Szewczuk, M. R. and Siskind, G. W. (1977). *J. Exp. Med.* **145**, 1590.
Teale, J. M., Howard, M. C. and Nossal, G. J. V. (1978). *J. Immunol.* **121**, 2561.
Waters, C. A., Diener, E. and Singh, B. (1980). *J. Exp. Med.* (in press).

10

Diversity 1980

MELVIN COHN, RODNEY LANGMAN and WILLIAM GECKELER

Developmental Biology Laboratory, The Salk Institute, San Diego, California

Would that GOD were not constructed from minutely composed particulars!
Mechkonik

This work has been supported by Allergy and Infectious Disease Grant (A-105875) to Dr M. Cohn.

What is an antibody?

An antibody is an effector molecule with specific recognition capabilities, the expression of which is inducible or paralysable. This latter property, referred to as the "self–nonself discrimination", distinguishes antibodies from other specific binding proteins of protective value found in invertebrates and plants. This definition makes no assumptions about the chemistry of antibodies, some of which are known to be immunoglobulins while others are of an as yet unknown nonimmunoglobulin structure.

Why is antibody not a universal glue?

Antibody must have a sufficient specific recognition capability to make the self–nonself discrimination. The necessity to make the self–nonself discrimination is the unique evolutionary selection pressure which drives the immune system to increase the specificity of antibodies.

Why is antibody not absolutely specific?

As specificity increases, the number of different antibodies required to deal with the universe of antigens must increase (Perelson and Oster, 1979). This in turn means that more genes must be carried in the germ line. As the number of germ line genes increases, the concomitant evolution of a regulatory system becomes exponentially more difficult. In addition, the selective pressures for the maintenance of each and every gene as the numbers increase becomes less and less effective. Hence, a counterselection is set up which limits the total number. As a consequence the actual number of genes carried in the germ line is determined by a balance between a selective pressure tending to increase specificity (driven by the self–nonself discrimination) and one tending to

Abbreviations
The nomenclature in this chapter differs from other chapters in the use of lower case roman letters (v) for genes and capital letters for regions (V).

decrease specificity (driven by difficulties due to the complexity of conserving the structure and of regulating the expression of germ line genes). The antibody molecule, therefore, is a compromise determined by these counter selective forces and it ends up with a degree of cross-reactivity compatible with a non-crippling level of autoimmunity. Clearly it is a sophism to conclude that "self-reactive cells cannot be deleted without the complete loss of the immune system" (Coutinho, 1979). Evolution may not have yielded the perfect solution but, unlike "Big A" it did provide one.

Why are there two classes of antibody: humoral and cell-mediated?

Antibody carries out 2 roles: protective and regulatory. The protective role requires 2 classes of antibody to deal with 2 classes of infectious disease. The regulatory functions determine the self–nonself discrimination as well as the class and magnitude of the response.

Humoral antibody is immunoglobulin secreted by induced bone marrow-derived B cells, i.e. plasmacytes. This antibody is the best characterized and has as its major protective role, defence against extracellular pathogens, e.g. bacteria, fungi, protozoa, helminths. Cell-mediated antibody is non-immunoglobulin acting as the receptor on effector cells which are thymus-derived. T cells are concerned with ridding intracellular pathogens, e.g. viruses, rickettsia, certain bacteria, tumourigenic cells.

TABLE I
Effector function—restricting element relationships

Effector T cell	*Category*	*H-2 encoded restricting element*[a]
T^S (suppressor)	Regulatory	K/D
T^K (killer)	Protective	K/D
T^H (helper)	Regulatory	I
T^{DH} (delayed hypersensitive)	Protective	I

[a] See discussion, Cohn and Epstein (1978).

Humoral antibody plays its regulatory role via antigen-specific feedback which can enhance or inhibit immune responsiveness. However, because of a fundamental asymmetry, i.e. T cells are required for the induction of B cells, not vice versa, the hegemony of regulatory T cells is undisputed in controlling the induction of responsiveness, i.e. the self–nonself discrimination and the class of the response. The key to understanding their function whether protective or regulatory (Table I) is that they mediate precisely controlled cell–cell signalling interactions.

These fundamentally different roles account for the distinct structural properties of humoral and cell-mediated antibody, one being immunoglobulin and the other nonimmunoglobulin in nature.

What properties must the humoral and cell-mediated antibody classes possess in common?

The above considerations dictate that:

(1) For each class, the effective range of specificities as well as the effective degree of specificity of individual antibodies must be the same. However, the dictionaries may be different. It is generally assumed, that the T cell repertoire is "both smaller than the B cell repertoire and less complete" (Jerne, 1979). It is hard to see why this idea is so popular since it is neither experimentally nor biologically based (Cohn, 1972, p. 17).

(2) Within each class, any specific recognition site must be capable of being physically coupled to any given effector function, protective or regulatory. Since the number of effector functions are few and the number of specific recognition sites are many, mechanisms for coupling them must be envisaged. Although the understanding of this mechanism has been the major triumph of recent biochemical studies, we will not consider this aspect. Rather we wish to concentrate on the origin of the combining site repertoire, a problem only partially solvable by biochemistry.

In order to do this we must first take a look at a stylized humoral immunoglobulin antibody and compare it with a stylized cell-mediated antibody.

What are the key structural elements of humoral antibody?

This molecule (with variations) is the antigen-specific receptor on B cells as well as the humoral antibody product which interact both with antigen and a variety of effector systems, e.g. complement, macrophages, basophils, etc.

The following elements of its structure are relevant to our discussion (Fig. 1).

(1) Humoral antibody is a polymer of 2 nonidentical subunits, L and H. Its unit structure is $(LH)_2$. Each subunit is comprised of domains which at the protein level are functional units of folding (Gally and Edelman, 1970) and at the DNA level are units of coding (exons) separated by intervening sequences (introns) from other exons which comprise the transcription unit (Tonegawa *et al.*, 1978; Sakano *et al.*, 1979).

(2) Humoral antibody possesses 2 or more identical combining sites. Multivalence of the immunoglobulin molecule has two consequences:

(a) The selectivity for a given antigen is greatly increased by multiple identical interactions. While a monovalent interaction with 2 cross-reacting antigens might show but little selectivity for one of them,

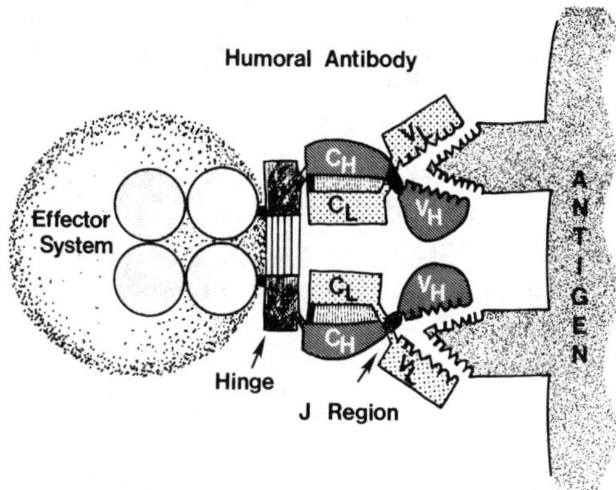

FIG. 1. *A stylized (Jaws 2 model) humoral (immunoglobulin) antibody.*

polygamous interactions greatly increases the selectivity or ability to discriminate (Ehrlich, 1979). Thus, low intrinsic affinity can still be important.

(b) Any effector function mediated by aggregation of the immunoglobulin requires at least bivalency.

(3) The combining site is made up of 2 nonidentical domains (V_LV_H). This allows, in principle, an expansion of the repertoire by $pv_L \times qv_H$ germ line encoded combinations which also act as starting points for somatic evolution. However, in fact, the starting repertoire is less than $pv_L \times qv_H$ because not all V_L regions function well with all V_H regions. There is a preferential V_LV_H fit (dePreval and Fougereau, 1976).

(4) The V regions are made up of complementarity-determining (CD) and framework (FW) residues. FW residues encoded by any given v gene are as invariant as those encoded by the c gene, i.e. the observed replacements in FW residues are due to mutations in the germ line whereas those in CD residues are due to mutations in the soma.

(5) The J region which joins V and C has been singled out by the discovery that it is encoded by a j gene separated in the germ line by noncoding sequences both from the v and c genes (Brack *et al.*, 1978; Bernard *et al.*, 1978). It was never revealed as a structurally important entity (domain?) by X-ray crystallographers or immunochemists until Tonegawa *et al.* (1978) proposed the concept that domains in a protein are encoded by exons which evolve separated by intervening sequences (introns). Ohno (1980) has suggested that the j gene was derived, during germ line evolution, from a leader sequence which was separated by an intron from the c gene but expressed at the protein level as part of the C region, e.g. at a time in evolution when the C region encoded a $\beta 2$ microglobulin. This permits an analogy between the J sequence (joiner) and the H sequence (hinge). The hinge domain was derived in

evolution from a larger ancestral domain, the present day derivative of which is still present in 2 classes of immunoglobulin, IgM and IgE (Tucker *et al.*, 1978).

There are several roles we might attribute to the J sequence:

(a) It might contribute directly to the repertoire of combining sites by introducing amino acid diversity in CD residues by combinational joining (pV × mJ) (Weigert *et al.*, 1978) as well as by intracodonic recombination at the vj junction in what might be part of the CD3 region (Bernard *et al.*, 1978).

(b) It might modulate the combining site by introducing rotational and angular flexibility in the interaction of V_LV_H domains with an antigenic determinant.

(c) It might be homologous in function to the hinge region which links C_{H1} to C_{H2} in *cis* and stabilizes H–H interactions in *trans*. The J region might play a similar role for V–C linking in *cis* and LH interactions in *trans* (Stevens *et al.*, 1980).

(d) It might play its principal role at the DNA and RNA level; its role at the level of protein structure being simply framework.

These roles are not mutually exclusive. Rather their relative importance in contributing to the combining site repertoire should be considered. We will argue that the contribution to the combining site repertoire as a consequence of an effect on primary (immunodominant) ligand interactions by combinatorial and junctional amino acid replacements in CD residues, is second order compared to somatic mutation (postulated role (a)). The contribution due to effects on the size and flexibility of the combining site is probably significant (postulated role (b)). Roles (c) and (d) make no contribution to combining site diversity but are major for the production of a functional molecule.

The question we must consider is whether given amino acid residues contribute to combining site recognition in a sufficiently unique way to add that antibody to the count of the size of the repertoire. The V_L and V_H domains sense unrelated structures in different relative geometries on the antigenic determinant. Since there is no way that the immune system can predict the stereochemical or topological relationship between the 2 unrelated subsites which V_L and V_H sense, a given pair of V_L and V_H domains must have rotational and angular flexibility in their interaction with antigenic determinants. If this is the primary contribution of the J region to the repertoire of combining sites, most of its effect would be equivalent to that of a framework region i.e., a second-order contribution.

(6) The C_LC_{H1} *trans* interaction stabilizes the V_LV_H *trans* interaction. The Fab is linked to the Fc region via the H domain (hinge) which links the LH monomers together as $(LH)_2$ in a way which permits angular and rotational flexibility in the interactions of Fab with antigen. The Fc region is responsible for effector function interactions.

The v gene is carried in the germ line as a contiguous coding sequence of some 300 bases. The j gene to which to the v gene is transposed encodes 10–15 amino acid residues (Brack *et al.*, 1978). The c gene encodes the remainder of the subunit.

The j gene is that remarkable segment of DNA which, at its 5′ end, carries splicing sequences for v–j fusion, a DNA level event, and at its 3′ end carries splicing sequences for intron excision, an RNA level event (Bernard *et al.*, 1978; Max *et al.*, 1979; Perry *et al.*, 1979). Ohno (1980) has introduced the captivating idea that the DNA level v–j fusion mechanism was derived during evolution from the RNA intron excision mechanism.

The leader sequence has not been considered in our analysis because it plays no role in the problem of combining site diversity.

What are the key structural elements of cell-mediated antibody?

Cell-mediated antibody, acting as a receptor on the effector T cell, must solve a problem quite different from that of humoral antibody. The cell-mediated system is concerned with cell–cell interactions which lead to signals to the target, be they lytic (to a virus infected cell, i.e. protective) or inductive/suppressive (to an antigen-sensitive cell which has bound antigen, i.e. regulatory).

There is no biochemistry of cell-mediated antibody so that we must derive its structure from physiology. This is most easily illustrated with the cytotoxic T cell but the arguments are applicable equally to regulatory T cells, such as helpers and suppressors.

The simplest interaction one can envisage is between an antigen specific receptor on the effector T cell and a surface bound determinant, e.g. a virus, on the target. As illustrated (Fig. 2A), the cell–cell interaction, requiring an antibody–antigen interaction only, leads to a lytic signal from the effector T cell to the target. Clearly, this formulation is incomplete. The efficiency and the specificity of delivery of the signal would be too low because:

(1) The effector T cell would waste its signalling function on free antigen which also would compete with cell-bound antigen.

(2) The signal would be delivered to innocent bystanders if no special mechanism is envisaged.

Consequently, all target cells must carry a flag which says "I am a cell". This flag which is referred to as a restricting element, R, must be recognized by the T cell receptor (Fig. 2B). It is this interaction which distinguishes the B cell receptor (humoral antibody) from the T cell receptor (cell-mediated antibody). We know that the restricting element is encoded in the major histocompatibility complex (MHC) and that a fundamental dichotomy in function exists between T cells recognizing K/D or I (Table I). Even as pictured in Fig. 2B, the model remains incomplete in a fundamental way. In order to

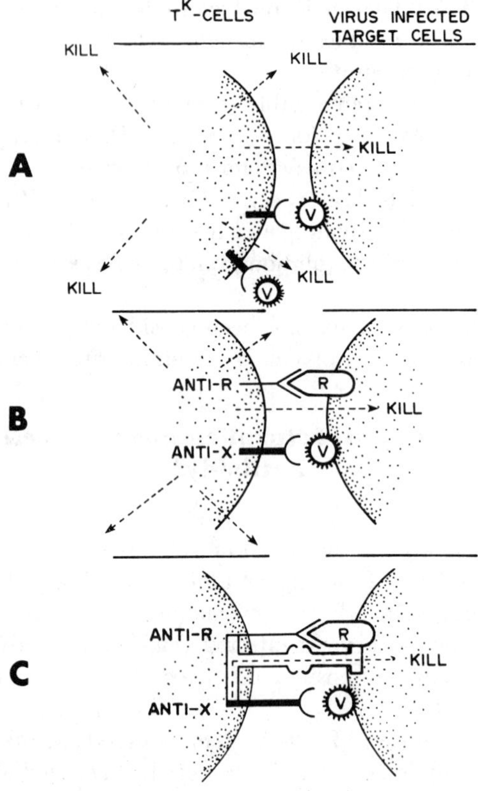

FIG. 2. *A stylized (Jaws 1 model) cell-mediated (nonimmunoglobulin) antibody. Stages A, B and C in analysing the effector mechanism of restrictive recognition of antigen by the T^K cell. V = virus; R = restricting element (in mouse H-2 encoded K/D or I): Note that anti-R (thin line) and anti-X (thick line) have different constant regions.*

maintain the specificity of the signal, i.e. avoid an innocent bystander effect, we must complete our picture of the T cell receptor (Fig. 2C) (Langman, 1978; Cohn and Epstein, 1978) as follows:

The effector T cell receptor must consist of 3 physically linked elements, anti-R, anti-X and a signal donor. The anti-R and the anti-X sites must be nonoverlapping and be coupled to different constant regions since the separation of their functions must be maintained.

The target or antigen-sensitive cell must possess 2 elements which are physically independent, an R element linked to a signal acceptor and an antigen-X bound to the target cell membrane directly or to the receptor on the antigen-sensitive cell.

The function of anti-R is to bring R coupled to its acceptor into a signalling channel or synapse. The function of anti-X is to activate the signal donor when it interacts with antigen X.

Unbound or free X does not inhibit significantly because (1) the signal donor–signal acceptor interaction is irreversible and (2) anti-R interacting with R is not inhibitable by free X making competition by free X for the receptor structure unfavourable.

Whether or not one accepts this particular formulation, all models require that R be linked to a signal acceptor and that the two sites anti-R and anti-X be physically linked, associated with different constant regions and non-overlapping.

TABLE II
Characterization of effector antibody

	Humoral antibody	*Cell mediated antibody*
Definition	Secreted from cell which makes it	Receptor of cell which makes it
Number of combining sites per unit	$\geqslant$2 *identical* sites	Two *nonidentical* sites physically linked; one anti-R and one anti-X
Number of subunits per combining site	Two ($V_L V_H$)	One (V_R or V_X)
Effector function	Property of C_H domains interacting with an effector system	Property of cell in which the relationship between the R-class (K/D or I) and effector function ($T^{K(S)}$ or $T^{H(DH)}$) is programmed during ontogeny
Signal transduction	Conformational change in many cases leading to activation of effector system via aggregation	Conformational change activating T cell to deliver a signal from donor to an R-linked acceptor on target
Genetic encoding	Known v_L and v_H gene loci	Locus not known. Unlikely to be any of those encoding humoral antibody
Germ line encoded combining specificities	Antipathogen (extracellular bacteria to helminth)	Antispecies-R and antipathogen (intracellular virus to bacteria)
Somatic encoded combining specificities (anti-X)	Derived by mutation and selection from germ line $pv_L \times qv_H$ encoding $V_L V_H$	Derived by mutation and selection from germ line genes encoding the monomer antiallo-R and antipathogen

A comparison of the humoral and cell-mediated antibodies might be made as shown in Table II. The humoral system was derived in evolution from the cell-mediated system, yet today these 2 systems have properties different enough to make us envisage that they are encoded by distinct loci. Although we can expect similar pathways of diversification, we will conclude that cell-mediated antibody has each of its combining sites, anti-R and anti-X, made up of a single subunit or V region, unlike humoral antibody which has a combining site comprised of two subunits, V_L and V_H. The consequences of this for the control of expression and generation of diversity in each class of antibody is the theme of our discussion.

What is the relationship between amino acid and combining site diversity?

The fundamental distinction between complementarity-determining (CD) and framework (FW) residues has been overlooked (Kindt and Capra, 1978; Seidman *et al.*, 1978a, b, 1979; Schilling *et al.*, 1980; Weigert *et al.*, 1978, 1980) in the recent flurry following the discovery that amino acid sequence diversity can be generated (1) by intracodonic recombination at vj or vdj junctions and (2) by combinatorial joining (pV × mJ) of a given V with several J's.

An analysis of the data on amino acid sequence diversity requires criteria for determining which residues are complementarity-determining (CD) and which are framework (FW). A complementarity-determining (CD) residue is one for which the pattern of replacements results in changes in the combining specificity without affecting the integrity of the molecule as a functional antibody. In principle, replacements in CD residues can affect specificity directly by *contact* with the ligand or indirectly by a *conformational* change in the combining site.

A framework (FW) residue is one for which the pattern of replacements has no effect (to be qualified later) on combining specificity. Given the nature of our available assays, replacements in the framework appear as neutral. We have no way at present to detect improved or deleterious effects on effector function as the consequence of a FW replacement.

This has led to a rather naïve view of the arrangement of CD and FW residues but it has given yeoman's service. It is usual to refer to CD regions which are viewed as contiguous stretches of residues comprising the combining site itself. There are 6 such regions, 3 contributed by the light and 3 by the heavy chain. The CD regions are linked coherently by contiguous FW regions, 4 contributed by the light and 4 by the heavy chain. The homologous FW regions in different antibodies are viewed as equivalent in their function which is

(1) to position CD residues in the combining site while allowing structural flexibility.
(2) to provide *trans* interactions between V_L and V_H.
(3) to provide *cis* interactions between V and C.
(4) to permit the transmission of signals that a combining site–ligand interaction has occurred.

The idealized picture is that any given set of CD segments when sewn into any set of homologous FW segments would result in absolutely equivalent antibodies both with respect to function and combining specificity. However, this picture is too simple because CD residues are the units of variation which generate combining site diversity, not CD regions. Further the FW regions must (1) contribute in determining which positions are CD, and (2) influence the topology (size, flexibility, contour) of the combining site.

These subtleties of structure make it all the more important that we understand the criteria for deciding which residues are CD and which are FW so that we can weigh the contribution of each ot the diversity of the repertoire. Three criteria have been used:

(1) The Kabat-Wu variability analysis (Kabat, 1978; Kabat *et al.*, 1979).

(2) X-ray analysis (Poljak *et al.*, 1976; Padlan, 1977; Amzel and Poljak, 1979).

(3) Pedigree analysis (Weigert *et al.*, 1970; Cesari and Weigert, 1973; Weigert *et al.*, 1978; McKean and Potter, 1979; Weigert *et al.*, 1980).

Pioneering in 1970, the Kabat–Wu variability plot is of limited value today. The reason is that this type of analysis is inherently unable to provide a criterion as to whether a given residue in a given V region is CD or FW. The variability analysis averages out the role of different FW's in determining which residues are CD and reveals, therefore, regions of "hypervariability" rather than discrete positions. Only under a somatic mutation model would residues in hypervariable regions be expected to be CD on *a priori* grounds (Weigert *et al.*, 1970; Cohn, 1973). In order to account for hypervariability of CD residues, *the* germ-line model requires selection on the FW and neutral drift in CD regions (Smith, 1973). This prediction is known now to be wrong. Other models do not *per se* predict hypervariability of CD residues with respect to FW. However, even under a somatic mutation model, while a CD position would be hypervariable with respect to its framework, the converse (i.e. a hypervariable position would be CD) is of limited validity (Cohn, 1974). Nevertheless, with a certain amount of judgement in equating "hypervariability" and CD and keeping in mind the theory that this equation depends upon, the variability plot has been a helpful tool.

The X-ray studies, in principle, should give us precise data. Unfortunately, they are too few and must be extended by model building which is dependent on many guesses that are not uninfluenced by the variability and pedigree analyses. Further (and probably the major limitation), no site-filling ligands have been studied and of course there is no way to derive what this ligand would be, given the X-ray defined topology of the combining site. Therefore, while X-ray analysis reveals contact residues as distinct from conformational residues (both of the CD category) it underestimates them. How accurate and how general, i.e. how framework-independent, contact residue designations are, remains to be seen. Nevertheless, X-ray studies leave us with a general picture similar to that arrived at by variability analysis.

Lastly, we have pedigree analysis which provides the most clear-cut and general criteria but it depends on a theory which, to date, has limited its acceptance by the immunological community.

For a pedigree analysis, one must start with the germ line v gene. In practice, if an amino acid sequence of a V region produced by independently isolated clones (plasmacytomas or hybridomas) has occurred several times, it is assumed to be encoded by a germ line v gene. Of course the larger the number of repeat sequences, the greater the certainty. In the case of $v_{\lambda 1}$, $v_{\kappa 21B}$ and $v_{\kappa 21C}$, this criterion has been confirmed by DNA sequencing of the germ line v gene (Bernard *et al.*, 1978; Heinrich and Tonegawa, pers. comm.).

Under a somatic mutation model, a CD position may be defined by pedigree analysis because it is assumed that an amino acid replacement would have a low probability of being seen unless it were selected for by antigen. Thus, CD positions should be revealed if the somatic variants of a single germ line gene are analysed. The $v_{\lambda 1}$ and $v_{\kappa 21}$ germ line genes and their somatic variants are examples.

These points are illustrated in Fig. 3 where data derived from the 3 analyses are compared.

While the variability plot (Kabat *et al.*, 1979) defined CD regions (indicated by 3 solid lines under plot) in an average FW sequence, the criterion which relates "variability" to a given CD position in a given FW sequence is imprecise. Our arbitrary cut-off value of variability equal to 45 that excludes all likely FW positions is indicated to illustrate this. We will use this as our criterion for "hypervariability" aware of course that more sophisticated statistical analyses are available to us.

The positions in $V_{\lambda 1}$ designated as contact residues by X-ray analyses and model building are dashed vertical lines (Poljak *et al.*, 1976). All CD positions defined by X-ray analyses are hypervariable but not all hypervariable positions are CD by X-ray criteria. In fact no positions in CD2 are defined as contact residues by X-ray analyses. In the case of V_κ only position 96 has been designated tentatively as a contact residue (Padlan, 1977). In both λ and κ this position is encoded by the first codon of the j gene. From the point of view of X-ray analysis, this is the only residue, out of the 13 encoded by the j gene, which might contribute to combining site diversity. Direct binding evidence for this is lacking. In any case an argument can be made from X-ray data that junctional, not combinatorial, amino acid diversity contributes to the repertoire of combining sites.

How do the somatic descendents of a single germ line v gene behave?

Considering $v_{\lambda 1}$ first (Fig. 3), the germ line $v_{\lambda 1}$ gene codes for such a distinct light chain that its somatic derivatives are easy to identify particularly since most differ by only 1 or 2 bases.

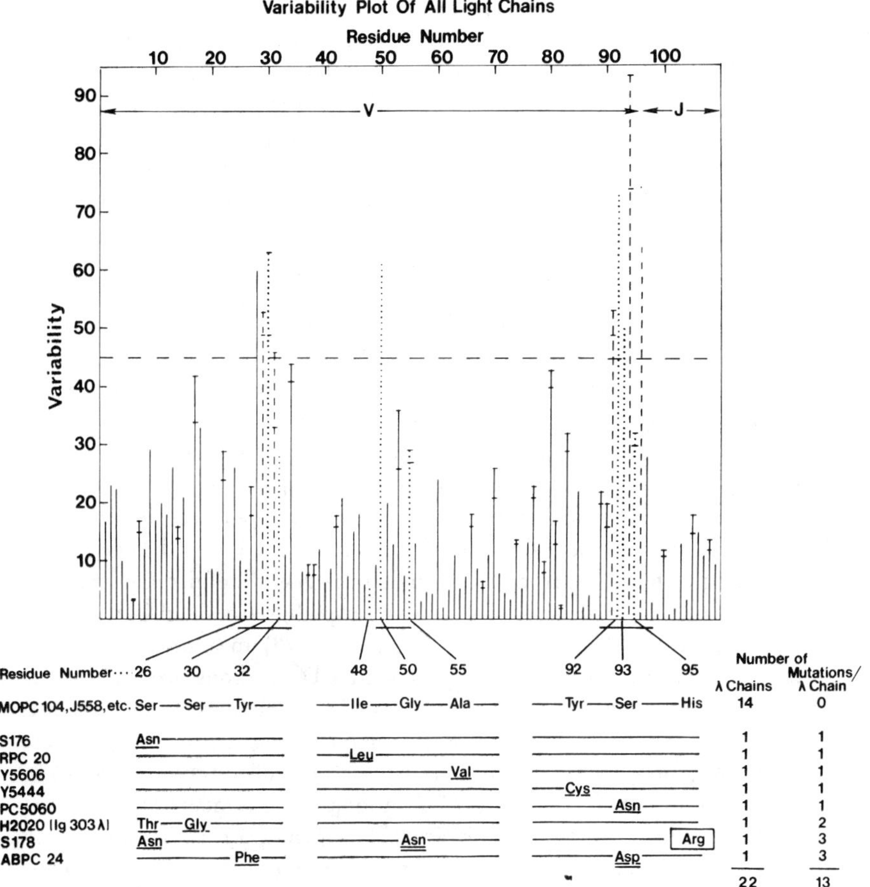

FIG. 3. *The comparison of a variability, X-ray and pedigree determination of complementarity-determining residues.*

Variability analysis (*Kabat* et al., *1979*). *Number of different amino acids at a given position; variability = frequency of the most common amino acid at that position.*

X-ray analysis (*Poljak* et al., *1976*). *The X-ray assignment of CD positions are indicated by vertical dashed lines* (---).

Pedigree analysis (*Weigert* et al., *1970; Cesari and Weigert, 1973*). *The assignment of CD residues by pedigree analysis are indicated by vertical dotted lines* (....). *The underlining of the amino acid replacements indicates the required number of base changes (mutational steps) in the germ line v gene codon. The placing of Arg (position 95) in a box indicates that it was derived by somatic vj recombination not mutation.*

Ig303λ is a DNA clone of the $v\lambda_1$ *region of myeloma H2020 sequenced by Bernard* et al., *1978. The myelomas from which the sequences were derived, are indicated on the left.*

The conclusions are:

(1) The $\lambda 1$ locus contains one germ line $v_{\lambda 1}$, $j_{\lambda 1}$, and $c_{\lambda 1}$ gene. The germ line $v_{\lambda 1}$ gene encodes to position 95; the germ line $j_{\lambda 1}$ gene encodes positions 96–108, the $c_{\lambda 1}$ gene encodes the remainder. The germ line $v_{\lambda 1}$ gene encodes the amino acid sequence which has been found 14 times out of 22 independent isolates. Since the nucleotide sequence of the germ line $v_{\lambda 1}$ and $j_{\lambda 1}$ gene is known (Bernard *et al.*, 1978) there is no doubt that the 14 repeats are germ line encoded. This interpretation of repeat sequences ia a central assumption of pedigree analyses.

(2) The $j_{\lambda 1}$ gene has been expressed invariant in 22/22 chains; identical in behaviour to the $c_{\lambda 1}$ gene.

(3) Thirteen base replacements due to somatic mutation have been detected by sequencing the 8 variant $\lambda 1$ chains. This has been confirmed by sequencing the DNA of the germ line $v_{\kappa 1}$ gene and somatic variant H2020 (Ig 3032) (Bernard *et al.*, 1978). In addition there is one amino acid replacement encoded by the last codon 95 of $v_{\lambda 1}$ which was varied by recombination during translocation of v to j.

(4) The 13 mutational replacements in the $v_{\lambda 1}$ gene are in "regions" defined both by X-ray and variability analysis as CD but the correlation at close quarters is far from good. In fact the X-ray defined CD positions (Poljak *et al.*, 1976) do not coincide with the pedigree defined CD positions (Weigert *et al.*, 1970; Cesari and Weigert, 1973) in a single case. Surprisingly, in all cases, the X-ray defined CD positions are adjacent to the pedigree defined CD positions. Since X-ray defines contact residues and pedigree defines complementarity-determining residues (contact and conformational), this one position displacement of assignments could be fundamental (implying that conformational replacements are more important in contributing to repertoire diversity than contact replacements) or artefactual (implying that the X-ray assignments derived from model building or the pedigree assignments derived from somatic mutation theory are incorrect).

(5) The 13 mutational replacements are argued to be CD. At the extremes either a low frequency "uniform", or a high frequency "CD specific" mutation mechanism operates on v genes. In the first case, the only way to see a mutant would be by antigenic selection for a change in combining specificity; in the second case the assumption itself defines CD positions.

(6) Since somatic replacements in FW would appear unselected or deleterious, they would be too rare to be detected. This essentially is the argument that the FW is germ line encoded. It is the same argument used to explain why somatic replacements in the C region are not found and why replacements in the C region are interpreted as germ line encoded i.e. allotypes, isotypes.

(7) Some positions such as 26, 50 and 93 have been replaced repeatedly, 3,2, and 3 times respectively, making them very convincing candidates for the CD category (X-ray and variability analyses disagreeing).

(8) It cannot be determined by pedigree analysis whether position 95, encoded by the $v_{\lambda 1}$ gene (not $j_{\lambda 1}$ gene) and likely varied by vj recombination, is CD or not. Position 95 is not CD either by variability or X-ray analysis.

Junctional diversity is certainly of high frequency compared to mutation but it is the consequence of another independently functionally important event, namely vj fusion to form a transcription unit. Whether this concomitantly contributes to combining site diversity is an open question. In any case, it is a minor contribution since only 1 of the 14 replacements can be due to vj joining; 13/14 are a consequence of mutation in the CD regions of the v gene itself. No replacement ($<1/22$) has been found at position 96, the first amino acid encoded by the j gene and identified as a contact residue by X-ray analysis (Poljak *et al.*, 1976).

Lastly, there is a preferred cross-over position which results in the His Trp sequence at the vj junction 21/22 times. If cross-over between the 6 nucleotides comprising v codons 95 (His) and $95+1$ and j codons 96 (Trp) and $96-1$ were random then the primotype would show amino acid replacements of either His or Trp with a frequency 0·57; in fact 0·05 is found. This shows that the mechanism of joining v to j by recombination has not been optimized during evolution to generate vj junctional amino acid diversity (see below). Consequently, its contribution to combining site diversity is also far from optimized.

Can the pedigree analyses of the $v_{\lambda 1}$ gene be extended to individual v_κ genes?

It is generally argued that the pattern of variation of the $v_{\lambda 1}$ and $j_{\lambda 1}$ genes (because there is one of each) cannot be extrapolated to v_κ (or v_H) where there are many germ line v genes and several j genes. The argument is that there is a qualitatively different behaviour between the $v_{\lambda 1}$ gene and any one (or given) v_κ or v_H gene. This argument has been pressed by those who believe that all genes expressed by an animal are germ line encoded or that the major somatic diversification mechanism is recombination between v gene sets or episomal insertion (minigene assembly) or a permuted combination of all of these. Clearly, $V_{\lambda 1}$ is varied in amino acid sequence almost exclusively by mutation ($>90\%$) and an extrapolation to other v gene loci would be incompatible with germ line (Dreyer and Bennett, 1965; Hood and Talmage, 1970; Williamson, 1976; Seidman and Leder, 1978; McKean and Potter, 1979), recombination (Gally and Edelman, 1970, 1972), episomal or minigene (Kabat, 1978; Kindt and Capra, 1978) and permuted predestination (Klinman *et al.*, 1975) models.

However, this argument has been interred for we know now that the extension of the pedigree analysis to the v_κ gene reveals the same rules of somatic diversification (Fig. 4).

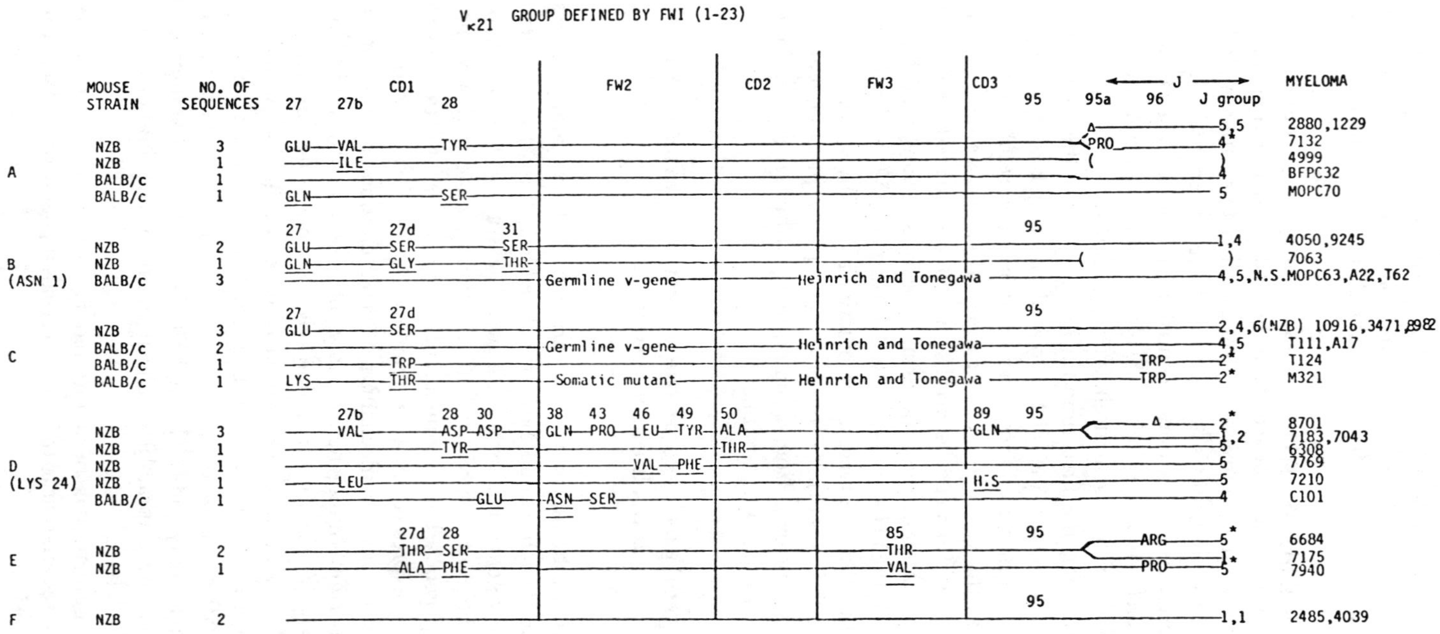

$V_{\kappa 21}$ GROUP DEFINED BY FWI (1-23)

	MOUSE STRAIN	NO. OF SEQUENCES	CD1	FW2	CD2	FW3	CD3	J (95, 95a, 96)	J group	MYELOMA
A	NZB	3	27 GLU, 27b VAL, 28 TYR					95a Δ / PRO	5,5; 4*	2880,1229; 7132
	NZB	1	27b ILE					(	)	4999
	BALB/c	1							4	BFPC32
	BALB/c	1	27 GLN, 28 SER						5	MOPC70
B (ASN 1)	NZB	2	27 GLU, 27d SER, 31 SER					95	1,4	4050,9245
	NZB	1	27 GLN, 27d GLY, 31 THR					(	)	7063
	BALB/c	3		Germline v-gene		Heinrich and Tonegawa			4,5,N.S.	MOPC63,A22,T62
C	NZB	3	27 GLU, 27d SER					95	2,4,6(NZB)	10916,3471,8982
	BALB/c	2		Germline v-gene		Heinrich and Tonegawa			4,5	T111,A17
	BALB/c	1	27d TRP					96 TRP	2*	T124
	BALB/c	1	27 LYS, 27d THR	Somatic mutant		Heinrich and Tonegawa		96 TRP	2*	M321
D (LYS 24)	NZB	3	27b VAL, 28 ASP, 30 ASP	38 GLN, 43 PRO, 46 LEU, 49 TYR	50 ALA		89 GLN	95; 96 Δ	2*; 1,2	8701; 7183,7043
	NZB	1	28 TYR		50 THR				5	6308
	NZB	1		46 VAL, 49 PHE					5	7769
	NZB	1	27b LEU				89 HIS		5	7210
	BALB/c	1	30 GLU	38 ASN, 43 SER					4	C101
E	NZB	2	27d THR, 28 SER			85 THR		95; 96 ARG	5*; 1*	6684; 7175
	NZB	1	27d ALA, 28 PHE			85 VAL		96 PRO	5*	7940
F	NZB	2						95	1,1	2485,4039

Data from Weigert et al (1978); McKean and Potter (1979).

* = Replacement by Recombination

38,43 = Possible polymorphism NZB vs BALB/c

46,49,85 = FW or CD? New germ-line v-gene or not?

(   ) or N.S. = not sequenced.

FIG. 4 *A pedigree analysis of germ line $v_{\kappa 21}$ genes.*

The experimental approach has been to sequence *in toto* independently derived κ-chains with identical (or similar) sequences in their *N*-terminal 23 amino acids (FW1).

Using the same rule as was used for $v_{\lambda 1}$, i.e. $\geqslant 2$ repeat V sequences defines a germ line v gene, 6 germ line v genes are identified and designated $v_{\kappa 21A-F}$ (Weigert *et al.*, 1978; McKean and Potter, 1979; Weigert *et al.*, 1980).

The individual germ line v_κ genes which encode identical FW1s are $v_{\kappa 21A}$, $v_{\kappa 21C}$, $v_{\kappa 21E}$ and $v_{\kappa 21F}$. Two genes, $v_{\kappa 21B}$ and $v_{\kappa 21D}$, encode FW1s which differ by one residue from the above group. The germ line v_κ gene encodes the sequence to position 95 after which vj joining introduces amino acid sequence differences both by combinatorial joining (pv × mj) and junctional recombination.

The conclusions from these V_κ sequences are as follows:

(1) The germ line v_κ genes defined by $\geqslant 2$ repeats are confirmed in the case of the $v_{\kappa 21B}$ BALB/c MOPC63/A22/T62 and $v_{\kappa 21C}$ BALB/c T111/A17 germ line sequence by DNA sequencing (Heinrich and Tonegawa, pers. comm.). The somatic variant of germ line $v_{\kappa 21C}$ is M321 which has been shown to have base replacements corresponding to the amino acid replacements, GLU→LYS and SER→THR (Heinrich and Tonegawa, pers. comm.). The remainder of the DNA sequence of the $v_{\kappa 21C}$ somatic mutant (M321) is identical to its germ line sequence (no silent mutations); a situation similar to that found for the $v_{\lambda 1}$ somatic mutant H2020 (Ig303λ). In fact for 3 pairs of sequences (germ line v gene (from embryonic DNA) *v.* myeloma expressed v gene), no silent mutations have been found (Bernard *et al.*, 1978; Seidman *et al.*, 1979; Nishioka and Leder, 1980; Heinrich and Tonegawa, pers. comm.). If mutations resulting in amino acid replacements in the FW (like silent mutations) are not selected for, their frequency per v gene expressed must be low. If there is uniform random mutation in the v gene, it must be sufficiently low that selection for a CD replacement by antigen has a negligible probability of entraining a FW replacement (or a silent mutation). This assumption puts a major emphasis on antigenic selection in the soma in increasing the range of diversity. If there is a specialized mechanism increasing the mutation frequency in CD codons relative to that in FW codons, as the precision and activity of this postulated mechanism increases, the requirement for antigenic selection to drive the diversification of the repertoire decreases. It would not be surprising if the frequency of mutation in CD codons is higher than that in FW codons but it will probably never be high enough to make the contribution to the repertoire by sequential antigenic selection negligible (Cohn, 1971).

(2) Some ambiguity in defining CD and FW positions is evident. In v gene group $v_{\kappa 21D}$, NZB 7769 differs from all other NZB $v_{\kappa 21D}$ sequences at positions 46 and 49 generally classified as FW. The same is true in the $v_{\kappa 21E}$ gene group where NZB 7940 differs from the other $v_{\kappa 21E}$ sequences by a 2 base replacement at position 85 generally classified as FW. We have minimized the number of postulated germ line $v_{\kappa 21}$ genes by assuming them to CD positions in proteins of these particular framework sequences. (Errors in sequence or in their publication are not being entertained as an explanation.)

Only one κ class immunoglobulin has been analysed by X-ray to date i.e. MOPC603, antiphosphorylcholine (Padlan, 1977). No positions in the V_L region are assigned as contact residues except possibly position 96 which is encoded by the j_L gene and varied by vj junctional recombination. Since the antiphosphorylcholine specificity is dependent on the light chain (Bhattacharjee and Glaudemans, 1978) and since the homologous λ_1 does have X-ray defined contact residues in nonjunctional CD1 and CD3 (Poljak *et al.*, 1976), this assignment of contact residues to only one position in kappa, is unlikely to be general.

(3) The NZB and BALB/c strains have surprisingly similar $v_{\kappa 21}$ genes given their large differences in other v_κ genes. This v gene group controlling the expression of about 7% of total light chain seems to code for an as yet unknown but important class of combining specificities. Some hints of polymorphism may be found, e.g. in $v_{\kappa 21D}$, BALB/c (C101) differs from the other NZB $v_{\kappa 21D}$ sequences at positions 38 and 43 believed to be FW.

A summary of the data shown in Figs 3 and 4 is compiled in Table III and Fig. 5. It can be seen that:

TABLE III

A comparison of the contribution of somatic mutation and VJ recombination to amino acid sequence diversity

	$V_{\lambda 1}$	$V_{\kappa 21}$	J_κ type (1 2 4 5)	$V_{\lambda 1}$ *and* $V_{\kappa 21}$ *composite data*
Total V sequences	22 (100%)	31 (100%)		53 (100%)
Germ line	14 (64%)	22 (71%)		36 (68%)
Somatic mutants	8 (36%)	9 (29%)		17 (32%)
Amino acid replacements in:				
CD regions	13 (100%)	18 (100%)		31 (100%)
CD_1	5 (38%)	14 (78%)		19 (61%)
CD_2	4 (31%)	3 (17%)		7 (23%)
CD_3 (to pos. 95)	4 (31%)	1 (5%)		5 (16%)
Total VJ joining regions	22 (100%)	28 (100%)		50 (100%)
V + J (germ line)	21 (95%)	22 (78%)	5 2 7 8	43 (86%)
V + J (somatic variant)	1 (5%)	6 (22%)	0 3 1 2	7 (14%)
			5 5 8 10	
Total amino acid replacements	14 (100%)	24 (100%)		38 (100%)
CD mutation	13 (93%)	18 (75%)		31 (82%)
V + J recombination	1 (7%)	6 (25%)		7 (18%)

Combinatorial joining (pv × mj) is not included in the calculations. Junctional diversity due to translocational recombination (V + J somatic variant) is included. The distribution of J_κ types in the V + J (germ line) and V + J (somatic variant) classes are shown.

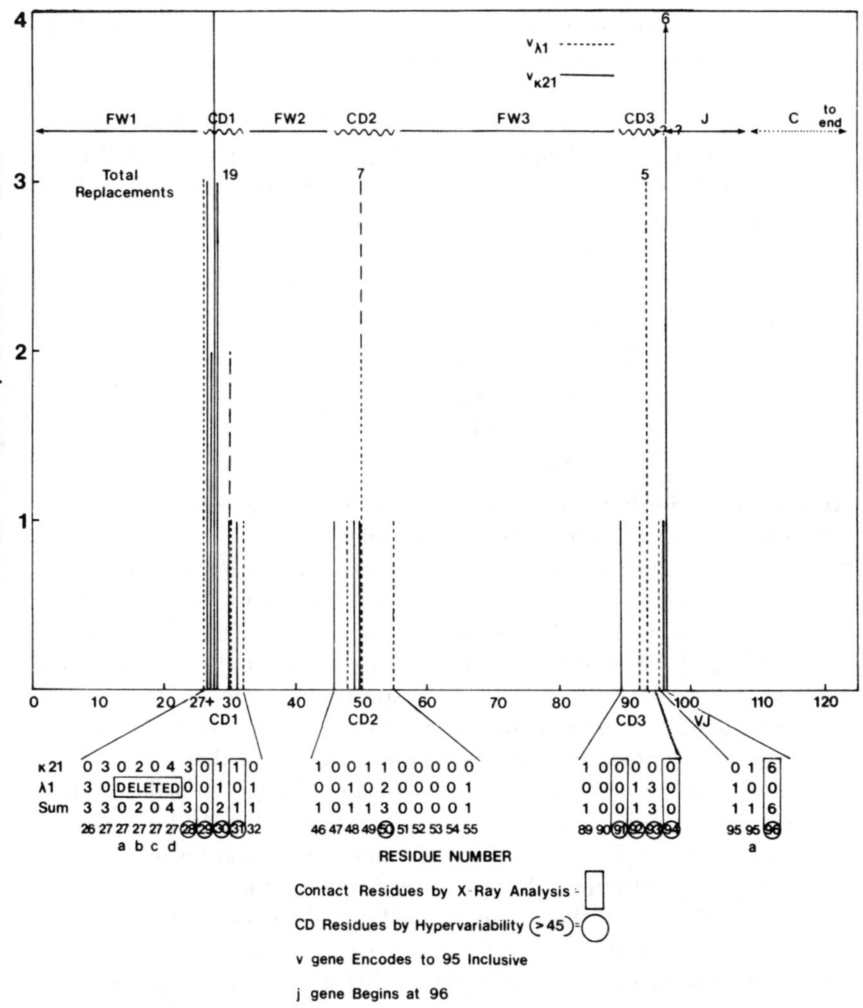

FIG. 5. *CD positions determined by pedigree analysis compared with those determined by variability and X-ray analyses.*

The "?" refers to the doubt as to whether VJ junctional or J residues are CD. The dashed vertical line at positions 30 and 50 sums up the λ1 and κ21 replacements at these positions, the only ones where both λ1 and κ21 replacements occur. At positions 95, 95a and 96 the replacements refer to amino acids not bases as indicated on the ordinate because the replacements are due to recombination. The digital read-out is the number of somatic replacements in $v_{\kappa 1}$ *and* $v_{\kappa 21}$ *at each indicated position. A circled position (○) indicates that it is hypervariable and a boxed position (□) indicates that it is a contact residue by X-ray analysis.*

(1) $v_{\kappa 21A-F}$ and $v_{\lambda 1}$ genes vary following identical patterns.

(2) In the pool of cells from which plasmacytomas are derived, a germ line v gene encoded subunit sequence has a 68% chance of being expressed. Thus if v_L and v_H genes vary similarly, on an average a germ line encoded $V_L V_H$ combination will appear ~50% of the time [$(0{\cdot}68)^2$]; a somatic variant in one or the other subunit, V_L or V_H, ~40% of the time [$2(0{\cdot}32)(0{\cdot}68)$]; a somatic variant in both subunits, V_L and V_H, ~10% of the time [$(0{\cdot}32)^2$]. To the extent that the normal composition of serum immunoglobulin reflects the distribution in the plasmacytoma precursor pool, 50% is expected to be germ line encoded and 50% mutationally derived.

The data (Table III) permit us to estimate with what frequency the following categories of light chain are expressed in the clonotype:

$$V_{\text{germ line}}\ VJ_{\text{germ line}} = 0{\cdot}58$$
$$V_{\text{germ line}}\ VJ_{\text{variant}} = 0{\cdot}09$$
$$V_{\text{mutant}}\ VJ_{\text{germ line}} = 0{\cdot}28$$
$$V_{\text{mutant}}\ VJ_{\text{variant}} = 0{\cdot}05$$

If, as we will argue later, the germ line is selected upon to encode specificities of immediate survival value to the animal, then

(1) germ line encoded VJ sequences are expected to dominate the available repertoire in frequency but contribute minimally to its size, and

(2) the contribution to the combining site repertoire, of combinatorial and junctional diversity due to vj fusion, is expected to be second order. Seidman *et al.* (1978a, 1979) confirm this expectation based on amino acid sequences and genetics by showing that a whimsically chosen "κ gene is formed by site-specific recombination without further somatic mutation", an inference which illustrates the use of the crystal ball to support their persuasion that the repertoire is essentially all germ line encoded.

(3) The major proportion (~80%) of amino acid replacements is due to somatic mutation affecting CD regions encoded by the v gene. A minor proportion (~20%) is at the vj junction and due to recombination. Whether the latter are CD remains to be seen. In most cases of vj gene fusion (~90%), v and j are juxtaposed with no replacements at the joining junction i.e. $VJ_{\text{germ line}}$. The probability of a VJ_{variant} being expressed in the primotype is 0·6 assuming recombination at any nucleotide in v gene positions 95 and 95 + 1 and in j gene positions 96 and 96 − 1 is equally probable. The clonotypes (Table III) show that the probability of being a VJ_{variant} is 0·14. Therefore, as pointed out for $\lambda 1$ earlier, either there is a preferred cross-over position (more likely) or VJ recombinational variants are counterselected. Both explanations imply that VJ amino acid junctional variation is not optimized to contribute to combining site diversity.

This argument might be countered by pointing out that the junctional first residue (position 96) encoded by the germ line j gene is different for J1 Leu, J2 Phe, J4 Tyr, J5 Trp. This could imply that the position was optimized during germ line evolution for amino acid diversity because it is CD. However, this is not a unique reason for the germ line encoded amino acid diversity at position 96. Since this codon (position 96) is involved in recombination which does not occur always at a precise nucleotide and itself generates new codons, there is weak (if any) selection pressure to maintain, at position 96, a given codon in the germ line, and it drifts. This supports our point that junctional amino acid diversity is a byproduct of the fusion mechanism and is not optimized as a contributor to the combining site repertoire.

Since one j gene is sufficient to permit the functioning of a locus e.g. $\lambda 1$, we must ask why there is more than one in the κ and H loci. Given that these loci are approximately 2000 Kb long, the most obvious answer is that it increases the rate of successful vj fusion. A modest increase in the "concentration" of j genes can increase the rate of fusion to a point where it occurs within a reasonable time. Those who argue that the j genes are a mechanism of combining site diversification by combinatorial joining (pV × mJ) might ask why there are so few of them.

As a first-order approximation, there is no J sequence preference in the $V_{\kappa 21}$ group compared with other V_{κ} sequences. In the $V_{\kappa 21}$ group, J1, J2, J4, and J5 has been expressed 5, 5, 8 and 10 times, respectively, whereas in non-$V_{\kappa 21}$ sequences the distribution is 4,2,5 and 5 times respectively (Kabat *et al.*, 1979). There might be a slight gradient of joining probability from J5 (closest to v) to J1 (farthest from v) since overall J1, J2, J4, and J5 has been expressed 9, 7, 13 and 15 times respectively.

If the 4 germ line J sequences contribute to the combining site diversity (i.e. are part of CD3 not FW4), this effect is, on an average, equivalent for all germ line v genes no matter what specificities they were selected to encode. Further the j genes of NZB and BALB/c are identical except possibly for one addition which is designated J6 NZB 8982 in Fig. 4. This J6 NZB sequence could have resulted either from a somatic mutation in the j1 gene of NZB in which case it might define a CD residue (unlikely) or from a germ line duplication of the j1 gene which subsequently diverged by mutation to become the j6 gene. The result is that both the j1 and j6 genes are expressed in NZB. Thus the j genes appear to be quite conserved in evolution compared to v genes and the nonjunctional residues which distinguish them in an individual are few, conservative and in FW positions uniquely.

Consequently, we conclude that the contribution by combinatorial joining (pV × mJ) is a second order source of combining site diversity. A more precise conclusion might be that the J segment contributes indirectly to combining site diversity as a FW4, not as a CD3 region. It affects which residues are CD, in large measure by determining the rotational and angular relationships between the $V_L V_H$ jaws of the combining site. This is the only framework we can analyse with subtlety thanks to combinatorial VJ joining. It is because the λ_1 locus has only one $j_{\lambda 1}$ gene that its role as a FW was evident by pedigree analysis. If light chains could be made with varied FW1's, FW2's or FW3's then we could analyse them as we did FW4 (J segment) and subtle or second-order effects on antibody activity would be revealed.

(4) The pedigree analysis gives precise criteria for CD residues compared to variability analysis (compare Figs 3 and 5). Of the 16 positions in which V region replacements have occurred, only 2 of them are common to $V_{\lambda 1}$ and $V_{\kappa 21}$. All, however, are clustered in 3 regions sharply defined by pedigree analysis. We recall that of the 18 positions in the V + J region where somatic replacements have been shown to occur, 16 positions are varied by mutation in the v gene itself and 2 are varied by recombination at the vj junction. The former are CD by the definition of a pedigree analysis; the latter are unresolved.

(5) The term "subgroup" has been avoided because its use is ambiguous. It varies in meaning from a group of sequences bearing family resemblances (Gally and Edelman, 1970, 1972; Rabbitts *et al.*, 1980; Seidman *et al.*, 1978, 1978a; Kabat *et al.*, 1979) to a group of sequences derived from a single germ line v gene (Cohn, 1973; Cohn *et al.*, 1974). For example, the $V_{\kappa 21}$ sequences could be referred to as a "subgroup" meaning that they bear family resemblances or as 6 "subgroups", $V_{\kappa 21A\text{-}F}$ meaning that they are encoded by 6 germ line v genes. Under the latter more rationale definition they should be numbered independently $V_{\kappa 21}$–$V_{\kappa 27}$. Their relatedness in frameworks reflects evolutionary history not a special relationship between members of this group of genes to the process of somatic diversification.

Can we extrapolate the behaviour of v_L to v_H genes?

The data are too meagre to assess the mutational contribution to v_H gene diversity. The general picture based on variability plots and limited X-ray data indicate the existence of 3 CD regions analogous to those discussed for v_L genes. The fusion event is somewhat more complicated than that seen for v_L genes. There is an additional feature, a D region defined by an amino acid sequence not encoded by the germ line v gene or j gene (Schilling *et al.*, 1980; Early *et al.*, 1980). This sequence is postulated to contribute to combining site diversity, particularly CD3, and has been viewed as an extension of the recombinational diversity as seen in $v_L j_L$ joining (Bernard *et al.*, 1978; Max *et al.*, 1979; Weigert *et al.*, 1980). The degree to which this source of amino acid diversity contributes to combining site diversity is an open question.

If one allows for the amino acid diversity generated at the 2 new junctions, vd and dj, it becomes evident that there is a precise control over which d gene is expressed with a given v gene. This invalidates calculations on the contribution to combining site diversity based on combinatorial (pv × nd) joining of v and d genes. For example $v_{H\lambda 1}^{\alpha(1,3)DEX}$ genes are associated with one set of d genes; $v_{H\kappa}^{\beta(1,6)GAL}$ genes are associated with another d gene set; v_H^{PC} genes with a third set; and so on. (Schilling *et al.*, 1980; Early *et al.*, 1980). This then implies two fusion events, $v_H \rightarrow d_H$ and $v_H d_H \rightarrow j_H$; as well as a grouping of splicing signals relating a given set of v_H genes with corresponding d_H genes. Putting aside the junctional diversity, the amino acid sequence variability in the D region itself could be due to one germ line d gene per sequence or to "mutation" in a given germ line d gene. If the former prevails, nothing can be said about the role of the D region in combining site diversity. If the latter prevails, the D region must contain CD residues using the argumentation of a pedigree analysis.

Out of the 5 contact residues determined for the MOPC603 antiphosphorylcholine heavy chain by X-ray analyses (Padlan, 1977) 4 are in CD1 and CD2 regions while 1 is the second residue encoded by the j_H gene if we are permitted to use the j_{H107} gene (Early *et al.*, 1980) as a model. None are in the D segment.

Poljak *et al.* (1980), by contrast, argue from model-building studies that the D segment occupies "a central position at the combining site" which is "X-ray" jargon taken to mean that the D segment is a sequence of or contains several contact residues. The variability analysis also favours a major role for the D segment as CD3 (the J segment is FW4) (Kabat *et al.*, 1979). However, both arguments are weak, "model building" because it is *a posteriori*; the variability analysis because it is *non sequitor* (p. 163) and, in any case, overestimates variability by not allowing for the non-randomness of vd joining.

The direct evidence that D_H and J_H play a CD role must come from binding studies. Poljak *et al.* (1980) and Schilling *et al.* (1980) understandably stretch the available data. Poljak *et al.* (1980) cite that antiphosphorylcholine heavy chains vary at position 102, the second residue in J_H (defined by Padlan (1977) as contact) and at position 100 the second residue in D_H (defined by Poljak *et al.* (1980), but not Padlan (1977), as contact). Then, they argue that variations in the amino acids at these positions are reflected in the different binding constants of myeloma proteins to phosphorylcholine and its analogues. However, the antibodies showing these D_H and J_H variations differ in V_LJ_L as well as in other residues in V_HD_H (S107, MOPC603 and M511 are encoded by different germ line v_H^{PC} genes). This makes it difficult to sustain any independent argument that would be based only on correlations between binding and replacements at positions 100 and 102 specifically. Schilling *et al.* (1980) cite 2 investigations on anti-α(1,3) dextran myeloma proteins, MOPC104 (Leon *et al.*, 1970) and J558 (Lundblad *et al.*, 1972) which differ in sequence by 2 residues only, Tyr Asp in MOPC104 is replaced by Arg Tyr in J558 at position 99, the only residue in D_H and 101 the first and junctional residue in J_H. A comparison of the findings of these 2 groups of workers indicated that the apparent size of the binding site was 1–2 sugar residues larger for J558 than for MOPC104. However, this is too small a difference for these 2 studies to be used as an argument. They are not comparisons of J558 and MOPC104 in one laboratory under identical conditions. The studies were carried out 2 years apart, each laboratory investigating 1 of the 2 proteins under different conditions with different assays. Even if this caution is put aside, the only assay one might compare in the 2 studies was inhibition of precipitation. In the case of MOPC104 (Table III in Leon *et al.*, 1970) the carbohydrate used for precipitation was B1254L which contains no α(1,3) linkages detectable by chemistry ($<5\%$) whereas in the case of J558 (Fig. 2 in Lundblad *et al.*, 1972) the carbohydrate used for precipitation was B1498S which contains 27% $\alpha(1,3)$ linkages. In the case of MOPC104 nigerotetraose was a slightly better inhibitor than nigerotriose placing the binding site between 3 and 4 sugar residues. In the case of J558 nigerohexaose was a slightly better inhibitor than nigeropentaose placing the binding site between 5 and 6 sugar residues. However, there is no way of knowing whether this difference in the findings of the 2 laboratories is a property of the precipitating carbohydrate (B1254L *v.* B1498S) or of the antibody (J558 *v.* MOPC104). Oddly, in none of these studies did large excess of inhibitor block precipitation completely. It is not clear why complete inhibition of a monoclonal antibody was not found but this fact further clouds the interpretation of differences in specificity because it shows that no site filling ligands were studied. Lastly, MOPC104 is IgM (a pentamer of $(LH)_2$) and J558 is IgA (a mixture of monomer $(LH)_2$, dimer and some trimer). The interaction of each protein with a repeating carbohydrate polymer will show a different co-operativity which might affect the apparent size of a binding site measured by inhibition of precipitation by ligands consisting of sugar residues added to the prime (immunodominant) determinant, nigerose. However, these extra (local environment) sugars show no specificity in binding, a general finding in studies of this kind that is difficult to evaluate in terms of its quantitative contribution to the diversity of the combining site repertoire. In any case even if we grant that J558 and MOPC104 show an apparent combining site size difference, the effect of the 2 amino acid replacements in question could fall into the category of FW variation effects not directly related to somatic diversification. It would not be surprising if the 4 FW regions controlled the interaction between V_L and V_H in a way which modulated, across all specificities, the combining site contour. In this sense D and J are FW's specialized to link functionally the V and C domains but which contribute concomitantly in a general and relatively nonspecific way to interactions with the local environment of a prime determinant and permit combining site flexibility both angular and rotational. In fact one might ask why the d gene which is argued to be of major importance (Schilling *et al.*, 1980; Early *et al.*, 1980; Poljak *et al.*, 1980) in generating combining site diversity is lacking in light chains? Is there a fundamental asymmetry in the relative contributions of v_L and v_H genes to the repertoire or does the d gene play another role unique to the function and/or expression of heavy chains in B cells. Consequently we conclude that it is an open question whether the nom de plume "d gene" is a framework metaphor.

What specificities expressed by humoral antibodies are encoded in the germ line?

This question is central to our views on the origin of diversity of humoral and cell-mediated antibodies. This is a question never posed by those of the germ line, recombinational, minigene (episomal), or permuted predestination persuasions because the selection pressures maintaining the germ line genes cannot be the combining specificities they encode. This was seen clearly by Smith (1973) who proposed that, under a germ line theory, the FW would be strongly selected upon but the CD residues would be unselected and allowed to drift. Thus, the germ line theory explains "hypervariability" on grounds which cannot account for the genetics of antigen-specific responsiveness (Cohn, 1974). In fact, none of the above theories do this. Rather, they keep us honest by challenging the existence of the phenomenon.

Under a somatic mutation theory the germ line v genes are maintained by the usefulness of the antibody combining specificities they encode (Cohn, 1971, 1974; Jerne, 1971).

The first hints of this came from the high frequency of antibody activity found among plasmacytoma proteins directed towards phosphorylcholine, levans, galactans, dextrans, flagellar proteins, etc. (reviewed by Potter, 1977). The high frequency of identical immunoglobulins of these specificities led us to propose that they were germ line encoded and that the evolutionary selection pressure maintaining these specificities was that they were directed against determinants present on the surface of extracellular pathogens (bacteria, fungi, protozoa, helminths, etc.) of prime importance to the survival of the newborn (Cohn, 1971, 1973).

Jerne (1971) starting from the premise that the repertoire is derived somatically in each individual from that subset of germ line v genes encoding antiself and focusing on the high frequency of alloreactive T cells, argued that the germ line encoded specificities were anti-MHC of the species. His assumption, still dominant today, was that humoral and cell mediated antibodies are encoded by the same loci. Jerne's hypothesis led us to screen plasmacytoma immunoglobulins against MHC products and other self-constituents (Hirst *et al.*, 1971). None which reacted were found. Anti-MHC showed a very much lower frequency in the humoral repertoire than anticarbohydrate and a very much higher frequency in the cell mediated than in the humoral repertoire.

The Jerne (1971) assumption that the germ line v gene pool is selected to encode antispecies-MHC is essentially disproven for humoral antibody, but it is most likely correct for cell-mediated antibody. However, this latter conclusion cannot be derived from his premise on somatic diversification in the absence of a reason as to why the antiself set should be anti-MHC. His assumption in no way implies the recognition or existence of a locus with the special properties of the MHC. This seems obvious today, for we know now that the germ line genes encoding the T cell receptor are selected during evolution to encode anti-MHC specificities because of their role in restrictive recognition, not because of their role in a process of somatic diversification by mutational escape from tolerance (Langman, 1978). It is the requirement for restrictive recognition that makes the MHC special. We make this point emphasizing that it is independent of whether Jerne's (1971) assumption regarding somatic diversification is right or wrong.

Returning now to the humoral antibody system, the evidence confirming that the germ line v genes encode anticarbohydrate specificities (probably of key protective value when the animal is born), comes from studies on the genetics of humoral responsiveness.

Our studies (Blomberg *et al.*, 1972; Weigert and Riblet, 1978; Geckeler *et al.*, 1978; dePreval *et al.*, 1979) with the humoral response to α(1,3) dextran are the most comprehensive and we will make 2 points with them.

(1) There is a germ line genetics of humoral responsiveness due to alleles of the regulatory and structural gene loci encoding V_L and V_H.

(2) As the germ line genes encoding a given specificity are dissected away, it is possible to reveal germ line genes which by somatic evolution (mutation and selection) acquire the given specificity, in this case recognition of the α(1,3) dextran determinant.

The findings are summarized in Fig. 6. The kinetics of anti-α(1,3) dextran responsiveness is illustrated for 3 cases; a fast responder, a slow responder,

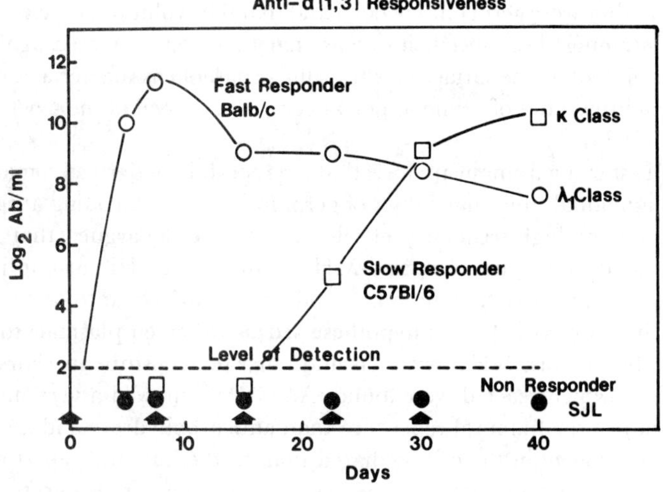

Prototype of mouse strain	$r_{\lambda 1}$ control of $V_{\lambda 1}$	$V_{\kappa}^{\alpha(1,3)}$ (chromosome 6)	$V_{H\lambda 1}^{\alpha(1,3)}$ (chromosome 12)	$V_{H\kappa}^{\alpha(1,3)}$	Anti-α (1,3) response
BALB/c (Ig^a)	+	−	+	−	λ1; fast (germ-line)
C57BL/6 (Ig^b)	+	+	−	+	κ; slow (somatic)
SJL (Ig^b)	lo	−	−	+	No response
SJA (Ig^a)	lo	−	+	−	λ1; patchy

FIG. 6. *Genetic dissection as a way of analysing immune responsiveness.*

Haemagglutinin assay of the anti-α(1,3) dextran activity expressed in log_2 *units. The arrows indicate repeated injections of α(1,3) dextran (dePreval* et al.*, 1979).* Ig^a *and* Ig^b *are the allelic heavy chain loci. +, − or lo refer to v or* $r\lambda_1$ *gene alleles, present, absent or leaky.*

and a nonresponder. The fast response is due uniquely to a germ line encoded $V_{\lambda 1}V_{H\lambda 1}^{a(1,3)}$ (e.g. (BALB/c) (Blomberg *et al.*, 1972; Weigert and Riblet, 1978). The slow response, revealed when either the $v_{\lambda 1}$ or $v_{H\lambda 1}^{a(1,3)}$ genes are mutationally inactivated, is derived from a pair of germ line genes $v_{\kappa}^{a(1,3)}$ $v_{H\kappa}^{a(1,3)}$ (e.g. C57BL/6). If both the fast λ1 and the slow κ class of response is deleted, the animal is a nonresponder. Presumably when the pair of genes encoding the fast λ1 class response are dissected away, the slow response in the κ class is revealed by selection for somatic mutants (dePreval *et al.*, 1979). If these latter genes are also dissected away, the animal has no way of responding because too many mutational steps are required to derive anti-α(1,3) dextran specificity from the residual v_L and v_H genes (e.g. SJL). The most informative response is that found with SJA. This strain has a fast responder heavy chain locus derived from BALB/c i.e., it possesses the $v_{H\lambda 1}^{a(1,3)}$ gene, but its λ1 locus is defective, not in its structural $v_{\lambda 1}$ gene but in some regulatory gene ($r_{\lambda 1}$) operating at the DNA level, e.g. one affecting the frequency of successful fusion of the $v_{\lambda 1}$ gene to the $j_{\lambda 1}$ gene. As a consequence the number of anti-α(1,3) dextran antigen-sensitive B cells is more than 10-fold below that of the fast responder (e.g. BALB/c). This leads to a Poisson distribution of responsiveness (referred to as "patchy") in which 21% of SJA mice are nonresponders and 79% responders (to various stepwise levels). This implies that the average number of anti-α(1,3) dextran responding units per SJA mouse is 1·6; one responding unit is about 50 antigen-sensitive B cells per mouse (Geckeler *et al.*, 1978).

These studies imply that there is only one (or very few) v genes in the germ line which encode the given specificity. If there were many ways to derive anti-α(1,3) specificity, no genetics of responsiveness would be seen. It is this fact which permits us to understand the strong germ line selection for given specificities of survival importance.

There is little doubt that germ line v genes are maintained by the antibody specificities that they encode, a fact which is accounted for almost uniquely by the somatic mutation theory.

How many functional v genes are carried in the germ line?

This is a major question to be answered when considering the origin of diversity. Here the principle of the argument as well as the sufficiency of the data are under discussion.

There is good evidence (Bernard *et al.*, 1978; Tonegawa *et al.*, 1978) that an intact v gene is carried in the germ line, i.e. there is coevolution of FW and CD regions as one v gene (Cohn *et al.*, 1974; Cohn, 1974). This might be stressed because our analysis of the function and number of germ line v genes would not be pertinent if they were comprised of minigenes (Kabat, 1979, 1980).

The first approximation was made (Weigert *et al.*, 1970) as follows:

The ratio of κ/λ varies widely in different species. In the mouse where there is one $v_{\lambda 1}$ gene this ratio is 67. Assuming uniform antigenic selection on all functional germ line v genes it was argued (Weigert *et al.*, 1970) that there is of the order of 10^2 v_κ genes, a crude but informative calculation. This calculation can be extended to the $V_{\kappa 21}$ group (described in an earlier section). It comprises about 7% of total kappa light chain and is encoded by 5–10 germ line $v_{\kappa 21}$ genes (Weigert *et al.*, 1978). This implies that the total number of germ line v_κ genes is 70–140 [100/7 × (5–10)]. Both estimates agree within a factor of 2 that the total germ line v_κ gene pool is of the order of 10^2.

Another approximation was made (Cohn, 1973, 1974; Cohn *et al.*, 1974; Weigert and Riblet, 1976) as follows:

The sequences of the V_κFW1 were grouped so as to determine the frequency of unique and repeat sequences. From the distribution, the size of the pool of V_κFW1 was estimated to be between 50–100. This pool size for V_κFW1 was multiplied by 2 (Cohn *et al.*, 1974) to estimate the total functional V_κ pool since it was known that, during evolution, germ line recombination (unequal crossing over) could assort FW segments (Kabat, 1979). However, since the frequency of this event cannot be high, the factor by which one must multiply the number of FW1's per individual to get the total number of v genes could never exceed a value of 2 on an average. The result was an estimate between 100–200 which we have referred to as "the order of 10^2".

There has been every reason to assume that the same estimate would apply to the germ line v_H gene pool also (Cohn *et al.*, 1974; Cohn, 1974) and some evidence supporting this has appeared (Rabbitts *et al.*, 1980).

These estimates of the number of functional germ line v genes have met with sharp criticism of 2 kinds:

(1) The sample derived from plasmacytoma immunoglobulins does not reflect what is in the germ line v gene pool (Hood *et al.*, 1974, 1976).

(2) The factor of 2 used to derive the total number, from the number in the pool of FW1's is too low. Values closer to 10 are suggested (Seidman *et al.*, 1978a, b; Valbuena *et al.*, 1978).

The first criticism has been dealt with in part elsewhere (Cohn, 1974). However since then a new argument has been proposed (Hood *et al.*, 1976). It is derived from the fact that random FW1 sequences from BALB/c and NZB mice exhibit few identical sequences (Weigert and Riblet, 1976). This has been taken to suggest that there is differential regulation of a large pool of germ line v_κ genes common to both BALB/c and NZB which results in the expression of different small subsets of v_κ genes in each strain. This new argument can be answered in 2 ways:

(a) In light of the extensive polymorphism of alleles at other genetic loci in mice, it is more likely that the structural v genes are highly polymorphic than that NZB and BALB/c have allelic regulatory genes which control different subsets of a single pool of structural germ line v genes common to both strains. Besides it would be a *reductio ad absurdum* to extend this argument to the other mouse strains which presumably also express large sequence differences from both BALB/c and NZB.

(b) Even were this latter hypothesis to be correct, our argument was used to count functional germ line v genes and a defect in regulation which effectively deletes the expression of a portion of the germ line v gene pool is equivalent to functionless structural genes.

The second criticism only illustrates how little DNA hybridization has contributed thus far to counting germ line v genes.

In the early studies, the stringent conditions of hybridization used to generate C_0t curves led to the conclusion, one mRNA–one($\leqslant 3$) germ line v gene. The only study for which this finding had any interpretation was the case of the λ_1 light chain because it solidly established the conclusion that the germ line $v_{\lambda 1}$ gene was varied by somatic mutation (Tonegawa *et al.*, 1974; Tonegawa, 1976). In the case of the κ locus nothing could be concluded until we could divine by what factor to multiply *one* to obtain the total. This problem is not solved by substituting restriction fingerprints (Southern Blots) for C_0t curves. As an example, a cloned, sequenced MOPC149 v region probe detects ~ 10 related v_κ sequences in a restriction fingerprint of embryonic DNA. The total number of germ line v_κ genes was estimated by multiplying the number of FW1's counted by amino acid sequence by the number of cross-hybridizable v_κ sequences detected in the restriction fingerprint (Seidman *et al.*, 1978a, b). Thus, $\sim 10^2$FW1 $\times$ $\sim 10^1$ cross-hybrids per probe = $\sim 10^3$(300–3000) germ line v_κ genes, leading Seidman *et al.* (1978a, b) to the conclusion that somatic diversification contributes negligibly to the total repertoire which is essentially germ line encoded.

This calculation is questionable on *a priori* grounds because it implies that on an average for every FW1 identified by amino acid sequence, there are in the germ line of the order of 10 v_κ replicates which have diverged from one another while preserving the sequence of FW1. It is also questionable on experimental grounds, for, in order to justify such a calculation, it must be assumed that the v_κ probe counts v genes which are identical to MOPC149 in the FW1's that they encode but which differ in codons determining the amino acid sequence of subsequent FW positions. Since the sequences of MOPC149 as well as 2 of the hybridizable restriction fragments, K2 and K3, differ in their FW1's (Seidman *et al.*, 1978a, b; Nishioka and Leder, 1980), this assumption is known to be incorrect. Therefore, most of the cross-hybridizable sequences have already been counted in the estimate of total FW1's (Cohn *et al.*, 1974; Weigert and Riblet, 1976). Consequently, the parameter $n > 5$ used by Seidman *et al.* (1978a, b) is much too high to adjust the estimates of total germ line v_κ genes made on the basis of an estimated FW1 pool of 50–100. The same argument also applies to the use of saturation hybridization experiments to get the average multiplier (Valbuena *et al.*, 1978).

It might be stressed that none of these estimates are independent of the one made by counting FW1's from amino acid sequence (Cohn, 1974). The DNA-hybridization studies only deal with whether the factor by which to multiply the estimated FW1 pool size is 2 or 10.

Given our present knowledge of the V_κ sequence distribution, the factor by which the number of germ line v gene encoded FW1's should be multiplied, could be as high as 5 for the $v_{\kappa 21}$ genes encoding identical FW1's (Fig. 4) or as low as one for the v_κ gene encoding anti-β(1,6) galactan (Rao *et al.*, 1978) or the $v_{\lambda 1}$ gene encoding anti-α(1,3) dextran (Fig. 3). The mean however does not seem to be larger than the original estimate of 2 (Cohn *et al.*, 1974).

Thus we are left with an important question. In principle, is there any way to derive the total number of functional germ line v genes from both data, i.e., amino acid sequences and DNA-hybridization?

Clearly, we would hope that each could give an independent count, the difference between them being due to nonfunctional germ line v genes. If there were (and there probably never will be) a sufficient number of complete V region (not just FW1) amino acid sequences, the total number of functional v genes would be counted as equal to the total number of frameworks (defined by a single amino acid replacement as different). This of course assumes the validity of the pedigree analysis. The ambiguity in the count would be in the distinction between FW and CD but this is at most a minor source of error (Fig. 4). In the case of DNA-hybridization, the degree of stringency used in a C_0t-, saturation-, or blot-hybridization determines the number of genes counted. Allowing for this source of arbitrariness, blot-hybridization could never be used to obtain an independent estimate of the total germ line v gene pool (functional and nonfunctional) until the overlap frequency of a large number of randomly chosen v probes were known. Depending on the nature of such data, a statistical calculation to derive the total might be made. However, it is not certain there will ever be a valid independent estimate from such data or that such data will ever be available.

Consequently, it is reasonable to try and combine the data based on FW1 (not complete) sequences and on DNA-hybridization to arrive at an estimate. Here, one uses judgement and taste (not uninfluenced by the espoused theory). This involves the use of the concept "subgroup" defined now as a group of sequences bearing family resemblances. In principle, a single FW replacement defines a germ line v gene. If the number of FW differences used to define a "subgroup" is $\geqslant 2$, no direct calculation of the number of germ line v genes is possible because the relationship between the genes and the "subgroup" disappears. In this case, it is argued that the total number of germ line v genes can be calculated as the number of "subgroups" times the number of DNA-hybridizable blots. As one increases the number of FW differences used to define a "subgroup", their total number decreases. Since as we have discussed, the calculation of the number of germ line v genes based on the number of FW's or "subgroups" (defined by single amino acid differences) times the number of DNA-hybridizable blots, is a gross overestimation due to the latter, decreasing the calculated total number of FW's or "subgroups" (defined by $\geqslant n$ amino acid differences) corrects for this, thus decreasing the total. Seidman *et al.* (1978, 1978a) use Potter's (1977) definition of a "subgroup" as one which comprises FW1's differing by $\geqslant 3$ amino acid residues. Under this definition there are ~ 30 $V\kappa$ "subgroups" which multiplied by 10

(DNA-hybridizable blots) gives ~300 germ line vκ genes. This brings the total more into line with that calculated from sequence alone but it requires an argument as to why ⩾3 amino acid differences were chosen. If one uses ⩾5 amino acid differences, the number of Vκ "subgroups" falls to 10–15 making the total 100–150. Potter (1977) chose the criterion of ⩾3 intuitively in order to correct for errors in sequence, ambiguities in distinguishing FW and CD residues, and possible somatic mutations affecting the FW which might be seen by entrainment during antigenic selection for CD residues. This, he felt was a more realistic datum on which to base a calculation for the total germ line v gene pool. The extreme form of this calculation is used by Rabbitts *et al.* (1980). They derive the size of the human germ line v_H gene pool to be 80 by referring the reader to Kabat *et al.* (1979) who distinguished 4 human V_H "subgroups" which is multiplied by 20 DNA-hybridizable blots per "subgroup". In the mouse this value would be ~40 which given the nature of the calculation is ~10^2.

None of these (FW × Blot)F_1 calculations contribute hybrid vigour to the discussion. The original estimate of ~10^2 based only on counting FW1's (defined rationally by single amino acid differences) is still the most reliable (Weigert and Riblet, 1976). It is not much of a comfort to make our original estimate of ~10^2 agree with the composite value (i.e., number of "subgroups" × number of blots) by a tailored definition of a "subgroup" as one in which the FW differences are ⩾*n*, some arbitrarily chosen number between 3 and 7. If it is argued that the principle of our estimate based on the pedigree analysis is incorrect, then an objective or at least rationalized competing criterion relating the total number of germ line v genes, "subgroups" defined by amino acid sequences, and "subgroups" defined by DNA-blots, or saturation-hybridization is required.

What is the status of the generation of diversity in the humoral antibody class?

Jerne (1979) has made a distinction between the available repertoire ("clonotype" in Gally and Edelman (1970) terminology) and the potential repertoire ("primotype" in Gally and Edelman (1970) terminology). The available repertoire of combining sites (clonotype) equals the number of V_LV_H pairs expressed somatically which upon appropriate interaction with antigen leads to induction.

We have estimated that there are of the order of 10^2 functional germ line v genes per locus which are maintained functional because they encode approximately 10^2 selected for nonself specificities (see Cohn, 1974 for a discussion of this selection).

We have argued that of the total of ~10^4 germ line encoded V_LV_H pairs only a proportion are starting points for somatic diversification. This is a consequence of V_LV_H preferential fit, which, if a property of the J segment even in part (Stevens *et al.*, 1980; Poljak *et al.*, 1980), implies that J complementation decreases the number of units of V_LV_H participating in somatic diversification. The repertoire is generated largely by a process of mutation followed by antigenic selection for v gene encoded CD mutants (Table III, Fig. 5) (Weigert *et al.*, 1970; Cohn *et al.*, 1974; Cohn, 1973, 1974).

There remains the question of how much of a contribution to the total repertoire is made by somatically replaced amino acids as a consequence of the fusion mechanism. From an analysis of the data, we conclude that the contribution to the diversity of the combining site by combinatorial joining (pv × mj) is of second-order importance, i.e., the J sequence contributes no more than that of a FW sequence. Hence like the C region there are few of them. Similarly, the junctional amino acid diversity due to intracodonic recombination is at best a minor contributor ($<10\%$) to the total repertoire compared to that of somatic mutation in v gene encoded CD1,2,3 codons.

Given this we consider the following models now ruled out:

(1) Somatic models in which there is

(a) Mutation operating on $\sim 10^1$ germ line v genes per locus (Cohn, 1970). (As an aside, in essence this starting point for somatic diversification is postulated for the cell-mediated or T cell repertoire (see later, discussion of von Boehmer *et al.*, 1978)).

(b) Recombination among "v gene sets" (Gally and Edelman, 1970, 1972).

(c) Translational variation (Potter *et al.*, 1965) or transcriptional variation (yet to be proposed).

(d) Episome (HVGS) insertion or minigene permutations (Kindt and Capra, 1978; Kabat, 1979).

(e) Germ line models (Dreyer and Bennett, 1965; Hood and Talmage, 1970; Wigzell, 1973; Klinman *et al.*, 1976; Williamson, 1976; Seidman *et al.*, 1978a, b; McKean and Potter, 1979).

Stated in this way, many feathers are certain to be ruffled. However, it is best to start future discussion at another level. Since many elements of the various theories are common, were any one to be correct then the others would have elements which are correct. However, this is not a clarifying way to view the problem today. It is the general tenor of each of the above listed theories which is ruled out.

There are several formulations which future discussions might try to keep clear.

(1) The use of the term "clonotype" needs precision. We are interested here in the repertoire of combining sites not of immunoglobulin molecules. The same combining site (V_LV_H pair) on 10 different heavy-chain isotypes does not permit us to multiply combinatorially by 10 in deriving the size of the relevant "clonotype". Similarly any arguments involving combinatorial joining of v, d and j (pv × mj etc.) must be made after evaluating quantitatively and qualitatively in what way a given V_LV_H pair linked to different J_LJ_H pairs affects combining specificity. If, for example, the various J sequences

function as FW4, the combining site repertoire would not be increased by combinatorial joining (subtleties discussed earlier) although the isoelectric focusing and idiotypic repertoire i.e., "clonotype" *à la* Klinman *et al.* (1976), could be increased 20-fold. Thus an estimate of 5×10^7 antibodies in the available "isoelectric focusing" repertoire might imply only 5×10^5 antibodies in the available combining site repertoire.

(2) It is like putting one's money in the mattress to equate *a* multigene which *the* germ line theory (Hood *et al.*, 1974, 1976; Klinman *et al.*, 1976) because, by pleading poverty, it conceals a wealth of queries concerning the selection pressures (germ line and somatic) determining the diversity of the combining site repertoire and the origin of the requirement for a vc joining mechanism. Consequently, it is no surprise that the only theories of germ line evolution which considered the selection pressures (Cohn, 1971; Jerne, 1971) came from those who proposed somatic not germ line models (see discussion Cohn, 1974). Further, a mechanism for joining v to c is mandated by all multigene theories and for the same reasons whether they be germ line (Dreyer and Bennett, 1965) or somatic (Lennox and Cohn, 1967; Gally and Edelman, 1970, 1972; Cohn, 1973, 1974). Likewise it locks the coop after the logic has flown, to equate paucigene and somatic theories (Klinman *et al.*, 1976) because the predicted number of germ line v genes is a consequence of the theory, somatic or germ line, not an assumption of it. This point concerning enumeration of germ line v genes usually evokes the comment that "those who espouse somatic mutation models" have increased the calculated number of germ line v genes from $\sim 10^1$ (Cohn, 1970) to $\sim 10^2$ (Cohn, 1973). This is correct but it neglects the distinction between "the principle of the argument" and "the sufficiency of the data". While it is the latter, not the former, which has changed, an incorrect estimate of $\sim 10^1$ (i.e., 25) from the early limited data (Cohn, 1970) is duly acknowledged.

(3) There is a fundamental problem of the relationship between how v genes vary and how they are selected (both germ line and somatic) which will continue to incite logomachy. In general, germ line theorists have always simply equated "*the* germ line theory" with the statement that all combining specificities expressed by an individual are germ line encoded. Unless the selection pressures determining the germ line are considered, this is an incomplete theory. We have argued that germ line v genes are selected for the combining specificities they encode. The germ line v genes encoding humoral antibody are selected for their antipathogen (extracellular) specificities (Cohn, 1971) whereas those encoding cell-mediated antibody are selected for two activities, their antispecies-R specificity (Jerne, 1971) because of restrictive recognition (Langman, 1978) and for certain antipathogen (intracellular) specificities. This minimizes nonfunctional v genes which nevertheless must be present like "selfish" DNA (Orgel and Crick, 1980) in numbers which will affect the interpretation of all estimates of germ line v genes using DNA technology. Only functional germ line v genes can contribute to the repertoire. The analogies between v gene loci and ribosomal or histone gene loci so

popular in the past have always been and still are derouting for they ignore the differential selection pressures which drive v genes to be many but different as contrasted to ribosomal genes which are many but identical (see discussion, Cohn, 1971).

(4) The importance of the contribution of antigenic selection in increasing the combining site repertoire depends upon the rate and the specificity (i.e., affect on CD relative to FW positions) of the proposed somatic mechanism. At one extreme is a category of somatic mutation model which because of a relatively low frequency uniform mutation in v genes requires sequential (stepwise) antigenic selection to amplify and stabilize the available repertoire. As the rate of mutation increases and as it affects CD residues preferentially, the requirement for antigenic selection to amplify the available repertoire diminishes but could never be negligible. At the other extreme is a germ line model (or its derivative, permuted predestination) which unfolds the total repertoire with no antigenic selection (primotype = clonotype). In this case, the germ line genes themselves cannot be selected upon for the antibody specificities they encode.

Germ line genes can be selected upon for the combining specificities they encode only if the loss or gain of that activity is of survival value. As the number of different germ line genes from which a given combining specificity can be generated by somatic diversification increases, the selective pressure to keep a given germ line gene encoding that specificity, becomes less effective. If there were many distinct clonotypes with overlapping specificities, programmed to be expressed somatically from a pool of permuted "minigenes" then specific antigenic selection could not maintain any given germ line gene set because it encoded a specificity of survival value.

The fact that the germ line loci are comprised of structural v genes which encode unique antibody specificities demonstrates that the selection pressure on germ line v genes is for that activity. This conclusion is incompatible with "*the* germ line model" or its derivative, permuted predestination (Klinman *et al.*, 1976).

Most workers are preoccupied with what appears to be (1) an order in the appearance of antigen-specific responsiveness; (2) a rapid antigen-independent expression of the repertoire; (3) an *absolutely* identical repertoire in every individual of an inbred strain; and (4) an enormous available repertoire ($\sim 10^8$). This for them precludes mutational variation and immunogenic selection as the major source of combining site diversification. The importance of these 4 preoccupations is debatable. First, whether germ line v genes are expressed during differentiation in a programmed order is not in question; it has always seemed likely. However, this argument against mutational diversification applies only to somatically derived v genes. Even were an order in their expression to be established (and no hint of this exists), the argument would be weak because (a) a germ line time-ordered expression could impose a loose somatic mutational time-ordered pattern, and (b) tolerance patterns vary as the embryo matures and this could indirectly create the illusion of an order in the appearance of somatically antigen-specific responsiveness. Second, the repertoire is often sampled with hydrophobic haptens such as DNP, TNP, fluorescein or with determinants recognized by germ line encoded combining specificities and present on erythrocytes (SRBC) or carbohydrates. The hydrophobic haptens bias the sampling because they can be recognized by combining sites that are derived from a large number of different $V_L V_H$ pairs i.e., they react with a wide variety of antibodies with totally different normally functional combining specificities. The erythrocytes and carbohydrates are recognized by germ line encoded antibodies and therefore provide no test of the rate of somatic diversification. It was precisely this latter problem that led us to analyse how an animal would respond to a given antigen by somatic evolution if its germ line v genes encoding recognition of that antigen were dissected away by genetic surgery. Third, identity of the combining site repertoire (clonotype) in various individuals cannot be established by the presently available crude methods, e.g. anti-idiotypic reagents or isoelectric focusing patterns. Fourth, the size of the available combining site repertoire expressed by an individual is unlikely to be larger than 10^6, which is about 10^2-fold less than the "isoelectric focusing" repertoire (see above). A viable theory must account for 10^5 which is sufficient to explain immune behaviour, e.g. that of a tadpole; somatic theories account for 10^6, and given the data presented here, none account for $> 10^7$ which is an upper limit of concern to those who might like to reflect upon idiotype network theory.

How is diversity generated in cell-mediated antibody?

There is at present only physiological data on which to base a discussion. Yet the problem can be defined with precision and the number of solutions are few. We will discuss the generation of diversity using the model of cell-mediated antibody which we presented earlier and return afterwards to a consideration of 2 other formulations which are variations of this theme (von Boehmer *et al.*, 1978; Williamson, 1980). Thus far, we have assumed that the germ line v_T genes encoding cell-mediated antibody (T cell receptor) are organized in a single locus distinct from the v_L and v_H loci encoding humoral antibody (B cell receptor). Now we will discuss the basis for this as well as its consequences for the generation of the T cell repertoire.

What combining specificities are encoded by the gene locus determining the T cell receptor?

The germ line v_T gene locus is assumed to encode two classes of combining specificity one antispecies-R, the other antipathogen (e.g., viruses). The postulated germ line encoded anti-X (pathogen) repertoire is a reasonable assumption based on the same arguments used for humoral antibody above.

There is no evidence at the moment for this anti-X pool and until we come to the final section, we will treat it as a second-order consideration.

We recall from an earlier section that the germ line encoded anti-R (K, D and I) combining specificities are directed against allele specific determinants on the highly polymorphic R molecules. Normally the anti-R combining site which recognizes self-R is selected in the thymus (Zinkernagel and Doherty, 1979) where we postulate that the relationship between effector function and restricting specificity (Table I) is also learned (Cohn and Epstein, 1978). These anti-R specificities are assumed to be germ line encoded for an experimental reason (i.e., alloreactivity or the relationship between anti-R and anti-X implied by the high proportion of cells whose anti-X receptors recognize allele specific determinants on the species-R) and for an *a priori* reason (i.e., anti-R combining specificities are maintained in the germ line of a random mating population because any animal whose precursor T cell population could not recognize its own restricting element (self-R) with high probability would be eliminated due to its lack of a functioning immune system). The pool of germ line v_T genes must be sufficiently large to make it highly probable that a random mating will produce a viable match between antiself-R and self-R and yet small enough to make the frequency of antiself-R specific precursor T cells sufficiently high to generate a responsive immune system in a limited time during ontogeny.

If there are $\sim 10^2$ alleles of R in a mating pool, then one might estimate the number of functional germ line v_T genes encoding monomeric antispecies-R and anti-X (pathogen) to be as large as $2–3 \times 10^2$.

How is the anti-X combining site determined?

The answer to this question requires first that we consider alloreactivity, in particular its high frequency. Under the model for cell-mediated antibody presented earlier (Fig. 2C), alloreactivity is mediated by the anti-X receptor (Langman, 1978). Why?

Allo-R is a special case of a foreign X antigen. It is special because R is the site where the signal is accepted. Allo-R is not special because of any antigenic relationship to self-R.

When an effector T cell (illustrated with T^K) interacts with a target expressing allo-R (Fig. 7) its antiself-R receptor cannot be occupied (no self-R is present). Consequently, allo-R must react with anti-X, to deliver a signal in the absence of an interaction with antiself-R because allo-R is itself complexed with the signal acceptor. Alloreactivity is apparently unrestricted, i.e. antiself-R need not be occupied, but a restricting element is nonetheless involved. Since alloreactive antigen-sensitive cells are of high frequency ($>10^{-3}$) and since allo-R must be recognized by anti-X, we conclude that anti-X is encoded by the same locus that encodes anti-R. Thus the locus encoding cell-mediated antibody is selected during germ line evolution largely

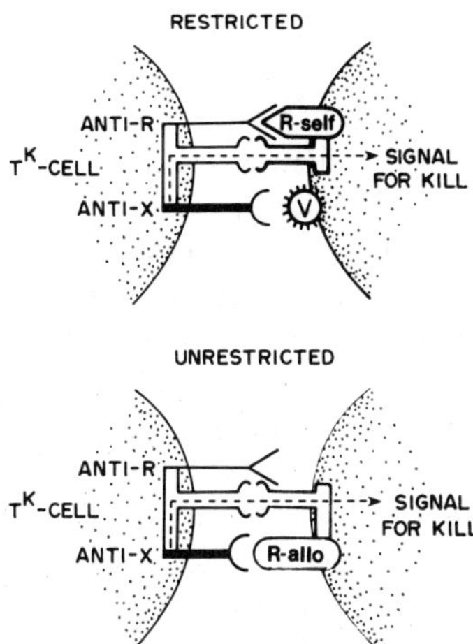

FIG. 7. *The cell–cell interactions with allorestricting elements (R) as target determinants. The cycotoxic T^K cell is used as an illustrative case (see legend Fig. 2).*

for antispecies-R specificity, whereas that encoding humoral antibody is selected essentially for anticarbohydrate (pathogen) specificity. This implies 2 different germ line starting points for somatic evolution.

Since alloreactivity is mediated by the anti-X receptor, antiallo-R must be a major source of the anti-X repertoire. The model requires that two v_T genes be expressed per cell, one encoding antiself-R (selected in thymus) and the other antiallo-R (diversified somatically to anti-X). Each v_T gene must be attached to a different constant region (anti-R = V_RC_R; anti-X = V_XC_X) to account for the different roles of the two receptors. Since the J segment is involved largely in V_LV_H pairing, the monomer T cell combining site is not expected to express J. In order for the same gene locus to express 2 different v genes properly related to 2 different c genes, both allelic loci must be expressed, i.e. haplotype inclusion must operate. Further, the linking of $V \rightarrow C$ must occur at the DNA level, otherwise the products C_R and C_X would associate randomly with V_R and V_X to destroy restrictive recognition. This is illustrated in Fig. 8 and represents a revision of our previous formulation (Cohn and Epstein, 1978; Langman, 1978). In addition, we have guessed that this locus is H-2 linked (Cohn and Epstein, 1978). This is not required by

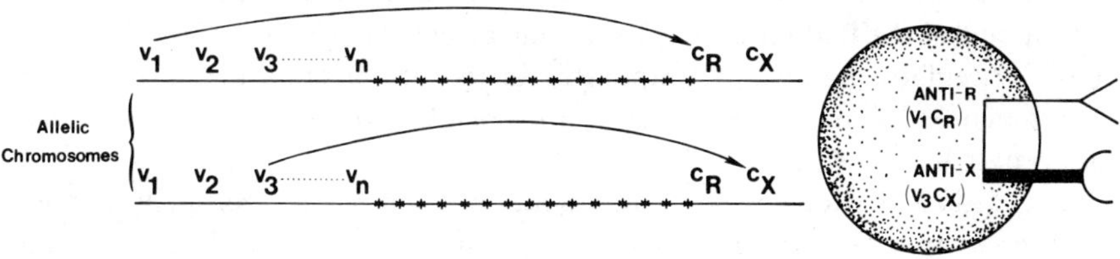

FIG. 8. *A model of v gene expression in T cells.*

the theory nor is it disproven. What is a consequence of our argument, is that the locus encoding the T cell receptor be distinct from that encoding the B cell receptor.

The assumption that R is polymorphic as an unavoidable consequence of the existence of a multigene system for its recognition (anti-R) (Langman, 1978), is necessary but insufficient. A selective pressure is required to maintain the polymorphism and this must operate on the germ line v_T genes encoding anti-R. Since these v_T genes determine the repertoire of anti-X specificities which arise by somatic mutation, selection, based both on the generation of the repertoire and restrictive recognition, is expected to optimally disperse and maintain the germ line encoded anti-R pool.

Lastly as an aside, since either Helper/Delayed Hypersensitive or Suppressive/Killer signals can be delivered via K/D or I when they are allotarget determinants, the signal acceptor linked to K/D or I must be the same and capable of registering either signal depending on which one the donor delivers.

How is the germ line encoded anti-X (antiallo-R) somatically diversified?

Since the humoral antibody system was derived during germ line evolution from the cell-mediated antibody system (Makela *et al.*, 1976; Langman, 1978), it is a reasonable guess that similar rules of somatic diversification apply. In this case, $\sim 10^2$ germ line v genes encoding antispecies-R (allo-R) vary by mutation and are selected upon by antigen-X. We have argued that the range (not the dictionary) of specificities of humoral and cell-mediated antibodies must be the same. Since they start from distinctly different germ line genes, this is understandable.

The anti-X (as well as anti-R) site of cell-mediated antibody must be monomeric. The consequence of having two receptor sites of different function and specificity is that they cannot each be comprised of two complementing subunits analogous to V_L and V_H, because phenotypic mixing of the subunits with the consequent drastic alteration of specificities would be unavoidable. In addition, the $p \times q$ rule cannot operate if we wish to account for the high frequency of alloreactive cells. A monomeric anti-X receptor appears to put a serious limit on its rate of diversification. There are several solutions of varying degrees of outrageousness. As an example, the V_T region comprising anti-X (as well as anti-R) could be longer (150–200 amino acids) than the one used by a humoral antibody subunit (100 amino acids). Therefore it could comprise 4–6 CD regions making it comparable in its rate of somatic diversification to a given $V_L V_H$ pair; the mutation rate per CD residue is independent of the gene which encodes it.

The antiself-R site selected in the thymus does not vary somatically because (1) there is no possible positive selection by antigen for anti-X variants derived from the genes encoding the antiself-R receptor, and (2) any somatic mutant which lost antiself-R recognition could not function in restrictive recognition.

How does our formulation compare with those which postulate similar effector mechanisms?

All formulations are basically incomplete, if no mechanism of effector T cell function is proposed. However, there are two models which we can complete in terms of the herein proposed effector mechanism. These will be compared now (Table IV).

The von Boehmer–Haas–Jerne model (1978) starts with the assumption that the total cell-mediated antibody repertoire is derived from those germ line v_T genes encoding the antiself-R receptor by mutational escape from tolerance (paralysis) (see discussion of Jerne (1971) earlier). This assumption has as its consequences:

(1) It accounts admirably for the genetics of antigen-specific responsiveness, so well in fact that it cannot single out which findings to treat with circumspect. Clearly, all of the examples of T cell unresponsiveness are unlikely to have a unique origin.

(2) There must be two gene loci encoding cell-mediated antibody: one has as its product anti-K/D of the species, the other anti-I of the species. The relationship between effector function and restricting specificity is not learned but is germ line encoded. T cells expressing anti-K/D become Suppressor/Killers; T cells expressing anti-I become Helper/Delayed Hypersensitors by a germ line gene locus regulated differentiation not by learning.

(3) Each cell must be born with its two sites, anti-R and anti-X, of similar combining specificity. The effector mechanism has not been analysed by von Boehmer *et al.* (1978) but it is reducible to the Langman–Cohn (1978) model because the expressed germ line v_T gene must be duplicated and coupled to two different c genes, c_R and c_X, one of which encodes anti-R function and the other anti-X function (including diversification). If the v_T genes were v_H genes, either a new mechanism of fusion would have to operate or each of the duplicated v genes would have to be fused to a different dj gene pair, the protein products of which would differ in amino acid sequence but be similar in combining site specificity. Coupling of one v to two c's at the level of RNA processing (a mechanism possible for IgM/IgD expression in B cells) is ruled out in the von Boehmer *et al.* (1980) model because the somatic mutational process affects only the v_T gene encoding anti-X.

(4) Alloreactivity is mediated by cells which express germ line encoded antiallo-R receptors. However, alloreactive T cells unlike all others must be induced "helper" independent.

(5) The alloreactive cell has a recognition specificity independent of the antiself-R selected for restrictive recognition because both sites on its

TABLE IV

A comparison of three related theories of the structure of cell-mediated antibody T cell receptor

	Langman–Cohn (*1978*)	*von Boehmer–Haas–Jerne* (*1978*)	*Williamson* (*1980*)
Structure of receptor	[Antiself-R / Antiallo-R][a] → anti-X	[Antiself-R / Antiself-R] → anti-X + [Antiallo-R / Antiallo-R]	[Antiself-R / Anti-X (Ig) + Antiallo-R / Anti-X (Ig)]
Origin of:			
Anti-R	Germ line encoded	Germ line encoded	Germ line encoded
Anti-X	Somatic diversification of antiallo-R	Somatic diversification of antiself-R	Same as for humoral antibody
Explanation of high frequency alloreactivity	Antiself-R / Antiallo-R	Antiallo-R / Antiallo-R	Antiallo-R / Antiminors
IR-1 genes	Several explanations: (1) affinity of antiself-R and anti-X (2) Antiallo-R-//→anti-X	Antiself-R-//→anti-X	X and self-R cross-react with antiself-R
Assumption that $v_L v_H$ encodes			
Anti-R	Incompatible	Incompatible	Incompatible
Anti-X	Incompatible	Incompatible	Postulated

	Langman–Cohn (1978)	*von Boehmer–Haas–Jerne (1978)*	*Williamson (1980)*
Haplotype exclusion of expression of receptor			
Anti-R	Anti-R and anti-X must each be encoded by a different allele[b]	Required[c]	Does not operate.
Anti-X		Required[c]	Assumed same as for humoral antibody
Relationship between anti-R (K/D or I) specificity and effector function	Learned somatically e.g. in thymus	Germ line encoded	Learned but few per cent possess wrong relationship
Assumption that idiotype network operates	Incompatible	Incompatible	Compatible

[a] Boxes indicate a cell bearing the postulated receptor.
[b] Since anti-R and anti-X are comprised of different V and C regions, one allelic locus must be activated to express $V_R C_R$ (anti-R) and the other must be activated to express $V_X C_X$ (anti-X) (Fig. 8).
[c] Since anti-R and anti-X are initially identical, expression by somatic gene duplication of only one v gene/cell is required to form the VC_R and VC_X receptors.

receptor are identical, antiallo-R. This consequence of the model has been shown to be untenable (Hunig and Bevan, 1980) but it can be modified to assume that alloreactivity is in large measure derived by somatic mutation of the genes encoding the antiself-R receptor as part of their diversification to encode the anti-X repertoire. This modification forces the model into a framework proposed many times by others and needs an independent justification (see below).

It is based upon three postulates which we deem unlikely to be correct:

(1) The anti-X repertoire is derived somatically from $<1\%$ of the germ line v gene pool encoding anti-R.

(2) The dictionary of the repertoires used by Helpers/Delayed-hypersensitors must be different from that used by Killers/Suppressors since the former is derived somatically from germ line encoded antiself-I whereas the latter is derived somatically from germ line encoded antiself-K/D. Given the limitations due to a derivation of the repertoire from $<1\%$ of the germ line v gene pool, this decreases still further the size of the repertoire possible for each cell type. We recall that under the Langman–Cohn (1978) model, a single gene locus encodes the total anti-K/D and I of the species, i.e., antispecies-R (Fig. 8) and serves as the starting point for somatic diversification to anti-X.

(3) There must be two mechanisms of paralysis; one which drives diversification of antiself-R to anti-X and the other which permits the self–nonself discrimination without contributing to diversification. $(A \times B)F_1 \rightarrow P_A$ chimaeras are restricted to A only, but tolerant to both A and B haplotypes.

The Williamson (1980) model puts two receptors on each T cell one [antiself-R + anti-X], and the other, [antiallo-R + anti-X]. Each receptor can be envisaged to function as in the Langman–Cohn (1978) model. The anti-X site identical in both receptors, is immunoglobulin encoded by the known $v_L v_H$ gene loci, while the anti-R is encoded elsewhere. This model has the unrationalized feature (i.e., added on *a posteriori* grounds) that the humoral and cell-mediated antibody anti-X repertoire are encoded by the same loci but it is incomplete in that the pathway of diversification in each category humoral and cell-mediated is not dealt with, although Williamson (1976) has always been an ascetic germ-line theorist. It, too, is based upon 3 postulates unlikely to be correct:

(1) The expression of both antiself-R and antiallo-R in each cell is looked upon as a failure of haplotype exclusion to operate (i.e. the cell-mediated system never evolved haplotype exclusion as did the humoral system). This postulate then gives no independent or *a priori* rationale to alloreactivity. It simply restates the fact. Further it treats the failure to find normal restriction to allo-R as a matter of limited (insensitive) experimentation (less than 5% of the total activity restricted to antiself-R, would not be detected) rather than a fundamental principle.

This formulation is to be contrasted with that of Langman–Cohn (1978) where any haplotype inclusion (Fig. 8) must be the consequence of a selected for mechanism because the anti-X repertoire is derived from the total germ line encoded antispecies-R pool.

(2) Alloreactivity is accounted for as due to a recognition of foreign minors restricted to allo-R. Under this assumption the number of alloreactive antigen-sensitive cells should be sharply dependent on the number of non-MHC encoded gene products (foreign minors) which the stimulating or target cell expresses. Alloreactivity assayed between strains (e.g. BALB/c anti-C57BL/10) should be much greater than that assayed between congenics (e.g. BALB/c anti-BALB.B). This, in fact, is not found. It is essential to point out that a difference between "strains" and "congenics" is not expected under the original "altered self" or "new antigenic determinant" version of this assumption (Matzinger and Bevan, 1977).

(3) IR-1 controlled genetic unresponsiveness is due to competition between a given self-R and the antigen-X for antiself-R. This assumption, hazardous as an explanation of unresponsiveness linked to one allele, becomes untenable when unresponsiveness is associated with 3 or 4 non-cross-reacting alleles. Further, a functional effector T cell receptor requires that the competitive effects of free (not cell-bound) antigen-X be minimized.

The various models which we have not considered in this discussion are based on the following assumptions which we believe to be untenable:

(1) The origin of restrictive recognition is an *obligatory* interaction between R and X (Janeway *et al.*, 1976; Matzinger and Bevan, 1977; Paul and Benacerraf, 1977). The reasons are analysed elsewhere (Cohn and Epstein, 1978). This assumption does not contribute to an analysis of the structure of cell-mediated antibody. *The use of the terms "one receptor" or "two receptors" to distinguish between theories where the origin of the restriction is [R + X] or [anti-R + anti-X] respectively, saddles the wrong horse.*

(2) Somatic selection for low affinity antiself-R entrains (unselected) a cross-reactivity of high affinity for allo-R (Janeway *et al.*, 1976) and at high frequency (Blanden and Ada, 1978) even including the anti-X set (Hoffmann, 1980; Klinman *et al.*, 1980; modification of von Boehmer *et al.*, 1978). No selection pressure can be rationalized which, driven only by an affinity-dependent recognition of *allele-specific* determinants on either self K, D or I, concomitantly co-opts a high frequency specific recognition of allo-R (as well as in some models, the universe of X-antigens); all of this occurring in the absence of these allo-R and X-antigens.

Where does the problem of the generation of diversity in the immune system, humoral or cell-mediated, go from here?

A large part of immunological thinking is guided by the network concept. While anti-idiotypic reagents are useful experimental tools in analysing immune responsiveness, there are no data which lead uniquely to the conclusion that antigen-specific responsiveness (the self–nonself discrimination or regulation of class) is governed normally by self-idiotypic interactions. The lack of a decisive experiment is certain to be considered a weak argument but it becomes stronger in view of the absence of a network theory of antigen-specific responsiveness which has both molecular level plausibility and the potential to be mapped onto known regulatory cell–cell interactions. Most of the findings purporting to show network regulation are predictable and understood under the associative recognition model which although not discussed here, underlies our thinking.

The generally accepted conclusion that cell-mediated and humoral antibody are encoded by the same germ line v gene loci, has been based on its common-sense appeal and on a massive accumulation of observations involving the use of anti-idiotypic (and anti-V_H) reagents. The first argument (Cohn, 1971) was reasonable in the era prior to the discovery of restrictive recognition but it is no longer valid. The second argument is based on experimental systems of such great complexity that many interpretations are possible and reproducibility becomes a luxury. Three generally drawn conclusions from the experiments, of importance to us in the present context, are commented upon below:

(1) That T cells anti-X express a v_H encoded idiotype because pretreatment of an animal with a foreign anti-idiotype changes responsiveness to antigen-X (which is characterized as being recognized by humoral antibodies bearing the reference idiotype). More likely is that tolerance to the self-idiotype is broken, i.e., regulatory T cells recognizing the self-idiotype are induced by the (self-idiotype–anti-idiotype) complex. These T cells anti-idiotype react with the B cells bearing the idiotype and modulate their responsiveness. Since T cells anti-idiotype cannot express the idiotype, the general conclusion that cell-mediated and humoral antibodies are encoded by the same v gene loci is unwarranted. Furthermore, under the associative recognition model an "idiotype network" only exists when self-idiotypes are complexed with foreign anti-idiotypes (i.e., when a hapten-carrier immunogen is present); therefore, self-idiotypes cannot be a factor distinct from any other self-component in driving the generation of diversity.

(2) That antigen-specific products of "T cells" react with anti-idiotypic (or anti-V_H) sera, and therefore, T cell repertoires are v_H gene-encoded. Even if the antisera assay "what their labels imply", these findings cannot tell us where the T cell receptor is encoded until it is known (a) whether the same T cell showing restricted effector function synthesizes the factor (product) and (b) how the factor and the effector mechanism are related. In essence, T cells show restricted effector function; the factors (which are believed to carry v_H encoded idiotypic determinants) do not (although this is disputed).

(3) That antigen-driven regulatory cell–cell interactions, e.g., T–B,

require "idiotype-matching" or "idiotype-restriction". This is ruled out on the *a priori* grounds that, if generalized, the assumption requires self-complementation of idiotypes.

In order to explain the specificity of immune responsiveness to an antigen, a functioning network requires an almost one to one relationship between the given antibody and the specificities of its two interactants, anti-Id and antigen. It is generally overlooked that (a) anti-idiotypic interactions are highly degenerate and (b) each step back into the chain of successive levels of regulatory anti-idiotypic interactions is increasingly uncoupled from the original antigen–antibody interaction that triggers the immune response which must be regulated. In experimental systems, anti-idiotypic sera are most often directed to FW determinants, some of which are close to the combining site (inferred from ligand modifiability); and, in all cases, they are very insensitive to single (or even double) amino acid replacements in CD residues which comprise most of the repertoire (Carson and Weigert, 1973). Consequently, we see no reason to believe that anti-idiotypic interactions can be mapped onto antigen-driven responsiveness with sufficient specificity to provide a requisite immune regulation.

The concepts referred to as "network" are so delusive that models of T cell induction and function (restrictive recognition) ignoring or incompatible with network regulation are proposed by network theorists (Janeway *et al.*, 1976; von Boehmer *et al.*, 1978; Hoffmann, 1980; Klinman *et al.*, 1980). If, as required under network regulation, the self–nonself discrimination were determined uniquely by a suppressive anti-idiotypic recognition of the anti-X receptor with antiself specificity, the cell-mediated system would be inoperative because suppression would operate per force on the anti-R receptor with antiself-R specificity. Further, the repertoire could not be derived by mutational escape of the antiself-R receptor from suppression (i.e., the network formulation of the von Boehmer–Haas–Jerne (1978) model) without the suppressive anti-Id (antispecies-R) itself being germ line encoded and that assumption will have to run the gauntlet. This is why paralysis, as defined by the associative recognition model, not suppression as defined by the network model, has been assumed to drive diversity in the thymus.

Returning now to our framework for the discussion of combining site diversity, in the absence of immunogenic selection the available repertoire (clonotype) of the naive immune system in an individual would consist of approximately:

(1) 10^2 germ line selected humoral antibodies.

(2) 10^3 ($<10^4$) V_LV_H pairs (which are useful only as starting points for mutational diversification).

(3) 10^2 germ line selected cell-mediated antibodies.

(4) 10^2 germ line selected antispecies-R specificities (which are useful only as starting points for mutational diversification).

(5) 10^5 somatic mutants in both classes humoral and cell-mediated.

The available repertoire in this system would be $10^5 \geqslant \mathcal{N} \geqslant 10^2$ in each class.

The somatic mutants would be generated in 10 days assuming a mutation rate of 10^{-4}/division in CD codons of the receptor, a division rate of 2–3/day and a steady state population of 10^8 in the dividing pool (Cohn, 1973). The assumed rate of mutation is sufficiently unusual that a "special" mechanism for a differential mutation rate in CD and FW codons is hinted. It need not be very exotic. In the absence of repair, the mutation rate per base pair in bacteria is 10^{-7}. If there are 50 CD bases in the genes encoding a receptor, the mutation rate per receptor would be 5×10^{-6}. A 10-fold increase in this basal rate could be accomplished in many ways, e.g., by "stuttering" excision-repair systems, by spontaneous deamination of methylated cytosine to thymine, etc.

In order for these single step mutants to be maximally different, i.e., cover as wide a range as possible, the starting germ line encoded receptor pool must be maximally diverse. For example, if the germ line encoded 10^2 identical v genes/locus (like ribosomal genes) then the resultant 10^5 mutants would comprise only $\sim 10^2$ different combining specificities (20 CD codons/receptor × 3–5 replacements/codon).

Thus there are 2 future problems:

(1) What is the selection pressure on the germ line to disperse the starting or parental pool so that it is optimized to give a range of different specificities?

(2) How does the system respond to immunogen it encounters initially?

We will not dwell on either of these problems. For humoral antibody it might be argued that the secondary source of variation due to combinatorial complementation, $pV_L \times qV_H$, is sufficient to provide the initial dispersion that maximizes the range of the single step mutationally derived repertoire. For cell-mediated antibody it might be argued that either the germ line encoded anti-X set and/or the germ line encoded antispecies-R set are selected so that the initial pool would be optimally dispersed. If this is a factor in the germ line selection of antispecies-R then the see-sawing polymorphism between the anti-R and R is selected upon not only for restrictive recognition (necessary) but also for the somatic descendants generated from anti-R by mutation. The selection pressure maximizing the dispersion results in a germ line antispecies-R repertoire directed largely at allele-specific determinants on R. This is explained only by the model presented here (Figs 2 and 7). Any germ line encoded anti-R specificities directed at common determinants on R could function perfectly well in restrictive recognition but be unable to act as a significant source of somatic variants. Paralysis would keep the cells expressing antiself-R in the anti-X position at a very low level compared to those expressing antiallo-R specificities which are allele specific. Therefore, germ line encoded anticommon determinants on R could not contribute efficiently to the anti-X repertoire. Consequently, germ line encoded allele-specific antispecies-R and anti-X provide dispersion for generating a cell-mediated repertoire in the same way that germ line encoded $pV_L \times qV_H$ pairs provide dispersion for generating a humoral repertoire.

The problem of initiating induction in the primotype involves many factors to which we will only allude. The commonly encountered immunogens (pathogens) are polymeric and therefore use co-operating ("helper") activity very efficiently. Further they are most likely recognized by germ line encoded combining specificities. Any immunogen which has determinants recognized by germ line encoded "helper" antibody will lead to the induction of any mutant in other T and B classes which recognizes another determinant on that immunogen. This will exponentially enlarge the available repertoire as mutants increase in number due to induction and second step variants can now arise with sufficient frequency to provide a totally adequate available repertoire (Cohn, 1970).

This last point shows that no matter how the discussions continue, the origin of the humoral and cell-mediated repertoires is one problem the solution to which has changed in emphasis from how do genes vary to how do we select them. GOD has become a problem of cellular immunology, alas!

References

Amzel, L. M. and Poljak, R. J. (1979). *Ann. Rev. Biochem.* **48**, 961.

Bhattacharjee, A. K. and Glaudemans, C. P. J. (1978). *J. Immunol.* **120**, 411.

Bernard, O., Hozumi, N. and Tonegawa, S. (1978). *Cell* **15**, 1133.

Blanden, R. V. and Ada, G. L. (1978). *Scand. J. Immunol.* **7**, 181.

Blomberg, B., Geckeler, W. and Weigert, M. (1972). *Science* **177**, 178.

von Boehmer, H., Haas, W. and Jerne, N. K. (1978). *Proc. Natn. Acad. Sci. U.S.A.* **75**, 2439.

Brack, C., Hirama, M., Lenhard-Schuller, R. and Tonegawa, S. (1978). *Cell* **15**, 1.

Carson, D. and Weigert, M. (1973). *Proc. Natn. Acad. Sci. U.S.A.* **70**, 235.

Cesari, I. M. and Weigert, M. (1973). *Proc. Natn. Acad. Sci. U.S.A.* **70**, 2112.

Cohn, M. (1970). *Cellular Immunol.* **1**, 461.

Cohn, M. (1971). *Ann. N.Y. Acad. Sci.* **190**, 529.

Cohn, M. (1972). *Cellular Immunol.* **5**, 1.

Cohn, M. (1973). *In* "Biochemistry of Gene Expression in Higher Organisms" (J. K. Pollak and J. W. Lee, eds) pp. 574–592. D. Reidel Publishing Co., Dordrecht, Holland.

Cohn, M. (1974). *In* "Progress in Immunology II" Vol. 2. (L. Brent and J. Halborow, eds) pp. 261–283. North-Holland Publishing Company, Amsterdam.

Cohn, M. and Epstein, R. (1978). *Cellular Immunol.* **39**, 125.

Cohn, M., Blomberg, B., Geckeler, W., Raschke, W., Riblet, R. and Weigert, M. (1974). *In* "The Immune System: Genes, Receptors, Signals" (E. Sercarz and A. Williamson, eds) pp. 99–117. Academic Press, London and New York.

Coutinho, A. (1979). *Ann. Immunol. (Inst. Pasteur)* **130C**, 781.

dePreval, C. and Fougereau, M. (1976). *J. Mol. Biol.* **102**, 657.

dePreval, C., Blomberg, B. and Cohn, M. (1979). *J. Exp. Med.* **149**, 1265.

Dreyer, W. J. and Bennett, J. C. (1965). *Proc. Natn. Acad. Sci. U.S.A.* **54**, 864.

Early, P., Huang, H., Davis, M., Calame, K. and Hood, L. (1980). *Cell* **19**, 981.

Ehrlich, P. H. (1979). *J. Theoret. Biol.* **81**, 123.

Gally, J. A. and Edelman, G. M. (1970). *Nature* **227**, 341.

Gally, J. A. and Edelman, G. M. (1972). *Ann. Rev. Genetics* **6**, 1.

Geckeler, W., Faversham, J. and Cohn, M. (1978). *J. Exp. Med.* **148**, 1122.

Hirst, J. W., Jones, G. G. and Cohn, M. (1971). *J. Immunol.* **107**, 926.
Hoffmann, G. W. (1980). *In* "Contemporary Topics in Immunology", Vol. 11, Plenum Press, New York (in press).
Hood, L. and Talmage, D. W. (1970). *Science* **168**, 325.
Hood, L., Barstad, D., Loh, E. and Nottenberg, C. (1974). *In* "The Immune System: Genes, Receptors, Signals" (E. Sercarz and A. Williamson, eds), pp. 119–139. Academic Press, London and New York.
Hood, L., Loh, E., Hubert, J., Barstad, P., Eaton, B., Early, P., Fuhrman, J., Johnson, N., Kronenberg, M. and Schilling, J. (1976). *Cold Spring Harbor Symp. Quant. Biol.* **41**, 817–836.
Hunig, T. and Bevan, M. (1980). *J. Exp. Med.* **151**, 1288.
Janeway, C. A., Wigzell, H. and Binz, H. (1976). *Scand. J. Immunol.* **5**, 993.
Jerne, N. K. (1971). *Eur. J. Immunol.* **1**, 1.
Jerne, N. K. (1979). Basel Institute for Immunology, Introduction to Annual Report.
Kabat, E. A. (1978). *Adv. Protein Chemistry* **32**, 1.
Kabat, E. A. (1979). *In* "Cells of Immunoglobulin Synthesis" (B. Pernis and H. J. Vogel, eds), pp. 33–44. Academic Press, London and New York.
Kabat, E. A. (1980). *J. Immunol.* (in press).
Kabat, E. A., Wu, T. T. and Bilofsky, H. (1979). *In* "Sequences of Immunoglobulin Chains", NIH Publication No. 80-2008.
Kindt, T. J. and Capra, J. D. (1978). *Immunogenetics* **6**, 309.
Klinman, N. R., Press, J. L., Segal, N. H. and Gearhart, P. J. (1976). *In* "The Generation of Antibody Diversity" (A. J. Cunningham, ed.), pp. 127–149. Academic Press, London and New York.
Klinman, N. R., Wylie, D. E. and Cancro, M. P. (1980). This publication.
Langman, R. E. (1978). *In* "Rev. Physiol. Biochem. Pharmac." **81**, pp. 1–37. Springer-Verlag, New York.
Leon, M. A., Young, N. M. and McIntire, K. R. (1970). *Biochemistry* **9**, 1023.
Lennox, E. S. and Cohn, M. (1967). *Ann. Rev. Biochem.* **36**, 365.
Lundblad, A., Steller, R., Kabat, E. A., Hirst, J. W., Weigert, M. G. and Cohn, M. (1972). *Immunochem.* **9**, 535.
Makela, O., Koskimies, S. and Karjalainen, K. (1976). *Scand. J. Immunol.* **5**, 305.
Matzinger, P. and Bevan, M. (1977). *Cellular Immunol.* **29**, 1.
Max, E. E., Seidman, J. G. and Leder, P. (1979). *Proc. Natn. Acad. Sci. U.S.A.* **76**, 3450.
McKean, D. J. and Potter, M. (1979). *In* "T and B Lymphocytes: Recognition and Function" (F. H. Bach, B. Bonavida, E. S. Vitetta, C. F. Fox, eds) ICN-UCLA Symp. on Molec. and Cell. Biol. XLI, pp. 63–71. Academic Press, London and New York.
Nishioka, Y. and Leder, P. (1980). *J. Biol. Chem.* **255**, 3691.
Ohno, S. (1980). *Differentiation* (in press).
Orgel, L. E. and Crick, F. H. C. (1980). *Nature* **284**, 604.
Padlan, E. A. (1977). *Qt. Rev. Biophys.* **10**, 35.
Paul, W. E. and Benacerraf, B. (1977). *Science* **195**, 1293.
Perelson, A. S. and Oster, G. F. (1979). *J. Theoret. Biol.* **81**, 645.
Perry, R. P., Kelley, D. E. and Schibler, U. (1979). *Proc. Natn. Acad. Sci. U.S.A.* **76**, 3678.
Poljak, R. J., Amzel, L. M., Chen, B. L., Chiu, Y. Y., Phizarkerly, R. P., Saul, F. and Yserm, X. (1976). *Cold Spring Harbor Symp. Quant. Biol.* **41**, 639–645.
Poljak, R. J., Amzel, L. M., Saul, F. (1980) (in press).
Potter, M., Appella, E. and Geisser, S. (1965). *J. Mol. Biol.* **14**, 361.
Potter, M. (1977). *Adv. Immunol.* **25**, 141.
Rabbitts, T. H., Matthyssens, A. and Hamlyn, P. H. (1980). *Nature* **284**, 238.
Rao, N. D., Rudikoff, S. and Potter, M. (1978). *Biochemistry* **17**, 5555.

Sakano, H., Rogers, J. H., Huppi, K., Brack, C., Traunecker, A., Maki, R., Wall, R. and Tonegawa, S. (1979). *Nature* **277**, 627.

Schilling, J., Clevinger, B., Davie, J. M. and Hood, L. (1980). *Nature* **283**, 35.

Seidman, J. G. and Leder, P. (1978). *Nature* **276**, 790.

Seidman, J. G., Leder, A., Edgell, M. H., Polsky, F., Treghman, S. M., Tiemeier, D. C. and Leder, P. (1978a). *Proc. Natn. Acad. Sci. U.S.A.* **75**, 3881.

Seidman, J. G., Leder, A., Nau, M., Norman, B. and Leder, P. (1978b). *Science* **202**, 11.

Seidman, J. G., Max, E. E. and Leder, P. (1979). *Nature* **280**, 370.

Smith, G. P. (1973). "The Variation and Adaptive Expression of Antibodies". Harvard University Press, Cambridge, Mass.

Stevens, F. J., Westholm, F. A., Solomon, A. and Schiffer, M. (1980). *Proc. Natn. Acad. Sci. U.S.A.* **77**, 1144.

Tonegawa, S., Steinberg, C., Dube, S. and Bernardini, A. (1974). *Proc. Natn. Acad. Sci. U.S.A.* **71**, 4027.

Tonegawa, S., Maxam, A. M., Tizard, R., Bernard, O. and Gilbert, W. (1978). *Proc. Natn. Acad. Sci. U.S.A.* **76**, 1485.

Tonegawa, S. (1976). *Proc. Natn. Acad. Sci. U.S.A.* **73**, 203.

Tucker, P. W., Marcu, K. B., Newell, N., Richards, J. and Blattner, F. R. (1979). *Science* **206**, 1303.

Valbuena, O., Marcu, K. B., Weigert, M. and Perry, R. P. (1978). *Nature* **276**, 780.

Weigert, M. G., Cesari, I. M., Yonkovich, S. and Cohn, M. (1970). *Nature* **228**, 1045.

Weigert, M. and Riblet, R. (1976). *Cold Spring Harbor Symp. Quant. Biol.* **41**, 837–846.

Weigert, M. and Riblet, R. (1978). *In* "Springer Seminars in Immunopathology", Vol. 1, pp. 133–169. Springer-Verlag, Berlin and New York.

Weigert, M., Gatmaitan, L., Loh, E., Schilling, J. and Hood, L. (1978). *Nature* **276**, 785.

Weigert, M., Perry, R., Kelley, D., Hunkapiller, T., Schilling, J. and Hood, L. (1980). *Nature* **283**, 497.

Wigzell, H. (1973). *Scand. J. Immunol.* **2**, 199.

Williamson, A. R. (1976). *Ann. Rev. Biochem.* **45**, 467.

Williamson, A. R. (1980). *Nature* **283**, 527.

Zinkernagel, R. M. and Doherty, P. C. (1979). *Adv. Immunol.* **27**, 51.

Theme 3: Summary

Expression of Antigen Receptors in Lymphocytes and Cellular Activation Mechanisms

F. MELCHERS

Basel Institute for Immunology, Basel, Switzerland

Cloning of genes and cloning of lymphocytes are quite clearly the most powerful instruments which have helped and will help us to understand the principles of structures and cells involved in the reception and transmission of signals initiated by antigen in an immune response. It is now evident that clones of functional helper and killer T cells can be propagated for months and years and that, with the stimulating action of colony-stimulating factors, functional macrophage clones can be obtained. What we still do not have and badly need, are functional B cell clones.

Immunoglobulin, in particular IgM and IgD, on the surface of B cells forms the site where binding of antigen initiates the reactions which lead to the proliferation and maturation of Ig secretion and, therefore, to an immune response of B cells. It is now clear that binding of antigen to Ig on the surface of B cells does not suffice to elicit this immune response. Nevertheless the importance of Ig in the selection of antigen-specific B cell clones should be recognized if we accept the clonal selection hypothesis.

Understanding the way in which Ig inserts into the surface membrane of B cells, hopefully, will clarify the manner in which antigen binding signals a B cell how and where to go.

The highlight of the first workshop of this theme was the elucidation of the structural differences between membrane-bound and secreted μ-chains. The secreted and the membrane-bound form of μ have identical constant region domains ($C_{\mu1}$, $C_{\mu2}$, $C_{\mu3}$, $C_{\mu4}$) but differ at their COOH-end. The secreted form has a peptide of 20 amino acids, containing a carbohydrate group, while the membrane-bound form contains, at the same location, a different, quite hydrophobic peptide, 41 amino acids long, which does not contain carbohydrate. The hydrophobic stretch of the membrane-bound form of the peptide is sufficiently long to span the lipid bilayer of the surface membrane, leaving some amino acids sticking out on the inner side of the lipid bilayer. On the DNA level information for V_H and $C_{\mu1}$, $C_{\mu2}$, $C_{\mu3}$, and $C_{\mu4}$, all interrupted by introns, is followed first by a stretch of DNA complementary to the secreted form (20 amino acids), followed by an intron of 1800 nucleotides, followed by the information for the membrane-bound-peptide of 41 amino acids, followed by an intron of over 5000 nucleotides, followed by the domains of C_δ. This all is transcribed in B cells into a primary transcript RNA which is then differently processed to yield either μ secreted or μ membrane or δ, all with the same V_H. The regulation of the processing of this primary RNA transcript into the different forms of mRNA for μ secreted, μ membrane of δ, done probably by RNA splicing enzymes, is in the centre of future interest in the biochemical reactions which B cells must perform in order to express IgM only, or simultaneously IgM and IgD on the surface membrane and which they must alter when they are stimulated by antigens or mitogens to secrete IgM.

It is already evident that most, if not all other classes and subclasses of heavy chains will have similar peptides which are distinct in their secreted and membrane-bound forms, and that the information for them in the DNA will be arranged quite similarly. The localization of IgM within the surface membrane is obviously such, that the antigen-binding V_H/V_L regions can be approached and bound by antigen from the outside. Antibodies directed against the different domains of μ have been used to probe those domains which can be approached by binding from outside the cell. It appears that $C_{\mu 1}$, and $C_{\mu 2}$ stick out of the membrane sufficiently to allow binding of antibodies, while $C_{\mu 3}$ and $C_{\mu 4}$ do not. Next-neighbour analyses of proteins near IgM or IgD molecules in the surface membrane, using bivalent cross-linking reagents, detect 2 proteins with mol. wts 56 000 and 46 000 near IgM, but none near IgD. The minimal statement derived from such studies is that the molecular environment of surface IgM and surface IgD appears to be different.

This leaves us with many unanswered questions. It seems clear that such molecules as Ia antigens, in particular the ones encoded for by the *I-A* and *I-E/C* region of the H-2 complex, Fc-receptors, C′ receptors, mitogen receptors for external, bacterial mitogens such as LPS or LPP, and growth factor receptor, e.g. for BRMF or TRF are functionally associated with antigen-binding Ig-molecules. How, then, are they structurally associated with each other? The complex of molecules which functionally can exist in different conformations, is certainly a fascinating problem to be solved by molecular genetics and biochemistry.

The clonal selection hypothesis states that one lymphocyte makes one antibody molecule. Since the statement is so radical many people are continuously tempted to challenge or at least to redefine it. This theme was full of such redefinitions and even challenges.

The switch of a B cell from the expression of one Ig class to another, at least for the time of the switching event, appeared to challenge the hypothesis, at least for the expression of more than one C_H gene. DNA-analyses, however, quite clearly show that at any given time there exists only one DNA sequence to be transcribed into RNA and translated into protein. That is so for the V-rearranged chromosome. For the present time the second chromosome of a normal cell remains not rearranged in a way meaningful for the expression of Ig H or L chains. Variant myeloma cells which rather frequently switch back and forth between the expression of different classes and subclasses of Ig are one problem in this switch scheme on the DNA level.

Another problem is raised by the well documented triple-class producers within the many subpopulations of B cells, expressing—as seen in immunofluorescence—IgM, IgD and other classes and subclasses of Ig. Short of casting doubt on a generally valid mechanism of DNA class-switch by DNA deletions in C_H they at least suggest "unorthodox" mechanisms such as extremely long-lived mRNA species or activation of the second chromosome.

A different situation prevails for μ and δ chains. Here, as mentioned above, a primary transcript of RNA including V_H,C_μ and C_δ exists, which is processed by splicing enzymes in the cell to yield V_H,C_μ and V_H,C_δ. However as shown by cellular studies, idiotypes and antigen-binding properties of these IgM and IgD molecules produced by one B cell are the same, preserving the clonal selection hypothesis not for C_H but for V_H. Simultaneous expression of more than one C_H, in a way, also exists in cells expressing C_μ membrane-bound and C_μ-secreted. As elaborated above, this again is due to posttranscriptional regulation, probably in the splicing of RNA to yield two mRNA species for membrane-bound IgM and secreted IgM. It is very likely, that a resting B cell producing mainly membrane-bound IgM, and an activated plasma cell mainly secreting IgM will not entirely produce only one of the two forms but, due to the inaccuracy of the regulation of the splicing processes of the primary RNA transcript, both forms in varying ratios.

Variants, or mutants, of normal B cells, most often detected as variants of myelomas or hybridomas, are, in a way, redefinitions of the original version of the clonal selection hypothesis stating that one B cell makes one heavy and one light chain. B cells can certainly make incomplete Ig molecules. These include deletions as well as point mutations. On the DNA level not every variant appears to be a deletion which is later detected as a smaller deleted protein. Insertions of extra pieces of DNA and false processing of transcribed RNA are amongst the more fascinating new possibilities by which phenotypic expression of a given *Ig* gene can be altered. As bewildering as the variety of variants may appear at the present, they may offer keys to our understanding of the requisites of gene structure for expression of functional Ig chains and of other proteins.

Another fascinating variation of the clonal selection hypothesis are pre B cells. One very early form of pre B cells expresses only μ, but no L. In the DNA of these cells V_H is rearranged to J_H and C_μ, but all L-chain genes appear in the germ-line form and, therefore, not rearranged. Apparently, the μ chains of these pre B cells are not expressed at the surface of the cells, but only intracellularly. They, nevertheless, offer the exciting possibility that the original repertoire of V_H may expose itself separately from V_L to the antigenic universe. This may allow original specificities towards germ line antigens directed by V_H or V_L *alone*, and not by the free (or possibly restricted) combinations of all V_H with all V_L. It, thereby, may reduce the number of antigens recognized by the germ-line repertoire of V_H and V_L quite drastically. This only points to the very interesting lack of information on the antigen recognition capacities of single V regions, in particular of isolated V_H. Two sets of antigenic determinants for such germ line encoded recognition by V gene product appear particularly attractive: endogenously those encoded in the H-2 complex and exogenously, but by symbiosis "quasi endogenously", those carried by the most common bacteria, viruses and parasites.

Pre B cells, quite clearly, can also express L-chain genes. The cell line 70Z is such an example, in which normally only μ-chains are detectable. After stimulation by LPS, synthesis of full IgM molecules is induced. Before stimulation, however, the DNA for L chains is already rearranged to form a transcribable and translatable V_L–J–C_L DNA. The simplest consequence of these findings is that postreorganizational control in pre B cells can control the expression of *Ig* genes. A series of other forms of pre B cells also exist; these include cells with high-turnover synthesis of IgM, cells with delayed responsiveness to antigenic and mitogenic triggering, and all of such cells with varying physical parameters such as e.g. size. The involvement of all of these various forms of pre B cells in the physiology of B-cell development and their interdependence remains unclear at present.

So far one essential rule of clonal selection has been carefully kept up, namely the expression of only *one* V_H and/or V_L in one lymphocyte. There is however some evidence that one B cell produces several different V_H/V_L combinations with several different antigen-binding properties.

Clearly T cells have the best chance of finally disproving the simple form of the clonal selection hypothesis, i.e. that one lymphocyte produces only one antibody molecule. The capacity to recognize antigen *and* to recognize with it H-2 antigens, for some of us indicates that there may be two V_H regions expressed in one T cell, one binding antigen, the other binding H-2. In the search for the antigen-specific and H-2 specific receptors of T cells two findings may lead us on. The one is that antisera have now been raised against factors which react with a variety of antigen-specific suppressor factors, all around 70 000 in mol. wt but not with antigen-specific helper factors. These antibodies may, therefore, be directed against constant regions of antigen-specific, T-cell derived molecules, and that may give us an assay to be employed in the identification of any possible products of *in vitro* translated mRNA or of cloned genes expressed in bacteria. The prediction would be that antigen-specific T cell factors are, in fact, the receptors normally located on T cells and that T cells with different functions (killer, suppressor, helper) produce receptors, and therefore factors, with different constant regions. It is also predictable that the constant regions of the H-2 specific restricting receptors are different from those of the antigen-recognizing receptors.

The other finding relevant to the identification of the T cell receptor is that amongst a series of antigen-specific, H-2 restricted T cell clones several have *not* rearranged their V_H genes as do B cells. If T cells use V_H genes, then this finding points us to the site where the constant region genes of T cell receptor molecules should be found. They should be located downstream, i.e. at the 3′ end of the cluster of V_H genes in the embryonic, nonarranged form of DNA. We will, however, only be able to find them if we are able to identify and determine the protein structure of the constant regions of T cell receptors of helper, killer and suppressor cells with the aid of such antibodies as described above.

An immune response of lymphocytes is brought about by the proliferation and/or maturation to effector functions of antigen-specific cells. The facts that 1) such immune responses depend on co-operative interactions of different cell types and 2) these interactions are restricted by the antigen encoded in the H-2 complex clearly indicate that binding of antigen to V_H/V_L containing Ig receptors of lymphocytes *alone* is *insufficient* to effect such an immune response. That is not contradicting the clonal selection hypothesis, it rather indicates that a split of labour has occurred in the immune system, separating clonally antigen specificity mediated by V-regions, from nonclonal cellular growth control. Experiments using antisera specific for the various Ig classes, subclasses and chains as surface Ig-probing devices for understanding the role of the different classes and subclasses expressed on the surface of different B cell subpopulations are highly confusing at the present time. Even with the aid of monoclonal antibodies different experimenters still obtain almost opposing results. *In vivo* and *in vitro* conditions of these experiments are still apparently too variable from case to case. Relief may come finally, from using clones of cells involved in these lymphocyte regulations.

Work with clones of helper T cells has helped to clarify the minimal requirements of antigen-specific, H-2 restricted co-operative interactions. Different steps can be distinguished. In the first step histocompatible macrophages, displaying *I*-region antigens and "processed" antigen, activate antigen-specific helper T cells. This may, in fact, be preceded by the activation of macrophages by antigen, possibly via antigen–antibody complexes, where natural serum antibody may play the crucial role. Once the helper T cells are activated they (or the macrophages) produce factors effective in replication (BRMF) and/or maturation (TRF) of B cells and T killer cells (TCGF). Since a series of T cell hybridomas produce such TCGF it has been argued that the T cells and not the macrophages produced such factors.

In the second step of T–B collaboration, the same helper T cells now interact with histocompatible small resting B cells. They recognize antigen, bound on B cells by surface Ig, and Ia antigen, expressed on the B cell surface. This excites the small B cell to an activated state where it now expresses functionally, receptors for growth factors (produced in the first step) which drive the B cells into cell cycle. Similar mechanisms may operate for T cells. It would be predicted that killer T cells have antigen-binding receptors and express Ia-antigens when they are resting and must be excited. Once doubly occupied they can respond to TCGF, and on the T cell side much discussion concerned how resting cells can be excited. Concanavalin A certainly does it, allo-H-2-reactive interactions also certainly do. The hope remains that, with all the experimental results quoted, some things would *not* excite a resting cell.

The excited activated cells lose all H-2 restrictions and antigen-specificity and can be driven into cell cycle by antigen unspecific factors. The cells are likely to use up the factors, and it seems that the factors are required early in the Gl-phase of each successive cell cycle. It is, therefore, the resting stage of lymphocytes which safeguards the immune system against unspecific activation. The many examples of unspecific responsiveness in the wake of a specific response only demonstrates that this safeguard is not foolproof.

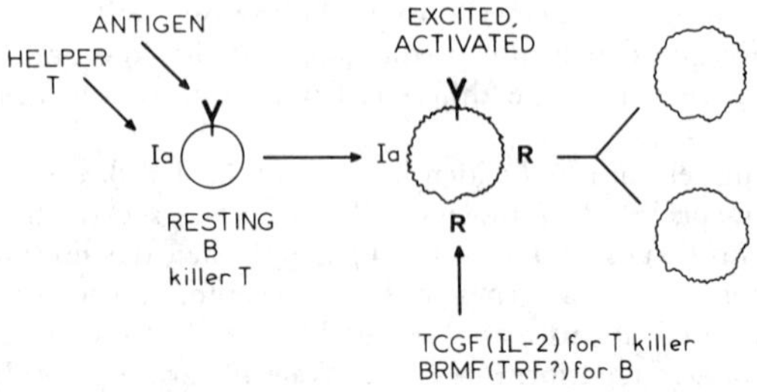

This simple scheme of H-2 restricted, antigen specific cell co-operation, however, is certainly incomplete. For once there are suppressive actions on lymphocytes which must be explained. Certainly Fc receptors are sites where Ig–Fc mediated inhibitory actions are conveyed. It is also clear that there is not only one B cell, one killer T cell and one helper T cell, but that there are subpopulations of each.

On the side of the B cell Lyb markers, complement receptors, Fc receptors, mitogen reactivities, reactivities to T-independent and T-dependent antigens and the Ig class expression form the basis for a bewildering heterogeneity. It can safely be said that not all B cells can respond equally well to all co-operative signals. On the side of helper T cells subpopulations also cause complications. In addition to antigen-specific, I-A or I-E/C region antigen-restricted helper T cells there is now evidence for idiotype-specific, allotype-specific and Ig-class-specific helpers, for which restrictions are not yet worked out. We clearly need clones of such cells representing the different T and B cell subpopulations, to understand better their activity. The finding of another gene separate from I-A coding for the classical Ia, namely for the W39 antigen, encoded by a structurally very similar gene, linked closely to I-A, may signal the discovery of more T-helper cell restricting elements within the chromosomal region of *Ir* genes, which could guide the co-operation of such additional helper T cells, which are probably effective in secondary T cell dependent responses.

The complexity of the system certainly justifies the 15 000–30 000 immunologists studying it. The breakthrough of new techniques such as those of cloning will certainly help our experimental approaches, allowing a clearer view and more accurate conclusions.

Theme 4

Nonantigen-specific Receptors

Presidents:
N. L. WARNER
J. L. PREUD'HOMME

Symposium chairman:
H. G. KUNKEL

11

Biochemical Properties of Nonimmunoglobulin, Non-MHC Lymphocyte Surface Components

PAUL D. GOTTLIEB

Department of Microbiology, University of Texas at Austin, Austin, Texas, USA

Introduction

Many of the important functions of lymphocytes are likely to be initiated at the cell surface and mediated by effector molecules that are integral

Abbreviations
B: bone marrow derived; T: thymus derived; Ig: immunoglobulin; H: heavy chain; L: light chain; MHC: major histocompatibility complex; NP-40: nonidet P-40 detergent; mol. wt: molecular weight; NEPHGE: nonequilibrium pH gradient electrophoresis; SDS-PAGE: polyacrylamide gel electrophoresis in the presence of sodium dodecyl sulphate; K (as in 35K): thousand; Con A: concanavalin A; NK: natural killer.

components of the lymphocyte surface. Studies of the biochemistry of lymphocyte surface components should therefore shed light on the mechanisms that underlie immune function. Because functional assays for cell interactions are complex, the traditional biochemical approach of isolating pure molecules and assessing their function is not feasible. A major approach therefore has been to identify new cell surface molecules and to try to obtain clues to function on the basis of molecular characteristics or by perturbing immune function with antibodies specific for such components.

Antigen recognition by B cells is mediated by cell surface Ig determined by H and L chain genes, and there is evidence that T cells employ receptors related in structure to Ig. A variety of lymphoid cell interactions and effector–target interactions require that the interacting cells be compatible at the MHC, and while the mechanisms are still obscure, advances have been made in the biochemistry of MHC products. In addition, a growing number of additional cell surface components has been described whose functions are unknown, but whose presence on unique cell subsets or at a restricted time in development suggests association with specific functions. Also, components unique to lymphocytes but not restricted to any one subset have been described. In the present communication, the properties of several non-Ig, non-MHC cell surface components will be described to provide an account of the classes of such molecules and their relationships, both spatial and structural, to other molecules of the cell surface.

Lyt-2 and Lyt-3 alloantigens

The Lyt-2 and Lyt-3 alloantigens (Boyse *et al.*, 1968a, 1971) have been very useful as markers of functional subsets of T lymphocytes. These antigens are present on cytotoxic killer and suppressor cells and their precursors, but not on helper T cells (Cantor and Boyse, 1977). The *Lyt-2* and *Lyt-3* loci are closely linked to each other on chromosome 6 (Itakura *et al.*, 1972), and the nature of the molecules bearing these antigenic determinants and their relation to each other are of great interest. That interest has been generated by the finding that binding of anti-Lyt-2 or anti-Lyt-3 sera to these antigens on effector cells will inhibit cytotoxic killing of targets in the absence of complement (Nakayama *et al.*, 1979; Shinohara and Sachs, 1979). Thus these components may participate in the binding of effector T cell to target or, alternatively, they may be topologically adjacent to cell interaction sites and be involved in some aspect of the killing mechanism. The very close linkage of the *Lyt-2* and *Lyt-3* loci to genes governing the κ L chain repertoire (Gottlieb, 1974) raised the intriguing possibility that these molecules might be related to L chains and perform analogous functions on T cells. However, structural studies of Lyt-2 and Lyt-3 antigens described below indicate that as they are isolated from thymocytes, they do not appear to have sufficient polypeptide molecular heterogeneity to suggest a role in determining differences in antigen binding specificity (Reilly *et al.*, in press).

Studies using the antibody blocking test (Boyse *et al.*, 1968b, 1971; see below) have indicated that Lyt-2 and Lyt-3 are topologically adjacent on the cell surface. This and their close genetic linkage prompted the suggestion (Itakura *et al.*, 1972) that Lyt-2 and Lyt-3 may be different antigenic determinants on the same glycoprotein molecule. Biochemical studies of Lyt-2 and Lyt-3 antigens suggest, however, that these determinants reside on different glycoprotein species which are closely related to each other in structure and which are noncovalently associated with each other in detergent extracts of cells and probably on the cell surface as well (Durda and Gottlieb, 1976, 1978; Reilly *et al.*, in press).

Biochemical studies have primarily involved labelling the cell surface of thymocytes with ^{125}I and lactoperoxidase or NaB^3H_4 and galactose oxidase, extracting with NP-40 detergent and precipitating with conventional or monoclonal anti-Lyt antibodies. Thymocytes from pairs of Lyt-congenic strains differing only in the region of the *Lyt-2* and *Lyt-3* loci were employed to control for nonspecific precipitation. Results of one- and two-dimensional polyacrylamide gels, the latter involving nonequilibrium pH gradient electrophoresis (NEPHGE) in the first dimension, indicate:

(a) ^{125}I-labelled material specifically precipitated with anti-Lyt-2 and anti-Lyt-3 antibodies consists of basic glycoprotein species with apparent mol. wts of 35 000 (35K), 30K and <30K under reducing conditions.

(b) The 35K and 30K species (especially the latter) exhibited considerable charge heterogeneity which was eliminated when extracts were treated with neuraminidase before precipitation. Thus the charge heterogeneity reflected variations in the number of terminal sialic acid residues.

(c) Two-dimensional NEPHGE under nonreducing conditions yielded basic species of apparent mol. wt 65K and higher aggregates. The 65K species could be resolved poorly into two closely spaced bands by SDS-PAGE.

(d) Reduction and re-electrophoresis of the higher mol. wt band yielded 35K components, and similar treatment of the lower mol. wt. 65K species yielded 30K components. Both 65K species yielded some <30K material upon reduction. Thus it appears that the 65K species consist of homodimers of 35K and 30K components, i.e. $(35K)_2$ and $(30K)_2$.

(e) Precipitates obtained with either anti-Lyt-2 or Lyt-3 conventional or monoclonal antibodies always contained both 35K and 30K species. Thus if one bears Lyt-2 determinants and the other, Lyt-3, then the homodimers of these species must be associated with each other in the cell extracts. Such association on the cell surface as well would account for the close topological relationship suggested by the antibody blocking method (see above).

(f) Treatment of ^{125}I-labelled cells with trypsin before NP-40 extraction greatly diminished precipitates subsequently obtained with anti-Lyt-3 but not anti-Lyt-2 sera. Thus Lyt-3 antigenic determinants are labile to trypsin on the cell surface.

(g) Results of sequential precipitation with anti-Lyt-2 and anti-Lyt-3 antibodies indicated that molecules bearing these antigenic determinants are associated with each other in the cell extracts. Interestingly, pretreatment of B6 extracts with some anti-Lyt-3·2 sera resulted in enhanced precipitation, particularly of 30K components, in subsequent treatment with anti-Lyt-2 sera. This suggested that Lyt-2·2 determinants might be associated with 30K components or $(30K)_2$ dimers (Reilly *et al.*, in press), but further study is required to verify this suggestion.

(h) Recovery of 35K and 30K species from polyacrylamide gels, digestion with trypsin and electrophoresis on highly cross-linked gels yielded peptide maps which allowed examination of the species for possible relatedness. The preliminary maps obtained were remarkably similar, suggesting that these basic glycoproteins with similar molecular properties may be related at the level of primary structure (Reilly and Gottlieb, in prep.).

If one of the glycoprotein species described bears Lyt-2 determinants and the other, Lyt-3, then the apparent structural homology and the close genetic linkage of *Lyt-2* and *Lyt-3* loci would suggest that they might be descended from a common ancestral gene, probably by a tandem gene duplication. It is possible, however, that the 30K and 35K components may contain identical polypeptides but may differ in the nature and/or extent of glycosylation. That heterogeneity in glycosylation exists within each species is indicated by the varying amounts of sialic acid. The meaning of this carbohydrate heterogeneity, whether functional or adventitious, is unknown, as is the precise function of these molecular species.

The possible role of Lyt-2 and Lyt-3 components in events associated with cytotoxic lysis, suggested by the blocking of lysis by antibodies directed against them (Nakayama *et al.*, 1979; Shinohara and Sachs, 1979), is intriguing. However, as is discussed further below, these workers have shown that antisera specific for Lyt-4 (previously called Ly-5) (Komuro *et al.*, 1975) also blocked cytotoxic killer activity. It would be of great interest to determine whether anti-Lyt-4 and anti-Lyt-2 or anti-Lyt-3 antibodies interfere with each other in the antibody blocking test, as this would implicate complexes of molecules bearing these determinants as part of or adjacent to the killing and/or binding mechanism. Experiments with chemical cross-linking reagents might help to determine whether such molecules are adjacent on the cell surface. However, both types of experiment must be interpreted with caution, since treatment with any reagent may cause perturbations of the cell surface which do not exist on untreated cells (see below).

T200 and related species

Trowbridge *et al.* (1975a, b; 1977) have assigned the name T200 to a glycoprotein of apparent mol. wt approximately 200K on the surface of mouse thymocytes, peripheral T cells and T lymphoid tumours. T200 can be labelled with ^{125}I and lactoperoxidase and NaB^3H_4 and galactose oxidase, and it binds to the lectins ricin, pea lectin and Con A. T200 can be resolved into at least two components by SDS-PAGE and is one of the major T cell components precipitated by rabbit antilymphocyte serum. Trowbridge (1979) has prepared a rat monoclonal antibody (I3/2) reactive with T200. Mouse B cells also contain a glycoprotein of slightly higher apparent mol. wt called T220 with properties similar to T200 and which is reactive with both antilymphocyte serum and I3/2 antibody. Omary *et al.* (1980) have shown that alloantisera to Lyt-4 (Komuro *et al.*, 1975), which are reactive with a surface component of T cells and natural killer (NK) cells (Kasai *et al.*, 1979) can precipitate T200 from thymocyte extracts, suggesting that Lyt-4 antigenic determinants reside on that molecule. The presence of T200 on NK cells, suggested by their reactivity with anti-Lyt-4 sera, has not been investigated. As described earlier, Nakayama *et al.* (1979) have presented evidence that binding of anti-Lyt-4 antibodies, probably to effector and not target cells, can block cytotoxic T cell killing, and this suggests that T200 may lie close to and possibly play a role in mechanisms of target cell binding and/or lysis.

Omary and Trowbridge (1980) have shown that T200 is a transmembrane glycoprotein with two distinct regions: a relatively protease-insensitive portion of apparent mol. wt 100K, which is exposed on the cell surface and includes the mannose-containing oligosaccharides and the antigenic determinant reactive with the monoclonal anti-T200 antibody; and a protease-sensitive portion exposed on the cytoplasmic side of the plasma membrane, which contains serine residues which can be labelled with $^{32}PO_4$ *in vivo*. The transmembrane disposition of T200 raises the possibility that it may serve to transfer signals which impinge on the cell surface to structures within the cell to bring about a cellular response. Protein phosphorylation is known to be a mechanism for regulation of a variety of cellular processes (Rubin and Rosen, 1975) and has been implicated in cell transformation (Collett and Erickson, 1978). Decker *et al.* (1977) have suggested that a glycoprotein of apparent mol. wt 150K to 200K may be the receptor for the proliferative signal of Con A, but Trowbridge has demonstrated that binding of the anti-T200 monoclonal antibody does not stimulate cell proliferation.

Capping of some cell surface antigens as a result of binding antibody to the cell is accompanied by accumulation of contractile elements of the cytoplasm at the capped pole (Schreiner and Unanue, 1977; Schreiner *et al.*, 1977). Cytoskeletal and contractile structures are known to be associated with the cytoplasmic face of the plasma membrane (Geiger and Singer, 1979), and the relocation of contractile structures with capping is likely to reflect either direct or indirect association of that antigen with these structures. Transmembrane components like T200 might mediate that association, and there is evidence that capping of T200 can affect the behaviour of other cell surface glycoproteins (Bourgignon *et al.*, 1978).

Kamarck and Gottlieb (in press) have demonstrated the presence of T200-like molecules on the surface of foetal mouse thymocytes on day 13 of gestation. On those cells, the lower mol. wt species of adult T200 was absent, and a species of apparent mol. wt >200K (called $T200^+$) was present. As gestation progressed, the $T200^+$ component disappeared and the doublet pattern characteristic of adult T200 appeared. This and other studies discussed above indicate that T200-related molecules are present on T cells, B cells and probably on NK cells, and that the apparent mol. wt of T200-like glycoproteins on thymocytes change during ontogeny. It is possible that the T200-like components present on different cell types or at different times in ontogeny are determined by different but closely related genes. Alternatively, they may all share the same polypeptide component which has post-translational modifications characteristic of the cell type in which it is expressed. Differences in glycosylation could generate the mol. wt differences observed, and there is evidence that glycosylation patterns of T200 may differ in different T cell lineages (Trowbridge *et al.*, 1977).

Thy-1

The Thy-1 alloantigen (previously called theta or θ) was originally defined by Reif and Allen (1964) using antithymocyte alloantisera, and it has been extremely useful as a marker for T lymphocytes. In the mouse it is found in two allelic forms, Thy-1·1 and Thy-1·2, and it is determined by a locus on chromosome 9 (Itakura *et al.*, 1971). Thy-1 antigenic determinants have also been detected on brain, epithelial cells and fibroblasts in the mouse (Hilgers *et al.*, 1975; Scheid *et al.*, 1972; Stern, 1973), but on lymphoid cells it is diagnostic for T lymphocytes. The antigen density of Thy-1 on thymocytes is somewhat greater than on peripheral T cells. Xenoantisera produced in rabbits against mouse brain are also reactive with Thy-1 on T cells (Golub, 1971), but such sera do not distinguish between allelic Thy-1 products and also contain other antibody activities. Thomas and coworkers (1978) have provided evidence that mouse Thy-1 antigen may be serologically heterogeneous, and that this heterogeneity may serve as a temporal marker for T cell differentiation. Both conventional anti-Thy-1 alloantisera absorbed with two- to three-day-old neonatal spleen cells and a rat anti-AKR/J mouse brain serum were unreactive with a subpopulation of peripheral T cells, which the authors suggested was comprised of young T cells which had recently left the thymus and which served as helper and killer cells in primary responses. Monoclonal anti-Thy-1 alloantibodies have also shown reactivity with subpopulations of

T cells (Fink and Bevan, in press), though in this instance as well as the above, the results may reflect difference in antigen density or distribution. Isolation and characterization of molecular species reactive with these antibody reagents should reveal whether or not the molecules recognized are structurally different.

Trowbridge *et al.* (1975b) have shown that the Thy-1 antigenic determinants on thymocytes reside on glycoprotein species of apparent mol. wt approximately 25K which they have designated T25. It represents one of the major T cell components which can be labelled with ^{125}I and lactoperoxidase and precipitated with heterologous antilymphocyte serum. T25 can be resolved into several closely spaced bands by SDS-PAGE, suggesting that it is heterogeneous in structure. Letarte-Muirhead *et al.* (1975) have demonstrated that rat thymocyte Thy-1 can be resolved into components of apparent mol. wt 25K and 27K on the basis of lectin affinity, and Trowbridge *et al.* (1977) have shown this for mouse Thy-1. These results suggest that the heterogeneity may represent differences in glycosylation. Monoclonal rat antimouse Thy-1 antibodies produced by Ledbetter and Herzenberg (1979) precipitated a family of glycoproteins of apparent mol. wt 25K to 30K with extensive charge heterogeneity from detergent extracts of ^{125}I-labelled thymocytes. As revealed on two-dimensional polyacrylamide gels, digestion of cell extracts with neuraminidase greatly reduced the charge heterogeneity, indicating that, as described above for Lyt-2 and Lyt-3, the charge heterogeneity reflected variable amounts of terminal sialic acid. When extracts of surface-radiolabelled thymocytes were fractionated into lentil lectin binding and nonbinding fractions, the bound fraction contained Thy-1 components of apparent mol. wt 25K, while nonbound fractions had higher apparent mol. wt (26K to 30K). It is therefore likely that the size heterogeneity observed reflects differences in the amounts of neutral sugars on the several molecular species.

Hyman and coworkers have produced Thy-1-negative mutants of lymphoma cell lines by immunoselection with antibody (Hyman and Trowbridge, 1978), and these could be grouped into 5 complementation classes on the basis of cell fusion studies. None of the mutants expressed Thy-1 antigenic determinants on the cell surface, but 4 of the 5 classes synthesized aberrant Thy-1 glycoproteins. On the basis of studies on T25 glycopeptides in these mutants, these workers concluded that normal T25 contains both complex and high mannose oligosaccharides. Analysis of mutants of the class E complementation group demonstrated structural alterations in many cell surface glycoproteins, and showed that high mannose oligosaccharide units were smaller than those of wild type cells. In contrast, with the exception of the T25 glycoprotein, the sizes of complex oligosaccharide units were not detectably different in mutant and wild type cells. The complex type oligosaccharides of T25 from class E mutants were incomplete. This could be a consequence of the failure of T25 to proceed to the cell surface in the mutant cells. The T25 glycoprotein may be more sensitive to changes in its oligosaccharide content than other cell surface glycoproteins because, by analogy with the comparable protein in the rat, T25 is approximately 30% carbohydrate by weight (Barclay *et al.*, 1976). Thus its physical properties and passage intracellularly to later stages of maturation may be greatly affected by its oligosaccharide content. Further studies of the glycosylation defect of class E mutants has shown that there is a block in the synthesis of the lipid-linked oligosaccharide precursor (Robbins *et al.*, 1977) of asparagine-linked oligosaccharides (Trowbridge and Hyman, 1979), and the specific enzymatic defect has been characterized (Chapman *et al.*, 1979).

The precise chemical nature of the Thy-1 antigenic determinants has not yet been determined, and the question of whether they reside on either protein or carbohydrate moieties (or both) has not been answered. Wang and co-workers (1978) have presented evidence that Thy-1 antigenic determinants can reside on both glycolipids and glycoproteins, and that Thy-1·1 and Thy-1·2 determinants are present on a ganglioside fraction that contaminates GM1 gangliosides isolated from thymocytes and brain from appropriate strains of mice. These investigators therefore suggest that the Thy-1 antigenic determinants, detected in their case by noncongenic mouse alloantisera, are carbohydrate in nature, and like many blood group substances (Hakomori *et al.*, 1977) they can reside on both protein and lipid carriers. Analysis of such glycolipid fractions with monoclonal anti-Thy-1 antibodies will be of considerable interest. As discussed above, different monoclonal rat antimouse (Ledbetter and Herzenberg, 1979) and mouse antimouse (Fink and Bevan, in press) antibodies have different reactivities, and this may reflect specificity for different portions of the antigen (i.e. carbohydrate or protein) or for different molecular species. Gangliosides have been implicated as receptors for toxins, viruses, interferon and hormones (Svennerholm *et al.*, 1980), and if gangliosides comprise a portion of Thy-1, it is interesting to consider the possibility that Thy-1 may function as some form of passive receptor on T cells.

Campbell *et al.* (1979) have determined the amino acid sequence of the polypeptide portion of rat brain Thy-1. The unglycosylated polypeptide of rat brain and thymocyte Thy-1 had been shown to have a mol. wt of 12·5K, and the amino acid sequence showed restricted but significant homology with immunoglobulin molecules. Like β-2 microglobulin, which is also homologous to Ig, the size is similar to that of the basic repeating unit of Ig chains (Edelman, 1970). This suggests a distant evolutionary relationship between the Thy-1 polypeptide and Ig, but in the light of the profound dissimilarity in overall structure, there is unlikely to be any functional similarity. It is apparent that the basic structure used for Ig domains has been used for a number of molecules associated with cell surfaces, and it must therefore provide significant advantages.

Lyt-1

Thy Lyt-1 alloantigen described by Boyse *et al.* (1968a) is determined by a genetic locus on chromosome 19 of the mouse (Itakura *et al.*, 1971). It has been very useful as a marker for subsets of T cells which mediate helper function and delayed type hypersensitivity (Cantor and Boyse, 1977). However, recent evidence has shown that Lyt-1 is also present on cytotoxic killer cells but probably in lesser amounts, thus accounting for the decreased sensitivity of such cells to lysis by anti-Lyt-1 serum and complement (Nakayama *et al.*, 1979).

Durda *et al.* (1978) have labelled thymocytes at the cell surface with ^{125}I and lactoperoxidase, prepared cell extracts with NP-40, precipitated with conventional anti-Lyt-1·1 serum and analysed the precipitates by SDS-PAGE. Electrophoresis with and without reduction revealed a component of apparent mol. wt 67K from extracts of B6-Lyt-1^{a} thymocytes (Lyt-1·1^{+}) but not from B6 thymocytes (Lyt-1·2^{+}) suggesting that this molecular species, which apparently exists as a monomer on the cell surface, bears Lyt-1·1 antigenic determinants. When thymocytes were labelled with $NaB^{3}H_4$ and galactose oxidase, a labelled 67K component was specifically precipitated and in addition, an 87K component not seen with ^{125}I labelling was precipitated. The relationship, if any, between these components is not known. Treatment of ^{125}I-labelled thymocytes with trypsin prior to NP-40 extraction resulted in little reduction in subsequent precipitation of the 67K component with anti-Lyt-1·1 serum, indicating that it is much less labile to trypsin on the cell surface than Lyt-3 (see above). Finally, precipitates obtained with an anti-Lyt-1·1-specific IgG2a mouse monoclonal antibody, 7–20·6/3, also yielded the 67K component (Hogarth *et al.*, in press).

Ledbetter and Herzenberg (1979) have employed a rat antimouse monoclonal anti-Lyt-1 antibody, 53–7·3, to precipitate and characterize the Lyt-1 antigen on two-dimensional polyacrylamide gels. The antibody employed did not distinguish between Lyt-1·1 and Lyt-1·2 alloantigens. In agreement with the above studies, a labelled component of apparent mol. wt 70K was observed under reducing and nonreducing conditions, and like Lyt-2, Lyt-3 and Thy-1, this component also exhibited extensive charge heterogeneity. This heterogeneity may also reflect variable numbers of terminal sialic acid residues, but this has not been tested.

Ly-9

A cell surface alloantigen present on both B and T cells has been described which appears to correlate with a glycoprotein component of apparent mol. wt 100K. This glycoprotein was detected by contaminating antibodies present in conventional anti-Lyt-2·1 serum (Durda *et al.*, 1979), confirming the need for caution in using complex alloantisera (Shen *et al.*, 1975). It also reacts with a monoclonal rat antimouse antibody, H30-C7 (Ledbetter *et al.*, 1979). Since this glycoprotein, previously called T100 (Durda *et al.*, 1979) and Lgp-100 (Ledbetter *et al.*, 1979), also bears the Ly-9·1 antigenic determinants detected by Mathieson *et al.* (in press) using alloantisera, this cell surface component has been designated Ly-9. The latter investigators have also described antisera which detect the product of the *Lyt-9^b* allele (Lyt-9·2), but the precipitation studies have not yet been performed. The *Ly-9* locus resides on chromosome 1 with a crossover distance of approximately 0·03 from the *Mls* locus (Ledbetter *et al.*, 1979). Expression of approximately 50% as much Lyt-9·1 and Lyt-9·2 on heterozygous as compared with homozygous cells suggests codominant expression of allelic products.

Studies employing the fluorescence activated cell sorter (FACS) have shown that the Ly-9 antigen resides on essentially all thymus, lymph node and peripheral blood lymphocytes, approximately 80% of spleen cells, approximately 40% of bone marrow cells and on B and T cell tumours (Ledbetter and Herzenberg, 1979; Mathieson *et al.*, in press). Immunofluorescence analyses indicated that peripheral lymphocytes expressed densities of Ly-9 antigen similar to thymocytes. Mathieson *et al.* (in press) have shown in adoptive transfer experiments that Ly-9 is present on at least two functional subsets of T cells (helpers and suppressors). All of these results indicate that Ly-9 is not unique to any functional subset of lymphoid cells, but rather is a general feature of lymphocytes with no known function.

The Ly-9 glycoprotein precipitated with anti-Lyt-2·1 serum can be labelled at the cell surface with ^{125}I and lactoperoxidase and with NaB^{3}H$_4$ and galactose oxidase, the latter demonstrating that it contains terminal galactose residues (Durda *et al.*, 1979). It is readily stripped from the cell surface of intact thymocytes by trypsin. Two-dimensional polyacrylamide gel analysis of Ly-9 precipitated by the H30-C7 monoclonal antibody demonstrated that the antigen exhibited considerable charge heterogeneity (Ledbetter and Herzenberg, 1979). Treatment of cell extracts with neuraminidase prior to immunoprecipitation eliminated this heterogeneity, indicating that the native molecule contained variable numbers of terminal sialic acid residues. The neuraminidase-treated 100K component migrated as a very basic species upon NEPHGE. A higher mol. wt component was precipitated by the H30-C7 monoclonal antibody from extracts of labelled thymocytes but not spleen cells. On the basis of preliminary studies, Ledbetter and Herzenberg (1979) suggest that this may be a more highly glycosylated form of the 100K component, but further studies are needed. The reason for its absence from spleen cells is not known, but as shown by mixing experiments, it is not due to excessive proteolysis in spleen cell extracts.

Asialo GM1 ganglioside

Natural killer (NK) cells are lymphocytes present in unprimed mice which are cytotoxic for a number of tumour cell lines *in vitro* (Kiessling *et al.*, 1975), and they are of great interest as possible mediators of antitumour immunity. In general, they lack the cell surface phenotype of B and T cells, but they do appear to bear the Lyt-4 alloantigen (Kasai *et al.*, 1979), a specificity called NK-1 detected by contaminating antibodies in conventional anti-Lyt-1·2 serum (Glimcher *et al.*, 1977), and possibly a very low density of Thy-1 (Herberman *et al.*, 1978).

Habu *et al.* (1979) have demonstrated that rabbit antimouse brain serum (anti-BAT)—an antiserum known to contain anti-Thy-1 antibodies and to be reactive with haematopoietic stem cells and T cells (Golub, 1971)—has cytotoxic activity for NK cells. Absorption with thymocytes removed all cytotoxic activity against T cells but left anti-NK activity intact. Since anti-BAT serum was produced by immunization with crude brain tissue and was likely to contain antibodies to brain lipids as well as proteins, Kasai *et al.* (1980) tested whether the anti-NK activity might be directed against brain glycolipids. They found that absorption of anti-BAT serum with asialo GM1 but not with other gangliosides removed 50% of the cytotoxic activity for NK cells but left anti-T cell activity intact. Furthermore, a rabbit antiserum raised against and specific for asialo GM1 completely abolished NK activity and showed much lower activity against Ig-negative cells of lymph node and spleen. Alloreactive cytotoxic T cell activity generated *in vitro* was unaffected by the antiasialo GM1 serum and complement, and *in vivo* activity was only slightly decreased. Thus asialo GM1 is much more prominent on the surface of NK cells than on cytotoxic T cells, and antiserum against this component would appear to be an important reagent for distinguishing these cell populations.

Recent studies by Habu *et al.* (in press) have shown that antiasialo GM1 serum is also reactive with the majority of thymus lymphoid cells very early in gestation (days 12–13) when characteristic T cell surface markers are not yet expressed (Kamarck and Gottlieb, 1977). The proportion of asialo GM1-positive cells decreased strikingly as gestation progressed and antigens such as Thy-1, Lyt-1 and Lyt-2 appeared. Double immunofluorescent staining analysis indicated that asialo GM1-positive cells lacked Thy-1 and vice versa, and it is likely (though not strictly proven) that asialo GM1-positive cells are precursors of Thy-1-positive cells. These investigators also observed a small proportion of asialo GM1-positive cells in foetal liver and adult bone marrow. Since NK cells have not been demonstrated in foetal liver but cells that home to the thymus are known to be present (Owen, 1972), it is possible that the cells reactive with antiasialo GM1 may be committed to the T cell lineage. NK cells may be ontogenically related to such pre-T cells.

Most adult thymocytes and peripheral T cells have been shown to bear the ganglioside GM1 (Stein *et al.*, 1978). It is therefore possible that the asialo GM1 present on early foetal thymocytes may be converted to or replaced by GM1 during embryonic thymus maturation and perhaps in the intrathymic maturation of T lymphocytes that continues into adult life. As discussed earlier for the T25 and T200 glycoproteins, this may be another instance where significant differences in glycosylation patterns may exist among different types of lymphoid cells and at different times in development. It is not known whether asialo GM1 performs any special function on early foetal thymocytes, but the known activity of certain gangliosides (including GM1) as receptors for various biological effectors (Svennerholm *et al.*, 1980) is of considerable interest.

Functions and spatial relationships of cell surface components

The biochemistry of several prominent non-Ig, non-MHC cell surface components has been briefly discussed. Unfortunately, detailed structural studies are not very far advanced, and no assignment of function has been made for any of these components. There are likely to be hundreds of additional unidentified glycoprotein and other components present either on all lymphocytes or on subpopulations of cells. Many of these may be present in minute amounts too low for detection by the methods described in this communication. The findings that conventional and monoclonal antibodies specific for Lyt-2, Lyt-3 and Lyt-4 antigens can block cytotoxic activity of killer T cells (see above) raises the possibility that those components may either play a role in the killing or are closely associated with molecules that do. The killing process is likely to be mechanistically complex—perhaps analogous to complement mediated lysis but involving membrane-bound precursors—and the number of different cell surface molecules that must interact to achieve a single killing event may be very large. Similarly, molecular mechanisms by which helper and suppressor T cells are stimulated to develop and perform their effector functions may be highly complex and require interaction of many surface constituents.

As described briefly above, clues concerning the interaction of cell surface components with each other can be obtained by means of the antibody blocking test described by Boyse *et al.* (1968b) and extended by Flaherty and Zimmerman (1979). The approach involves determining the effect of saturation of the cell surface with antibodies to one surface constituent upon the subsequent binding of antibody to another cell surface component. This can be performed on untreated cells or on cells fixed with paraformaldehyde to prevent reorganization of the cell surface as a result of binding the first antibody. Data obtained permit construction of a crude topological map of the cell surface. Such data have suggested that Lyt-2 and Lyt-3 must be very tightly associated on the thymocyte surface, and that Lyt-1 and Lyt-2 antigens show small but significant associations with H-2K and H-2D components, respectively. They also demonstrate that the association of TL and H-2D components observed on unfixed cells is not seen with paraformaldehyde-treated cells, suggesting that that association was brought about by binding the first antibody. This type of induced alteration may be analogous to the type of molecular rearrangements that may occur when lymphocytes encounter other cells or molecules *in vivo*, and the co-capping of several surface components with T200 seen by Bourgignon *et al.* (1978) and so-called syn-capping of vesicular stomatitis virus proteins and H-2K^b antigens described by Geiger *et al.* (1979) are probably similarly induced. Use of reversible cross-linking reagents should provide further information on cell surface topology and permit recovery of separate molecular species. Such analyses involving the components described in this report and additional biochemically characterized cell surface constituents defined by allo- and xenoantisera, monoclonal antibodies, lectins or other approaches may provide clues to the mechanisms by which cells perform their characteristic effector functions upon antigen-binding and/or interaction with other cells.

References

Barclay, A. N., Letarte-Muirhead, M., Williams, A. F. and Faulkes, R. (1976). *Nature (Lond.)* **263**, 563.

Bourgignon, L. Y. W., Hyman, R., Trowbridge, I. and Singer, S. J. (1978). *Proc. Natn. Acad. Sci. U.S.A.* **75**, 2406.

Boyse, E. A., Miyazawa, M., Aoki, T. and Old, L. J. (1968a). *Proc. R. Soc. Lond. B Biol. Sci.* **170**, 175.

Boyse, E. A., Old, L. J. and Stockert, E. (1968b). *Proc. Natn. Acad. Sci. U.S.A.* **60**, 886.

Boyse, E. A., Itakura, K., Stockert, E., Iritani, C. A. and Miura, M. (1971). *Transplantation* **11**, 351.

Campbell, D. G., Williams, A. F., Bayley, P. M. and Reid, K. B. M. (1979). *Nature (Lond.)* **282**, 341.

Cantor, H. and Boyse, E. A. (1977). *Cold Spring Harbour Symp. Quant. Biol.* **41**, 23.

Chapman, A., Trowbridge, I. S., Hyman, R. and Kornfeld, S. (1979). *Cell* **17**, 509.

Collett, M. S. and Erikson, R. L. (1978). *Proc. Natn. Acad. Sci. U.S.A.* **75**, 2021.

Decker, J. M., Warr, G. W. and Marchalonis, J. J. (1977). *Biochem. Biophys. Res. Commun.* **74**, 1536.

Durda, P. J. and Gottlieb, P. D. (1976). *J. Exp. Med.* **144**, 476.

Durda, P. J. and Gottlieb, P. D. (1978). *J. Immunol.* **121**, 983.

Durda, P. J., Shapiro, C. and Gottlieb, P. D. (1978). *J. Immunol.* **120**, 53.

Durda, P. J., Boos, S. C. and Gottlieb, P. D. (1979). *J. Immunol.* **122**, 1407.

Edelman, G. M. (1970). *Biochemistry* **9**, 3188.

Fink, P. J. and Bevan, M. J. *J. Immunol.* (in press).

Flaherty, L. and Zimmerman, D. (1979). *Proc. Natn. Acad. Sci. U.S.A.* **76**, 1990.

Geiger, B. and Singer, S. J. (1979). *Cell* **16**, 213.

Geiger, B., Rosenthal, K. L., Klein, J., Zinkernagel, R. M. and Singer, S. J. (1979). *Proc. Natn. Acad. Sci. U.S.A.* **76**, 4603.

Glimcher, L., Shen, F-W. and Cantor, H. (1977). *J. Exp. Med.* **145**, 1.

Golub, E. S. (1971). *Cell. Immunol.* **2**, 353.

Gottlieb, P. D. (1974). *J. Exp. Med.* **140**, 1432.

Habu, S., Hayakawa, K., Okumura, K. and Tada, T. (1979). *Eur. J. Immunol.* **9**, 938.

Habu, S., Kasai, M., Nagai, Y., Tamaoki, N., Tada, T., Herzenberg, L. A. and Okumura, K. *J. Immunol.* (in press).

Hakomori, S., Watanabe, K. and Laine, R. A. (1977). *Pure Appl. Chem.* **49**, 1215.

Herberman, R. B., Nunn, M. E. and Holden, H. J. (1978). *J. Immunol.* **121**, 304.

Hilgers, J., Haverman, J., Nusse, R., Van Blitterwijk, W. J., Cleton, F. J., Hegeman, P. C., van Nie, R. and Calafat, J. (1975). *J. Natn. Cancer Inst.* **54**, 1323.

Hogarth, P. M., Potter, T. A., Cornell, F. N., McLachlan, R. and McKenzie, I. F. C. *J. Immunol.* (in press).

Hyman, R. and Trowbridge, I. S. (1978). *Conf. Cell Prolif.* **5**, 741.
Itakura, K., Hutton, J. J., Boyse, E. A. and Old, L. J. (1971). *Nature New Biol.* **230**, 126.
Itakura, K., Hutton, J. J., Boyse, E. A. and Old, L. J. (1972). *Transplantation* **13**, 239.
Kamarck, M. E. and Gottlieb, P. D. (1977). *J. Immunol.* **119**, 407.
Kamarck, M. E. and Gottlieb, P. D. *Molec. Immunol.* (in press).
Kasai, M., Leclerc, J. C., Shen, F-W. and Cantor, H. (1979). *Immunogenetics* **8**, 153.
Kasai, M., Iwamori, M., Nagai, Y., Okumura, K. and Tada, T. (1980). *Eur. J. Immunol.* **10**, 175.
Kiessling, R., Klein, E. and Wigzell, H. (1975). *Eur. J. Immunol.* **5**, 112.
Komuro, K., Itakura, K., Boyse, E. A. and John, M. (1975). *Immunogenetics* **1**, 452.
Ledbetter, J. A. and Herzenberg, L. A. (1979). *Immunol. Rev.* **47**, 64.
Ledbetter, J. A., Goding, J. W., Tsu, T. T. and Herzenberg, L. A. (1979). *Immunogenetics* **8**, 347.
Letarte-Muirhead, M., Barclay, A. N. and Williams, A. F. (1975). *Biochem. J.* **151**, 685.
Mathieson, B. J., Sharrow, S. O., Bottomly, K. and Fowlkes, B. J. *J. Immunol.* (in press).
Nakayama, E., Shiku, H., Stockert, E., Oettgen, H. F. and Old, L. J. (1979). *Proc. Natn. Acad. Sci. U.S.A.* **76**, 1977.
Omary, M. B. and Trowbridge, I. S. (1980). *J. Biol. Chem.* **255**, 1662.
Omary, M. B., Trowbridge, I. S. and Scheid, M. P. (1980). *J. Exp. Med.* **151**, 1311.
Owen, J. J. T. (1972). *In* "Ontogeny of Acquired Immunity", Ciba Foundation Symposium, p. 35. Associated Scientific Publishers, Amsterdam.
Reif, A. E. and Allen, J. M. V. (1964). *J. Exp. Med.* **120**, 413.
Reilley, E. B., Auditore-Hargreaves, K., Hämmerling, U. and Gottlieb, P. D. *J. Immunol.* (in press).
Robbins, P. W., Hubbard, S. C., Turco, S. J. and Wirth, D. F. (1977). *Cell* **12**, 893.
Rubin, C. S. and Rosen, O. M. (1975). *A. Rev. Biochem.* **44**, 831.
Scheid, M., Boyse, E. A., Carswell, E. A. and Old, L. J. (1972). *J. Exp. Med.* **135**, 938.
Schreiner, G. F. and Unanue, E. R. (1977). *J. Immunol.* **119**, 1549.
Schreiner, G. F., Fujiwara, K., Pollard, T. D. and Unanue, E. R. (1977). *J. Exp. Med.* **145**, 1393.
Shen, F-W., Boyse, E. A. and Cantor, H. (1979). *Immunogenetics* **2**, 591.
Shinohara, N. and Sachs, D. H. (1979). *J. Exp. Med.* **150**, 432.
Stein, K. E., Schwarting, G. A. and Marcus, D. M. (1978). *J. Immunol.* **120**, 676.
Stern, P. L. (1973). *Nature New Biol.* **246**, 76.
Svennerholm, L., Mandel, P., Dreyfus, H. and Urban, P-F. (Eds) (1980). *Structure and Function of Gangliosides*, Plenum Press, New York.
Thomas, D. B., Calderon, R. A. and Blaxland, L. J. (1978). *Nature* (*Lond.*) **275**, 711.
Trowbridge, I. S. (1979). *J. Exp. Med.* **148**, 313.
Trowbridge, I. S. and Hyman, R. (1979). *Cell* **17**, 503.
Trowbridge, I. S., Ralph, P. and Bevan, M. J. (1975a). *Proc. Natn. Acad. Sci. U.S.A.* **72**, 157.
Trowbridge, I. S., Weissman, I. L. and Bevan, M. J. (1975b). *Nature* **256**, 652.
Trowbridge, I. S., Nilsen-Hamilton, M., Hamilton, R. and Bevan, M. J. (1977). *Biochem. J.* **163**, 211.
Wang, T. J., Freimuth, W. W., Miller, H. C. and Esselman, W. J. (1978). *J. Immunol.* **121**, 1361.

12

T Cell Fc Receptors as Markers of Functional Human Lymphocyte Subsets

L. MORETTA, M. C. MINGARI, A. MORETTA, B. F. HAYNES,* and A. S. FAUCI*

Unit of Human Cancer Immunology, Ludwig Institute for Cancer Research, Epalinges sur Lausanne, Switzerland
Istituto de Microbiologia, University of Genoa, Genoa, Italy
**National Institutes of Health, Bethesda, Maryland, USA*

Introduction

Although lymphocytes show little morphologic differences, they display a high degree of functional heterogeneity. Major advances in the understanding of

Supported in part by a CNR/PFCNN Grant to L. Moretta.

the complex events taking place in the immune response have been provided by improved and more sophisticated techniques of identification, isolation and functional characterization of various subsets of immunocompetent cells.

Two major groups of lymphoid cells were primarily recognized by clinical observations and by ablative experiments in laboratory animals (Cooper *et al.*, 1966; Miller and Osoba, 1967; Good *et al.*, 1962; Werner, 1965). Thus, neonatal thymectomy as well as the study of patients with congenital thymic aplasia showed that lymphocytes derived from the thymus (T cells) are responsible for so called cell-mediated immunity (Di George, 1968). These original studies also indicated that T cells are required for co-operation with B cells in antibody responses to the large majority of antigens. B cells themselves, the other major class of lymphoid cells, are directly responsible for antibody production and are thymus independent (Glick *et al.*, 1956; Owen *et al.*, 1974).

A major effort of immunologists was then directed towards the identification of surface markers specific for the two principal lymphoid cell populations. This line of research appeared particularly appealing since it seemed reasonable to assume that structures incorporated in the cell surface could mediate some of the functions of the cells themselves and the interactions among cells. Thus, for example, it became evident that surface immunoglobulins (Ig), the principal marker of the mature B cells, are involved in antigen induced B cell activation (Pernis *et al.*, 1970; Raff *et al.*, 1970). On the other hand, the generally accepted prototype of human T cell surface markers, the receptor for sheep erythrocytes (E) (Jondal *et al.*, 1972), does not seem to be involved in any of the *in vitro* measurable T cell functions. Nevertheless, this surface marker has been successfully employed to define the total T cell population in humans since all of the T cell functional properties measurable *in vitro* are generally restricted to the E rosetting population. Additional markers for identifying the total T cell population in humans include surface antigens recognized by heteroantisera (Balch *et al.*, 1977; Greaves and Janossy, 1976), as well as hybridoma monoclonal antibodies.

The availability of a number of additional markers, not necessarily restricted to T or B cells, allowed the further dissection of immunocompetent cells into subpopulations. Thus, for example, subsets of human T cells could be recognized by different markers such as receptors for autologous erythrocytes (Palacios *et al.*, 1980), various lectins (Hammarstrom *et al.*, 1973) and histamine (Saxon *et al.*, 1977), expression of Ia antigens (Greaves *et al.*, 1979; Reinherz *et al.*, 1979), etc. However, only certain of these markers have been reported to define functional subsets of cells, such as "suppressor" T cells which have surface receptors for histamine. Other markers, such as Ia only appear on activated T cells.

Surface antigens on T cell subsets recognized by heteroantisera bind to cell fractions with defined functions (Evans *et al.*, 1977). The TH_2 antigen(s) falls into this category and is present on cells with *in vitro* measurable suppressor activity (Evans *et al.*, 1977; Reinherz *et al.*, 1979). However, these antigens do not seem to be directly involved in the actual functional capability of the cells. The same applies to recently developed monoclonal antibodies specific for T cell subsets having certain measurable *in vitro* functional activity.

Another type of surface marker has been shown to define functional T cell subsets. These membrane components are in fact sites which bind Ig (Dickler, 1976). In view of the obvious functional relevance of Ig in the immune response, these sites may themselves play a role in the T cell functional activities. Indeed, it has been shown that both effector cell functions such as antibody dependent cellular cytotoxicity (ADCC) (Perlmann *et al.*, 1972; MacLennan, 1972) and immunoregulatory activities, such as suppression of T or B cell activation and proliferation in certain *in vitro* systems (Moretta *et al.*, 1977a; Ballieux *et al.*, 1979) are directly mediated via surface Fc receptors. In the present chapter, we shall briefly review the general characteristics of the Fc receptors present on T cells and discuss their importance in defining different T cell lineages and/or cells at different stages of maturation or activation. The cellular functional activities in which Fc receptors are directly involved will be also briefly discussed.

General characteristics of Fc receptors on human T cells

Receptors with affinity for Ig have been detected on mononuclear cells of different animal species. Following the original observation by Lo Buglio *et al.* (1967) that certain lymphocytes can bind immune complexes (IC) by a mechanism which does not involve complement, a more precise analysis of the mononuclear cell population(s) involved has shown that receptors for Ig are expressed by monocytes, macrophages and lymphocytes (Dickler, 1976). Studies of lymphocyte subpopulations have demonstrated that T cells (Lee and Paraskevas, 1972; Yoshida and Andersson, 1972; Ferrarini *et al.*, 1975; Moretta *et al.*, 1975; Winchester *et al.*, 1975), B cells (Basten *et al.*, 1972; Dickler and Kunkel, 1972), and a third subset of non-T, non-B cells (null cells) (Froland and Natvig, 1972; Kurnik and Grey, 1975) may have surface receptors for Ig. In the earlier studies FcR for IgG were predominantly investigated, but receptors for other Ig isotypes have been subsequently described. Thus, receptors for IgM have been detected on normal and leukaemic T lymphocytes and on certain T cell lines (Moretta *et al.*, 1975; McConnell and Hurd, 1976; Gmelig-Meyling *et al.*, 1976; Moretta *et al.*, 1977c; Preud'homme *et al.*, 1979), on normal and neoplastic B lymphocytes, and on certain B cell lines (Pickler and Knapp, 1977; Ferrarini *et al.*, 1977; Preud'homme *et al.*, 1979). Receptors for IgA, IgE and IgD have also been recently detected on various fractions of T and B lymphocytes (Strober *et al.*, 1978; Lum *et al.*, 1979; Yodoi and Ishizaka, 1980; Sjoberg, 1980).

Principal methods of detection of FcR

FcR for Ig present on lymphocytes can be detected by different techniques which vary both for the type of complex utilized and the method used for measuring the binding.

Immune complexes formed of *antibodies bound to soluble antigens* have been used and have been detected by techniques such as radioautography or fluorescence. Direct fluorescence has proven especially useful. Either the antibody (Forni and Pernis, 1975), or the antigen (Dickler *et al.*, 1974) or both (Winchester *et al.*, 1975) have been conjugated with the fluorochrome. Fluorescence microscopy and more recently the fluorescence activated cell sorter (FACS) have been used to analyse the lymphoid populations binding the complexes. Both B and T cells have been shown to bind such complexes (Dickler, 1976; Stout and Herzenberg, 1975). It is of note that this type of molecular antigen–antibody complex occurs naturally *in vivo* and therefore these particular *in vitro* observations may well be relevant to *in vivo* phenomena.

Aggregated Immunoglobulins have been also extensively used for detection of $Fc_{\gamma}R$. They bind to the same surface site to which Ag-Ab complexes bind, as shown by inhibition studies. Aggregated IgG (or IgG immune complexes) appear to have much greater avidity for FcR than native IgG. This is probably the consequence of the potentially multiple binding interactions which occur between FcR and Fc fraction of IgG when the latter are aggregated in the complex. However, molecular changes in the Fc portion of IgG leading to a higher affinity for the FcR cannot be excluded as a cause of this increased avidity of binding. In the preparation of aggregated IgG, it is important to determine that the starting native IgG does not contain antibodies against the cell population to be tested. Both radioautography and fluorescence can be used for detection of aggregated IgG bound to lymphoid cells. This method mainly detects binding of aggregates to B cells (Dickler and Kunkel, 1972; Preud'homme and Seligmann, 1972).

Immune complexes formed with cellular antigens have also been used to evaluate interactions between lymphocytes and antibody-coated cells. This method is based on the formation of "rosettes" between the lymphocytes bearing FcR and indicator cells coated with antibodies. This type of complex may be present in various *in vivo* circumstances such as transplantation, blood transfusions, pregnancy, bacterial infections, etc. In this regard also, *in vitro* studies are likely relevant to *in vivo* conditions. Rosetting techniques have been widely used for detection of FcR on human T cells. FcR for IgG and IgM have been detected in most cases by rosette formation with erythrocytes coated with purified IgM and IgG antibodies made in rabbit (Ferrarini *et al.*, 1975; Moretta *et al.*, 1975). This method has proved to be reliable and simple. In addition, it offers a major advantage over other techniques in that the rosette forming cells can be easily isolated from nonrosetting cells. Bovine erythrocytes are especially suitable for detection of FcR due to their poor agglutinability. Erythrocytes can therefore be coated with relatively large amounts of antibody (Uhlenbruck *et al.*, 1967). Other indicator red cells successfully used include human Rh+ erythrocytes sensitized with anti-Rh antibody (Van Oers *et al.*,

1977) or chicken erythrocytes coated with rabbit antibodies.

Whereas FcR for IgG can be detected on freshly isolated lymphocytes, FcR for IgM can be demonstrated especially on cells which have been incubated *in vitro* for at least 4–6 h in media supplemented with IgM-free sera (such as FCS). Lower proportions of cells expressing FcR for IgM can be demonstrated in cultures containing human AB or autologous serum and generally the proportions of rosettes detectable varied inversely with the percentage of serum added. This observation, together with the results of inhibition experiments using purified human IgM, show that FcR for IgM can easily be blocked *in vitro* by small amounts of native IgM. It is likely that FcR for IgM are present on freshly isolated T lymphocytes, but cannot be detected because they are masked by serum IgM. This view is substantiated by the detection of free FcR for IgM on T lymphocytes freshly isolated from patients with severe hypo-γ-globulinaemia with low or undetectable serum IgM (Moretta *et al.*, 1977b). It should be pointed out that the incubation of normal T cells, necessary for optimal expression of FcR for IgM could thus allow the cells to shed both the $Fc_{\mu}R$ and the IgM bound to them and to express new receptors.

Specificity of Fc_{μ} and Fc_{γ} receptors present on T cells

The specificity of FcR for IgM on human T cells has been studied by analysing the inhibitory capacity of purified human Ig or Ig fragments in the rosette assay. These experiments have shown that the FcR for IgM has specificity for the Fc fragment of IgM molecules (Moretta *et al.*, 1975; Ferrarini *et al.*, 1976; McConnell and Hurd, 1976; Gmelig-Meyling *et al.*, 1976). More precisely, the CH_4 homology domain was identified as the portion for which the receptor has affinity (Conradie and Bubb, 1977). Preud'homme *et al.* (1979) demonstrated that native monomeric IgM bound to the $Fc_{\mu}R$ with an even greater efficiency than pentameric IgM. Reports from different laboratories have indicated that relatively low concentrations of IgM are required for saturation of the receptors and consequent inhibition of IgM rosette formation. This, together with the fact that $Fc_{\mu}R$ can be detected by using indicator erythrocytes coated with relatively low amounts of rabbit IgM antibodies suggest that human T cells are equipped with a low number of relatively high avidity receptors.

Detailed studies of the specificity of FcR for IgG on isolated T cells have not yet been carried out. Inhibition studies (Moretta *et al.*, 1975) indicate that these receptors recognize molecules of the IgG class only, bind preferentially to IgG aggregated by antigen or other means, and have a low avidity for the substrate. Many of the characteristics of these receptors are similar to those of the $Fc_{\gamma}R$ present on B cells and on the so called "third population" or "null cells". If indeed a common membrane molecular structure serves as the $Fc_{\gamma}R$ of various lymphoid populations, the $Fc_{\gamma}R$ on T cells would have affinity for the Fc portion of all human IgG subclasses (Dickler, 1976). It is of note, however, that as mentioned above, the different methods used to detect $Fc_{\gamma}R$ preferentially reveal these receptors on different cell populations.

Turnover of Fc receptors for IgM and IgG present on T cells

The turnover of FcR has been investigated in experiments in which T cells were treated with proteolytic enzymes and receptor expression *in vitro* was determined as a function of time. Mingari *et al.* (1978) have shown that FcR for IgM are highly susceptible to both trypsin and pronase, whereas FcR for IgG were resistant to trypsin and sensitive only to high concentrations of pronase. In this connection, it is of interest that FcR for IgG present on monocytes, granulocytes and on a variable fraction of the "null cells" are also pronase-resistant. This may reflect structural differences in the FcR or the presence on these cells of two different types of $Fc_{\gamma}R$, as shown on mouse macrophages (Silverstein *et al.*, 1977; Sulica *et al.*, 1979a, b). After removal with pronase the $Fc_{\mu}R$ on the cell surface were detectable within 2 h and the resynthesis was completed in 6 h. $Fc_{\gamma}R$ were detectable in 4–6 h and complete expression took 12 h (Mingari *et al.*, 1978). In another series of experiments (Mingari *et al.*, 1978; Moretta *et al.*, 1978) the consequences of interactions with IgG or IgM-IC on the turnover of the receptors was investigated. Whereas interaction of IgG-IC with the $Fc_{\gamma}R$ was shown to induce a modulation of the receptors (Moretta *et al.*, 1978), contact with antigen-IgM antibody complexes did not alter the mode of re-expression of FcR for IgM. This suggests that contact with IgG-IC may act as a "switch off" signal for synthesis and/or membrane insertion of $Fc_{\gamma}R$ of T_G cells. If this is the case, it could have a significant effect on the modulation of the normal immune response and on the impaired immunologic reactions which may be observed in the course of diseases with circulating immune complexes (Fauci, 1980). As we shall discuss later, modulation of FcR present on T cells can have indeed important consequences on certain functional capabilities of the cells.

Fc receptors discriminate between T cell populations with different *in vitro* functional activities

As mentioned above human peripheral blood T cells have surface receptors for Ig of different classes. FcR for IgG and IgM ($Fc_{\gamma}R$ and $Fc_{\mu}R$) have been studied in great detail and have proven useful for identification and fractionation of T cell subsets with different functional properties. They are virtually absent on thymocytes and are present in different proportions on peripheral blood T cells; in this respect they represent markers for T cell maturation. $Fc_{\gamma}R$ and $Fc_{\mu}R$ define two sets of peripheral blood T cells which may represent two distinct cell lineages or cells at different stages of maturation or activation. Analysis of certain *in vitro* properties of isolated T cell subsets, has shown that it is feasible to attribute certain T cell activities to T_M or T_G subpopulations, as summarized in Table I.

TABLE I
In vitro *measurable activities of peripheral blood* T_M *and* T_G *cells*

Function	T_M	T_G
Helper activity for antibody production (irradiation resistant)	+	−
Suppressor activity for antibody production, T cell proliferation, and CFU-c (irradiation sensitive)	−[a]	+[b]
Response in MLR	+	±
Response to PHA and Con A	+	±
Cytotoxicity in ADCC and NK	−	+

[a] T_M populations do contain cells that can be induced to suppress, i.e. suppressor precursors
[b] Refer to naturally occurring or spontaneous suppressor cells

Thus, in the pokeweed mitogen (PWM) driven B cell differentiation T_M and T_G cells play an antithetical role, T_M cells acting as inducers of B cell activation and T_G cells as suppressors (Moretta *et al.*, 1977a). Analysis of the mechanism leading to the induction or to the suppression of B cell differentiation demonstrated that T_M helper activity was resistant to irradiation, whereas irradiation of T_G cells completely abrogated their suppressor ability. Both help and suppression are mediated by soluble factors. Helper factors act at the B cell level inducing cell maturation. On the contrary suppressor factors act on T_M cells by preventing them from helping B cells (Moretta *et al.*, 1979).

T_M and T_G cells differ also in their proliferative responses to T cell mitogens such as Con A and PHA (Moretta *et al.*, 1979). Similar dose response curves to Con A were observed for the two T cell subsets. On the contrary, consistent differences were observed in PHA responses. Thus, T_M cells only responded to high concentrations of the mitogen, whereas minimal responses were observed by using mitogen doses which elicited maximal responses in infractionated T cells. T_G cell responses were lower than those of unfractionated T cells at all of the mitogen concentrations tested.

The ability to proliferate in response to allogeneic cells has been studied in the one way mixed lymphocyte reaction (MLR) using a pool of allogeneic irradiated T depleted cells as targets. These experiments showed that T_G cells responded poorly whereas T_M and T null cells gave responses comparable to (or higher than) those of unfractionated T cells (Moretta *et al.*, 1980 and Moretta A. *et al.*, submitted). Low responses elicited by T_G cells could be consequent to the interaction of their FcR with ox-IgG-IC, a routine step necessary for positive selection of these cells. Modulation of $Fc_{\gamma}R$ has been shown to have important influences on the expression of certain functional capacities of T_G cells. Thus, following modulation of surface $Fc_{\gamma}R$, T_G cells lose their cytotoxic capacity on ADCC (Moretta *et al.*, 1978); in addition, rosetting of T_G cells with IgG-IC serves as an "off signal" for the cells and inhibits their blastogenic responses to T cell mitogens (Samarut *et al.*, 1979). It is possible that irreversible modulation of $Fc_{\gamma}R$ could also involve surface structures necessary for alloantigen recognition. Indeed, $Fc_{\gamma}R^+$ PBL purified under conditions in which $Fc_{\gamma}R$ modulation did not occur, gave proliferative responses much higher than those elicited by the same "modulated" population; the responses were comparable to those of $Fc_{\gamma}R^-$ cells (Samarut *et al.*, 1979). Mingari and colleagues have studied the proliferative responses of purified T_G cells isolated in conditions leading to or not leading to $Fc_{\gamma}R$ modulation. Unmodulated T_G cells responded 5 to 20 times more than modulated T_G cells. Their responses were about one-third of those of purified T_M cells (unpublished).

In addition to the suppression observed in the PWM—driven B cell differentiation system, T_G cells are also capable of exerting inhibitory activity in other experimental models. It has been shown that human lymphocytes precultured for 15–20 h with PHA are capable of forming colonies in semisolid media (Rosenszajn *et al.*, 1975). This technique provides an easy method for a quantitative evaluation of lymphocytes capable of proliferative responses to PHA. Ability to form colonies is restricted to T cells and is greatly enhanced by the presence of adherent cells or their soluble factors. Among T cell subsets, only T_M and T null cells form colonies whereas T_G do not (Pistoia *et al.*, submitted). It has been shown that T_G can sharply suppress colony formation by other cell fractions. T_G cells inhibit colony formation only after having been exposed to IgG-IC and their suppressive effect is radiosensitive. Suppression of T lymphocyte proliferation by naturally occurring suppressor cells present in the T_G cell population can also occur in physiologic conditions such as pregnancy. Indeed T_G cells from cord blood of human newborns show an antimitotic effect on adult PB lymphocytes (Oldstone *et al.*, 1977).

T cells have been recently shown to play an important role in the regulation of normal haematopoiesis (Parkman *et al.*, 1978). Thus, a promoting activity of T lymphocytes on haematopoiesis has been suggested by a number of experimental approaches (Trainin *et al.*, 1969; Wictor-Jedrzejczak *et al.*, 1977; Zipori and Trainin, 1975). T lymphocytes have also been shown to produce colony stimulating factors after stimulation with PHA or Con A (Parker and Metcalf, 1974). It was less clear whether T lymphocytes were also normally involved in the suppression of haematopoiesis since bone marrow T lymphocytes from normal individuals enhance rather than suppress colony formation (CFU-c) when cocultured with normal bone marrow cells (Singer *et al.*, 1980). On the contrary, suppressor activity of BM T lymphocytes is quite clear in some patients with severe aplastic anaemia (SAA). Thus, a group of patients with idiopathic SAA in complete haematologic remission induced by immunosuppressive therapy, had suppressor T_G cells which spontaneously inhibited CFU-c in both autologous and allogeneic combinations (with bone marrow of normal individuals). Other cell populations such as adherent cells (AC) had no suppressive effects themselves, nor did they significantly enhance the suppressor effect of T_G cells. T_G cells from normal marrows, on the other hand, were unable to suppress CFU-c of autologous or allogeneic marrows. It is of note that as few as 10^4 T_G cells had the same suppressor activity as 10^5 T_G cells when cocultured with $2{\cdot}5 \times 10^5$ normal marrow cells. Further analysis has shown that suppression is completely abrogated by irradiation of T_G cells and is mediated by soluble factors.

In vitro T cell activities directly involving surface FcγR

Antibody dependent cellular cytotoxicity (ADCC)

Cytotoxicity against antibody-coated target cells by freshly isolated lymphocytes can be detected either by incubating lymphocytes with target cells pretreated with antibody or with target cells in the presence of antiserum (Perlmann *et al.*, 1972). Target cell damage is usually assessed by labelling the target cells with radioactive chromium and measuring its release in the supernatants. The FcR on the effector cells appear directly involved in the phenomenon since $F(ab')_2$ fragments of the antitarget antibodies will not mediate ADCC. Intact IgG, but not their $F(ab')_2$ fragments added to the cytotoxic assay inhibit ADCC. An additional proof of the direct involvement of $Fc_\gamma R$ on ADCC was provided by the finding that modulation of surface $Fc_\gamma R$ induced by the interaction of cells with IgG-IC or aggregated IgG leads to a complete loss of cytotoxic activity (Cordier *et al.*, 1977; Moretta *et al.*, 1978). The presence of FcR on the effector cells is necessary but not sufficient for ADCC to occur. Effector cells also require a cytotoxic potential and an active metabolic activity since ADCC can be inhibited by various antimetabolites (reviewed by Perlmann *et al.*, 1972; Cerottini and Brunner, 1974).

It has been shown that among lymphocytes isolated from human PB, the cells cytotoxic in ADCC are included in both T and "null cells". In addition $Fc_\gamma R$ positive T cells generated in MLR are extremely efficient in mediating ADCC.

Suppression of B cell differentiation induced by PWM

As mentioned above, T_G cells, but not other T cell populations, sharply suppress B cell differentiation induced either by PWM (Moretta *et al.*, 1977a) or by specific antigens (Ballieux *et al.*, 1979). Further analysis of the suppressor mechanism of T_G cells has shown that suppression is mediated by soluble factors (Moretta *et al.*, 1979; Ballieux *et al.*, 1979). The factors which inhibit polyclonally induced B cell differentiation in the PWM assay are clearly nonspecific and are likely acting at the level of helper T cells. Of particular interest is the fact that release of suppressor factors occurs within a few hours and only when T_G cells have been exposed to both IgG-IC and PWM. IgG-IC or PWM alone are not sufficient to induce suppressor factor release. Thus, two combined signals are required for triggering normal T_G cells to release soluble suppressor factors and surface $Fc_\gamma R$ themselves play a direct role in triggering the cells. Since IgG antibodies likely have a homeostatic role in the immune response (Uhr and Moller, 1968), it is possible that T_G cells can be activated in a similar manner *in vivo*. In this case, the second signal (PWM *in vitro*) would be provided by a specific antigen and would therefore be effective only on T_G cells belonging to a specific clonotype. In view of the relatively low avidity of the $Fc_\gamma R$, T_G cells would bind IgG only when aggregated by antigen or other means. This could imply that binding of IgG to $Fc_\gamma R$ and consequent T_G cell triggering would occur only at particular stages of an antibody response. Modulation of $Fc_\gamma R$ induced by IgG-IC, in turn, could serve as a regulatory device which would render cells less susceptible or unsusceptible to activation by IC. Abnormal modulation of $Fc_\gamma R$ with possible consequences on cell functions could occur in the course of diseases with high levels of IC. Although FcR play probably an important role in triggering certain mechanisms of suppression, there are other mechanisms by which suppressor cells present within the T_G cell fractions can be activated. For example, con A activated T cells suppress B lymphocyte responses without need for binding IC (Haynes and Fauci, 1978). Con A-induced suppression, however, is not restricted to T_G cell populations (Hayward *et al.*, 1978; Haynes and Fauci, 1978); in addition, cell proliferation is required to generate suppressor cells indicating that, in this case, the mitogen can induce precursors of suppressor cells also present among $Fc_\gamma R$ negative cells, to become active suppressor cells.

Changes of the FcR phenotype of T cells

In view of the reproducibility of *in vitro* measurable activities which can be attributed to T_G or T_M cells isolated from human PB, we had originally suggested that T_M and T_G cells could possibly represent separate sublines of T cells derived by post-thymic activation of already committed cells. However, a group of subsequent observations has suggested that T cells with FcR for either IgG or IgM can derive from a common precursor. Furthermore, there is now clear evidence that a change of the FcR phenotype can indeed occur under particular *in vitro* conditions. The first point was shown by studies on a malignant T cell clone marked by a chromosonal translocation in a patient with ataxia telangiectasia (Saxon *et al.*, 1979). Cells with both T_M and T_G phenotype had the translocation. The second point was demonstrated by the fact that peripheral T cells with surface $Fc_\gamma R$, upon interaction with IgG-IC lost $Fc_\gamma R$ and could express new receptors with affinity for IgM (Pichler *et al.*, 1978; Perlmann *et al.*, unpublished). In addition, we have recently shown (Moretta *et al.*, 1980 and Moretta, A. *et al.*, submitted) that peripheral T cells, upon activation in MLR progressively lose $Fc_{\mu}R$ and acquire $Fc_{\gamma}R$. The change of the FcR phenotype is not the consequence of a preferential proliferative response of T_G versus T_M cells, but is due to a *de novo* expression of $Fc_{\gamma}R$ by cells lacking detectable FcR (T null) and also to the sequential loss of $Fc_{\mu}R$ and expression of $Fc_{\gamma}R$ by T_M cells. Thus, human T cells under appropriate *in vitro* conditions can subsequently express different surface FcR. This might suggest that peripheral T cells with a different FcR phenotype do not necessarily belong to a different T cell lineage, but may in part represent cells at different stages of activation. It is of note that peripheral T null cells, upon activation in MLR express FcR; Astaldi *et al.* (1978) showed that thymocytes (lacking both $Fc_{\mu}R$ and $Fc_{\gamma}R$) express $Fc_{\mu}R$ following culture with thymic factors. In view of the sharp change of the proportions of cells expressing $Fc_{\mu}R$ or $Fc_{\gamma}R$ in the MLR, it might be possible to observe a similar imbalance also in analogous *in vivo* conditions. Suitable candidates for these studies were patients who had undergone BM transplantation who developed graft versus host disease (GVHD). Indeed, dramatic changes of T cell subsets (2–5 fold increase of T_G and 2–20 fold decrease of T_M cells) occurred in these patients when clinical symptoms of GVHD appeared (Bacigalupo *et al.*, submitted). Another obvious question to ask was whether T cells which have undergone a phenotypic change of their surface FcR also undergo a complete functional transition. Preliminary experiments by Mingari *et al.* have shown that T_G cells which have expressed $Fc_{\mu}R$ after modulation of $Fc_{\gamma}R$ do not acquire *in vitro* activities of T_M lymphocytes, since they do not provide help to B cells for Ig production nor do they respond efficiently to PHA or allogeneic cells. Furthermore, $Fc_{\gamma}R$ bearing cells generated in MLR have only some of the functional characteristics of the conventional T_G cells isolated from PB. Thus, they mediate ADCC and NK activity but do not suppress Ig production in different *in vitro* systems. Hence, cells which perform NK and ADCC activities are included within the "total" peripheral T_G cells, and it is possible that the latter indeed include different cell types. This view is further supported by recent data using alloantisera specific for T cell fractions obtained by planned immunizations involving HLA-A and B compatible donors (Ferrara *et al.*, 1979). Some of these antisera recognize large proportions, but not all of T_G cells (Ferrara *et al.*, submitted).

Proportions of circulating T_G and T_M cells in disease states

Alterations in proportions and/or absolute numbers of T_G or T_M subsets have been reported in a number of disease states, usually those which are at least associated with aberrations in immunological reactivity (reviewed in Fauci, 1980). Certain representative diseases with well documented abnormalities in T cell subsets as determined by FcR are listed in Table II. The most well

TABLE II

Immune disorders with altered proportions of circulating T_G and T_M cells

Immunodeficiencies (certain diagnostic groups)	Lack or low proportions of T_M cells and/or high proportions of T_G cells (Moretta *et al.*, 1977b; Gupta and Good, 1977)
Systemic lupus erythematosus	Lack or low proportions of T_G cell especially in the active phases of the disease (Fauci *et al.*, 1978; Moretta *et al.*, 1979)
Atopic diseases	Low proportions of T_G cells (Canonica *et al.*, 1979)
Hodgkin's disease	High proportions of T_G cells with or without altered proportions of T_M cells (Romagnani *et al.*, 1978; Moretta *et al.*, 1979)
Sarcoidosis	Frequent increase of T_G cell proportions (but not absolute numbers)
Multiple sclerosis	Frequent alterations of T_G cells proportions (Santoli *et al.*, 1978)
Graft versus host disease	Great increase of T_G cells with sharp decrease (or disappearance) of T_M cells (Bacigalupo *et al.*, in press)

studied and in essence the prototype of an immunologically mediated disease with abnormalities in proportions and absolute numbers of FcR bearing T cells is systemic lupus erythematosus (SLE). In this disease there is a relative and selective decrease in the proportion as well as the absolute number of circulating T_G cells (Fauci *et al.*, 1978; Moretta *et al.*, 1979). Since patients with SLE have circulating antibodies specific for T cells, it is likely that the depletion of T_G cells is at least in part explained by the action of these antibodies in either clearing T_G cells from the circulation and/or depleting them by a cytotoxic mechanism. However, as mentioned above, since circulating IC can clearly modulate T_G cells with a resulting loss of expression of the $Fc_\gamma R$, it is also likely that the circulating IC in SLE further influence the observed proportion of T_G cells by modulating the expression of the $Fc_\gamma R$ on the T_G cells that are not removed by specific antibody. In certain of the other diseases listed in Table II, it is possible that the increase in proportion of T_G cells results from the *in vivo* activation of T cells with resultant expression of $Fc_\gamma R$. Since multiple factors and circumstances may influence the expression or lack of expression of $Fc_\gamma R$ on T_G cells, data referable to the relative proportions of T_G cells in various diseases should be interpreted with this realization in mind and diminution of T_G cells or of the expression of $Fc_\gamma R$ should not invariably be extrapolated to represent a deficiency of suppressor T cell function merely because T_G cells have been demonstrated to be the suppressor cells in certain systems of *in vitro* lymphocyte function. It should be remembered that it is highly likely that T_G cells are a heterogeneous population, only a proportion of which may express suppressor cell function.

FcR bearing T cells and monoclonal antibodies

Analysis of FcR bearing T cell subsets with various hybridoma monoclonal antibodies which react with cell surface antigens on T cell subsets as well as other mononuclear cell subsets supports the concept that T_G cells are indeed a heterogeneous population of cells. At present, there are no reported monoclonal antibodies which exclusively recognize T cell subsets according to the expression of FcR. There has been some question as to the T cell origin of T_G cells (Reinherz *et al.*, 1980). Different monoclonal anti-T cell antibodies from independent laboratories recognize variable proportions of T_G cells ranging from 5% to as high as 90% (Haynes *et al.*, 1979; Reinherz, *et al.*, 1980; Gupta, pers. comm.). Using the 3AI monoclonal antibody which recognizes approximately 85% of PB T cells in man, it was found that the 3AI positive cells contained the helper cells for PWM-induced Ig secretion by B cells. In addition, 3AI positive cells contained the mitogen (Con A)-inducible suppressor cells for B cell function (Haynes *et al.*, 1979). The vast majority of the 3AI positive population were T_M cells. However, enough of the 3AI positive cells were T_G cells to result in a large proportion (up to 50–80%) of the total T_G cells being 3AI positive. On the other hand, most of the 3AI negative population were T_G, but since the 3AI negative population was a relatively small proportion of the total T cell population (approximately 15%), this still was compatible with the observation that the majority of the T_G cells were in fact 3AI positive. It should be noted that studies with a monoclonal antibody which binds to adherent cells (OKMI) showed that large proportions of T_G cells bind with low affinity to this antibody suggesting that these cells may belong to the monocyte lineage, perhaps being a promonocytic cell (Reinherz *et al.*, 1980). However, other preliminary studies have demonstrated that other monoclonal antibodies which react with PB monocytes do not bind to T_G cells (Haynes and Fauci, unpublished observations). It is clear that at least a proportion of this heterogenous T_G population are T cells. In this regard, there is little doubt that exclusive T cell functions such as response in the MLR and specific and nonspecific suppression argue in favour of the T cell nature of at least a fraction of PB T_G cells.

Subsets of T cells defined by FcR will surely overlap with populations of T cells as determined by binding with monoclonal antibodies. Using both of these markers as well as other markers of T cell subsets in a complementary manner should prove useful in delineating functionally distinct T cell subsets determined by an antigen that may be unrelated to function as well as T cell subsets whose functions may directly relate to the receptor marker in question.

Conclusion

Despite the fact that major advances in cell surface markers have been and will continue to be extremely important in delineating lymphoid cell fractions in humans, it is essential to realize certain important limitations. a) An immediate source of artifact in human experimentation is that of sampling only a small representation of a complex system since only PBL and BM are routinely available. b) The problem of clearly defining the "starting definition" of a given lymphoid population is still critical. c) A given activity measurable by *in vitro* assays may not necessarily nor precisely reflect *in vivo* functions. d) It is likely that the cell responsible for a certain activity which is detectable in a subset of cells defined by a given surface marker may represent only a small fraction of the subset in question.

References

Astaldi, A., Astaldi, G. C. B., Wijermans, P., Groenewoud, M., Van Bemmel, T., Schellekens, P. Th. A. and Eijsvoogel, V. P. (1978). *In* "Cell Biology and Immunology of Leukocyte Function" (Proc. 12th Leukocyte Culture Conference). (M. R. Quastel, ed.) p. 221. Academic Press. New York.

Bacigalupo, A., Podesta, M., Mingari, M. C., Moretta, L., Van Lint, M. T. and Marmont, A. (1980). *J. Immunol.* (in press).

Balch, C. M., Dougherty, P. A., Dagg, M. K. *et al.* (1977). *Clin. Immunol. Immunopathol.* **8**, 448.

Ballieux, R. E., Heijnen, C. J., Uytdehaag, F. and Zegars, J. M. (1979). *Immunol. Rev.* **45**, 3.

Basten, A., Miller, J. F. A. P., Sprent, J. and Pye, J. (1972). *J. Exp. Med.* **135**, 610.

Canonica, G. W., Mingari, M. C., Melioli, G., Colombatti, M. and Moretta, L. (1979). *J. Immunol.* **124**, 112.

Cerottini, J. C. and Brunner, K. T. (1974). *Adv. Immunol.* **18**, 67.

Conradie, J. D. and Bubb, M. D. (1977). *Nature* **265**, 160.

Cooper, M. D., Peterson, R. D. A., South, M. R., *et al.* (1966). *J. Exp. Med.* **123**, 75.

Cordier, G., Samarut, C., Revillard, J. P. (1977). *J. Immunol.* **119**, 1943.

Dickler, H. B. (1976). *In* "Advances in Immunology" (F. J. Dixon and H. G. Kunkel, eds) p. 167. Academic Press, New York.

Dickler, H. B. and Kunkel, H. G. (1972). *J. Exp. Med.* **136**, 191.

Dickler, H. B., Adkinson, N. F. and Terry, W. D. (1974). *Nature* **247**.

Di George, A. M. (1968) *In* "Immunologic Deficiency Diseases in Man" (D. Bergsma and R. A. Good, eds) pp. 116–121. The National Foundation, New York.

Evans, R. L., Lazarus, H., Penta, A. C. and Schlossman, S. F. (1977). *J. Immunol.* **120**, 1423.

Fauci, A. S. (1979). *Immunol. Rev.* **45**, 93.

Fauci, A. S. (1980). *J. All. Clin. Innumol.* (in press).

Fauci, A. S., Steinberg, A. D., Haynes, B. F., and Whalen, G. (1978). *J. Immunol.* **121**, 1473.

Ferrara, G. B., Strelkauskas, A. J., Longo, A., McDavell, J., Yunis, E. J. and Schlossman, J. F. (1979). *J. Immunol.* **123**, 1272.

Ferrarini, M., Moretta, L., Abrile, R. and Durante, M. L. (1975). *Eur. J. Immunol.* **5**, 70.
Forni, L. and Pernis, B. (1975). *In* "Membrane Receptors of Lymphocytes" (M. Seligman, J. L. Preud'homme and F. M. Kouzilsky, eds) pp. 193–201, North–Holland Publishing Co., Amsterdam.
Froland, S. S. and Natvig, J. B. (1973). *Transplant. Rev.* **16**, 114.
Glick, B., Chang, T. S. and Jaap, R. G. (1956). *Poultry Sci.* **35**, 224.
Gmelig-Meyling, F., van der Ham, M. and Ballieux, R. E. (1976). *Scand. J. Immunol.* **5**, 487.
Good, R. A., Dalmasso, A. P., Martinez, C., *et al.* (1962). *J. Exp. Med.* **116**, 773.
Greaves, M. F. and Janossy, G. (1976). *In* "*In Vitro* Methods in Cell Mediated and Tumor Immunity" (B. Bloom and J. David, eds) p. 89, Academic Press, New York.
Greaves, M. F., Verbi, V., Festenstein, H., Pajorsteriadis, C., Jaraquemada, D. and Hayward, A. (1979). *Eur. J. Immunol.* **9**, 365.
Hammarstrom, S., Hellstrom, V. Perlmann, P., *et al.* (1973). *J. Exp. Med.* **138**, 1270.
Haynes, B. F. and Fauci, A. S. (1978). *J. Immunol.* **121**, 559.
Haynes, B. F., Eisenbarth, G. S. and Fauci, A. S. (1979). *Proc. Natn. Acad. Sci. U.S.A.* **76**, 5829.
Haynes, B. F., Mann, D. L., Hemler, M. E., Schroer, J. A., Schelhamer, J. H., Eisenbarth, G. S., Strominger, J. L., Thomas, C. A., Mostowski, H. and Fauci, A. S. (1980). *Proc. Natn. Acad. Sci. U.S.A.* **77**, 2914.
Hayward, A. R., Layward, L., Lydyard, P., Moretta, L., Dagg, M., Lawton, A. R. (1978). *J. Immunol.* **121**, 1.
Ko, H-S., Fu, S. M., Winchester, R. J., Yu, T. Y. D. and Kunkel, H. G. (1979). *J. Exp. Med.* **150**, 246.
Jondal, M., Holm, A. and Wigzell, H. (1972). *J. Exp. Med.* **136**, 207.
Lee, S. T. and Paraskevas, F. (1972). *J. Immunol.* **109**, 1262.
Lo Buglio, A. F., Cotran, R. S. and Jadl, J. H. (1967). *Science* **158**, 1582.
Lum, L. G., Muchmore, A. V., Keren, D., Decker, J., Koski, I., Strober, W., Blaese, R. M. (1979). *J. Immunol.* **122**, 65.
MacLennan, I. C. M. (1972). *Transplant. Rev.* **13**, 67.
McConnell, I. and Hurd, C. M. (1976). *Immunology* **30**, 835.
Miller, J. F. A. P. and Osoba, D. (1967). *Physiol. Rev.* **47**, 437.
Mingari, M. C., Moretta, L., Moretta, A., Ferrarini, M. and Preud'homme, J. L. (1978). *J. Immunol.* **121**, 767.
Moretta, L., Ferrarini, M., Durante, M. L., and Mingari, M. D. (1975). *Eur. J. Immunol.* **5**, 565.
Moretta, L., Webb, S. R., Grossi, C. E., Lydyard, P. M. and Cooper, M. D. (1977a). *J. Exp. Med.* **146**, 184.
Moretta, L., Mingari, M. C., Moretta, A. and Lydyard, P. M. (1977b). *Clin. Immunol. Immunopathol.* **7**, 405.
Moretta, L., Mingari, M. C., Webb, S. R., Pearl, E. R., Lydyard, P. M., Grossi, C. E., Lawton, A. R. and Cooper, M. D. (1977c). *Eur. J. Immunol.* **7**, 696.
Moretta, L., Mingari, M. C. and Romanzi, C. A. (1978). *Nature* **272**, 618.
Moretta, L., Mingari, M. C. and Moretta, A. (1979). *Immunol. Rev.* **45**, 163.
Moretta, L., Bacigalupo, A., Moretta, A., Canonica, G. W. and Mingari, M. C. (1980). *In* "Suppressor T Cell in Humans" (B. Serrou and C. Rosenfeld, eds) (in press). Elsevier/North Holland Publishing Co.
Oldstone, M. B. A., Tishon, A. and Moretta, L. (1977). *Nature* **269**, 333.
Osmond, D. G., Nossal, G. J. V. (1974). *Cell. Immunol.* **13**, 132.
Owen, J. J. T., Cooper, M. D., Raff, M. C. (1974). *Nature* **249**, 361.
Palacios, R., Lorente, L., Alarcon-Segovia, D. *et al.* (1980). *J. Clin. Invest.* **65**, 1527.
Parker, J. W., Metcalf, D. (1974). *J. Immunol.* **112**, 502.

Parkman, R. (1978). *Clin. Hematol.* **7**, 482.
Perlmann, H., Perlmann, P. and Wigzell, H. (1972) *Transplant. Rev.* **13**, 3.
Pernis, B., Forni, L. and Amante, L. (1970). *J. Exp. Med.* **132**, 1001.
Pichler, W. J., Lum, L. and Broder, S. (1978). *J. Immunol.* **121**, 1540.
Preud'homme, J. L. and Seligman, M. (1972). *Proc. Natn. Acad. Sci. U.S.A.* **69**, 2132.
Preud'homme, J. L., Gonnot, M., Fellous, M. and Seligmann, M. (1979). *Scand. J. Immunol.* **10**, 207.
Raff, M. C., Sternberg, M. and Taylor, R. (1970). *Nature* **225**, 553.
Reinherz, E. L., and Schlossman, S. F. (1979). *J. Immunol.* **122**, 1335.
Reinherz, E. L., Kung, P. C., Pesando, J. M., Ritz, J., Goldstein, G. and Schlossman, S. F. (1979). *J. Exp. Med.* **150**, 1472.
Reinherz, E. L., Moretta, L., Mingari, M. D., Roper, M., Breard, J. M., Kung, P. C., Goldstein, G., Cooper, M. D. and Schlossman, S. F. (1980). *J. Exp. Med.* **151**, 969.
Romagnani, S., Maggi, E., Biagiotti, R., Giudizi, M. G., Amadori, A. and Ricci, M. (1978). *Scand. J. Immunol.* **7**, 511.
Rozenszajn, L. A., Shoham, D. and Kalechman, I. (1975). *Immunol.* **29**, 1061.
Samarut, C., Revillard, J. P. (1979). *Transplant.* **27**, 283.
Samarut, C., Cordier, G. and Revillard, J. P. (1979). *Cellular Immunol.* (in press).
Saxon, A., Morledge, V. D., Bonavida, B. (1977). *Clin. Exp. Immunol.* **28**, 324.
Saxon, A., Stevens, R. H. and Gold, D. W. (1979). *New Engl. J. Med.* **300**, 700.
Silverstein, S. C., Steinman, R. M., and Cohn, Z. A. (1977). *Annu. Rev. Biochem.* **46**, 669.
Singer, J. W., Brown, J. E., Doney, K., Warren, R., Storb, R., Thomas, E. D. (1980). *Blood* (in press).
Sjoberg, O. (1980). *Scand. J. Immunol.* **11**, 377.
Stout, R. D. and Herzenberg, L. A. (1975). *J. Exp. Med.* **142**, 611.
Strober, W., Hague, N. E., Lum, L. G. and Henkart, P. A. (1978). *J. Immunol.* **121**, 2440.
Sulica, A., Gherman, M., Madesan, C., Sjoquist, J. and Ghetie, V. (1979a). *Eur. J. Immunol.* **9**, 979.
Sulica, A., Gherman, M. Madesan, C., Ghetie, V. and Sjoquist, J. (1979b). *Eur. J. Immunol.* **9**, 985.
Trainin, N., Resnitzky, P. (1969). *Nature* **221**, 1154.
Uhlenbank, K. G., Seaman, G. V. F. and Coombs, R. R. A. (1967). *Vox. Sang.* **12**, 420.
Uhr, J. W. and Moller, G. (1968). *Adv. Immunol.* **8**, 81.
Van Oers, M. H. J., Zeijlemaker, W. P. and Schellekens, P. Th. A. (1977). *Eur. J. Immunol.* **7**, 143.
Warner, N. L. (1965). *Aust. J. Exp. Biol. Med. Sci.* **43**, 439.
Winchester, R. J., Fu, S. M., Hoffman, T., and Kunkel, H. G. (1975). *J. Immunol.* **114**, 1210.
Wiktor-Jedrzejczak, W., Sharkis, S., Ahmed, A. and Sell, K. (1977). *Science* **196**, 313.
Yodoi, J. and Ishizaka, K. (1980). *J. Immunol.* **124**, 934.
Yoshida, T. O. and Andersson, B. (1972). *Scand. J. Immunol.* **1**, 401.
Zipori, D., Trainin, N. (1975). *Experimental Hematology* **3**, 1.

13

Generation of Diversity at MHC Loci: Implications for T Cell Receptor Repertoires

JAN KLEIN

Max-Planck-Institut für Biologie, Abteilung Immungenetik, Tübingen, West Germany

Alle fine et cetera

According to his biographers, Giuseppe Verdi was in such a feverish haste to write all his operas that while collecting musical ideas for *La Traviata*, he just jotted down the first bars of the melody for *Sempre libera degg'io folleggiare di gioja in gioja* without bothering to write the rest of the aria. Instead, he merely added to these few bars, *Alle fine et cetera*. Comments Verdi's biographer Carlo Gatti: "One of the greatest melodies ever composed and Verdi just writes 'to the end, et cetera' as though everyone knew it already. *Et cetera*

I thank Drs Donald V. Cramer, Dietrich Götze, Joseph H. Nadeau, and Uzi Ritte for their critical reading of this manuscript, Ms Rosemary Franklin for editorial work, and Ms Korinna Bartels for secretarial help. The experimental work on which this manuscript is based was supported by grants from the Volkswagen Siftung and from the National Institutes of Health, Bethesda, Maryland, USA (AI 14736).

for whom, I ask you? Not for you, and not for me and not for anyone except a genius like Verdi. Fortunately, in a later draft, he took time to write out the whole melody" (cited by Wechsberg, 1974.)

In the study of the major histocompatibility complex (MHC) function, we are just about as far as that Verdi sketch. We are tantalized by a few bars that promise to develop into one of the most beautiful melodies ever written, yet no one seems to be able to write out this melody to its end. We know that any time a T lymphocyte recognizes an antigen, it simultaneously recognizes MHC molecules (it sometimes recognizes MHC molecules alone but, apparently, never the conventional antigen alone). We surmise from this knowledge that T lymphocytes bear receptors specifically recognizing MHC molecules—but that is about where the melody ends. We do not know *what* the receptors are, *how* they recognize MHC molecules, whether there are separate receptors for antigens and for MHC molecules, what process selects the right combinations of receptor, how the MHC molecules function, *alle fine et cetera.*

Of the few clues that we have regarding the MHC–T-cell receptor relationship, the most promising are those relating to properties that set the MHC apart from other genetic systems. The most striking of these properties is the polymorphism of the MHC loci. Hence, when considering the relationship of the MHC to its receptors, the MHC polymorphism is a good point to start.

What is so special about the MHC polymorphism? The best way of answering this question is by reminding ourselves that in any population some 70% of all genetic loci do not vary (i.e., they are monomorphic), and that of the 30% that do vary, most occur in only 2 forms (alleles), usually one relatively frequent and one relatively rare (Lewontin, 1974). Only a few loci occur each in 3, 4 and, rarely, more than 4 forms. Furthermore, the 2 or more alleles at each of the polymorphic loci code for products that differ from one another very little structurally, usually only in a single amino acid.

The MHC loci defy the general rules of population genetics in that they are *always* polymorphic and in that allelic products differ in *several* amino acids (Klein, 1979). The latter observation more than anything else proves the uniqueness of the MHC loci in terms of population behaviour. It also represents a strong argument against the oft considered possibility that MHC loci are not more polymorphic than other loci—what makes them *seem* to be more polymorphic is the availability of sensitive methods which detect more variation at these loci than other methods do at other loci. The fact that allelic MHC products have accumulated multiple amino acid differences fits in well with the antigenic variation detected by serological methods.

Polymorphism of hamster, rat and human MHC

The available data suggest that the degree of MHC polymorphism varies from species to species. Among the species thus far studied, the polymorphism appears to be lowest in the Syrian hamster, extensive in the rat, high in man and extremely high in the mouse. In the hamster, Duncan and Streilein (1977) have identified what appears to be the homologue of the MHC in other species. It is not yet clear how many loci the hamster MHC consists of but no matter what this number is, the loci are apparently not highly polymorphic: Only two alleles (haplotypes, i.e. *Hm-1*^{a} and *Hm-1*^{b}) have been identified at these loci. Until recently, one could argue that the MHC polymorphism in the hamster merely *appears* low because most of the animals bred in captivity derive from the same founding pair. But typing of animals clearly not derived from this pair, including animals recently captured in Syria, suggests that the MHC polymorphism of this species may indeed be low.

In the rat, the *RT1* complex is composed of one class I (*A*) and one class II (*B*) locus cluster.* There are apparently at least two loci in each of the two clusters, but recombinants between loci of a single cluster have not been found (Günther and Štark, 1979). The *A* locus is known in 12 forms ("alleles") present in the laboratory rat; 8 of these 12 alleles have also been found in wild rats (Cramer *et al.*, 1978; Wagener *et al.*, 1979). In the largest population studied, 7 alleles were identified and their frequencies ranged from 5 to 35%. Less than 10% of the tested haplotypes code for products not detectable with the available typing reagents. These "blanks" presumably code for thus far unidentified antigens and hence represent new alleles. The low frequency of blanks suggests that the majority of the class I alleles occurring among wild rats has already been identified so that the total polymorphism can be estimated at approximately 10–12 alleles. At the *B* locus, 9 alleles have been identified in inbred strains using the mixed lymphocyte reaction (MLR) assay, 5 of which have also been found in wild rats. However, since there are about 25% of *B* locus blanks present in wild rats, several alleles still need to be identified and hence the total number of *B* alleles may approach that of *A* alleles. How these numbers will change once it is possible to identify true alleles at the two presumed *A* and the two presumed *B* loci remains to be seen.

In man, 3 class I MHC loci have been identified, *HLA-A*, *-B* and *-C* (Bodmer *et al.*, 1977). The numbers of allele at the *A, B* and *C* loci are 17, 20 and 7, respectively; the frequencies of blanks at these three loci in well characterized populations (e.g., European Caucasians) are 2·2, 2·4 and 46%, respectively. These figures suggest that virtually all the polymorphic variation of the *A* and *B* loci, at least in the well characterized populations, has been identified; at the *C* locus, one could still expect to uncover 5–7 more alleles. However, it is still possible that these figures represent significant underestimates of true polymorphic variation at the *HLA* loci primarily for the following reason. Although the serological identification of *HLA* alleles has

* Class I loci are loci coding for a 44 000 dalton polypeptide chain which associates with β_2 microglobulin in the plasma membrane; class II are loci coding for either 33 000 or 28 000 dalton polypeptides which, in the membrane, associate noncovalently to form dimers. The 2 classes of loci differ also in their functional properties.

greatly improved since the early days of HLA serology, one could still argue that the presently available typing reagents identify allelic families rather than single alleles. Simple checks for allele identity, such as peptide-mapping comparisons of serologically indistinguishable class I molecules isolated from geographically distant regions of the globe, have not yet been made. Until such checks are carried out, the estimates of *HLA* class I loci polymorphism must be taken with a grain of salt.

The situation at class II loci is far from clear. At present, there are two kinds of human class II loci defined by different methods, *D*, defined by MLR typing and *D*-related (*DR*), defined serologically. The genetic relationship between the *D* and the *DR* loci is still unresolved; however, the experience with homologous loci in other species, particularly in the mouse, suggests that considerable if not complete overlap between the loci is to be expected. Unresolved is also the question of the number of loci in the *D* region; if there is more than one *D* locus, which is very likely, then the presently known polymorphism (11 *D* alleles and 39% blanks and 7 *DR* alleles and 26% blanks) will need to be re-evaluated.

It should also be mentioned that most of the present knowledge about the *HLA* polymorphism is based on the use of typing reagents produced against antigens from Caucasian populations. Such reagents are inadequate for the characterization of polymorphisms in other races and ethnic groups. Additional polymorphism at both class I and class II loci may, therefore, turn up when reagents specific for different populations are used more extensively.

Polymorphism of the mouse MHC

In the mouse, there are three class I loci, *K*, *D* and *L*, and two serologically easily identifiable class II loci, *A* and *E* (Klein, 1979). In addition there is a family of loci referred to as *Qa* and *Tla* which are, at present, poorly characterized but which show some resemblance to the class I loci (molecular weight 45 000 daltons and association with β_2 microglobulin-like molecules). Eventually these loci may well be included in the class I category.

In the mouse, as in the rat, there are two ways of counting alleles at the MHC loci: by isolating the alleles and identifying them in inbred strains and congenic lines, and by determining gene frequencies in wild mouse populations. Alleles carried by inbred and congenic lines are well defined serologically and often also biochemically and functionally. In most instances, there is no doubt that the alleles are distinct from one another. In the classical inbred strains one finds 11 *K*, 9 *D*, 3 *L*, 10 *A* and 4 *E* alleles. We have increased these numbers by isolating additional *H-2* alleles from wild mice, putting them on the C57BL/10Sn strain background and so producing 34 new B10.W lines. Analysis of the B10.W lines enriched the collection of alleles maintained in the laboratory by 19 *K*, 28 *D*, 3 *L*, 11 *A* and 2 *E* alleles (Klein, 1972; Zaleska-Rutczynska and Klein, 1977; Duncan and Klein, 1980; Wakeland

and Klein, 1979a; Huang *et al.*, 1979). Thus, the total number of *H-2* alleles in the laboratory collection is 30 *K*, 38 *D* 6 *L*, 21 *A* and 6 *E* alleles (Table I). These numbers give the minimal estimates of the MHC polymorphism in the mouse, provided of course that all these laboratory alleles can also be found with appreciable frequencies in natural populations—which, as we shall see shortly, is indeed the case.

TABLE I
Laboratory collection of alleles at H-2 *loci*

Locus	*Allele (private antigen, if known)*	*Total number*
K	*b* (33), *d* (31), *f* (26), *j* (15), *k* (23), *p* (16), *q* (17), *r* (18), *s* (19), *u* (20), *v* (21), *w3* (103), *w7* (132), *w9* (101), *w13* (113), *w15* (115), *w16* (116), *w17* (111), *w27* (138), *w6, w23, w28, w29, w30, w31, w32, w33, w34, w35, w36*	30
D	*b* (2), *d* (4), *f* (9), *k* (32), *p* (22), *q* (30), *r* (10), *s* (12), *s* (14), *z* (114), *w3* (118), *w4* (104), *w7* (131), *w8* (110), *w12* (112), *w13* (133), *W16* (117), *w21* (130), *w26* (27), *w1, w5, w6, w9, w10, w11, w18, w23, w24, w27, w28, w29, w30, w31, w32, w33, w34, w35, w36*	38
A	*b, d, f, j, k, p, r, s, u, v, w3, w4, w5, w6, w7, w9, w13, w17, w23*	21
E	*b, d, p, k, w4, w27*	6

A better estimate of the extent of *H-2* polymorphism can be obtained from frequencies of individual *H-2* alleles in wild mice. The determination of these frequencies has been slow in comparison with similar studies in man. While HLA typing is carried out by hundreds of people in dozens of laboratories all over the world, ours is virtually the only laboratory that does *H-2* typing of wild mice. We have typed samples of wild mice from North America (Michigan, Texas), South America (Chile), North Africa (Egypt), and many localities in Europe, from Spain and Italy to Scotland (Duncan *et al.*, 1979a; Götze *et al.*, 1980; Nadeau *et al.*, 1980; Figueroa and Klein, 1980). I shall consider the typing results in two forms, as pooled data from all the populations ("global population"), and separately for the individual populations.

In the global population, we have found all the *H-2* alleles present in the laboratory collection. There are no great variations in the frequency of alleles at the individual loci (since most mice are heterozygous for *K*, *D* and *A* loci (Duncan *et al.*, 1979b; Nadeau *et al.*, 1980), gene frequencies can be obtained by dividing private antigen frequencies by two). At the class I loci, there are only three alleles K^d, K^p and D^d) which occur with a frequency higher than 6%; the frequency of all other alleles is one to 3% (see Fig. 1; only data for *K* and *D* loci are shown; no information is available on the frequency of *L* alleles in wild mice). However, the frequencies are getting smaller as we test more mice from additional geographical regions and so, until a saturation point is reached, all the estimates of allele numbers must be considered as

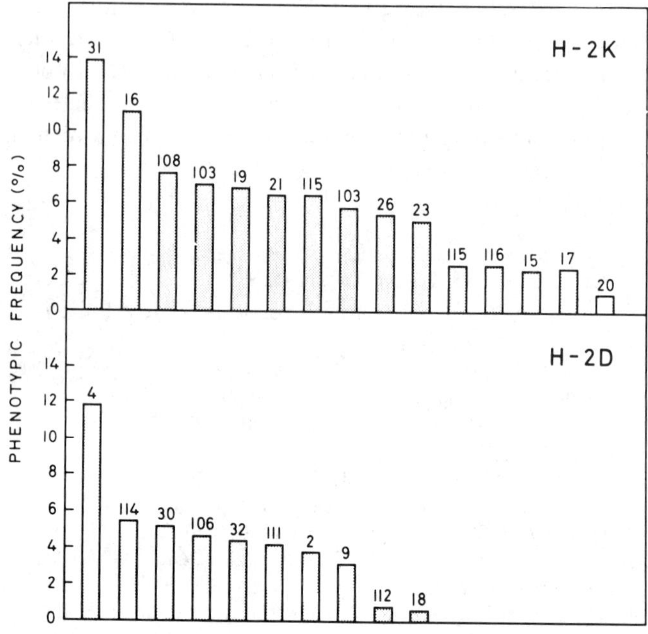

FIG. 1. *Frequency of H-2 antigens in global mouse populations.*

minimal. The high frequency of blanks (50% at the *K* locus and 50% at the *D* locus) suggests that there are still many more alleles to be identified. Assuming an average allele frequency of 2%, there must be a minimum of 50 alleles at the *K* and 50 alleles at the *D* loci (we do not find any evidence for a difference in the extent of polymorphism at these two loci). Should further typing halve the present gene frequency estimates (which I consider likely to happen), the number of alleles at the *K* and *D* loci may easily reach 100 or more per locus.

Similar data concerning class II loci are also available but are less reliable than the class I locus data, mainly because of the poor quality of the available class II typing reagents. Only very few class II allele-specific reagents could be used for testing wild mice. Assuming that some of these reagents are truly allele-specific, which is by no means certain, the frequency of an average *A* allele can be estimated to range from 10 to 15% and that of an *E* allele from 25 to 35%. If these data could be trusted, they would indicate that the polymorphism of the *A* locus is lower than that of the *K* and *D* loci and that the *E* locus may not be more polymorphic than some of the polymorphic non-MHC loci. However, before making far reaching conclusions about these lower class II polymorphisms, 2 things need to be taken into account. First, very likely the so-called *A* locus is in fact a composition of at least 3 loci, and similarly the *E* locus may also be a group of loci rather than a single locus (review in Klein, 1979); at present the distribution of polymorphisms among these loci is unclear. And second, some of the *A* loci co-operate with some of the *E* loci in the construction of class II molecules: one chain of the molecule is contributed by one locus and the other chain by another locus (Jones *et al.*, 1978). Recent evidence indicates that the combination of chains controlled by different loci results in hybrid determinants (Lafuse *et al.*, 1980). The formation of hybrid molecules may thus add another dimension to the polymorphism of the class II loci.

Structural correlates of antigenic variation

Although structural studies of the MHC molecules have been spectacularly successful in the last few years, the information that they have provided is still sketchy. Two human MHC class I polypeptide chains have been completely sequenced in their portions extending to the exterior of the plasma membrane (about 270 amino acids corresponding to about two-thirds of the molecule which is estimated to contain some 350 amino acids; see Orr *et al.*, 1979); in the mouse, complete sequence is known for one class I chain and almost complete sequence for another chain (Coligan *et al.*, 1979). Furthermore, several class I and class II chains of different species have been sequenced in their N-terminal segments (reviewed by Vitetta and Capra, 1978). Complete sequences of human, mouse, dog and rat β_2 microglobulin molecules are also available (reviewed by Poulik and Reisfeld, 1975). In the mouse, the products of several MHC genes have been finger-printed (Brown *et al.*, 1974). These studies are summarized elsewhere in this volume and also in numerous review articles; here I would like to draw attention only to a few points that are pertinent to the discussed topic.

The most important point for consideration of MHC polymorphism is the number of amino acid differences between two allelic products. Although no two allelic MHC molecules have been sequenced in their entirety, the number of amino acids in which they differ can be estimated indirectly. The N-terminal sequences of two allelic mouse class I molecules differ in 2 amino acids per 20 sequenced residues. If this degree of variation were to exist throughout the molecule (or at least throughout its external portion), there should be about 10 amino acid substitutions per 100 residues (and about 35 substitutions per MHC molecule). Another way of estimating the number of interallelic differences is by comparing interlocus differences. The human HLA-B7 and HLA-A2 molecules differ in 25 of the total 150 residues sequenced which comes to about 14 substitutions per 100 residues. Since peptide mapping comparisons indicate that there is about the same structural difference between molecules controlled by two class I loci as there is between alleles of a single class I locus, the estimate 14/100 should roughly apply to interallelic differences as well.

Interspecies comparisons reveal that, for example, human HLA-B7 and mouse H-2K^b molecules differ in 40 of the 160 sequenced residues, that is in about 25 amino acids per 100 residues.

The estimates of *H-2* gene frequencies in wild mouse populations are based on the assumption that whenever a typing reagent reacts with cells from a given mouse, this mouse carries an allele identical with that carried by the immunizing cells used for the production of this reagent. One may challenge this assumption on the grounds that the alleles may *seem* to be identical only because their products share one antigenic determinant, and that these products may differ in other determinants for which one does not type. In addition, some allelic products may be so similar to one another that they may be difficult to distinguish serologically. Taking into account the high degree of MHC polymorphism and the claimed high mutation rate of some of the MHC loci (reviewed by Klein, 1978), one might even question whether

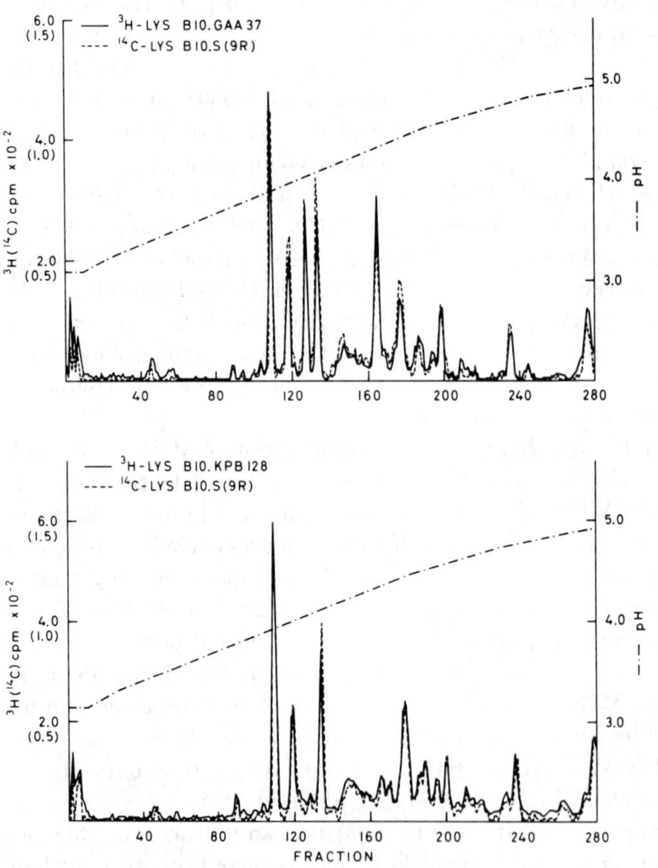

FIG 2. *Ion-exchange chromatography of tryptic peptides from lysine-labelled H-2K glycoproteins. B10.S(9R) is compared with B10.GAA37 (upper panel) and B10.KPB128 (lower panel). (From Arden* et al., *1980.)*

the same allele occurs repeatedly in populations separated in time and space. To answer this question, we have randomly selected several groups of serologically indistinguishable alleles of class I and class II loci and compared them by tryptic peptide mapping (Wakeland and Klein, 1979b; Arden *et al.*, 1980). Figure 2 shows an example of such a comparison. The 2 *K* alleles compared here are clearly of different origin. The K^s allele of the B10.S(9R) strain has been maintained in the laboratory for at least 50 years and is derived from mice originally imported to the USA from Switzerland. The serologically indistinguishable. K^s allele of the B10.GAA37 and B10.KPB128 strains has recently been extracted from wild mice captured in Michigan. Figure 2 shows that the peptide maps of the molecules controlled by these 3 alleles are the same. We have obtained similar data for one other group of class I alleles and one group of class II alleles. In every case where the alleles were serologically indistinguishable, they were also chemically identical, although they were clearly of different origin. Although tryptic peptide mapping has its limitations and so this method may miss some amino acid differences, for all practical purposes the alleles may be considered identical (for obvious reasons, it is not possible to compare the complete amino acid sequence of the serologically indistinguishable class I or class II molecules). The conclusion from these studies, therefore, is that identical alleles of both class I and class II loci occur repeatedly in unrelated populations.

Origin of the MHC polymorphism

The high variability of the MHC loci may tempt one to regard the MHC polymorphism as a more or less continuous spectrum of variants. One can view the MHC genes as mutating at a high rate, rapidly accumulating these mutational differences, and thus differentiating into a great number of alleles. According to this view, the MHC polymorphism should be in a dynamic state in which alleles constantly change into one another and in which transitional forms span the entire variability spectrum. If this view were correct, the probability of finding identical alleles in unrelated populations would be extremely low. The fact that we have found, without really trying, a number of identical alleles in different populations strongly suggests that this view is incorrect.

In a search for an alternative explanation for the origin of the MHC polymorphism, we shall start with Dobzhansky's oft quoted "Nothing in biology makes sense except in the light of evolution", and ask the question: How could loci like those composing the MHC have evolved? Before attempting to answer this question, let us first briefly recapitulate what is known about the evolution of non-MHC loci, and let us do so using the locus coding for the haemoglobin (*Hb*) α chain as an example.

Although many variants have been isolated at the *Hb* α locus, most of them could be demonstrated to be the result of recent mutations (White, 1978a).

These variants occur in the population only fleetingly and the locus remains monomorphic. Only occasionally, a second allele established itself in a population so that in these populations the locus becomes polymorphic. An example of the latter situation is the Melanesian population of a Pacific island in which the α-chain variant Hb Tongariki, is carried by 10% of individuals (Gajdusek *et al.*, 1967). Haemoglobin Tongariki differs from the standard haemoglobin in that alanine is replaced by asparagine at position 115 in the α chain.

It is not unreasonable to assume that a similar situation existed at the *Hb* locus in the common ancestor of mouse and man so that when these ancestors split into two lineages, one lineage leading to primates and the other to rodents, the evolution in the lineages started from identical, homogeneous gene pools. The genes then mutated at a rate of about 10^{-7} mutations/generation but most of the mutations were lost soon after their appearance, either because of random drift or because of selection working against them. However, approximately once every 5·6 M years, a mutation became established in a population—again either by chance or because it provided the species with some selective advantage. The mutation probably coexisted for some time in the population with the original allele but eventually, completely replaced this allele. Some 5·6 M years later another mutation became fixed so that the haemoglobin molecule then differed from the starting molecule of the ancestors in 2 amino acids, and this process then continued all the way to the present-day forms (Goodman *et al.*, 1975). Because of the randomness of the mutation process, randomness of the drift, and different selective pressures, different mutations were fixed in the 2 evolving lineages, and the haemoglobin genes of the 2 lineages drifted further and further apart. Human and mouse haemoglobins accumulated a total of 18 amino acid differences in the 143 residues composing the α chain, which comes to about 16 amino acid substitutions/100 residues. The accumulation of so many differences took about 50–75 M years (it was 50–75 M years ago that the lineages leading to man and the mouse separated).

The evolution of the MHC genes might have proceeded in a similar way with one exception. Since the MHC loci in both man and the mouse are highly polymorphic, it again seems reasonable to assume that they were also polymorphic in the common ancestors of these two species. Consequently the evolution of the MHC drew not on pools of identical genes, as in the case of haemoglobin, but on pools of already differentiated (diversified) genes (the extent of this diversification depended on several factors, most importantly on the age of the MHC loci and on the time for which the diversification had been going on before the stage of the common mouse–man ancestor). Hence, in contrast to haemoglobin where evolution always operates with only one or two types of gene, at the MHC loci evolution operates with a group of already diversified genes (Fig. 3). In other words, the MHC genes (alleles) behave during evolution as if they were representatives of different loci although in fact they are representatives of a single locus.

Speciation is probably always initiated by segregation of a single gene pool

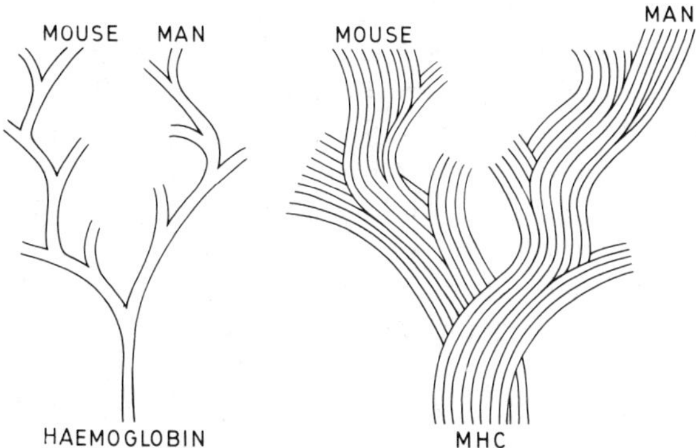

FIG. 3. *Differences in the evolution of* Hb *and* MHC *genes. In the case of Hb, evolution operated with a homogeneous pool of genes; in the case of MHC, the gene pools are heterogeneous and alleles evolve independently of one another.*

into two, an event occurring as a result of isolation (e.g., geographical; see White, 1978b). When a group of individuals separates from another group, it may not receive all the different MHC genes present in the original population, so that 2 species derived from a common ancestor may start their evolution with different MHC gene pools. If one of the separated groups were relatively small, it could contain only a limited selection of all the MHC genes present in the original population. The species evolving from this group may then have to make do with this small number of alleles at a given MHC locus for millions of years. Hence, depending on the size of the founding population, there could be considerable differences in the degree of the MHC polymorphism, as indeed there seem to be. The degree of polymorphism may then, in turn, influence the adaptability of a species. Perhaps one of the reasons why mice and not hamsters have conquered the world is that in the former but not in the latter the MHC loci are highly polymorphic.

It is of course possible that MHC genes evolve more rapidly than the haemoglobin gene. Significant differences in the rate of accumulation of amino acid substitutions in protein molecules during evolution have indeed been reported (reviewed by Fitch, 1973). For example, fibrinopeptides require "only" 1·1 M years to fix one amino acid substitution in their molecules; cytochrome c, on the other hand, requires 20 M years for this fixation. There is some evidence suggesting that the mutation rate of some MHC loci may be higher than that of, for example, the haemoglobin locus. But, as I have argued elsewhere (Klein, 1978), this difference in the mutation rate may be more seeming than real. However, even if MHC loci were to evolve as fast as the fibrinopeptide loci, or even faster, it would still take millions of years to differentiate alleles at a single locus to the degree that they are known to be differentiated today. If the *K* locus in the mouse or the *A* locus in man evolved with the speed of haemoglobin, the known alleles at either of these 2 loci must have diverged from a common ancestral gene some 20 M years ago. But even if they diverged 10 or 5 M years ago, it still is a very long time, longer than the age of the human or mouse species. The history of the present-day MHC alleles thus reaches far beyond the time of the establishment of a given species. The MHC polymorphism must, therefore, be discrete rather than continuous, composed of a mosaic of alleles with a long history, most of the alleles separated from one another for periods longer than the age of the species. This discreteness has little to do with selection; it simply reflects the evolutionary history of the genes.

These speculations are not meant to argue that MHC alleles are no longer diversifying. Of course they are, but it is totally unrealistic to think that polymorphic alleles are produced within a few generations, and that adaptive mechanisms select from these alleles the ones most suitable for given conditions. Such a degree of plasticity may not be possible even in so highly variable loci as the MHC loci undoubtedly are. Selection must probably make do with alleles that have been around for thousands, if not millions of years and may still be around long after immunologists' preoccupation with the MHC has become an unimportant footnote in the annals of science.

MHC polymorphism and the T cell receptor

Why are MHC loci so polymorphic? Before attempting to answer this question, we must first consider what the function of the MHC loci might be. The available evidence strongly suggests that the MHC is intimately involved in the body's defence mechanisms and it will be this involvement that we shall now consider.

The defence system of an organism must solve one basic problem: how to distinguish self from nonself. The seemingly simplest solution to this problem was proposed by Burnet (1969) who speculated that an organism possesses lymphocytes with receptors for both self and nonself but that the self-recognizing lymphocytes are eliminated during ontogeny, at the time when they first come in contact with self. However, Burnet's hypothesis has several weak points. For example, it has never been clear to me how a lymphocyte manages within a relatively short period to come into contact with all the individual's own molecules distributed throughout the body—all while remaining confined to more or less predetermined pathways. Also, it seems to me that by eliminating lymphocytes with receptors for self the body is depriving itself of the possibility to recognize self molecules of damaged tissues.

A better solution to the self–nonself distinction problem might be one in which the body:

(a) *selects* for lymphocytes recognizing self, and

(b) delegates the function to serve as markers of self to one *group* of molecules, namely the molecules controlled by the MHC.

According to this alternative to Burnet's hypothesis, the body actively recognizes self via specific lymphocyte receptors. Recognition of self alone results in either a tolerizing signal or no signal at all; recognition of self and nonself together results in a stimulatory signal.

Formally, one can argue that the MHC molecules must vary, otherwise they could not serve as markers of individuality. However, such an argument is meaningless unless accompanied by a specific explanation. One basic assumption of the explanation I favour is that there is no fundamental difference between T lymphocyte receptors for self and nonself. There is only one world of epitopes and corresponding to it one world of receptors. If organisms were to operate with 2 receptor worlds, one for self and the other for nonself, they would run into all kinds of problems, not to mention the fact that solving the same problem twice would be an awfully uneconomical way of doing things.

The second assumption of the explanation is that MHC molecules are unusually rich in epitopes. One can view an MHC molecule as a mosaic in which each stone represents one epitope recognized by one corresponding receptor (all the stones being different from one another). If the epitope world were to be finite and the number of epitopes carried by a single MHC molecule very large (as indeed experimental data suggest it is, see Melief *et al.*, 1977), each molecule would carry a fair portion of all possible epitopes and all MHC molecules of all individuals could cover most of the possible epitope spectrum.

In ontogeny, an individual may start with a pool of lymphocytes that carry receptors for most of all conceivable epitopes. At a certain stage of ontogeny, however, these lymphocytes may have to pass through a sieve, represented probably by the thymus, which matches the receptors against the individual's own MHC molecules. Lymphocytes with matching receptors are allowed to pass; all other lymphocytes are retained. Since the MHC molecules contain many epitopes, lymphocytes with many different receptors are allowed to enter the body. Then, as the lymphocytes circulate, they constantly "feel" certain other cells (macrophages, other lymphocytes?) for epitopes exhibited by these cells in a fashion that allows recognition by the T cell receptors. If the presenting cells exhibit only matching epitopes of these cells' own MHC molecules, no signals or only tolerizing signals are passed to the lymphocyte. But when the presenting cells also exhibit other epitopes in a fashion favouring recognition, these "foreign" determinants are recognized by cross-reacting receptors and the "dual recognition" activates the corresponding lymphocytes.

Organisms cannot do without the sieve because then they would consider everything as self. For the same reason, the MHC molecules of a single individual cannot cover the entire spectrum of epitopes (because then the sieve would allow all lymphocytes to pass through and the net result would be the same as if the organism operated without a sieve). Thus the organism must strike the right balance between what it does and what it does not pass through the sieve, and this balance is determined by the sieve itself.

However, an organism pays a certain price for this sort of arrangement. Since the sieve takes a cut of the receptor spectrum, it inadvertently leaves out receptors for some nonself epitopes so that the organism becomes vulnerable to parasites carrying these epitopes: the organism becomes a non-responder to such epitopes. This situation may have potentially catastrophic consequences: if all individuals in a given population were to have the same MHC molecules, the emergence of a parasite carrying epitopes for which the individuals are "blind", could result in the extinction of this population. The organisms' answer to this danger is the MHC polymorphism. In a situation where different individuals possess different MHC molecules and thus different thymic sieves, different individuals also have different cuts of the receptor spectrum and hence different blind spots in their defence mechanisms. While an individual may be endangered because of the particular blind spot it carries, the population as a whole is safe; it always contains some individuals that lack the particular blind spot which makes other individuals vulnerable to the attack by a particular parasite. However, populations need not *always* be polymorphic. A population occupying a relatively small and relatively constant environmental niche and exposed to a certain relatively constant spectrum of parasites may be adapted to these conditions to the degree that it can do well with only a few MHC variants. But, in the long run, the evolutionary success of the species might depend, to a certain degree, on what potential this species has, in terms of MHC polymorphism, to adapt itself to changing environmental conditions.

Hence the answer to the question posed at the beginning of this section could be: the MHC loci are highly polymorphic because there is strong environmental selective pressure on them to vary. This selective pressure might have been strongest when the present-day MHC genes began their evolution from unknown progenitor genes, presumably in the vertebrates' ancestors. But the pressure probably persists throughout evolution and acts together with the mechanisms of MHC evolution described in the preceding section.

All this may, however, be futile speculations. There are hundreds of melodies that can be written out from a few bars but there is only one melody for the *Sempre libera degg'io* aria. We will not know which of the proposed melodies is the correct one until we learn a few more bars of the sketch that we are working with.

References

Arden, B., Wakeland, E. K. and Klein, J. (1980). *J. Immunol.*, submitted.

Bodmer, W. J., Batchelor, J. R., Bodmer, J. G., Festentein, J. G. and Morris, P. J. (eds) (1977). "Histocompatibility testing 1977." Munskgaard, Copenhagen.

Brown, J. L., Kato, K., Silver, J. and Nathenson, S. G. (1974). *Biochemistry* **13**, 3174–3178.

Burnet, F. M. (1959). "The Clonal Selection Theory of Acquired Immunity." Cambridge University Press.

Coligan, J. E., Kindt, T. J., Ewenstein, B. M., Uehara, H., Martinko, J. M. and Nathenson, S. G. (1979). *Mol. Immunol.* **16**, 3–8.

Cramer, D. V., Davis, B. K., Shonnard, J. W., Štark, O. and Gill III, T. J. (1978). *J. Immunol.* **120**, 179–187.

Duncan, W. R. and Klein, J. (1980). *Immunogenetics* **10**, 45–65.
Duncan, W. R. and Streilein, J. W. (1977). *J. Immunol.* **118**, 832–839.
Duncan, W. R., Wakeland, E. K. and Klein, J. (1979a). *Immunogenetics* **9**, 261–272.
Duncan, W. R., Wakeland, E. K. and Klein, J. (1979b). *Nature* **281**, 603–605.
Figueroa, F. and Klein, J. (1980). *Tissue Antigens*, submitted for publication.
Fitch, W. M. (1973). *Ann. Rev. Genetics* **7**, 343–380.
Gajdusek, D. C., Guiant, J., Kirk, R. L., Carrell, R. W., Irvine, D., Kynoch, P. A. M. and Lehman, H. (1967). *J. Med. Genet.* **4**, 1.
Goodman, M., Moore, G. W. and Matsuda, G. (1975). *Nature* **25**, 603–608.
Götze, D., Nadeau, J., Wakeland, E. K., Berry, R. J., Bonhomme, F., Egorov, I. K., Hjorth, J. P., Hoogstraal, H., Vives, J., Winking, H. and Klein, J. (1980). *J. Immunol.* (in press).
Günther, E. and Štark, O. (1979). *Transplant. Proc.* **11**, 1550–1553.
Huang, C-M., Huang, H-J. S. and Klein, J. (1979). *Immunogenetics* **9**, 173–182.
Jones, P. P., Murphy, D. B. and McDevitt, H. O. (1978). *J. Exp. Med.* **148**, 925–936.
Klein, J. (1972). *Transplantation* **13**, 291-299.
Klein, J. (1978). *Adv. Immunol.* **26**, 55–146.
Klein, J. (1979). *Science* **203**, 516–521.
Lafuse, W. P., McCormick, J. F. and David, C. S. (1980). *J. Exp. Med.* **151**, 709-715.
Lewontin, R. C. (1974). "The Genetic Basis of Evolutionary Change." Columbia University Press, New York.
Melief, C. J. M., van der Meulen, M. Y. and Postma, P. (1977). *Immunogenetics* **5**, 43–56.
Nadeau, J. Wakeland, E. K., Götze, D. and Klein, J. (1980). *Genet. Res.* (*Camb.*) (in press).
Orr, H. T., De Castro, J. A. L., Parham, P., Ploegh, H. L. and Strominger, J. L. (1979). *Proc. Natn. Acad. Sci. U.S.A.* **76**, 4395–4399.
Poulik, M. D. and Reisfeld, R. A. (1975). *Contemp. Topics Mol. Immunol.* **4**, 157–204.
Vitetta, E. S. and Capra, J. D. (1978). *Adv. Immunol.* **26**, 147–192.
Wagener, D. K., Cramer, D. V., Shonnard, J. W. and Davis, B. K. (1979). *Immunogenetics* **9**, 157–164.
Wakeland, E. K. and Klein, J. (1979a). *Immunogenetics* **8**, 27–39.
Wakeland, E. K. and Klein, J. (1979b). *Immunogenetics* **9**, 535–550.
Wechsberg, J. (1974). *Verdi.* Putnam, New York.
White, J. M. (1978a). *In* "The Biochemical Genetics of Man" (2nd edn) (J. H. Brock and O. Mayo, eds) pp. 561–631. Academic Press, London.
White, M. J. D. (1978b). "Modes of Speciation." Freeman, San Francisco.
Zaleska-Rutczynska, Z. and Klein, J. (1977). *J. Immunol.* **119**, 1903–1911.

14

Cell Surface Receptors for Lectins: Markers of Murine and Human Lymphocyte Subpopulations

NATHAN SHARON

The Weizmann Institute of Science, Rehovoth, Israel

Abbreviations
FITC, fluorescein isothiocyanate; GVH, graft-versus-host; HP, *Helix pomatia* agglutinin; MLR, mixed lymphocyte reaction; PHA, phytohaemagglutinin; PNA, peanut agglutinin; SBA, soybean agglutinin; WGA, wheat germ agglutinin. All sugars are of the D-configuration.

Studies in our laboratory were supported in part by a National Institutes of Health Contract, number NO1-CB-74163, and by a grant from the Leukaemia Research Foundation, Chicago.

Introduction

Research carried out during the last two decades has revealed that the lymphoid system is comprised of numerous cell subpopulations (or subsets) with different functions, and that in many immunological processes several subpopulations participate and interact with each other in a variety of complex ways. Thus, within the major class of T lymphocytes, there are different types of helper, suppressor and killer cells. In spite of their functional heterogeneity, the various cells are as a rule morphologically similar, and are often found together in the same lymphoid tissue. For example, in a suspension of mononuclear cells from blood, it is not easy to discriminate one cell type from another by conventional techniques such as microscopic examination of the cells, unstained or stained. The discovery, in the late 1960s, that mouse T cells have a specific surface marker, the θ (or Thy-1) antigen, made it possible for the first time to identify these cells directly, to determine their distribution in the lymphoid organs of the mouse and their development in and migration from the embryonic thymus gland (Raff, 1976). It also permitted the study of T cell functions more directly than before.

Over a dozen distinct surface antigens have now been defined that distinguish between murine lymphocyte subpopulations (Benacerraf and Unanue, 1979). Several such antigens have also been found on human lymphocyte subpopulations (Moretta *et al.*, 1979), very recently with the aid of monoclonal antibodies (Reinherz and Schlossman, 1980). Antibodies against cell-surface antigens serve not only to identify cell types, but also to separate them. Such separations can be achieved either by the use of immobilized antibodies, by fluorescein labelled antibodies in a fluorescence activated cell sorter, or with the aid of complement, which leads to lysis of the antibody binding cells. In the latter case, only the cells which do not bind the antibody are recovered.

Knowledge of lymphocyte surface antigens has played a major role in the explosive advance of cellular immunology in the past decade. It is apparent, however, that for further progress in this area, many more surface markers for lymphocytes must be identified. In particular, surface markers are required which can be used for the investigation of pathways of lymphocyte differentiation, both in normal and pathological conditions, and for the separation of different cell subpopulations. Such separations should preferably be simple and should afford cells in good recovery, high purity and without alteration of their biological functions.

Lectins in immunology

A new technique with a great potential for detection and identification of lymphocyte surface markers is the use of lectins. These are proteins (or glycoproteins) of nonimmune origin, that bind carbohydrates and agglutinate cells. They combine noncovalently with mono- and oligosaccharides, both simple and complex (e.g. in glycoproteins, glycolipids), in the same way that antibodies bind antigens. Binding may involve several forces, mostly hydrophobic and hydrogen bonds, but only rarely electrostatic ones since most monosaccharides with which lectins interact are devoid of electrical charge. Because lectins are multivalent with respect to their sugar binding sites, they precipitate polysaccharides and glycoproteins from solution and agglutinate cells. Both reactions can be competitively inhibited by carbohydrates, the specificity of a lectin being defined in terms of the best mono- or oligosaccharide inhibitor. Lectins are thus excellent surface probes, in that they attach tightly to specific carbohydrate moieties on cell surfaces, and in most cases can be readily removed by suitable monosaccharides. In this respect they offer an important advantage over antibodies to cell surface constituents, since it is not always possible to remove the latter from cells to which they are bound. The properties of lectins commonly employed in immunology are listed in Table I (this is reviewed in Lis and Sharon, 1977).

TABLE I

Lectins used for immunological studies

Lectin	*mol. wt.*	*Sugar specificity*	*Combining sites/mol*	*Main application*
Con A	108 000	Mannose, glucose	4	Mitogenic stimulation
HP	79 000	*N*-Acetylgalactosamine	6	Cell separation
PNA	110 000	Galactosylβ1→3-*N*-acetyl-galactosamine	2	Cell identification and separation
PHA	120 000	(*N*-Acetylgalactosamine)		Mitogenic stimulation
SBA	120 000	*N*-Acetylgalactosamine	2	Cell separation
WGA	36 000	*N*-Acetylglucosamine	4	Cell separation

Abbreviations

Con A, concanavalin A; HP, *Helix pomatia* (snail); A, agglutinin; PNA peanut agglutinin; PHA, phytohaemagglutinin; SBA, soybean agglutinin; WGA, wheat germ agglutinin.

For further data on these lectins, see Lis and Sharon (1977).

Note that HP and WGA are not mitogenic at all; PNA and SBA are mitogenic only in their polymerized form, and do not stimulate mouse or human lymphocytes unless the cells have been treated with sialidase.

Since the 1960s, lectins such as phytohaemagglutinin (PHA) and concanavalin A have been of interest to immunologists mainly because of their mitogenic properties, i.e. the ability to induce blastogenesis and to stimulate proliferation of resting lymphocytes. Unlike most antigens, lectins are polyclonal mitogens; nevertheless, they are useful in studies of the mechanism by which an antigen triggers proliferation of a certain class of lymphocytes. Both

PHA and concanavalin A stimulate T cells but not B cells, so they also serve as an aid in identifying the major lymphocyte subpopulations.

Schnebli and Dukor (1972) were the first to demonstrate that lectins may specifically bind to and agglutinate certain murine lymphocyte subpopulations. They found that splenocytes of nude mice (B cells) and cortisone resistant thymocytes (T cells) were agglutinated equally well by soybean agglutinin (SBA), whereas thoracic duct cells (mainly T cells) were not agglutinated. They also showed that B cells were agglutinated at considerably lower concentrations of wheat germ agglutinin (WGA) than either cortisone resistant thymocytes or thoracic duct cells, and suggested that this lectin may serve as a new specific marker for B cells. The different behaviour of the two T cell preparations used was taken as further evidence for the existence of subpopulations of thymus derived lymphocytes.

Murine lymphocyte subpopulations

Studies with peanut and soybean agglutinins

The first clear-cut demonstration that subpopulations of T cells carry distinct lectin receptors was made in the course of our studies on the interaction of peanut agglutinin (PNA) with mouse thymocytes (Reisner *et al.*, 1976a). Two lymphocyte subpopulations are easily distinguished in the thymus, one located in the cortex and the other in the medulla. The medullary thymocytes, which in the past could be isolated in sufficient quantities only from mice that had been treated with cortisone or radiation, comprise about 10% of the total number of thymus cells. They exhibit immunological reactivity of the cellular type (e.g. they react in the mixed lymphocyte reaction (MLR) and possess the ability to induce graft-versus-host (GVH) disease) and also respond to PHA, showing that they are immunologically mature or immunocompetent. In addition, the medullary thymocytes express a low density of the θ antigen and a high density of the H-2 antigen. In contrast, the cortical thymocytes, which comprise the majority of the thymus cells ($\sim$90%) and which are eliminated by treatment of the animal with hydrocortisone or radiation, are immunologically immature. Thus, they are inactive in cell mediated immune reactions (MLR and GVH) and are not stimulated by PHA. They also differ from the medullary cells by a high level of θ antigen and a low level of H-2 antigen. The medullary thymocytes are believed to be the maturation product of the cortical ones, although it is possible that the two subpopulations develop independently.

Examination by fluorescence microscopy of thymocytes treated with fluorescein isothiocyanate-labelled PNA (FITC-PNA) revealed that the majority of the cells were stained, whereas a small portion ($\sim$10%) was not; galactose, a sugar which binds to PNA, completely inhibited staining. No staining of hydrocortisone-resistant thymocytes by FITC-PNA was observed. It was further found that whereas the latter cells were not agglutinated by PNA, most of the untreated thymus cells were. Following treatment of thymocytes with PNA, the clumps formed were separated from the unagglutinated single cells by sedimentation at unit gravity. Addition of galactose to the cell clumps led to their dissociation and removal of the lectin (Reisner *et al.*, 1976a). The procedure is illustrated in Fig. 1.

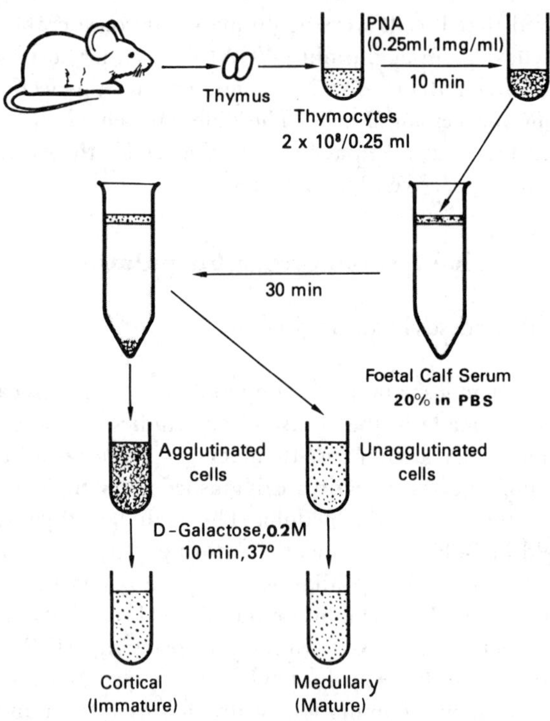

FIG. 1. *Fractionation of mouse thymocytes by peanut agglutinin.*

The separated cells, which were obtained in good yield (up to 80%), were fully viable (>95% in each fraction). In all the properties tested by us (level of θ and H-2 surface antigens, stimulation by PHA and GVH activity), the cells agglutinated by PNA (PNA^+) were essentially identical with the cortical thymocytes, whereas the unagglutinated fraction (PNA^-) consisted of cells which were similar to the hydrocortisone-resistant medullary thymocytes, as well as to spleen T cells.

Soon afterwards we were able to confirm and extend the earlier observations of Schnebli and Dukor (1972) that mouse B lymphocytes are more susceptible to agglutination by SBA than T lymphocytes. Under suitable conditions only B splenocytes were agglutinated by this lectin (Reisner *et al.*, 1976a). Using the same procedure developed for the isolation of PNA^+ and PNA^- thymocytes, SBA agglutinated (SBA^+) and unagglutinated (SBA^-) subpopulations of spleen cells were obtained. The two subpopulations were characterized by their surface antigens (IgG, IgM and θ), the GVH reaction and the mitogenic response of the cells to PHA and concanavalin A (T mitogens) and to lipopolysaccharide (a B cell mitogen). The results showed that the SBA^+ fraction consisted mainly of B cells and the SBA^- fraction of T cells, with some cross-contamination.

Fractionation of lymphocytes by the method described offers many advantages over other techniques: it is inexpensive, simple, rapid, reproducible, and efficient for large numbers of cells. Furthermore, it permits recovery of both the unagglutinated and agglutinated cell populations in high yield (Sharon, 1979b; Reisner and Sharon, 1980).

The difference between the lectin binding properties of the lymphocyte subpopulations examined could be rationalized on the basis of the specificity of the lectins used, and the limited information available on the structure of carbohydrates present on lymphocyte surfaces. PNA is specific for Galβ1→3GalNAc, but may also combine with nonreducing terminal galactose residues in other compounds (Lotan *et al.*, 1975; Pereira *et al.*, 1976). The disaccharide Galβ1→3GalNAc is present in many soluble glycoproteins and has also been identified in the few membrane glycoproteins examined (e.g. in glycophorin), in membrane glycolipids (e.g. ganglio-*N*-tetraosylceramide or asialo-GM_1) and on lymphocytes (Sharon and Lis, 1980). In general, however, sialic acid residues are attached to the disaccharide, so that its interaction with PNA is precluded. SBA, in addition to interacting with galactose, binds more strongly to *N*-acetylgalactosamine residues (Lis *et al.*, 1970; Pereira *et al.*, 1974), so that the two lectins do not necessarily combine with the same carbohydrate structures in glycoconjugates. It has also been reported that cortisone-resistant thymocytes and spleen T cells are more negatively charged and have a higher content of sialic acid than unfractionated thymocytes (Despont *et al.*, 1975).

We have therefore proposed a simple model which incorporates our findings (Fig. 2) and have made the following tentative conclusions (Sharon, 1979a; Sharon and Reisner, 1979):

(a) Cell surface receptors for PNA and SBA change in an orderly manner during murine lymphocyte differentiation and maturation.

(b) The change involves the attachment of sialic acid residues to galactose and *N*-acetylgalactosamine residues on the cell surface.

(c) The PNA receptor is a marker for undifferentiated, immature cells.

(d) Haemopoietic stem cells that are devoid of GVH activity may be PNA^+SBA^+; such cells may be isolated with the aid of the lectins.

(e) Results of experiments in mice may be applicable to man. Further work carried out in our laboratory and elsewhere has provided strong support for the above assumptions, and has established the use of PNA and SBA as important tools for the study of murine lymphocytes.

The new methods have permitted better characterization of lymphocyte subpopulations in terms of their surface properties, effector functions and differ-

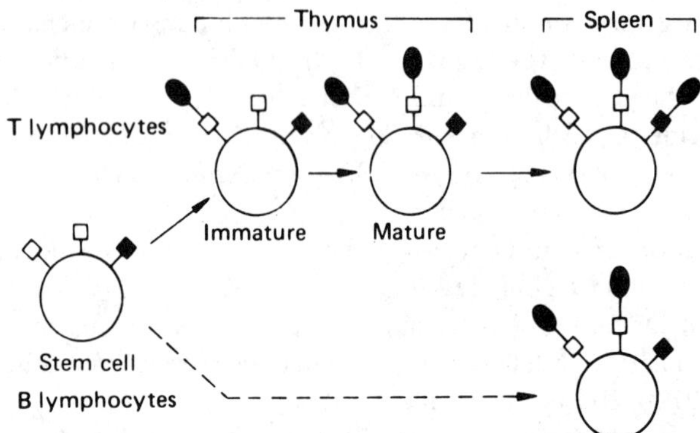

FIG. 2. *Sequential changes in lectin receptors during lymphocyte differentiation.* □, *Receptor for SBA and PNA;* ■, *receptor for SBA only;* ●, *sialic acid (from Sharon and Reisner, 1979).*

entiation patterns. The number of publications in this area, mostly on the application of PNA, is now so large that an exhaustive coverage is not possible within the space allotted. I shall therefore limit myself to selected examples dealing with methodology, the distribution of PNA$^+$ cells in different organs, their surface markers and functional properties.

Methodology

Lectin binding cells are most readily detected with the aid of fluorescent lectin derivatives. Other derivatives, such as those commonly employed for the detection of cell surface antigens by antibodies, can also be used. Thus, horseradish peroxidase conjugated with PNA has been used by Rose *et al.* (1980) to study the distribution of PNA$^+$ cells in sections of mouse lymphoid organs, and ferritin-labelled PNA has been employed by Skutelsky (see Lis and Sharon, 1977) to demonstrate by electron microscopy the presence of PNA receptors on immature thymocytes and their absence on the mature cells. In all cases, it is essential to test for the specificity of the reaction, by including controls in which a suitable inhibitory sugar is present.

Selective agglutination is the technique of choice when working with mixtures of cells that differ markedly in their lectin binding properties and when a high proportion of the cells is agglutinated, as is the case with murine thymocytes and PNA, or murine splenocytes and SBA. Other approaches may be necessary in different situations (Sharon, 1979b; Reisner and Sharon, 1980). For example, separation of PNA$^+$ cells from mouse spleen in which their level is low (about 5%), is best achieved with the aid of rabbit erythrocytes. Such erythrocytes possess receptors for PNA, and in the presence of the lectin form mixed rosette-like aggregates with the PNA$^+$ splenocytes, which facilitates isolation of the latter (Reisner *et al.*, 1978, 1980a). Rosetting with sialidase (neuraminidase) treated sheep erythrocytes was used by Berrih *et al.* (1979) for the fractionation by PNA of murine thymocytes and splenocytes. Separation of mouse T spleens into PNA$^+$ and PNA$^-$ subpopulations using FITC-

PNA was achieved in a fluorescence activated cell sorter (Imai *et al.*, 1979); the major disadvantages of this technique are the length of time required to separate large numbers of cells, and the high cost of the equipment.

Thymocytes treated with subagglutinating doses of PNA were fractionated by affinity chromatography on a column of Sepharose to which anti-PNA antibodies were covalently attached (Irlé *et al.*, 1978); the PNA$^+$ cells that bound to the column were eluted with galactose.

Recently, a procedure for cell fractionation by beads to which lectins are covalently bound has been developed in our laboratory (M. Rosenberg, unpublished results).

Distribution

Data from several laboratories on the distribution of PNA$^+$ cells in different mouse organs, as examined mostly by staining with FITC-PNA, are summarized in Table II. It can be seen that the agreement between the results is remarkable. PNA$^+$ lymphocytes in mice are not confined to the thymus; as expected, however, their level in most other organs is much lower. Although peripheral blood was reported to have a high level of PNA$^+$ cells, the intensity of the fluorescence of the FITC-PNA stained cells was much weaker than that of the thymocytes, suggesting that the number of PNA receptors on these cells is low.

TABLE II

Distribution of PNA$^+$ cells in mouse organs

	PNA$^+$ *cells* (%)			
References:	*a*	*b*	*c*	*d*
Thymus	90	85	82	86
Peripheral lymph node		16	3·5	
Spleen	15	6	5·5	13
Bone marrow	20	19	4	20
Peyer's patch			24	
Peripheral blood lymphocytes		36		25[e]
Foetal liver				19

[a] Reisner *et al.* (1976), Reisner, Ph.D. thesis (1979). [b] London *et al.* (1978), Roelants *et al.* (1979). [c] Rose *et al.* (1980). [d] Newman and Boss (1980). [e] Weak intensity of staining by FITC-PNA.

Confirming our findings that hydrocortisone-resistant cells are PNA$^-$, London *et al.* (1978) have further examined the changes in the number of PNA$^+$ cells in mouse thymus following treatment of the animals with hydrocortisone acetate or with irradiation. Three days after irradiation (450 rads), 99·4% of the PNA$^+$ thymocytes and 66% of the PNA$^-$ thymocytes disappeared (Fig. 3). There was a rapid increase in the number of PNA$^+$ cells upon thymic regeneration, accompanied by a much smaller rise in the PNA$^-$ cells.

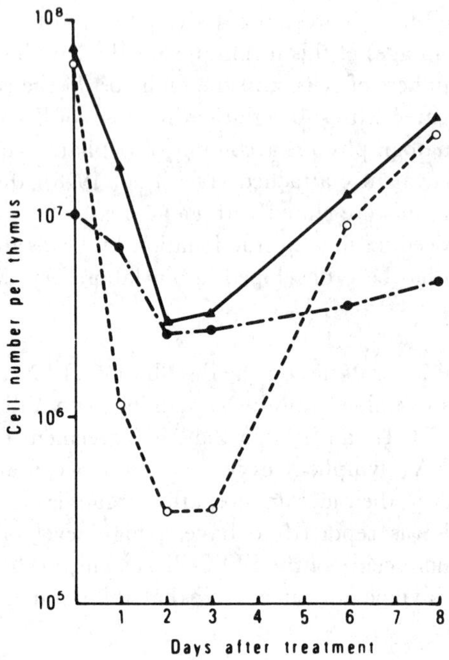

FIG. 3. *Changes in mouse thymocyte subpopulations following irradiation. Cells:* ▲——▲, *total;* ○---○, *PNA⁺;* ●-.-●, *PNA⁻.* (*From London* et al., *1978.*)

A study of PNA binding during ontogenesis revealed that PNA$^+$ cells appear very early during the development of liver, thymus and spleen (London *et al.*, 1978, 1979a). In thymus, the appearance of PNA$^+$ cells correlated well with that of θ^+ cells; on day 14, both PNA$^+$ and PNA$^-$ cells were present but, in contrast to the mature thymus, the proportion of PNA$^-$ cells was higher than that of PNA$^+$ cells. Some PNA$^+$ cells were found in foetal liver before the thymic rudiment became fully colonized. The early onset of PNA$^+$ cells in embryonic organs, and in particular the finding of such cells in foetal liver before their appearance in the thymus, would suggest that PNA binds to prothymocytes or lymphoid stem cells. However, the finding of high levels of PNA$^-$ cells in the foetal liver, coupled with other observations, has led London *et al.* (1979a) to postulate that two different pathways exist for the formation of functional T lymphocytes: in thymus, immunoincompetent thymocytes and immunocompetent thymocytes may develop from separate lineages, without maturation from PNA$^+$ to PNA$^-$ cells; in the periphery, adult functional T cells (mostly PNA$^-$ cells) could arise from nonfunctional PNA$^+$ cells present in large amounts in the perinatal period.

Rose *et al.* (1980) have reported that PNA bound to cells in murine germinal centres (Peyer's patches) but not to those in other areas containing activated lymphocytes. There was a good correlation between the presence of PNA$^+$

cells in germinal centres in sections of lymphoid organs, and in cell suspensions from the same organs. Although the anatomic origin of PNA^+ germinal centre cells is not clear, there is preliminary evidence that some or all of them are lymphocytes. It was further proposed that these observations, together with our suggestion that the PNA receptor is a marker for immaturity among T cells and cells of the haemapoietic stem cell population, again raise the possibility that germinal centres harbour a population of immature B cells (Rose *et al.*, 1980). The use of PNA to separate germinal centre cells should allow further characterization of their properties and functions.

PNA has been employed to distinguish preleukaemic cells from end stage leukaemia cells in mice. Preleukaemic bone marrow and spleen cells of irradiated C57BL/6 mice, that had been inoculated with the radiation-induced leukaemia virus D-RadLV, were PNA^+ whereas the end stage leukaemia cells were PNA^- (Reisner *et al.*, 1980b). This observation provides further evidence that preleukaemic cells possess surface markers similar to those of the prothymocyte. Both *in vivo* and *in vitro*, the cells in the thymus susceptible to the viral transformation were present mainly among the PNA^+ thymocytes.

Surface markers

Results of measurements of the binding of PNA and SBA to mouse lymphocytes, both before and after treatment with sialidase, are summarized in Fig. 4 and corroborate the model presented by us (Fig. 2).

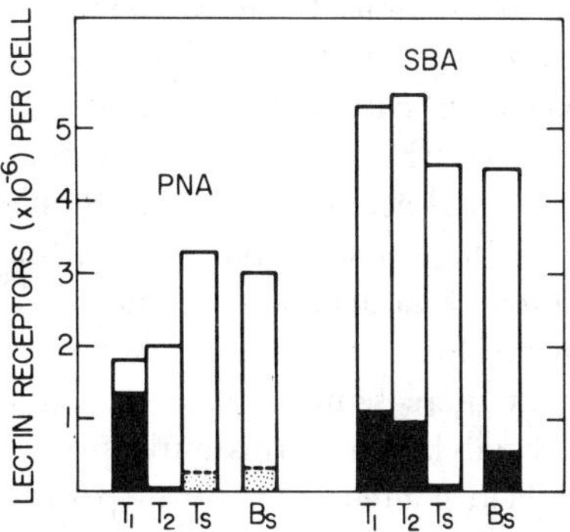

FIG. 4. *Binding of* ^{125}*I-labelled PNA and SBA to mouse lymphocytes before and after the cells have been treated with sialidase:* T_1 *and* T_2*—immature and mature thymocytes, respectively;* T_s *and* B_s*—T and B splenocytes, respectively. Columns indicate total binding before (■) and after (□) sialidase treatment; stippled area, a small proportion or* PNA^+ *cells without sialidase treatment. (Data from Prujansky, 1977.)*

An inverse relationship between the PNA-binding ability and the electrophoretic mobility of thymocytes from normal and cortisone-treated mice was found by Dumont and Nardelli (1979) (Fig. 5). Thymocytes recovered from the fractions with the lowest electrophoretic mobility were all strongly PNA^+, whereas those with the highest electrophoretic mobility were all PNA^-. Of the thymocytes recovered 2 days after treatment of the mice with cortisone

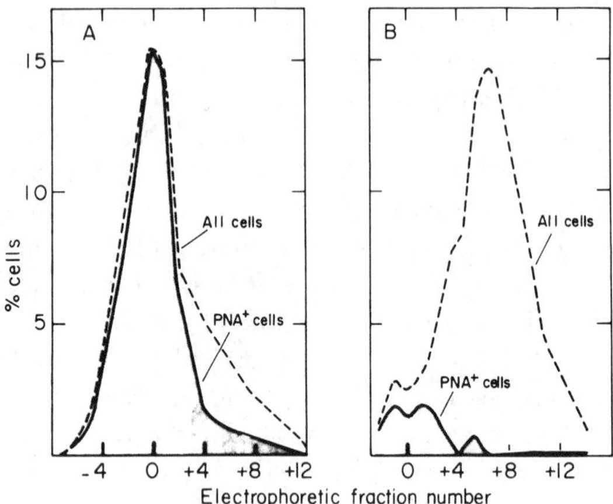

FIG. 5. *PNA binding and electrophoretic mobility of cells from adult C3H mice* (*A*) *before and* (*B*) *2 days after treatment with cortisone acetate, 200 mg/kg body weight.* (*Data from Dumont and Nardelli, 1979.*)

acetate, only a small proportion (5%) were PNA$^+$. Eight days after the treatment, the thymus started to regenerate and the majority of the thymocytes exhibited dull staining with FITC-PNA. By day 14 most of the cells were strongly PNA$^+$, as in normal thymus. Reciprocal experiments in which normal thymocytes were separated by selective agglutination with PNA according to Reisner *et al.* (1976a), definitely established that PNA$^+$ cells are of lower electrophoretic mobility than the PNA$^-$ cells, and that these two cell types also differed in size. These findings support our suggestion that the difference in PNA binding between the cell subpopulations is the result of masking of the corresponding receptors by attachment of sialic acid residues. It has indeed very recently been shown (Hoessli *et al.*, 1980) that T lymphocyte differentiation is accompanied by an increase in the sialic acid content of the θ antigen. However, the increased sialylation of this antigen cannot by itself account for the increased sialic acid content of mature (peripheral) T cells, mainly because they carry less θ than do immature thymocytes. Therefore changes in other glycoproteins and/or glycolipids must also occur.

The distribution and quantitative expression of various surface antigens was most thoroughly examined in PNA$^+$ and PNA$^-$ thymocytes, using fluorescent antibodies and differential cytotoxicity caused by specific antisera and complement. The results obtained by the various techniques are summarized in Table III. Clearly, PNA$^+$ and PNA$^-$ cells differ significantly in their surface phenotypes. Such studies have also led to the identification of two new and distinct subsets of T cells; cells that are PNA$^-$ and Lyt-1$^+$23$^-$ (Betel *et al.*, 1980), and those that are PNA$^+$ and Lyt-6$^+$ (London and Horton, 1980). It has been suggested that the latter cell type may represent an intermediate form along one of the T cell lineages within the thymus (presumably for the

TABLE III
Surface antigens of mouse lymphocytes

Cells and Markers	*PNA*$^+$	*PNA*$^-$	*References*
Thymocytes			
θ	High	Low	Reisner *et al.* (1976a)
H-2	Low	High	Reisner *et al.* (1976a)
TLa	+	–	Roelants *et al.* (1979) Zeicher *et al.* (1979)
Lyt 1^+23^+	+	+, –	Betel *et al.* (1980)
Lyt 1^+23^-	–	+	Betel *et al.* (1980)
Lyt 6·2	+	+, –	London and Horton (1980)
Splenocytes			
θ	–	+	Roelants *et al.* (1979)
Ig	–	+, –	Roelants *et al.* (1979)

generation of Lyt-1^+23^- cells). Accordingly, PNA binding is progressively, though incompletely, lost during maturation, and Lyt-1^+23^- cells gain the Lyt-6 antigen before their emigration from the thymus (London and Horton, 1980).

Functional properties

Following our initial report that PNA$^+$ and PNA$^-$ mouse thymocytes differ in their response to PHA and in their GVH activity (Reisner *et al.*, 1976a) and that SBA$^+$ and SBA$^-$ splenocytes exhibit similar differences, it was found that PNA$^+$ thymocytes (Umiel *et al.*, 1978), as well as PNA$^+$ and SBA$^+$ splenocytes, are nonresponsive in the MLR (Reisner *et al.*, 1980a) (Fig. 6).

We have also shown that the two thymocyte subpopulations have different effects on tumour growth in mice (Umiel *et al.*, 1978). The PNA$^+$ cells

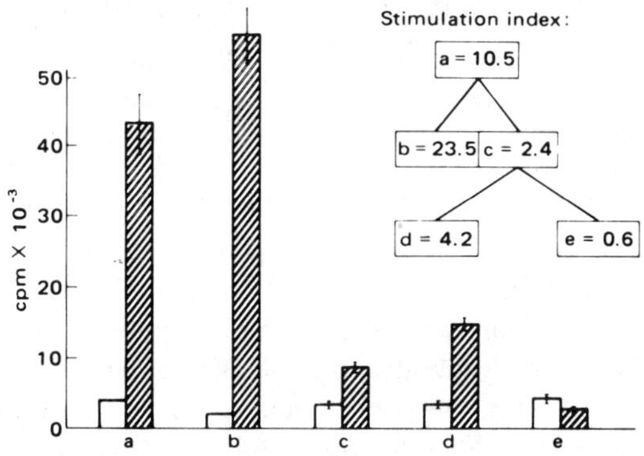

FIG. 6. *MLR response of fractionated mouse splenocytes:* □, *C57BL/6 spleen cells as stimulator; hatched area, C3H/HeJ spleen cells as stimulator. Cells: a, unseparated; b, SBA*$^-$*; c, SBA*$^+$*; d, SBA*$^+$*, PNA*$^-$*; SBA*$^+$*, PNA*$^+$. (*Reisner* et al., *1980a.*)

accelerated the growth rate and increased the number of takes of 3LL tumours in mice more than the unfractionated thymocytes, thus acting as suppressor cells. The PNA$^-$ cells, on the other hand, caused pronounced inhibition of tumour growth and a decrease in the number of tumour takes, similar to that observed with spleen cells, indicating that they act as helper cells. In another study, we have found that PNA$^+$ cells from embryonic mouse liver were enriched in suppressor activity, as evidenced by their effect in the MLR of adult murine spleen cells, and the response of the latter to different mitogens (Globerson *et al.*, 1979; Rabinovich *et al.*, 1979) (Fig. 7).

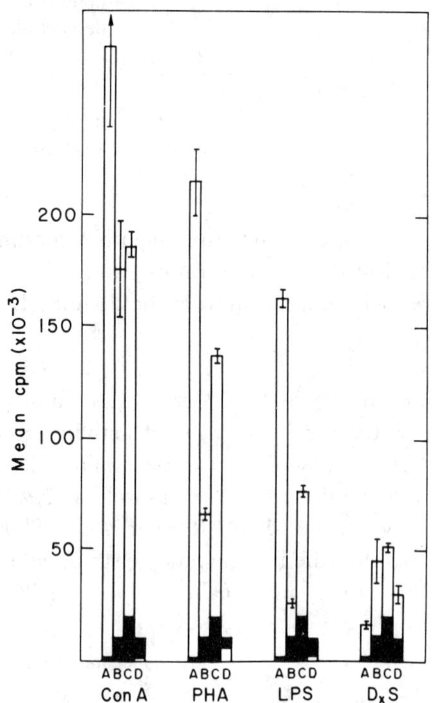

FIG. 7. *Suppression of adult spleen cell response to mitogens by embryonic liver cell preparations.* □, + *Mitogen;* ■, — *mitogen; A, spleen; B, spleen and liver, unfractionated; C, spleen and liver PNA$^-$ cells; spleen and liver PNA$^+$ cells. LPS, lipopolysaccharide; DxS, dextran sulphate. Ordinate:* [^3H] *thymidine incorporation expressed by mean ct/min.* (*From Globerson* et al., *1979.*)

PNA$^+$ cells isolated from T splenocytes (obtained from mice injected with concanavalin A) were found to exert a marked suppressive effect on primary antisheep red blood cell antibody response *in vitro*, whereas the PNA$^-$ cells did not affect the antibody response (Imai *et al.*, 1979). Here too, the suppressor cells were in the PNA$^+$ fraction. Both PNA$^+$ and PNA$^-$ thymocytes were required, however, for the *in vitro* generation of suppressor cells, as assayed by their effect on the MLR (Eisenthal *et al.*, 1979). Although there were previous indications for the requirement of cell co-operation in the generation of suppressor cells, the PNA fractionation technique provided direct evidence for it. In another study it was shown that cytotoxic lymphocyte precursors are contained in the PNA$^-$ thymocyte subpopulation (Mathieson *et al.*, 1979).

Fractionation of thymocytes by PNA has been used in several studies aimed at demonstrating that PNA$^+$ cells can be made to mature *in vitro*. Irlé *et al.* (1978) have shown that when PNA$^+$ thymocytes were cultured in the presence of concanavalin A and a supernatant from 24 h concanavalin A treated lymphoid cultures, they acquired new cell membrane markers characteristic of mature thymocytes, including the loss of the PNA receptor. The treated cells also acquired other properties characteristic of mature, immunocompetent thymocytes, such as the response to PHA.

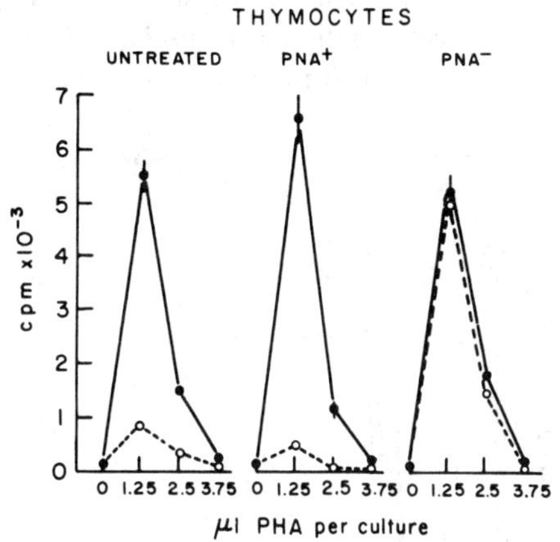

FIG. 8. *Effect of thymic epithelial culture supernatant on* ^{14}*C-thymidine incorporation into mouse thymocytes stimulated with PHA, before and after separation with peanut agglutinin.* —, *Thymic epithelial culture supernatant;* ----, *control.* (*Kruisbeek and Astaldi, 1979.*)

Maturation of PNA$^+$ thymocytes, but not of the corresponding PNA$^-$ cells, could also be induced by thymic epithelial supernatants (Kruisbeek and Astaldi, 1979) (Fig. 8), and by a thymic hormone known to potentiate T cell differentiation (Umiel *et al.*, 1980). These findings strongly support the idea of a differentiation pathway in which PNA$^+$ thymocytes are the precursors of PNA$^-$ thymocytes.

Marked differences were observed in the migration patterns of PNA$^+$ and PNA$^-$ thymocytes after their injection into syngeneic hosts (Madyashta *et al.*, 1980). The PNA$^+$ cells migrated preferentially to the spleen, whereas the PNA$^-$ cells were lymph node seeking. Upon treatment of the PNA$^+$ cells with galactose oxidase, they became unagglutinable by PNA and their propensity to localize in the spleen of syngeneic animals was drastically curtailed. Structures resembling the PNA receptor are known to be involved in phenomena related to biological recognition. Most importantly, Ashwell and Morell (1974) have demonstrated that sialidase treatment of certain serum glycoproteins, which leads to the exposure of galactosyl residues, caused their prompt removal from the circulatory system via a specific receptor on the surface membrane of hepatocytes. Sialidase treatment of rabbit and human erythrocytes also caused their rapid disappearance from the blood. The PNA receptor present on most thymocytes may thus be responsible for their prompt removal from circulation and sequestration in the liver (Berney and Gesner, 1970).

Application to bone marrow transplantation

A key prediction of our model (Fig. 2) is that haemopoietic stem cells are PNA^+SBA^+. Since GVH disease is the major obstacle encountered in attempts to achieve bone marrow transplantation across histocompatability barriers, the isolation of such PNA^+SBA^+ cells seemed highly desirable. We have indeed found that sequential fractionation of mouse spleen cells by PNA and SBA afforded a fraction enriched in stem cells as measured by spleen colony assay *in vivo*. The PNA^+SBA^+ cell fraction was also devoid of GVH activity, as evidenced by its ability to reconstitute lethally irradiated allogeneic mice.

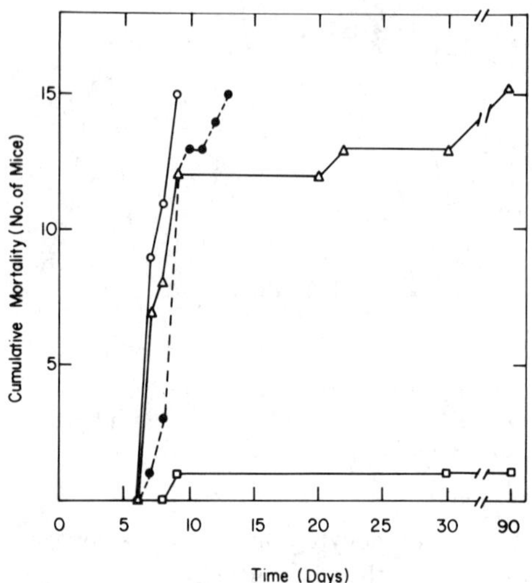

FIG. 9. *Cumulative mortality of irradiated* (*BALB/c* × *C57BL/6*)F_1 *mice after transplantation with splenocytes* (*10^7 cells per animal*) *from SWR mice, starting with 15 mice in each group. Grafts:* △——△, *unfractionated splenocytes;* □——□, *splenocytes sequentially agglutinated by SBA and PNA;* ○——○, *splenocytes unagglutinated by SBA;* ●– – –●, *control without graft.* (*From Reisner* et al., *1978.*)

The results of a typical experiment are shown in Fig. 9. Grafting lethally irradiated allogeneic mice with unfractionated splenocytes or with cells unagglutinated by SBA resulted in high mortality (13/15 and 15/15, respectively) within the first 30 days after irradiation. The 2 mice surviving the first 4 weeks were suffering from secondary disease (delayed GVH reaction) and died within the second month after transplantation. In a parallel experiment, the few surviving mice were sacrificed 4 and 5 weeks after transplantation. Spleen histology and bone marrow differential count revealed typical GVH symptoms. Among the mice grafted with the twice-agglutinated fraction, only one out of 15 died. The remaining mice survived more than 6 months. Spleen histology and bone marrow differential count taken 4 and 5 weeks after transplantation in a parallel experiment, revealed that in the reconstituted mice both spleen and bone marrow were completely restored. These results are in line with the previous reports (Reisner *et al.*, 1976a, b) in which the GVH activity of fractionated splenocytes and thymocytes was tested in newborn mice. The implications of these findings to bone marrow transplantation in humans are obvious.

Other lectins

Many other lectins have been examined for differential binding to or agglutination of lymphocyte subpopulations, and in attempts to identify new subpopulations. Satisfactory results were obtained only in a limited number of cases.

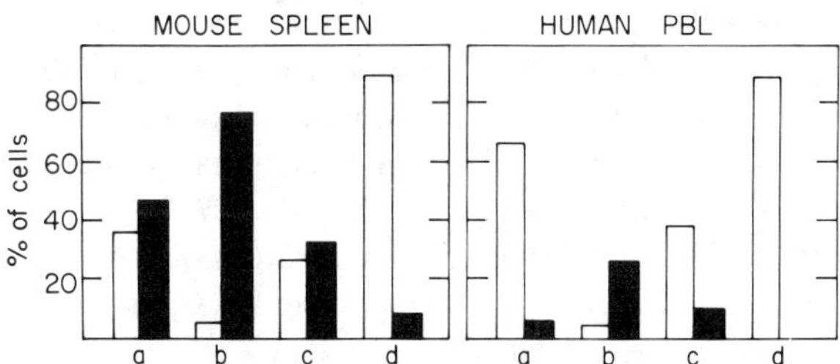

FIG. 10. *Fractionation of lymphocytes by affinity chromatography on sepharose bound* Helix pomatia *lectin: a, unfractionated cells; b, unadsorbed to column; c, eluted with 0·1 mg/ml* N-*acetylgalactosamine; d, eluted with 1 mg/ml* N-*acetylgalactosamine. Unshaded bars indicate* Helix pomatia *positive cells; shaded bars indicate cells with surface immunoglobulin.* (*From Hammarstrom* et al., *1978.*)

The lectin from the snail *Helix pomatia* (HP) specific for *N*-acetylgalactosamine, has been shown to be a useful reagent for the identification and isolation of T cells in several species, including mouse and man (Hammarström *et al.*, 1978). Treatment of the cells with sialidase is, however, required to unmask the receptor sites for this lectin. HP^+ lymphocytes were separated from HP^- lymphocytes on columns charged with HP covalently bound to sepharose, to yield a B cell enriched fraction (Fig. 10). The intermediate fraction contained both B and T cells, in a ratio similar to that of the unfractionated splenocytes. The total cell yield was typically between 60 and 70%, and the fractionated cells exhibited functional integrity as shown by their response to mitogens and in the assay for antibody dependent cell mediated cytotoxicity.

Affinity chromatography on HP-sepharose has permitted the isolation for the first time of a cell fraction highly enriched in mouse natural killer (NK) cells, for which no conventional surface marker was previously known (Haller *et al.*, 1978). NK activity was highest in the intermediate fraction eluted from HP-sepharose and was somewhat enriched in the last fraction (cf. Fig. 10). Separation between NK activity and alloreactive cytotoxic activity was also achieved, showing that while NK cells are HP^+, their lectin binding properties seem to differ from those of alloreactive cytotoxic T cells. HP receptors thus represent the first simple and reliable marker detected on NK cells and may be useful for purification of this cell type.

A single membrane glycoprotein, with an apparent mol. wt of 130 000, appeared to be responsible for the bulk of the binding of HP to sialidase treated lymphocytes (Axelsson *et al.*, 1978). This glycoprotein was expressed on mouse T lymphocytes, both normal and malignant, but not on B cells.

As mentioned earlier, mouse B cells are agglutinated more strongly by WGA than T cells (Schnebli and Dukor, 1972). Bourguignon *et al.* (1979) have now reported the separation of mouse spleen B and T cells by selective agglutination with this lectin. The aggregates formed upon treatment of mouse splenocytes with WGA were separated from the monodisperse T cells by gravity sedimentation and subsequently dissociated into single cells by treatment with the inhibitory monosaccharide *N*-acetylglucosamine to yield a B cell enriched fraction. Approximately 10–15% cross-contamination of the resultant T and B cell fractions was observed, which is higher than that obtained when splenocyte separation is done with SBA (Reisner *et al.*, 1976b).

Immobilized WGA has been used to separate mouse bone marrow cells into fractions enriched in different cell types; elution of the cells was achieved with *N*-acetylglucosamine (Nicola *et al.*, 1978).

Binding of surface labelled glycoproteins from cytotoxic mouse T lymphocytes to a panel of immobilized lectins has been examined (Kimura *et al.*, 1979). Evidence was obtained for specific interaction of this glycoprotein (designated as T 145, mol. wt 145 000) with a lectin derived from seeds of *Vicia villosa*. Cytotoxic T lymphocytes bearing the T 145 marker were isolated by adsorption to columns of sepharose-bound *Vicia villosa* lectin, and elution with the inhibitory sugar *N*-acetylgalactosamine.

Preliminary results on interaction of a partially purified lectin from the Maine lobster (*Homarus americanus*) with murine lymphocytes have been reported (Hartman *et al.*, 1976, 1977). The lectin, specific for sialic acid residues, agglutinated cortisone-resistant thymocytes and spleen T cells; however only a small percentage of normal thymocytes were agglutinated. It was suggested that the lobster agglutinin covalently linked to sepharose could be used for the separation and isolation of cortical lymphocytes. Such separations, if successful, would be complementary to the separation with PNA. In any event, the above results provide further support to the findings that mature and immature T cells differ in their content of surface sialic acid.

TABLE IV
Distribution of PNA⁺ lymphocytes in human tissues

	% of PNA⁺ cells (average)		
	a	*b*	*c*
Peripheral blood	1	1	1
Thymus	70	52	50
Spleen		5	
Tonsils		14	13
Cord blood	18		24

[a] Reisner *et al.* (1979) Lis *et al.* (1979). [b] London *et al.* (1979b). [c] Ballet *et al.* (1980).

Human lymphocyte subpopulations

nteraction with peanut and soybean agglutinins

Because of the many similarities between the lymphoid systems of mouse and man, it seemed to us reasonable to assume that the findings described above with PNA and SBA would be applicable also to human lymphocytes. We did indeed find that the majority of human thymocytes (60–80%) bound FITC-PNA (Reisner *et al.*, 1979). Similar values were reported from other laboratories (Table IV). Upon removal of sialic acid with sialidase, all the cells bound the lectin. The PNA⁺ subpopulation was separated from the PNA⁻ cells by differential agglutination with the lectin (Reisner *et al.*, 1979). The former cells responded poorly to the mitogenic stimulation of PHA and in the MLR, whereas the latter subpopulation responded strongly to both stimuli. Thus it seems that in humans, as in mice, the PNA⁺ thymocytes are functionally immature. In support of this conclusion is the report of London *et al.* (1979b) that upon separation of human thymocytes on a discontinuous Ficoll gradient, the PNA⁺ cells were found mainly in the layers corresponding to the immunoincompetent cells. In the mouse this subpopulation is sensitive to hydrocortisone treatment and can be selectively eliminated. Since no such manipulations are possible in humans, PNA provides a unique tool for the separation of mature from immature human thymocytes.

In both human thymocyte subpopulations, more than 90% of the cells formed E rosettes. The finding that immature, PNA⁺ thymocytes bear the receptor for E rosette formation suggests that the masking of the PNA receptor by sialic acid occurs at a later stage of T cell maturation than the expression of the E rosette receptor; therefore, PNA is a more sensitive marker of T cell immaturity than E rosetting.

In tonsils, some 10–15% of the cells were PNA⁺ (London *et al.*, 1979b; Ballet *et al.*, 1980; see also Table IV). In contrast to peripheral blood, most of these PNA$^+$ cells did not ingest latex particles and thus are not monocytes but lymphocytes. Only a small percentage of the PNA$^+$ lymphocytes in tonsils formed E rosettes, suggesting that the PNA$^+$ cells are B lymphocytes. The difference in PNA receptors between thymocytes, tonsil lymphocytes and peripheral blood lymphocytes, may reflect their degree of maturation, as also indicated by other surface markers (Chess and Schlossman, 1977) and by the enzyme terminal deoxynucleotidyltransferase.

We have also investigated the binding of FITC-PNA to peripheral blood mononuclear cells of normal donors and leukaemic patients (Reisner *et al.*, 1979). Examination of the peripheral blood lymphocytes of normal donors showed that less than 2% of lymphocytes bound the lectin. This residual binding is largely to monocytes, that are as a rule PNA$^+$. Upon treatment of the cells with sialidase, binding occurred to all the cells; both B and T lymphocytes had on the average $3{\cdot}8 \times 10^6$ PNA binding sites per cell (Newman *et al.*, 1978).

Pathologic cells of different types of leukaemia varied in their PNA binding properties (Reisner *et al.*, 1979). Blast cells from most patients with acute lymphatic leukaemia, stem cell leukaemia and myeloid leukaemia, were PNA$^+$. Several cases of Burkitt tumours and one case of IgG positive acute leukaemia were tested and were also found to be PNA$^+$. In contrast, the lymphocytes of the majority of chronic lymphatic leukaemia patients tested did not bind PNA. However, a subpopulation of PNA$^+$ lymphocytes was found in 3 of the chronic leukaemia patients, all of whom had low and stable cell counts. Our results are summarized in Fig. 11. The presence of PNA$^+$ cells in the peripheral blood of 13 out of 25 patients with childhood acute

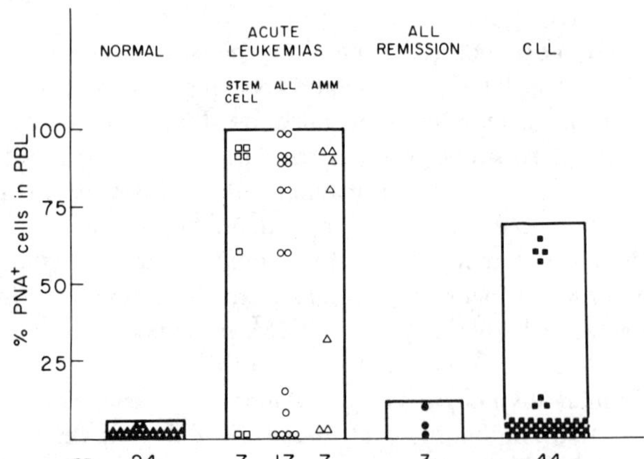

FIG. 11. *PNA$^+$ cells in normal and leukaemic human peripheral blood. Peripheral blood mononuclear cells (PBL) isolated from either normal donors or patients suffering from various leukaemias, were stained with FITC-PNA and the percentage of PNA$^+$ cells was determined. ALL, acute lymphatic leukaemia; CLL chronic lymphatic leukaemia; n = the number of individuals examined in each group. AMM, acute myeloid monocytic leukaemia. (Data from Reisner* et al., *1979 and unpublished results.)*

lymphoblastic leukaemia was also reported by Levin *et al.* (1980). It was further suggested that a high level of PNA$^+$ lymphocytes may serve as an indication for poorer prognosis among these patients. No correlation, however, can as yet be discerned between PNA binding and the expression of T cell characteristics by the various leukaemic cells examined (see also Boumsell *et al.*, 1979).

The finding that the PNA receptor may also be a marker for immature lymphocytes in man, made it likely that foetal cells could be detected and isolated with the lectin. As a first step, we examined the interaction of PNA with human umbilical cord lymphocytes (Lis *et al.*, 1979). About 15–25% of these cells were PNA$^+$, a value much higher than that found in human peripheral blood. Following separation by selective agglutination with PNA, the PNA$^+$ cells responded poorly to PHA and concanavalin A, suggesting that they are immunologically immature, whereas the PNA$^-$ cells gave a good response to both mitogens, indicating that they are mature.

Work in progress in our laboratory is aimed at fractionation of human peripheral blood lymphocytes by SBA. Under suitable conditions, two fractions were obtained: the SBA$^+$ cells were depleted of T cells and were enriched 5-fold in B lymphocytes compared to the SBA$^-$ cells (M. Barzilay, unpublished results). Although the fractions did not differ in their response to PHA or concanavalin A, Reisner *et al.* (1980d) have now obtained evidence that they differ markedly in antibody production stimulated by pokeweed mitogen; the SBA$^-$ cells responded poorly to this mitogen whereas the SBA$^+$ cells gave a high response. It was further shown that this difference may be ascribed to the separation, by SBA, of the major regulatory T cell subpopulations: antibody helper that are SBA$^+$ and antibody suppressor cells (SBA$^-$). In human bone marrow, Reisner *et al.* (1980c) have found that the bulk of the cells (80–90%) were agglutinated by SBA, similarly to mouse bone marrow cells. However, in contrast to the latter, the agglutinated human bone marrow cell subpopulation was highly depleted of stem cells, whereas the minor, unagglutinated subpopulation was enriched (5–10-fold) in stem cells in comparison with the unfractionated bone marrow cells. Therefore most of the human myeloid precursors were SBA$^+$, unlike mouse stem cells.

In passing, mention should be made of the proposal to use PNA as a marker for human breast epithelial cell differentiation (Newman *et al.*, 1979).

Other lectins

Treatment of human peripheral blood lymphocytes with sialidase has been shown to uncover receptors for the *Helix pomatia* lectin (Hammarström *et al.*, 1973; Hellström *et al.*, 1976a). Since the receptors appeared mainly on T lymphocytes, these cells could be separated from B cells, using HP-sepharose (Hellström *et al.*, 1976b). The majority of the B cells were recovered in the fraction that was not bound to the column; the bound T cells were eluted in good yield with *N*-acetylgalactosamine (Fig. 10). In a modification of the original technique, a highly enriched B cell population was isolated with a purity of 80%, and a yield of 65% (Schrempf-Decker *et al.*, 1980). A major cell surface glycoprotein (apparent mol. wt 150 000 under reducing conditions) was responsible for almost all the binding of HP to sialidase treated human lymphocytes, as has been found with mouse T cells (Axelsson *et al.*, 1978). The glycoprotein was present on normal and malignant T lymphocytes and on chronic lymphocytic leukaemia cells, but not on various B cells.

It should be noted, however, that a minor fraction of B lymphocytes in normal peripheral blood was HP$^+$; this fraction constituted about 10% of the total number of HP$^+$ lymphocytes in the blood (Hellström *et al.*, 1978). The HP receptors on the B cells were different from those on the majority of T cells, and indications were obtained that these structures were expressed on an immature variety of B cells. Therefore, the HP receptor seems to fall into the category of differentiation markers, and may constitute a useful tool for characterization and separation of human lymphocytes within both the T and B compartments.

Human peripheral blood T lymphocytes were separated by chromatography on sepharose-bound WGA into two subpopulations that differed in their response to PHA and concanavalin A. Elution of the WGA$^+$ cells was performed with *N*-acetylglucosamine (Hellström *et al.*, 1976c).

Separation of human peripheral lymphocytes into fractions that differ in binding to lentil lectin has been described (Boldt and Lyons, 1979a). In these experiments, the lymphocytes were incubated in plastic tubes or Petri dishes coated with a gelatin layer to which lentil lectin had been coupled. Adherent cells (approximately 25–50% of the total) were recovered by melting the gelatin, and the bound lectin was removed by treating the cells with mannose. However, no functional differences were observed between the two fractions, except that the cells which bound to lentil lectin responded better to stimulation by this lectin than the unbound cells. Using the above technique, separation of human peripheral blood lymphocytes by WGA was also carried out (Boldt and Lyons, 1979b). The WGA$^+$ cells responded less well to PHA than the WGA$^-$ cells (Boldt and Lyons, 1980).

Concluding remarks

We have demonstrated that cell surface carbohydrates, detectable by lectins, are characteristic markers of lymphocyte subpopulations, normal and leukaemic, in mouse and man. We have also shown that lymphocytes are inseparable by lectins into biologically distinct subpopulations. Very little is known about the structure of the lectin receptors, nor are their functions understood. One attractive hypothesis is that the specific acquisition of components at the cell surface occurring during differentiation affects cell location by providing surface receptors for interaction with lectins in certain tissues, for example in the thymic cortex (Hughes and Pena, 1980). Other surface sugars may be required for cell activation or co-operation in the immune system.

Isolation of the receptors and elucidation of their structure and biosynthesis may help in clarifying their biological functions. Whatever these functions are, there is no doubt that lectins have become an important and most useful tool for cell separation, as is evidenced by the following cartoons (Fig. 12). It is also apparent that studies with lectins are leading to the identification of new lymphocyte subpopulations, and are providing deeper insights into the role of cell surface sugars in the ontogeny of the immune system. Last but not least, based on our findings, a new approach to the isolation of human stem cells for bone marrow transplantation can be envisaged.

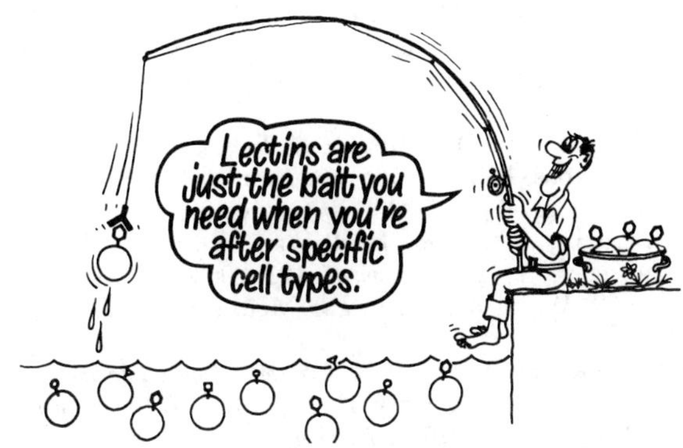
Lectins are just the bait you need when you're after specific cell types.

Why fish in the dark?

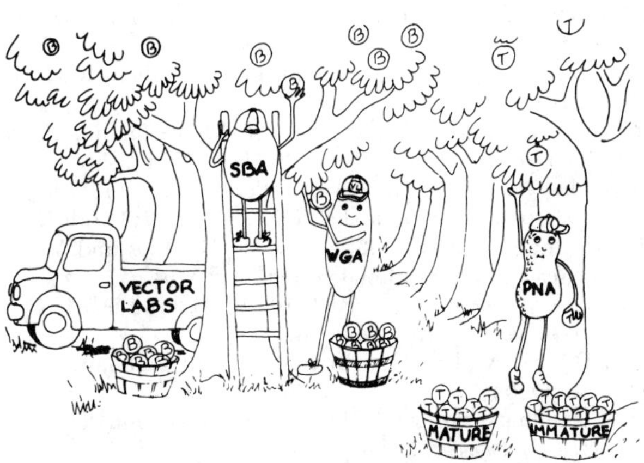

FIG. 12. *Two artists' views of the benefits accrued from the use of lectins for cell fractionation. Courtesy of Boehringer Mannheim (top) and Vector Laboratories (bottom).*

References

Ashwell, G. and Morell, A. G. (1974). *Adv. Enzymol.* **41**, 99–128.

Axelsson, B., Kimura, A., Hammarström, S., Wigzell, H., Nilsson, K. and Mellstedt, H. (1978). *Eur. J. Immunol.* **8**, 757–764.

Ballet, J.-J., Fellous, M., Sharon, N., Reisner, Y. and Agrapart, M. (1980). *Scand. J. Immunol.* **11**, 555–560.

Benacerraf, B. and Unanue, E. R. (1979). "Textbook of Immunology", Chapter 5, pp. 6–98. Williams and Wilkins, Baltimore and London.

Berney, S. A. and Gesner, B. M. (1970). *Immunology* **18**, 681.

Berrih, S., Bonavida, B. and London, J. (1979). *Protides Biol. Fluids* **27**, 551–555.

Betel, I., Mathieson, B. J., Sharrow, S. O. and Asofsky, R. (1980). *J. Immunol.* **124**, 2209–2217.

Boldt, D. H. and Lyons, R. D. (1979a). *Cell. Immunol.* **43**, 82–93.

Boldt, D. H. and Lyons, R. D. (1979b). *J. Immunol.* **123**, 808–816.

Boldt, D. H. and Lyons, R. D. (1980). *Immunology* **39**, 519–527.

Boumsell, L., Bernard, A., Coppin, H., Richard, Y., Penit, C., Rouget, P., Lemerle, J. and Dausset, J. (1979). *J. Immunol.* **123**, 2063–2067.

Bourguignon, L. Y. W., Rader, R. L. and McMahon, J. T. (1979). *J. Cell. Physiol.* **99**, 95–99.

Chess, L. and Schlossman, S. F. (1977). *Contemp. Topics Immunol.* **7**, 303.

Despont, J. P., Abel, C. A. and Grey, H. M. (1975). *Cell. Immunol.* **17**, 487–494.

Dumont, F. and Nardelli, J. (1979). *Immunology* **37**, 217–224.

Eisenthal, A., Nachtigal, D. and Feldman, M. (1979). *Transplant. Proc.* **11**, 904–906.

Globerson, A., Rabinowich, H., Umiel, T., Reisner, Y. and Sharon, N. (1979). *In* "Function and Structure of the Immune System" (W. Muller-Ruchholtz and H. K. Muller-Hermelink, eds) pp. 345–350. Plenum, New York.

Haller, O., Gidlund, M., Hellström, U., Hammarström, S. and Wigzell, H. (1978). *Eur. J. Immunol.* **8**, 765–771.

Hammarström, S., Hellström, U., Perlmann, P. and Dillner, M.-L. (1973). *J. Exp. Med.* **138**, 1270–1275.

Hammarström, S., Hellström, U., Dillner, M.-L., Perlmann, P., Perlmann, H., Axelsson, B. and Robertsson, E.-S. (1978). *In* "Affinity Chromatography" (Hoffmann-Ostenhof *et al.*, eds), pp. 273–286. Pergamon Press, Oxford.

Hartman, A. L., Despont, J.-P. and Abel, C. A. (1976). *In* "10th Leucocyte Culture Conference, Amsterdam" (V. R. Eijsvoogel, D. Roos and W. P. Zeijlemaker, eds) p. 115. Academic Press, London and New York.

Hartman, A. L., Campbell, P. A., Richard, B. M. and Abel, C. A. (1977). *J. Supramol. Struct., Suppl.* **1**, 187 (Abstr. 885).

Hellström, U., Dillner, M.-L., Hammarström, S. and Perlmann, P. (1976a). *Scand. J. Immunol.* **5**, 45–54.

Hellström, U., Hammarström, S., Dillner, M.-L., Perlmann, H. and Perlmann, P. (1976b). *Scand. J. Immunol.* **5**, Suppl. 5, 45–55.

Hellström, U., Dillner, M. L., Hammarström, S. and Perlmann, P. (1976c). *J. Exp. Med.* **144**, 1381–1385.

Hellström, U., Perlmann, P., Robertsson, E. S. and Hammarström, S. (1978). *Scand. J. Immunol.* **7**, 191–197.

Hoessli, D., Bron, C. and Pint, J. R. L. (1980). *Nature* **283**, 576–578.

Hughes, R. C. and Pena, S. D. J. (1980). *In* "Carbohydrate Metabolism and its Disorders" (P. J. Randle, D. F. Steiner and W. J. Whelan, eds) Vol. 3. Academic Press, London and New York (in press).

Imai, Y., Oguchi, T., Nakano, T. and Osawa, T. (1979). *Immunol. Commun.* **8**, 495–503.

Irlé, C., Piquet, P.-F. and Vassalli, P. (1978). *J. Exp. Med.* **148**, 32–45.

Kimura, A., Wigzell, H., Holmquist, G., Ersson, B. O. and Carlsson, (1979). *J. Exp. Med.* **149**, 473–484.

Kruisbeek, A. M. and Astaldi, G. C. B. (1979). *J. Immunol.* **123**, 984–991.

Levin, S., Russell, E. C., Blanchard, D., McWilliams, N. B., Maurer, H. M., and Mohanakumar, T. (1980). *Blood* **55**, 37–39.

Lis, H. and Sharon, N. (1977). *In* "The Antigens" (M. Sela, ed.) Vol. IV, pp. 429–529. Academic Press, London and New York.

Lis, H., Sela, B., Sachs, L. and Sharon, N. (1970). *Biochim. Biophys. Acta* **211**, 582–585.

Lis, H., Garnett, H., Rotter, V., Reisner, Y. and Sharon, N. (1979). Abstr. Meeting of Society of Complex Carbohydrates, Toronto, July 1979.

London, J. and Horton, M. A. (1980). *J. Immunol.* **124**, 1803–1807.

London, J., Berrih, S. and Bach, J.-F. (1978). *J. Immunol.* **121**, 438–443.

London, J., Berrih, S. and Papiernik, M. (1979a). *Devel. Compar. Immunol.* **3**, 343–352.

London, J., Perrot, J. Y., Berrih, S., Laroche, L. and Niaudet, P. (1979b). *Scand. J. Immunol.* **9**, 451–459.

Lotan, R., Skutelsky, E., Danon, D. and Sharon, N. (1975). *J. Biol. Chem.* **250**, 8518–8523.

Madyastha, K. R., Baker, M. A. and Taub, R. N. (1980). *Transplantation* **29**, 252–254.

Mathieson, B. J., Mage, M., Betel, I. and Sharrow, S. O. (1979). *Protides Biol. Fluids* **27**, 535–538.

Moretta, L., Mingari, M. C. and Moretta, A. (1979). *Immunol. Rev.* **45**, 163–193.

Newman, R. A., Uhlenbruck, G., Schumacher, K., Mil, A. V. and Karduck, D. (1978). *Z. Immun. Forsch.* **154**, 451–462.

Newman, R. A., Klein, P. J. and Rudland, P. S. (1979). *J. Natl. Canc. Inst.* **63**, 1339–1346.

Newman, R. R. and Boss, M. A. (1980). *Immunology* **40**, 193–200.

Nicola, N. A., Burgess, A. W., Metcalf, D. and Battye, F. L. (1978). *Austral. J. Exp. Biol. Med. Sci.* **56**, 663–679.

Pereira, M. E. A., Kabat, E. A. and Sharon, N. (1974). *Carbohyd. Res.* **37**, 89–102.

Pereira, M. E. A., Kabat, E. A., Lotan, R. and Sharon, N. (1976). *Carbohyd. Res.* **51**, 107–118.

Prujansky, A. (1977). M.Sc. thesis, Weizmann Institute of Science.

Rabinovich, H., Umiel, T., Reisner, Y., Sharon, N. and Globerson, A. (1979). *Cell. Immunol.* **47**, 347–355.

Raff, M. C. (1976). *Scient. Am.* **234(5)**, 30–39.

Reinherz, E. L. and Schlossman, S. F. (1980). *Cell* **19**, 821–827.

Reisner, Y. (1979). Ph.D. thesis, Weizmann Institute of Science.

Reisner, Y. and Sharon, N. (1980). *Trends Biochem. Sci.* **5**, 29–31.

Reisner, Y., Linker-Israeli, M. and Sharon, N. (1976a). *Cell. Immunol.* **25**, 129–134.

Reisner, Y., Ravid, A. and Sharon, N. (1976b). *Biochem. Biophys. Res. Commun.* **72**, 1585–1591.

Reisner, Y., Itzicovitch, L., Meshorer, A. and Sharon, N. (1978). *Proc. Natn. Acad. Sci. U.S.A.* **75**, 2933–2936.

Reisner, Y., Biniaminov, M., Rosenthal, E., Sharon, N. and Ramot, B. (1979). *Proc. Natn. Acad. Sci. U.S.A.* **76**, 447–451.

Reisner, Y., Ikehara, S., Hodes, M. Z. and Good, R. A. (1980a). *Proc. Natn. Acad. Sci. U.S.A.* **77**, 1164–1168.

Reisner, Y., Sharon, N. and Haran-Ghera, N. (1980b). *Proc. Natn. Acad. Sci. U.S.A.* **77**, 2244–2246.

Reisner, Y., Kapoor, N. O'Reilly, R. J. and Good, R. A. (1980c). (In preparation).

Reisner, Y., Pahwa, S., Chiao, J. W., Sharon, N., Evans, R. L. and Good, R. A. (1980d). *Proc. Natn. Acad. Sci.* (in press).

Roelants, G. E., London, J., Mayor-Withey, K. S. and Serrano, B. (1979). *Eur. J. Immunol.* **9**, 139–145.

Rose, M. L., Birbeck, M. S. C., Wallis, V. J., Forrester, J. A. and Davies, A. J. (1980). *Nature* **284**, 364–366.

Schnebli, H. P. and Dukor, P. (1972). *Eur. J. Immunol.* **2**, 607–609.

Schrempf-Decker, G. E., Baron, D. and Wernet, P. (1980). *J. Immunol. Meth.* **32**, 285–296.

Sharon, N. (1979a). *In* "Structure and Function of Biomembranes" (K. Yagi, ed.) pp. 63–82. Japan Scientific Societies Press, Tokyo.

Sharon, N. (1979b). *In* "Affinity Chromatography and Molecular Interactions: Biochemical and Biomedical Applications" (J. Egly, ed.) pp. 197–206. Colloq. Inserm 86.

Sharon, N. and Lis, H. (1980). *In* "The Proteins" (3rd edn) (H. Neurath and R. L. Hill, eds), Vol. V. Academic Press, London and New York (in press).

Sharon, N. and Reisner, Y. (1979). *In* "Molecular Mechanisms of Biological Recognition" (M. Balaban, ed.), pp. 95–106. Elsevier-North Holland Biomedical Press, Amsterdam.

Umiel, T., Linker-Israeli, M., Itzchaki, M., Trainin, N., Reisner, Y. and Sharon, N. (1978). *Cell. Immunol.* **37**, 134–141.

Umiel, T., Klein, B., Dröge, W., Sharon, N. and Trainin, N. (1980). (In preparation.)

Zeicher, M., Mozes, E., Reisner, Y. and Lonai, P. (1979). *Immunogenetics* **9**, 119–124.

Theme 4: Summary
Nonantigen-specific Receptors

GÖRAN MÖLLER

Department of Immunobiology, Karolinska Institutet Medical School, Stockholm, Sweden

At the Second International Congress of Immunology at Brighton it was thought that all known lymphocyte receptors had no known function and all functional receptors were unidentified. This is not so today. In order to summarize the present knowledge of nonimmunoglobulin receptors it is necessary to distinguish between receptors on T and B lymphocytes.

Receptors on B lymphocytes

Fc receptors. These receptors are present on most B cells. Several attempts to determine their mol. wts have been made but the mol. wts have varied from 28 000 to 255 000. It has been reported that treatment of B cells with antibodies against β_2-microglobulin, Ia antigens and IgM receptors lead to cocapping of Fc receptors (Moretta, Chapter 12). The function of the Fc receptors appears to be the delivery of negative signals to B cells. The addition of immune complexes to B cells *in vitro* has been found to cause stimulation, suppression or to have no effects. The stimulatory effects of complexes is caused by macrophages and thus not relevant to this discussion. Whether immune complexes can or cannot suppress activation of B cells by polyclonal B cell activators (PBA) appears to depend on the physical form of the complexes: insolubilized complexes are inhibitory, whereas soluble complexes have no effect, suggesting that the affinity between the Fc receptor and Fc part of the Ig molecules is low. The finding that immune complexes (e.g. sheep red cells and antisheep red cell antibodies) can specifically suppress PBA induced activation of the antigen-specific (antisheep red cell) B cells have been interpreted as follows: Antigen-specific B cells bind the antigen via their high affinity Ig receptors. Doing so the B cells interact with the antibodies complexed with the antigen. Due to high affinity binding of the Ig receptors to the antigen, the specific B cells receive a strong negative signal via their Fc receptors, a signal which cannot be overcome even by strong PBA substances.

B cell activating receptors. The receptors responsible for B cell activation (PBA receptors) have been studied intensively. Ten years ago radiolabelled LPS was found to bind weakly but equally to T and B cells. In the workshops to this theme, three reports on binding of LPS to lymphocytes were presented. In one (Gregory *et al.* 7.3.05)* it was found that radiolabelled lipid A bound to about 20% of Ig positive B cells, but not to Ig negative cells. However, B cells from LPS high-responder mice bound as much as cells from nonresponder strains. Jacobs and Rosenspire (7.3.06) found that radiolabelled LPS bound better to cells from high-responder strains and Nylén *et al.* (personal communication) observed strong binding to B cells from LPS

*Reference numbers indicate Abstract numbers in: Abstracts 4th International Congress of Immunology, Paris, 1980.

responder strains only when low concentrations of horseradish peroxidase labelled LPS were added. Taken together, the findings suggest the existence of a genetically determined LPS receptor. So far only Coutinho *et al.* have directly demonstrated this receptor by the use of a specific antibody.

The early events of lymphocytes activation and the nature of transmembrane triggering signals remain unknown.

Receptors on T cells

A variety of receptors have been described on T cells, such as receptors for sheep red cells, histamin, various lectins, measles virus, Fc parts of immunoglobulin molecules. In addition, T cells have several different antigens, such as Thy-1, Ly-1,2,3 and T-200. Since there are some differences between human and mouse lymphocytes they will be dealt with separately.

Mouse T cells. The most important question is whether distinct functions can be ascribed to different receptors. The conventional belief is that Ly-1 antigens define helper T cells, Ly-2,3 antigens (specified by genes on chromosome 6) cytotoxic effector cells and suppressor cells and Ly-1,2,3 antigens precursor T cells. Although this may be basically correct, the analytical tools are still blunt and new findings changing this picture are likely to emerge. Already Ly-1 positive cells have been described as cytotoxic effector cells.

A major intellectual dilemma is that there appears to be a linkage between expression of Ly antigens and the antigen-specific receptors on the T cells. Thus, Ly-1 helper cells recognize antigen in conjunction with Ia antigens, whereas Ly-2,3 cells see antigen in association with H-2 K and D structures.

Fc receptors on murine T cells. It was shown first by B. Andersson that T cells could bind the Fc part on Ig molecules. Before that, it was known that lymphocytes could be activated into cytotoxicity by binding to antibody-coated target cells (the ADCC reaction), although the nature of the effector cells was unknown. Now Andersson and collaborators (Skoglund *et al.*, 7.1.29) show that T cells having Fc receptors for IgM antibodies can kill IgM, but not IgG, coated target cells. Furthermore, these T cells function as helper cells and they possess Ly-1 antigens. Depletion of Ly-1 antigen positive T cells does not affect the response of the remaining T cells to con A or PHA.

The precise nature of the K cells executing the ADCC reaction remains obscure, except for their ability to interact with and be activated by the Fc part of Ig molecules. Lamon *et al.* (7.1.11) found that part of the ADCC effector cells carry Thy-1 antigens, identifying them as T cells. Although the ADCC reaction *in vitro* is potent and easy to induce, it is still not known whether the reaction has any function *in vivo*. When antibody-coated nucleated cells are injected into allogeneic animals they are protected from cell-mediated destruction, instead of being killed by K cells, as predicted from the ADCC reaction *in vitro*.

Human T cells. It is generally accepted that human T cells having receptors for the Fc part of IgG molecules (Tγ cells) are cytotoxic effector cells and those with receptors for IgM (Tμ cells) are helper cells. However, the situation is probably more complex. Thus, it has been found that the phenotypes of the Fc binding T cells are not stable (Moretta, Chapter 12). Thus, Tγ cells that have interacted with an immune complex containing IgG lose their receptors for IgG and gain receptors for IgM. Contrariwise, Tμ cells activated in a mixed lymphocyte culture reaction lose the receptors for IgM, which are replaced by receptors for IgG. However, at any given time each T cell is characterized by binding either IgM or IgG. It has been suggested that these receptors are not necessarily markers for cell function, but rather markers for differentiation stages or activation markers. Thus, Tμ cells would be helper cells and precursors for suppressor cells, whereas Tγ cells would be active suppressor cells.

Lectin receptors and triggering sites. Although T cells are easily activated by many lectins with known specificity for different saccharides the triggering receptors have been elusive. Several groups have attempted to characterize the activation receptor by isolating unique lectin binding proteins on activated cells. Marked progression has occurred in this area. Although the approach is straightforward it may not give the information needed, because T cell activation may not occur by the lectins binding to unique proteins on the T cells. This is illustrated by the finding by U. Persson (personal communication) that purified T cells cannot be activated by con A in serum free medium, although con A binds to the T cells. T cell activation by con A requires helper factors present in macrophages and serum. Actually, these helper factors may be the triggering substances interacting with receptors on T cells and the role of con A may be only to stabilize the interaction between the activating substances and the corresponding receptors. Although most students of MHC restriction are eagerly discussing whether one or two receptors are needed for recognition of antigen in association of MHC products, they do not seriously consider the possibility that recognition and activation are carried out as separate events. It is my belief that the general scheme of activation found in B cells, namely that one set of clonal receptors recognizes the antigen and another set of nonclonal receptors is responsible for activation, will be generally true also for T cells. However, the nature of the receptors on T and B cells must be drastically different. The T cell recognition of antigen plus MHC products and the totally different polyclonal activators of T and B cells argue in this direction.

Although much knowledge has accumulated concerning the function of many receptors on T and B cells we do not yet understand the details of B cell activation and remarkably little of the mechanism of T cell activation.

Theme 5

Ontogeny and Differentiation of T and B Lymphocytes

Presidents:

J. J. T. OWEN

J. F. BACH

Symposium chairman

M. FELDMAN

15

Homing of Lymphoid Stem Cells to the Thymus and the Bursa of Fabricius Studied in Avian Embryo Chimaeras

N. M. LE DOUARIN and F. V. JOTEREAU

Institut d'Embryologie du CNRS et College de France, Nogent-sur-Marne and Laboratoire de Biologie du Développement, Faculté des Sciences de Nantes, Nantes, France

Introduction

Although it has long been a matter of controversy, it is now unequivocally established that lymphoid precursor cells (LPC) have an embryonic origin

Abbreviations
LPC: lymphoid precursor cells; PLR: primary lymphoid rudiments; HC: haemopoietic cells; CAM: chorioallantoic membrane; CFU-C: colony-forming units-culture; CFU-S: colony-forming units-spleen.

extrinsic to the rudiments of primary lymphoid organs. This was achieved through the use of various cell marking techniques which allow the migration streams and ultimate fates of primitive cells to be observed throughout ontogeny (Moore and Owen, 1965, 1967a, b; Le Douarin and Jotereau, 1973, 1975; Houssaint *et al.*, 1976). The concept of extrinsic origin of LPC, first presented in the haematogenous hypothesis of blood forming organ ontogeny by Metcalf and Moore (1971), in itself raises a number of issues. For example, does a precommitment of the LPC precede their colonization of the primary lymphoid rudiments (PLR)? Our studies with avian embryos suggest that the first immigrants to the epithelium of the bursa of Fabricius are not restricted to B lymphocyte differentiation alone. However, it remains to be determined if these precursors could follow nonlymphoid avenues of differentiation. A second question relates to the site or sites where LPC arise. If they emerge both within the embryos and in extraembryonic tissues, it is important to know which populations are essential to the development of the immune systems. Although this may have been well clarified in the avian embryo, the question still remains open in mammals. Finally, it is important to define the dynamics of stem cells entry in primary lymphoid organs at various stages of development precisely before considering mechanisms which might regulate these events.

All of these ontogenetic problems can be efficiently approached by the use of chimaeras constructed with quail (*Coturnix coturnix japonica*) and chick (*Gallus gallus*) tissues according to methods which have been described in detail in our previous publications (Le Douarin, 1969, 1973, 1978, 1979). The unique features of this model are that the embryonic tissues of the two species are completely compatible and the structure of interphase nuclei of their cells differs in such a way that they can be unambiguously distinguished in histological preparations.

The various points which will be considered in this review concern modalities of the colonization of the thymus and of the bursa of Fabricius by haemopoietic cells (HC) and the mechanisms underlying these events. Recent investigations on the role of the thymic and bursic microenvironments on the differentiation of LPC into either the T or the B cell lineages will also be discussed.

Colonization of the primary lymphoid organs by haemopoietic cells in avian embryo

Timing of the first influx of HC into the developing thymic and bursic rudiments

In previous studies, we showed that the first influx of HC into the thymus and the bursa of Fabricius begins at a precise stage of embryonic development according to the chronology indicated in Fig. 1. The nonintrusion of HC into the thymic and bursal primordia before this stage is not due to the lack of

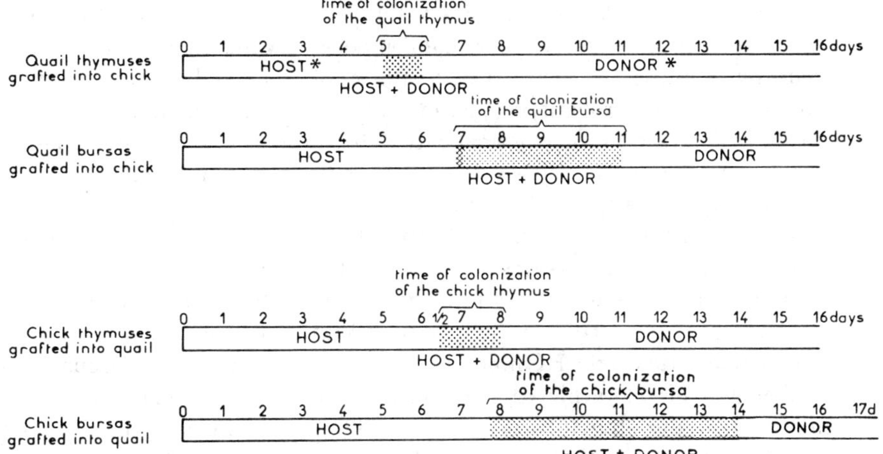

FIG. 1. *Time of development at which the first colonization of the thymus and the seeding of the bursa of Fabricius by LPC take place in chick and quail embryos. * Type of lymphocytes found in thymuses and bursas from quail and chick embryos of different ages grafted until they reach the age of 14 days for the thymus and 19 days for the bursa.*

"competent" HC in the blood of younger embryos. On the contrary, we showed unequivocally that cells able to colonize the thymus and to differentiate along the T cell lineage are present in the blood stream 2–3 days prior to the stage at which the thymus normally becomes seeded during embryogeny. This permitted us to define "prereceptive" and "receptive" periods in the early stages of thymus ontogeny and their respective durations. The ability to receive HC appears to result from specific maturation of the thymic epithelium (Le Douarin and Jotereau, 1975). The latter, grafted alone (after being isolated from the 3rd and 4th branchial arch mesenchyme) into the somatopleural mesenchyme of a 3-day host embryo, is capable of pursuing its differentiation (i.e. of becoming seeded by HC) and giving rise to normally developed thymic tissue in that ectopic situation (Le Douarin *et al.*, 1968). In such a case, the development of thymic tissue results from the co-operation of the somatopleural mesenchyme of the host which forms the connective component of the organ, the grafted endodermal thymic rudiment, and the host HC which invade it.

The developmental behaviour of the tissue components in the bursa of Fabricius is somewhat different; the digestive (cloacal) endoderm which is at the origin of the lymphoid follicles does not develop if it is separated from the bursal mesoderm. Substitution of the latter by any kind of mesenchymal tissue, used until now for this purpose, prevented formation of the follicles and seeding by HC. This therefore precluded the bursal epithelium from accomplishing its role in the ontogeny of B cells. Another method that has been used to arrest the evolution of the bursa of Fabricius is the treatment of embryos at any stage of development with high doses of androgens (Kirkpatrick and Andrews, 1944; Glick, 1955; Höhn, 1956; Le Douarin *et al.*, 1980).

This was recently shown to be the result of deleterious hormonal action specifically directed to the endodermal component of the organ. The latter, taken from a bursal rudiment treated with testosterone and associated with nontreated bursal mesoderm of the same age, did not evolve into lymphoid follicles. In contrast, the mesodermal part of the androgen-treated bursa could still promote the development of lymphoid follicles in a nontreated bursal endoderm (Le Douarin *et al.*, 1980).

The arrest of the stem cell influx into the PLR does not seem to be stage-dependent in the same way as its onset. Although the normal period for seeding the thymus is about 24 h in the quail and 36 h in the chick (see Fig. 1), the receptivity for HC can be maintained in the thymic rudiment for a longer period of time if the HC influx is experimentally prevented (Le Douarin, 1978, 1979). This was achieved by culturing quail or chick thymic rudiments before their seeding by HC *in vitro*, or in a diffusion chamber on the chorio-allantoic membrane (CAM), for several days. If the rudiments were grafted after the culture period, they could still receive HC and give rise to thymic tissue. The duration of the influx depends therefore on the number of cells which invade the epithelium.

Evolution of thymus and bursa following the first influx of HC

The next question we considered was whether the first influx of HC into the thymus and the bursa of Fabricius was followed by other waves of LPC entering these organs.

Thymus: evidence for a second wave of stem cell influx

The fact that the initial early and rapid influx of HC is followed by a refractory period during which no cells enter the rudiment was established by several types of experiments. Firstly, when the thymus was taken from the embryo at day 6 or 7 for the quail and 8 or 9 for the chick and grafted heterospecifically, the lymphoid population observed when the thymus had reached 14 days of age was entirely of the donor type. Secondly, a double transplantation experiment already described (Le Douarin and Jotereau, 1975) was also significant in this respect. It consisted of grafting a 4-day quail thymic rudiment into a 3-day chick embryo for 2 days and then its retransplantation into a 3-day quail for 8 days. In such a case, the quail thymus which reached its "receptive" period during its graft time in the chick developed a lymphoid population that was entirely of the chick type, which means that no LPC entered it immediately after its transplantation into the second chick host.

By using serial transplantations of thymic rudiments into successive hosts alternatively hetero- and homospecific, we demonstrated that the seeding of the quail thymic rudiment by LPC is a cyclic phenomenon (Jotereau and Le Douarin, in prep.) (Fig. 2, Table I). The quail thymic rudiment was taken at 7 and 8 days of development and grafted into a 3-day chick embryo for a period of 3–5 days. It was then transplanted into a quail for 3–10 days. Chimaerism analysis was done on serial sections of the explant stained for

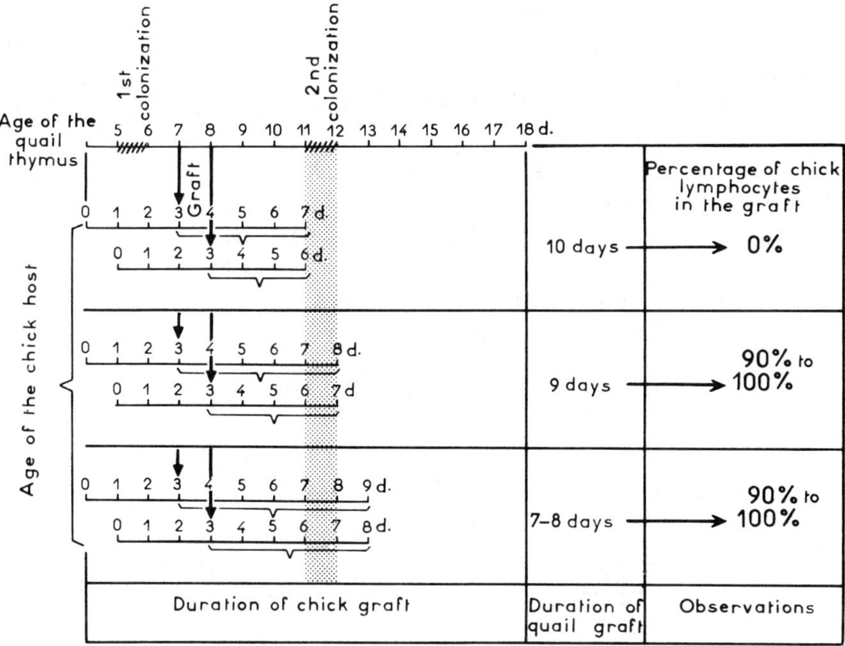

FIG. 2. *Double transplantation experiments of 7- and 8-day quail thymic rudiments showing that a second wave of LPC colonize the grafted thymus when it reaches day 11 of incubation. When the thymus is 19–20 days the quail lymphocytes have practically all been replaced by chick lymphocytes.*

TABLE I

Seeding of a quail thymus by chick cells in double transplantation experiments. (The quail thymic rudiment is successively grafted into chick and quail embryos for various periods of time.)

Duration of the graft in the first host (chick)	*3 days*	*4 days*	*5 days*
Age of the quail donor			
7 days		0/12[a]	11/17
8 days	0/9	5/7	18/22

[a] Proportion of thymuses in which chick (first host) lymphocytes develop.

DNA with the Feulgen–Rossenbeck's technique. Lymphoid cells of the chick were counted and their localization (in cortex or medulla) and degree of maturation were assessed. Large haemopoietic cells with a clear nucleus were distinguished from the various types of lymphocytes according to the nuclear characteristics defined earlier (Le Douarin and Jotereau, 1975; see also Sugimoto *et al.*, 1977).

A renewal of the quail lymphoid population by the progeny of chick LPC took place in the graft, provided that the latter was in a chick host when it was 11–12 days old (Fig. 2, Table I). Within 24 h (from day 11 to day 12) it was seeded by enough stem cells to renew totally the quail lymphoid population during its stay in the second (quail) host. This indicates that the second influx of LPC takes place during the 12th day of incubation in the quail and lasts, like the first one, about 24 h. In addition, it appears that the time necessary for the second wave of LPC to divide and renew the lymphocytes originating from the first wave was about 8 days. When the age of the thymus reached 19–21 days, quail lymphocytes had been practically totally replaced by chick cells (Fig. 3). It was also observed that the seedings of the external

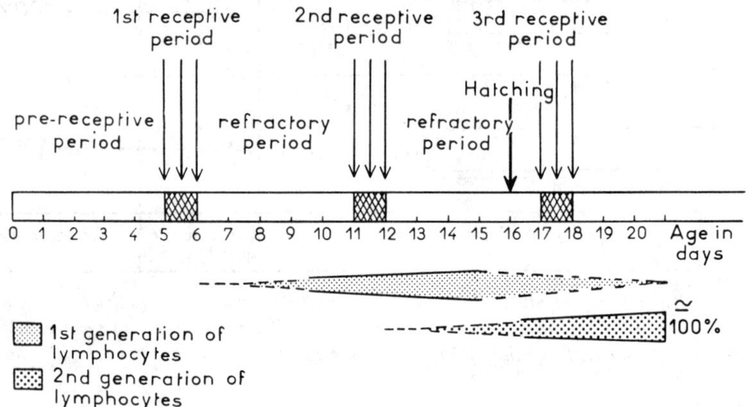

FIG. 3. *Cyclic seeding of the embryonic and postnatal quail thymus by LPC. Short receptive periods alternate with 5-day refractory periods during which no LPC enter the thymus. Each wave of LPC gives rise to a lymphoid population the maximum development of which is reached around 8 days after the influx of the precursor cells.*

cortex and of the medulla by HC take place simultaneously. Therefore, the lymphocytes populating these two different regions of the thymus are derived from different stem cells. This indicates that most lymphocytes of the medulla are not derived from cortical cells as was proposed by some authors (Weissman, 1967, 1973; Fathman *et al.*, 1975).

Other types of experimental designs were devised to control these results:

(1) Instead of two successive graftings, only one was performed with 7- and 8-day quail thymuses implanted into a single 3-day chick host. The replacement of the lymphoid population was also shown to take place when the quail thymus had reached about 19 to 21 days of total age.

(2) Since the transplantations may have disturbed the renewal of LPC, we compared the chimaerism in 8-day quail thymuses in which two successive transplantations were performed at various times. One was performed first into a 3-day chick for 5 days and then into a 3-day quail for 5 days (total duration of the grafts was 10 days). The other was

performed successively into two 3-day chick hosts for a period of 3 days in the first and 7 days in the second (total duration of the graft was 10 days). Then the chimaerism was compared in both types of explants. In the second type of experiment (successive transplantation into two chick embryos), the quail thymus was colonized only in the second host soon after its transplantation (see Table 1), and not during the first as in the other kinds of grafts. No significant differences were found in the chimaerism, showing that the chronological pattern of transplantation does not modify the LPC influx.

Thymus: evidence for a third wave of stem cell influx

When the chronological pattern of grafting was that represented in Fig. 2, signs of a third wave of invasion by HC into the quail thymus could be detected. An example is the experiment involving a first graft of 7- and 8-day quail thymuses for 5 days in the chick, followed by a second graft for 7 days into a quail (total age of the explant, 19–20 days). The lymphoid population was practically all chick cells but a fringe of large HC with the quail nuclear marker was seen in the external cortex.

If retransplanted into a 3-day chick for 6 days (third graft), such a thymus shows mainly chick lymphocytes in the internal cortex and a majority of quail lymphocytes in the external cortex. The former were derived from the LPC belonging to the second invasion and taken from the first chick host, while the latter arose from the quail LPC which penetrated the explant during the second transplantation in the quail.

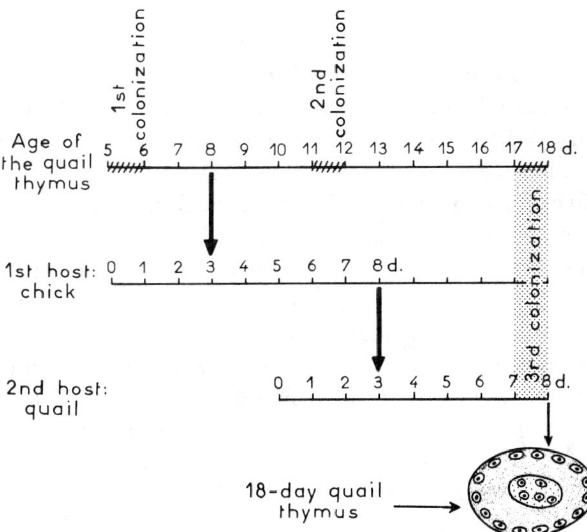

FIG. 4. *Transplantation experiment designed to precise the stage of the third wave of LPC into the quail thymus. An 8-day quail thymus is grafted into a first chick host for 5 days and then for another period of 5 days into a second quail host. Quail LPC are seen in the medulla and in the external cortex of the explant in which the lymphocytes are all (or nearly all) of the chick type.*

Another pattern of transplantation was the one represented in Fig. 4. An 8-day quail thymus was transplanted into a 3-day chick host for 5 days and then into a quail for 5 days. The total age of the thymus was 18 days at the time of fixation and cells of the third wave were also present in this experimental series.

It therefore appears that a third wave of HC influx into the thymus takes place after a refractory period of about 6 days and has a duration of about 24 h like the first two. The invasion of the thymic rudiment by LPC during the embryonic and postnatal life is therefore a cyclic process with a regular periodicity of phases refractory for HC invasion which last about 5 days and are separated by receptive periods of about 24 h (Fig. 3).

In all the experiments reported above, a total of 46 explants were observed and indications of a cyclic renewal of lymphocytes was found in 34 of them. In the others, the seeding process by the host HC was delayed for reasons which remain unclear but which may be related with the chronological or spatial patterns of vascularization of the graft.

The results discussed above concern the thymus of the quail. Investigations are presently in progress on the chick and our preliminary observations indicate that a second wave of HC also takes place after a refractory period in that species, the duration of which is about 6 days.

This suggests that the capacities of proliferation of the HC which colonize the thymus are limited to a certain number of cell cycles. According to such an interpretation, a self-renewing pool of stem cells would not exist in the thymus.

Bursa of Fabricius

The time of colonization of the quail and chick bursal primordium by HC was established through interspecific grafting experiments in which chimaerism analysis was carried out when the total age of the organ had reached 19–20 days (see Le Douarin and Houssaint, 1974; Le Douarin *et al.*, 1975; Houssaint *et al.*, 1976). In recent experiments, Houssaint (unpublished results) protracted the duration of the graft in one single host and also carried out double transplantations into two successive hosts, as described for the thymus, in order to see whether a second wave of colonization could be observed at later stages of development. No indications were found that such a phenomenon takes place. It has to be noted that bursal tissue does not tolerate successive transplants as well as thymic tissue; some grafts were found to be healthy after 20 days in graft while others degenerated during the second transplantation period. In any case, no phenomenon analogous to the cyclic renewal of the thymus was demonstrated for the bursa.

Mechanisms of the seeding of the thymus and the bursa of Fabricius by HC

The data reported above suggested that the influx of HC into the PLR might be regulated by some type of chemotactic mechanism. This hypothesis, formulated some time ago (Le Douarin, 1978, 1979) and summarized in Fig. 5, prompted several series of experiments in which a traffic of LPC from a "colonized" PLR to a noncolonized PLR could be induced.

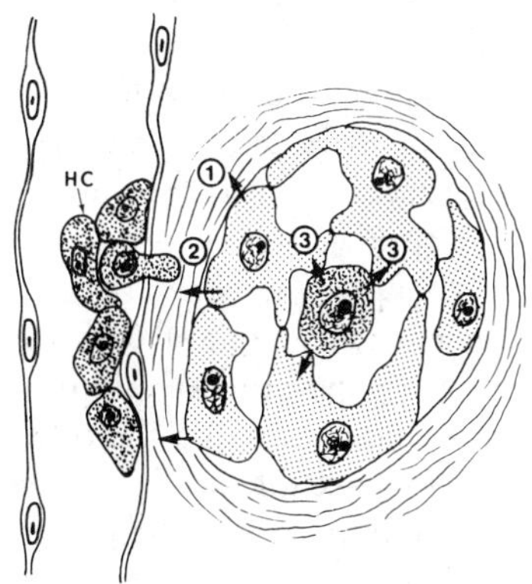

FIG. 5. *Hypothesis according to which a chemotactic mechanism could account for the seeding of primary lymphoid organs (here, the thymus rudiment) by lymphoid precursors. Three steps are proposed to explain the onset and the arrest of stem cell invasion. 1. Production of a diffusible "attractive" substance. 2. Invasion of the thymic rudiment by haemocytoblasts (HC). 3. Feedback inhibition of the production of the diffusible "attractive" substance by the haemocytoblasts.*

TABLE II

Number of quail bursa cells crossing the filter and found in the upper compartment of the culture 5, 10, 16 and 72 h after the onset of culture

	Type of culture[a]			
Duration (h)	*6·5-day Ch. Thymus 11-day Q. Bursa*	*6·5-day Ch. Liver 11-day Q. Bursa*	*6·5-day Ch. Meso. 11-day Q. Bursa*	*10-day Ch. Thymus 11-day Q. Bursa*
5 m	58·10 ± 9·20	3·33 ± 1·28	1·00 ± 0·35	
n	10	6	5	ND
C.V.	47·50%	86·3%	70·7%	
10	111·75 ± 50·5			
	4	ND	ND	NC
	78·2%			
16	268·33 ± 39·78	5·60 ± 2·39	2·50 ± 1·37	22·50 ± 8·17
	9	5	4	8
	41·9%	85·3%	95·2%	96·1%
72	432·00 ± 68·28	29·40 ± 7·43	30·00 ± 3·86	26·55 ± 6·53
	10	5	5	11
	47·4%	50·6%	25·7%	77·8%

[a] m = mean ± standard error; n = number of observations; C.V. = coefficient of variation in %; ND = not determined; Ch., Q = chick, quail; Meso. = mesonephros.

Transfilter experiments were performed in which the chick thymus was taken at day 6·5 of incubation and cultured on the upper side of a Nuclepore filter (Nuclepore, General Electric) with a 5 μm pore size, while an 11-day quail bursa was placed underneath the filter according to a method already described (Jotereau *et al.*, 1980). As controls, liver and mesonephros taken at day 6·5 of incubation and 10-day chick thymus were also confronted to the bursa. The number of quail cells which crossed the filter was counted after various periods (Table II).

It is clear that besides a random migration of cells which occurs in control cultures (including the already "colonized" 10-day chick thymus) the presence of 6·5-day thymus on the upper side of the filter induces a noticeable flow of quail cells from the bursa. Those were shown to be mostly composed of LPC since they differentiated into lymphocytes when the duration of the culture was protracted for 7–9 days or when the explant was transplanted into a 3-day chick host. In this case a mixed population of lymphocytes of quail and chick types developed in the organ, indicating that the cells coming from the bursa were not in sufficient number to make the thymus unreceptive. In consequence, chick host LPC entered the rudiment after the graft until the completion of the seeding process was achieved.

Another type of experiment also supports the "chemotactic" hypothesis. It consisted of grafting side by side in the chick somatopleure a quail organ supposed to contain HC ("donor explant") and a receptive thymus of the chick (taken at day 6·5 of incubation: "receptor" explant). (See Le Douarin, 1978 for details of the technique) (Table III).

TABLE III

Association in graft of various kinds of quail donor organs with 6·5-day chick thymuses. Chimaerism analysis was done after Feulgen-Rossenbeck's staining

Donor organ	*Number of grafts*	*Chimaeric thymuses*	%
Yolk sac	10	6	60
Bone marrow	4	3	75
Spleen	6	5	83
Thymus	10	6	60
Bursa	18	10	56
TOTAL	48	30	668

Results between groups are homogeneous: $\chi^2 = 1{\cdot}81$ for 4 degrees of freedom; $P > 0{\cdot}50$.

The results presented in Fig. 6 show that stem cells competent to home to a thymus rudiment are present in all the quail organs tested, i.e. the yolk sac (head process to 5 somites stage); the bone marrow (14 days); spleen (14 days); thymus (10 days); and bursa of Fabricius (11 days). However, the extent of the chimaerism within 14-day chick thymus is higher in associations with yolk sac and bone marrow than with bursa of Fabricius and thymuses. The former group of tissues either provide the receptive thymus with more

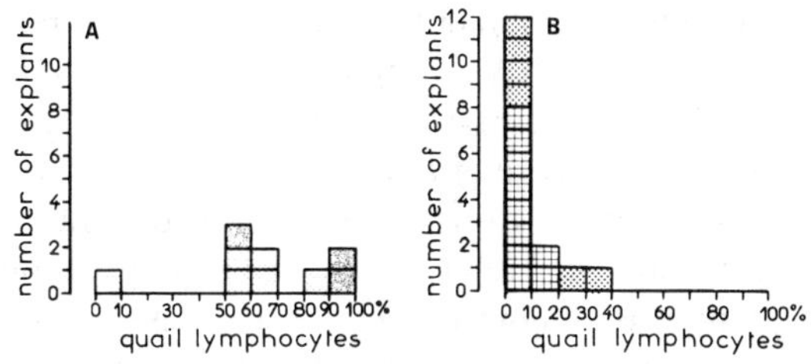

A: Bone marrow ▦ and yolk sac ☐; B: bursa of Fabricius ▦ and thymus ▦.

FIG. 6. *Distribution of percentages of quail lymphocytes counted in 6·5-day chick thymuses associated for 9 days in graft with several quail donor organs. Bone marrow and yolk sac provide the thymus with a larger contribution of lymphocytes than the primary lymphoid organs, bursa and thymus. The two distributions are highly different* ($\chi^2 = 20$ *for 1 degree of freedom,* P $< 0{\cdot}01$) (*Jotereau* et al., *1980*).

LPC or they contain stem cells with higher proliferation rates than the ones coming from the PLR. Investigations are presently in progress to answer this question.

In conclusion, these experiments, like those of Pyke and Bach (1979), support the hypothesis that the PLR actually produce an attractant which is responsible for their seeding by HC. They also show that once it has been seeded with a sufficient number of cells, it is no longer attractive for HC. Presumably the production of the chemotactic factor by epithelial cells has stopped.

The first step of stem cell seeding is very likely the adhesion of LPC to the endothelium of the blood vessels irrigating (for the bursa) or lining (for the thymus) the primary lymphoid organ rudiments. This phenomenon can be easily observed in normal embryos at the time of thymic colonization by LPC and also in the vessels irrigating a grafted thymic rudiment in the somatopleure. Similar processes of adhesion mediated by specific membrane molecules have been demonstrated to occur between lymphocytes and the specialized lymph node venules (Butcher *et al.*, 1979). This type of mechanism may be a general feature of the lymphoid (and possibly of the haemopoietic) system and could be an important aspect of the specific homing of circulating blood cells in the various compartments of the haemopoietic system. Confirmation of this hypothesis would require the identification of the factor(s) responsible for the attraction as well as their specific receptors on the LPC.

Analysis of the role of microenvironments in lymphocyte differentiation

One interesting aspect of the experiments described above is that they show that haemopoietic cells which have first colonized a bursal rudiment can then be induced to migrate into a thymus when the bursa is at a "postreceptive" and the thymus at a "receptive" period of development. It was therefore tempting to look at differentiation of LPC coming from the bursa and homing secondarily to a thymus. This was achieved in two different experimental systems. In one, 11-day quail bursas and 6·5-day chick thymuses were grafted side by side in the somatopleure of a 3-day host and the lymphocytes of the thymic explant were treated with an antibody raised in rabbit against quail thymocytes (see Jotereau *et al.*, 1980 for protocol of preparation of the serum). The thymic explant was removed from the host after 9-day engraftment. About 70% of the thymocytes were found to be fluorescent in these grafts whether they were of quail or of chicken type.

The second way to approach this question was to associate 11-day quail bursa and 6·5-day chick thymus in transfilter cultures as described earlier. The culture time was 7–9 days and the lymphoid cells present in the thymus were assayed with the antibody against thymocytes. In this case, most quail cells were found to bear thymic surface antigens. In contrast, in none of these experiments were cells with surface Igμ ever found in the thymus after either 10 days in graft or 7–9 days in culture.

It therefore appears that at day 11 of incubation in the quail, the bursa of Fabricius contains cells able to differentiate along the T cell pathway if they are transferred into the thymic environment. In addition, the ability of cells which have already homed to a bursa to migrate secondarily into a thymus shows that the HC respond to the signals arising from both bursal and thymic rudiments. This suggests that the HC responsible for the early seeding of the PLR are pluripotent rather than already committed towards just the T or the B cell lineages. However, one cannot consider this to be an undisputably demonstrated fact since alternative explanations are possible. Precommitted B and T cells could exist, as has been proposed by some authors (Weber and Mausner, 1977), provided that both cell types respond similarly to bursal and thymic attractive signals. The latter factors may actually be identical and, in such a case, the cells might leave the PLR if they happened to seed the microenvironment for which they were not precommitted. Such an interpretation is unlikely however for the following reason. Lymphoid rudiments (thymus or bursa), either in the course of, or just after their colonization by HC, were grafted into the somatopleure of a chick host and observed at regular intervals following the graft on serial sections stained according to the Feulgen–Rossenbeck's technique. Very few quail HC could be seen around the graft in the somatopleural mesenchyme or in the blood vessels. This means that a centrifugal movement of HC from the PLR to the periphery does not take place, as probably would happen if the hypothesis proposed above were true. Another possibility, however, is that pre T cells homed to the bursa finally die and vice versa.

It is interesting to notice that the chronological pattern of HC homing to the thymus and bursa shows that the two processes occur as successive events. No competition exists for stem cell seeding between thymus and bursa since the first colonization of the former is completed when the latter becomes receptive. And the second wave of HC inflow in the thymus seems to occur once homing of HC to the bursa ends (see Figs 1 and 3).

Another series of experiments supports our hypothesis that the cells which colonize the PLR are actually pluripotential or bipotential (i.e. lymphoid precursors able to differentiate along either the B or the T cell lineages). In previous experiments it was obvious that the mesenchyme and the endoderm of the bursa could not only not be seeded by HC and evolve separately, but, once seeded, could not retain the HC when grown apart either in graft or in culture. Maintenance of HC homing in these tissues appeared to be dependent upon tissue interactions occurring between the two initial components of the rudiment. It seemed therefore of interest to separate bursal mesenchyme and follicles by trypsinization of 14- to 16-day quail bursas or even 1-day post-hatching quails. Quail bursal mesenchyme and follicles contain at this stage numerous Ig positive cells, but also stem cells with a basophilic cytoplasm (unpub. data; Houssaint *et al.*, 1976). When confronted with a 6·5-day chick thymus in transfilter cultures, both mesenchyme and follicles provided the thymus with numerous quail cells. Their migration to the upper compartment of the system was very active from the onset of the culture and cells with the quail marker could be seen in the pores of the filter. After 8–9 days of explantation, about 50% of them bear T cell surface antigens but none was found to be Igμ positive. One can therefore conclude from these experiments that cells competent to differentiate along the T cell line are still present in the bursa around hatching time. Whether those are pluripotent uncommitted cells or reversibly committed B cells cannot be inferred from these observations. It would be most interesting to know whether cells bearing cytoplasmic or surface Ig can respond to thymus attraction and migrate through the filter. If not, this would strongly suggest that the cells which colonize the thymus belong to the pool of nondifferentiated HC contained in the bursa at the end of embryonic development.

Embryonic origin of the HC responsible for the colonization of the early thymic and bursic rudiments

According to the hypothesis of Moore and Owen (1965, 1967), intraembryonic haemopoietic organs are seeded by blood-borne stem cells originating in the yolk sac. In cultures of presomite mouse embryos deprived of yolk sac, normal development of the haemopoietic organs occurred, but no evidence of haematopoiesis or haemopoietic stem cell development was obtained. In contrast, cultures of presomite yolk sac showed marked erythropoiesis with increased numbers of colony-forming units—culture (CFU-C) and colony-forming units—spleen (CFU-S). On the other hand, in intact presomite embryos maintained *in vitro*, normal development of haemopoiesis occurred in both the intraembryonic organs and in the yolk sac (Moore and Metcalf, 1970; Moore and Johnson, 1976). In the avian embryo, suspensions of cells from the yolk sac were shown to be able to reconstitute the blood cell populations when they were injected into sublethally irradiated embryos (Moore and Owen, 1967c).

However, the idea that HC arise exclusively in the yolk sac was challenged recently by Dieterlen-Lièvre (1975; Dieterlen-Lièvre *et al.*, 1976), who grafted quail embryos onto chick yolk sacs in chick eggs at a stage preceding circulation. Vascular connections were rapidly established between embryo and yolk sac and, in successful grafts, normal quail embryos developed. Their haemopoietic organs were found to be predominantly—and even exclusively in most cases—colonized by quail HC. This indicates that haemopoietic foci able to provide haemopoietic stem cells exist inside the embryo and are probably responsible for the colonization of intraembryonic blood-forming organs in normal conditions. In Moore and Owen's experiments where yolk sac cells were injected into irradiated hosts, the cells were taken from 7-day-old embryos. At that stage, cellular traffic between intra- and extraembryonic stem cell compartments has occurred and, in view of Dieterlen-Lièvre's results, one wonders whether stem cells of intraembryonic origin were not solely responsible for the repopulation of intraembryonic haemopoietic organs.

In fact, there is structural evidence of haemopoietic processes in the embryo, and intraembryonic blood islands in the mesoderm of chick embryo were described long ago (see Le Douarin, 1966 for a review and Miller, 1913). These haemopoietic foci were especially associated with the developing lymphatic vessels. Extensive studies of these structures were recently performed by Dieterlen-Lièvre and Martin (in prep.) in both quail and chick embryos and also in yolk sac chimaeras. In the chick, haemopoietic foci were most prevalent within the dorsal mesentery at the level of the lung and in the neck at 6–9 days of development. Their sizes and positions varied extensively from one individual to another. In the quail, at the same period of development, they were mostly located close to the bifurcation of the canal of Cuvier. Significantly, in yolk sac chimaeras, where the intraembryonic foci were always composed of quail HC, circulating stem cells were all (or nearly all) of the chick type up to day 4 of development. It was only from 5–6 days that quail cells arising from the intraembryonic foci were peripheralized and seen in the bloodstream. The bursa and thymic rudiments are not receptive for stem cells until days 5 and 7 respectively. It is therefore easy to understand why in these embryos the thymus and bursal rudiments were colonized by quail cells.

Apparently, the pool of basophilic cells of yolk sac origin which are still in the bloodstream when the haemopoietic organs become receptive are incompetent to seed them. Most of them may in fact already be committed to the erythroid differentiation pathway. It therefore appears that yolk sac stem cells emerge, enter the circulation and then become exhausted within the first third of the incubation period.

Whether for a while in development yolk sac stem cells have multiple differentiation capabilities is a very crucial question. Several approaches to this problem have demonstrated that such is indeed the case. There have been investigations on the capacity of yolk sac stem cells to differentiate along various pathways *in vitro*, and after transplantation into irradiated recipients. Multipotential stem cells (CFU-S) and committed granulocyte–monocyte progenitor cells (CFU-C) are detectable in mouse yolk sac blood islands as early as days 7–8 of gestation, whereas they appear only at days 9–10 in the circulation and at day 10·5 in the foetal liver (Metcalf and Moore, 1971; Johnson *et al.*, 1976). Yolk sac cell suspensions transferred from normal embryos into syngeneic, lethally irradiated, adult recipients produce spleen colonies (Perah and Feldman, 1977; Metcalf and Moore, 1971).

In our avian system, yolk sac stem cells have been shown to be able to colonize a thymus anlage *in vitro* (Jotereau *et al.*, 1980) and also *in vivo* when a presomite yolk sac of quail was associated with a "receptive" chick thymus (Jotereau and Houssaint, 1977). In both cases there was a delay of 2–3 days before yolk sac cells colonized the thymus, whereas in other types of associations (with bursa of Fabricius, spleen or bone marrow) the movement of cells to the receptive thymus took place within hours. A similar difference in the behaviour of yolk sac and foetal liver cells was observed by Stutman (1976) using a kidney capsule grafting technique to study thymus colonization.

The capacity for yolk sac cells to generate B cells, T cells, myeloid cells and CFU-S in irradiated CBA/N recipients was recently demonstrated. The particular advantage of this strain of mice is that it has a genetically determined immunodeficiency restricted to certain functional B cell sets. This made it possible to enumerate carefully newly formed B cells. Yolk sac grafts were far less efficient than foetal liver in this model where even the equivalent numbers of stem cells (CFU-S) were transferred. It was suggested that a majority of the B cells formed in irradiated, grafted recipients derive from precommitted cells which are absent in yolk sac. Still to be excluded is the possibility that yolk sac stem cells are intrinsically different from their multipotential counterparts in foetal liver and adult marrow (Paige *et al.*, 1979).

Conclusions and discussion

The results that we have presented above show that the process of stem cell seeding of the primary lymphoid organs depends upon their "receptivity". The latter is very likely due to the production of substance(s) by the epithelial part of the rudiment to which the circulating haemopoietic cells are sensitive and respond by a migration along an increasing concentration gradient. A kind of feedback loop is suggested by the finding that entry of HC rather than the stage of the rudiment determines when the receptive period terminates. New cycles of attractions might be initiated when numbers of undifferentiated cells fall below some critical level. The homing process by itself seems to stop the production of the chemoattractant making the number of HC which have homed to an organ the factor which regulates its production.

Our studies of the quail thymus clearly demonstrate that receptivity for HC is a recurrent phenomenon which reappears periodically during ontogeny.

The progeny of each HC influx seems completely to replace the preceding one(s). This results in a periodical and complete renewal of the lymphocyte population of the thymus during embryonic and early postnatal life.

Certain of our observations address the question of the precommitment of HC which populate primary lymphoid organs. We were able to induce T lymphocyte development from cells from the embryonic bursa by allowing them to populate thymic rudiments. Assuming that there were destined originally to become B cells, they are at least bipotential. No doubt, monoclonal antibodies will be developed to an increasing number of structures on B and T cells and their precursors. Use of these to characterize more precisely the HC which populate the bursa and thymus should extend our understanding of the time in the genetic programme when the differentiation options become restricted.

Examples from neural development suggest that some differentiation events may be reversible. Bipotentiality and lability of determination have been demonstrated in the development of the nervous system and, more precisely, in the differentiation of the autonomic neurons. Environmental cues arising from nonneuronal embryonic tissues have actually been shown to influence the chemical differentiation of autonomic neuroblasts into either cholinergic or adrenergic neurons. In addition, reversibility from one to the other phenotype is inducible during a long period of development by monitoring the environmental factors (see Patterson, 1978 and Le Douarin, 1980a, b for reviews on this question).

Another question raised in this article that deserves some comment concerns the embryonic origin of the HC which colonize the intraembryonic organ and therefore constitute the pool of stem cells functioning throughout life. The analysis carried out in birds by using the quail–chick (and also the chick–chick) chimaera system (see Dieterlen-Lièvre, 1980) clearly demonstrates their intraembryonic origin. For the mammalian embryo, however, the question remains open. In the development of mammals, the haemopoietic activity of the yolk sac is very transitory in comparison with birds because of their adaptation to viviparity and the lack of vitellus in the egg. It is of primary importance to discover whether the HC of the yolk sac which do not participate in primitive erythropoiesis become peripheralized at the time when foetal liver, thymus, spleen and bone marrow become receptive. On the other hand, a careful analysis of possible intraembryonic blood island and their contribution to the stem cell pool of adults would be of great interest.

The question of heterogeneity of HC is also mentioned and the possible differences between those found within the embryo or in yolk sac suggests that maturational stages within the multipotential stem cell compartment may essentially be resolved.

References

Butcher, E., Scollay, R. and Weissman, I. (1979). *Nature* **280**, 496.

Dieterlen-Lièvre, F. (1975). *J. Embryol. Exp. Morph.* **33**, 607–619.

Dieterlen-Lièvre, F. (1980). *In* "XXVIIIth International Congress Physiological Sciences", Budapest. (In press.)

Dieterlen-Lièvre, F., Beaupain, D. and Martin, C. (1976). *Ann. Immunol.* (*Inst. Pasteur*) **127C**, 857–863.

Fathman, C. G., Small, M., Herzenberg, L. A. and Weissman, I. L. (1975). *Cell Immunol.* **15**, 109–128.

Glick, B. (1955). Ph.D. dissertation. Ohio State University, Columbus.

Höhn, E. O. (1956). *Can. J. Biochem. Physiol.* **34**, 90–101.

Houssaint, E., Belo, M. and Le Douarin, N. M. (1976). *Devl. Biol.* **53**, 250–264.

Johnson, G. R., Metcalf, D. and Wilson, J. W. (1976). *Immunology* **30**, 907–915.

Jotereau, F. and Houssaint, E. (1977). *In* "Developmental Immunobiology" (J. B. Solomon and J. D. Horton, eds), pp. 123–131. Elsevier/North Holland Biochem. Press, Amsterdam.

Jotereau, F. V., Houssaint, E. and Le Douarin, N. M. (1980). *Eur. J. Immunol.* (in press).

Kirkpatrick, C. M. and Andrews, F. N. (1944). *Endocrinology* **34**, 340–345.

Le Douarin, N. (1966). *Ann. Biol.* **5**, 105–171.

Le Douarin, N. (1969). *Bull. Biol. Fr. Belg.* **103**, 435–452.

Le Douarin, N. (1973). *Devl. Biol.* **30**, 217–222.

Le Douarin, N. M. (1978). *In* "Differentiation of Normal and Neoplastic Hematopoietic Cells", pp. 5–31. Cold Spring Harbor Lab., New York.

Le Douarin, N. M. (1979). *In* "Mechanisms of Cell Change" (J. E. Ebert and T. S. Okada, eds), pp. 293–326. John Wiley and Sons, New York.

Le Douarin, N. M. (1980a). *Nature* (in press).

Le Douarin, N. (1980b). *In* "Current Topics in Developmental Biology" (in press).

Le Douarin, N. and Houssaint, E. (1974). *C.R. Acad. Sci.* **278**, 2975–2978.

Le Douarin, N. and Jotereau, F. (1973). *C.R. Acad. Sci.* **276**, 629–632.

Le Douarin, N. and Jotereau, F. (1975). *J. Exp. Med.* **142**, 17–40.

Le Douarin, N., Bussonnet, C. and Chaumont, F. (1968). *Ann. Embryol. Morph.* **1**, 29–40.

Le Douarin, N. M., Houssaint, E., Jotereau, F. V. and Belo, M. (1975). *Proc. Acad. Nat. Sci.* **72**, 2701–2705.

Le Douarin, N. M., Michel, G. and Baulieu, E. E. (1980). *Devl. Biol.* **75**, 288–302.

Metcalf, D. and Moore, M. A. S. (1971). *In* "Haemopoietic Cells". North-Holland Publ. Co., Amsterdam.

Miller, A. M. (1913). *Am. J. Anat.* **15**, 131–198.

Moore, M. A. S. and Johnson, G. R. (1976). *In* "Stem Cells of Renewing Cell Populations" (A. Cairnie, P. Lala and D. Osmond, eds), pp. 323–330. Academic Press, New York and London.

Moore, M. A. S. and Metcalf, D. (1970). *Br. J. Haematol.* **18**, 279–296.

Moore, M. A. S. and Owen, J. J. T. (1965). *Nature* **208**, 956, 989–990.

Moore, M. A. S. and Owen, J. J. T. (1967a). *J. Exp. Med.* **126**, 715–723.

Moore, M. A. S. and Owen, J. J. T. (1967b). *Lancet* **ii**, 658–659.

Moore, M. A. S. and Owen, J. J. T. (1967c). *Nature* **215**, 1081–1082.

Paige, C. J., Kincade, P. W., Moore, M. A. S. and Lee, G. (1979). *J. Exp. Med.* **150**, 548–563.

Patterson, P. H. (1978). *Ann. Rev. Neurosci.* **1**, 1–17.

Perah, G. and Feldman, M. (1977). *J. Cell Physiol.* **91**, 193–200.

Pyke, K. W. and Bach, J. F. (1979). *Eur. J. Immunol.* **9**, 317–324.
Stutman, O. (1976). *Ann. Immunol.* (*Inst. Pasteur*) **127C**, 943.
Sugimoto, M., Yasuda, T. and Egashira, Y. (1977). *Devl. Biol.* **56**, 281–292.
Weber, W. T. and Maunser, R. (1977). *In* "Avian Immunology" (A. A. Benedict, ed.), pp. 47–59. Plenum Press, New York.
Weissman, I. L. (1967). *J. Exp. Med.* **126**, 291–304.
Weissman, I. L. (1973). *J. Exp. Med.* **137**, 504–510.

16

B Cell Development

J. J. T. OWEN

Department of Anatomy, Medical School, Birmingham, UK

Introduction

Any amount of B cell development should contain some discussion about certain commonly used terms which are applied to differentiating B cell types. I have chosen to begin with this topic because of its central importance to

Abbreviations
c μ cells: cells with low levels of cytoplasmic μ; sIg: surface immunoglobulin; CFU-S: colony forming unit-spleen.

an understanding of the subject. I will attempt to provide definitions of the terms used, noting how they relate to the assays employed. I will then try to review critically recent experimental evidence concerning structural and functional characteristics of mammalian B cell development. Many of these data have been obtained in rodents but studies on human material suggest that the broad conclusions are applicable to Man.

Multipotential stem cells

The continuous production of blood cells is thought to be based on a population of haemopoietic stem cells which are capable of self-renewal and maturation into all of the various blood cell types. Detection of these cells is still based on the spleen colony assay (Till and McCulloch, 1961). Individual (CFU-S) stem cells form discrete splenic nodules when grafted into lethally irradiated recipients, but no new lymphocytes are formed in these colonies. A recent report has claimed to demonstrate the differentiation of clonable B cells (i.e. B cells capable of proliferating to form colonies in agar) within spleen colonies derived from a single CFU-S stem cell (Lala and Johnson, 1978). However, in a system in which CBA/N immunodeficient mice, which lack clonable B cells, were used as recipients of normal cells, clonable B cells were found to be derived, not from donor CFU-S cells, but from other donor precursors (Paige *et al.*, 1979). In view of the superior design of the latter experiments, where recipients were chosen, which lacked any background clonable B cell activity, more weight must be placed on the results. Furthermore, in immunofluorescent studies, pre B cells have not been detected within spleen colonies (Owen, 1979).

It seems doubtful, therefore, whether B cells differentiate within spleen colonies and the only evidence which is available to relate spleen colonies to B cell differentiation is derived from experiments which have shown that spleen colonies contain cell precursors which can mature into B cells after transfer into irradiated hosts. The inadequacies of this data have been discussed by Abramson *et al.* (1977) and although these authors have provided some experimental data to support the role of multipotential stem cells in B cell differentiation, it must be concluded that evidence for a direct link between CFU-S stem cells and B cells is inconclusive.

Pre B cells

Attempts to identify more immediate precursors of B lymphocytes have been based on various assays. Unfortunately, the same term, pre B cell, has been applied to the cells identified in each instance. Since it is by no means certain that comparable cells are identified in each assay, considerable confusion has resulted. I will take this opportunity, therefore, to review briefly and evaluate critically the assays used. This information should be of value in assessing the results of experiments on pre B cells which are described in later sections.

Assays for pre B cells have been of 3 main types:

(a) Assays which measure the functional maturation of precursor cells *in vivo*: Lafleur *et al.* (1972a) grafted irradiated mice with various fractions of bone marrow cells separated by velocity sedimentation plus T cells. Antigen (sheep red blood cells) was injected at various times after grafting and plaque-forming cell responses were measured. Immunization of the recipients immediately after grafting was found to give the distribution of B lymphocytes in marrow, but if the grafted cells were allowed to differentiate for 7 days in recipients before immunization, a new profile of precursor activity was detected in a larger cell population. These larger cells which require a longer period for maturation than B cells were identified as pre B cells.

The main disadvantage of this assay is the fact that it takes little account of the ability of host B cells to participate in the result despite heavy irradiation. The fact that this may be a significant factor has been shown in the experiments of Pilarski and Cunningham (1975) and in those of Paige *et al.* (1979) where host B cell recovery after 1350 rads was demonstrated.

(b) Assays which measure the functional maturation of precursor cells *in vitro*: Melchers (1977) tested the ability of foetal liver pre B cells to mature *in vitro* into B lymphocytes which could then be detected by the fact that in the presence of mitogens they will differentiate into antibody secreting cells. The latter are demonstrated by a nonspecific plaque assay which enables all antibody forming cells to be identified. Limiting cell dilution assays can be used to estimate precursor cell frequency.

Although this method has obvious advantages over the *in vivo* assay in providing control over the environment in which cell maturation takes place and in eliminating host cell contributions, a disadvantage is that precursor cells are detected only indirectly after maturation and/or proliferation over an extended culture period. Thus, if B cells as well as pre B cells are present in the cell population under test, their contribution to the result can only be avoided by fractionating the cells so as to remove the small lymphocyte population. Of course, only large pre B cells are then demonstrated and there is a danger of applying the circular argument that all pre B cells are therefore large cells. In addition, if a proportion of pre B cells die during the culture period, their presence in the starting population will be missed.

(c) Immunofluorescence assays: Raff *et al.* (1976) used two-colour immunofluorescence to discriminate between B lymphocytes and pre B cells. Sequential staining for surface and cytoplasmic immunoglobulin with anti-μ antibodies conjugated with different fluorochromes showed that pre B cells have low amounts of cytoplasmic μ but lack surface μ (c μ cells). Thus they can be distinguished from B cells with surface Ig and from plasma cells which may contain large amounts of cytoplasmic μ. A major advantage of the assay is that it detects a variety of c μ cells, irrespective of size, without an intervening *in vivo* or *in vitro* maturation phase. On the other hand, the intensity of cytoplasmic fluorescence is low and suitable reagents and careful controls are required. In addition, the functional capabilities of the cells are not tested and a formal proof of their pre B nature has still to be obtained. However, their early appearance in ontogeny and presence in marrow favours this function.

In summary, various assays are available for the detection of pre B cells. It would be surprising if they all identified the same set of cells, although presumably the sets are overlapping. It is important, therefore, that when the term pre B cell is used, the assay employed for the detection of these cells is stated.

Primary sites of B lymphocyte differentiation

Although a number of early reports showed that B precursor cell activity could be demonstrated in various foetal organs, assays were carried out in irradiated recipients and sufficient time elapsed between cell injection and assay to allow differentiation of multipotential stem cells (Tyan and Herzenberg, 1968). More direct evidence for the differentiation of B lymphocytes within foetal organs was obtained by demonstrating the generation of B lymphocytes in organ cultures of foetal liver and foetal spleen removed at a stage of ontogeny before B lymphocytes had appeared (Owen *et al.*, 1974, 1975). There seems little doubt, therefore, that multifocal development of B lymphocytes occurs in ontogeny but foetal liver is probably the major B lymphopoietic site.

If an analysis of sites of pre B cell differentiation is made, the situation becomes more complex. Pre B cells as detected by immunofluorescence assays have been found in mouse foetal liver and in foetal blood as early as the eleventh day of gestation (Andrew and Owen, 1978). Functional *in vitro* assays have demonstrated pre B cells in placenta as early as the tenth day of gestation (Melchers, 1979). It is doubtful if 1 day's difference in gestation is significant, especially since it is not always clear how carefully gestation time is measured. The fact that pre B cells are detected in blood at these early stages means that it is impossible to define precisely the exact site of initial pre B cell differentiation; the cells found in liver and placenta might easily have migrated from some other source. It does seem, however, that yolk sac, although containing multipotential stem cells (Moore and Metcalf, 1970), is not a site of pre B cell differentiation. No pre B cells have been detected in yolk sac either before or after organ culture (Andrew and Owen, 1978).

In summary, B cell differentiation is multifocal in ontogeny but foetal liver is the major site of production prior to the takeover of activity of bone marrow in late foetal and postnatal life (Osmond and Nossal, 1974; Owen *et al.*, 1977).

Pre B cells

Kinetics

Most studies on pre B cell kinetics have been performed on bone marrow.

Osmond and Nossal (1974) used thymidine uptake studies to demonstrate a proliferating lymphocyte population in marrow. These cells were identified on a morphological basis alone, i.e. on their appearance as lymphocytes. Cells with sIg and so identified as B cells were found not to be proliferating. In a later study, Owen *et al.* (1977) identified the proliferating population as pre B cells on the basis of combined immunofluorescence and thymidine uptake studies. Indeed, the rate of entry of c μ cells into DNA synthesis was such that almost 30% of these cells were labelled within 5 h of radioactive thymidine injection. On the other hand, in agreement with the conclusions of Osmond and Nossal, B lymphocytes did not show rapid entry into DNA synthesis.

Although Lau *et al.* (1979), using a functional *in vitro* assay for bone marrow pre B cells, suggested that the shape of the velocity sedimentation profile for pre B cells is not consistent with a rapidly proliferating population, in a subsequent study using the same assay, Rusthoven and Phillips (1980) showed that hydroxyurea, a cycle specific drug which kills proliferating cells, had an immediate effect on marrow pre B cells but not on B cells.

In summary, at least a proportion of pre B cells are in active cell cycle. It seems likely that many of these proliferating B cell precursors are expressing cytoplasmic μ as demonstrated by immunofluorescence assays. Paige *et al.* (1979) have shown that normal marrow contains a population of cells which are neither multipotential stem cells nor B lymphocytes, which can proliferate and reconstitute the clonable B cell compartment of CBA/N mice. Although it is not known whether these precursor cells contain cytoplasmic μ, this data does support the notion that some pre B cells have considerable proliferative capabilities.

Size

In view of the proliferating nature of pre B cells it would not be surprising to find that they are heterogeneous in size. Cell size estimates based on velocity sedimentation studies and ocular micrometer measurements have confirmed this prediction (Owen *et al.*, 1976, 1977; Yoshida and Osmond, 1971). Pre B cells detected by immunofluorescence have cell diameters ranging from 6 to 16 μm. In functional studies, it has been concluded that pre B cells are predominantly large cells (Miller *et al.*, 1975; Lau *et al.*, 1979). However, in order to distinguish between pre B from B cell activities, velocity sedimentation techniques were used to separate large cells which could then be tested without contamination by small B cells. Thus, the small cell fractions could not be adequately examined for pre B activity. In addition, it is possible that only large pre B cells mature sufficiently slowly to be identified as B cell precursors in these assays; small pre B cells as identified by immunofluorescence may mature *in vitro* or *in vivo* quite rapidly.

In conclusion, pre B cells assayed by immunofluorescence are heterogeneous in size. However, it may be that only the larger pre B cells mature slowly over a period of days, and so will be identified by functional assays.

Immunoglobulin synthesis

There is general agreement that μ chains are synthesized by pre B cells but controversy has surrounded two issues namely (i) whether light (L) chains are synthesized as well and (ii) whether these molecules are expressed on the cell surface. For reasons that will be discussed later, both are important questions.

Immunofluorescence studies on pre B cells initially indicated that L chains as well as μ chains could be detected within the cell cytoplasm (Raff *et al.*, 1976). Studies on the biosynthesis of Ig within pre B cells using radioactive amino acids also suggested that both μ and L chains are synthesized (Melchers *et al.*, 1976). However, later immunofluorescence studies using the same reagents as before failed to detect L chains in pre B cells (Levitt and Cooper, 1980). Furthermore, these authors were also unable to demonstrate L chain synthesis in pre B cells by immunochemical analyses, in circumstances where L chains can readily be detected on newly formed B cells. The argument that pre B cells do not synthesize L chains has been strengthened by observations that hybridomas made from murine foetal liver cells and a non-producing myeloma variant synthesize μ chains only (Burrows *et al.*, 1979) and that a number of murine lymphoblastoid cell lines thought to be derived from pre B cells synthesize μ chains only (Bosset *et al.*, 1979; Siden *et al.*, 1979). Thus the balance of evidence suggests that murine pre B cells synthesize μ chains only. Some information is available to suggest that the same situation exists in human pre B cells (Levitt and Cooper, 1980), but not in rabbits where κ light chains have been shown to be allelically excluded (Hayward *et al.*, 1978).

With regard to the question as to whether or not Ig molecules are expressed in the surface of pre B cells, conflicting data is also available. Melchers *et al.* (1976) claimed that they could demonstrate IgM molecules in pre B cells after labelling with ^{125}I and lactoperoxidase. Rosenberg and Parish (1977) were able to use a rosetting technique to demonstrate IgM on early foetal liver cells and Lafleur *et al.* (1972b), using a functional *in vivo* maturation assay, were able to inactivate pre B cells with anti IgM antisera. On the other hand, immunofluorescence assays have suggested that μ chains are cytoplasmic in pre B cells (Raff *et al.*, 1976) and the development of pre B cells in organ cultures of foetal liver is not affected by the presence of anti μ antibodies, whereas the development of newly formed B cells expressing sIg is inhibited (Raff *et al.*, 1975). Levitt and Cooper (1980) have been unable to repeat the earlier observations showing ^{125}I labelling of surface Ig on pre B cells; instead, immunochemical analysis of murine foetal liver cells in culture showed that pre B cells secrete free μ chains rapidly into the culture medium. Perhaps, it was these secreted chains which were detected as surface Ig in earlier studies.

In conclusion, it is likely that pre B cells synthesize μ chains only and that these molecules are not inserted into the cell membrane. As Levitt and Cooper

(1980) have pointed out, the asynchronous synthesis of heavy (H) and L chains and the lack of surface expression of either during B cell development allows pre B cells to express a specific *H* gene without the external influence of antigen which might accompany the presence of a surface receptor. In addition, each member of a clone of B cells derived from a single pre B precursor expressing a particular V_H gene can select a different V_L gene for expression so contributing to the diversity of cells generated. Of course, this proposal begs the question as to whether or not V region sequences are expressed in pre B cells. This question is by no means settled although immunofluorescence data is available to suggest that c μ cells in human marrow express idiotypes (Kubagawa *et al.*, 1979).

Newly formed B cells

Assays

Just as a variety of assays has been designed to detect pre B cells, so a number of assays are used for identifying newly formed B cells. Immunofluorescence, radioisotope or rosetting techniques can be used to detect B cells in foetal tissues or adult bone marrow (Owen *et al.*, 1974; Osmond, 1979). Functional assays based on the ability of B cells to mature *in vitro* or *in vivo* into antibody secreting cells are also available. Thus *in vitro*, newly formed B cells can be stimulated by mitogens to differentiate into plasma cells giving a peak response at about 4 days' culture (Lau *et al.*, 1979). Transfer of newly formed B cells into lethally irradiated recipients has been used in various studies as an assay system for demonstrating the functional capability of virgin B cells. A modification of the more usual assay in which antibody forming cell progeny of the transferred cells are identified in whole spleen, is the splenic focus assay (Metcalf and Klinman, 1976). In this assay limiting cell dilutions are transferred to lethally irradiated, carrier primed recipients so that each of 48 fragment cultures of spleen derived from these animals contains one or no B cells specific for the hapten determinant used for *in vitro* stimulation. The culture fluids are then assayed for specific antihapten antibody.

In summary, caution is required in interpreting and comparing data derived from these varied assays. Identical cell populations are unlikely to be detected in each case.

Kinetics

Newly formed B lymphocytes show no DNA synthesis although they become labelled after tritiated thymidine infusion due to replacement from proliferating pre B precursors (Osmond and Nossal, 1974; Owen *et al.*, 1977). Thus, newly formed B cells are not in active cell cycle and they are rapidly replaced by new cells. The rate of production is considerable and it seems likely that many cells are short lived. Perhaps this apparent over-production is not surprising, if the generation of antibody specificities is dependent on pre B cell proliferation. In other words, a constant rate of new cell production may be required to ensure that the repertoire of specificities is always available to the individual.

Expression of V region genes

The notion expressed in the last section, namely that generation of the antibody repertoire may depend in large part on pre B cell proliferation, is only credible if newly formed B cells express distinct antibody specificities. Evidence that they do has been obtained in a number of studies. Assays which measure the antigen binding capability of cells have suggested that a broad repertoire of specificities is present as soon as B cells have been generated in foetal liver (Cohen *et al.*, 1977). Such studies are, however, open to the criticism that they do not measure functional ability to produce antibody. Studies designed to test the latter have suggested that the repertoire develops more gradually in terms of both specificity (Klinman *et al.*, 1976) and range of affinities (Goidl and Siskind, 1974). However, these studies employ transfer of foetal cells to irradiated recipients before function is tested and it may be argued that as a result, the complete repertoire is not examined.

It seems clear that the antibody repertoire is developed, at least in part, as soon as B cells appear. Recent studies employing organ culture of foetal liver in combination with the splenic focus assay have shown that not only are B cells specific for the hapten DNP present in foetal liver at 17 days gestation in the mouse embryo, but that DNP specific cells are detected at day 14 when only pre B cells are present (Teale and Mandel, 1980). This result suggests that distinct specificities are already developed at the pre B stage as discussed earlier. Furthermore, these studies showed that an increase in the frequency of clonable DNP precursors could be obtained in organ cultures of foetal liver, thus opening the way to experimental manipulations.

In summary, there is ample evidence to suggest that V region gene expression occurs at the level of newly formed B cells and probably at the level of pre B cells as well.

Tolerance

Recent experiments from a number of laboratories have indicated that newly formed B cells are extremely sensitive to tolerance induction (Nossal and Pike, 1978; Metcalf and Klinman, 1976; Cambier *et al.*, 1977; Elson, 1977). Most of these studies have been performed, at least in part, *in vitro*. However, Kay *et al.* (1980) have now shown that tolerance to the hapten fluorescein can be induced *in vivo* by much lower concentrations in newborn mice than in adult mice and that this effect is evident in nude mice and so is not dependent on T cell influences. Thus the ideas of Burnet (1957) and Lederberg (1959) suggesting clonal deletion as a mechanism of tolerance to self antigens are gaining recent experimental support. However, most of this work utilizes oligovalent antigens as tolerogens. It remains to be seen whether monovalent antigens have the same effect.

Another interesting finding which may relate to the observations above is the difference in behaviour between newly formed B cells and mature B cells in response to anti-Ig antibodies. The sIg on newly formed B cells is more readily "capped" by anti-Ig antibodies (Sidman and Unanue, 1975) and incubation of organ cultures of foetal liver with anti-Ig antibodies results in a complete suppression of sIg expression on developing B cells (Raff *et al.*, 1975). These observations suggest that there may be fundamental differences between the behaviour of mature and immature B cells and taken together with the studies in tolerance induction in immature cells, they emphasize the importance of further studies in this field.

Expression of C region genes

The concept of a switch in isotype synthesis within a single line of developing B cells, while retaining V region specificity, is now well known (Cooper *et al.*, 1976). There is general agreement that the first immunoglobulin isotype synthesized during ontogeny is IgM but there has been uncertainty about the order in which other isotypes follow. These problems are now being studied using cloned immunoglobulin DNA molecules and the results suggest that lymphocytes clones switch expression of C_H genes by successive gene deletions. This subject and the question of the functional significance of Ig isotype expressed on newly differentiated B cells are topics of considerable recent debate. Many questions, especially concerning the role of surface IgD (Kettman *et al.*, 1979), remain open and will be considered elsewhere in this volume.

B cell subsets

Although the general subject of B lymphocyte subsets is outside the scope of this paper, it is worth emphasizing the point that distinct B cell subsets may be formed during ontogeny at the earliest stages of B cell differentiation. Thus, in immunodeficient CBA/N strain mice, a subset of clonable B cells is absent from the embryo as well as from the adult (Kincade, 1977). Newly formed B cells express Fc receptors, Ia antigen and a proportion at least, express C3 receptors (Osmond, 1979). The extent to which these properties relate to maturation of function and/or define cell subsets is still a matter of debate.

Factors controlling B cell development

The factors (local or general) which may regulate the production of B cells remain unknown. An influence of environmental antigens has been suggested by the observations of reduced marrow lymphocyte production in germ-free animals (Osmond, 1979) and by the stimulatory influence of environmental antigens on "preprogenitor" B cells (Howard *et al.*, 1978). It seems most likely that there must be other regulatory influences but little progress has been made in defining them. A role for factors operating via cyclic nucleotides has been suggested in studies in which treatment of developing B cells with agents known to influence levels of intracellular cyclic AMP has been shown to produce phenotopic conversion of cells from Ia negative to Ia positive, from sIg negative to sIg positive and from C3 receptor negative to C3 receptor positive (Hammerling *et al.*, 1976). A recent novel idea is that during B cell development, pre B cells express idiotype-cross-reactive structures to which physiological mitogens bind and so trigger differentiation and proliferation (Forni *et al.*, 1979).

Summary

Despite the importance of the topic to basic problems of immunology, many questions regarding the development of B cells remain unanswered. The initial site(s) of primary differentiation of pre B cells during embryogenesis have not been defined nor have the factors which regulate their production. Although there is evidence to support the notion that pre B cells are in active cell cycle, the cell kinetics of B development requires further analysis.

Pre B cells produce μ chains and, although there is support for the notion that light chains are only synthesized and expressed at the sIg B cell stage, the matter requires further investigation. Likewise the fate of the synthesized μ chains in pre B cells, whether expressed on the surface or not, is an important topic for future work.

A substantial body of evidence supports the notion that newly formed B cells are more susceptible to tolerance induction by antigen than are mature B cells. The importance of this mechanism in the maintenance of the tolerant state to self antigens is an important subject for future work. The development of the antibody repertoire in terms of both specificity and isotype is intimately linked to studies on B cell development. It seems likely that rapid progress may be made in this area by the combination of molecular and cellular approaches.

To conclude, it is likely that answers to some of the basic issues of immunology will emerge from studies on B cell development.

References

Abramson, S., Miller, R. G. and Phillips, R. A. (1977). *J. Exp. Med.* **145**, 1567.
Andrew, T. A. and Owen, J. J. T. (1978). *Develop. Comp. Immunol.* **2**, 339.
Boss, M., Greaves, M. F. and Teich, N. (1979). *Nature* **278**, 551.

Burnet, F. M. (1957). *Aust. J. Sci.* **20**, 67.
Burrows, P., Le Jeune, M. and Kearney, J. F. (1979). *Nature* **280**, 838.
Cambier, J. C., Vitetta, E. S., Uhr, J. W. and Kettman, J. R. (1977). *J. Exp. Med.* **145**, 778.
Cohen, J. E., D'Eustachio, P. and Edelman, S. M. (1977). *J. Exp. Med.* **146**, 394.
Cooper, M. D., Kearney, J. F., Lawton, A. R., Abney, E. R., Parkhouse, R. M. E., Preud'homme, J. L. and Seligmann, M. (1976). *Ann. Immunol.* (*Inst. Pasteur*) **127C**, 573.
Elson, C. J. (1977). *Eur. J. Immunol.* **7**, 6.
Forni, L., Cazenave, P., Cosenza, H., Forsbeck, K. and Coutinho, A. (1979). *Nature* **280**, 241.
Goidl, E. A. and Siskind, G. W. (1974). *J. Exp. Med.* **140**, 1285.
Hammerling, V., Chin, A. F. and Abbott, J. (1976). *Proc. Natn. Acad. Sci. U.S.A.* **73**, 2008.
Hayward, A. R., Simons, M. A., Lawton, A. R., Mage, R. G. and Cooper, M. D. (1978). *J. Exp. Med.* **148**, 1367.
Howard, M. C., Fidler, J. M., Hamilton, J. and Shortman, K. (1978). *J. Immunol.* **120**, 911.
Kay, T. W., Pike, B. L. and Nossal, G. J. V. (1980). *J. Immunol.* **124**, 1579.
Kettman, J. R., Cambier, J. C., Uhr, J. W., Ligler, F. and Vitetta, E. S. (1979). *Immunol. Rev.* **43**, 69.
Kincade, P. W. (1977). *J. Exp. Med.* **145**, 249.
Klinman, N. R., Sigal, N. H., Metcalf, E. S., Pierce, S. K. and Gearhart, P. J. (1976). *Cold Spring Harbor Symp. Quant. Biol.* **41**, 165.
Kubagawa, H., Vogler, L. B., Capra, J. D., Conrad, M. E., Lawton, A. R. and Cooper, M. D. (1979). *J. Exp. Med.* **150**, 792.
Lafleur, L., Miller, R. G. and Phillips, R. A. (1972a). *J. Exp. Med.* **135**, 1363.
Lafleur, L., Underdown, B. J., Miller, R. G. and Phillips, R. A. (1972b). *Ser. Hematol.* **5**, 50.
Lala, P. K. and Johnson, G. R. (1978). *J. Exp. Med.* **148**, 1468.
Lau, C. Y., Melchers, F., Miller, R. G. and Phillips, R. A. (1979). *J. Immunol.* **122**, 1273.
Lederberg, J. (1959). *Science* **129**, 1649.
Levitt, D. and Cooper, M. D. (1980). *Cell* **19**, 617.
Melchers, F. (1977). *Eur. J. Immunol.* **7**, 476.
Melchers, F. (1979). *Nature* **277**, 219.
Melchers, F., Andersson, J. and Phillips, R. A. (1976). *Cold Spring Harbor Symp. Quant. Biol.* **41**, 147.
Metcalf, E. S. and Klinman, N. R. (1976). *J. Exp. Med.* **143**, 1327.
Miller, R. G., Gorczynski, R. M., Lafleur, L., MacDonald, H. R. and Phillips, R. A. (1975). *Transplant. Rev.* **25**, 59.
Moore, M. A. S. and Metcalf, D. (1970). *Br. J. Haematol.* **18**, 279.
Nossal, G. J. V. and Pike, B. L. (1978). *J. Exp. Med.* **148**, 1161.
Osmond, D. G. and Nossal, G. J. V. (1974). *Cell Immunol.* **13**, 132.
Owen, J. J. T. (1979). *In* B "Lymphocytes in the Immune Response" (M. Cooper, D. E. Mosier, J. Scher and E. S. Vitetta, eds), p. 63. Elsevier/North Holland.
Owen, J. J. T. (1979). *In* "Lymphocytes in the Immune Response" (M. Cooper, D. E. Mosier, J. Scher and E. S. Vitetta, eds), p. 71. Elsevier/North Holland.
Owen, J. J. T., Cooper, M. D. and Raff, M. C. (1974). *Nature* **249**, 361.
Owen, J. J. T., Raff, M. C. and Cooper, M. D. (1975). *Eur. J. Immunol.* **5**, 468.
Owen, J. J. T., Jordan, R. K., Robinson, J. H., Singh, U. and Willcox, H. N. A. (1976). *Cold Spring Harbor Symp. Quant. Biol.* **41**, 129.
Owen, J. J. T., Wright, D. E., Habu, S., Raff, M. C. and Cooper, M. D. (1977). *J. Immunol.* **118**, 2067.

Paige, C. J., Kincade, P. W., Moore, M. A. S. and Lee, G. (1979). *J. Exp. Med.* **150**, 548.
Pilarski, L. M. and Cunningham, A. J. (1975). *J. Immunol.* **114**, 138.
Raff, M. C., Owen, J. J. T., Cooper, M. D., Lawton, A. R., Megson, M. and Gathings, W. E. (1975). *J. Exp. Med.* **142**, 1052.
Raff, M. C., Megson, M., Owen, J. J. T. and Cooper, M. D. (1976). *Nature* **259**, 224.
Rosenberg, Y. J. and Parish, C. R. (1977). *J. Immunol.* **118**, 612.
Rusthoven, J. J. and Phillips, R. A. (1980). *J. Immunol.* **124**, 781.
Siden, E. J., Baltimore, D., Clarice, D. and Rosenberg, N. E. (1979). *Cell* **16**, 389.
Sidman, C. L. and Unanue, E. (1975). *Nature* **257**, 149.
Teale, J. M. and Mandel, T. E. (1980). *J. Exp. Med.* **151**, 429.
Till, J. E. and McCulloch, E. A. (1961). *Radiat. Res.* **14**, 213.
Tyan, M. L. and Herzenberg, L. A. (1968). *J. Immunol.* **101**, 446.
Yoshida, Y. and Osmond, D. G. (1971). *Blood* **37**, 73.

17

Generation and Propagation of Thymus-dependent Lymphocytes in Continuous Culture:

Characterization of cloned populations bearing cell surface glycoproteins of immature and mature cells sets within the thymus-dependent lineage

GARY NABEL, MANUEL FRESNO, LAILA McVAY-BOUDREAU, ALEC CHESSMAN, RANDY BUCALO and HARVEY CANTOR

Department of Cell Biology and Pathology, Harvard Medical School and Farber Cancer Institute, Boston, Massachusetts, USA

Abbreviations
BM: bone marrow; C: centigrade; CCM: complete conditioned medium; CFU-C: colony forming units-culture; CFU-S: colony forming units-spleen; CE: cloning efficiency; Ci: curie; CM: conditioned medium; con A: concanavalin A; ^{51}: Crchromium-51; DME: Dulbecco's modified Eagles media; DMSO: dimethyl sulphoxide; FACS: fluorescence activated cell sorter; FCS: foetal calf serum; FL: foetal liver; HCl: hydrochloric acid; ^{3}H-T: ^{3}H-methylthymidine; Ig: immunoglobulin; IL-II: interleukin-II; 2ME: 2-mercaptoethanol; MEM: minimum essential media; mM: millimolar; mol. wt: molecular weight; N_2: nitrogen; NK cells: natural killer cells; PAS: periodic acid-Schiff; pp IL-II: partially purified interleukin II: SRBC: sheep red blood cells; R: rads; TdT: terminal deoxynucleotidyl transferase; μ: micron; μg: microgram.
Supported by: NIH Grants #5 T32 GM07753–01, AI–12184, AI–13600.

Introduction

Mammalian lymphocytes are divisible into 2 major classes. One class requires the presence of an intact thymus gland for normal maturation (T cells) while a second class (B cells), develops elsewhere. Fully differentiated T cells and B cells both carry, at their membrane surface, receptor molecules capable of binding to different chemical determinants, and are responsible for initiating specific immunologic responses. Recently neoplastic clones of B cells (myeloma cells) have been used to analyse the genes that govern immunoglobulin synthesis, with particular emphasis on genetic mechanisms that might account for immunoglobulin diversity (Sakano *et al.*, 1979; Schilling *et al.*, 1980; Seidman and Leder, 1978).

Thymus-dependent lymphocytes have several features that make them a more attractive model for analysis of genetic mechanisms that govern cellular differentiation. First, glycoproteins expressed at the surface of cells within the thymus-dependent lineage have been identified using both conventional and monoclonal antibodies (Cantor and Boyse, 1977). Many of the genes coding for these glycoproteins have been precisely mapped, and are expressed exclusively on cells undergoing thymus-dependent differentiation. Assessment of the immunologic function of several mature T cell populations, each carrying unique molecular labels at their membrane surface, has demonstrated that each is specialized to carry out a particular immunologic activity (Cantor and Boyse, 1977).

These glycoproteins have also been used to partially delineate several immature cell types that represent early stages of thymus-dependent differentiation. This analysis has indicated that stem cells migrate from yolk sac and liver in the embryo (Owen and Ritter, 1969) and from bone marrow in the adult (Ford *et al.*, 1966) into the thymus where they differentiate to thymocytes (Owen and Raff, 1970); one result of intrathymic differentiation is the export of different T cell sets that are specialized to mediate one or another immunologic activity (Cantor and Boyse, 1977).

Although this approach has successfully delineated cells at different stages of thymus-dependent maturation, analysis of each of these populations has been difficult. First, many cell types are difficult to isolate and expand to significant numbers in long term *in vitro* cultures. Second, mature T lymphocyte sets that carry distinctive cell surface glycoprotein markers often do not represent homogenous populations, and thus are liable to confound biochemical analysis.

We describe here a general method for producing cloned populations of cells bearing surface glycoproteins found at different stages of thymus-dependent differentiation. The procedure does not require hybridization to tumour cells. We reasoned that expression of receptors for a T cell specific growth factor (Gillis *et al.*, 1978) might be part of the genetic programme of all cells within the thymus-dependent lineage, including precursor populations; therefore, this growth factor might selectively stimulate proliferation of these cells from a heterogeneous cell population. In addition, particular types of irradiated cells monolayers are necessary to initiate efficient clonal growth of cells at different stages of thymus-dependent differentiation. This approach has resulted in the production, *in vitro*, of cloned populations that are stable with respect to expression of unique patterns of cell surface glycoproteins, histochemical reactions, and immunologic function and can be expanded in culture to numbers $> 10^8$. These cell populations represent a unique source of material for biochemical analysis of the cellular events required to generate specialized cellular progeny from precursor populations and, in some cases, the specialized differentiated functions of these cells.

Materials and methods

Animals

C57BL/6 "B6" (T lymphocyte surface phenotype: Ig^-, Lyb-2·2^-, TL^-, Thy-1·2^+, NK^+, Ly-1·2^+, Ly-2·2^+, 5·1) BALB/c and B6-Thy-1·1 mice were obtained from the Jackson Laboratory, Bar Harbor, ME. The congenic inbred mouse strains: B6-Ly-5·2, B6-Ly-1·1, B6-TL^+, B6-Ly-2·1, B6-Lyb-2·1, were kindly provided by Dr E. A. Boyse from Memorial Sloan-Kettering Research Center.

Antisera

The production and use of antisera specific for Ly-1·2, Ly-2·2 (Shen *et al.*, 1975) Ly-5·1 (Komuro *et al.*, 1975) TL (Boyse *et al.*, 1969) and Lyb-2 (Sato and Boyse, 1976) have been previously described. With the possible exception of Lyb-2, each of the genes for these antigens is expressed as one of the two alternative alleles in all inbred mouse strains that have been studied. These antisera were kindly provided by Dr F. W. Shen. The following monoclonal antibodies were used: αThy-1·2 was the generous gift of Dr Ed Clark; Ly-1 was provided by Drs J. Ledbetter and L. Herzenberg; αLy-2·2 was the generous gift of Dr F. Fitch, and αQat-5 was produced by Dr U. Hammerling. Antiserum specific for the enzyme terminal deoxynucleotidal transferase (anti-TdT) was purchased from Bethesda Research Laboratories, Bethesda, MD. The specificity of this antiserum was confirmed using a biochemical assay, kindly performed by Dr W. McCaffrey.

Analysis of cell surface antigens

Specificity of antibody reactions against cell-surface antigens using immunofluorescence To ensure specificity of the antisera used for immunofluorescence, each antiserum was divided into 2 aliquots and incubated at a final dilution of 1:5 with an equal volume of lymphoid cells (thymocytes, bone marrow cells and spleen cells) at 4° C × 20 min. One aliquot was incubated with cells from B6 mice expressing the relevant gene product at the cell surface. The second aliquot was incubated with cells from a congenic inbred "partner" strain that differs only at the gene locus coding for the relevant cell surface marker glycoprotein. The comparison of immunofluorescence of the antiserum after absorption with cells obtained from these congenic mouse pairs provides a stringent test of specificity. In addition, with the exception of αLyb-2 and αLy-5·1 antisera, the reactions were verified using appropriate monoclonal antibodies.

Measurement of fluorescence

After incubation of cells with monoclonal or conventional antibodies, the cells were washed ×2 and incubated ×20 min at 4° C with a rabbit anti-immunoglobulin conjugated to fluorescein. A fluorescence activated cell sorter (FACS) was used to measure intensity of fluorescence.

Analysis of cell surface glycoprotein by complement fixation: anti-Ly-5·1

This antisera recognizes 2 cell populations: one is detected by antibodies that fix complement and lyse the cell. These cell populations include so-called natural killer cells, thymocytes and a portion of peripheral T cells but do *not* include cells that give rise to CFU-S or CFU-C (Komuro *et al.*, 1975; Michaelson *et al.*, 1979; Lemke *et al.*, 1979; Minato *et al.*, in press). Therefore reactions with this antiserum were monitored by the release of a radioactive label, ^{15}Cr, from lysed cells in the presence of complement rather than by immunofluorescence. A cell population was considered positive if >90% lysis occurred.

Surface antigens expressed on different cell sets in heterogeneous populations

Patterns of cell surface glycoproteins expressed on selected T cell sets within heterogeneous cell populations have been defined using the above techniques. The following surface glycoprotein patterns are associated with populations belonging to early stages of differentiation within the thymus-dependent lineage:

(1) Immature (pre-thymic) cells: Ig$^-$Lyb-2$^-$/Thy-1$^-$TL$^-$Ly-1$^-$2/Ly-5$^+$Qat-5$^+$NK-1$^-$Tdt$^-$/Qat-5$^+$Ly-5$^+$ (Cantor and Boyse, 1977; Boyse *et al.*, 1969; Silverstone *et al.*, 1978). These cells do not give rise to CFU-S, CFU-C or B cell colonies, but are present on cells within the T cell lineage (Komuro *et al.*, 1975; Michaelson *et al.*, 1979; Minato *et al.*, in press).

(2) Immature thymocytes: Ig$^-$Lyb-2$^-$/TL$^+$Thy-1$^+$2$^+$/Ly-5$^+$Qat-5$^+$ NK-1$^+$/Tdt$^+$ or Tdt$^-$ (Cantor and Boyse, 1977; Boyse *et al.*, 1969; Silverstone *et al.*, 1978).

(3) Natural killer (NK) cells: Cell populations that mediate this activity express two sets of surface glycoprotein patterns (Glimcher *et al.*, 1977; Herberman *et al.*, 1975b; Kasai *et al.*, 1979).

(a) Ig$^-$Lyb-2$^-$/Thy-1$^-$TL$^-$Ly-1$^-$2$^-$/Ly-5$^+$Qat-5$^+$NK-1$^+$/TdT

(b) Ig$^-$Lyb-2$^-$/Thy-1$^+$TL$^-$Ly-5$^+$Ly-1$^-$2$^-$/Ly-5$^+$Qat-5$^+$NK-1$^+$ TdT (Seidman and Leder, 1978; Cantor and Boyse, 1977; Michaelson *et al.*, 1979; Glimcher *et al.*, 1977; Herberman *et al.*, 1975b; Kasai *et al.*, 1979).

'ell culture

Preparation of conditioned media (CM) and cell culture conditions for initiation of clonal growth and expansion of cloned cells are described in detail elsewhere (Nabel et al., *in press).*

Preparation of partially purified T cell growth factor

Interleukin-II was obtained after incubation of spleen cells with con A using culture conditions described earlier (Nabel *et al.*, in press) but in the absence of FCS. IL-II in supernates was partially purified (pp IL-II) after ammonium sulphate (80%) precipitation, followed by Sephadex G-100 column chromatography. The ability of this material to support cell growth was measured according to a ^{3}H-methylthymidine (^{3}H-T) incorporation assay.

Use of supernatant material of cloned inducer T cells to support cell growth

Ly-1-D9·1 is a cloned population of T cells expressing the Thy-1^{+}Ly-1^{+}2^{-} surface glycoprotein pattern. This clone has been grown in CCM at concentrations of 0·5–3 × 10^{5}/ml in continuous culture for 10 months. Supernatant material was filtered through a 0·22 μ Swinnex filter after incubation of 5 × 10^{5} Ly-1-D9·1 cells/ml in DME-4% FCS × 24 h at 37° C in a humidified atmosphere. The fraction of supernatant material supporting long-term cell growth had an apparent mol. wt of 30 000 as determined by Sephadex G-100 column chromatography.

'reincubation

In some cases, cells were incubated in CCM × 7–10 days before initiation of the cloning procedure. These cells were incubated at 10^{6}/ml for the first 2–3 days and subsequently maintained at concentrations of 5 × 10^{4}–3 × 10^{5}/ml.

Preparation of selected heterogeneous lymphoid populations

Ly-1^{+}2^{-} spleen T cells were obtained as follows: single cell suspensions from spleen were incubated on rabbit α mouse Ig coated plates to remove Ig^{+} cells (Mage *et al.*, 1977) and incubated with anti-Ly-2·2 (5 × 10^{7} cells/ml) × 1/2 h at 4°, followed by 40 min incubated with anti-Ly-2·2 (5 × 10^{7} cells/ml) × 1/2 h at 4°, followed by 40 min incubation with selected rabbit complement at 37° C as described previously (Shen *et al.*, 1975). Contamination of these cells by B cells was assessed by enumerating (a) Ig^{+} cells in the initial population and (b) cells secreting Ig after incubation × 5 days at 37° C *in vitro*. In most experiments, the initial cell population was <5% Ig^{+} and, after incubation *in vitro* × 5 days, did not contain any Ig secreting cells. Purified B cells were obtained by incubating spleen cells with αLy-1·2, αLy-2·2 and monoclonal anti-Thy-1·2

× 30 min at room temperature before incubation with rabbit complement at 37° C × 40. To ensure depletion of all T cells, this treatment was followed by incubation of remaining cells with monoclonal anti-Thy-1·2 and rabbit complement at 37° C for 30 min. These cells did not secrete significant amounts of Ig *in vitro*, unless small numbers of purified T cells were added at the onset of incubation.

Stimulation of lymphocytes *in vitro*

Activation of immunoglobulin secretion

A modification of the cell culture technique of Mishell and Dutton (1967) was used to induce B cells to secrete immunoglobulin. Briefly, 10^6 nonimmune B cells, or Ly-1 cells (2×10^5) plus B cells (8×10^5), were incubated in 0·2 ml of modified DME media supplemented with 4% FCS, glutamine and 5×10^{-5} M 2-mercaptoethanol (2ME) × 4 days.

Enumeration of Ig secreting cells

Ig secreting cells were enumerated using a modification of a haemolytic plaque assay that has been described in detail (Molinaro *et al.*, 1974; Strelkauskas *et al.*, 1976): 25 μl of a 12% suspension of horse erythrocytes (which were coated with rabbit-antimouse Fab_2 and 25 μl of lymphocytes from the cell culture were pipetted into 12 × 75 mm glass test tubes containing 450 μl of a 0·8% solution of Sea-plaque agarose (Maine colloids, Rockland, ME) in special balanced salt solution (SRSS). The tubes were mixed and layered over 2 ml of gelled 1% Sea kem agarose (Maine colloids) in a 30 × 10 mm Petri dish. After incubation × 1 h at 37° C in a humidified atmosphere containing 5% CO_2, 0·35 ml of rabbit-antimouse Fab_2 developing sera (final dilution 0·05 mg/ml in SBSS) was pipetted onto the Petri dishes. After an additional incubation for 1 h at 37° C, 0·34 ml of reconstituted guinea-pig complement (Grand Island Biological Co.) diluted 1:10 was added. Plaques were enumerated 2 h later.

Assay of cell proliferation

10^6 cells were incubated in 0·1 ml CCM at 37° C in flat-bottom wells of a 96-well microtitre plate (Falcon plastics 3040). Wells were pulsed daily with 0·2 or 1 μCi ^{3}H-methylthymidine (20 Ci/mM, New England Nuclear, Boston, MA) overnight before harvesting. Data is expressed as the arithmetic mean of cts/min as detected by liquid scintillation counting of triplicate cell cultures.

"Natural killer" (NK) assay

Lysis of the YAC-1 lymphoma, an NK sensitive tumour (Kiessling *et al.*, 1975a, b) (35% specific kill at effector: target ratio of 1:1) and lack of lysis against the RL-12 lymphoma, an NK resistant tumour, was used to define

NK activity. Briefly, 2×10^4 ^{51}Cr-labelled YAC-1 lymphoma cells were incubated in MEM + 10% FCS alone or with various cloned cell populations × 3·5 h at 37° C in a humidified atmosphere of 95% air and 5% CO_2 according to the method of Glimcher *et al.* (1977). The amount of γ radioactivity released from triplicate was measured. Cytotoxicity is expressed as % specific lysis according to the formula

$$\% \text{ lysis} = \frac{\text{experimental release-spontaneous release}}{\text{maximal release (HCl)-spontaneous release}} \times 100$$

Karyotype

Cells were incubated with colcemid (GIBCO, Grand Island, New York) (0·1 μg/ml for 45 min at 37° C) and processed according to the method of Moorhead *et al.* (1960), substituting 0·075 M KCl for distilled water during hypotonic lysis.

Cryopreservation

Cloned cells can be frozen in liquid N_2 and thawed with complete recovery of growth and immunologic function, using a modification of Lionetti *et al.* (1978). Cells were pelleted and resuspended in a 2 ml provial (Cooke 235–1) with 0·5 ml of cold FCS at 10^6 cells/ml. An equal volume of media containing cold FCS, 10% DMSO and 12% hydroxyethyl starch was added dropwise to the provial immersed in ice. Cells were frozen in a controlled cooling chamber (Union Carbide Biological Freezer) at a rate of −1° C/min. At −50° C; they were transferred for storage in liquid N_2. To recover cells, provials were quickly thawed, transferred to test tubes, diluted dripwise with cold DME, and washed × 3. The cells were then dispersed into microtitre plates (Falcon 3040) containing 8×10^5 irradiated (1500 R) spleen cells at a final concentration of 1–2 × 10^5 cells/ml in 0·15 ml of CCM. Medium was changed daily. When colonies were observed (2–10 days), cells were expanded as described above.

Results

Generation of cloned populations that express differentiated function

Distribution compared with heterogeneous sets (*Table I*)

Cloned cells expressing inducer activity

All Thy-1$^+$Ly-1$^+$2$^-$ cloned populations tested (total of 5) augmented the secretion of immunoglobulin by B cells 10–100 fold. Cloned cells expressing the Ly-1$^+$2$^+$ or Ly-1$^-$2$^+$ surface phenotype did not (Table II).

Cloned cells expressing inhibitory activity

All Thy-1$^+$Ly-1$^-$2$^+$ cloned populations suppressed Ig secretions. A portion

TABLE I

Expression of different Ly glycoproteins on heterogeneous spleen

Cell populations	Thy-1+ Ly-1+2−	Thy-1+ Ly-1+2+	Thy-1+ Ly-1−Ly-2+	Thy-1+ Ly-1−2−
	T cells and colonies derived from this population	*Surface phenotype (% positive)*		
Ig− Spleen cells	25	40–50	5–10	10–20
Colonies derived from Ig− spleen cells	20	46	13	20

The proportion of cells within heterogeneous spleen T cell population expressing different Ly glycoproteins was determined by immunofluorescein on the FACS-I (see Materials and methods): 15 colonies derived from this starting population were similarly tested for expression of different Ly surface glycoproteins.

TABLE II

Cloned populations expressing the Ly-1$^+$2$^-$ phenotype

	No. of cloned cells/culture ($\times 10^4$)	*Immunologic function — No. of immunoglobulin-secreting cells in culture after incubation with:* B cells	Ly-1 cells + B cells
Expt 1	0	320 ± 29	2520 ± 197
	1	3040 ± 413	4240 ± 357
	5	4680 ± 423	4280 ± 482
Expt 2	0	500 ± 72	7400 ± 592
	2	2600 ± 210	8300 ± 913
	5	5600 ± 632	7232 ± 774

Isolated B cells or mixtures of Ly-1 and B cells were incubated × 4 days *in vitro* with increasing numbers of cloned Ly-1$^+$2$^-$ cells. The number of Ig-secreting B cells was then enumerated. This activity of Ly-1-D-9·1 is representative of the activities of 4 other Ly-1$^+$2$^-$ clones.

(4/7) of Ly-1$^+$2$^+$ clones, the surface phenotype associated with precursors of suppressive cells also inhibited secretion of Ig. By contrast, none of the 5 Ly-1$^+$2$^-$ clones suppressed the response (Tables III, IV).

Cloned cells expressing natural cytolytic activity (Table V)

Spleen cells from nonimmune mice (or blood lymphocytes from humans) can lyse or damage a variety of target cells, notably malignant cells, *in vitro*, and have been termed natural killer (NK) cells (Kiessling *et al.*, 1975a, b; Greenberg and Playfair, 1974; Herberman *et al.*, 1975). This activity is independent of antibody and complement and does not reflect conventional phagocytic activity. Cells responsible for this reaction are said to resemble small lympho-

TABLE III

Cloned populations expressing the Ly-1$^-$2$^+$ phenotype

	No. of cloned cells/culture ($\times 10^4$)	Immunologic function: No. of immunoglobulin secreting cells after incubation of: Ly-1 + B cells	B cells
Expt 1	0	7233 ± 770	2100 ± 452
	2	7100 ± 640	n.d.
	5	1600 ± 173	1600 ± 321
Expt 2	0	2601 ± 302	500 ± 221
	2	2408 ± 133	n.d.
	5	799 ± 98	800 ± 133

Immunologic function of Cl.Ly-1$^-$2$^+$/6: immunoglobulin secretion was detected using the haemolytic plaque assay described. Ly-1 cells + B cells or B cells alone were incubated × 4 days *in vitro* in the presence or absence of the indicated numbers of cloned cells. This activity is representative of the activity of 3 additional Ly-1$^-$2$^+$ clones.

TABLE IV

Cloned populations expressing the Ly-1$^+$2$^+$ phenotype

	No. of cloned cells/culture ($\times 10^4$)	Immunologic function: No. of immunoglobulin secreting cells after incubation of: Ly-1 + B cells	B cells
A. *Clone Ly-1$^+$2$^+$-B-12*			
Expt 1	0	7233 ± 940	1600 ± 192
	1	12600 ± 1285	1100 ± 198
Expt 2	0	1133 ± 181	500 ± 65
	1	1000 ± 150	700 ± 56
B. *Clone Ly-1$^+$2$^+$-D-11*			
Expt 1	0	1476 ± 221	390 ± 35
	10	260 ± 13	104 ± 13
Expt 2	0	5700 ± 456	3000 ± 302
	0·2	2600 ± 364	n.d.
	10	1600 ± 96	550 ± 61

Immunologic function of 2 representative Ly-1$^+$2$^+$ clones (a total of 7 were tested) are shown: A. Cl. Ly-1$^+$2$^+$-12 and B. Cl. Ly-1$^+$2$^+$-11. Immunoglobulin secreting B cells were enumerated after 4 days *in vitro* incubation in the presence of Ly-1 cells (as a source of inducer activity) or in their absence. Two patterns of activities were observed: 3 of 7 Ly-1$^+$2$^+$ clones expressed the regulatory properties of Cl. Ly-1$^+$2$^+$-12 while two were similar to Cl. Ly-1$^+$2$^+$-11.

TABLE V

Cytolytic activity against YAC-1 and RL-12

	Lymphoma target cells % Specific lysis YAC-1 lymphoma target Effector: target ratio				R12 lymphoma target Effector: target ratio
Source of cells tested:	*50 : 1*	*12·5 : 1*	*6·25 : 1*	*·5 : 1*	*6·25 : 1*
Spleen	29	10	< 1	< 1	0
$Ig^-Ly\text{-}5^+$ fraction of spleen	n.d.	28	14	< 1	0
Clone NK-2 ($Thy\text{-}1^+Ly\text{-}1^-2^-5^+$)	n.d.	39	40	28	0
Clone FL-1 ($Thy\text{-}1^-Ly\text{-}1^-2^-5^+$)	n.d.	0	0	0	0
Clone BM-I-1 ($Thy\text{-}1^-Ly\text{-}1^-2^-5^+$)	n.d.	0	0	0	0

Heterogeneous cell populations from spleen and the $Ig^-Ly\text{-}5^+$ fraction of spleen cells were prepared as previously described (Kasai *et al.*, 1979). Cloned population NK-2 was derived by positive selection from spleen cells; FL-1 clone was derived from foetal liver; BM-I-1 clone was derived from a colony from bone marrow cells. All populations were tested for cytolytic activity against the NK sensitive YAC-1 lymphoma and the NK resistant RL-12 lymphoma.

cytes morphologically, and are found mainly in spleens of young animals. Numerous studies have indicated that this cell set represents an immature cell within the thymus lineage (Minato *et al.*, in press; Herberman *et al.*, 1978), although the possibility that at least a portion of NK cells represents monocyte/macrophage precursors has not been ruled out. The surface phenotype of cells carrying NK activity in heterogeneous spleen cell populations is TL^-, $Ly\text{-}1^-2^-Ig^-Ly\text{-}5^+Qat\text{-}5^+NK\text{-}1^+$ and a substantial fraction may also express Thy-1 (Minato *et al.*, in press). Cells mediating NK activity were enriched from heterogeneous spleen cell suspensions before initiation of the cell growth in cultures containing irradiated spleen cell monolayers. Cloning efficiency of cells that (a) expressed the NK glycoprotein pattern and (b) expressed lytic (NK) function, was 27%. Lytic activity of cloned NK cells was 100-fold more potent than unselected spleen cell populations. Cl.NK/11 was also tested for its ability to lyse several cellular targets. Lysis (≥50%) was seen at effector to target rations of less than 1 (Table V). Conventional targets YAC-1 and MBL2 lymphomas were susceptible. In addition, P815 mastocytoma and EL-4 lymphoma cells, targets of activated NK cells, were also lysed. Syngeneic LPS-activated B lymphocytes were very susceptible to NK lysis (>50% lysis at E/T = 1); con A activated T lymphocytes, thymocytes and bone marrow cells were relatively resistant. No activity was observed against an NK resistant radiation-induced lymphoma (R12) or the K562 erythroleukaemia, a human NK target cell.

Cl.NK/11 mediates antibody-dependent cellular cytotoxicity

In heterogeneous populations, cells which mediate antibody dependent cellular cytotoxicity (ADCC) express the same cell surface glycoproteins as NK cells. To test whether a cloned population bearing this glycoprotein pattern could mediate both activities, Cl.NK/11 was incubated in the presence of antibodies to mouse lymphocytes and the NK-resistant lymphoma RL-12. Addition of this antibody resulted in 50% lysis at effector:target ratios of 1:1. No lysis was observed in the absence of antibody or in the presence of antibodies directed against an irrelevant target (data not shown).

Generation of cloned populations at early stages of lymphocyte differentiation (Table VI)

TABLE VI

Cloning efficiency of immature and mature cells within the thymus-dependent lineage

Source of irradiated cell-monolayer:	*Source of cloned cell-populations: Mean cloning efficiency (%)* Foetal liver		*Bone marrow*		*Thymus*		*Spleen*	
	A	*B*	*A*	*B*	*A*	*B*	*A*	*B*
None	<0·05	0·1	<0·05	0·1	<0·05	0·1	<0·01	n.d.
Foetal liver	0·16	n.d.	0·10	n.d.	<0·05	n.d.	7·0	n.d.
Bone marrow	0·63	33·0	0·61	10·0	<0·05	0·45	6·0	n.d.
Spleen	0·42	<1	1·24	n.d.	<0·03	85·0	23·4	48·0
Thymus	n.d.		2·35	n.d.	<0·05	6·1	15·0	n.d.

A. Single cell suspensions prepared from the indicated tissues were incubated at estimated final concentrations of 10^3–10^0 in microtitre wells containing different irradiated cell monolayers. Colonies arising at clonal frequency appeared 10–17 days later. Each value was calculated from a minimum of 96 wells.

B. Single cell suspensions were incubated *in vitro* for 10 days prior to initiation of the cloning procedure as outlined above.

Cloned populations from foetal liver cells

Cell suspensions obtained from the liver of day 13 mouse foetuses were distributed at limiting dilution into microwells containing 0·1 ml CM and monolayers of irradiated cells from either foetal liver, bone marrow or spleen (see Materials and methods). The mean cloning efficiency of cultures containing these 3 types of cell monolayers was 0·16%, 0·63% and 0·42% respectively; preincubation of foetal liver cells before cloning on irradiated bone marrow cells resulted in a CE of 33%. Examination of 10 randomly selected clones from 3 experiments showed that all expressed the glycoprotein pattern of cells within the thymic lineage ($Ig^-Lyb\text{-}2^-/TL^-Th\text{-}1^-Ly\text{-}1^-2^-/Ly\text{-}5^+NK\text{-}1^-$). No other surface pattern was observed.

Cloned populations from bone marrow cells

Two types of colonies were detected after initiation of growth on irradiated BM monolayers. These cells were first identified by their distinctive morphology (Table VII-legend). Type I cells accounted for approximately 60% of colonies and expressed surface glycoproteins identical to the pattern of clones from F.L. Type II cells expressed the surface glycoproteins characteristic of immature thymocytes ($Ig^-Lyb\text{-}2^-/Thy\text{-}1^+TL^+Ly\text{-}1^+2^+/Ly\text{-}5^+$). These cells did not contain detectable levels of the enzyme terminal deoxynucleotidyl transferase (TdT) by chemical assay, although slight positivity was detected by immunofluorescence. Growth on irradiated thymocyte or spleen monolayers increased the proportion of Type II (thymocyte) colonies to 80–90%. In all cases, cloned populations derived from Type I or II colonies maintained the cell surface glycoprotein pattern and TdT activity of the parent colony.

Cloned populations of thymocytes from heterogeneous thymocyte suspensions

TABLE VII
Influence of irradiated monolayer cells upon development of Type I and Type II lymphocyte cell colonies

Source of irradiated cell monolayer	*Colony type* (%) *Type I*	*Type II*
Foetal liver	100	0
Bone marrow	60	40
Bone marrow[a]	100	0
Thymus	20	80
Spleen	17	83

Type I colonies were initially identified by their smooth, round appearance in contrast to the irregular shape and rough borders of Type II colonies. The cell surface glycoprotein patterns of those two cell types are described in the text.
[a] Single cell suspensions were preincubated *in vitro* for 10 days prior to initiation of the cloning procedure.

Attempts to initiate efficient cell growth on thymocytes using different irradiated cell monolayers failed (C.E. + 0·03%). However, preincubation of thymocytes *in vitro* before initiation of clonal growth was initiated on irradiated spleen cell monolayers. All cloned populations tested expressed the glycoprotein markers characteristic of immature thymocytes. Whether a portion of these cloned lines contains TdT is currently being tested.

Analysis of material synthesized by cloned inducer cells

Cl. $Ly\text{-}1^+2^-/p$ cell-free supernatant material activates B cells to secrete Ig

Cloned $Ly\text{-}1^+2^-$ inducer cell activates B cells to secrete immunoglobulin. Cell-free material substituted for activity of the intact cells. Supernatant material diluted approximately 10^{-3} stimulated B cells to secrete Ig: addition

TABLE VIII
Cl. Ly-1$^+$2$^-$ cell-free supernatant fractions activate B cells to secrete immunoglobulin

Dilution of cell-free supernatant fraction	*Source of supernatant fraction* Cl. Ly-1$^+$2$^-$/9	Cl. Ly-1$^-$2$^+$/16	Medium alone
0	120, 40	100, 60	120, 40
10^{-3}	720, 880	n.d.	n.d.
10^{-2}	3040, 3080	n.d.	n.d.
10^{-1}	5240, 4960	80, 40	40, 100

Cell-free supernatant material from Cl. Ly-1$^+$2$^-$/9, Cl. Ly-1$^-$2$^+$/16 or a control media was added at day 0 to 10^6 B cells. Ig-secreting cells were enumerated after 4 days incubation *in vitro*.

of higher concentrations resulted in a 50–70 fold increase in Ig secretion. By contrast, other cloned T lymphocyte populations that did not bear Ly-1$^+$2$^-$ inducer phenotype did not stimulate B cells to secrete Ig (Table VIII).

Cl. Ly-1$^+$2$^-$/9 cell-free supernatant material stimulate GM-CFU-C colony formation in semisolid medium

In collaboration with Dr Joel Greenberger, we tested the ability of cloned inducer T cell populations to induce granulocyte/macrophage colonies. Supernatant material from Cl.Ly-1$^+$2$^-$/9 cloned cells (but not cloned cells that did not express the Ly-1$^+$2$^-$ phenotype) also supported colony growth (Table IX). Analysis of the cells found in these colonies indicate that the majority (approximately 77%) of colonies were comprised of homogeneous macrophage populations; 20% of the colonies contained a mixture of granulocyte and

TABLE IX
Cl. Ly-1$^+$2$^-$/9 cell-free supernatant fractions stimulate granulocyte-macrophage colony formation

Source of supernatant material	*Final dilution of supernatant in culture*	*Colonies (per 10^5 cells)*	*Clusters (per 10^5 cells)*
Media alone	0	0, 0	0, 0
Ly-1$^-$2$^-$/11	1:10	0, 0	0, 0
Ly-1$^-$2$^+$/16	1:10	0, 0	0, 0
Ly-1$^+$2$^+$/4	1:10	0, 0	0, 0
Ly-1$^+$2$^-$/9	1:10	24, 24	68, 48
L929 CSF[a]	1:10	120, 88	100, 80

Cell-free supernatant material in serum free media was derived from T cell clones and added directly to culture dishes on day 0. Colonies and clusters were enumerated on day 7 using a Unitron inverted microscope.
[a] Positive control-L929 derived colony stimulating factor.

macrophages, and very few contained homogeneous granulocyte populations.

Cell-free supernatant material from Ly-1$^+$2$^-$/9 cells stimulates T cell and mast cell proliferation

IL-II, a factor having an apparent mol. wt of 30 000 stimulates proliferation of T cells *in vitro* (Watson *et al.*, 1979). This molecule has been identified in supernatant fluid of con A stimulated MLC activated spleen cells. We tested supernatant material derived from Cl.Ly-1$^+$2$^-$/9 for its ability to induce T cell proliferation, as determined by ^{3}H-thymidine incorporation. The proliferative response of 3 cloned T cell populations, and 2 cloned mast cell populations were examined. Addition of cell-free supernatant material resulted in 5–13 fold increase in ^{3}H-T uptake. An example of this enhancement of ^{3}H-T incorporation is shown (Fig. 1). Activity resided in a supernatant fraction

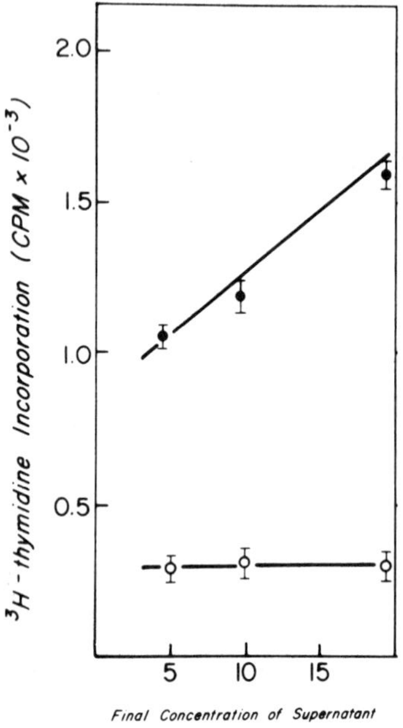

FIG. 1. *Cl. Ly-1$^+$2$^-$/9 synthesizes cell-free supernatant material that stimulates proliferation of other cloned T cell lines. Supernatant fractions, generated in serum-free media were added in graded concentrations to clones bearing (A.) Ly-1$^+$2$^+$ glycoprotein patterns. ^{3}H-Thymidine incorporation was measured after 24 h. Supernatant fractions from Cl. Ly-1$^+$2$^-$/9 (●) and Cl. Ly-1$^-$2$^+$/16 (○) were tested.*

having an apparent mol. wt of 30 000 according to Sephacryl S 200 chromatography (Fig. 2) and could be eluted from DEAE-cellulose with 130 mM phosphate. Interestingly, activation of mast cells resided in fractions having a slightly higher apparent mol. wt on Sephacryl S 200 (data not shown).

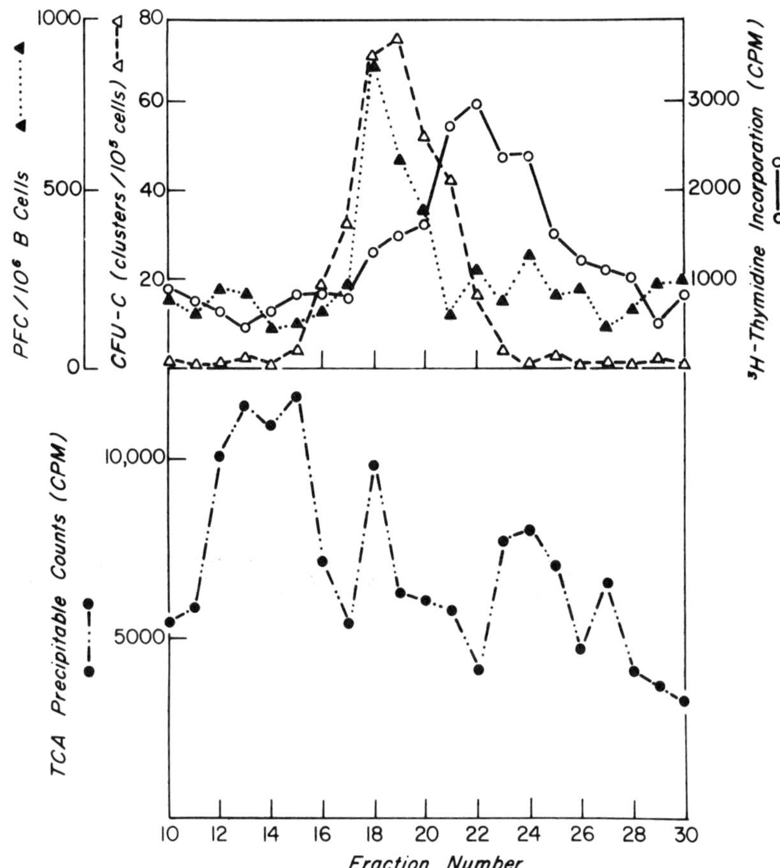

FIG. 2. *Separation of biologic activities in Cl. Ly-1*$^{+}$*2*$^{-}$*/9 supernatant material. Cell-free supernatant material was prepared in serum free media with* ^{3}*H-1-leucine, concentrated 20-fold by vacuum dialysis and applied to Sephadex G-100. Fractions were passed through 0·22 μ Swinnex filters after addition of bovine serum albumin (final concentration: 0·1 mg/ml). Each fraction was tested for CSF (△), T cell proliferative (○), B cell stimulatory activity (▲) and trichloroacetic acid precipitable counts (●).*

Definition of an antigen-specific suppressor glycoprotein produced by cloned suppressor T cells

Activation of antibody forming (B) lymphocytes to most antigens requires induction by thymus-derived (T) lymphocytes. In addition, analysis of T cells has shown that this class of lymphocytes is capable of exerting specific suppressive effects, and that these 2 functions are mediated by different sets of T lymphocytes that each express a different and characteristic pattern of cell-surface glycoprotein (Sakano *et al.*, 1979). In addition, unlike antigen-specific T helper cells, antigen-specific suppressor T cells bind to antigen-coated columns. Recently, supernates of cultures containing T cells have been shown to mimic the action of T suppressor cells (Schilling *et al.*, 1980). However, so far, analysis of supernate material has not allowed insight into the structural basis of antigen-specific suppression.

We have produced several clones of Ly-2^+ T suppressor cells from donors immunized with sheep red blood cells (SRBC); each binds specifically to sheep glycophorin, a major erythrocyte membrane protein. All of these clones secrete a polypeptide that binds specifically to SRBC and this binding is inhibited by glycophorin purified from sheep erythrocytes but not other erythrocytes. Analysis by column chromatography shows the polypeptide runs slightly slower than bovine serum albumin (68 000). After elution with 0·2 M sodium phosphate pH 7·2, from DEAE-cellulose and preparative flat bed isoelectrofocusing (IEF), an internally labelled polypeptide responsible for antigen binding and specific suppression has been purified to virtual homogeneity. The purified protein has an apparent mol. wt of 70 000 under reducing as well as nonreducing conditions, and shows 2 very close bands in analytical IEF (pI = 5·0). It is likely that one of the two represents a post-transcriptional modification (Fig. 3).

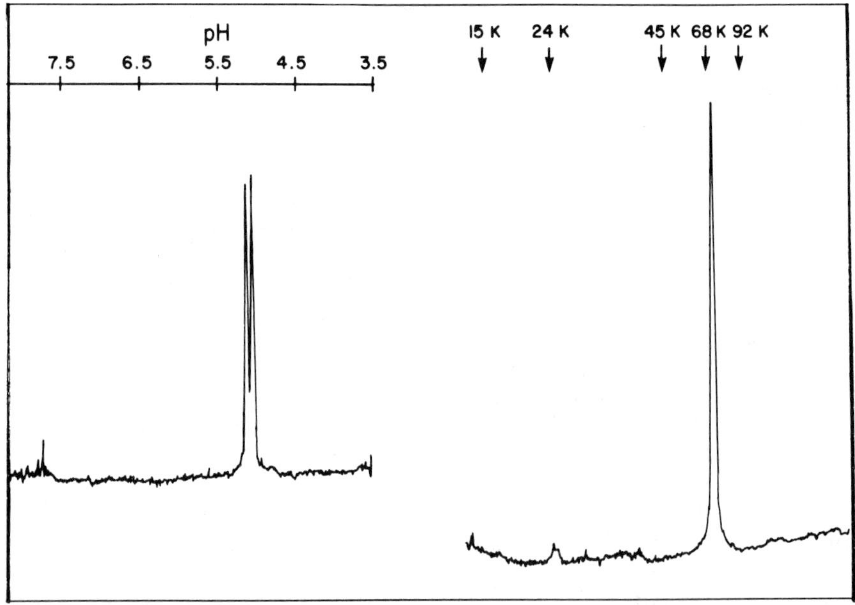

FIG. 3. *Densitometric scans of fluorograms of purified* ^{35}*S-methionine labelled suppressor peptide. Right, SDS-polyacrylamide gel electrophoresis. Left, isoelectrofocusing on polyacrylamide gels, pH gradient 3–8.*

Of this internally labelled material 95% binds to sheep erythrocyte but not to horse or burro erythrocytes. Binding to SRBC is completely inhibited by

TABLE X
Immunological characteristic of purified suppressor polypeptide

Immunoadsorbent	^{35}S *methionine labelled SF bound (% ct/min added)*
A. lentil-lectin-sepharose	100
R anti MIg sepharose	0
anti I-J^b sepharose	0
B. SRBC	100
HRBC	5
BRBC	3
C. SRBC + Sheep glycophorin	0
SRBC + Horse glycophorin	95
SRBC + Sheep glycophorin (asialo)	33

1000 ct/min of purified suppressor polypeptide were incubated with: A) 1 ml sepharose beads/ml B) 10^7 RBC/ml C) 10^7 SRBC/ml in presence of 10 μg/ml of indicated glycophorins.

glycophorin from sheep but not horse or human erythrocytes, nor neuraminidase-treated sheep erythrocyte glycophorin, strongly suggesting that the factor recognize glycophorin determinants in the surface of the erythrocyte membrane and that the sugar moiety plays a very important role in this recognition (Table X). In addition, the polypeptide is retained by sheep glycophorin but not human glycophorin-coated sepharose columns. This purified antigen binding material is retained by lentil-lectin-sepharose columns, but not by columns coupled with antisera directed against the *I*-region or *I-J* subregions of the major histocompatability locus. Sepharose columns coupled with antisera raised against immunoglobulins from mice, also failed to retain the factor. Taken together the above data indicate that the purified antigen binding material is glycoprotein in nature and does not bear either conventional *Ig* or *I* region determinants.

Incubation of Ly-1 cells from SRBC-immune donors with the purified 70K glycopeptide (final concentration 100 pcg/ml) × 18 h results in 90% reduction in the ability of these helper cells to induce B cells to secrete anti-SRBC immunoglobulins. Identical incubation of Ly-1 cells from donors immune to burro erythrocytes (BRBC) has no effect on anti-BRBC specific helper function (Table XI). Antigen is required for the 70K glycopeptide to suppress T_H activity: preincubation of Ly-1 cells with the 70K molecule in the absence of antigen (or in the presence of the wrong antigen) has no effect on subsequent SRBC specific T helper activity (Table XI). Because preincubation of B cells under identical conditions does not inhibit B cell secretion of anti-RBC antibodies, the main target of the 70K glycopeptide appears to be antigen-specific inducer T cells.

These data show that a cloned T cell population synthesizes (and probably

TABLE XI

Effect of the suppressor polypeptide on inducer T cells and B cells: specific inhibition of inducer T cell activation in the presence of antigen

	First incubation (24 h)	Anti-SRBC Ig secretion	(% suppression)
A) Ly-1 target	$Ly\text{-}1_{is}$ + SRBC	675 ± 33	(—)
	$Ly\text{-}1_{is}$ + SRBC + SF-70K	54 ± 8	(92)
	$Ly\text{-}1_{is}$	650 ± 51	(—)
	$Ly\text{-}1_{is}$ + SF-70K	459 ± 40	(29)
	$Ly\text{-}1_{ib}$ + BRBC	850 ± 85[a]	(—)
	$Ly\text{-}1_{ib}$ + BRBC	1000 ± 100[a]	(0)
B) B cell target	B	302 ± 18	(—)
	B + SF-70K	300 ± 37	(1)
	B + SRBC	720 ± 56	(—)
	B + SRBC + SF-70K	630 ± 48	(12)

Cells were incubated for 24 h in the first culture in the presence or absence of purified 70 000 dalton suppressor molecule, washed and transferred to a second culture containing the indicated cells. After a further 72 h incubation, anti-SRBC or anti-BRBC specific ([a]) Ig secretion by B cell enumerated. $Ly\text{-}1^+$ cells (10^5) immune to SRBC ($Ly\text{-}1_{is}$) or to BRBC ($Ly\text{-}1_{ib}$), nonimmune B cells (10^6) and RBC (10^6) were included in culture.

secretes) a glycopeptide of 70 000 daltons and pI of 5·0 that binds specifically to sheep erythrocyte glycoprotein and that this single polypeptide pre-empts the T helper response to the whole erythrocyte. The structural basis of T cell recognition has been the object of many studies. Two main approaches have been followed: analysis of extracts from suppressor cells or analysis of supernatants from heterogeneous populations of T cells. These have not provided insights into the biochemical structure of T cell molecules that directly suppress immune function due to the lack of homogeneity of the preparations. More recently, T cell hybrids have been analysed. However, in general T cell hybrids rapidly lose chromosomes and express as mainly the phenotype of the tumour partner: it is extremely difficult to demonstrate biological significance of hybrid T cell products. Nonetheless, the above approaches have indicated a major type of suppressor factor. It can be obtained from suppressor cell extracts, or supernates, and T cell hybridomas. The factor has a mean size of 45–50K, bears I-J regions products, and suppresses by recruiting more suppressor cells from precursor $Ly\text{-}1^+2^+$ populations.

The suppressive molecule described here directly suppresses T_H activity. The use of cloned T cell populations has allowed us to purify this molecule to virtual homogeneity and will provide a more clear insight into the biochemical basis of the structure of antigen-specific T cell products. The data

TABLE XII

Presence of two different domains in the suppressor factor molecule

	Mol. wt	PI	Antigen binding	Suppression Antigen-specific	Nonspecific	Reaction αTSF	αFv
Purified TSF	70K	5·0	+	++	−	+	+
Peptide A	45K	5·6	−	−	+	+	−
Peptide B	24K	?	+	−	−	−	+

summarized in Table XII are instructive in this regard. The molecule is very sensitive to proteolytic as well as spontaneous degradation; it gives rise to 2 main peptides of apparent mol. wt 45 000 and 24 000 according to SDS polyacrylamide gel electrophoresis. The 45K moiety (Peptide A) cannot bind antigen but retains suppressive activity which is no longer specific for SRBC. By contrast, the 24K peptide (Peptide B) retains SRBC specific binding activity, but lacks suppressor function. These 2 molecules can be distinguished by serological criteria. Antisera directed against a suppressor factor specific for TNP, which, after appropriate absorption seems to bind to "constant regions" suppressor molecules reacts strongly with peptide A (45K) but very poorly with peptide B (24K). A rabbit antimouse Fab antisera that recognizes Ig framework regions, reacts with peptide B but not with peptide A. Taken together, these data strongly indicate that the 70K suppressor molecule is composed of 2 biological domains: a constant domain that mediates suppression and probably is present on suppressor molecules directed against all antigens and a variable domain that probably carries V_H-like structures which serve to focus suppression exerted by the constant domain.

Discussion

In heterogeneous populations, T cells mediating different immunologic functions display characteristic surface Ly gene products. Some of these glycoproteins may play a role in specialized function: treatment of Ly-1^-2^+ cytotoxic T cells with anti-Ly-2 antiserum can inhibit cytolysis. This correlation of glycoprotein expression with function has now been extended to individual clones of cells: cloned populations of Ly-1^+2^- cells, (but not Ly-1^+2^+ or Ly-1^-2^+ cells), induce B cells to secrete Ig but do not suppress Ly-1 induction of B cell secretion. These cloned populations have maintained this function and their associated Ly surface glycoproteins after 15 months in continuous culture. Like heterogeneous populations of Ly-1^-2^+ cells, Ly-1^-2^+ clones inhibit B cell immunoglobulin secretion; a proportion of Ly-1^+2^+ cloned populations studied also suppress B cell activation. In some cases, these cloned populations suppressed the background response of B cells below control levels.

This background was most likely the result of small numbers of residual T cells contaminating the B cell population.

Previous experiments using heterogeneous populations suggest that Ly-1$^+$2$^+$ cells can differentiate into Ly-1$^-$2$^+$ cytotoxic or suppressor effector cells. Whether these Ly-1$^+$2$^+$ cells are induced by Ly-1 cells to acquire the Ly-1$^-$2$^+$ phenotype and associated suppressor function is yet to be established. Nonetheless, different activities have been found here in Ly-1$^+$2$^+$ clones grown under identical condition. Their presence suggests that at least 2 functional subpopulations can be defined in the Ly-1$^+$2$^+$ set.

In these studies, assays of immunologic function were chosen to avoid the bias of antigen specificity. Because precursor frequencies of cells that react with a given chemical determinants may differ among T cell sets and because the specificities of T cell clones were unknown, total immunoglobulin secretion was measured without regard to specificity. Nonspecific activation or inhibition of Ig secretion is dependent on certain specialized T cells and their gene products: these assays therefore represent an unbiased measure of differentiated T cell function. In addition, whether cells were grown in the presence or absence of con A containing media, the same functional activities were seen in these assays. Con A can, however, affect the initial cloning efficiency, improving it 10–100 fold in spleen T cells.

The molecular basis of the T cell functions described above is currently unknown. By contrast, the biochemical basis of the function and specificity of antibodies has been well characterized using myelomas as a source of large amounts of homogeneous immunoglobulin. An analogous effort has been made to define the molecules responsible for specific T cell functions. Unfortunately, "T cell lymphomas" have not proven as useful as neoplastic B cells: they do not constitutively secrete functionally active molecules. In addition, efforts to immortalize normal T cells by fusion with T cell tumours have been, on the whole, disappointing. With few exceptions, the hybrid expresses the phenotype of the tumour partner, rapidly loses chromosomes and cannot maintain immunologic function. Functionally active continuously propagatable T cell clones provide a new source of cellular material for such an analysis. Cell-free supernatant material can be generated from these cloned populations in serum-free conditions. These molecules can mediate inducer or suppressor activities and are available to biochemical and functional analyses.

These experiments extend the findings of previous studies in several ways. First, cloned populations of all major Ly$^+$ T cell sets can be maintained in continuous culture. Studies of Ly-1$^+$2$^+$ cloned cells indicate functional heterogeneity within this population. Second, these and other experiments extend the range of growth-promoting activity of Ly-1 cells and their products. First, cloned and Ly-1 cells synthesize polypeptides that support growth of cells bearing glycoproteins characteristic of both immature and mature thymus-dependent lymphocytes (TCGF) resembles IL-LL (Gillis *et al.*, 1978; Aaarden *et al.*, 1979). These data formally show that TCGF is directly synthesized by inducer T cells. Cloned inducer cells synthesize a second sized molecule, (45K according to sephacryl chromatography) that activates differentiation of macrophage granulocyte precursors; activation of B cells to secret Ig is not distinguishable from CFU activity by sephacryl chromatography.

In general these experiments represent a new approach to determine the steps in a cell's differentiative path that results in the synthesis of a new pattern of proteins and acquisition of a specialized function. Defining the molecular basis of these differentiative steps requires (a) identification of a cloned population of mature cells that synthesizes large amounts of a polypeptide that mediates a specialized function and (b) a method for generation of large numbers of cloned precursor cells and mature cells within this lymphocyte lineage.

Each of these cloned cell populations can be expanded to large numbers ($\geq 10^8$) to provide large quantities of homogeneous material for biochemical analysis. In addition, these cloned populations represent a normal cell at particular stages of thymus-dependent differentiation, as defined by their pattern of cell surface glycoproteins and, in fully differentiated cells, specialized function. We have not yet demonstrated that these clones maintain precursor function *in vitro*; i.e. they give rise to thymocytes and mature T lymphocytes. However, preliminary experiments indicate that some immature clones acquire glycoproteins of more mature cells after culture on irradiated thymic monolayers.

One molecule described here appears to be secreted only by inducer T cells. It has an apparent mol. wt of 45 000 and is sensitive to treatment with protease. Further analysis of this 45K polypeptide has demonstrated that it activates a limited set of target cells; e.g. it activates GM-CFU-C formation of B cells to secrete Ig but it does not activate other types of thymus-derived lymphocyte or fibroblasts to either divide or differentiate. The mechanism of activation are not yet understood in molecular terms. However, the following point is central to the present discussion: *extensive analysis of clones of prethymic cells, thymocytes, suppressor and inducer cells has indicated that this polypeptide is expressed only in cloned inducer cells.* This means that the step-wise development from thymus-processed lymphocyte precursors to differentiated progeny expressing specialized function (inducer activity) is marked by the selective activation of a gene controlling synthesis of this specific peptide within the differentiated inducer cell type but not other cell types.

T inducer cells probably freely recirculate, and act as sentinal cells that are activated by determinants recognized as foreign (Seidman and Leder, 1978). Stimulation of inducer cells to produce molecules described in this report can result in activation of macrophage precursors to divide and differentiate, and as well activation of B cells to secrete Ig. This allows for rapid expansion of immunologic cells at a site containing foreign determinants, resulting in efficient inflammatory reactions.

These studies suggest an explanation for the failure of specifically activated inducer cells to prevent *in vivo* growth of lymphomas which display unequivocally foreign determinants at their membrane surface (Leclerc and

Cantor, 1980). Although inducer cells are specifically stimulated by lymphoma cells (as judged by amounts of ^{3}H-thymidine incorporation by Ly-1 cells from immunized animals), coinoculation of these inducer cells and lymphoma cells does not retard progressive growth of tumour cells *in vivo* despite activation of a small inflammatory response. In some cases, tumour growth is actually enhanced by small numbers of inducer cells. By contrast, coinoculation of tumour-specific cytotoxic T cells efficiently prevents *in vivo* tumour growth. Possibly growth of lymphomas, like other malignancies derived from hormone dependent cells, remains dependent on hormone-like molecules secreted by inducer lymphoid cells for optimal growth.

The findings reported here suggest that the effects of activated immunologic inducer cells upon *in vitro* growth of lymphoid (and nonlymphoid) tumours should be determined before designing protocols for immunologic protection against tumour growth *in vivo*.

References

Aazden L. A. *et al.* (1979). Letter to the Editor, *J. Immunol.* **123**, 2928.

Bernard, O., Hozumi, N. and Tonegawa, C. (1978). *Cell* **15**, 1133.

Boyse, E. A., Stockert, E. and Old, L. J. (1969). *In* "International Convocation on Immunology, Buffalo" (N. R. Rose and F. Milgrove, eds), p. 353. Karger, Basel.

Cantor, H. and Boyse, E. A. (1977). *Immunol. Rev.* **33**, 105.

Ford, C. E., Micklem, H. S., Evans, E. P., Grax, J. G. and Ogden, D. A. (1966). *Ann. N.Y. Acad. Sci.* **229**, 283.

Gillis, S., Ferm, M. M., Ou, W. and Smith, K. A. (1978). *J. Immunol.* **120**, 2027.

Glimcher, L., Shen, F. W. and Cantor, H. (1977). *J. Exp. Med.* **145**, 1–9.

Greenberg, A. M. and Playfair, J. H. (1974). *Clin. Exp. Immunol.* **16**, 99.

Herberman, R. B., Nunn, M. E., Holden, H. T. and Lauria, D. H. (1975). *Cancer* **16**, 230.

Herberman, R. B., Nunn, M. E. and Holden, H. T. (1978). *J. Immunol.* **121**, 304–309.

Kasai, M., Leclerc, J.-C., Shen, F. W. and Cantor, H. (1979). *Immunogenetics* **8**, 153–9.

Kiessling, R., Klein, E. and Wigzell, H. (1975a). *Europ. J. Immunol.* **5**, 112.

Kiessling, R., Klein, E., Pross, H. and Wigzell, H. (1975b). *Europ. J. Immunol.* **5**, 117.

Komuro, K., Itakura, K., Boyse, E. A. and John, M. (1975). *Immunogenetics* **1**, 452.

Leclerc, J. C. and Cantor, H. (1980). *J. Immunol.* **124**, 15.

Lemke, H., Hammerling, G. and Hammerling, U. (1979). *Immunol. Rev.* **47**, 175.

Lionetti, F. J., Hunt, S. M., Mattaliano, R. J. and Valeri, C. R. (1978). *Transfusion* **18**, 685.

Mage, M. G., McHugh, L. and Rothstein, T. L. (1977). *J. Immunol. Meth.* **15**, 47.

Michaelson, J., Scheid, M. and Boyse, E. A. (1979). *Immunogenetics* **9**, 193.

Minato, N., Reid, L., Langyel, P., Cantor, H. and Bloom, B. Regulation of NK activity by interferon. *J. Exp. Med.* (in press).

Mishell, R. I. and Dutton, R. W. (1967). *J. Exp. Med.* **126**, 423.

Molinaro, G. A., Maren, E. and Dray, S. (1974). *Proc. Natn. Acad. Sci., U.S.A.* **71**, 1229.

Moorhead, P. S., Nowell, P. C., Mellmen, W. J., Battips, D. M. and Hungerford, D. A. (1960). Chromosome preparation of leukocytes developed from human peripheral blood. *Exp. Cell. Res.* **20**, 613.

Nabel, G., Fresno, M., Greenberger, J. and Cantor, H. Biologic activities of cloned inducer T-cells. *Proc. Natn. Acad. Sci.* (in press).

Omary, M., Trowbridge, I. and Scheid, M. (1980). *J. Exp. Med.* **151**, 1311.

Owen, J. J. T. and Raff, M. C. (1970). *J. Exp. Med.* **132**, 1216.
Owen, J. J. T. and Ritter, M. A. (1969). *J. Exp. Med.* **129**, 431.
Sakano, H., Huppi, K., Heinrich, G. and Tonegawa, S. (1979). *Nature* **280**, 288.
Sato, H. and Boyse, E. A. (1976). *Immunogenetics* **3**, 565.
Schilling, J., Clevinger, B., Davie, J. and Hood, L. (1980). *Nature* **283**, 35.
Seidman, J. and Leder, P. (1978). *Nature* **276**, 790.
Shen, Fung-Win, Boyse E. A. and Cantor, H. (1975). *Immunogenetics* **2**, 591.
Silverstone, A. E., Rosenberg, N., Baltimore, D., Sato, V. L., Scheid, M. P. and Boyse, E. A. (1978). *In* "Differentiation of Normal and Neoplastic Hematopoietic Cells" Book A (B. Clarkson, P. Marks and J. Till, eds), p. 433. Cold Spring Harbor Laboratory, USA.
Strelkauskas, A. J., Eby, W. E., Molinaro, G. A. and Dray, S. (1976). *Clin. Immunol. Immunopathol.* **6**, 334.
Watson, J., Gillis, S., Marbrook, J., Mochizuki, D. and Smith, K. A. (1979). *J. Exp. Med.* **150**, 849.

18

T Cell Differentiation and T Cell Restriction

ROLF M. ZINKERNAGEL

Division of Experimental Pathology, Institute of Pathology, Universitätsspital, Zurich, Switzerland

Introduction

Several experimental findings have shaken our ideas on cellular immunity quite profoundly during the past 8 years. Firstly, T cells have been found to express a double specificity for self–major transplantation antigens coded by the major histocompatibility gene complex (MHC, H-2 in mice, HLA in humans) and foreign antigenic determinants (X), i.e. T cells are restricted (reviewed in Möller, 1976; Paul and Benacerraf, 1977; Katz, 1977; Shearer and Schmitt-Verhulst, 1977; Zinkernagel and Doherty, 1979). The restriction specificity defines the effector function of T cells (H-2K, D or HLA-A, B restricted T cells are lytic, H-2I or HLA-D restricted T cells induce differentiation in the cells they interact with). The fact that T cells are double specific for self and antigen has a profound influence on their capacity for responding to antigens, i.e. T cell responsiveness is regulated by the genes that code for the restricting element. Thus, all *H-2K, D* (Schmitt-Verhulst and Shearer, 1975, 1976; Gomard *et al.*, 1977; Simpson and Gordon, 1977; von Boehmer, 1977; Zinkernagel *et al.*, 1978; Doherty *et al.*, 1978) and *I* (McDevitt *et al.*, 1972; Benacerraf and Germain, 1978) or *HLA-A*, *B* and *D* are immune response or *Ir* genes.

Secondly, antigenic determinants must be presented together with a "signal" to be immunogenic (Lafferty and Woolnough, 1977; Schwartz, 1978; Rosenthal, 1978); antigen-presenting cells which express certain H-2I or HLA-D self-determinants probably release such signals.

Thirdly, T cell specificity for self-MHC determinants is selected and expanded preferentially in favour of self-MHC recognition (Katz, 1977); thymus- and antigen-presenting cells are involved in this learning process (Bevan, 1977; Bevan and Fink, 1978; Zinkernagel *et al.*, 1978a, b; Zinkernagel, 1978). In parallel with the restriction specificity, the capacity of T cells to respond to antigen which is under the influence of MHC-coded immune response (*Ir*) gene is selected (von Boehmer *et al.*, 1978; Kappler and Marrak, 1978; Zinkernagel *et al.*, 1978b). This, together with the finding that the same *MHC*-regions code for the restricting element as well as for *Ir* genes, suggests that gene products of restricting and *Ir* genes are either intimately linked or *identical*.

All of these phenomena obviously hang together and seem to simplify our ideas on lymphocyte interactions and recognitions. They have theoretical implications for the understanding of T cell differentiation and recognition, and practical consequences for attempts to reconstitute immunodeficient patients and for our understanding of mechanisms leading to MHC-disease associations.

What and how do T cells recognize and how is specificity for self acquired?

The dual specificity of T cells has been explained with 2 competing models: the single v. dual recognition models (reviewed in Zinkernagel and Doherty, 1979). According to the former, T cells possess a single recognition site that does not recognize either the self-MHC antigen or the foreign antigenic determinant X themselves, but a neoantigenic determinant formed by the complexing self-MHC and X antigens. The implication of this model is that MHC-antigen and X interact with a certain degree of specificity.

The dual recognition model proposes that T cells express 2 separate recognition sites, one for self and one for X. The crucial characteristic is that the 2 recognition sites are separable, the one for self having a more constant quality than the much more variable anti-X receptor site. According to this model, the need for closeness or interaction between self and X is only determined by the 3 dimensional arrangement of the 2 receptor sites. Whether one of these 2 models is adequate, or whether an as yet unimagined new model (see the controversial somatic mutation v. germ line theories for the generation of immunoglobulin diversity and the related recent developments of molecular biology) would explain the phenomenology best is completely open at this time. Since the T cells' capacity to react with X is influenced by their restriction specificity, *Ir* phenomena have been explained within the 2 proposed models.

According to the single receptor model, *Ir* phenomena are put at the level of antigen-presentation, i.e. the restraint is determined by the "specific" interaction between X and self; if no such interaction or complexing occurs, no T cells are triggered. This was first proposed as a consequence of the "altered self" model (Doherty and Zinkernagel, 1975). Recently it has been formulated in a more extreme form to reflect the interaction of 3 amino acids of X via van der Waal's forces with 3 appropriate amino acids on the self-MHC-antigen (Benaceraff, 1978).

Within a dual recognition model, *Ir* phenomena are explained by considering there to be a defect (or blind spot) in the T cell repertoire for X. Three proposals exist. One explains the defect by the possibility that anti-X is selected after antiself has been chosen; accordingly anti-X is chosen out of the total germ line potential minus antiself, selection of antiself recognition leaving a blind spot (Langman, 1978; Cohn and Epstein, 1978). The second explanation is symmetrical with the first. Here, T cells express 2 identical anti-MHC receptors, one of which is driven to diversify upon encounter of self in the thymus; therefore anti-X must be derived by somatic mutation from one of the antiself receptors, otherwise a nonresponder situation results (von Boehmer *et al.*, 1978). The third proposal argues that, for biochemical/genetic reasons, antiself may not be able to complex with all possible anti-X, similar to the allotype's effect on the combination of constant with hypervariable regions in immunoglobulins (Zinkernagel and Doherty, 1979).

It is quite unknown what T cells actually recognize; this is true for all; self-MHC, X or for the complex neoantigen.

The apparent clarity and simplicity of using haptenic X to define T cell recognition has so far been an illusion; and attempts to define viral antigens with biochemical purification procedures or monoclonal antibodies have not been convincing and/or successful as yet. Despite excellent immunogenetics and transplantation antigen serology, we do not know what T cells recognize as self-MHC determinant. In mice the correlation between the T cells' restriction specificity and the serologically defined "private" transplantation antigens is of the order of 99%. Nevertheless, examples such as the K^{b}–$K^{bml(ba)}$ mutant pairs are very provoking; they are serologically virtually indistinguishable, but differ greatly with respect to restriction (Blanden *et al.*, 1976; Zinkernagel, 1976; McKenzie *et al.*, 1977; Klein, 1978). This and the "background" of HLA-nonrestricted killing or interaction in human test conditions (McMichael *et al.*, 1977; Shaw *et al.*, 1978; Shaw and Biddison, 1979; Biddison and Shaw, 1979) indicate clearly that the discrepancy is real and may still hide a great deal of crucial information.

This basic information (or rather the lack of it) sets the stage for the discussion of studies and their interpretation on the question of how do T cells acquire the specificity for self?

The basic problem: cellular immunology is still an inexact science

Whenever T cell immunologists think of new biological (i.e. phenomenological and *not* biochemical/molecular biological) experiments to distinguish the 2 alternative models of T cell recognition, there are generally 2 inherent major problems that sooner or later destroy the strength of the theoretical arguments and/or the discriminating value of the experimental result:

(1) immunological phenomena, even if defined biochemically are never static and absolute in physicists' terms. Relative specificity is defined by a factor derived by comparison which is usually not very large (e.g. H-2^k restricted T cells lyse infected H-2^k targets some 30- to 300-fold better than infected H-2^b targets, reviewed in Zinkernagel and Doherty, 1979), and is often limited for experimental/technical reasons; in addition, any such comparative value may change with time during an immune reaction. A key to the better understanding of immunophenomena, therefore, is meticulous time-dependent quantitation of measured parameters.

(2) immunological cell interactions are complex and are often referred to as cellular network interactions (Cantor and Boyse, 1977; Cantor and Gershon, 1979). A particular cell that reacts or interacts may trigger various counter-balancing cell reactions. Since we do not understand the simpler types of cell interactions between 2 cells, it follows that multicellular equilibria are understood even less.

Both these problems lead to the following well known and realized dilemma: because of the relative nature of specificity and experimental differences one may not perceive their real quantitation; in addition, because of the complexity of cell interactions and of experimental protocols, it becomes disquietingly feasible that an expected or unexpected "answer" or result may be found for many "wrong" reasons (including experimental artifacts and mistakes, or interpretational bias). The fact that cellular immunology does not have, at this time, the facts and tests available to make it an exact science where differences can be expressed in association constants and affinities (i.e. physically or physicochemically defined parameters), any discussion of the subject automatically becomes very vague indeed. We all know the consequences well: discussions are endless, emotional, evoke ideological wars, and involve the use of mythological terms (e.g. "altered self", "neoantigenic determinants", "physiological interactions", "adaptive differentiation", etc.).

The experimental results and their interpretation

There are 2 sets of experimental results that need to be reviewed here: experiments which indicate that there is a selection of some sort during T cell differentiation strongly in favour of self-MHC, and other experiments which say T cells—although restricted individually—are as a population not biased towards self. Amongst the experiments demonstrating *a priori* bias towards self-recognition are those which suggest that the thymus and its MHC has something to do with the differentiation of the restriction specificity, and other experiments which suggest that the thymus has nothing to do with it and that this selection is promoted solely by lymphohaemopoietic cell interactions themselves.

The proposals that T cells are not biased towards self and that T cells' restriction specificity is not selected in the thymus are often discussed together. It is clear, however, that they differ fundamentally with respect to T cells' degree of bias towards self-recognition.

T cells as a population not biased towards recognition of self-MHC

The evidence in favour of the notion that T cell populations are biased towards self-recognition stems mainly from 3 sets of experiments:

Neonatally tolerant mice

T cells from mice A that have been made neonatally tolerant of B are not able to respond to B + X in certain model systems (Zinkernagel *et al.*, 1977), but can do so in others (Forman *et al.*, 1977). Therefore, tolerance alone does not seem to be sufficient to allow expression of possibly pre-existent and expressed restriction specificity that usually cannot be demonstrated because of alloreactivity.

Negative selection experiments

Negative selection can be obtained *in vitro* by the so-called suicide technique; here, lymphocytes of strain A are mixed with irradiated B or (A × B) lymphocytes and then pulsed with heavily labelled DNA precursors or analogues. This procedure has mainly been applied to TNP and proliferative responses (Schmitt-Verhulst and Shearer, 1977; Thomas and Shevach, 1977; Janeway *et al.*, 1978). It was shown that A(anti-B) lymphocytes were able to respond not only to A-TNP but also to B-TNP. Since it is not quite clear how much of an anti-TNP response is classically restricted and how much of it is an alloresponse, this result is equivocal. This protocol has not been used in the virus or minor histocompatibility systems as yet and these findings therefore cannot be generalized.

Alternatively, unresponsiveness to an allogenic haplotype can be achieved via acute depletion of alloreactive T cells. Usually, this is done by filtration of lymphocytes from donor A through an irradiated homozygous strain B or heterozygous (A × B) (Wilson *et al.*, 1977). This protocol has been applied to TNP-specific or virus-specific cytotoxic T cell responses as well as to T helper responses (Bennink and Doherty, 1978a, b; Sprent, 1978a, b; Doherty and Bennink, 1979). For TNP the results are compatible with those from the suicide experiments: A (anti-B) lymphocytes react against B-TNP. The situation is partially different for virus-specific responses. A(anti-B) lymphocytes may respond to B + virus in certain haplotype combinations (e.g. H-2^b(anti-K^k)) but not in others (e.g. H-2^k(anti-K^b)). Nevertheless, it appears that in the combinations where "abnormally" restricted T cells can be generated, the response restricted to self is considerably greater; however at this time this is more a feeling than a fact since proper filtration and determination of precursor frequencies have not been performed as yet. Similar experiments assaying T helper against sheep red blood cells (SRBC) failed to show any appreciable T restriction for the haplotype against which the lymphocytes had been selected (Sprent, 1978a).

Nevertheless, more recently yet a third approach was used to study this question—negative selection *in vitro*, where lymphocytes A anti-B are absorbed onto a B-macrophage monolayer (Wagner *et al.*, 1980). Limiting dilution techniques revealed high frequencies for virus or TNP-specific T cells restricted to B. If truly repeatable and generalizable, these results may profoundly change our thinking on restriction.

Several possibilities have been discussed as to how to explain the positive or the negative results obtained with this technique (for a review see Zinkernagel and Doherty, 1979). Positive results may be caused by natural killer cell activity, low level alloreactivity, nonspecific "stickiness" caused by haptenization or certain viruses, etc. Negative results may be due to excessive negative filtration of T cells expressing a restriction receptor for the particular alloantigens, or the acute induction of pre-existent suppressive mechanisms, or the possibility that T cell populations are in fact biased towards recognition of self-MHC.

T cells as a population biased towards recognition of self-MHC

As may be seen from the previous section, the fact that T cells are restricted is not in serious doubt. However, at the level of T cell populations, views differ substantially. The results that suggest an *a priori* bias of a T cell population towards recognition of self-MHC derive partially from the experiments that have been discussed above, and partly from a series of experiments where unreactivity to a foreign haplotype is achieved via long-term lymphohaemopoietic and/or thymic chimaerism.

Experiments indicating a crucial role of the thymus in the selection of anti-self recognition Acute tolerance experiments after negative selection *in vivo* A(anti-B), at least in some examples of haplotype combinations, have failed to reveal whether T cells of A type could respond to B + X. The results from the virus model have already been discussed. In all tested combinations where T help for antisheep red blood cells has been analysed no restriction could be demonstrated for the tolerated B. Since this protocol has not been extended to academic antigens, where environmental priming may be much less common than for SRBC, one might argue that in the case of SRBC the bias is caused by natural priming rather than by an *a priori* bias of the T cells for self-MHC.

Chronically tolerant mice have been constructed in several ways. Neonatally tolerant mice A (tolerant of B) have been tested in a few examples and found not to respond to B plus virus (Zinkernagel *et al.*, 1977), whereas similar mice did respond to TNP-B (Forman *et al.*, 1977) or B plus minor histocompatibility antigens. Because of the limited data available on this model the results cannot be generalized as yet. Many more data have been published about restriction specificities expressed by irradiation bone marrow chimaeras (von Boehmer and Sprent, 1976; Bevan, 1977; Zinkernagel *et al.*, 1978a, b; Waldmann *et al.*, 1978; Katz *et al.*, 1978; Miller *et al.*, 1979). These chimaeras are formed by lethally irradiating recipient mice (e.g. A) and subsequently reconstituting them with T cell depleted stem cells of bone marrow or foetal liver origin from A × B donors; some 6–8 weeks later these chimaeras express immune competence and usually are reconstituted >95% by donor lymphocytes. Such composite mice are designated (A × B) → A chimaeras. When infected with virus, confronted with minor histocompatibility antigens or with a lesser effect confronted with TNP, such chimaeric (A × B) → A lymphocytes are predominantly restricted to A. If instead of using stem cells, (A × B) spleen cells are transferred into irradiated A recipients, such irradiation spleen cells chimaeras will express both restriction specificities. Therefore, selection of the restriction specificity must have been influenced by the radioresistant part of the host during T cell maturation.

This was shown more directly with thymus chimaeras. Adult thymectomized, lethally irradiated and bone marrow reconstituted (ATXBM) (A × B)F_1 mice were transplanted with irradiated (Zinkernagel *et al.*, 1978a, b) or neonatal (Fink and Bevan, 1978) thymus grafts of A or B origin. In each case tested (except for one instance which was poorly controlled in several ways), the thymic H-2 determined the restriction specificity.

Although in most laboratories (A × B) → A types of chimaeras have been found to be very heavily if not exclusively biased towards the host's H-2A type, other laboratories have reported that this is not the case; accordingly some B-restricted reactivity may be found (Blanden and Andrew, 1979), particularly upon appropriate restimulation with B + virus. Therefore, the restrictedness in (A × B) → A chimaeras may not be absolute, but certainly highly biased towards A (but then, as stated in the earlier sections, restriction itself is not absolute).

The major criticism against the general validity of these results is that in long term lymphohaemopoietic chimaeras mechanisms that modulate or suppress certain restriction specificities—via antibody or lymphocytes—may be responsible for the restriction phenotype observed (Zinkernagel *et al.*, 1978a, b; Zinkernagel *et al.*, 1979; Bevan and Fink, 1978; Zinkernagel and Doherty, 1979). For example, in (A × B) → A chimaeras (A × B) lymphocytes may generate antibodies or suppressor cells directed against the anti-B receptors on irradiated recipient A lymphocytes. Similar arguments can be made in thymus chimaeras (ATXBM) (A × B) with an A thymus. Several experiments have attempted to examine this possibility. Most of them have failed to demonstrate such antireceptor modulation, but because it is difficult to control these experiments properly, this negative answer may not be meaningful. For example, (A × B) → A lymphocytes have been mixed with normal (A × B) lymphocytes in adoptive transfer experiments over a limited dose range without obvious influence on B restricted effector T cell responses (Bevan and Fink, 1978; Zinkernagel and Althage, 1979). When (A × B) → A lymphocytes were mixed with (A × B) T cell depleted stem cells and used to reconstitute lethally irradiated (A × B) recipients, B-restricted responses developed some 8–12 weeks later, suggesting that anti-anti-B suppression was either absent or only short lived (Zinkernagel and Althage, 1979). However, there is one report that (A × B) cells transferred to irradiated (A × B) → A chimaeras were impaired in their capacity to express B-restricted delayed-type hypersensitivity (Smith and Miller, 1980).

Suppression by modulation has not yet been found in thymus chimaeras. Since in thymus chimaeras either recipient or stem cells may be influenced by the thymus, the following protocol was tested (Zinkernagel, unpublished). ATXBM (A × B) mice were transplanted with thymus grafts from both parental A and B, both thymuses functioned and both restriction specificities were expressed; if thymus A had modulated B-restricted responses, and thymus B modulated the A-restricted responses, one would expect that immunoincompetence should result; alternatively if one or the other of the thymuses had dominated, then only one restriction specificity would be expressed. This was clearly not the case and therefore renders the postulated type of modulation unlikely.

Histoincompatible irradiation bone marrow chimaeras or thymus chimaeras survive very poorly if raised under conventional conditions (Zinkernagel *et al.*, 1980a, b); in fact only a few per cent of the chimaeras survived the necessary 8–10 weeks so that immunocompetence could be measured. This contrasts sharply with the survival rate of $F_1 \rightarrow P$ or $P \rightarrow F_1$ irradiation bone marrow or thymus chimaeras. The few surviving chimaeras tested in various laboratories have yielded various results. Primary antiviral responses were found to be poor (Zinkernagel *et al.*, 1980a, b), as were primary anti-SRBC responses (Onoe *et al.*, 1980). However, when lymphocytes from primed allogeneic chimaeras were restimulated *in vitro* an appreciable degree of immunocompetence was found (Wagner *et al.*, 1980b), in most cases restricted to donor rather than recipient H-2 type. These experiments seem to indicate that in histoincompatible thymus–stem cell combinations, immunocompetence does not seem to develop at all, or only poorly, and much more slowly than in histocompatible combinations. Whether this is caused by modulating or other suppressive influences or whether this reflects a need for thymic and lymphohaemopoietic cells to be histocompatible for optimal T cell differentiation to occur, remains to be seen.

Experiments on the role of lymphohaemopoietic cells in promoting T cell maturation
Several experiments indicate that either thymic selection of restriction is not necessary at all or, although necessary may not alone be sufficient. Accordingly, lymphocyte interactions themselves may promote selection of T cells' restric-

tion specificity or are involved in the promotion of full T cell maturation.

This became obvious, when ATXBM or nude A mice were reconstituted with foetal, neonatal or irradiated thymus grafts $(A \times B)F_1$ (Zinkernagel *et al.*, 1980a, b). When the mature lymphocytes were sensitized adoptively in infected and irradiated $(A \times B)F$ recipients, no B-restricted reactivity was measurable. It therefore seemed as if thymic H-2 was not enough to promote that restriction specificity. Although no convincing experiment has been achieved that could demonstrate a 2-step differentiation—first selection at the level of the thymus and subsequent expansion upon contact of environmental or self-antigen on antigen-presenting cells—this might be a reasonable sequence of events (Zinkernagel *et al.*, 1979). Whether the second step occurs within or without the thymus is not crucial to the argument. From this point of view, earlier experiments with $A \rightarrow (A \times B)$ irradiation chimaeras that showed some T cells restricted to B, if sensitized appropriately in infected and irradiated $(A \times B)F_1$, might have to be reinterpreted (Zinkernagel *et al.*, 1978b). Probably in these chimaeras sufficient numbers of antigen-presenting cells survived long enough (or some lymphoreticular cells might even have survived irradiation altogether) to promote measurable T cell maturation. Recent experiments using more severely irradiated $A \rightarrow (A \times B)$ support this interpretation (unpublished observation).

None of the above experimental evidence and its interpretation fits the results obtained with nude mice reconstituted with foetal or neonatal thymus grafts. Nude mice A with a foetal or neonatal thymus grafts B become immunocompetent within 6 weeks and their T cells express restriction for A only (Zinkernagel *et al.*, 1980a, b; Kindred, 1979). Since irradiated 3- to 4-week old allogeneic thymus grafts do not reconstitute nude mice readily, one might be tempted to interpret the previous result to mean that allogeneic effects and/or the production of soluble mediators may make T cell maturation possible in an "abnormal" way. Attempts to induce this maturation in nude mice with allogeneic T cells or thymocytes or T cell growth factors alone without thymus graft have failed. Similarly, this interpretation does not readily fit the fact that $(A \times B)$ nude mice with a foetal or neonatal thymus graft A do not express restriction specificity for B. An allogeneic effect may be exerted by thymic cells A onto $(A \times B)$ cells; under the condition where syngeneic thymic maturation is possible, this other pathway may be much less attractive. The nude mice definitely are different from irradiation bone marrow or thymus chimaeras. When irradiated thymuses are used to reconstitute nude mice, they seem to behave in a way similar to the other models.

At first glance, one might be tempted to take these results to indicate that maturation of the T cell restriction specificity is independent of the H-2 of the thymus. In view of the poor definition of the baseline from which T cell differentiation starts in nude mice, this interpretation remains equivocal.

Conclusion: what next?

The various experimental results summarized in this review leave us with a picture that is still very incomplete and subject to future changes. Because of the vastly differing results that are in several instances contradictory, we must weigh up the various facts and try to come to a conclusion that will be shaky, but still gives a basis for further experiments and questions.

Overall, there is no doubt that T cells of an individual mouse express a certain, though varying degree of bias towards recognition of self. The fact that restriction is relative, and that certain overlaps can be found and selected for under certain experimental conditions, does not negate this bias. The very fact that *Ir* gene phenomena exist tells us that restriction is real, because without the link between restriction specificity and blind spots in T cell reactivity polymorphism of MHC products becomes meaningless, and vice versa. Part of our lack of understanding, and therefore inability to predict "cross-reactivities" or "overlaps" of restriction specificities as revealed in negative selection or some chronic tolerance models, may be that we do not really understand the relationship between restriction specificities and serologically defined MHC-products. Although in inbred mice the correlation between so-called private specificities and restriction specificities is great, this may be meaningful in a way that may be completely "wrong" from tomorrow's point of view.

What is the thymus' v. lymphoreticular cells' role in selecting the restriction specificity of maturing T cells? Again results are found supporting all arguments. Overall, there is still a strong case for the thymus' role in directing selection. Whether this direction is exerted by the thymic epithelial cells or lymphoreticular cells within the thymus remains to be shown. The recently described thymic nursing cells of epithelial nature that seem to contain many rapidly dividing lymphocytes are attractive candidates for such contact-mediated specific differentiation and/or selection under the influence of high local hormone levels. The experiments with nude mice may be very revealing, but probably by illustrating an *abnormal* way of inducing T cell maturation rather than by documenting normal differentiation. I feel that the present situation leaves open a few avenues for research on varying aspects of T cell immunology. For example, if most of the chimaera data should turn out to be due to modulating influences of antireceptor for restriction antigen reactivities, the old seminal ideas of Lindenmann and Ramseier's network idea may be revitalized. But there is no doubt that we need to find the T cell receptor(s), must become able to measure precursor frequencies, and should conceptualize and, it is hoped, explain the relationship between restriction and *Ir* genes. Once this is known, we will certainly be able to understand T cell differentiation much better.

Whatever the outcome of the present discrepancies, the results from experiments in mice have suggested improved rationales and rules for how possibly to improve therapeutic protocols for reconstituting immunodeficient patients. Obviously, the rather strict rules derived from inbred mice may be much more relaxed in outbred populations, where the relationship is between serologically defined transplantation antigens (the only parameter besides mixed lymphocyte reactions to assess immunological parameters relevant for restriction) and restriction specificities as expressed by mature T cells. What the present experiments indicate clearly is that immunologically $P \rightarrow F_1$ and $F_1 \rightarrow P$ chimaeras function excellently. Once the problem of graft v. host can be solved by the availability of proper anti-T cell antisera to eliminate mature T cells from donor bone marrow, such bone marrow donor and recipient combinations should be readily available within families. Whether fully histoincompatible bone marrow chimaeras become immunocompetent at all or to what degree, remains an interesting question that has been answered only partially as yet; a better understanding is again linked to the many open questions of basic cellular immunology; what is the receptor, how specific is restriction, what is the relationship between serologically defined transplantation antigens, restriction specificities and *Ir* genes?

References

Benacerraf, B. (1978). *J. Immunol.* **120**, 1809–1812.

Benacerraf, B. and Germain, R. (1978). *Immunol. Rev.* **38**, 70–119.

Bennink, J. R. and Doherty, P. C. (1978a). *J. Exp. Med.* **148**, 128–135.

Bennink, J. R. and Doherty, P. C. (1978b). *Nature (Lond.)* **276**, 829–831.

Bevan, M. J. (1977). *Proc. Natn. Acad. Sci. U.S.A.* **74**, 2094–2098.

Bevan, M. J. and Fink, P. J. (1978). *Immunol. Rev.* **42**, 4–19.

Biddison, W. E. and Shaw, S. (1979). *J. Immunol.* **122**, 660–664.

Blanden, R. V. and Andrew, M. E. (1979). *J. Exp. Med.* **149**, 535.

Blanden, R. V., Dunlop, M. B. C., Doherty, P. C., Kohn, H. I. and McKenzie, I. F. C. (1976). *Immunogenetics* **3**, 541–548.

von Boehmer, H. (1977). Basel Institute of Immunology, Basel.

von Boehmer, H. and Sprent, J. (1976). *Transplant. Rev.* **29**, 3–23.

von Boehmer, H., Haas, W. and Jerne, N. K. (1978). *Proc. Natn. Acad. Sci. U.S.A.* **75**, 2439–2442.

Cantor, H. and Boyse, E. (1977). *In* "Contemporary Topics in Immunobiology" (O. Stutman, ed.) Vol. 7, pp. 47–67. Plenum, New York.

Cantor, H. and Gershon, R. K. (1979). *Fed. Proc.* **38**, 2058–2064.

Cohn, M. and Epstein, R. (1978). *Cell. Immunol.* **39**, 125–153.

Doherty, P. C. and Bennink, J. R. (1979). *J. Exp. Med.* **149**, 150–157.

Doherty, P. C. and Zinkernagel, R. M. (1975). *Lancet* **i**, 1406–1409.

Doherty, P. C., Biddison, W. E., Bennink, J. R. and Knowles, B. B. (1978). *J. Exp. Med.* **148**, 534–543.

Fink, P. J. and Bevan, M. J. (1978). *J. Exp. Med.* **148**, 766–775.

Forman, J., Klein, J. and Streilein, J. W. (1977). *Immunogenetics* **5**, 561–567.

Gomard, E., Duprez, V., Reme, T., Colombani, M. J. and Lévy, J. P. (1977). *J. Exp. Med.* **146**, 909–922.

Janeway, C. A., Jr, Murphy, P. D., Kemp, J. and Wigzell, H. (1978). *J. Exp. Med.* **147**, 1065–1077.

Kappler, J. W. and Marrack, P. (1978). *J. Exp. Med.* **148**, 1510–1522.

Katz, D. H., ed. (1977). "Lymphocyte Differentiation, Recognition, and Regulation". Academic Press, New York.

Katz, D. H., Skidmore, B. J., Katz, L. R. and Bogowitz, C. A. (1978). *J. Exp. Med.* **148**, 727–745.

Kindred, B. (1979). *Cell. Immunol.* (in press).

Klein, J. (1978). *Adv. Immunol.* **26**, 55.

Lafferty, K. and Woolnough, J. (1977). *Immunol. Rev.* **35**, 231–262.

Langman, R. E. (1978). *Rev. Physiol. Biochem. Pharmacol.* **81**, 1.

McDevitt, H. O., Deak, B. D., Shreffler, D. C., Klein, J., Stimpfling, J. H. and Snell, G. D. (1972). *J. Exp. Med.* **135**, 1259–1278.

McKenzie, I. F. C., Pang, T. and Blanden, R. V. (1977). *Immunol. Rev.* **35**, 181–230.

McMichael, A. J., Ting, A., Zweerink, H. J. and Askonas, B. A. (1977). *Nature (Lond.)* **270**, 524–526.

Miller, J. F. A. P., Gamble, J., Mottram, P. and Smith, F. I. (1979). *Scand. J. Immunol.* **9**, 29–38.

Möller, G., ed. (1976). *Transplantation Rev.* **29**.

Onoe, K., Fernandes, G. and Good, R. A. (1980). *J. Exp. Med.* **151**, 115.

Paul, W. E. and Benacerraf, B. (1977). *Science* **195**, 1293–1300.

Rosenthal, A. S. (1978). *Immunol. Rev.* **40**, 136–152.

Schmitt-Verhulst, A.-M. and Shearer, G. M. (1975). *J. Exp. Med.* **142**, 914–927.

Schmitt-Verhulst, A.-M. and Shearer, G. M. (1976). *J. Exp. Med.* **144**, 1701–1706.

Schmitt-Verhulst, A.-M. and Shearer, G. M. (1977). *J. Supramol. Struct.* **6**, 206.

Schwarz, R. H. (1978). *Scand. J. Immunol.* **7**, 3–10.

Shaw, S. and Biddison, W. E. (1979). *J. Exp. Med.* **149**, 565.

Shaw, S., Nelson, D. L. and Shearer, G. M. (1978). *J. Immunol.* **121**, 281–289.

Shearer, G. M. and Schmitt-Verhulst, A.-M. (1977). *Adv. Immunol.* **25**, 55–91.

Simpson, E. and Gordon, R. D. (1977). *Immunol. Rev.* **35**, 59–75.

Smith, F. I. and Miller, J. F. A. P. (1980). *J. Exp. Med.* **151**, 246.

Sprent, J. (1978a). *J. Exp. Med.* **147**, 1838–1842.

Sprent, J. (1978b). *J. Exp. Med.* **148**, 478–489.

Thomas, D. W. and Shevach, E. M. (1977). *Proc. Natn. Acad. Sci. U.S.A.* **74**, 2104–2108.

Wagner, H., Röllinghoff, M., Rodt, H. and Thierfelder, S. (1980). *Eur. J. Immunol.* (in press).

Waldman, H., Pope, H., Brent, L. and Bighouse, K. (1978). *Nature (Lond.)* **274**, 166–168.

Waldman, H., Pope, H., Bettles, C. and Davies, A. J. S. (1979). *Nature (Lond.)* **277**, 137–138.

Wilson, D. B., Lindhal, K. F., Wilson, D. H. and Sprent, J. (1977). *J. Exp. Med.* **146**, 361–367.

Zinkernagel, R. M. (1976). *J. Exp. Med.* **143**, 437–443.

Zinkernagel, R. M. (1978). *Immunol. Rev.* **42**, 202.

Zinkernagel, R. M. and Althage, A. (1979). *J. Immunol.* **122**, 1742–1749.

Zinkernagel, R. M. and Doherty, P. C. (1979). *Adv. Immunol.* **27**, 52–177.

Zinkernagel, R. M., Callahan, G. N., Streilein, J. W. and Klein, J. (1977). *Nature (Lond.)* **266**, 837.

Zinkernagel, R. M., Althage, A., Cooper, S., Callahan, G. N. and Klein, J. (1978a). *J. Exp. Med.* **148**, 805–810.

Zinkernagel, R. M., Callahan, G. N., Althage, A., Cooper, J., Klein, P. A. and Klein, J. (1978b). *J. Exp. Med.* **147**, 882–896.

Zinkernagel, R. M., Althage, A., Waterfield, E. M. and Pincetl, P. (1979). *Proc. Symp. Cell Lineage Stem Cell Determination, Seillac, France* (in press).

Zinkernagel, R. M., Althage, A., Callahan, G. and Welsh, R. M. (1980a). *J. Immunol.* **124**, 2356–2365.

Zinkernagel, R. M., Althage, A., Waterfield, E., Kindred, B., Welsh, R. M., Callahan, G. and Pincetl, P. (1980b). *J. Exp. Med.* **151**, 376.

Theme 5: Summary

Ontogeny and Differentiation of T and B Lymphocytes

A. J. S. DAVIES
Chester Beatty Research Institute, London, UK

Ontogeny and differentiation have proved at the same time the most intricate and the most perplexing of studies in contemporary biology. The lymphoid system is a special case in that its moving parts are among the few cells in the metazoan body which are peripatetic and which retain the capacity to divide: this latter facility is only rarely exercised when the cells involved are in transit.

In the last 20 years or so we have learned that the lymphocytes originate from precursor cells, which may or may not be committed to the lymphocyte way of life before they get into the lymphocyte-differentiating environments. In my mind this issue is not resolved. Environments are basically of 2 kinds, exemplified by the thymus and the bursa of Fabricius, within which some kind of differentiational processing occurs. The exact identities of the novitiates, prior to entry to these monastic places, the details of the inducing rituals and the restrictions on the behaviour of the fully fledged brotherhood of lymphocytes are our present concern. Once outside their inductive environments, the cohorts of processed cells, perhaps according to their individual specific potentialities, interact in a complex manner in response to antigenic stimuli. This interaction and its various consequences occupy a large part of the minds of contemporary immunologists. The methods involved in improving our understanding of the orders of lymphocytes are of necessity analytic—as Richard Gershon (Chapter 20) put it, "fishing things out of the black box". We should always remember that the last act in the model building which is the proper end of scientific activity, is to put the pieces back together.

This Theme shows four quite disparate approaches to the problem. Nicole Le Douarin (Chapter 15) was concerned with the migration of novitiate stem cells into the differentiating monasteries in the chick and the quail. She felt that there were chemical angelus bells which operated prior to the intake of a new batch of beginners. When the monastery was full the bell stopped ringing. This is an attractive idea and my only reservation is that chicken and quail stem cells may interact with each other and the relevant reticular cells because they are so different in addition to responding to the various signals relating to the induction process. It would be nice to know, for example, if chick cells emerging from a quail bursa or thymus behave as good lymphocytes should. John Owen (Chapter 16) considered the problem of the nature of the cells in mammals which appear to have small amounts of cytoplasmic μ chains and which are thought to precede the more mature B cell which has surface immunoglobulin. It was intriguing to note that no light chains appear to be contained in these supposedly early cells. It is also worthwhile recalling that some of the idiotypic suppressor factors mentioned by Nisonoff (Chapter 4) are also lacking in light chains. I wonder to what extent these so-called pre B cells are antigen responsive and whether they can initiate the sequence of interaction with T cells which culminates in the expression of immunity—perhaps they would need surface immunoglobulin to do this.

Harvey Cantor (Chapter 17) described his careful pursuit of the T-suppressor substance based on T cell lines with defined antigenicities. The material itself appears to be part of an immunoglobulin molecule and has some of the characteristics of an antibody. However, how a single molecule can suppress the response to such a complex antigen as sheep red blood cells is a problem, unless perhaps the *in vitro* IgM response to SRBC is already idiotypically restricted. Putting these complex bits back into the black box is, I suspect the next task.

Rolf Zinkernagel's exposition (Chapter 18) of the MHC restriction of cytotoxicity with which he is so much identified, was, as always, illuminating, but the mechanisms remain elusive. It may be that interaction of thymic macrophages with lymphocytes, with which they seem to be able to associate in large numbers, as Pulvertaft showed many years ago, will tell us something useful. MHC restriction could mean some kind of exposure to MHC antigens or an environment in which their differentiation can occur. Thus, studies of the development of cell surface characteristics in relation to the timing of receipt of the thymic imprimatur may be helpful. It is also mildly inconsistent that experts on tolerance talk of elimination of self-reactive clones in the thymus, whereas Zinkernagel believes that the development of bias towards active recognition of self develops in the same organ.

The ontogeny of T cells

The thymus, as you have heard, is regarded as a staging house within which cells from such a source organ as the bone marrow or foetal liver can undergo maturation. Recently there has arisen the notion that the cells which enter the thymus to undergo this processing are pre-T or prothymocytes, the differentiational fate of which is determined prior to entry into the organ itself. This idea has depended largely on the demonstration that cells in the bone marrow or foetal liver, either have, or can be induced to have, some of the characteristics by which thymocytes or T cells are commonly recognized (Cohen *et al.*, 3.1.03*; Hanna *et al.*, 3.1.08; Jankovic *et al.*, 3.1.10; Maryanski and Cerottini, 3.1.16; Mukhopadhyay *et al.*, 3.1.20; Nabel *et al.*, 3.1.21). As John Owen pointed out, other studies, based on the repopulation of genetically anaemic mice, are consonant with the same idea (S. Abramson, R. G. Miller and R. A. Phillips, *J. Exp. Med.* **145**, 1567; 1977). The argument for pre-T cells is good but one paper in the present workshop casts a different light on the problem (Lightowlers *et al.*, 3.1.14). A neonatally thymectomized marsupial (the quokka) seems to develop normal numbers of T cells in the complete absence of a thymus, and it is claimed that these cells are fully functional. Assuming that the ablative surgery during these experiments left no thymic remnants, we must take seriously the idea that there are extrathymic environments for T cell maturation from cells which may be haematopoietic precursors common to all blood cells, rather than necessarily precommitted to the pathway of thymic development. If this is true, the properties of the T cells produced in the putative alternative environment(s) will prove of interest as will the extent to which this pathway of development is followed under normal circumstances in the presence of the thymus.

It is also being claimed (Goldschneider and Bollum, 3.1.06; Kruisbeck, 3.1.12; Piguet *et al.*, 3.1.23; Salmon, 3.1.29) as has Shortman previously, that populations of cells in the cortex and the medulla of the thymus are not necessarily sequentially related but can be thought of as independent. In similar vein, Mathieson and colleagues (3.1.18) show that Ly-1^+23^- cells can be found in the thymus at an earlier gestational age than Ly-123^+ cells. It seems that we need to know even more about the signifi-

* Reference numbers indicate Abstract numbers in: Abstracts 4th International Congress of Immunology, Paris, 1980.

cances of the variously described antigenicities of thymocytes in relation to their functional maturation.

T cell antigens

The plasma membrane of lymphoctes, the interface they have with the various ecological niches they can occupy, is being increasingly heavily explored. The adoption of such powerful analytic techniques as are available from monoclonal antibodies and fluorescent activated cell sorters, is creating a tower of information. Antigens which characterize malignant and/or normal lymphocyte populations are multiplying in number. One might well ask if this is O.K., and the answer must be that unless some steps are taken soon to co-ordinate the approach, confusion may ensue. A number of papers illustrate this point (Boumsell *et al.*, 3.2.03; Dalchau *et al.*, 3.2.06; Ferrara *et al.*, 3.2.07; Hansen *et al.*, 3.2.10; Horton, 3.2.13; Potter and McKenzie, 3.2.23; Spitz *et al.*, 3.2.26; Van der Reyden, 3.2.28). A further workshop specifically intended to reconcile the different types of discovered molecules might be helpful.

The glycoprotein present on mixed lymphocyte reaction blast cells but not on other transformed cells (Andersson *et al.*, 3.2.01) is reminiscent of that described by Faulk as a trophoblast antigen. A T cell antigen present on many B-CLL lymphocytes but not on normal B cells (Boumsell *et al.*, 3.2.03) is very thought-provoking, and we should look at B lymphocytes more carefully to determine whether at some stage of their ontogeny, perhaps under the influence of antigen, they express T cell characteristics. An antigen on T cells and polymorphs is described (Dalchau *et al.*, 3.2.06), the functional significance of which should be entertaining; the polymorph is a cell long ignored by immunologists.

A "thy" type alloantigen in man (Spitz *et al.*, 3.2.26), if confirmed, will promote much further work. The carefully documented structural similarity between TL and histocompatibility antigens is thought provoking. Most exuberant was the paper of Potter and McKenzie (3.2.23) describing the identification of no less than 8 new Ly alloantigeneic systems—now that's travelling.

Factors of T cell differentiation

Many years ago, Grobstein investigated the interaction of epithelial and mesenchymal elements in differentiation using tissue culture methods as his analytic tool. These studies were extended to the thymus by Auerbach, one of his students. It has emerged that interactions between the 2 initiating cell populations are to be thought of as a complex sequence of changes of action and interaction. Contemporary thymologists are involved in various simplified versions of the same approach. More than half of the papers in the workshop on factors of T cell differentiation utilize thymic epithelial cells in one way or another in an endeavour to understand the nature of their interactions with the stem cells from which, in the thymus, T lymphocyte populations derive. The epithelial cells possess FTS (Dardenne *et al.*, 3.3.05) and thymosin alpha 1 (Hirokawa and Saitoh, 3.3.14) though the exact role of these agents and their uniqueness in relation to the exercise of epithelial function *in vivo* remain to be determined. Dardenne notes *en passant* that thymosin fraction V of thymic origin, includes a material similar to FTS.

Several papers (Jenkinson *et al.*, 3.3.16; Rouse *et al.*, 3.3.23; Thomas *et al.*, 3.3.28; van Ewijk *et al.*, 3.3.30) record the timing of appearance of MHC antigens on the stromal elements of the thymus, a finding thought to be relevant to the epithelial–stem cell interactions involved in the establishment of MHC restrictions of activity which is proposed by Zinkernagel to occur in the thymus and to which I have already alluded.

Interleukin-2 (Heeg *et al.*, 3.3.13) is shown by one group to promote the development of potentially cytotoxic cells in nude mice and also partially to overcome the unresponsiveness of certain normal mice to mount H-2 restricted cytotoxic responses. Although the utility of agents such as interleukin-2 will be greater when their identity is more clearly established, it may well be that they point to the general nature of the biochemical milieu within the thymus.

T cell subsets in relation to T cell differentiation

The notion that lymphocytes are of 2 different anatomic origins is less than 20 years old. All small lymphocytes seemed alike to the haematologist in those days but things have changed greatly. T cells and B cells exist in a bewildering variety of so-called subsets, sometimes defined on orthodox morphological criteria, sometimes on the basis of cell surface properties, occasionally by demonstration of functional peculiarities. Many of these schismatic observations have been made only in tissue culture. It would be wrong to quote the philosopher who was of the opinion that given 4 independent variables he could epistemologically derive an elephant, but the immunologist faced with an experimental result may now call up the innumerable cohorts of cells by way of explanation and thus perhaps create his own white elephant.

In this workshop on T cell subsets most emphasis was placed on thymocyte populations, the responses of which to a variety of stimuli have been determined (Banga *et al.*, 3.4.02; Bartlett *et al.*, 3.4.03; Habu *et al.*, 3.4.08; Kisielov and Draber, 3.4.11; Lattime *et al.*, 3.4.12) and to an extent the topics of discussion overlapped with earlier workshops. From a careful developmental study, it seems that the thymus is unlikely to release only Ly-$1^{+}2^{+}$ positive cells.

Work on the lectin binding characteristics of lymphocytes used in conjunction with labelling of antigenicities (Banga *et al.*, 3.4.02; Berrih and London, 3.4.04; Habu *et al.*, 3.3.08; London *et al.*, 3.4.13) may help us to understand better the role of sugars on the surfaces of the various definable cell populations. CFU-s cells may be distinct from thymocyte precursors (Boersma, 3.4.05). It will be useful in time to be able to establish which characteristics are sequential stages in the differentiation of individual cells and which indicative of basic heterogeneity.

Ontogeny of B cells

A number of papers in this session (Coutinho *et al.*, 3.5.06; Durkin *et al.*, 3.5.08; Ekino *et al.*, 3.5.10; Francus and Siskind, 3.5.13; Hayward, 3.5.16; Kim *et al.*, 3.5.21; Toivanen and Vainio, 3.5.38) either explicitly or implicitly indicated that the system of B lymphocytes is driven by antigenic stimuli. Thus, the work of Durkin *et al.* (3.5.08) shows that in Peyer's patches the ratios of IgM to IgA and IgE bearing cells are drastically altered in germ-free animals in favour of the latter pair. The studies of Kim and his colleagues (3.5.21) make it clear that the state of responsiveness of B cells to nonspecific B cell activators was very much determined by the dietary and microbial status of the gnotobiotic miniature swine that they studied.

The mechanisms by which B cells switch towards the expression of single isotypes of immunoglobulin, characteristic of their late stage of development, is the subject of several papers of which that by Gandini *et al.* (3.5.15) may be used as an example. From their analysis of the B cell populations of neonatal humans and mice, using a method enabling them to identify up to 3 immunoglobulin isotypes on individual cells, they conclude that the products of up to 3 C_H genes can be expressed by single cells. It is tempting to postulate that on individual "virgin" B cells the products of all the C_H genes are expressed, albeit to a variable degree. Differentiation in response to specific or nonspecific stimulus would then proceed by progressive restriction and amplification of specific isotypes, perhaps different locations favouring one isotype rather than another. Hijmans has espoused such a view for some years.

Other studies showed that immature B cells may be PNA^{+} as are thymocytes and some cells in the bone marrow (Osmond *et al.*, 3.5.28; Rose *et al.*, 3.5.35). In a beautiful study Toivanen (3.5.38) and his colleagues, following Dieterlen-Lievre (Lassila *et al.*, 3.5.24) seem to have shown that lymphoid stem cells (if such there be) originate in the embryo and only migrate secondarily to the yolk-sac—another sacred cow bites the dust.

Circulation and homing of lymphocytes

Part of the difficulty experienced by those working on the recirculatory property of lymphocytes has been the inaccessibility of the HEV lymphocyte interface. The work of Woodruff and her colleagues, enthusiastically adopted in California by Weissman and his associates, on the binding characteristics of HEV in frozen sections, is perhaps circumventing this problem. Butcher *et al.* (3.6.04) demonstrate that, *in vitro*, Peyer's patch lymphocytes stick better to the HEV of Peyer's patches than lymph node lymphocytes—a comparable result emerged from *in vivo* homing studies. In 2 further papers, a glue and an antiglue are postulated to be involved with the process of lymphocyte-endothelial recognition (Carey and Woodruff, 3.6.05; Woodruff and Chin, 3.6.28).

In vivo, Degos *et al.* (3.6.06) describe how lymphocyte recirculation requires identity at the *H-2* locus for its full-flowering. Shields and Parrott (3.6.23) showed that the localization of blast cells in skin lesions may have a similar requirement for self-recognition. Ford (3.6.24) and his coworkers conclude from a study involving serial transfer of unstimulated cells starting with T.D.L. that "homing" of cells from lymph nodes and spleen back to their organ from which they were obtained does not occur. The same group (3.6.10) studied the flat HEVs of nude mice, and concluded that their slow transmission of cells was partly due to the quality of the HEVs and partly that of the lymphocytes in nude mice.

The work of Koch and Benner (3.6.16) on the migration patterns of B lymphocytes, based on parabiosis of mice congenic for an immunoglobulin allotype gene, illustrates migration of B cells to the marrow, probably from the spleen, in the late stages of immune responses. Their general conclusion that the maintenance of persistent antibody production is largely a property of the bone marrow should be more widely recognized.

Phylogeny of immunoreceptors: cellular and molecular aspects

Phylogenetic studies are not a popular approach to immunological phenomena but they may prove to have much to tell us. The T cells and thymocytes in certain fish (Van Loon *et al.*, 3.7.08; Warr, 3.7.10) carry immunoglobulin molecules which may lack light chains. And although the heavy chains are in some respects different from those found in mammalian cells, it is difficult not to hope that some of the secrets of T-cell receptors in mammalians will emerge from a study of their more cold-blooded antecedents. Seasonal variations in immunological responsiveness can be found in rainbow trout and tolerance can be induced in *Xenopus laevis* by flank-skin. Both phenomena which ought to interest the homoiothermophilic immunologists.

Invertebrate studies seem to show analogies with vertebrate immunology in that there are "complement-related" activities in the silkworm (Noguchi, 3.7.06) and T- and B-like cells in starfish. The grafting of skin in *Lumbricus terrestris* leads to proliferative responses which are reminiscent of those in mammals following homografting. Colony formation in *Botryllus* is controlled by multiple alleles of which the products should be of interest to those generally interested in cell-to-cell interaction. My feeling about the invertebrate immunology is that it could be better related to defence against invasion and would thus perhaps give us some idea of the biological significance of the lymphoid system of vertebrates.

The immunobiology of ageing

The notion that immunological responsiveness reduces with old age is seductive. It carries the implication that the decline in immunological responsiveness is in some way responsible for ageing. This in turn raises the possibility that by modulation of immune mechanisms ageing might be arrested. In any case it might just explain the age/incidence of cancer. One might add, cynically, that ideas such as these are coincident with ageing of the science of immunology. That aside, all the paraphernalia of the descriptive immunologists has been employed to show that aged organisms (mice and men mainly) are immunologically deficient. Macrophage functions change with age it is said; helpful macrophages become suppressive (*in vitro*) with increasing age of the donor (Bash, 3.8.01). The liver fails to take up quite so much antigen in older animals (Garvey *et al.*, 3.8.14) which it is thought could alter the pattern of immunological responsiveness. Mixed lymphocyte reactivity is diminished in mice (Zharhary and Gershon, 3.8.37) and men (Bátory *et al.*, 3.8.03; Klajman *et al.*, 3.8.24) presumably indicating a decline in cell-mediated immunological capacity. More interestingly, in a number of studies, MHC genetic status seems definitely to be involved in ageing (Bátory *et al.*, 3.8.03; Popp, 3.8.31; Proust *et al.*, 3.8.32). Autoanti-idiotypic antibodies are plausibly proposed to be more easily produced in aged individuals (Goidl *et al.*, 3.8.17; Szewczuk, 3.8.34)—i.e. the network becomes tighter (Klinman, 3.8.25). Autoimmune status is not so noticeably changed (Proust *et al.*, 3.8.32) though autorosetting frequencies may alter (Fournier and Charreire, 3.8.12). Responses *in vitro* to Con A and PHA are reduced in old mice (Joncourt *et al.*, 3.8.21). T cell growth factor production is down in aged mice (Gillis *et al.*, 3.8.15) as is the density of receptors for the factor. Peanut agglutinin positive (PNA^+) cells increase in number in aged mice as do PNA^+ suppressor cells (Globerson *et al.*, 3.8.16). T cell helper activity is reduced in old mice but happily it can be restored with extracts of thymus (Frasca *et al.*, 3.8.13). Natural killer cells are up in old mice (Bátory *et al.*, 3.8.02; Bruley-Rosset *et al.*, 3.8.07) but can be reduced by bestatin or levamisole (Bruley-Rosset *et al.*, 3.8.07) as can tumour incidence. The consequences of injection of levamisole into aged humans, however, seems less happy in that B cells are unaffected and T cells slightly increased.

The lymphoid system as a whole ages in chickens (Isakovic *et al.*, 3.8.20) and the thymus epithelium perhaps changes with age in man (Oosterom *et al.*, 3.8.30)—a conclusion which I suspect Jean-Francois Bach would relate to declining FTS production. The neuroendocrine axis is thought to decay in turn leading to diminution of the lymphoid system (Muzzioli and Fabris, 3.8.27)—thyroxine injections are said to stop all this.

For all this activity, the extensive and careful studies of the group at the Faculty of Medécine Pitié-Salpêtrière (Devillechabrolle *et al.*, 3.8.11; Proust *et al.*, 3.8.32) indicate that in man age-related decline in immune functions may often be a consequence of various exogenous factors; malnutrition, infection, inflammation, renal failure and the like. Others in the field should remember this work in their search for tired T cells.

Theme 6

Cellular Co-operation

Presidents:
J. F. A. P. MILLER
W. H. FRIDMAN

Symposium chairman:
D. W. TALMAGE

19

MHC Restrictions in Cellular Co-operation

J. F. A. P. MILLER

Walter and Eliza Hall Institute of Medical Research, Melbourne, Australia

Introduction

An immune response does not occur only as a result of a simple encounter between immunocompetent lymphocyte and antigen. On the contrary, there are many complex cellular interactions which take place and determine the outcome of such an encounter. In addition, each response is a highly amplified reaction and, as is the case with other amplification systems, each step has to be subjected to a multitude of rigorous controls. This presentation is not intended to discuss the entire network of cell-to-cell interactions which is involved in immunity. It will rather focus on one aspect of such interactions which has been documented in the last few years, namely the influence of gene products of the major histocompatibility complex (MHC) in controlling various interactions. It is not possible, in the space allotted, to refer to the work of all investigators in this field. Only a few topics relevant to the present discussion will be selected. Further details will be found in several extensive reviews on MHC restriction in series such as "Immunological Reviews" and "Advances in Immunology".

A modest beginning was made in unravelling the complexities of immune induction some 12 years ago when the existence of cell-to-cell interactions in antibody responses was unequivocally documented. It was originally shown that T cells were essential to assist B cells produce antibody to a variety of antigens (Miller and Mitchell, 1968, 1969; Mitchell and Miller, 1968; Miller, 1972). Later, other investigators showed the reverse: a suppressive influence of T cells on B cell responsiveness (Gershon, 1974). Evidence then accumulated for a functional heterogeneity in the T cell pool: distinct subsets of T lymphocytes performed distinct immunological tasks (Cantor and Weissman, 1976).

T cell subsets

Subsets of T cells can be distinguished according to distinct differentiation antigens on the cell surface identifiable by specific antisera, such as anti-Ly sera. They may also be classified according to the differential expression of antigens coded by the MHC and to the restrictions on their activities imposed by the MHC as discussed later. In addition, of course, they can be characterized by the various roles they play in the immune response. Thus, for example, helper T cells (T_H) usually assist B cells produce IgG antibody in response to the so-called "T dependent" antigens. T_H cells are also involved in assisting other T cells perform their various tasks. These helper cells are Ly-1^+ and generally lack Ia determinants, although a distinct subset of T_H cells exists which does bear Ia (Tada *et al.*, 1978). In addition, factors claimed to be produced by T_H cells are said not only to be antigen-specific and thus possess a binding site for antigen, but also to bear Ia determinants (Munro and Taussig, 1975; Shiozawa and Diener, 1980). T cells involved in delayed-type hypersensitivity (DTH, T_D cells) are Ly-1 and lack Ia determinants (Vadas *et al.*, 1976). It is possible, however, that T_D cells require some interaction with and Ia^+ T_H cell or that they bind Ia antigen complexes after activation. The occurrence of T-T cell interaction in DTH has been suggested (Bullock *et al.*, 1975). Cytotoxic T cells (T_C), which can directly kill targets for which they possess an immunospecific receptor, are Ly-23^+ and usually Ia^+. Here, again, some experiments suggest that a T_H cell may be required for the activities of T_C cells and that such helper cells must recognize Ia on the surface of T_C cells (Zinkernagel *et al.*, 1978b). Suppressor T cells (T_S), which inhibit T or B cell functions are Ly-23^+ and bear Ia determinants; generally coded by *I–J*. Factors released from such T_S cells are said to possess a specific antigen-binding site and MHC determinants, e.g. I-J or, in some cases, I-C (Tada *et al.*, 1977; Rich and David, 1979). Some T cells are involved in feedback suppression and express both Ly-1 and Ly-23 antigens as well as the surface component Qal coded by an *MHC* gene mapping between *H-2D* and *Tla* (Eardley *et al.*, 1978). These Ly-123 cells are thought to be relatively recently derived from the thymus and nonrecirculating in contrast to Ly-1 and Ly-23 cells which are long lived and recirculating from blood to lymph. There are thus numerous T cell subsets and some appear well characterized (Table I). The exact extent to which the various differentiation antigens, such as Ly or Ia antigens, are represented on each subset is not always clear. Thus, some Ia molecules may be acquired passively from body fluids or serum, having been shed from other cell types, e.g. macrophages (Mph) or antigen-presenting cells (APC). It is hoped that future work utilizing more extensively purified T cell subsets, preferably carried as lines *in vitro*, and monoclonal antibody reagents, will help clarify the situation.

TABLE I

Properties of T cell subsets in mice

T cell subsets	*Function*	*Cell surface markers*	*MHC region imposing restriction*
T_H	Assist B cells produce IgG antibody	Ly-1$^+$; some are Ia$^-$ some are Ia$^+$	I-A
T_D	Involved in delayed-type hypersensitivity	Ly-1$^+$ Ia$^-$	I-A
T_C	Kill specific targets after contact	Ly-23$^+$ Ia$^-$	H-2K, H-2D
T_S	Suppress response of other lymphocytes	Ly-23$^+$ Ia$^+$ (coded by I-J)	None in some cases I-J in some cases H-2D in some cases
T_F	Exert potent feedback inhibitory effects by activating T_S cells	Ly-123Qa-1$^+$ Ia$^-$	

For further details see Eardley *et al.* (1978), Katz and Benacerraf (1975), Sprent (1978), Tada *et al.* (1977, 1978), Vadas *et al.* (1976, 1977).

The MHC exerts a profound influence on T cell functions. The frequency of alloreactive T_C cells (i.e. those directed against H-2 antigens) is generally said to be 100 to 1000 times as high as the frequency of T cells reactive to non-H-2 antigens (e.g. Lindhal and Wilson, 1977). This has led to much speculation about the origin of the T cell repertoire (Jerne, 1971). Unfortunately, most frequency estimates are based on work employing strains of mice which differ at the entire *H-2* region—a region which can accommodate numerous genes, many of which could code for a distinct private or several public specificities. Little work has been done on the frequency of T_C cell precursors specific for only one determinant coded by some single *H-2* gene. Even then, one H-2 molecule can express different antigenic specificities (one private and several public) and, if each specificity is recognized by a separate T_C clone, allogeneic stimulation will activate multiple clones.

MHC restriction

Apart from its influence on alloreactive T cells, the MHC restricts the activities of a large number of T cell subsets. This phenomenon, also known as H-2 restriction, may be defined as the requirement for identity at certain MHC gene products between APC involved in initiating T cell activation and targets of immune T cells. Examples of MHC restriction are to be found in T cell dependent immune responses such as cytotoxic responses, DTH and helper functions. For example, mice recovering from virus infections generate T_C cells which, *in vitro*, can kill targets infected by the same virus, only if the target cell and the mice from which the T_C cells were obtained are identical at *H-2K* or *H-2D* (Doherty *et al.*, 1976). Likewise, T_C cells directed against chemically modified cell surface antigens or minor histocompatibility antigens are restricted by *H-2K* or *H-2D* (Shearer *et al.*, 1976; Bevan, 1975; Gordon *et al.*, 1975). By contrast, T cells involved in DTH are restricted by I-A. Thus, to achieve successful transfer of DTH, there is a requirement for I-A matching between donors of sensitized T cells and naive recipients (Vadas *et al.*, 1977). Further experiments showed the requirement for such a matching between antigen-pulsed Mph used for sensitization and those used for elicitation *in vivo* (Miller *et al.*, 1977; Smith *et al.*, 1979). This is in line with observations of other investigators showing a requirement for Ia matching between antigen-pulsed Mph and sensitized T cells to allow these to proliferate *in vitro* (Yano *et al.*, 1977; Brown *et al.*, 1979). In the case of T_H cells, it was originally observed that T_H and B cells had to share I-A gene products for successful co-operation in antibody responses (Katz and Benacerraf, 1975). The restriction of T_H cells was soon shown to occur both at the level of induction (presumed to reflect activation of T_H cells by Mph-associated antigen) and during T and B cell co-operation (Sprent, 1978). T cell recognition of MHC-associated antigen on Mph and on specific B cells may thus be identical or very similar. Finally, in the case of T_S cells, restriction was observed in some cases, not in others. When observed, it involved *I-J* (Tada *et al.*, 1977) or *H-2D* (Miller *et al.*, 1978) depending on the experimental system.

In addition to restrictive elements summarized briefly above, the MHC codes for genes which govern the strength of T cell dependent immune responses. These genes are localized in the *I* region (MHC linked *Ir* genes), although recent findings indicate that responsiveness of T_C cells may be governed by genes in the *H-2K* and *H-2D* region of the MHC. It seems very likely, as discussed below, that MHC-linked *Ir* genes and MHC restrictive elements may be identical. Finally, there are MHC-coded determinants on the so-called cell interaction molecules which appear to be released from various T cell subsets (T_H and T_S cells) and also from APC.

The results obtained in studies of MHC restriction indicate that the major stimulus for the activation of many T-cell subsets is not antigen alone, but antigen in association with one or the other of the gene products of the MHC. These products are present on the surface of the body's own cells and some, such as Mph or APC, appear particularly well equipped to present antigen in the appropriate form to T cell and deliver the activating signal. In addition, some MHC components (e.g. Ia) may be released or shed from cells, such as APC, into body fluids or serum and may associate with antigen or mitogen on the surface of T cells which possess appropriate receptors for these substances. Examples of this are to be found with T_H cells and "processed" antigen in material containing Ia determinants (Erb and Feldmann, 1975; Puri and Lonai, 1980) and in T cells which proliferate in response to concanavalin A (con A), only if a source of Ia is available (Möller *et al.*, 1979). It is this requirement for the recognition of both MHC component and antigen which accounts for MHC restriction and, very likely, *MHC*-linked *Ir* gene effects (see below).

Some aspects of MHC restrictions operating in cellular interactions in the immune response will now be examined in more detail.

APC (which may include some subset of Mph) play a crucial part in the activation of T lymphocytes. A role for Mph-associated antigen in the induction of T_H cells was evident some time ago in experiments utilizing the technique of "hot antigen suicide" (Basten *et al.*, 1975). Suicide of B cells could be achieved simply by incubating cells with radioactive antigen in soluble form, in the presence of azide and at 4°C. The cells could be protected by preincubation with anti-immunoglobulin (Ig) reagents but not with antisera directed against MHC components (alloantisera). On the other hand, T-cell suicide required the radioactive antigen to be presented not in soluble form, but on the surface of other cell types, presumably some type of APC, possibly Mph. It also required active metabolism since it occurred only at 37°C and was prevented by metabolic inhibitors. However, the most pertinent finding was that T cells could be protected by preincubation of the mixed cell population, not with anti-Ig sera, but with alloantisera. These early findings implied that T cell activation required the participation of actively metabolizing APC and also hinted at some crucial role of MHC gene products.

Other investigators showed that sensitized lymphocytes from a variety of animal species, including man, guinea-pigs, rats and mice, could be induced to proliferate *in vitro* when incubated with the appropriate antigen (Rosenthal, 1978). This reaction is generally accepted to represent an *in vitro* correlate of cell-mediated immunity, i.e., it is a T cell response. It is dependent on antigen processing and antigen presentation by Mph. Functionally significant interaction of sensitized T cells with native soluble antigen failed to occur. On the contrary, during the inductive phase of this response, antigen had to be presented in association with Mph. This *in vitro* system enabled the investigators to determine the role played by antigen and MHC components in stimulating sensitized T cell proliferation (Schwartz *et al.*, 1978; Thomas *et al.*, 1978). Incubation of T cells, themselves, with anti-Ia antibody had no effect. Antibody directed to Ia antigens, of the appropriate specificities present on Mph, blocked the ability of the antigen-pulsed Mph to stimulate proliferation.

By contrast, antibody to native antigen failed to block proliferation (although somewhat different results have been obtained very recently in some systems with monoclonal antibody). In general, it may be stated therefore that the antigenic determinants which stimulated T cells did so in association with Ia determinants but were not readily accessible to antibodies directed against native soluble antigen. The implications of these observations are crucial to our understanding of how T cells perceive antigen. They all point to one important conclusion: native antigen is not effectively recognized as such, or in isolation, by most T cell subsets; an MHC component must be involved in this recognition (by "effective" recognition is implied recognition followed by activation of the cell).

TABLE II

Involvement of Ia molecules in T cell activation

T cell subset	*Stimulating material*	*Reference*[a]
Antigen-specific T cell proliferating *in vitro*	Antigen presenting Ia^+ Mph	Thomas *et al.* (1978)
Mitogen-reactive T cell proliferating *in vitro*	Con A plus a source of Ia molecules	Möller *et al.* (1979).
Antigen-binding T cell	"IAC", a complex of Ia and "processed" antigen	Puri and Lonai (1980).
Helper T cell	"GRF" containing Ia and antigen	Erb and Feldmann (1975).
DTH T cell	Antigen-pulsed Ia^+ Mph	Mottram and Miller (1980).

[a] Space does not allow a complete list of references.

Many other observations substantiate this general conclusion (Table II). Thus, Ia molecules appear essential for the ability of con A to activate purified T cells. It was hypothesized that T cells must contain receptors for Ia molecules and that con A would activate T cells by binding to the sugars present on Ia molecules and stabilize their interaction to the receptors for Ia on T cells (Möller *et al.*, 1975). Likewise, in antigen-induced T cell activation, specific antigen-binding T cells would bind antigen on Ia containing APC or B cells and triggering would result from the binding of an appropriate concentration of Ia molecules. Some time ago, Erb and Feldmann (1975) invoked the operation of a factor containing Ia and antigen: it was released from antigen-pulsed Mph and was able to trigger antigen-specific T cells. More recently, a similar factor, containing Ia and antigen, has been implicated in antigen-binding by T_H cells and in their effective activation (Puri and Lonai, 1980). Similarly, in DTH responses, only antigen-pulsed Ia^+ Mph were capable of eliciting DTH, Ia^- Mph being ineffective (Mottram and Miller, 1980). It seems likely that neither antigen or mitogen molecules on their own, nor

Ia molecules on their own, can bind sufficiently well to T cells to activate them. Perhaps the receptors on T cells are of low avidity and perhaps an interaction between Ia, antigen, and the respective receptors on the surface of the appropriate T cells is required to stabilize the complex prior to activation of the cell.

Whatever the case may be, it would seem that such interactions of Ia and of antigen molecules with T cells constitute the basis of MHC restriction. Once activated, the T cells proliferate and the effector cells recognize only an identical complex of the same Ia and antigen molecules. Such a restriction thus appears to be induced as a result of priming. Certainly, this must be the case when one considers the situation in an F_1 animal. Thus, for example, F_1 mice between two MHC-incompatible strains (say P_1 and P_2) can be sensitized to antigen and lymphoid cells from the sensitized F_1 can transfer DTH to naive recipients of both parental strains. If, however, the F_1 is sensitized by antigen-pulsed Mph derived from one of the parental strains (say P_1), lymphoid cells from such F_1 mice will transfer DTH only to naive P_1 recipients, not to P_2 (Miller *et al.*, 1976). This suggests that in the F_1 immunized to antigen in the usual way (i.e. by antigen given in complete Freund's adjuvant in the footpads), some T cells are responding to antigen in association with a P_1 MHC component, whereas others respond to antigen in association with P_2 MHC products (both P_1 and P_2 products being expressed in every F_1 APC). If the F_1 is immunized by antigen-pulsed Mph derived from one parental haplotype, only one of these two populations of T cells will be induced, and transfer will be possible only with that population recognizing that haplotype combination. Clearly in this situation the restriction has been imposed as a result of priming. Similar results have been obtained in other F_1 experiments in which priming by antigen associated with one haplotype was shown to restrict T_C cells (Zinkernagel and Doherty, 1974), T_H cells (Sprent, 1978) and T cells proliferating *in vitro* to antigen-pulsed Mph (Paul *et al.*, 1977).

If MHC restriction is imposed as a consequence of priming, then it should be possible to demonstrate allogeneic restriction: i.e. T cells restricted by antigen in association with a foreign *H-2* haplotype. To determine whether this is so, alloreactive T cells must first be removed. One technique employed antigen-driven 5-bromodeoxyuridine and light suicide. By this method, T cells reactive to *H-2* incompatible cells could be eliminated and the residual cells tested for their capacity to respond to antigen on allogeneic stimulator cells. Another method employed the selective absorption of alloreactive T cells on allogeneic cell monolayers which leaves the nonadherent cells unable to respond to *H-2* incompatible cells. A third method utilized the "negative selection" procedure in which parental strain lymphocytes were depleted of alloreactive cells by "filtration" from blood to lymph in irradiated F_1 hybrids. Several studies using such procedures showed that T cells could indeed respond to antigens presented on allogeneic stimulator cells and were restricted by the particular *MHC* haplotype of the stimulator cells (Thomas and Shevach, 1977;

Wilson *et al.*, 1977; Stockinger *et al.*, 1980). Unfortunately, however, other investigators showed the opposite; deletion of alloreactive cells left a population with little or no reactivity specific for modified allogeneic stimulator cells (Janeway *et al.*, 1978; Schmitt-Verhulst and Shearer, 1977). If this is true, one might be tempted to conclude that T cells are committed to recognizing only self-H-2 specificities and that this precedes intentional immunization. Further investigations are thus required to establish unequivocally what is in fact the case.

Some experiments employing chimaeric mice have supported the idea of some commitment of T lymphocytes to MHC components expressed prior to immunization (Bevan, 1978; Zinkernagel *et al.*, 1978a). F_1 mice between two H-2 incompatible strains (say P_1 and P_2) were thymectomized, irradiated and protected with F_1 bone marrow. An epithelial thymus (preirradiated to remove lymphocytes) from one of the parental strains (say P_1) was grafted and the mice allowed to regenerate their haemopoietic system. They were then infected with virus (Zinkernagel *et al.*, 1978a), or immunized with antigen (Sprent, 1978; Miller *et al.*, 1979) and the T cells activated by such an immunization regime were then tested in appropriate systems: e.g. *in vitro* on virus-infected P_1 and P_2 targets, or *in vivo* after transfer with P_1 or P_2 B cells or in naive P_1 or P_2 mice. In all systems, the results were the same: the T cells could only respond to antigen presented in association with P_1 cells, not P_2. This is in contrast to the situation in ordinary (nonchimaeric) F_1 mice where T cells can respond to antigen in association with either P_1 or P_2 haplotypes. The essential difference between the chimaera and the F_1 experimental systems is that in the former, the F_1 stem cells have differentiated in a thymus expressing only one H-2 haplotype, whereas in the latter, differentiation occurred in a thymus expressing both H-2 haplotypes. The T cells must thus "learn" to recognize within the thymus which H-2 haplotype is expressed. Viewed in this way, H-2 restriction is primarily imposed by the H-2 type expressed in the thymus epithelium and commits the immature T cell whilst differentiating in the thymus. If this is so, T cells should not recognize antigen in association with an entirely foreign H-2 haplotype. The fact that they do in some systems, though not in others (see above), does not clarify the situation.

Experimental results obtained in normal homozygous mice, heterozygous F_1 and various chimaeras can be summarized as follows (see also Table III).

(1) Normal homozygous T cells of strain *a* consist primarily of a predominant population of anti-self-*a* (anti-*a*) T cells which recognize antigen presented by cells or APC of strain *a*; the question whether, in the normal *a* animal, T cells can recognize antigen presented by cells of strain *b* is unfortunately not clearly resolved even today.

(2) Normal heterozygous $(a \times b)F_1$ T cells consist of an approximately 50:50 mixture of anti-*a* and anti-*b* cells: their proportion can be altered by exposure to antigen on APC bearing only one of the haplotypes *a* or *b* (restriction imposed by priming).

(3) Heterozygous $(a \times b)F_1$ T cells derived from stem cells differentiating

TABLE III

Restriction specificities and alloreactivity in thymus grafted chimaeras and nude mice

Group	Stem cell	Thymus graft	Host	APC	Restriction specificity In host	Restriction specificity In a × b environment	Anti-b alloreactivity
1	*a*	*a*	*a*	*a*	*a*	—	present
2	$a \times b$	$a \times b$	$a \times b$	$a \times b$	*a,b*	—	absent
3	$a \times b$	irradiated *a*	irradiated $a \times b$	$a \times b$	*a*	—	absent
4	*a*	irradiated $a \times b$	irradiated $a \times b$	*a*	*a*	*a,b*	absent
5	*a*	irradiated $a \times b$	nude *a*	*a*	*a*	*a*	present
6	*a*	unirradiated $a \times b$	nude *a*	*a*	*a*	*a*	absent
7	*a*	unirradiated *b*	nude *a*	*a*	*a*	*a*	absent
8	*a*	irradiated *b*	nude *a*	*a*	—	—	incompetent

In group 3, the results apply to T_C (Zinkernagel *et al.*, 1978a), to T_H (Sprent, 1978) and to T_D (Miller *et al.*, 1979) cells. In group 4, the results apply to T_C cells (Zinkernagel *et al.*, 1978a, b) and to T_H cells (Sprent, 1978). The results in groups 5 to 8 apply to T_H (Kindred, 1980) and T_C cells (Zinkernagel *et al.*, 1980).

in an *a* thymus contain functional anti-*a* but not anti-*b* T cells (restriction imposed in thymus).

(4) Homozygous strain *a* T cells derived from strain *a* stem cells differentiating in an $(a \times b)F_1$ thymus apparently contain both anti-*a* and anti-*b* T cells. The anti-*a* cells may be revealed by appropriate stimulation within the chimaera. The anti-*b* cells can only be revealed after transfer to an irradiated F_1 (Zinkernagel *et al.*, 1978b), since the APC of the original chimaera are of strain *a* genotype only (having been derived from strain *a* stem cells). Recent experiments by Zinkernagel *et al.* (1980) in fact implicate a post-thymic maturation step dependent on the H-2 haplotype of the lymphohaemopoietic system. If this lacks the H-2 haplotype of one parental type (strain *b* in the present example) post-thymic expansion of only anti-*a* T cells will take place. This was clearly the case in strain *a* nude mice grafted with an $(a \times b)F_1$ thymus (Kindred, 1980; Zinkernagel *et al.*, 1980). Thus the thymus can select the restriction specificity but this, in itself, is not sufficient to promote T cell maturation: a second step dependent on exposure to lymphohaemopoietic cells (possibly involving priming to self or environmental antigen on APC) is necessary.

MHC-LINKED *Ir* genes

The next point to consider is the relationship between MHC restriction and *MHC*-linked *Ir* genes. H-2 restriction may be imposed either during priming, or prior to immunization when T cells differentiate in the thymus. Likewise, *MHC*-linked *Ir* genes may be considered to exert their effects either at the level of the APC or at the level of the generation of the T-cell repertoire during differentiation in the thymus. When responsiveness is under *MHC*-linked *Ir* gene control, the trait is dominant and an F_1 between responder (R) and low responder (LR) strains can respond. In DTH, it will be recalled that lymphocytes from F_1 mice sensitized to antigen not under *Ir* gene control, could transfer sensitivity equally well to naive recipients of both parental strains. If, however, the cells were obtained from a sensitized $(R \times LR)F_1$, transfer of sensitivity to the terpolymer L-glutamic acid^{60}-L-alanine^{30}-L-tyrosine^{10}(GAT) was successful in naive recipients of the F_1 and of the R but not of the LR haplotype (Miller *et al.*, 1977). The naïve recipients are essentially passive and only present antigens to the T cells which have been actively sensitized in the F_1 donors. The sensitized $(R \times LR)F_1$ behaves essentially as the $(P_1 \times P_2)F_1$ sensitized by antigen-pulsed P_1 Mph. The latter can transfer sensitivity to naïve P_1, not P_2, the former to naive R, not LR. It seems, therefore that in LR strains, APC fail to display antigen under *Ir* gene control in a form immunogenic for T lymphocytes. Support for this came from studies using GAT-pulsed Mph: both LR and R Mph could take up radioiodinated GAT but only RMph could sensitize and elicit sensitivity in F_1 mice *in vivo*; GAT-pulsed LR Mph were totally ineffective (Miller *et al.*, 1979). On the other hand, antigens like

GAT which fail to associate with the relevant MHC gene product on the surface of APC may be available in some other form to activate T_S cells. These in turn would suppress any response that may have been initiated by some minimal presentation of antigen to LR T cells involved in DTH or helper function. In fact GAT LR mice do have activated T_S cells (Benacerraf *et al.*, 1975).

An alternative possibility is that *Ir* genes exert their effect at the level of generation of the T-cell repertoire. For example, *a* strain mice are essentially LR to virus infected *b* targets. When, however *a* stem cells differentiate in an $(a \times b)F_1$ thymus, the *a* T cells can now lyse virus-infected *b* targets (in an F_1 environment as explained above). In other words, the LR *a* becomes an R if its cells can differentiate in an F_1 thymus, i.e. an R with respect to virus on *b* targets. Investigations were thus made of the responsiveness of LR derived T cells after differentiation in an $(R \times LR)F_1$ thymus. CBA (H-2^k) mice are R to GAT and A.SW (H-2^s) mice are LR. $(A.SW \times CBA)F_1$ mice were irradiated and repopulated with bone marrow cells from either A.SW or CBA. DTH response was observed in the CBA $\rightarrow$ $(A.SW \times CBA)F_1$ chimaeras, not in the A.SW $\rightarrow$ $(A.SW \times CBA)F_1$ chimaeras. If, however, these chimaeras were primed not by GAT given in Freund's complete adjuvant, but by GAT-pulsed F_1 Mph, DTH to GAT could be induced (Miller *et al.*, 1979). The lymphohaemopoietic system of the chimaeras not primed with Mph had only A.SW Mph. The results therefore do not allow us to distinguish between a defect at the level of the generation of anti-GAT receptors in A.SW T cells or a failure of effective association between GAT and Ia^s on A.SW Mph, as the reason why A.SW T cells cannot respond to GAT. When F_1 Mph are provided, T cells with reactivities against H-2^k are likely to be those cells activated to the complex antigen formed by Ia^k and GAT on the surface of F_1 Mph. Hence one cannot assume that the repertoire of the LR T cell has been "enlarged" by differentiation in a R thymus to include a reactivity which can recognize antigen in association with an LR MHC gene product.

Recently, persuasive evidence has been obtained which implicates the lesion of the LR as being at the level of antigen presentation by APC rather than at the level of the T cell repertoire (Longo and Schwartz, 1980). The cellular requirements for *Ir* gene expression in a T cell proliferative response under dual, complementing, *Ir* gene control was examined. The response to the linear polymer poly $(Glu^{55}Lys^{36}Phe^{9})_n$ (GLØ), requires two *R* alleles, which in the $(B10.A \times B10.A(18R))F_1$ map in *I-A^b* and *I-E^k/C^d*. Using a variety of thymus-grafted chimaeric mice, it was shown (a) that the gene products of the complementing Ir-GLØ *R* alleles functioned as a single restriction element at the level of the APC, and (b) that T cells that do not possess *R* alleles are not intrinsically defective, since they could be made phenotypic R if they developed in an environment in which R MHC products were learned as self and if antigen was presented to them by APC bearing R MHC products.

If the lesion of LR is at the level of antigen association with LR MHC products one would expect that the *Ir* genes controlling T_C cell reactions should be localized in the *K* and *D* regions of the MHC, since those regions restrict the activities of T_C cells. Evidence for this has been obtained in studies demonstrating an apparent inability of certain *H-2K* or *H-2D* alleles to associate effectively with a particular antigen to stimulate T_C cell activity, e.g. the defective response to influenza infected H-2K^b targets, to vaccinia infected H-2D^k targets (Zinkernagel *et al.*, 1978c) and to H-Y in association with H-2K^b, H-2K^d or H-2D^d (Simpson and Gordon, 1977). As a corollary, one would expect MHC molecules to have the ability to associate closely with other proteins on the cell surface. Evidence in favour of this is rapidly accumulating (e.g. viral antigens, Helenius *et al.*, 1978; Callahan *et al.*, 1979; bacterial antigens, Klareskeg *et al.*, 1978; parasite antigens, Sher *et al.*, 1978; allogeneic cell antigens, Preud'homme *et al.*, 1979). However, the question arises as to the type of association which takes place and how this accounts for the specificity of the *Ir* gene effect. These are major problems for which no biochemical solution has yet been offered.

T cell factors

Some cell to cell interactions in immune responses are thought to be mediated by T cell factors. Such factors have been extracted from both T_H and T_S cells. They are produced as a consequence of antigenic stimulation. They are antigen specific being absorbed by antigen-sepharose columns. They lack *Ig* constant regions gene products (of heavy and light chains), but possess V_H region determinants and some even carry the major idiotypes found on antibody produced by B cells. Their estimated mol. wt is of the order of 40 000 to 50 000 and they bear distinct *I* region determinants, helper factors bearing I-A and suppressor factor I-J. Further details are to be found in the vast literature on this subject (e.g. Tada *et al.*, 1977; Thèze *et al.*, 1977; Greene *et al.*, 1979; Rich and David, 1979; Munro and Taussig, 1975). In spite of the large amount of work done on these factors, there are still many fundamental questions which have not been answered unequivocally. Thus, for example, how do the factors act and what is their target cell? Do they in fact bear Ia antigens, or were the anti-Ia sera used contaminated with anti-idiotype antibodies (i.e. anti-anti-Ia)? If so the factors would have an anti-Ia specificity and this would make them analogous to the current models of specific receptors on the T cell from which the factors are claimed to be derived (Schrader, 1979). Are they MHC restricted in the same manner as the T cells which produce them? Finally and most importantly, what is their exact molecular nature and their relationship to T cell surface receptors and to antibody binding sites?

Idiotype–anti-idiotype interactions

In addition to interactions mediated via T cell factors, recent evidence points to co-operation within a network of idiotype-recognizing cells. A recognition system, involving the variable portions of Ig receptors, would enable a highly specific type of interaction between anti-idiotypic T cells and idiotype positive T or B cells. Several investigations have documented the existence of such interactions. For example, anti-idiotypic antibodies to the major cross-reactive idiotype (CRI) associated with anti-*p*-azobenzenearsonate (ABA) antibodies in A/J mice, when administered under differing conditions, can result in the production either of T_D cells (Sy *et al.*, 1980) or T_S cells (Sy *et al.*, 1979). Suppressor factor obtained from ABA-specific T_S cells bears the CRI (Greene *et al.*, 1979) and can, itself, induce the production of T_S cells which express anti-idiotypic receptors. Idiotype–anti-idiotype interactions have also been demonstrated in T and B cell co-operation. Thus, for example, recent studies with the T15 idiotype suggested the involvement of two types of carrier specific T_H cells in the induction of an antiphosphoryl choline antibody response dominated by the T15 clonotype. One required the hapten and carrier to be present on the same molecule and was presumably MHC restricted in the usual way (although this was not determined in the particular study). The other appeared to be specific for idiotype, as it induced the selective activation of T15-bearing B cells, but it also showed specificity for the priming carrier, although it did not require physical linkage of hapten to carrier (Bottomly and Mosier, 1979). This second T_H cell must thus have had dual specificity both for carrier and for idiotype. It would seem imperative to determine whether it is also MHC restricted. Likewise in the system where ABA-specific DTH is induced by anti-CRI antibodies, it would be important to know whether the T_D cells, activated in this way, display the same MHC restriction as do T_D cells induced by ABA. If it is not MHC restricted, one might conclude that anti-idiotype can trigger T cells directly (without prior presentation via APC) and that normal T cells are not all self-H-2 restricted. If so, T cells must be able to recognize antigen on allogeneic stimulator cells. This is clearly an area for extensive investigation.

Conclusion

Speculations on the origin of the T cell repertoire have often used as their basis the high frequency of alloreactive T cells and the phenomenon of thymus-dictated self-MHC restriction. They have often ignored the reservations made above concerning frequency estimates across entire *H-2* regions. They have accepted as dogma the learning of self-H-2 recognition by T cells developing within the thymus, even though it is still not excluded that T cells might recognize antigen on allogeneic stimulator cells, as mentioned above. Recent work with thymus-grafted nude mice does indeed lead one to question whether new restriction specificities are acquired by T cells within the thymus. Thus, although immunocompetence was restored to homozygous nude mice by a completely allogeneic thymus graft, the T cells could recognize antigen, not on APC bearing the same H-2 as the thymus graft, as might have been expected, but on APC syngeneic with the nude host (Kindred, 1980; Zinkernagel *et al.*, 1980). Therefore, the whole question of the learning of restriction specificities in the thymus requires re-examination and all the theories which imply that thymic H-2 alone drives the diversification of the T cell repertoire (Jerne, 1971; von Boehmer *et al.*, 1978) must either be discarded or radically modified. Clearly the time has come to review such speculations and even to abandon complex and indirect grafting and chimaeric experiments. We should concentrate our efforts on more direct approaches to study the specificities of T lymphocytes, approaches based on cloning antigen-specific T cells and utilizing DNA recombinant techniques with defined tools such as V_H gene probes.

References

Basten, A., Miller, J. F. A. P. and Abraham, R. (1975). *J. Exp. Med.* **141**, 547–560.
Benacerraf, B., Kapp, J. A., Debré, P., Pierce, C. W. and de la Croix, F. (1975). *Transpl. Rev.* **26**, 21–38.
Bevan, M. J. (1975). *J. Exp. Med.* **142**, 1349–1364.
Bevan, M. J. (1978). *Nature (Lond.)* **269**, 417–418.
Bottomly, K. and Mosier, D. E. (1979). *J. Exp. Med.* **150**, 1399–1409.
Brown, E. R., Singh, B., Lee, K. C., Wegmann, T. G. and Diener, E. (1979). *Immunogenetics* **9**, 33–43.
Bullock, W. W., Katz, D. H. and Benacerraf, B. (1975). *J. Exp. Med.* **142**, 275–287.
Callahan, G. N., Allison, J. A., Pellegrino, M. A. and Reisfeld, R. A. (1979). *J. Immunol.* **122**, 70–74.
Cantor, H. and Weissman, I. (1976). *Progr. Allergy* **20**, 1–64.
Doherty, P. C., Blanden, R. V. and Zinkernagel, R. M. (1976). *Transpl. Rev.* **29**, 89–124.
Eardley, D. D., Hugenberger, J., McVay-Boudreau, L., Shen, F. W., Gershon, R. K. and Cantor, H. (1978). *J. Exp. Med.* **147**, 1106–1115.
Erb, P. and Feldmann, M. (1975). *Eur. J. Immunol.* **5**, 759–766.
Gershon, R. K. (1974). *Contemp. Top. Immunobiol.* **3**, 1–40.
Gordon, R. D., Simpson, E. and Samelson, L. E. (1975). *J. Exp. Med.* **142**, 1108–1120.
Greene, M. I., Bach, B. and Benacerraf, B. (1979). *J. Exp. Med.* **149**, 1069–1083.
Helenius, A., Morein, B., Fries, E., Simons, K., Robinson, P., Schirrmacher, V., Terhorst, C. and Strominger, J. (1978). *Proc. Natn. Acad. Sci. U.S.A.* **75**, 3846–3850.
Janeway, C. A., Murphy, P. D., Kemp, J. and Wigzell, H. (1978). *J. Exp. Med.* **147**, 1065–1077.
Jerne, N. K. (1971). *Eur. J. Immunol.* **1**, 1–19.
Katz, D. H. and Benacerraf, B. (1975). *Transpl. Rev.* **22**, 175–195.
Kindred, B. (1980). *Cell Immunol.* **51**, 64–71.
Klareskeg, L., Banck, G., Forsgren, A. and Peterson, P. A. (1978). *Proc. Natn. Acad. Sci. U.S.A.* **75**, 6197–6201.
Lindahl, K. F. and Wilson, D. B. (1977). *J. Exp. Med.* **145**, 508–521.
Longo, D. L. and Schwartz, R. H. (1980). *J. Exp. Med.* (in press).
Miller, J. F. A. P. (1972). *Intern. Rev. Cytol.* **33**, 77–130.
Miller, J. F. A. P. and Mitchell, G. F. (1968). *J. Exp. Med.* **128**, 801–820.
Miller, J. F. A. P. and Mitchell, G. F. (1969). *Transpl. Rev.* **1**, 3–42.
Miller, J. F. A. P., Vadas, M. A., Whitelaw, A. and Gamble, J. (1976). *Proc. Natn. Acad. Sci. U.S.A.* **73**, 2486–2490.

Miller, J. F. A. P., Vadas, M. A., Whitelaw, A., Gamble, J. and Bernard, C. (1977). *J. Exp. Med.* **145**, 1623–1628.

Miller, J. F. A. P., Gamble, J., Mottram, P. and Smith, F. I. (1979). *Scand. J. Immunol.* **9**, 29–38.

Miller, S. D., Sy. M. S. and Claman, H. N. (1978). *J. Exp. Med.* **147**, 788–799.

Mitchell, G. F. and Miller, J. F. A. P. (1968). *J. Exp. Med.* **128**, 821–837.

Möller, G., Hammarström, L., Möller, E., Persson, U., Smith, E., Waterfield, D. and Waterfield, E. (1979). *Haematologia* **12**, 37–45.

Mottram, P. and Miller, J. F. A. P. (1980). *Eur. J. Immunol.* **10**, 165–170.

Munro, A. J. and Taussig, M. J. (1975). *Nature (Lond.)* **256**, 103–106.

Paul, W. E., Shevach, E. M., Thomas, D. W., Pickeral, S. F. and Rosenthal, A. S. (1977). *Cold Spring Harbor Symp. Quant. Biol.* **41**, 571–578.

Prud'Homme, G., Shon, U. and Delovitch, T. L. (1979). *J. Exp. Med.* **149**, 137–149.

Puri, J. and Lonai, P. (1980). *Eur. J. Immunol.* **10**, 273–281.

Rich, S. S. and David, C. S. (1979). *J. Exp. Med.* **150**, 1108–1121.

Rosenthal, A. S. (1978). *Immunol. Rev.* **40**, 136–152.

Schmitt-Verhulst, A-M. and Shearer, G. M. (1977). *J. Supramol. Struct. Suppl.* **1**, 206.

Schrader, J. W. (1979). *Scand. J. Immunol.* **10**, 387–393.

Schwartz, R. H., Yano, A. and Paul, W. E. (1978). *Immunol. Rev.* **40**, 153–180.

Shearer, G. M., Rehn, T. G. and Schmitt-Verhulst, A-M. (1976). *Transpl. Rev.* **29**, 222–248.

Sher, A., Hall, B. F. and Vadas, M. A. (1978). *J. Exp. Med.* **148**, 46–57.

Shiozawa, C. and Diener, E. (1980). *J. Immunol.* (in press).

Simpson, E. and Gordon, R. D. (1977). *Immunol. Rev.* **35**, 59–75.

Smith, F. I., Mottram, P. L. and Miller, J. F. A. P. (1979). *Scand. J. Immunol.* **10**, 343–347.

Sprent, J. (1978). *J. Exp. Med.* **147**, 1159–1174.

Stockinger, H., Pfizenmaier, K., Rölinghoff, M. and Wagner, H. (1980). *Proc. Natn. Acad. Sci. U.S.A.* (in press).

Sy, M. S., Bach, B. A., Dohi, Y., Nisonoff, A., Benacerraf, B. and Greene, M. I. (1979). *J. Exp. Med.* **150**, 1216–1228.

Sy, M. S., Brown, A. R., Benacerraf, B. and Greene, M. I. (1980). *J. Exp. Med.* **151**, 896–909.

Tada, T., Taniguchi, M. and Okumura, K. (1977). *Progr. Immunol.* **3**, 369–377.

Tada, T., Toshitada, T., Okumura, K., Nonaka, M. and Tokuhisa, T. (1978). *J. Exp. Med.* **147**, 446–458.

Thèze, J., Kapp, J. A. and Benacerraf, B. (1977). *J. Exp. Med.* **145**, 839–856.

Thomas, D. W. and Shevach, E. M. (1977). *Proc. Natn. Acad. Sci. U.S.A.* **74**, 2104–2108.

Thomas, D. W., Clement, I. and Shevach, E. M. (1978). *Immunol. Rev.* **40**, 181–204.

Vadas, M. A., Miller, J. F. A. P., McKenzie, I. F. C., Chism, S. E., Shen, F. W., Boyse, E. A., Gamble, J. R. and Whitelaw, A. M. (1976). *J. Exp. Med.* **144**, 10–19.

Vadas, M. A., Miller, J. F. A. P., Whitelaw, A. M. and Gamble, J. R. (1977). *Immunogenetics* **4**, 137–153.

von Boehmer, H., Haas, W. and Jerne, N. K. (1978). *Proc. Natn. Acad. Sci. U.S.A.* **75**, 2439–2442.

Wilson, D. B., Lindahl, K. F., Wilson, D. H. and Sprent, J. (1977). *J. Exp. Med.* **146**, 361–367.

Yano, A., Schwartz, R. H. and Paul, W. E. (1977). *J. Exp. Med.* **146**, 828–843.

Zinkernagel, R. M. and Doherty, P. C. (1974). *Nature (Lond.)* **251**, 547–548.

Zinkernagel, R. M., Callahan, G. N., Althage, A., Cooper, S., Klein, P. A. and Klein, J. (1978a). *J. Exp. Med.* **147**, 882–896.

Zinkernagel, R. M., Callahan, G. N., Althage, A., Cooper, S., Streilein, J. W. and Klein, J. (1978b). *J. Exp. Med.* **147**, 897–911.

Zinkernagel, R. M., Althage, A., Cooper, S., Kreeb, G., Klein, P. A., Sefton, B., Flaherty, L., Stimpfling, J., Shreffler, D. and Klein, J. (1978c). *J. Exp. Med.* **148**, 592–606.

Zinkernagel, R. M., Althage, A., Waterfield, E., Kindred, B., Welsh, R. M., Callahan, G. and Pincetl, P. (1980). *J. Exp. Med.* **151**, 376–399.

20

Suppressor T Cells: A Miniposition Paper Celebrating A New Decade

RICHARD K. GERSHON

Laboratory of Cellular Immunology
Howard Hughes Medical Institute at Yale, New Haven, Connecticut, USA

Introduction

The organizers and editors of the 4th International Congress of Immunology have requested me to write a "position paper" on the subject of suppressor T cells. Having recently refused several requests to write reviews on the subject because the voluminous number of publications on the subject would make a literature search so arduous, that little time would be left for writing grant proposals which have already left little time for doing research which—(I leave the rest to the reader's imagination), I start this "position paper" with an *apologia* and a caveat; what follows must be considered neither a review nor a position paper. Rather, it can be considered a "miniposition paper" or, for all those whose original and important contributions I have neglected to cite, this may even be considered to be a "microposition paper."

What then do we know about suppressor T cells that we didn't know at the time of the 1st International Congress and/or was not documented in the publication of its proceedings:

The existence of suppressor T cells

Suppressor T cells exist; i.e. they are now an entity and not a concept. This knowledge stems from the elegant studies of Cantor and Boyse (1977) using antisera against polymorphic determinants on a series of glycoproteins called Ly antigens, that are expressed only on T cells and thus can be considered to be candidates for true "differentiation antigens." That is the presence of these antigens on the cells surface indicates the nature of the gene programme that has been switched on during the cells differentiative life history. Cantor and Boyse and their colleagues (see Cantor and Boyse, 1977 for specific references) showed that a small proportion of T cells express an Ly cell surface profile of Ly-1^-;23^+. Within that group of T cells resides a cell "set" that has (a) no helper activity and (b) potent suppressive activity.

This observation allowed workers who had previously demonstrated T cell mediated suppression, to show that the phenomena they were describing were actually mediated by a distinct cell type with, as far as could be told, a unique function. Quantitative arguments (e.g. suppression = too much help) which had "raged" in the early 1970s were ruled out. The existence of a cell set that has the specialized job of suppressing immune responses was firmly established. It is highly unlikely that any new findings will challenge this point.

The precise phenotype of the suppressor cell is not yet completely settled.

Several workers using monoclonal antibodies have claimed that all murine T cells are Ly-1 positive, denying the existence of an Ly-1^-23^+ T cell set. However, since many investigators, using many kinds of anti-Ly-1 sera +C′ to kill T cells, find an Ly-1^-; Ly-2^+ T cell with unique functions remaining after this treatment, the resolution of the apparent conflict between the "morphologists" and the "functionalists" will probably be of interest only to "specialists" and will not seriously alter the interpretation of the large body of data that says that suppressor T cells are a distinct cell set with a fully differentiated gene programme which allows them to perform a very specialized function.

It should also be noted that several investigators (including A. J. Schwartz in collaboration with my laboratory), have presented data to show that some forms of T cell mediated suppression can be removed by treatment with either anti-Ly-1 serum or anti-Ly-2 serum and that mixtures of the treated cells fail to return suppression. From this data they have inferred that some suppressor T cells do express the Ly-123 phenotype. Although this influence is likely to be true, until the activity of positively selected Ly-123 cells is tested directly (as opposed to inferentially), the relation of the 2 suppressor cells, separated by functionally detectable Ly-1 antigen, will remain unclear. It is my feeling that the Ly-123 phenotype on suppressor T cells will not be stable; that these cells will turn out to be precursors of "functionally" Ly-1^-;23^+ cells.

Heterogeneity of suppressor T cell activities

This discussion is more appropriate in a consideration of how many types of suppressor T cells there are; not of whether they exist. As the previous discussion has suggested the answer to this question is not at all clear. In fact, the information available to us, to help answer this question is roughly equivalent to that available for answering the first question I discussed, prior to the work of Cantor and Boyse (1977). Thus, in 1980 we can say that there probably is more than one type of suppressor T cell but that there are no available data sufficiently compelling to cause William of Occam to apply his caveat to his razor. It is not yet necessary to postulate more than one entity.

Claims for heterogeneity in suppressor T cell types are based on things like antigen specificity; some suppressor T cells work in an antigen specific way, some do not. Presentation of this kind of evidence to a disciple of Occam might bring forth the following rejoinder. Of course! The gene product used by the suppressor T cell, to inhibit the function of its target cell, is *not* likely to be encoded in the V_H region of the *Ig* locus wherein the specificity for antigen is likely to lie. Thus, suppressor T cells may release functional suppressor gene products, before they mature to the state where they can merge the "specificity" gene product with the "suppressor" gene product. That is why "nonspecific" suppressor T cells sometimes express more Ly-1 antigen than do specific suppressor cells (Schwartz *et al.*, 1979); the Ly-123 is likely to be the precursor of the Ly-23.

Other characteristics which suggest heterogeneity in the suppressor T-cell set include differential effects on the isotype of antibody being made, on delayed hypersensitivity versus antibody formation, on T cells *v.* B cells *v.* Ig secreting cells, etc. All these findings *could* be explained by postulating a differential sensitivity to the activity of a single type of suppressor T cell rather than by invoking multiple suppressor T cell types.

Differences in sensitivity to drugs and ionizing radiation of different suppressor T cell effects are even less compelling reasons for invoking more than one suppressor T cell entity. These agents are known to show cell cycle dependence in their efficacy of action and for these and other reasons are poor markers for identifying fully differentiated cells with unique gene programmes.

Lastly, some claims for suppressor T cell heterogeneity have been made on the basis of differential sensitivity of the suppression to cytotoxic alloantisera + C′. Interpretations of this type of data are so fraught with difficulty that when present day "Occamists" are presented with arguments for heterogeneity based on these considerations they respond only with a wry smile. Those "nonspecialists" who fail to understand why these arguments evoke such responses must read on to find the answer (for those in a hurry, I will deal with this point in the next section).

To sum up this section; the answer in 1980 to the question of how many separable suppressor T cell sets there are is: probably more than one, but the evidence is not sufficient to convince a hard core "one function : one cell" man.

Suppressor T cells' partner cells

The problem alluded to above, concerning phenotyping of suppressor cells stems from the fact that suppressor effector cells are not an autonomous group of cells; they depend on other cells (as well as antigen) to function (Cantor and Gershon, 1979). Thus when a given treatment removes suppression one is hard put, without the availability of several other data, to attribute the characteristic one has deleted with the specific treatment, to the suppressor cell itself rather than to another cell that may affect suppressor cell activity. Perhaps an illustrative example can help clarify this point. When Claman *et al.* (1966) added thymocytes to lethally irradiated bone marrow reconstituted mice and the mice made antibody, they did not conclude that the thymocytes made antibody; nor did Davies *et al.* (1967) or Mitchell and Miller (1968) conclude, when they removed T cells from a heterogeneous population of cells and found that the remaining cells did not make antibody, that the T cells they removed were antibody forming precursors.

What do we know at present about cells which influence the activity of suppressor cells? A suppressor circuit with a specialized inducer cell, an amplifier/precursor cell, another distinct amplifier cell and an effector cell has been defined (see Cantor and Gershon, 1979). Removal of any one of the cells in this circuit can reduce or even eliminate the ability to demonstrate T cell mediated suppression. It is even possible that the circuit could be activated by feedback products of cells which are not actually members of the circuit (e.g. see L'age-Stehr *et al.*, 1980). The murine cells that comprise this suppressor circuit express the following profile of cell surface alloantigens:

Inducer cell

The inducer cell is Ly-1$^+$;23$^-$;Qa-1$^+$;I-J$^+$.

Amplifier/precursor cell

The amplifier/precursor cell is Ly-123$^+$;Qa-1$^+$;I-J$^+$ and thus differs from the inducer cell only by the expression of Ly-23 alloantigens. The I-J determinant on the 2 cells is serologically identical (Eardley *et al.*, 1980).

Amplifier cell

The other amplifier cell is Ly-1$^-$;Ly-23$^+$;I-J$^+$;Qa-1? (see Tada *et al.*, 1977). The amplifying activity of this cell, like the inducing activity of the I-J$^+$Ly-1 cell mentioned above, is highly dependent on an I-J$^+$Ly-123 cell. Whether the same Ly-123 cell is involved in "transducing" the signal from the I-J$^+$Ly-1 inducer cell and the I-J$^+$Ly-23 amplifier cell is not known, nor is the relation of the I-J determinants to one another on the 2 cells known. Another I-J$^+$Ly-23$^+$ amplifier cell, which is Qa-1$^-$ has recently been described by McDougal *et al.* (1980). Whether this is an additional cell in the suppressor circuit or is the same Ly-23 amplifier cell described by Tada *et al.* remains to be determined.

Effector cell

Lastly, in collaboration with Donal Murphy, we have found that the effector cell of this circuit expresses the phenotype Ly-1$^-$;Ly-23$^+$;I-J$^-$;Qa-1$^-$. The finding that suppressor effector cells do not express I-J determinants may be surprising to some and should be viewed with scepticism by all. As far as I can tell, the only laboratories to ask the experimental question of whether *I-J* subregion controlled determinants are expressed on suppressor *effector* cells are Murphy's and my own. The only way to ask this question is to assay for suppression on cell populations that have no cells with potential suppressor activity present (e.g. the assay cells must be depleted of all Ly-2$^+$ cells). Without using this assay system, the possibility that the test cell acts by turning on suppressor cells in the assay cannot be discounted. When we have used such assay populations we have found that neither anti-Ly-2 nor anti-Qa-1 + C′ can diminish suppression (in addition we have found the biologically active product of suppressor effector T cells is I-J^- (Yamauchi *et al.*, in preparation)).

The reason I suggest the reader view these results with scepticism stems from the problem inherent in interpreting all "negative types" of results. Thus it is possible that suppressor effector cells are I-J^+ but express an *I-J* subregion controlled determinant that our antisera do not recognize. (Or, less likely, express an I-J determinant but in too low amounts to be killed by treatment with antibody +C′. I say less likely because the cells product is I-J^-, in contradiction to the product of the I-J^+ Ly-1 inducer cell.)

Communication between cells in the suppressor circuit

Having defined a suppressor circuit, composed of at least 4 distinct cell subsets, the question of how these subsets communicate with each other arises.

The use of V_H linked gene products

The use of gene products tightly linked to the locus that controls the variable portion of Ig heavy chains, for communication between cells in the suppressor circuit can be inferred from studies of Ig congenic mice (Cantor *et al.*, 1978). These studies have shown that Ly-1 inducer cells (or their biologically active cell free products (Yamauchi *et al.*, in preparation)) will not activate the suppressor circuit in mice which are identical except for a small region of the twelfth chromosome which contains the genes that control V_H expression. On the other hand these same cells will activate the suppressor circuit in mice which have identical V_H linked genes but lack identity at many other major gene loci, such as those encoded in the major histocompatibility complex (MHC). Thus it is likely that the polymorphic portions of gene products controlled by V_H linked genes are used by the suppressor inducer cell to communicate with its Ly-2^+ acceptor cell.

What could these gene products be? The most likely candidate would seem to be idiotype (id) making id anti-id reactions an important mode of communication within the suppressor circuit. However, there is a minor histocompatibility antigen which is linked to V_H (Rolink *et al.*, 1978) and is another gene product which is different in the Ig congenic mouse strains. There are several reasons for thinking that this gene product may be used for communication by the cells in the suppressor circuit. A "position paper" is not the appropriate place to discuss these reasons but it is at least important to point out that an id anti-id reaction is not the only mechanism by which V_H linked T cell expressed communication molecules may function.

The use of MHC controlled gene products

Another important communication molecule(s) in the suppressor circuit is (are) the gene product(s) controlled by the *I-J* subregion of the MHC. This conclusion is based on the finding of *I-J* controlled determinants on T suppressor "factors" (see Germain and Benacerraf, 1980). In contrast to the situation with V_H linked gene products, *I-J* controlled interactions are usually not restricted by the presence of different polymorphic determinants on the communicating molecules, although an important exception to this generalization has been noted (see Tada *et al.*, 1977). In particular, communication between the Ly-1$^-$;Ly-23$^+$;I-J$^+$ amplifying factor isolated by Tada's group will not work if its acceptor cell expresses a different I-J polymorphism.

The use of extrinsic antigen

Since many reported "suppressor factors" bind antigen, antigen bridges between cell sets must also be considered as an important possible mode of communication.

Speculative synthesis based on available data

Speaking of bridges, one must try to incorporate the isolated observations listed above into a theoretical scheme, so that a bridge between information and understanding can be made. I offer the following scheme for consideration.

Antigen bridging serves to focus the messenger cell (or its cell free product) on antigen specific acceptor cells. This focusing interaction is necessary but not sufficient to activate the acceptor cell. Activation requires a second signal which is delivered by an interaction between V_H linked and *I-J* controlled gene products. This notion stems from our observation (Yamauchi *et al.*, in preparation) that I-J$^+$ biologically active molecules in the suppressor circuit are restricted by V_H linked genes while I-J$^-$ molecules are MHC restricted in their function (i.e. an interaction between V_H linked and *I-J* controlled products is key for functional interactions). Exceptions to this "rule" exist. One already mentioned is that of Tada *et al.* (1977) who found MHC restrictions between an I-J$^+$ factor and an I-J$^-$ acceptor cell. Thus, if there is not another I-J$^-$ intermediary cell involved in this interaction it *might* be necessary to add to the notion expressed above, that complementary interactions between 2 *I-J* controlled determinants can serve the same activating function as do the interactions between *I-J* controlled and V_H linked gene products. (I have used the word "might" because more complex explanations could account for this finding but again, it is beyond the scope of this article to consider them.)

Another exception is the finding of an interaction in the suppressor circuit which is restricted by both *MHC* and *Ig* controlled gene products (Weinberger *et al.*, 1980). However, the possibility that this "dual" restriction is not the result of 2 "single" restrictions (i.e., that the read-out required more than one T cell interaction) was not ruled out and thus the explanation I have put forth above has not *yet* been ruled out either.

Intermediary cells

Up to now I have concentrated the discussion on the molecules T cells in the suppressor circuit use to communicate with one another. The question of how these molecules get together has been dealt with only *en passant*. There is a considerable body of evidence that suggests that cells in the macrophage lineage may be involved in passing signals along. This evidence has recently been reviewed (Gershon *et al.*, 1980). The basic logic is that macrophage like cells are specialized to present signals to T cells and that there are 2 major classes of signals; one is antigen which is an "extrinsic" signal and the other is T cell "factor" which is an "intrinsic" signal. The affinity of T cell "factors" for Fc like receptors on antigen presenting cells (see Gershon *et al.*, 1980) has been noted and is the cornerstone on which this notion is built.

Another important observation, which supports the notion, is that effector suppressor T cells definitely use macrophage like cells to inactivate target cells (Ptak *et al.*, 1978). This use of macrophage like cells for intercircuit communication reinforces the possibility that they are also used for intracircuit communication. The premise is that T cells in the suppressor circuit use "complementary" *I-J* controlled markers on macrophage to communicate with one another and use macrophages marked doubly with *I* region controlled gene products to exert their effect on cells in different circuits. Thus, helper cells will react with I-A$^+$ antigen presenting cells and when these I-A$^+$ cells have a passively acquired suppressor signal on their I-J controlled determinant, the helper cells will be knocked out instead of activated. Observations consistent with this scheme are: (1) the presence of I-J on macrophage like cells (Niederhuber and Allen, 1980); (2) the serologic difference of this I-J molecule from the ones on the T cells in the suppressor circuit, suggesting that the 2 I-J subregion products are controlled by different loci (Eardley *et al.*, 1980); (3) the finding that some I-J$^+$ macrophage like cells are I-A$^-$ and that some are not (Habu *et al.*, in prep.; Ptak *et al.*, in prep.).

Targets of suppressor T cells

Another important question concerning suppressor T cell function is "What cell is the target of the suppression?" As discussed above all the cells involved in the immune response: T cells, B cells and macrophages have been implicated as targets. In many cases the assignation of "suppressee" to the various target cells has been based on deduction rather than on direct data. Since so many facets of the antibody response are T dependent the question under consideration cannot be answered simply; one cannot mix suppressor and target cells together and get a clear answer. In regard to cell mediated immunity (CMI) the question is easier to answer since B cells are not required for these responses but the need for macrophage like cells in CMI still creates a problem.

cells

To my mind there is no better published evidence than that put forth by Herzenberg *et al.* (1976) that demonstrates a helper T cell as a target of suppressor cell. These workers showed that demonstrable "allotype specific" suppressor cells could be removed by treatment with anti-Ly-2 sera + C′ and that after suppression was removed the treated cells had no demonstrable "allotype specific" helper cells left, but did have activatable allotype specific B cells. The simplest explanation for these findings, assuming the treatment that removed the suppressor cell did not also remove helper cells, is that the suppressor cell inactivated the helper cell and that once the helper was inactivated there was no need for continued suppression to prevent responsiveness.

Eardley and Green (in preparation), working in my laboratory, have obtained results that support this interpretation and extend it to antigen specific cells as well. They have incubated immune Ly-1 cells with activated Ly-2 suppressor cells for 48 h, after which time they removed the suppressor cells by treatment with anti-Ly-2 + C′. The anti-Ly-2 treatment removed all detectable suppressor cells and did not in itself affect the control helper cells (those not incubated with suppressor cells). However, helper cells that had been incubated with the suppressor cells were unable to help B cells in a primary *in vitro* response to SRBC. Thus, it seems almost certain that Ly-1 helper cells are one target for T cell suppression.

What about other Ly-1 cells? Eardley and Green also noted that the suppressor cells could inactivate the I-J$^+$Ly-1 cell responsible for suppressor induction. In fact they found that this inducer cell was more easily suppressed than the Ly-1 helper cell. These findings bear significantly on the question discussed above concerning heterogeneity in the suppressor cell set. They indicate that apparent heterogeneity could stem from quantitative rather than qualitative differences. Of course, Eardley and Green's findings could also be due to qualitative effects. At this point the question of quantitative *v.* qualitative effects remains open.

B cells

The data suggesting that the B cell may also be a target of suppressor T cells are less direct than the data discussed above and require a greater number of assumptions to reach the conclusion. To the best of my knowledge no one has shown that B cells have lost responsiveness after a sojourn with the cells of the suppressor circuit, as has been shown with T cells.

In terms of studies using T cells to suppress thymus independent antibody responses, the work of Andersson and Blomgren (1975) suggests that B cells can be suppressor T cell targets. However, since these workers used unfractionated T cells to suppress the thymus independent response to polyvinyl pyrrolidone (PVP), and since Ordal *et al.* (1976) have shown that thymus independent responses are very sensitive to IgM feedback, it is not clear whether Andersson and Blomgren's findings were due to suppressor T cell function or due to helper cells inducing a precocious antibody response which was the suppressing agent.

Baker *et al.* (1974) have also presented a large quantity of elegant data concerning T cell regulation of the response to polysaccharide antigens. However, their findings are even more complex and cannot be used to say B cells are a target of suppressor T cells. In fact their results suggest quite the opposite; that the target of suppression is a T cell.

Warren and Davie's (1977) finding that T cells suppress plaque forming cells and the findings of Lynch *et al.* (1979) that T cells can suppress myeloma secretion and proliferation without being cytotoxic, can be viewed as strong arguments in favour of suppressor T cell effects on antibody producing cells. Lynch's work also showed the need for a macrophage accessory cell for suppression to be manifest. This is analogous to findings with suppressor T cells in other systems.

A series of experiments performed by J. Kemp in collaboration with Lynch and Rohrer, have shown that the cell interactions required to suppress myeloma secretion are similar to those found in the suppressor circuit defined above. Since the effector cell is not a killer cell it is likely to be a suppressor cell working on a cell in the B cell lineage.

Macrophages

Since some macrophage functions can be assayed for in the absence of all lymphocytes it has been relatively easy to demonstrate that at least one macrophage function (antitumour cell immunity) can be deleted by cells of the suppressor circuit (Rao *et al.*, 1980).

Why suppression and not help?

The technique used to generate the antimacrophage suppressor T cell mentioned above was by immunization with antigen–antibody complexes. This relates to another major question concerning the generation of suppressor T cells; what determines whether suppression or help will dominate after a certain form of immunization. Again, this is too large and complex a question to discuss adequately in a "miniposition" paper. However several major variables have been identified and deserve at least to be mentioned.

Role of Ig

As alluded to above, whether the antigen is seen by the T cells in connection with Ig is an important variable. Besides the study mentioned above, two other major series of studies bear on this point.

Janeway (1979) has identified a subgroup of T cells that "see" self Ig products, probably in lieu of recognizing self MHC. In a series of collaborative experiments we have shown that this subgroup of T cells that Janeway has defined, contains the major proportion of suppressor inducer cells.

L'age-Stehr *et al.* (1980) have defined an "antiself" suppressor circuit which is triggered by an Ig dependent structure on B cell blasts.

These and other studies (e.g. Gershon *et al.*, 1974b) indicate that preferential activation of suppression may be brought about by the initial presentation of antigen to the system in association with Ig in general or, perhaps with a certain Ig subclass.

Role of different lymphoid organs

Another important variable is the anatomical site at which antigen and the immune system meet. If the initial encounter takes place in the spleen there is a greater likelihood that suppression will be induced than if the initial encounter occurs in peripheral lymph nodes (Gershon *et al.*, 1974a).

Role of special antigen presenting cells

This observation is probably related to another that has shown that a special "class" of antigen presenting cells exist and that when only these cells present antigen to the system a major skewing towards "help" in the helper: suppressor competition can be achieved (Ptak *et al.*, 1980). This special class of antigen presenting cells includes Langerhans cells, splenic dendritic cells and complete Freund's adjuvant induced peritoneal exudate cells (J. Britz *et al.*, in prep.).

Miscellaneous factors

Numerous other variables including *Ir* genes, intrinsic and extrinsic adjuvants, antigen solubility, antigen dose and the ability to "digest" antigen have also been identified. It is possible that all these variables affect a common (or at least a limited number of common) denominator(s) but much more work must be done before definitive answers to the question being asked in this section can be achieved.

Regulation of suppressor T cell activity

The discussion to this point has focused on how suppressor T cells regulate other cells. The question of how other cells regulate suppressor T cells is perhaps of equal importance. According to our preliminary evidence (Eardley *et al.*, unpublished data) it appears that the suppressor T cells are "negatively regulated." That is to say their activity is highly dependent on a continuing source of inducer signals. In the absence of these signals the suppressor cells rapidly lose demonstrable activity. Since, as mentioned above, the cells which induce suppressor cell activity are themselves the target of the suppression, it is easy to see how suppressor cells can act as part of a "closed circuit"; by turning off the cells which are responsible for their activity they act to turn themselves off. Whether suppressor cell products act directly to suppress the suppressor cells themselves is a difficult question to answer; at present no evidence for this type of regulation exists.

It is worth underscoring the notion of what I have defined as "negative regulation." Perhaps a comparison with enzyme: substrate systems would be helpful. In this analogy the substrate acts like the Ly-1 inducer cell in that it activates the enzyme, which acts like the suppressor cell in that it removes its own inducing signal. That removal is the event that inhibits the continued activity of the enzyme or the suppressor cell. This point has important practical and theoretical implications.

Practical implications

In practice it means that assays for suppressor cells must always be done with a known source of cells or other agents that can act as inducers. Without a source of induction in the system, the presence of "latent" suppressor cells that have already shut off the cells that had originally induced them, could be missed in "mixing" type experiments. These findings make attempts to distinguish between "clonal deletion" and T cell suppression as mechanisms for specific immunological unresponsiveness almost meaningless. It is clear that suppressor cells can "delete" activity and then disappear, probably secondary to the "deleting" event. This sequence of events of course could appear to be (or actually be) clonal elimination.

Theoretical implications

Of theoretical importance, the "negative regulation" system allows for the possibility of microenvironmental immune regulation. If suppressor inducer cells (or the cells that induce these inducers) were concentrated in a certain anatomical site, this could allow local suppression to take place in the face of strong systemic immunity. One illustrative example of why this microenvironmental regulation might be useful could be in regulating the size of local granulomata that help contain the spread of micro-organisms, without compromising systemic immunity, which might also be needed to prevent dissemination of these organisms (as happens in miliary tuberculosis).

Role of suppressor T cell malfunction in autoimmunity and human disease

One last major area which I have not discussed is the status of our knowledge on the role of suppressor T cells in regulating immunity in man and in autoimmunity in any species. This subject is itself so large that it requires its own "position paper." I hope the editors and organizers agree. In brief, it could be said that many investigators have found "abnormal" suppressor T cell behaviour in disease states of mice and men. However, in no case has a clear cause and effect analysis been established in a fashion that has led to universal acceptance of the notion that lack of suppressor T cell control is a cause of autoimmune disease. For what it is worth, I am convinced.

Prospects for the future

If the pace of increase in our knowledge of suppressor T cell physiology proceeds at the same rate as it did between the 1st and 4th International Immunology Congresses, the editors of the proceedings of the 7th Congress will need more than one "position paper" on the subject.

References

Andersson, B. and Blomgren, H. (1975). *Nature* **253**, 5491.

Baker, P. J., Stashak, P. W., Amsbaugh, D. F. and Prescott, B. (1974). *J. Immunol.* **112**, 404.

Cantor, H. and Boyse, E. A. (1977). *Immunol. Rev.* **33**, 105.

Cantor, H., Hugenberger, J., McVay-Boudreau, L., Eardley, D. D., Kemp, J., Shen, F. W. and Gershon, R. K. (1978). *J. Exp. Med.* **248**, 871.

Cantor, H. and Gershon, R. K. (1979). *Fed. Proc.* **38**, 2058.

Claman, H. N., Chaperon, E. A. and Triplett, R. F. (1966). *Proc. Soc. Exp. Biol. Med.* **122**, 1167.

Davies, A. J. S., Leuchars, E., Wallis, V., Marchant, R. and Elliott, E. V. (1967). *Transplantation* **5**, 222.

Eardley, D. D., Murphy, D. B., Kemp, J. D., Shen, F. W., Cantor, H. and Gershon, R. K. (1980). *Immunogenetics* (in press).

Germain, R. N. and Benacerraf, B. (1980). *Springer-Seminars Immunopath.* **3**, 93.

Gershon, R. K., Lance, E. M. and Kondo, K. (1974a). *J. Immunol.* **112**, 546.

Gershon, R. K., Orbach-Arbouys, S. and Calkins, C. (1974b). *In* "Progress in Immunology II" (L. Brent and J. Holborow, eds) Vol. 2, pp. 123–134. North-Holland Publishing, Amsterdam.

Gershon, R. K., Naidorf, K. F. and Ptak, W. (1980). *In* "Macrophage Regulation of Immunity" (E. R. Unanue and A. S. Rosenthal, eds) p. 431. Academic Press, New York.

Herzenberg, L. A., Okumura, K., Cantor, H., Sato, V., Shen, F. W., Boyse, E. A. and Herzenberg, L. A. (1976). *J. Exp. Med.* **144**, 330.

Janeway, C. A. Jr. (1979). *Fed. Proc.* **38**, 2071.

L'age-Stehr, J., Teichmann, H., Gershon, R. K. and Cantor, H. (1980). *Eur. J. Immunol.* **10**, 21.

Lynch, R. G., Rohrer, J. W., Odermatt, B., Gebel, H. D., Autry, J. R. and Hoover, R. G. (1979). *Imm. Rev.* **48**, 45.

McDougal, J. S., Shen, F. W., Cort, S. P. and Bard, J. *J. Immunol.* (in press).

Mitchell, G. F. and Miller, J. F. A. P. (1968). *J. Exp. Med.* **128**, 821.

Niederhuber, J. E. and Allen, P. (1980). *J. Exp. Med.* **151**, 1103.
Ordal, J., Smith, S., Ness, D., Gershon, R. K. and Grumet, F. C. (1976). *J. Immunol.* **116**, 1182.
Ptak, W., Zembala, M. and Gershon, R. K. (1978). *J. Exp. Med.* **148**, 424.
Ptak, W., Rozycka, D., Askenase, P. W. and Gershon, R. K. (1980). *J. Exp. Med.* **151**, 362.
Rao, V. S., Bennett, J. A., Shen, F. W., Gershon, R. K. and Mitchell, M. S. (1980). *J. Immunol.* **125**, 63.
Rolink, T., Eichmann, K. and Simon, M. M. (1978). *Immunogenetics* **7**, 321.
Schwartz, A., Janeway, C. A. and Gershon, R. K. (1979). *In* "T and B Lymphocytes" (F. H. Bach, B. Bonavida, E. Vitetta and C. F. Fox, eds) pp. 589–598. Academic Press, New York.
Tada, T., Taniguchi, M. and David, C. S. (1977). *Cold Spring Harbor Symp. Quant. Biol.* **41**, 119.
Warren, R. W. and Davie, J. M. (1977). *J. Exp. Med.* **146**, 1627.
Weinberger, J. Z., Benacerraf, B. and Dorf, M. (1980). *J. Exp. Med.* **151**, 1413.

21

Antigen-specific Helper and Suppressor Factors

TOMIO TADA and KYOKO HAYAKAWA

Department of Immunology, Faculty of Medicine, University of Tokyo, Tokyo, Japan

Abbreviations

ABA: azobenzenearsonate; DNFB: dinitrofluorobenzene; DNP: 2,4-dinitrophenyl; GAT: L-glutamic acid^{60}-L-alanine^{30}-L-tyrosine^{10}; GT: L-glutamic acid^{50}-L-tyrosine^{50}; HGG: human γ globulin; Ia: *I* region associated antigen; KLH: keyhole limpet haemocyanin; MHC: major histocompatibility complex; NP: 4-hydroxy-3-nitrophenyl acetyl; SRBC: sheep red blood cells; TaF: antigen-specific augmenting T cell factor; (T_1G)-A-L: poly (L-tyrosine,L-glutamic acid)-poly(DL-alanine)—poly(L-Lysine); ThF: antigen-specific helper T cell factor; TsF: antigen-specific suppressor T cell factor; V_H: framework structure of heavy chain variable region; V_L: framework structure of light chain variable region.

We thank Drs M. Taniguchi, K. Hiramatsu, K. Okumura, T. Saito, G. Suzuki, R. Abe and S. Miyatani for their collaboration, and to Ms Yoko Yamaguchi for the secretarial assistance.

Introduction

Antigen-specific T cell factors (TFs) are defined on the basis of their specific regulatory functions in the immune response and their ability to bind antigen with an exquisite specificity comparable to that of antibodies (Tada and Okumura, 1979; Germain, 1980; Taussig, 1980). A number of TFs have been reported in different experimental systems, while there still exist several unexplained controversies. Nevertheless, TFs have been shown to share many functional and structural properties in common that distinguish them from other nonspecific lymphokines. The most important features are: 1) they possess determinants controlled by genes in the *I* region of major histocompatibility complex (MHC), and 2) no ordinary immunoglobulin (Ig) constant structures are detected despite their definite antigen specificity. TFs sometimes show genetic restrictions in their actions on target cells which are imposed by *MHC* or *Ig* genes. Many of the TFs have been found not to be the final effector molecules that directly inhibit the ultimate response, but to be the initiators of a consequence of cellular events that subsequently lead to the augmentation or suppression of the immune response. Thus, TFs lend important clues to determine the structures responsible both for the antigen recognition by T cells and for the genetically restricted interactions among different types of lymphocytes.

We will describe in this section some salient features of antigen-specific helper (ThF), augmenting (TaF) and suppressor (TsF) factors from only limited literatures. Some comparisons will be made on the structural, serological and functional features of TFs obtained in different experimental systems. A major purpose of this review is, however, to place these TFs within the regulatory circuit of the immune system.

Helper (ThF) and augmenting (TaF) T cell factors

Two types of antigen-specific T cell factors that finally augment the B cell response have been described. One is the helper or co-operative T cell factor (ThF) that can replace the function of the antigen-specific helper T cell (Taussig, 1974; Taussig and Munro, 1974; Mozes *et al.*, 1975; Howie and Feldmann, 1977). We do not have to reiterate its well known properties as it has been extensively reviewed by Munro and Taussig 1975) and to a lesser extent by Tada and Okumura (1979). Although people have been aware of the difficulty in obtaining ThF in the manner originally described, recent development of the hybridoma technique allowed the establishment of a hybrid cell line continuously secreting the molecule and having the same properties as ThF from immunized mice (Eshhar *et al.*, 1980). A similar factor is also obtainable in the primary culture supernatant of spleen cells with an optimal

TABLE I

Properties of antigen-specific helper (ThF) and augmenting (TaF) T cell factors

ThF

1. Secreted in the culture supernatant of *in vivo* educated T cells with antigen
2. Adsorbable to antigen by which T cells were educated
3. Acts on bone marrow cells *in vivo* and on primed or unprimed B cells *in vitro* to produce mostly IgM antibodies
4. Molecular weight: 60K; Ig constant structure
5. Contains Ia antigen encoded in *I-A* subregion
6. Production of ThF by T cells and/or acceptance of ThF by B cells are under *Ir* gene controls.

TaF

1. Extractable from antigen-primed T cells
2. Adsorbable to antigen
3. Acts on T cells of *I-A* subregion compatible strains
4. Not helper T cell-replacing, but augments the antibody response in the presence of helper T cells
5. Molecular weight: 60K; no Ig constant structure
6. Contains Ia antigen encoded in *I-A* subregion
7. Augments the *in vitro* antibody response only if it is added 25–48 h after the cultivation.

concentration of the stimulating antigen (Howie and Feldmann, 1977). Some essential properties are summarized in Table I.

The second category of the augmenting T cell factor is the TaF which augments the antibody response only in the presence of helper T cells having the same antigen specificity (Tokuhisa *et al.*, 1978). This factor, when added to the culture of primed spleen cells 1–2 days after the onset of cultivation, enhanced the antibody response in an antigen-specific fashion. If T cells were completely deprived from responding spleen cells, no augmenting activity was observed. We have recently established hybridoma cell lines which produce TaF with the same properties (Hiramatsu *et al.*, in prep.).

These two types of TF have the following common general properties: 1) mol. wt less than 70 000 (70K); 2) contain *I-A* subregion gene products; 3) have no Ig structure; and 4) have definite antigen specificities. Some comparisons can be made from the listed properties of these two types of TFs in Table I.

Suppressor T cell factors (TsF)

TsF has been described in many experimental systems in which suppression is directed at antibody formation against protein (Tada and Takemori, 1974; Jones and Kaplan, 1977; Taniguchi and Miller, 1978; Kontiainen and Feldmann, 1977), synthetic polypeptides (Kapp *et al.*, 1976; Waltenbough *et al.*,

1977; Kontiainen *et al.*, 1979), and haptens (Zembala and Asherson, 1974; Greene *et al.*, 1977a; Moorhead, 1977; Noonan and Halliday, 1980). The methods for obtaining TsF are also different depending on the type of the suppressed immune response, i.e., antibody formation (general suppression or tolerance), delayed type hypersensitivity, and the induction of cytotoxic T cells (Greene *et al.*, 1977b; Takei *et al.*, 1978). It is generally noted that TsF is more easily obtained by extracting from the cells than by culturing the cells with or without antigen.

The most important property of TsF is that it generally contains determinants coded for by genes in *I-J* subregion *H-2* complex. This is true for TsF specific for keyhole limpet haemocyanin (KLH), human γ globulin (HGG) and synthetic polypeptides. In the case of TsF obtained from a hybridoma specific for SRBC (Taussig and Holliman, 1979) and that in mixed lymphocyte reaction (Rich and Rich, 1975), the Ia structure is coded for by a gene mapped right to *I-J*, likely to be *I-C* subregion. Some general properties of TsF are summarized in Table II.

TABLE II

Properties of antigen-specific suppressor T cell factors

1. Extracted or secreted from antigen-primed suppressor T cells
2. Bind specifically to antigen, and suppress the immune response (Ab producing, DTH, cytotoxic T cell response) against the antigen by which they were generated
3. Lack conventional Ig determining
4. Carry determinants coded by genes in *I-J*, *I-C* (presumably) or exceptionally *I-A* subregion
5. IgV_H or idotypic determinants are detected
6. Molecular weight: 70K
7. Acts on T cells to induce a second type of suppressor T cells. In some cases acts directly on B cells
8. H-2 or idiotype restricted in their action in most cases.
9. Probably consists of 2 chains, one being a product of H-2, and the other containing IgV_H

Mechanism of action

It has been reported that there exist diverse modes of action of T helper cells in assisting the antibody synthesis by B cells via cell to cell contact or by soluble mediators (Dutton *et al.*, 1971). Besides the well known formula of collaborative interactions between carrier-specific helper T cells and hapten-specific B cells by an antigen link (Mitchison, 1971), helper effects are known to be manifested by a separate signal independently given to helper T and B cells (non-linked help) (Kishimoto and Ishizaka, 1973; Hamaoka *et al.*,

1973; Tada *et al.*, 1978). The latter effect may be conveyed at least in part by nonspecific helper factors termed "T cell replacing factors (TaF)" (Schimpl and Wecker, 1972). In addition, we are aware that there exists a type of helper T cell that recognizes idiotype or other immunoglobulin structures carried by B cells (idiotype-specific help) (Hämmerling *et al.*, 1976; Eichmann *et al.*, 1978; Woodland and Cantor, 1978; Julius *et al.*, 1980). The reported properties of ThF conform to the concept of "linked recognition" in that ThF will bind to the "carrier" portion of the antigen and the functional end of ThF is focused onto the reactive site ("acceptor") of B cells. In some experiments, it has been shown that antigens with repeated antigenic epitopes can do so much better than oligoepitope antigens due to their ability to focus ThF on B cell acceptor sites (Shiozawa *et al.*, 1977). If the factors as well as acceptor sites are products related to immune response (*Ir*) genes, some facets of *Ir* gene effects can be explained by the expression of these complementary molecules on T and B cells as proposed by Munro and Taussig (1975). The only known pharmacologic activity of ThF is to increase the level of cyclic nucleotide in B cells upon incubation with splenic B cells (Mozes, 1978).

The mechanism of TaF action is still largely unknown. One important distinction of TaF from ThF is that TaF can augment the antibody response only in the presence of T cells with the same carrier specificity (Tokuhisa *et al.*, 1978). It is not known what type of T cell is required for the TaF effect, but at least the presence of a minimal number of helper T cell is necessary for the augmentation of the immune response. It is known only that TaF manifests its maximal effect when added to the *in vitro* secondary antibody response 24–28 h after the onset of culture (Tada *et al.*, 1977). This suggests that TaF recruits a new type of helper T cells apart from originally existing helper T cells. The sites of action of ThF and TaF are assigned as shown in Fig. 1.

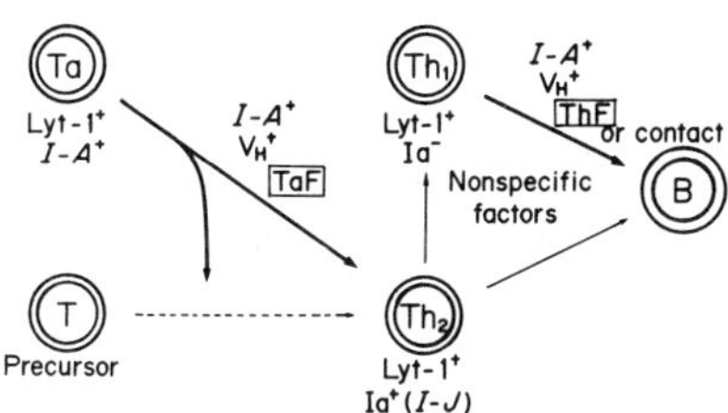

FIG. 1. *Possible site of action of antigen-specific helper (ThF) and augmenting (TaF) T cell factors in the helper circuit.*

The mechanism of action of TsF has been analysed better than the above mentioned augmenting factors. Reports have come from at least two independent laboratories that TsF induces new suppressor T cells (Ts_2) from the pool of precursor T cells (Germain, 1980; Tada and Okumura, 1979). Some other reports indicate that TsF, especially induced *in vitro* would directly suppress helper T or B cells (Kontiainen and Feldmann, 1978; Taussig *et al.*, 1979a).

In our own experimental system of KLH-specific suppression, TsF derives from Lyt-2^+,3^+ suppressor T cells, and acts on syngeneic or *H-2* compatible Lyt-1^+,2^+,3^+ T cells. The imposed restriction was found to be on the interaction between TsF and Lyt-1^+,2^+,3^+ "acceptor" cells. By using the mixture of spleen cells from Lyt-1 congenic and Lyt-2,3 congenic mice, we examined whether or not the Lyt-1^+,2^+,3^+ acceptor T cell itself suppresses the immune response as the second type of suppressor T cell (Ts_2). We found that Ts_2, which has Lyt-2^+,3^+ phenotype, derives from a pool of Lyt-2^+,3^+ precursors but not from Lyt-1^+,2^+,3^+ acceptor cells. Ts_2 thus generated by TsF suppresses antibody response across the *H-2* barrier by an antigen-nonspecific factor (Taniguchi and Tokuhisa, 1980).

The extensive studies with synthetic polypeptides, GAT (glutaminic acid^{60},alanine^{30},tyrosine^{10}) and GT (glutaminic acid^{50},tyrosine^{50}) showed a somewhat different pathway of Ts_2 generation (Germain, 1980). Originally, GAT-specific factor was obtained only from nonresponder strains, but with higher dose of antigen, responder strains also produced TsF. The GAT- and GT-TsF when inoculated into both nonresponder and responder strains resulted in the induction of Ts_2 which specifically suppress the GAT- and GT-specific antibody formation. The most noteworthy differences are 1) there is no *H-2* related restriction in the generation of Ts_2 by TsF, and 2) the specificity of Ts_2 action is always maintained through the course of suppression.

In a number of other experimental systems, the genetic restriction and targets of TsF action are still controversial. TsF induced in the *in vitro* culture shows no genetic restriction for KLH-, GAT- and (T,G)-A--L-specific TsF (Kontiainen and Feldmann, 1978; Kontiainen *et al.*, 1979). The hybridoma-derived TsF specific for SRBC (Taussig *et al.*, 1979b) also showed no *H-2* restriction. Such differences may be attributable to the different targets to which TFs act, as *in vitro* induced normal and hybridoma-derived TsFs apparently act on helper T cells or directly on B cells. In our hybridoma-derived TsF, the same rigorous *H-2* restriction was observed in the induction of Ts_2. In addition, our more recent data on the action of idiotype-bearing TsF indicate that the genetic restriction is imposed either by *H-2* or V_H genes (see below). The apparent lack of restriction in GAT system may be due to the prevalence of GAT idiotype among different haplotype strains (Thèze and Sommé, 1979).

TsF found in delayed-type hypersensitivity and cytotoxic T cell response probably act on different targets from those in the antibody response. Ptak *et al.* (1978) demonstrated that TsF for picryl chloride endows macrophages with nonspecific suppressor properties. On the other hand, in the suppression of contact sensitivity to dinitrofluorobenzene (DNFB) by DNP-specific TsF, the factor acts directly on DNP-primed T cells with *H-2K* or *H-2D* compatible mice (Moorhead, 1979). No *I* region compatibility was required even though the factor is an *I* region gene product. This apparently suggests that TsF in this system recognize DNP together with *H-2* products. The target of TsF in cytotoxic T cell response to tumour antigens can be either cytotoxic T cell itself (Greene *et al.*, 1977a; Fujimoto *et al.*, 1978) or its precursor (Takei *et al.*, 1977, 1978).

On the other hand, in the suppression of footpad reaction to ABA conjugated spleen cells, Greene *et al.* (1979) found that TsF induces second suppressor T cell (Ts_2) in a manner similar to that in the suppression of the antibody response. They found that Ts_1, the initial producer of ABA-specific TsF, carries the major cross-reactive idiotype, while Ts_2 does not have the same idiotype (Bach *et al.*, 1979). These different pathways and actions are illustrated in Fig. 2.

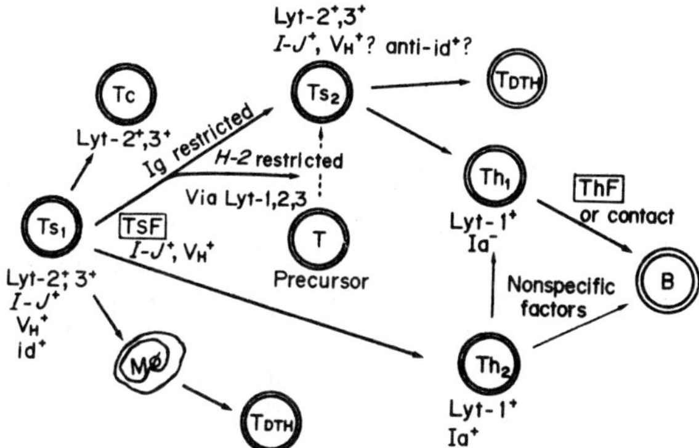

FIG. 2. *Different pathways in the effect of antigen-specific suppressor factors (TsF) in the regulation of immune response.*

The major points to be considered are: 1) whether they are all mediated by a single or multiple TsF; 2) what portion of the TsF effects is *MHC* or *Ig* gene restricted; and 3) whether the TsF effect examined by different investigators is via the same or different pathways. It is conceivable that Ts_1 and Ts_2 have different properties, and that the links between these two cell types may be restricted by the intermediary processes, i.e., idiotype–anti-idiotype, MHC anti-MHC and MHC-MHC interactions. In certain cases, I-J products, which are known to have a considerable heterogeneity, would serve as cell interaction elements, while Ig-V_H gene compatibility would be prerequisite in other experimental systems. Further important information will be published shortly (see also Chapter 20 by R. K. Gershon, in this publication).

Antigenic determinants

Ia antigen

Both ThF and TaF carry Ia determinants controlled by genes in the *I-A* subregion. The serological analyses with various anti-Ia reagents suggest that the determinants are entirely different from those detected on B cell Ia antigens which are also controlled by genes in the *I-A* subregion. Taussig *et al.* (1975)

showed that ThF can be absorbed with anti-Ia antisera raised against the haplotype from which ThF was obtained, but not with those having specificities against cross-reactive determinants which are shared by Ia antigens on B cells. Tokuhisa *et al.* (1978) demonstrated that anti-Ia antisera preabsorbed with B cells could still absorb TaF, while those preabsorbed with T cells failed to do so.

Definitive evidence was recently obtained with TaF from T cell hybridomas in our laboratory. Hiramatsu *et al.* (to be published) were successful in making hybridomas carrying Ia antigen encoded in the *I-A* subregion of $H\text{-}2^k$. TaF extracted from these hybridomas possessed an antigen-specific augmenting activity. They found that an anti-Ia antiserum preabsorbed with B cells failed to kill these Ia-bearing hybridomas. None of the monoclonal antibodies against private (Ia. 2) and public (Ia. 17) specificities of Ia^k was able to kill or stain the cells. The results indicated that Ia antigens on T cell factors are entirely different molecules than B cell Ia, and that they do not follow the general prototype of Ia molecules consisting of α and β chains.

It has generally been accepted that TsF carries determinants coded for by genes in the *I-J* subregion. *I-J* products are not detected at least on B cells (Murphy *et al.*, 1976). Since the suppressor T cells, both Ts_1 and Ts_2, are killed by anti-*I-J*, the question arose whether I-J determinants on these two cell types are the same or different. In addition, I-J determinants were also detected on some helper T cells (Th_2; Tada *et al.*, 1978) and macrophages (Niederhuber *et al.*, 1979), and thus the identity of I-J products on different cell types still has some ambiguity.

We have shown that I-J determinants expressed on Ts_2 and Th_2 are different by differential absorption of an anti-I-J antiserum with Lyt-1 (containing Th_2) and Lyt-2,3 (containing Ts) cells (Tada *et al.*, 1979a). More definitive evidence for the heterogeneity of I-J determinants was presented by the examination of functionally different T cell hybridomas. As reported previously, $I\text{-}J^+$ hybridomas were divided into three categories: 1) antigen-specific suppressor; 2) antigen-nonspecific suppressor; and 3) nonfunctional ones (Taniguchi and Miller, 1978; Tada *et al.*, 1979b). An anti-$I\text{-}J^b$ antiserum was absorbed by either one specific or nonspecific suppressor, and tested for its reactivity on the others. It was found that absorption by a specific hybridoma resulted in the diminution of reactivity to homologous and other specific suppressor hybridomas leaving the activity to kill nonspecific suppressor hybridomas. Conversely, the antiserum absorbed with nonspecific hybridomas was still capable of killing the specific hybridomas. These results suggest that the *I-J* subregion accommodates more than two loci which are expressed on functionally different subsets of T cells. It is obvious that antigen-specific hybridoma corresponds to Ts_1, and the nonspecific hybridoma to Ts_2.

The SRBC-specific suppressor hybridoma reported by Taussig *et al.* (1979b) also carries *I* region determinants, but the subregion assignment of Ia was entirely different from others. It is coded for by a gene mapped at least right to *I-J*, most probably in the *I-C* subregion as in the case of the suppressor factor generated by mixed lymphocyte reaction (Rich and Rich, 1976).

V_H and idiotype

The nature of the antigen-binding structure associated with TFs is still largely unknown. However, recent reports from various laboratories suggest that TFs utilize similar V_H gene products as an antigen-binding device. Eshhar *et al.* (1980) produced a hybridoma producing (T,G)-A--L-specific ThF. The basic properties of the hybridoma-derived ThF are similar to those of previously known normal ThF. The striking fact is that the cloned cell line-expressed determinants which can be detected by antibodies against the framework structure of V_H, were produced in rabbits by Ben-Neriah *et al.* (1978). Antibodies reactive to V_L were unable to stain the cells.

The same antisera were adopted to stain semi-purified Ts_1 (Tada *et al.*, 1980). Anti-V_H stained a substantial number of Ts obtained by adsorption to and elution from KLH-coated Petri dishes. Furthermore, KLH-specific TsF was successfully absorbed onto anti-V_H column, and was recovered in the acid eluate from the column. Anti-V_L was unable to do so.

This was recently confirmed by a similar experiment using hybridoma-derived TaF and TsF. Both antigen-specific factors bound to anti-V_H but not to anti-V_L columns. In addition, many of the T cell hybrids having antigen-specific suppressor or augmenting functions were killed or stained with anti-V_H but not with anti-V_L. Together with the reports of detection of V_H determinants on some T cells (Lonai *et al.*, 1978), these results indicate that V_H structure is responsible for the antigen-binding ability of T cell factors.

In accordance with the above results, idiotypic determinants have been detected in some T cells (Rajewsky and Eichmann, 1977; Eichmann, 1978; Binz and Wigzell, 1977), and on TFs. GAT-TsF was found to carry this idiotype shared by anti-GAT antibodies (Germain *et al.*, 1979). The major cross-reactive idiotype of anti-GAT is detected among all mouse strains (Thèze and Sommé, 1979). This may account for the apparent lack of genetic restriction in the suppression of GAT response (see below). Similarly, TsF specific for ABA that suppresses delayed type hypersensitivity in A/J mice also carries the major ABA idiotype (Bach *et al.*, 1979).

We ourselves have been working on the suppression of antibody response against a hapten, 3-nitro-4-hydroxy phenyl acetyl (NP) in mice carrying Igh^b allotype to which the major cross-reactive idiotype (NP^b) is associated. We have purified NP-binding T cells which contain a majority of NP-specific Ts_1. In collaboration with Drs K. Rajewsky and M. Reth, we tested the presence of NP^b idiotype using monoclonal anti-idiotype antibodies which react with idiotypes associated with framework (group 2) or antigen-binding structure (group 1) of anti-NP antibodies. It was found that a portion of NP-binding T cells carry NP^b idiotype detectable by these monoclonal antibodies. Such cells mostly belonged to $Lyt\text{-}1^-,2^+,3^+$ T cells. It is interesting that in order to suppress the secondary anti-NP antibody response, either *H-2* or Igh allotype matching was sufficient, but the matching in both gave a higher degree of suppression than in either one alone. No suppression was obtained in the entirely mismatched combination of TsF and responding cells. Furthermore, we were able to make NP-specific suppressor hybridomas, in which NP^b idiotype was detected. These results indicate that TF carries three entities of antigenic determinants, Ia, V_H and idiotype.

Possible structures of TF and their significance

Painstaking efforts to study the structure of TFs by biochemical means made by various laboratories have been unsuccessful—probably because of too small a yield of TFs for such studies. Even with high activity hybridoma factors, it has not been possible to isolate them by biochemical means. Since molecular weights of TFs are in most cases smaller than 70K, it may not have a structure similar to Igs. It should, however, contain at least two distinct gene products, Ig-V_H and *I* region products.

Taniguchi *et al.* (1979) made an interesting observation which implies that TsF from a hybridoma consists of two polypeptide chains. They obtained KLH-specific TsF from a hybridoma (9F181a) by sonication of cultured cells or from ascitic fluid of animals transplanted intraperitoneally with these hybrid cells. With extracted material, they found that the KLH-specific suppressor activity was completely absorbed either with an antigen (KLH) or with anti-I-J^b column. However, the 1 : 1 mixture of filtrates, which had been extensively absorbed through the KLH and anti-I-J columns, reconstituted the complete suppressor activity. This was only observable with the extracted material, and did not apply to the secreted TsF in ascetic fluid. This indicates that the extracted material contained at least three different molecules, i.e., a molecule having an antigen-binding site, an *I-J*-coded molecule, and the combination of these two. It also suggests that TsF consists of two chains carrying antigen-binding and I-J structures that are independently synthesized in the cytoplasm and secreted as a combined form, and that either one chain cannot produce the suppressor activity while the combination of both chains reconstitutes the activity. Taniguchi *et al.* have recently found that these two chains are disulphide linked when they are secreted.

We have also studied them using TsF from normal KLH-primed suppressor T cells of *H-2*^{k} mice. TsF was absorbed either with anti-I-J^k or anti-V_H instead of KLH column. After absorption, both filtrates had no suppressor activity, while the mixture of these filtrates reconstituted the suppressor activity. It implies that the TsF from normal Ts are also composed of two polypeptide chains, one containing V_H framework, and the other *I-J* product.

Similar observations had been made by Taussig and Holliman (1979) with their SRBC-specific hybridoma. Although this hybridoma (A-1) has several distinct features from those of Taniguchi *et al.* (1979), the essential findings are that the internally labelled TsF from A-1 consists of two noncovalently linked polypeptide chains of sizes about 85K and 25K, and that the antigen-binding structure resides on the "heavy" chain while the *H-2*-coded structures are on the "light" chain. The subregion specificity of the light chains is still not determined but is encoded to the right of the *I-J* subregion of *H-2* complex, most likely to be in the *I-C* subregion (Taussig *et al.*, 1979b).

Similar experimental procedures applied to KLH-specific TsF from 9F181a have not been successful in characterizing the chemical structure of the factor. Recent experiments by Saito *et al.* (unpublished) were, however, able to demonstrate two radioactive peaks with mol. wts 45K and 25K in SDS polyacrylamide gel with ^{125}I-labelled specifically purified TsF. With the extracted material from the hybridoma 9F181a, it was further found that a repeated absorption and elution procedure with the antigen column resulted in the dissociation of two chains, one of which could be precipitated by anti-I-J (mol. wt 25K) and the other by antigen (mol. wt 45K). However, the precise molecular weight of heavy chain cannot be predicted, as the 45K chain could be a degraded molecule by proteolytic cleavage.

All these results indicate that Ia antigens on T cell factors are distinct from B cell Ia antigens with respect to serological specificities and the mode of association with the second polypeptide chain. It is probable that Ia antigens associated with V_H structure not only determine the functional properties of Ia-bearing T cell factors, but also serve to maintain the tertial structure of antigen-binding sites which construct the idiotypic determinants.

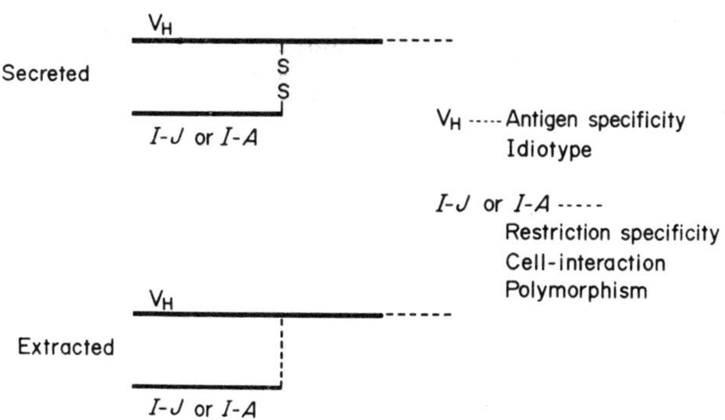

FIG. 3. *Possible structure of antigen-specific T cell factors.*

From the above and other findings, we would propose a possible minimal structure of Ia-bearing T cell factors as illustrated in Fig. 3. It is obvious that the molecule consists of two different chains, one containing the structure coded for by V_H genes and the other being an *I* region gene product. They are synthesized independently but combined when they are secreted. The constant structure which is associated with V_H is, at the moment, only negatively defined.

How then can we envisage the significance of the *I* region coded structures associated with V_H structure in the regulation of the immune response? Above observations indicate that T cell Ia antigens are a series of polymorphic cell surface molecules controlled by closely linked multiple *I* region loci whose expression is directly related to the function borne by the T cell subset. It is possible that these *I* region gene products by themselves have defined biologic activities as those of Fc portion of immunoglobulin molecules. Our presumption is, however, that the *I* region products may simply select the second cell type to be activated by virtue of their endowed restriction specificity, and that as a consequence the whole suppressor or enhancing process is begun by this simple selection of target cells. If we admit that T cell Ia antigens have some heterogeneity which are associated with the antigen-binding structure, it is predictable that the tertial structure of T cell receptor for antigen will have a considerable polymorphism that is recognized by other T cells. This would mimic the recognition by T cells of antigen presentation by macrophages in association with conventional Ia antigens, that imposes the genetic restriction in macrophage-T cell interactions. We can assume that the antigen bound to Ia-bearing T cell factor is focused on the second cell type to be activated, which does recognize antigen plus Ia-portion of the factor (or even the idiotype associated with Ia-bearing T cell receptor). The observed genetic restriction between the factor and responding T cells in our experimental system implies that the association of Ia antigen with the antigen receptor of T cells is of great significance in finding the right cell type to be activated in the circuitry regulation. Thus, it is assumed that the Ia antigen on T cells plays a critically important role in the accuracy of cell interactions, analogous to Ia antigen on macrophages in the antigen-presentation, which as a whole contributes to the genetic regulation in the immune response.

References

Bach, B. A., Greene, M. I., Benacerraf, B. and Nisonoff, A. (1979). *J. Exp. Med.* **149**, 1084.

Ben-Neriah, Y., Wuilmart, C., Lonai, P. and Givol, D. (1978). *Eur. J. Immunol.* **8**, 797.

Binz, H. and Wigzell, H. (1977). *Contemp. Top. Immunobiol.* **7**, 113.

Dutton, R. W., Falkoff, R., Hurst, J. A., Hoffman, M., Kappler, J. W., Kettman, J. R., Lesley, J. F. and Vann, O. (1971). *Prog. Immunol.* **1**, 335.

Eichmann, K. (1978). *Adv. Immunol.* **26**, 195.

Eichmann, K., Falk, I. and Rajewsky, K. (1978). *Eur. J. Immunol.* **8**, 600.

Eshhar, E., Apte, R. N., Ben-Neriah, Y., Givol, D. and Mozes, E. (1980). *Nature* (in press).

Fujimoto, S., Matsuzawa, T., Nakagawa, N. and Tada, T. (1978). *Cell. Immunol.* **38**, 378.

Germain, R. N. (1980). *Lymphokine Report* **1**, 7.

Germain, R. N., Ju, S.-T., Kipps, T. J., Benacerraf, B. and Dorf, M. E. (1979). *J. Exp. Med.* **149**, 613.

Greene, M. I., Fujimoto, S. and Sehon, A. H. (1977a). *J. Immunol.* **119**, 757.

Greene, M. I., Pierres, A., Dorf, M. E. and Benacerraf, B. (1977b). *J. Exp. Med.* **146**, 293.

Greene, M. I., Bach, B. A. and Benacerraf, B. (1979). *J. Exp. Med.* **149**, 1069.
Hamaoka, T., Katz, D. H. and Benacerraf, B. (1973). *J. Exp. Med.* **138**, 538.
Hämmerling, G. J., Black, S. J., Berek, C., Eichmann, K. and Rajewsky, K. (1976). *J. Exp. Med.* **143**, 861.
Howie, S. and Feldmann, M. (1977). *Eur. J. Immunol.* **7**, 417.
Jones, T. B. and Kaplan, A. M. (1977). *J. Immunol.* **118**, 1880.
Julius, M. H., Cosenza, H. and Augustin, A. A. (1980). *Eur. J. Immunol.* **10**, 112.
Kapp, J. A., Pierce, C. W., DeLa Croix, F. and Benacerraf, B. (1976). *J. Immunol.* **116**, 305.
Kishimoto, T. and Ishizaka, K. (1973). *J. Immunol.* **111**, 1194.
Kontiainen, S. and Feldmann, M. (1977). *Eur. J. Immunol.* **7**, 310.
Kontiainen, S. and Feldmann, M. (1978). *J. Exp. Med.* **147**, 110.
Kontiainen, S. and Feldmann, M. (1979). *Thymus* **1**, 59.
Kontiainen, S., Howie, S., Maurer, P. H. and Feldmann, M. (1979). *J. Immunol.* **122**, 253.
Lonai, P., Ben-Neriah, Y., Steinman, L. and Givol, D. (1978). *Eur. J. Immunol.* **8**, 827.
Mitchison, N. A. (1971). *Eur. J. Immunol.* **1**, 10.
Moorhead, J. W. (1977). *J. Immunol.* **119**, 315.
Moorhead, J. W. (1979). *J. Exp. Med.* **150**, 1432.
Mozes, E. (1978). *In* "Ir Genes and Ia Antigens" (H. O. McDevitt, ed.), p. 475. Academic Press, New York.
Mozes, E., Isac, R. and Taussig, M. J. (1975). *J. Exp. Med.* **141**, 703.
Munro, A. J. and Taussig, M. J. (1975). *Nature* **256**, 103.
Murphy, D. B., Herzenberg, L. A., Okumura, K., Herzenberg, L. A. and McDevitt, H. O. (1976). *J. Exp. Med.* **144**, 699.
Niederhuber, J. E., Allen, P. and Mayo, L. (1979). *J. Immunol.* **122**, 1342.
Noonan, F. P. and Halliday, W. J. (1980). *Cell Immunol.* **50**, 41.
Ptak, W., Zembala, M. and Gershon, R. K. (1978). *J. Exp. Med.* **148**, 424.
Rajewsky, K. and Eichmann, K. (1977). *Contemp. Top. Immunobiol.* **7**, 69.
Rich, S. S. and Rich, R. R. (1975). *J. Exp. Med.* **142**, 1391.
Rich, S. S. and Rich, R. R. (1976). *J. Exp. Med.* **143**, 672.
Schimpl, A. and Weckner, E. (1972). *Nature* **237**, 15.
Shiozawa, C., Singh, B., Rubinstein, S. and Diener, E. (1977). *H. Immunol.* **118**, 2199.
Sy, M.-S., Dietz, M. H., Germain, R. N., Benacerraf, B. and Greene, M. I. (1980). *J. Exp. Med.* **151**, 1183.
Tada, T. and Okumura, K. (1979). *Adv. Immunol.* **28**, 1.
Tada, T. and Takemori, T. (1974). *J. Exp. Med.* **140**, 239.
Tada, T., Taniguchi, M. and David, C. S. (1977). *Cold Spring Harbor Symp. Quant. Biol.* **41**, 119.
Tada, T., Takemori, T., Okumura, K., Nonaka, M. and Tokuhisa, T. (1978). *J. Exp. Med.* **147**, 446.
Tada, T., Nonaka, M., Okumura, K., Taniguchi, M. and Tokuhisa, T. (1979a). *In* "Cell Biology and Immunology Leukocyte Function" (M. Quastel, ed.), p. 353. Academic Press, New York.
Tada, T., Taniguchi, M. Saito, T. and Matsuzawa, T. (1979b). *Monogr. Allergy* **14**, 45.
Tada, T., Hayakawa, K., Okumura, K. and Taniguchi, M. (1980). *Molec. Immunol.* (in press).
Takei, F., Levy, J. G. and Kilburn, D. G. (1977). *J. Immunol.* **118**, 412.
Takei, F., Levy, J. G. and Kilburn, D. G. (1978). *J. Immunol.* **120**, 1218.
Taniguchi, M. and Miller, J. F. A. P. (1978). *J. Exp. Med.* **148**, 378.
Taniguchi, M. and Tokuhisa, T. (1980). *J. Exp. Med.* **151**, 517.
Taniguchi, M., Saito, T. and Tada, T. (1979). *Nature* **278**, 555.
Taniguchi, M., Takei, I. and Tada, T. (1980). *Nature* **283**, 227.
Taussig, M. J. (1974). *Nature* **248**, 234.

Taussig, M. J. (1980). *Cancer Immunology and Immunopathology* (in press).
Taussig, M. J. and Holliman, A. (1979). *Nature* **277**, 308.
Taussig, M. J. and Munro, A. J. (1974). *Nature* **251**, 63.
Taussig, M. J., Munro, A. J., Campbell, R., David, C. S. and Staines, N. A. (1975). *J. Exp. Med.* **142**, 694.
Taussig, M. J., Corvalàn, J. R. F., Binns, R. M. and Holliman, A. (1979a). *Nature* **277**, 305.
Taussig, J. J., Corvalàn, J. R. F. and Holliman, A. (1979b). *Ann. N.Y. Acad. Sci.* **332**, 316.
Taussig, M. J., Corvalàn, J. R. F., Binns, R. M., Roser, B. and Holliman, A. (1979c). *Eur. J. Immunol.* **9**, 768.
Thèze, J. and Sommé, G. (1979). *Eur. J. Immunol.* **9**, 294.
Tokuhisa, T., Taniguchi, M., Okumura, K. and Tada, T. (1978). *J. Immunol.* **120**, 414.
Waltenbough, C., Debré, P., Thèze, J. and Benacerraf, B. (1977). *J. Immunol.* **118**, 2073.
Woodland, R. and Cantor, H. (1978). *Eur. J. Immunol.* **8**, 600.
Zembala, M. and Asherson, G. L. (1974). *Eur. J. Immunol.* **4**, 799.

22

Nonantigen-specific T Cell Factors

A. SCHIMPL, L. HÜBNER, C. WONG and E. WECKER

Institut für Virologie und Immunbiologie, Würzburg, West Germany

Introduction

Overshadowed by the spectacular immunological hypothesis and results of recent years, e.g. the idiotype–anti-idiotype networks, and H-2 restriction of T cell–antigen interactions, the field of nonantigen-specific mediators active in the immune response has experienced slow growth. The lack of enthusiasm shown by immunologists towards this particular field is not surprising.

The phenomena involved are those of cell biology rather than phenomena particular to immunology. While one needs antigen-receptor interactions to produce these factors and, in most instances, antigen activated cells to receive the signals mediated by them, their existence does not teach us much about the details of receptor fine specificity. It does teach us, however, a great deal about the different stages a cell has to undergo to turn into an effector lymphocyte and about how cells communicate.

The title of this chapter and our personal experience restricts us to nonantigen-specific mediators operative in T–B cell co-operation. In practice we

Abbreviations
CASUP: Con A supernatant; LAF: lymphocyte activating factors; LPS lipopolysaccharide; MØ: macrophage; PFC: plaque forming cell; T_h: T helper cell; TCDF: T cell differentiation factor; TCGF: T cell growth factor; TRF: T cell replacing factor; SRBC: sheep red blood cell.

We thank Mrs C. Tony, Mr M. Clark and Mr A. Zant for expert technical assistance. This work was supported by the Sonderforschungsbereich 105 of the Deutsche Forschungsgemeinschaft.

looked for soluble mediators that could restore *in vitro* T cell deprived spleen cell cultures consisting of mostly B cells and macrophages to give a humoral immune response. Traditionally such cultures are obtained from anti-Thy-1 and complement treated spleen cultures of conventional mice or from spleen cells of congenitally athymic nu/nu mice. T cell deprived cultures of human peripheral blood cells have also been used but so far they have not provided evidence beyond that obtained in the mouse system. We shall not go into detail but shall restrict ourselves to the murine system.

Biology of T cell factors

If one speaks of factors operative in T–B cell collaboration, one should consequently only consider factors produced by T cells which act on B cells. This restriction would still be preserved if such factors acted via an intermediary third party cell, e.g. the macrophage, but no longer if they acted on residual T cells.

The actual situation is presented in Fig. 1. The model for T–B cell cooperation on which we based all further experiments is that proposed by Mitchison *et al.* (1970). Except for the obligatory inclusion of macrophage T cell interactions, this model has so far not been contradicted. If one depletes the system of T cells, one can restore their action in at least 3 ways: by a product directly acting on B cells or, if T cells are not totally removed, by

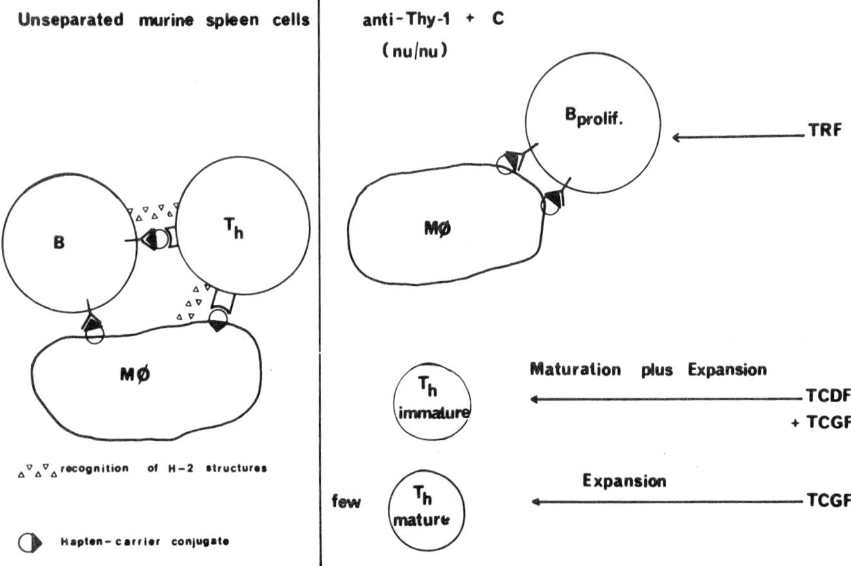

FIG. 1. *Schematic drawing of the three possibilities by which different factors can restore an antibody response to T dependent antigens in T cell depleted spleen cultures.*

replenishing residual T cell function, either by expanding the few remaining mature T cells, or by converting immature T cells into mature ones and expanding those. In other words, one would be dealing with *a* T cell replacing factor(s) or *a* T cell growth factor(s) or *a* T cell differentiation factor(s) in combination with *a* T cell growth factor(s). All of these factors have been reported to be operative in the appropriate systems and all of them seem to be produced by either alloantigen, mitogen or conventional antigen activated T helper cells (reviewed in Schimpl and Wecker, 1979). The producing T cells are predominantly of the Ly-1^+2^- phenotype (Pickel *et al.*, 1976; Shaw *et al.*, 1980), but possibly not exclusively so (Dutton *et al.*, 1978). From the beginning we concentrated our efforts on *a* factor(s) truly replacing T cells, since mere T cell replacement would still leave us with the question of what happened during T–B cell co-operation. Fortunately, the murine immune response to heterologous blood cells *in vitro* gave us a unique opportunity to pursue this interest. We, and other workers (Schimpl and Wecker, 1972; Hünig *et al.*, 1974; Dutton, 1975; Waldmann *et al.*, 1976) could show that in this system T cell help—mediated by nonantigen-specific mediator(s), which we called T cell replacing factor (TRF)—is only required during the maturation phase of antigen stimulated, already proliferating B cells into actively synthesizing and/or secreting plaque forming cells. The evidence for the late action of TRF inducing differentiation of proliferating B cells is presented in Table I. Why is the late action important in demonstrating T cell replacing rather than T cell replenishing activity? Figure 2 shows why one would expect different kinetics of response to a given factor, depending on whether such a factor acted on B cells or on residual T cells. Obviously, if a small compartment of residual mature T_h cells had to proliferate to reach functional levels, or if the equally rare immature T_h cells had to mature and proliferate, the time required would exceed the 72 h left after TRF addition to 48 h antigen stimulated B cell/MØ cultures.

The kinetics of the B cell response to TRF were thus helpful in showing that possible interference by T cell growth factor(s) and T cell differentiation-inducing factors, acting on the few T cells present in nu/nu spleen cultures (Gillis *et al.*, 1979) was minimal. Additional control experiments (Figs 3–5), however, eliminate the possibility that TRF might act via residual T cells:

TABLE I

Evidence for a late acting B cell differentiation factor (TRF)

(1) Kinetics of action (Schimpl and Wecker, 1972)
(2) Autoradiographic studies (Hünig *et al.*, 1974)
(3) Strong B cell proliferation after late addition of TRF is not obligatory (Askonas *et al.*, 1974)
(4) Hot pulse (Dutton, 1975)
(5) Limiting dilution experiments (Waldmann *et al.*, 1976)

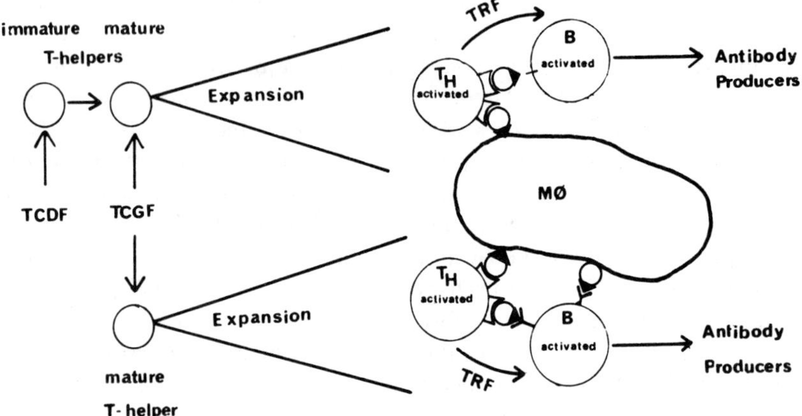

FIG. 2. *Schematic drawing of the consecutive action of different factors leading to the restoration of B cell responses to T dependent antigens.*

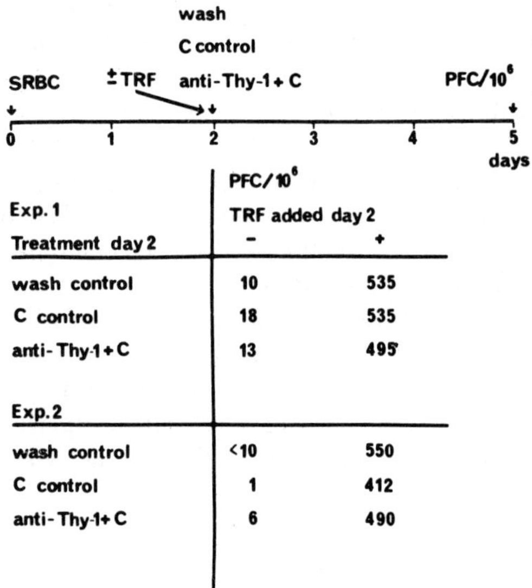

	PFC/10⁶ TRF added day 2	
Exp. 1 Treatment day 2	−	+
wash control	10	535
C control	18	535
anti-Thy-1+C	13	495
Exp. 2		
wash control	<10	550
C control	1	412
anti-Thy-1+C	6	490

FIG. 3. *Treatment of nu/nu cultures 2 days after addition of antigen with anti-Thy-1 and complement Monoclonal anti-Thy-1 and/or rabbit complement selected for low toxicity were added to the cultures. After 1·5 h of incubation all cells were washed once by centrifugation. The cells were resuspended in one half of the former volume in fresh medium and returned to half the number of the original wells. Where indicated, TRF was then added and all cultures were further incubated until day 5 when the plaques were scored. As TCGF, crude Con A supernatants were used, TRF was the supernatant of KLH-restimulated spleen cells of KLH-preimmunized mice. 20 × concentrated dialysis against PEG.*

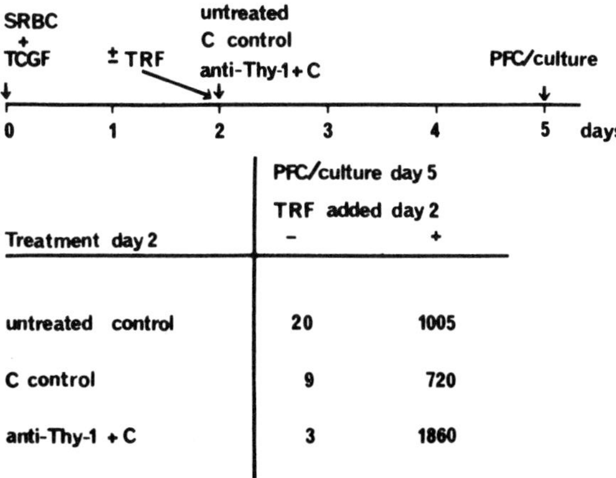

Treatment day 2	PFC/culture day 5 TRF added day 2 –	+
untreated control	20	1005
C control	9	720
anti-Thy-1 + C	3	1860

FIG. 4. *Treatment of nu/nu cultures 2 days after addition of antigen and TCGF with anti-Thy-1 and complement. Both SRBC and TCGF were added on day 0. All further procedures were as described in Fig. 4.*

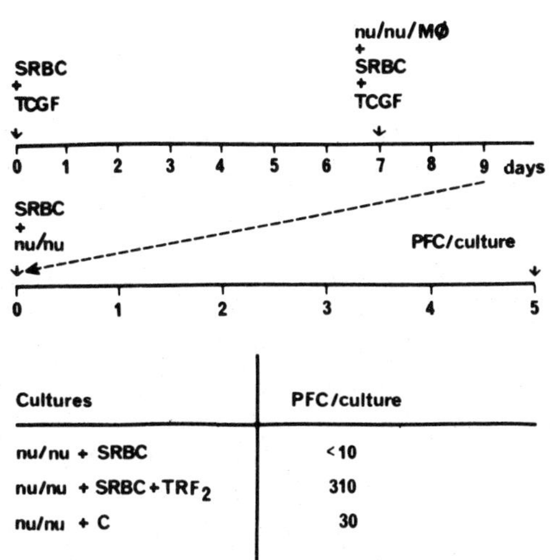

Cultures	PFC/culture
nu/nu + SRBC	<10
nu/nu + SRBC + TRF_2	310
nu/nu + C	30

FIG. 5. *Failure to generate functional T cells in 9 days nu/nu mouse spleen cultures in the presence of TCGF. Nu/nu spleen cultures received SRBC and TCGF on day 0. On day 7 they received nu/nu macrophages which had been exposed to SRBC and again TCGF. On day 9 these cells were added to fresh nu/nu cultures which were stimulated by the addition of SRBC.*

Fig. 3 shows that treatment with anti-Thy-1 and complement of nu/nu spleen cells 2 days after treatment with antigen, and the rigours of the culture system, does not influence their responsiveness to TRF. Thus, TRF does not seem to act on T cells induced in nu/nu spleen cultures, e.g. by endogenously formed LAF (Farrar and Koopman, 1979). Figure 4 demonstrates that adding a preparation containing TRF to nu/nu cultures on day 0, together with the antigen SRBC, does not induce T cells which might be obligatory for TRF action. Finally, Fig. 5 demonstrates that the BALB/c nu/nu mice used in our experiments do not generate antigen-specific T helper cells after being cultured in the presence of antigen, and T cell growth factor containing supernatants.

These experiments substantiate previous observations listed in Table I and show that a late acting factor derived from T_h cells, whose target is the proliferating B cell, is sufficient to induce antibody production in such cells. However, as mentioned above, this product is not the only one that results in antibody production in T cell depleted spleen cell cultures. Several groups have reported that early acting factors are operative in such systems (Waldmann and Munro, 1974; Farrar *et al.*, 1978; Watson *et al.*, 1979a; Hofmann and Watson, 1979; and references in Schimpl and Wecker, 1979). Some of them went on to show that these early acting factors were indistinguishable from factors acting on T cells, such as TCGF (Gillis and Smith, 1977), costimulator (Shaw *et al.*, 1980) and a putative T–T helper factor that leads to the generation of cytotoxic T cells in cultures of thymocytes (Farrar *et al.*, 1978) or nu/nu spleen. They concluded that all four activities were mediated by the same molecule (Farrar *et al.*, 1978; Watson *et al.*, 1979b). An alternative possible interpretation would be that in all cases they measured T cell growth, i.e. one and the same activity giving rise to different secondary phenomena. Farrar *et al.* found, in addition to this early acting mediator which they thought identical to thymocyte mitogenic factor (TMF), a late acting TRF, both contained in supernatants of Con A stimulated spleen cells and both produced by T cells. Using phenylsepharose chromatography they obtained a partial separation of the two activities. However, the late acting TRF was, as such, unable to restore plaque responses in T cell deprived cultures, and could do so only if early acting TMF was present from the beginning of the culture until addition of late TRF. This need for a synergism between early and late acting factors is in contrast to what we have found with our late acting TRF. Short of a more obvious explanation, e.g. that both factors investigated by Farrar *et al.* act on T cells, reconstituting them to functional levels, there is another possibility worth mentioning. It is tacitly assumed that in all assay systems in which the ability to restore a PFC response to T dependent antigens is tested, the B cells are capable of performing their part only if T cell help is provided. This, however, may not be so and we have good evidence that, in nu/nu mice up to the age of 7–8 weeks, the B cells are ontogenically not advanced enough to reach the TRF responsive state induced by antigen. Con A supernatants added to those cultures on day 0, together with the antigen, seem to possess the capability to render the immature B cells reactive to the antigen and thus to become intermediary B cells which then, on day 2, react to the late acting differentiation signal provided by TRF. In order to avoid the additional complication of B cell inadequacies on top of the complications so richly provided by the various T cell types still present in the assay systems, one ought to use spleens of nu/nu mice no younger than 8 weeks.

Indeed, Hoffmann *et al.* (1979) have described a macrophage produced T cell replacing factor, TRF_M, which induces phenotypic and functional differentiation of B cells. This factor increases the frequency of precursor B cells capable of interacting with helper cells or T cell replacing factors released by them. Consequently, TRF_M and TRF_T act synergistically in the generation of antibody-forming cells (Hoffmann and Watson, 1979). Chemical analysis can bring about a meaningful resolution only if (a) the two biological activities can be separated from one another, even though both are still not purified to homogeneity or if, (b) one molecular entity purified to homogeneity displays more than one biological activity. The latter case requires a completely defined and certain assay system.

Separation of TRF from TCGF

So far no one has succeeded in purifying a T cell helper factor to homogeneity. We have applied 4 different consecutive steps of purification to biosynthetically labelled TRF preparations (Müller *et al.*, 1978). The assay for TRF was always conducted in nu/nu spleen cell cultures. While the final product was void of conventionally detectable protein, it still possessed good biological activity and, on fluorography of SDS-PAGE, displayed at least 5 different bands. One of them was tentatively assigned to TRF on the grounds of molecular weight. These semi-purified preparations were used to raise an antiserum in a goat.

The antiserum inhibited the generation of anti-SRBC PFCs in normal mouse spleen cell cultures and it also inhibited the action of TRF in the nu/nu system without affecting LPS induced plaque response (Hübner *et al.*, 1980). In contrast, it did not interfere at all with TCGF activity. Therefore, it appears that TRF and TCGF are different molecules.

This serological evidence is confirmed using different purification steps. While sephadex G-75, hydrophobic chromatography on phenylsepharose and ion exchange chromatography usually lead to a poor resolution of the various activities, we have recently succeeded in totally separating TCGF from TRF by other means. Thus we found that in the murine system only TCGF binds to lentil lectin columns while TRF fails to do so (Fig. 6), as had already been reported by Waldmann *et al.* (1976). Another means of separating the two activities—although not completely—is Cu chelate affinity chromatography. Both TRF and TCGF bind to Cu columns. The affinity of TCGF for the metal is, however, higher than that of TRF, leading to fractions being

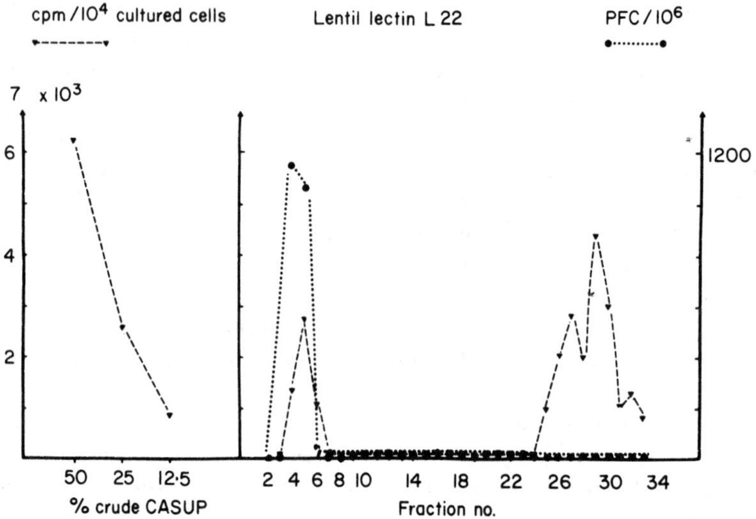

FIG. 6. *Separation of TCGF from TRF on lentil lectin sepharose. The eluting sugar* N-*acetyl-D-glucosamine was added after 21 fractions had been collected.*

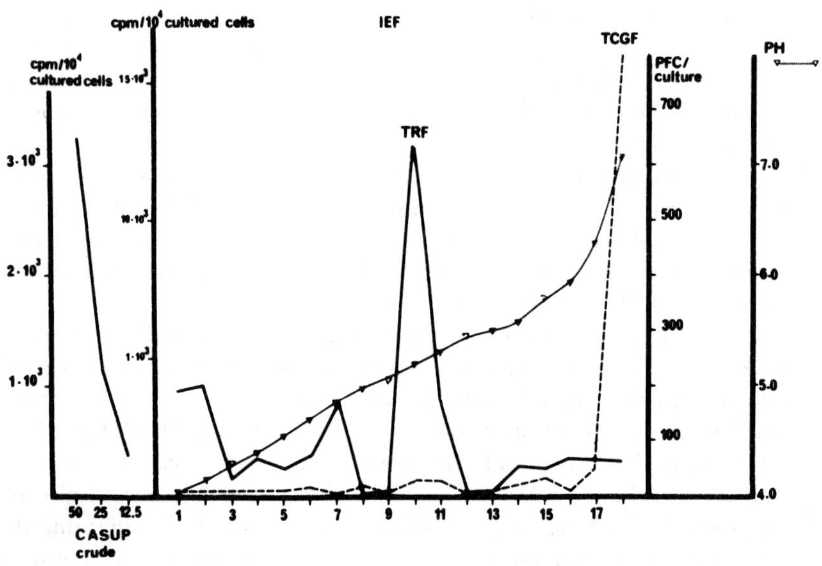

FIG. 7. *Separation of TRF and TCGF by IEF in the presence of 4* M *urea using a pH gradient from 4–7.*

highly depleted of the respective contaminants. A third way to separate TCGF and TRF is isoelectring focusing in 4 M area using very shallow pH gradients from 4–7 (Fig. 7). TRF focuses very sharply at pH 5·2, while TCGF can be found at a more alkaline pH. Preliminary evidence suggests that these separation techniques may not only separate factors acting on B cells from those acting on T cells, but also that factors affecting T cell growth may be distinct from those acting on T cell maturation and from those helping to convert precytotoxic T cells into T cells.

Conclusion

Obviously one can no longer assume that factors which lead to a common result, i.e. antibody production to a T cell dependent antigen, in T cell deprived cultures, are identical. In contrast, we have every reason to believe that such reconstitutions can be, and indeed are, brought about by distinct molecular moieties acting on distinct cells via different mechanisms. Consequently, it is no longer acceptable to lump together all biological activities, which restore the humoral immune response in so-called B cell cultures, simply by calling the activity TRF.

The greatest possible efforts should be made to simplify and to define the assay systems. A considerable advance in such endeavours is to be expected from the availability and use of long-term cultures or even permanent cell lines to assay biologically active factors. They offer the unique chance of obtaining cloned cell populations and thus assaying a defined biological response. This has already been achieved with respect to TCGF and we have preliminary evidence that late acting TRF can be assayed using appropriate and cloned populations of mouse plasmacytoma cell lines. This approach should finally make it possible to study the types of signals mediated by these factors in terms of molecular biology.

Of equal importance is the molecular characterization of the various biological activities using advanced biochemical techniques. Unfortunately, many of the so-called antigen nonspecific T helper activities, although in fact carried by different molecules, copurify when one applies only the more conventional techniques. Again, the possibility of obtaining permanent and cloned cell lines producing a particular mediator will prove helpful. Indeed, such cell lines have already helped to eliminate the possibility, favoured by some (Bernabé *et al.*, 1979), that the "nonantigen specific factors" are a mixture of anti-idiotypic factors. One must, however, keep in mind that even one defined type of cell may well produce more than one biologically active factor.

In spite of all the obstacles encountered so far, the demonstration of mediators which reconstitute humoral immune responses to T cell dependent antigens under various conditions has already greatly enriched our knowledge. We now know more about the means by which cells of the immune system communicate with one another, and we are learing which factor is operative on what cell. While all this is still somewhat remote from the main fascinations of classical immunology, it has no doubt contributed significantly to the understanding of immunological phenomena in particular and of cell biology in general.

References

Askonas, B. A., Schimpl, A. and Wecker, E. (1974). *Eur. J. Immunol.* **4**, 164.
Bernabé, R. P., Martinez-Alonso, C. and Coutinho, A. (1979). *Eur. J. Immunol.* **9**, 546.
Dutton, R. W. (1975). *Transpl. Rev.* **23**, 66.
Dutton, R. W., Panfili, P. R. and Swain, S. (1978). *Immunol. Rev.* **42**, 20.
Farrar, J. J. and Koopman, W. J. (1979). *In* "Biology of the Lymphokines" (S. Cohen, E. Pick and J. J. Oppenheim, eds), p. 325. Academic Press, New York and London.
Farrar, J. J., Simon, P. L., Koopman, W. J. and Fuller-Bonar, J. (1978). *J. Immunol.* **121**, 1353.
Gillis, S. and Smith, K. A. (1977). *Nature* **263**, 154.
Gillis, S., Union, N. A., Baker, P. E. and Smith, K. A. (1979). *J. Exp. Med.* **149**, 1460.
Hoffmann, M. K. and Watson, J. (1979). *J. Immunol.* **122**, 1371.
Hoffmann, M. K., Koenig, S., Mittler, R. S., Oettgen, H. F., Ralph, P., Galanos, C. and Hämmerling, U. (1979). *J. Immunol.* **122**, 497.
Hübner, L., Schimpl, A. and Wecker, E. (1980). *J. Mol. Immunol.* **17**, 591.
Hünig, Th., Schimpl, A. and Wecker, E. (1974). *J. Exp. Med.* **139**, 754.
Mitchison, N. A., Rajewski, K. and Taylor, R. B. (1970). *In* "Prague Symposium on Development Aspects of Antibody Formation and Structure" (J. Sterzl, ed.), p. 547.
Müller, G., Hübner, L., Schimpl, A. and Wecker, E. (1978). *Immunochemistry* **15**, 27.
Paetkau, V., Mills, G., Gerhart, S. and Monticone, V. (1976). *J. Immunol.* **117**, 1320.
Pickel, K., Hämmerling, U. and Hoffmann, M. K. (1976). *Nature* **264**, 72.
Schimpl, A. and Wecker, E. (1972). *Nature New Biol.* **237**, 15.
Schimpl, A. and Wecker, E. (1979). *In* "Biology of the Lymphokines" (S. Cohen, E. Pick and J. J. Oppenheim, eds), p. 369. Academic Press, New York and London.
Shaw, J., Caplan, B., Pretkau, V., Pilarski, L. M., Delovitch, T. L. and McKenzie, I. F. C. (1980). *J. Immunol.* **124**, 2231.
Waldmann, H. and Munro, A. (1974). *Immunology* **27**, 53.
Waldmann, H., Poulton, P. and Desaymard, C. (1976). *Immunology* **30**, 723.
Watson, J., Aarden, L. and Lefkovits, I. (1979a). *J. Immunol.* **122**, 209.
Watson, J., Aarden, L. A., Shaw, J. and Paetkau, V. (1979b). *J. Immunol.* **122**, 1633.

Theme 6: Summary

Cellular Co-operation

D. H. KATZ

Department of Cellular and Developmental Immunology, Scripps Clinic and Research Foundation, La Jolla, California, USA

The advances that have been made during the past two decades with respect to our understanding of various facets of the immune system have been remarkable. Consider, for example, that during that time-span studies in immunology have resulted in: (1) the elucidation of the structure of immunoglobulins; (2) definition of the components and mechanisms of the complement system; (3) identification of distinctions between the two major classes of lymphocytes and the fact that they interact with one another as well as with macrophages in the development of various immune responses; (4) elucidation of ontogenic events in the development of the immune system and appreciation of phylogenetic considerations; (5) demonstration of antigen-specific receptors on the surface membranes of B cells and T cells and the presence of other cell surface markers which coincide with various subclasses of lymphocytes and are expressed at distinct stages of differentiation; (6) the genetic, serologic and biochemical definition of the histocompatibility systems of man and certain experimental animals and the discovery that genes of the major histocompatibility complex (MHC) play a pivotal role in governing cell–cell communication in the immune system; and (7) definition of mechanisms by which the immune system can be triggered to result in pathologic processes that are deleterious to the individual and definition of an array of immunologic deficiency disorders that are either genetically inherited, or which result from consequences of other disease processes or the treatment of such diseases.

The past

The true roots of this theme date back nearly 20 years ago when Miller in Australia, and independently, Good in the USA discovered the immunologic role of the thymus. At present, when so many of us rely heavily on inbred mice, it is hard to imagine that much of the early groundwork in identifying the existence of 2 distinct lymphocyte systems came out of work in chickens by Warner and by Cooper working in Good's laboratory, and also out of the analysis of primary immune deficiency diseases of man studied so intensively by Good and coworkers in Minneapolis. One must also recall the even earlier dissection of specificities of cellular and humoral immune responses conducted by Benacerraf and Gell in guinea-pigs, leading ultimately to the discovery by Ovary and Benacerraf of the classical "carrier effect" in hapten-specific antibody responses, which ultimately was clarified by Rajewsky and Mitchison and by studies that I had the good fortune to carry out with Benacerraf and Paul some years ago, which demonstrated the collaborative contributions of carrier-specific helper cells and hapten-specific precursors of antibody-forming cells in such responses.

The existence of cellular co-operation between two distinct lymphocyte classes in mice, one contributed by the thymus and the other by bone marrow, was first reported in an obscure paper by Claman, although comparable evidence was being obtained independently by Davies. Then came the studies of Mitchell and Miller which identified bone marrow as the source of antibody-forming cell precursors and the thymus as the source of Claman's postulated "auxilliary" cells. All of this done in the sheep red blood cell system. This led to a virtual avalanche of work in many experimental systems including the previously mysterious hapten-carrier system, where Raff made use, for the first time, of antibodies to an alloantigen on T cells called theta by Reif and Allen (who discovered it 6 years earlier) to show directly that T cells in the mouse provided carrier-specific helper function for hapten-specific B cells in the Mitchison adoptive transfer model.

From a different vantage point cellular co-operation was unravelling another perplexing immunologic issue, namely the basis for immune response gene control. The use of synthetic polypeptide antigens, introduced and championed by Sela in Israel, resulted in the discovery of *Ir* genes in guinea-pigs by Benacerraf and colleagues and in mice by McDevitt and Sela. Having the advantage of congenic and recombinant inbred mice developed initially by Gorer and Snell and extended by Shreffler and Klein and many others enabled McDevitt and Benacerraf to establish linkage of *Ir* genes to the *MHC* and ultimately to map such genes in a distinct region of *H-2*.

The above brief summary of earlier work shows how things stood at the beginning of the 1970s.

The dominant theme at the 1st International Congress in 1971 in terms of cellular co-operation was the mystery of how T cells "helped" B cells to form antibodies. There was one detractor in the crowd—Dick Gershon who, stubbornly it seemed, kept bringing up "suppression". I think it is obvious how effective his stubbornness has been when you appreciate the fact that at this Congress, suppression and suppressor cells seem to grab at us from every angle.

The decade bringing us up to 1980 has been an exciting period for this theme, during which such things have come to light as (1) MHC-linked genetic restrictions on cell–cell interactions of all types, and the plasticity of the self-recognition repertoire so that cells can adapt to their environmental milieu; (2) identification of Ia and Dr antigens in *H-2* and *HLA* respectively, and their role in cell–cell recognition processes; (3) delineation of T–T cell co-operative interactions analogous to T–B cell co-operation; (4) the discovery of soluble lymphocyte products, nonimmunoglobulin in nature, some of which display antigen-binding capacity, and some of which display Ia determinants; (5) elucidation of new cell surface alloantigens whose expression appear to correlate with distinct stages of differentiation and functional phenotypes; and (6) the importance of macrophages, particularly those expressing Ia or Dr antigens in presenting antigens to trigger immune responses. These matters have all been detailed in this Theme.

The present

Viewing our present state of affairs, obviously from a personal perspective, three things strike me with particular emphasis. Firstly, it is obvious that we are becoming more and more sophisticated in our approaches both in terms of the reagents we develop and use and also in our experimental designs. The good that comes from this lies in the fact that we are hastening our chances to apply solid modern molecular biology to defining the molecules involved in cell–cell recognition and specific antigen recognition by T cells, macrophages and B cells (other than conventional immunoglobulins). I should not hesitate to state, however, that we must be cognizant of an inherent trap that could lie obscurely in all of this, which is as follows: the system is multicellular and normally closed; as such, the communication processes that operate normally could be considerably tighter than we are able to view by our increasingly sophisticated modern techniques. In other words, we may have to keep in mind the possibility that as we select further and further our cell types, subtypes and sub-subtypes for analysis we may unwittingly uncover phenotypic functions and perhaps molecular entities that are never behaving as such under normal circumstances. In a sense, we may be opening the window too widely in this respect, and I raise this point only as a matter of caution.

The second point that strikes me relates to the story evolving with respect to idiotype and anti-idiotype-specific collaborating T cells that are now being found in several laboratories. I have no personal difficulty in accepting as real the results that are being presented. I do, however, have some concerns about whether the interpretation of many investigators pertaining to the T cell nature of the main cells of interest is correct. It seems that if, for example, the PC-specific receptor on T cells is comprised of V_H genes encoding the T15 idiotype, then someone should be able to identify PC-specific cytotoxic T lymphocytes (CTL) with $T15^+$ receptors; to my knowledge this has not been found in the several idiotype systems in which it has been examined. Perhaps it is true that CTL express different V_H gene repertoires and, if so, my concerns are unjustified. However, the other side of the coin, and one perhaps worth greater exploration, is that we may be ignoring an important participation of B cells in these different systems and that these are the true targets of the many anti-idiotype reagents being used.

The third point, which is on a more optimistic note, is the very substantial growth of human lymphocyte biology in terms of experimentation pertaining to specific and nonspecific cellular co-operation among human lymphoid cells. One has occasionally heard in the past, sceptical comments made by less optimistic onlookers that simply because results of one kind or another are obtained in mice or other experimental animals does not mean that the same will be true in man. That is certainly a possibility. Therefore, it is particularly gratifying to see that the findings being made in cellular co-operation systems in man are virtually 100% in concordance with the basic principles derived from studies in experimental animals including MHC-linked genetic restrictions soluble factors and lymphocyte subset phenotypy. This should be extremely encouraging to those working in animal models to continue with great fervour and optimism with the awareness that what we learn from such work will be of benefit to mankind. Additionally, as more and more work is translated to human systems, we can expect that from such studies new breakthroughs will surface. Let us not forget that Fc receptor heterogeneity relationships to functionally distinct T cell subsets was established first with human, and not mouse, lymphocytes.

The future

This brings us to the last topic of my summary, namely what directions can we envisage this theme taking in the next 5 years? To continue with the point mentioned above, it is obvious that studies with human lymphocytes and lymphocyte products will be the next avalanche. This will be good not only for the new knowledge we will obtain, and especially in terms of what manipulations can be feasibly explored to develop new immunomodulatory therapies, but also because we can at last have an indisputable justification for continued growth of basic biomedical research support to counter arguments raised recently by certain elements of our society.

I feel intuitively that over the next years our previous one-sided fascination with T cells will mellow and more and more attention will be directed towards B cells. Particularly, I believe that the handful of us who have obtained evidence for the notion that B cells self-recognize partner cells in a manner analogous to T cells will be joined by many others using even better assay systems for demonstrating this. Instinctively, I am a symmetricist, as those who have worked with me know very well—and so it is difficult for me *not* to believe that B cells, like T cells, perceive "self" in the same sense. Additionally, I predict a wealth of new information demonstrating more sophisticated regulatory roles of B cells than has generally been recognized. Such studies will not be easy but they will be great fun and very educational. Remember how long the gestation period was for macrophages? I think the B cell story is nearing its delivery time.

Frankly, I think we are still on the threshold of soluble factor clarification. We must, however, be extraordinarily patient and flexible-minded on this subject. There is a trend to believe that T cell hybridoma and cloned line technology should make this an easy solution in the very near future. I think more caution must be exercised in this respect or we could make serious errors that will set us back—we cannot forget that we are limited by, and therefore at the mercy of, our biological assays for these soluble factors. We still have much valuable information that can be obtained even with factors that are not yet purified to homogeneity. After all, out of relatively dirty preparations came results which have placed a totally new and exciting perspective on Fc receptor molecules for IgG, and more recently IgE, and the important immunoregulatory effects such molecules have on physiologic immune responses.

Although nothing was presented publicly at this Congress about it, I will also predict that the next few years will witness the unfolding of an exciting story about the existence of responses against self-specific receptors; namely those which normally interact with cell interaction molecules. We are developing mounting evidence for the occurrence of such anti-self receptor responses in our own laboratory and it will be interesting to determine how such responses participate in normal immune regulation and whether they explain mechanisms of *Ir* gene function.

Finally, I think a point should be raised about energy conservation in cell interactions. Inherent in most evolutionary development of system specialization to higher orders of complexity is nature's drive to conserve biological energy. As I viewed some of the more up-to-date schemes of cellular interactions and the presumed molecular interactions involved in them, I was struck by the question "why?". If, in fact, these highly complicated circuits are correct, then we must accept the paradox that the immune system, unlike most other biological systems, has failed to conserve biological efficiency as it evolved from lower species. This confuses me, and so I tend to believe that, as we appreciate the limits to which we allow ourselves to open the "window" on these processes, we may find that our schemes will again revert to those of a few years ago which, for any given response, involved 3, or maybe 4, cells and 2, or maybe 3, factors operating in concert in a highly efficient and effective manner.

Theme 7

Genetic Regulation of Immune Responsiveness

Presidents:
B. BENACERRAF
G. BIOZZI

Symposium Chairman:
M. SELA

23

Genetic Control of the Specificity of T Lymphocytes and their Regulatory Products

B. BENACERRAF

Department of Pathology, Harvard Medical School, Boston, Massachusetts, USA

Two genetic regions regulate immune responses, the major histocompatibility complex (*MHC*) and the immunoglobulin V_H genes. These genes and their products mediate such regulations by controlling essential cell interactions involving helper and suppressor T cells and by determining the specificity of T lymphocyte clones that are stimulated following antigen administration. I propose to discuss the mechanism of these regulations and the manner in

Abbreviations
MHC: major histocompatibility complex; V_H: variable segment of immunoglobulin heavy chains; Ir: immune response; DTH: delayed type hypersensitivity; GLΦ: copolymer of L-glutamic acid, L-lysine and L-phenylalanine; PLL: poly-L-lysine; GAT: copolymer of L-glutamic acid^{60}, L-alanine^{30} and L-tyrosine^{10}; GT: copolymer of L-glutamic acid^{50} and L-tyrosine^{50}; CRI: cross-reactive idiotype; ABA: azobenzene-arsonate; T_s: suppressor T cell; T_sF: suppressor T cell factor.

which *MHC* and V_H genes contribute to these complex regulatory processes. We shall begin with an analysis of immune response gene function and demonstrate how the presentation of antigen in relation with Ia molecules on antigen presenting cells determines T cell responses. We shall then discuss the suppressor T cell systems which display well characterized cross-reactive idiotypes and which have been studied in our laboratory. Such systems afford a unique opportunity to demonstrate the respective contribution of V_H and *MHC* genes to the regulation of specific immune responses. Lastly, we shall discuss the commitment of T cells to MHC specificities and how this process is responsible for the origin of alloreactivity.

MHC-linked immune response genes

Immune response genes were described initially 17 years ago to control responsiveness to synthetic polypeptide antigens (Levine *et al.*, 1963; Benacerraf and McDevitt, 1972) and have been the object of extensive investigation. It is now well established that specific immune responses to T dependent antigens are controlled by *MHC*-linked *Ir* genes. The identification of *H*-linked *Ir* genes led to the following discoveries:

(1) the identification of a new region of the *MHC*, the *I* region, where *Ir* genes map (McDevitt *et al.*, 1972) and the demonstration that this region codes for glycoprotein antigens (Shreffler *et al.*, 1974; Schwartz and Cullen, 1978), Ia molecules, expressed selectively on macrophages, B cells and activated T cells;

(2) the demonstration of the commitment of T cell to *MHC* gene products and to T dependent antigens concomitantly (Paul *et al.*, 1977);

(3) the critical role of antigen presentation by macrophages to stimulate T cells (Rosenthal and Shevach, 1973) and the contribution of macrophage Ia molecules to the specificity of helper T cells (Kappler and Marrack, 1976) and delayed type hypersensitivity (DTH) T cells (Miller *et al.*, 1975);

(4) *I* region control of T–B cell interaction and its relationship to macrophage–T cell interaction (Katz *et al.*, 1973; Kindred and Shreffler, 1972);

(5) The discovery of T cell regulatory factors bearing *I* region controlled determinants (Katz and Amerding, 1976; Tada *et al.*, 1976 Thèze *et al.*, 1977).

Ia molecules

In an attempt to better understand *Ir* gene function, several laboratories prepared alloantisera against *I* region controlled gene products (Shreffler *et al.*, 1974), and it was soon demonstrated that 2 out of 3 of the regions where *Ir* genes have been mapped code for a new class of polymorphic glycoproteins expressed on macrophages, B lymphocytes and activated T lymphocytes, the Ia molecules. These molecules are made of 2 chains, respectively 33 000 and 28 000 mol. wt referred to as the α and β chains, the β chain being the most polymorphic (reviewed by Schwartz and Cullen, 1978).

The discovery of Ia molecules raised the question of whether they are indeed the functional *Ir* gene products. There is strong genetic evidence that this is the case and the most convincing data has been provided by the genetic control of the immune response of inbred mice to the terpolymer of L-glutamic acid, L-lysine and L-phenylalanine (GLΦ) (Dorf and Benacerraf, 1975), illustrated in Table I. The response to GLΦ requires the interaction of two *Ir* genes, one mapping in the *I-E* subregion (α gene) and the other mapping in the *I-A* subregion (β gene). It is now established, based on the work of Jones *et al.* (1978), of Cook *et al.* (1979), and of Silver and Russell (1979), that the *I-E* subregion codes for the α chain of a molecule whose β chain is coded for in the *I-A* subregion. Whereas, for an antigen under the control of the *I-A* subregion alone, both α and β chains are coded for by the *I-A* subregion. The evidence that Ia molecules are the *Ir* gene products is detailed in Table II.

TABLE I
Localization of the Ir-GLΦ *α and β genes*

		H-2 region formulae								
Strain	*H-2 haplotype*	*K*	*I-A*	*I-B*	*I-J*	*I-E*	*I-C*	*S*	*D*	*GLΦ response (% binding ± s.e.)*
B10	*b*	*b*	*b*	*b*	*b*	*b*	*b*	*b*	*b*	1 ± 3
B10.BR	*k*	*k*	*k*	*k*	*k*	*k*	*k*	*k*	*k*	5 ± 3
B10.S	*s*	*s*	*s*	*s*	*s*	*s*	*s*	*s*	*s*	−1 ± 1
B10.D2	*d*	*d*	*d*	*d*	*d*	*d*	*d*	*d*	*d*	61 ± 5
B10.A	*a*	*k*	*k*	*k*	*k*	*k* ⇐	*d*	*d*	*d*	4 ± 2
3R	*i3*	*b*	*b*	*b*	*b* ⇐|⇒	*k*	*d*	*d*	*d*	59 ± 7
5R	*i5*	*b*	*b*	*b* ⇐|⇒	*k*	*k*	*d*	*d*	*d*	73 ± 5
18R	*i18*	*b*	*b*	*b*	*b*	*b*	*b*	*b* ⇐	*d*	5 ± 2
7R	*t2*	*s*	*s*	*s*	*s*	*s*	*s*	*s* ⇐	*d*	4 ± 2
9R	*t4*	*s*	*s*	? ⇐|⇒	*k*	*k*	*d*	*d*	*d*	71 ± 10
A.TL	*t1*	*s* |⇒	*k*	*k*	*k*	*k*	*k*	*k*	*d*	4 ± 3
B10.HTT	*t3*	*s*	*s*	*s*	*s* ⇐|⇒	*k*	*k*	*k*	*d*	77 ± 7
			β			α				

Vertical bar indicates position of crossing-over

Determinant selection

The conclusion that the *Ir* genes code for Ia molecules still leaves much of

TABLE II
Ia Molecules are Ir *Gene Products*

(I) They map in the same genetic region
(II) Specific helper and DTH T cells bind antigen and are stimulated only when antigen is presented on cells (macrophages) together with the appropriate Ia molecule
(III) Stimulation of these T lymphocytes *in vitro* or *in vivo* is blocked by appropriately specific anti-Ia antisera
(IV) *Ir* gene complementation for GLΦ responses parallels closely interchain complementation between *I-E* controlled α chain and *I-A* controlled β chain
(V) The expression of Ia-7 specificity controlled by the *I-E* region correlates with the *Ir GLΦ* α gene

the puzzle of the mechanism of *Ir* gene function unresolved. We must consider how Ia molecules selectively and specifically restrict T cell immune responses. The contributions of many laboratories, starting initially with Shevach and Rosenthal (1973), then with Schwartz and Paul (1976), Singer *et al.* (1978) and ourselves (Germain and Benacerraf, 1978), have clearly shown that the major site of *Ir* gene function is at the level of the antigen presenting cell, a class of macrophage. Responding T cells have receptors for antigen and also for autologous Ia molecules and the two molecules have to be presented jointly, to the T cell, as shown diagrammatically in Fig. 1, for the T helper or DTH T cell to be stimulated. This phenomenon can best be analysed by studying the specific T cell proliferative response *in vitro* to antigen pulsed macrophages.

Such responses can be effectively blocked by anti-Ia antisera directed against these molecules on the antigen presenting macrophages (Shevach *et al.*, 1972; Schwartz *et al.*, 1978). In the GLΦ system controlled by complementing *Ir* genes, the proliferative response of immune T cells is blocked by an anti-Ia

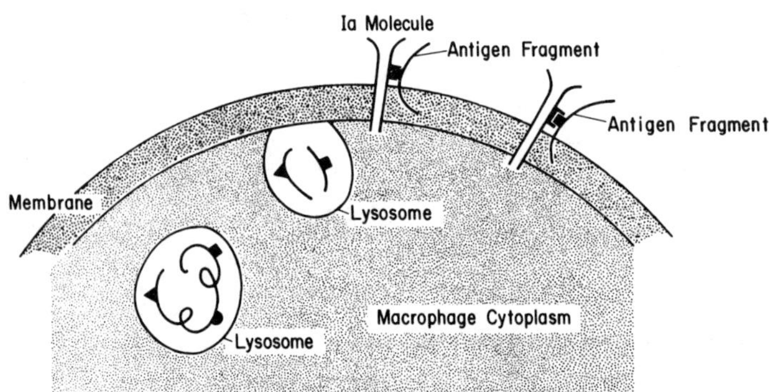

FIG. 1. *Processing of antigen and presentation of antigen fragment by Ia bearing macrophages to T cells. Note the postulated interaction between antigen and Ia molecules responsible for determinant selection.*

monoclonal antibody specific for conformational determinants contributed by the *I-E* controlled α chain and *I–A* controlled β chain (Janeway, pers. comm.). Moreover, in a series of elegant experiments in the same GLΦ system, Longo and Schwartz (1980) have established that both α and β complementing genes need to be expressed in the antigen presenting cell. In contrast, using chimaeric mice they showed that T cells lacking the appropriate T cell responder genotype can nevertheless be induced to respond to GLΦ on responder antigen presenting cells. There is no doubt, therefore, that in many *Ir* gene systems, of which GLΦ is a model, antigen presentation in relation to Ia molecules is responsible for the *Ir* gene restrictions observed.

Two distinct mechanisms can be evoked to explain the commitment of T lymphocytes to autologous Ia molecules in relation to thymus dependent antigens, exemplified by the GLΦ system and, therefore, for the specificity of *Ir* gene defects: (1) a specific interaction between macrophage Ia molecules and antigen or antigen fragments is postulated to permit the effective presentation of the complex antigen–Ia molecule to the appropriate T cell clones bearing receptors for antigen and Ia molecules; (2) in the course of T cell differentiation in the thymus, individual T lymphocyte clones are restricted to display receptors for certain antigens and Ia molecules selectively.

Different investigators have favoured one or the other of these two hypotheses (von Boehmer *et al.*, 1978; Benacerraf, 1978). In my opinion, however, there is indirect evidence in favour of the first hypothesis, based on the observation that the specificity of *Ir* genes does not match the specificity of the T cell responses controlled by the genes (Benacerraf, 1977, 1978). This is best illustrated in the experiments of Schlossman (1972) on the response of strain 2 guinea-pigs to DNP-oligolysine conjugates. Strain 2 guinea-pigs possess the PLL gene which controls responses to poly-L-lysine, oligolysines and hapten conjugates of these polymers. In earlier studies, Schlossman established that a minimal sequence of 7 lysines is required for immunogenicity in this system. However, strain 2 guinea-pigs will also respond to DNP-conjugates bearing a sequence of 4 lysines joined to 3 alanines and a lysine. The specificity of the T cell responses, as analysed by specific proliferation *in vitro*, are quite different for the various DNP-oligolysine compounds. The T cell receptors are therefore much more discriminating than the *Ir* gene products. Many other examples have been presented of the ability of *Ir* gene function to select antigen determinants reactive for T cells on thymus dependent antigens (Rosenthal *et al.*, 1977; Bluestein *et al.*, 1972; Berzofsky *et al.*, 1979). We have interpreted these data to indicate that Ia molecules on antigen presenting cells interact specifically with selected amino acid sequences, involving at most 3–4 amino acids, on antigen fragments from macrophage processed antigens (Benacerraf, 1978). These interactions should result in the selection of antigen determinants for interaction with T lymphocytes specific for such determinants presented in conjunction with autologous Ia molecules. To perform the function of antigen presentation, Ia molecules are expressed on macrophages in a non-clonal fashion. The issue must be considered whether the number of potential distinct Ia molecules expressed in a given animal is sufficient to permit this type of function for most protein antigens. There are in the mouse two distinct families of Ia molecules with similar two chain structure. These two molecules are controlled respectively by the *I-A* subregion and *I-A–I-E* subregion as discussed earlier. In a heterozygote if an α chain can interact with any β chain, as is probably the case, the number of different Ia molecules determined by the two loci concerned is 16, each capable of a specific interaction with a postulated amino acid sequence.

In addition, the Ia molecules on B cells and activated T cells may be considered to have the same function as those on antigen presenting cells. The T cell clone, initially selected for its specificity for the determinant presented in relation to autologous Ia molecules, is therefore specifically reactive with the B cell or the T cell that it is designed to regulate after that cell has bound antigen.

Suppressor T cell responses

I now propose to discuss *I* region control of suppressor T cell responses as an introduction to the analysis of T cell suppressor interactions. As shown first by Kapp *et al.* (1974) and then by Debré *et al.* (1975, 1976) and Waltenbaugh *et al.* (1977) in our laboratory, nonresponder strains immunized with the copolymers poly-(Glu^{60}, Ala^{30}, Tyr^{10}) (GAT) and poly-(Glu^{50}, Tyr^{50}) (GT) develop suppressor T cell responses. We then demonstrated (Benacerraf and Dorf, 1976) that wheras all nonresponder strains to GAT are suppressor strains, only some of the nonresponder strains to GT are suppressor strains and that the suppressor phenotype is controlled by two *I* region complementing genes mapping, respectively, in *I-A* and *I-C*. I will not pursue this line of evidence any further at this time except to point out that these data indicate that, whatever form of antigen presentation is required to stimulate the suppressor T cell circuits in the GT system, it involves as its initial step the activity of *I* region gene products probably on antigen presenting cells.

I region controlled factors

In addition to the antigen presenting role of a class of glycoprotein coded for by the *I* region, discussed earlier, this region has been shown to code for antigen determinants expressed on regulatory factors obtained from T cells with helper or suppressor activity for immune responses (Feldman *et al.*, 1979; Tada *et al.*, 1976; Thèze *et al.*, 1977). The most thoroughly studied materials have been the T cell suppressor factors. These have been shown by Tada *et al.* (1976) and ourselves (Thèze *et al.*, 1977; Germain *et al.*, 1979; Bach *et al.*, 1979; Greene *et al.*, 1979) to have the following properties:

(1) they are antigen specific,
(2) they lack Ig constant region determinants,
(3) they possess *I-J* coded determinants,
(4) they possess idiotype determinants of specific Ig,
(5) they have a mol. wt between 40 000 and 60 000 daltons.

Moreover, in the GAT system, as shown in our laboratory, the suppressor factor is able to induce a new class of suppressor T cells termed T_{s_2} (Waltenbaugh *et al.*, 1977) across *MHC* and V_H differences in both non-responder and responder strains (Pierres *et al.*, 1979).

Role of V_H and *MHC* genes in suppressor T cell circuits

A genetic analysis of idiotypic restriction that *V* region genes might impose on the suppressor T cell response to GAT was rendered impossible by our finding that the CGAT cross-reactive idiotype expressed on anti-GAT antibodies is present in all mouse strains (Ju *et al.*, 1978). We decided therefore to investigate more appropriate systems which exhibit V_H restricted cross-reactive idiotype (CRI). In collaboration with Nisonoff, we have carried out a study of DTH response to azobenzenearsonate (ABA) in A/J mice which express the ABA-CRI and investigated the suppression of this response (Greene *et al.*, 1979; Bach *et al.*, 1979). The administration intravenously of ABA coupled syngeneic cells previous to sensitization to ABA induces ABA specific suppressor T cells capable of transferring adoptive suppression against ABA-DTH. Such suppressor cells were studied in our laboratory by Sy *et al.* (1980)

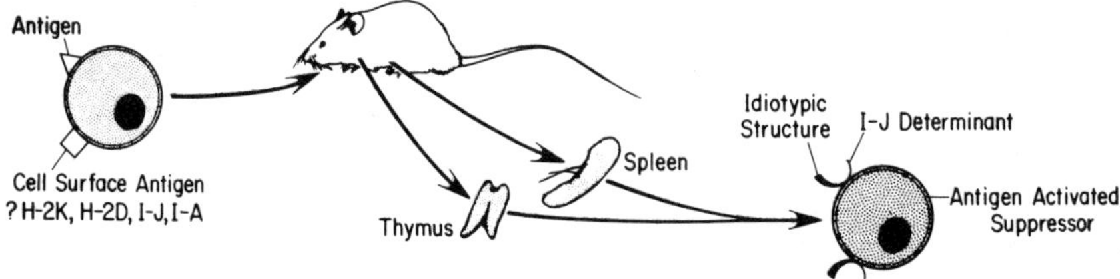

FIG. 2. Antigen conjugated to syngeneic spleen cells induces antigen specific suppressor T cells (T_{s_1}) in the thymus and spleen of mice. These T_{s_1} cells bear I-J and idiotypic determinants on their antigen receptors. From Greene and Sy (1981).

and were shown to be antigen specific and to possess both idiotypic and *I-J* coded determinants on their surface (Fig. 2). From such suppressor cells an antigen specific factor can be obtained which is ABA specific and bears both *I-J* and idiotypic determinants, as in the GAT system. This factor is indeed in every way similar to the GAT factor, except that it only suppresses DTH-ABA responses in V_H matched recipient mice which express the ABA–CRI.

The V_H restriction and the presence of ABA–CRI in the A/J strain permitted an analysis of the mode of action of suppressor factor and of its ability to stimulate suppressor T cells in this system, as shown in Fig. 3. Suppressor factor from T_{s_1} cells induces a second set of suppressor T cells, T_{s_2}, which are anti-idiotypic. An analysis was indeed made of the specificity of the suppressor T cells induced by ABA specific suppressor factor by adherence of these cells to antigen or idiotype coated plates. We observed that the antigen induced T_{s_1} cells are ABA specific, whereas the suppressor T cells induced by factor are anti-idiotypic. Moreover, the ABA specific cells suppress immune induction whereas the idiotype specific T_{s_2} cells suppress immune cells at the effector phase of the response. Similar results were obtained by Weinberger *et al.* (1980) in the NP haptenic system.

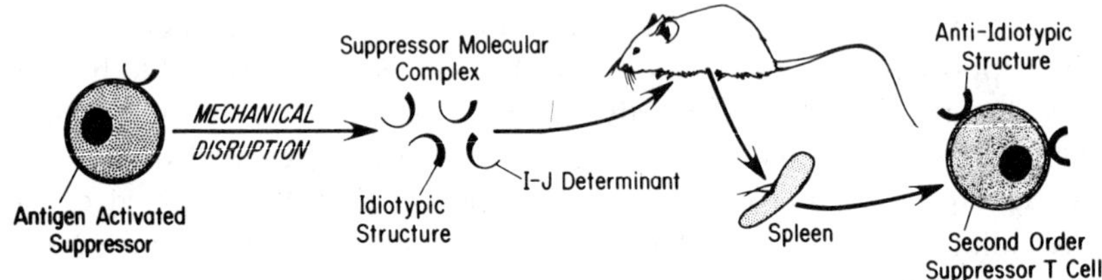

FIG. 3. *T_{s_1} cells and their suppressor factor, T_sF_1, induce a second order of suppressor T cells, T_{s_2}, which are anti-idiotypic and active on immune cells. From Greene and Sy (1981).*

The analysis of the suppressor circuit in the three model systems discussed—GAT, ABA, NP—into 2 phases involving 2 interacting suppressor T cells allows a definition of the genetic restrictions that govern the interaction of the 2 suppressor T cells and their factors at their respective stage of action. As we stated earlier, the antigen specific suppressor factor (T_sF_1) was shown not to be *MHC* restricted but to be functionally restricted by V_H genes. In contrast, the effector suppressor T cells (T_{s2}) and its factor (T_sF_2) are restricted in their activity by both V_H genes and *I* region genes, findings which were documented in both the ABA and NP systems. The V_H gene restriction was expected on the basis of the anti-idiotypic specificity of the effector suppressor T cells induced, but we cannot offer as yet an explanation for the *I* region restriction of effector suppressor T cells, nor can we account for how this restriction operates.

A model for the immune regulation of the suppressor circuits in the ABA, NP and GAT systems is presented in Fig. 4. An analysis of the suppressor T cell circuits depicted in Fig. 4 permits an appreciation of how *I* region and V_H genes and their products intervene at different stages of the complex regulation of the immune response in a correlated manner. The data also illustrate the important finding that the idiotypic network, postulated by Jerne to operate on antibodies and B cells, is even more important for the regulation of T cell responses in conjunction with *MHC* gene products.

In summary, I have attempted to demonstrate how, in selected systems,

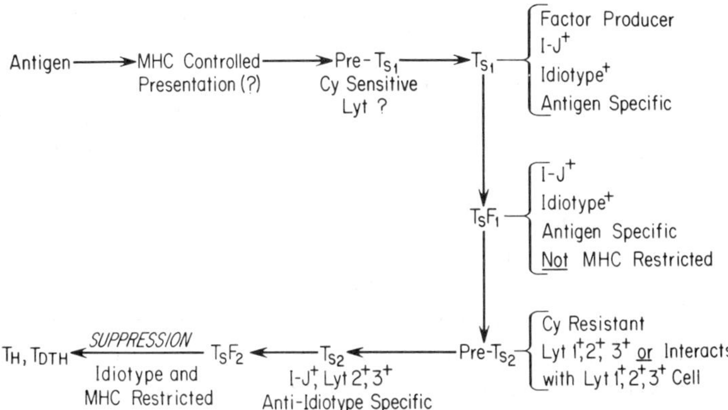

FIG. 4. *A model for the suppressor T cell circuit operative in the regulation of anti-ABA, NP and GAT murine immune responses. From Germain and Benacerraf (1981).*

I region and V_H genes intervene in the specific regulation of immune responses in correlated fashion, both in the generation of helper dependent T cells and also in the development of suppressor T cells which together regulate the complex interactions of lymphocyte clones that result in specific immunity and its normal homeostasis.

The commitment of T cells to MHC antigens

Jerne (1971) originally proposed a theory which was further elaborated by ourselves (Lemonnier *et al.*, 1977) to explain the generation in the thymus of T cells specific for MHC antigens. According to the theory, in the first stage T cells initially specific for self-*MHC* gene products are selected in the thymus to differentiate and proliferate. Then, in a second stage, only those T cells which bear low affinity receptors for self-MHC antigens are allowed to mature and leave the thymus as functional T cells. Such T cells, having low reactivity for self-MHC antigens, have concomitantly high affinity for variants of self-MHC antigens. These variants appear to be the same or similar to the allogeneic MHC antigens expressed in the same species. Simultaneously and independently these T cells develop receptors for determinants expressed on conventional thymus-dependent antigens.

The high degree of reactivity to MHC antigens which constitute the polymorphic population encountered in the same species (i.e., alloantigens) and the lower reactivity to xenogeneic MHC antigens may be accounted for by the fact that low affinity receptors for self-MHC antigens might be expected to react optimally with allogeneic MHC antigens, but much less so with xenogeneic antigens. This would account for the paradox that the strongest T cell responses are not elicited by antigens further removed phylogenetically from the responder. Two predictions from this theory would be: (a) that clones of T cells induced by xenogeneic MHC antigens should be highly cross-reactive with allogeneic MHC antigens, even to the extent that they may demonstrate a heteroclitic response. This has indeed been demonstrated when mouse antirat CTL were shown in our laboratory to be comprised of clones cross-reactive with allogeneic target cells (Burakoff *et al.*, 1977); (b) alloreactive T cells should be expected to be highly cross-reactive with modified syngeneic cells. This was also shown to be the case when we observed considerable cross-reactivity by alloreactive cells for TNP conjugated target cells syngeneic to the responder (Lemonnier *et al.*, 1977).

Since the T cell repertoire for MHC specificities is normally determined by the self-MHC antigens of the thymus, we should expect the T cell repertoire to vary according to the MHC of the thymus in which T cells differentiate. Recent experiments utilizing radiation chimaeras by Zinkernagel *et al.* (1978), Bevan (1978) and Billings *et al.* (1978) have demonstrated this to be the case. The postulate that alloreactive T cells are generated from T cells differentiating in the thymus that are strongly reactive for variants of self-MHC antigens leads to the expectation that immunization with virally infected syngeneic cells should result in the stimulation of T cell clones that are reactive with the virally infected syngeneic cells used to immunize and also reactive with uninfected allogeneic target cells.

We have recently shown that immunization of BALB/c ($H\text{-}2^d$) mice with Sendai coated syngeneic cells stimulates CTL which lyse Sendai coated BALB/c target cells and also lyse uncoated $H\text{-}2^b$, $H\text{-}2^q$, $H\text{-}2^k$, $H\text{-}2^s$ *and* $H\text{-}2^r$ allogeneic target cells to an appreciable degree (Finberg *et al.*, 1978). We further demonstrated by the cold target inhibition technique that the same clones that lysed BALB/c coated Sendai targets also cross-reactively lysed the allogeneic targets. Furthermore, it was observed that separate CTL clones lysed each of the different allogeneic targets. In addition, there was significantly less lysis of target cells bearing the $H\text{-}2^q$ haplotype than of target cells bearing the $H\text{-}2^k$ or $H\text{-}2^r$ haplotypes. This later finding suggests that the association of Sendai virus antigens with the $H\text{-}2^d$ gene products of BALB/c mice creates determinants which are more cross-reactive with $H\text{-}2^k$ and $H\text{-}2^r$ than with $H\text{-}2^q$ gene products. Our hypothesis would therefore predict that the T cell responses by BALB/c mice to other viruses or to Sendai virus by mice of different haplotypes should result in different patterns of cross-reactivity for allogeneic targets.

In another system, Bevan (1975) has reported that stimulation of mouse spleen cells by H-2 identical spleen cells bearing foreign minor H antigens results in the generation of T cells that lyse H-2 identical targets bearing the appropriate foreign minor antigens. Recently, he has found that repeated stimulation of such CTL with allogeneic cells results in selection of an effector population which lyses both allogeneic cells as well as H-2 identical target cells bearing the appropriate minor foreign H antigens with a similar efficiency (Bevan, 1977). These findings are consistent with our observations that autologous MHC antigens in association with non-MHC antigens are cross-reactive with allogeneic MHC antigens.

Recent experiments on the Ly phenotype of the precursors of alloreactive CTL are also in agreement with our hypothesis. Precursors of alloreactive CTL have been found to belong to the Ly-23 set, while precursors that respond to TNP-coupled syngeneic cells were found to reside in the Ly-123 set. We have found that alloreactive prekiller CTL in young mice reside initially in the Ly-123 pool but shift to the Ly-23 pool by 5 weeks of age. This suggests that the Ly-23 alloreactive prekiller T cells found in adult mice are actually 'memory' cells; these alloreactive precursor T cells shift from the Ly-123 pool to the Ly-23 pool when they encounter autologous MHC antigens in association with foreign antigens, such as virus (Finberg *et al.*, 1980).

In conclusion, we feel that the proposed hypothesis can account for several of the observations that have puzzled immunologists previously. It should be pointed out, however, that these data do not permit firm conclusions on the critical issue of whether cross-reactive recognition of MHC products and conventional antigens is mediated by T cells carrying a single receptor or two receptors. However, if, as proposed by many investigators, T cells bear two distinct receptors, one specific for MHC gene products and the other for conventional antigens, an analysis of the specificity of the receptors must account appropriately for the large number of alloreactive T cell clones. In this context, the data we have discussed strongly suggest that in a two receptor model, the receptor specific for MHC antigen is specific for variants of self rather than self, as proposed by Zinkernagel *et al.* (1978) and that the two receptors function in close relationship.

References

Bach, B. A., Greene, M. I., Benacerraf, B. and Nisonoff, A. (1979). *J. Exp. Med.* **149**, 1084.

Benacerraf, B. (1977). *Ann. Inst. Pasteur, Ann. Immunol.* **128C**, 385–392.

Benacerraf, B. (1978). *J. Immunol.* **120**, 1809.

Benacerraf, B. and Dorf, M. E. (1976). *Proc. Cold Spring Harbor Symp. Quant. Biol.* **41**, 465.

Benacerraf, B. and McDevitt, H. O. (1972). *Science* **175**, 273.

Berzofsky, J. A., Richman, L. K. and Killien, D. J. (1979). *Proc. Natn. Acad. Sci. U.S.A.* **76**, 4046.

Bevan, M. G. (1975). *Nature* **256**, 419.

Bevan, M. G. (1977) *Proc. Natn. Acad. Sci. U.S.A.* **74**, 2094.

Bevan, M. G. (1978). *Nature* **269**, 417.

Billings, P., Burakoff, S. J., Dorf, M. E. and Benacerraf, B. (1978). *J. Exp. Med.* **148**, 352.

Bluestein, H. G., Green, I., Maurer, P. H. and Benacerraf, B. (1972). *J. Exp. Med.* **135**, 98.

von Boehmer, H., Haas, W. and Jerne, N. K. (1978). *Proc. Natn. Acad. Sci. U.S.A.* **75**, 2439.

Burakoff, S. J., Ratnofsky, S. E. and Benacerraf, B. (1977). *Proc. Natn. Acad. Sci. U.S.A.* **74**, 4572.

Cook, R. G., Vitetta, E. S., Uhr, J. W. and Capra, J. D. (1979). *J. Exp. Med.* **149**, 981.

Debré, P., Kapp, J. A., Dorf, M. E. and Benacerraf, B. (1975). *J. Exp. Med.* **142**, 1447.
Debré, P., Waltenbaugh, C., Dorf, M. E. and Benacerraf, B. (1976). *J. Exp. Med.* **144**, 272.
Dorf, M. E. and Benacerraf, B. (1975). *Proc. Natn. Acad. Sci. U.S.A.* **72**, 3671.
Feldmann, M., Howie, S. and Kontianinen, S. (1979). *In* "Biology of the Lymphokines" (S. Cohen, E. Pick and J. J. Openheim, eds.) pp. 391–419. Academic Press, New York.
Finberg, R., Burakoff, S. J., Cantor, H. and Benacerraf, B. (1978) *Proc. Natn. Acad. Sci. U.S.A.* **75**, 5145.
Finberg, R., Cantor, H., Benacerraf, B. and Burakoff, S. J. (1980). *J. Immunol.* **125**, 1858.
Germain, R. N. and Benacerraf, B. (1978). *J. Exp. Med.* **148**, 1324.
Germain, R. N. and Benacerraf, B. (1981). *Springer Sem. Immunopathol.* (in press).
Germain, R. N., Ju, S-T., Kipps, T. J., Benacerraf, B. and Dorf, M. E. (1979). *J. Exp. Med.* **149**, 613.
Greene, M. I. and Sy, M. S. (1981). *Fedn. Proc.* (in press).
Greene, M. I., Bach, B. A. and Benacerraf, B. (1979). *J. Exp. Med.* **149**, 1069.
Jerne, N. K. (1971). *Eur. J. Immunol.* **1**, 1.
Jones, P. P., Murphy, D. B. and McDevitt, H. O. (1978). *J. Exp. Med.* **148**, 925.
Ju, S-T., Benacerraf, B. and Dorf, M. E. (1978). *Proc. Natn. Acad. Sci. U.S.A.* **75**, 6192.
Kapp, J. A., Pierce, C. W., Schlossman, S. and Benacerraf, B. (1974). *J. Exp. Med.* **140**, 648.
Kappler, J. W. and Marrack, C. P. (1976). *Nature* **262**, 797.
Katz, D. H. and Amerding, D. (1976). *In* "The Role of Products of the Histocompatibility Gene Complex in Immune Responses" (D. H. Katz, and B. Benacerraf, eds.) p. 541. Academic Press, New York.
Katz, D. H., Hamaoka, T., Dorf, M. E. and Benacerraf, B. (1973). *Proc. Natn. Acad. Sci. U.S.A.* **70**, 2024.
Kindred, B. and Shreffler, D. C. (1972). *J. Immunol.* **109**, 940.
Lemonnier, F., Burakoff, S. J., Germain, R. N. and Benacerraf, B. (1977). *Proc. Natn. Acad. Sci. U.S.A.* **74**, 1229.
Levine, B. B., Ojeda, A. and Benacerraf, B. (1963). *J. Exp. Med.* **118**, 953.
Longo, D. L. and Schwartz, R. H. (1980). *J. Exp. Med.* **151**, 1452.
McDevitt, H. O., Deak, B. D., Shreffler, D. C., Klein, G., Stimpfling, J. H. and Snell, G. D. (1972). *J. Exp. Med.* **135**, 1259.
Miller, J. F. A. P., Vadas, M. A., Whitelaw, A. and Gamble, J. (1975). *Proc. Natn. Acad. Sci. U.S.A.* **72**, 5095.
Paul, W. E., Shevach, E. M., Pickeral, S., Thomas, D. W. and Rosenthal, A. S. (1977). *J. Exp. Med.* **145**, 618.
Pierres, M., Benacerraf, B. and Germain, R. N. (1979). *J. Immunol.* **123**, 2756.
Rosenthal, A. S. and Shevach, E. M. (1973). *J. Exp. Med.* **138**, 1194.
Rosenthal, A. S., Barcinski, M. A. and Blake, J. T. (1977). *Nature* **267**, 156.
Schlossman, S. F. (1972). *Transplantation Rev.* **10**, 97.
Schwartz, B. D. and Cullen, S. E. (1978). *Springer Sem. Immunopathol.* **1**, 85.
Schwartz, R. H. and Paul, W. E. (1976). *J. Exp. Med.* **143**, 529.
Schwartz, R. H., Yano, A. and Paul, W. E. (1978). *Immunol. Rev.* **40**, 153.
Shevach, E. M. and Rosenthal, A. S. (1973). *J. Exp. Med.* **138**, 1213.
Shevach, E. M., Paul, W. E. and Green, I. (1972). *J. Exp. Med.* **136**, 1207.
Shreffler, D., David, C., Gotze, D., Klein, J., McDevitt, H. O. and Sachs, D. (1974). *Immunogenetics* **1**, 189.
Silver, J. and Russell, W. A. (1979). *Immunogenetics* **8**, 339.
Singer, A., Cowing, C., Hathcock, K. S., Dickler, H. B. and Hodes, R. J. (1978). *J. Exp. Med.* **147**, 1611.

Sy, M. S., Dietz, M. H., Germain, R. N., Benacerraf, B. and Greene, M. I. (1980). *J. Exp. Med.* **151**, 1183.
Tada, T., Taniguchi, M. and David, C. S. (1976). *J. Exp. Med.* **144**, 713.
Thèze, J., Kapp, J. and Benacerraf, B. (1977). *J. Exp. Med.* **145**, 839.
Waltenbaugh, C., Thèze, J., Kapp, J. A. and Benacerraf, B. (1977). *J. Exp. Med.* **146**, 970.
Weinberger, J. Z., Benacerraf, B. and Dorf, M. E. (1980). *J. Exp. Med.* **151**, 1413.
Zinkernagel, R. M., Callahan, G. N., Althage, A., Cooper, S., Klein, P. A. and Klein, J. (1978). *J. Exp. Med.* **147**, 882.

24

Genetic Selections for Relevant Immunological Functions

G. BIOZZI*, M. SIQUEIRA, C. STIFFEL*, O. M. IBANEZ, D. MOUTON* and V. C. A. FERREIRA

** Service d'Immunogénétique, Institut Curie, Paris, France and Seçao de Immunologia, Instituto Biologico, Sao Paulo, Brazil*

Abbreviations

H: high antibody responder; L: low antibody responder; F_0: foundation population; RT: total response; n: number of loci; Hi/PHA: high responder to PHA; Lo/PHA: low responder to PHA; KTH: high responder to triolein; KTL: low responder to triolein; K.BCG.H: high responder to BCG; K.BCG.L: low responder to BCG.

Introduction

The evident teleonomy of the immune system is the host defence against infections. This goal is achieved in every individual by a cybernetic control of complex interactions of cells and molecules participating in the various immunity functions. In genetically heterogeneous populations, there is a large quantitative variability, at the individual level, in the principal immunity functions: antibody response, cell mediated immunity and macrophage activity. Our original approach to study the genetic regulation of immunoresponsiveness is the modification of those immunological functions by bidirectional selective breeding. The selected High and Low responder lines proved to present large modifications in the resistance to different infections according to the defensive efficacy of the genetically modified function (Biozzi *et al.*, 1979a).

Our investigations demonstrate two principal findings: (1) all the immunological functions are subject to quantitative polygenic regulation; (2) each of these functions has an independent genetic regulation. As a consequence, a total immune deficiency is statistically a very rare event (Mouton *et al.*, 1980).

This arrangement in the genetic control of the immune system has a high selective value in the phylogeny since it is the most able to ensure an optimal protection to a population. Each immunological function constitutes the paramount protective device against certain types of infections, whereas it plays only a minor role against other infections. The polygenic regulation of each immunological function determines a normal frequency distribution of individual phenotypes. Therefore, a very large number of individuals present a median resistance to all types of mild endemic infections and at the same time a small number of individuals (distribution tails of each function) endowed with extremely strong defence mechanisms permit a partial survival of the population against any given severe epidemic infection (Biozzi *et al.*, 1979a).

The polygenic regulation concerns the global immunoresponsiveness to multideterminant natural immunogens. The response to each of their epitopes should be largely controlled by phenomena of cross-self tolerance. In fact, a variable degree of polymorphism of structural genes is present in genetically heterogeneous populations. The larger the polymorphism of a given locus is, the broader its impact on the regulation of specific immunoresponsiveness will be. It is therefore very probable that the large polymorphism of the MHC is responsible for its frequent association with the control of the immune responses to specific epitopes themselves or to new antigenic determinants constituted by the epitope association with an MHC product on the cell membrane.

Methods of genetic analysis

The immunologic parameters here described are all subject to polygenic regulation. The following methods of quantitative genetics were used:

Bidirectional selective breeding

Figure 1 gives a schematic representation of the bidirectional selective breeding process. This process consists of the assortative mating of the highest or lowest phenotypes for the character investigated starting from a genetically heterogeneous foundation population (F_0). The selective breeding continued in consecutive generations produced a high (H) and a low (L) line. In each line, 6–10 parental pairs were culled in each generation and the number of offspring produced varied between 45 and 65.

The 2 lines diverged progressively until the maximal interline separation was reached: selection limit. At this stage, the 2 lines are considered homozygous for all the independent loci intervening in the quantitative regulation of the character investigated (Fig. 1B). The phenotypic variance (V) of the 2 populations at the selection limit is therefore only due to an environmental effect: environmental variance (VE). The phenotypic variance of genetically heterogeneous populations such as F_0, F_2 interline hybrids and backcrosses is produced by both genetic and environmental factors. The genetic variance (VG) is therefore calculated by subtracting VE from the total phenotypic variance (Fig. 1A).

The response to selection (R) is the difference between the mean values ($\bar{x}$) of 2 successive generations of each line. It may be expressed either per generation (RG) or as the total response to selection at the selection limit (RT). The value of the selection differential (S) is measured as the difference between the mean of the selected parents and that of the total generation out of which they have been culled.

The mean realized heritability (h^2) is calculated by the least-squares linear regression of R/S in the generations between F_0 and the selection limit (Fig. 1C). The h^2 value results from the additive effect of homozygous loci occupied by either high or low effect alleles. The most accurate h^2 estimation is obtained with cumulated R and S values calculated for the interline divergence. In this way the impact of the environmental factors affecting both lines alike is eliminated and the h^2 value is the mean of the values in H and L lines. For the h^2 value calculated in each line, see Biozzi *et al.* (1979a).

Interline hybrids analysis

The following interline hybrids were produced from parents originated in H and L lines at the selection limit: $(H \times L) = F_1$, $(F_1 \times F_1) = F_2$, $(F_1 \times H) = BcH$, $(F_1 \times L) = BcL$.

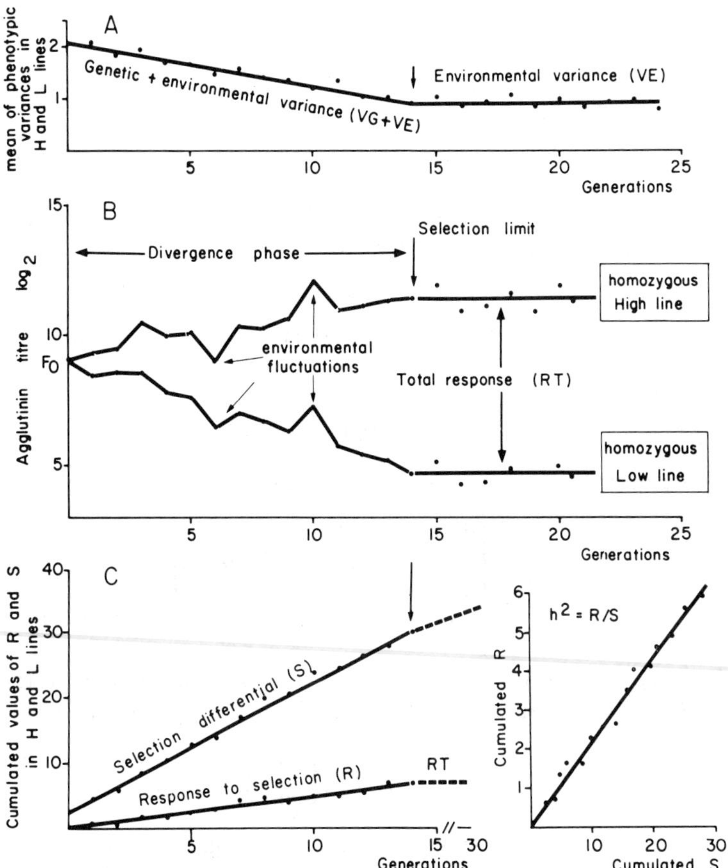

FIG. 1. *Schematic representation of the method of bidirectional selective breeding. (A) Phenotypic variances in successive generations (means of the 2 lines). (B) Means in successive generations of H and L lines. (C) Calculation of heritability (h^2): cumulated R and S and R/S regression (The values chosen for the parameters are mean results obtained in selections I, II, III and IV, see Table I).*

The genetic parameters are calculated as follows:

The total additive effect (a) of all the homozygous loci in H and L lines at the selection limit in the absence of dominance is given by

$$a = \frac{1}{2}(\bar{x}H - \bar{x}L).$$

The global dominance deviation (d) in F_1 hybrids is given by

$$d = \bar{x}F_1 - \frac{1}{2}(\bar{x}H + \bar{x}L).$$

The dominance effect, d/a.

The environmental variance,

$$VE = \frac{VH + VL + VF_1}{3} \tag{1}$$

The variance of F_2 hybrids,

$$VF_2 = VA + VD + VE \tag{2}$$

in which VA is the additive variance and VD the dominance variance.

The summed variance of the 2 backcrosses (VBcH + VBcL),

$$VBcs = VA + 2VD + 2VE \tag{3}$$

From variances,

$$VA = 2VF_2 - VBcs \tag{4}$$

The standard error of *VA* calculated by Eqn 4

$$\sqrt{2\left[\frac{4VF_2{}^2}{nF_2} + \frac{VBcH^2}{nBcH} + \frac{VBcL^2}{nBcL}\right]}$$

(in which *n* is the number of mice). Obviously, the VA value may be affected by a large sampling error.

There is another way of estimating VA, based on mean values rather than variances. Assuming that individual genes have an equivalent effect, then

$$\frac{VD}{VA} = \frac{1}{2}\left[\frac{d}{a}\right]^2 \tag{5}$$

The VA and VD values may therefore be calculated from VF_2 and VBcs according to Eqns 2 and 3 respectively. Knowing VA, it is possible to calculate the number of independent loci (n) controlling the quantitative character

$$n = \frac{a^2}{2VA} \tag{6}$$

The meaning of n calculated in this way is subject to several restrictions as stressed in classic references of quantitative genetics (Falconer, 1960; Cavalli-Sforza and Bodmer, 1971) and in our previous publications (Feingold *et al.*, 1976; Biozzi *et al.*, 1979a, b).

Selective breeding for antibody responsiveness in mice

Five different selections, referred to as selections I, II, III, IV and V, were carried out in mice up to the selection limit. The character selected for was maximal antibody response to an optimal dose of the various complex antigens used in the different selections. Except for selection II, 2 noncross-reacting antigens were alternated in consecutive generations in order to avoid the specific interference of maternal antibodies passively transmitted to the progeny. The antibody response was measured by direct or passive agglutination. In every population studied this character presented a normal frequency distribution when expressed as $\log_2$ of the highest doubling serum dilution giving a positive agglutination (agglutinin titre). All the results will therefore be given on that scale.

Results of selection

In selection I, initiated in 1965, the most thoroughly studied, the antigen used was sheep erythrocyte (SE) in the first 6 generations. Afterwards, SE and pigeon erythrocytes (PE) were alternated at each generation (Biozzi *et al.*, 1971).

All the generations of selection II were immunized with SE but the period

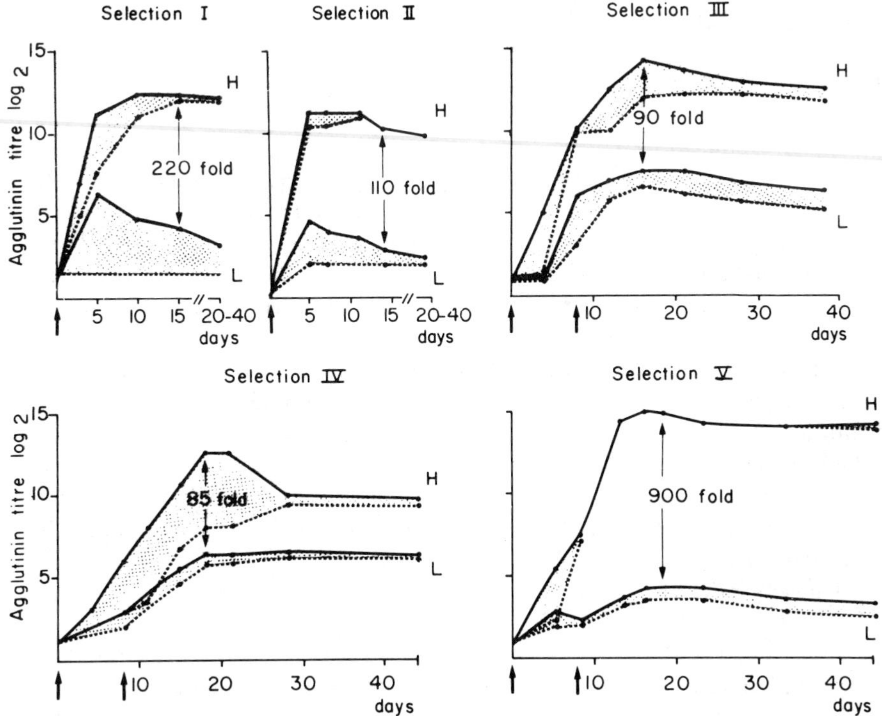

FIG. 2. *Kinetics of total (continuous line) and ME resistant (dotted line) agglutinin titres in H and L mice (at selection limit) of the 5 selections. Immunizations are those used for selective breeding (ags used for* F_0*). Arrows indicate injections of optimal doses of the various antigens: selections I and II,* 5×10^8 *SE i.v.; selections III and IV,* $3{\cdot}3 \times 10^8$ S. typhimurium *i.p.; selection V, 1 mg heat-aggregated BSA i.p. The interline difference is given at the time chosen for measuring the phenotypic character during the selective breeding and the responses in interline hybrids.*

between weaning and immunization was prolonged to eliminate the maternal antibodies (Biozzi *et al.*, 1979b).

Selections III and IV originated from a common foundation population and were carried out for responses to flagellar antigen, f ag. (selection III) or somatic antigen, s ag. (selection IV) of two noncross-reacting *Salmonellae: Salmonella typhimurium* (*S. typhimurium*) and *Salmonella oranienburg* (*S. oranienburg*), alternately (Siqueira *et al.*, 1976).

The antigens used for selection V were bovine serum albumin (BSA) and rabbit γ globulin (RGG) alternately (Passos *et al.*, 1977).

The immunization procedures and the time of agglutinin measurement chosen for phenotypic character in each selection are indicated in Fig. 2 which shows the kinetics of the agglutinin responses in H and L lines of the 5 selections.

In all the selections, the interline difference was very large during the whole response. It was calculated at the time chosen for estimating the phenotypic character. It is also obvious that the difference between H and L mice concerns both IgM and IgG antibody syntheses.

Comparison of the immunogenetic parameters in the five selections

Realized heritability (h^2)

Table I shows a remarkable similarity in the parameters of selections I, II, III and IV, in spite of the diverse origins of their F_0, the different natures of the antigens, and the various immunization procedures. The selection limit was attained after 13–16 generations. In selection V, only 7 generations were required to reach the selection limit. The h^2 value is the most important parameter since it results from 2 independent data: the mean and the variance of each population investigated. The identical value found in the 5 selections suggests that an heritability of about 20% is an immunogenetic constant of antibody responsiveness. The partition of VG and VE was nearly 50% in the F_0 populations except for selection V in which the genetic component was greater. These values underline the importance of the interaction of both genetic and environmental factors in the quantitative regulation of antibody responsiveness to all the antigens investigated.

Variance analysis and calculation of the number of independent loci

Table II shows the means and variances in large populations of homozygous H and L lines of the 5 selections at the selection limit, and in their interline hybrids. These data are used for the genetic analysis reported in Table III.

In the 5 selections the mean antibody response was slightly higher in females than in males (range 0·2–0·6). Because of this sex effect, the values reported in Table II were calculated as the average of the data obtained in each sex.

A maternal effect was observed in F_1 hybrids of some selections: the F_1 born from H line females made a higher response than those issued from L line females. This difference was due to maternal effect rather than to cytoplasmic inheritance since it was no longer observed in the subsequent generations (F_2).

TABLE I

Principal parameters of the 5 selective breedings for antibody responsiveness

Selection		Foundation[b] population	Selection differential per gen.	Response to selection		Selection limit	Heritability	Variance in foundation population	
No.	*Antigens*[a]	$\bar{x}$	*SG*	*Per gen. RG*	*Total RT*		h^2	*Total*	*Genetic* (%)
I	SE	9·7	2·5	0·48	7·8	F_{16}	0·20 ± 0·08	2·6	60
II	SE	10·1	2·2	0·43	6·7	F_{13}	0·21 ± 0·05	2·3	49
III	f ag. *S. typhimurium*	10·3	2·0	0·40	6·3	F_{16}	0·20 ± 0·04	1·5	51
IV	s. ag. *S. typhimurium*	6·4	2·4	0·49	6·5	F_{13}	0·21 ± 0·06	2·0	47
V	BSA	6·1	4·7	1·40	9·8	F_7	0·22 ± 0·06	15·2	76

[a] Antigens used for immunization of foundation populations and for calculations of immune parameters. (For immunization schedules and time of antibody measurement, see Fig. 2).

[b] The foundation population is different for each selection (except for selections III and IV) and composed of 50–75 outbred albino mice.

TABLE II

Antibody responses in H, L and interline hybrids of the 5 selections

	Agglutinin titres after immunization with selection antigens[a]														
	Selection I			*Selection II*			*Selection III*			*Selection IV*			*Selection V*		
	No. of mice	$\bar{x}$	*V*	*No. of mice*	$\bar{x}$	*V*	*No. of mice*	$\bar{x}$	*V*	*No. of mice*	$\bar{x}$	*V*	*No. of mice*	$\bar{x}$	*V*
H	472	12·5	0·7	466	11·6	1·0	128	12·8	0·5	198	11·4	1·1	293	14·2	3·8
L	497	4·7	1·3	455	4·9	1·5	93	6·5	0·6	207	4·9	1·5	269	4·4	4·3
F_1	211	9·6	1·6	88	10·1	1·5	86	10·1	0·4	73	8·6	0·9	52	7·4	7·8
F_2	363	8·6	2·0	171	9·5	4·2	88	10·7	1·4	63	7·9	3·0	195	6·0	10·0
BcH	166	11·4	1·0	88	10·3	1·8	69	11·7	0·8	46	10·8	2·6	72	13·0	4·2
BcL	168	7·6	2·3	146	7·5	5·9	84	8·9	0·9	69	6·0	2·1	68	5·2	10·2

[a] The antigens used for F_0 immunization. For immunization schedules and time of antibody measurement, see Fig. 2.

TABLE III

Interline hybrids analysis in the 5 selections[a]

Selection	Additive effect a	Global dominance d/a	VE (Eqn 1)	$VG\ F_2$ % of total variance	$VG\ F_2$ VA (Eqn 2)	$VG\ F_2$ VD (Eqn 2)	$VG\ Bcs$ VA (Eqn 3)	$VG\ Bcs$ VD (Eqn 3)	$VA \pm s.e.$ (Eqn 4)	Number of loci (Eqn 6)
I	3·9	0·26	1·2 ± 0·4	40	0·77	0·03	0·84	0·03	0·7 ± 0·4	9–11
II	3·35	0·55	1·3 ± 0·3	69	2·52	0·38	3·92	0·59	0·7 ± 1·0	2–8
III	3·15	0·14	0·5 ± 0·1	64	0·89	0·009	0·69	0·007	1·1 ± 0·4	4–7
IV	3·25	0·14	1·2 ± 0·3	60	1·78	0·018	2·25	0·02	1·3 ± 1·0	2–4
V	4·95	−0·39	5·3 ± 2·2	47	4·37	0.33	3·30	0·25	5·6 ± 2·7	2–4

[a] Calculated from results of Table II.

The maternal effect was variable. It was absent in selection III, rather small in selections I and IV (0·35 and 0·7 respectively) and quite strong in selection V (3·4). On account of the maternal effect, the data of F_1 hybrids reported in Table II were calculated as the average of the 2 reciprocal crosses. The results in Table III show that the additive effect (a) is roughly similar in the 5 selections. In contrast, the dominance deviation (d) differs. The dominance effect measured by the ratio d/a indicates that the high response character is incompletely dominant in selections I, II, III and IV whereas it is incompletely recessive in selection V.

The estimates of VF_2 and of its genetic component (Table III) are somewhat different from those obtained for the F_0 populations (Table I). This difference is due to the different ways of estimating VE: from Eqn 1 (Table III), or from the values in H and L lines only (Table I). Moreover, in F_2 hybrids, there is an equivalent frequency distribution of all the relevant alleles whereas the allele frequency distribution in the F_0 population is unknown. The contribution of the dominance variance (VD) to the total VF_2 is negligible is selections I, III, and IV, and quite small in selections II and V, about 12% and 5% respectively.

The most important variance component is the additive variance (VA) since it is used for the calculation of the number of loci (n). VA, according to Eqn 5 can be estimated from 2 different experimental data, VF_2 (Eqn 2) and VBcs (Eqn 3). Equation 4 gives another estimate of VA calculated directly from variances. When the 3 estimates are fairly concordant, the VA value may be considered as reasonably reliable. In view of the large standard error in Eqn 4, we may consider that the results of the three VA estimations are in agreement, except for selection II. Consequently, the number of independent loci controlling antibody responsiveness was estimated with a fairly good accuracy in selections I, III, IV and V. In selection II, the calculation of n was much less satisfactory (range 2–8). For reasons discussed elsewhere (Biozzi *et al.*, 1979b) the most probable value is closer to 8 than to 2.

The number of independent loci involved in the quantitative regulation of antibody responsiveness may differ in the 5 selections because of the different natures of the antigens used and of the various immunization procedures (primary response in selections I and II, and secondary response in the other 3 selections). The n values calculated from the variances obtained in interline hybrids (Table III) are somewhat smaller than those calculated from the VA of the F_0 population (estimated as the inheritable fraction of VF_0: $VA = h^2 \times VF_0$) (Biozzi *et al.*, 1979a).

Linkage with H-2 *locus*

The calculation of n (Table III) postulates that the loci are completely independent from each other and may be occupied by only "high" or "low" alleles endowed with equivalent effects. As a consequence, only one out of the loci regulating antibody responsiveness in each selection can be linked with the *H-2* locus and its quantitative effect should be $\frac{RT}{n}$.

So far the *H-2* linkage was investigated for SE in selection I and for the two selection antigens in selections III, IV and V. The determination of H-2 phenotypes was carried out using alloimmune sera raised against lymphoid cells from H or L mice. These immune sera were cytotoxic in presence of C′, for lymphoid cells isolated from every mouse of the immunizing line, and never cytotoxic for the cells of the other line mice. This cytotoxicity was essentially due to alloantibody directed against the *H-2* locus. In fact, the distribution of homozygous H/H, L/L and H/L phenotypes in large populations of F_2 hybrids is close to a monolocus Mendelian distribution. The alloimmune sera may detect the *H-2* locus corresponding to the H or L line in populations carrying a single or several H-2 serotypes. In selection I, a single phenotype has been found in each line and was recently identified (Colombani *et al.*, 1979).

The mean responses obtained in F_2 hybrids homozygous for either H or L H-2 phenotypes are shown in Table IV. In selection I, one of the genes regulating antibody responsiveness to SE was *H-2* linked. Its quantitative effect was equal to 14% of the total range of interline difference. A similar *H-2* linkage was found in selection V for both antigens, BSA and RGG. In selection IV the *H-2* linkage was significant only for the response to s ag. of *S. typhimurium*. No participation of *H-2* linked genes was observed in selection III.

Another linkage was demonstrated in selection I. The H and L lines have different immunoglobulin allotypes. In F_2 hybrids, the mice homozygous for H Ig allotype gave a mean agglutinin response to SE higher than those homozygous for L Ig allotype (difference: 0·95, $P < 0{\cdot}001$) (Lieberman *et al.*, 1972). The allotype linked gene contribution accounted for 12% of the total range of interline separation. The demonstration, in selection I, that *H-2* linked and *Ig* allotype linked genes contribute each about 10% of RT in a 10 loci model (Table III), constitutes a sound experimental support of the method of n calculation according to Eqn 6 which postulates that each locus has an equivalent effect. A similar consistency in the quantitative effect of the *H-2* linked gene, with n value according to the RT/n ratio, was also demonstrated in selection IV for the response to s ag. of *S. typhimurium* (*H-2* effect = 26%), and in selection V for the response to BSA (*H-2* effect = 26%). In contrast the effect of the *H-2* linked gene for the response to RGG was markedly smaller.

Nonspecific effect of the selections

In each selection, the difference between H and L lines was not restricted to antibody responses to selection antigens but was also observed for responses to unrelated antigens (nonspecific effect).

Many examples of the nonspecific effect of the selections have been reported, including responsiveness to antigens of very different natures (heterologous erythrocytes, bacteria, viruses, alloantigens, proteins, haptens) (Biozzi *et al.*,

TABLE IV

Participation of H-2 linked genes in the regulation of antibody responsiveness

Selection		Responses in F_2 hybrids homozygous				H-2 effect		
		H-2 phenotypes of H		H-2 phenotypes of L		Difference		
No.	Antigen [a]	No. of mice	$\bar{x} \pm s.d.$ (1)	No. of mice	$\bar{x} \pm s.d.$ (2)	(2) − (1)	(p)	% of RT
I [b]	SE	38	10·1 ± 1·3	51	9·0 ± 1·3	1·1	($\ll$0·001)	14
III	f ag. *S. typhimurium*	35	10·7 ± 1·1	19	10·3 ± 1·4	0·4	(n.s.)	—
	f. ag. *S. oranienburg*	26	10·5 ± 1·6	17	10·3 ± 0·9	0·2	(n.s.)	—
IV	s ag. *S. typhimurium*	14	9·0 ± 1·7	14	7·3 ± 1·7	1·7	(0·001)	26
	s ag. *S. oranienburg*	26	8·7 ± 1·8	13	8·5 ± 2·1	0·2	(n.s.)	—
V	BSA	49	7·8 ± 3·4	55	5·2 ± 2·1	2·6	($\ll$0·001)	26
	RGG	49	12·1 ± 1·7	58	11·2 ± 3·1	0·9	(0·05)	11

[a] For immunization schedules and time of antibody measurement, see Fig. 2.

[b] In selection I a part of the results are obtained in F_3 mice bred from F_2 homozygous for either H or L H-2 phenotypes (see Mouton *et al.*, 1979).

1979a). However the nonspecific effect of the selective breeding, though very large, cannot be considered as a general phenomenon since a few exceptions were observed in each selection. The few antigens giving equivalent antibody responses in H and L lines are: Dextran and Levan in selection I (Howard *et al.*, 1974); pigeon erythrocytes in selection III, sheep and human erythrocytes in selection IV; and s ag. of *S. typhimurium* in selection V (Biozzi *et al.*, 1979a).

The magnitude of the nonspecific effect depends on the nature of the immunogen and the immunization procedure. The nonspecific effect in selection I is probably due to modifications in macrophage activity. The phagocytic activity was similar in the 2 lines but the rate of intracellular catabolism of the phagocytized antigen was much higher in L responder than in H responder mice. Four days after an i.v. immunization with an optimal dose of SE, the antigen was no longer detectable in the spleen of L line whereas it persisted in immunogenic form for 14 days in H line spleen macrophages (Biozzi *et al.*, 1975). The difference in the persistence of the immunogen in H and L line macrophages is probably the principal phenomenon responsible for the nonspecific effect. In fact Levan and Dextran, which induced a similar response in both lines, were metabolized in the same way in H and L line macrophages (Howard *et al.*, 1974; Wiener and Bandieri, 1974).

The difference in antigen catabolism inside the macrophages of H and L mice explains the modification of the antibody responses to BSA according to the physical state of the antigen. When this antigen was injected in the form of molecular aggregates, the interline difference in antibody responses was as large as that observed for the selection antigen. When BSA was included in alum gel, the difference between H and L line antibody titres was smaller, particularly in the advanced phase of the response. The continuous BSA release from the site of antigen deposit delayed the antigen shortage due to the high rate of BSA catabolism in L line macrophages (Heumann and Stiffel, 1978).

Also related to the modification of antigen metabolism in macrophages is the difference in the threshold doses of antigen required for inducing detectable antibody responses. The threshold dose was markedly lower in H than in L line. This difference was about 100-fold for SE and hen egg albumin and 10 000-fold for BSA (Mouton *et al.*, 1980).

The minimal dose of BSA required for inducing immunological memory (secondary response) was also 100-fold lower in H than in L lines (Heumann and Stiffel, 1978).

Two examples of genetic analysis of the nonspecific effect are reported in Table V. They concern the antibody response to f ag. of *S. typhimurium* in selection I and to *Plasmodium berghei* (*P. berghei*) antigens in selection II.

Response to f. ag. of S. typhimurium (*Sant'Anna* et al., *1979*)

The interline difference in the peak agglutinin responses to f ag. of *S. typhimurium* was 5·9, i.e. 75% of the interline difference for selection antigen. The frequency distribution of the phenotypes in the L line was atypical, therefore the VF_1 was taken as the most probable estimate for VE. VA was 0·99

TABLE V

Genetic analysis of antibody responses to antigens unrelated with selection antigens

	Selection I—response to f ag. S. typhimurium [a]			*Selection II—response to* P. berghei *antigens* [b]		
	No. of mice	$\bar{x}$	*V*	*No. of mice*	$\bar{x}$	*V*
H	32	10·42	1·16	10	5·9	0·52
L	34	4·52	2·08	12	2·9	0·46
F_1	38	9·56	0·89	27	5·4	0·46
F_2	65	8·60	1·79	—	—	—
BcH	40	10·42	0·63	29	4·3	0·30
BcL	40	7·57	1·96	38	3·8	1·20

[a] Agglutinin titres 13 days after i.p. injection of $3{\cdot}3 \times 10^8$ *S. typhimurium*.
[b] Antibody titres measured by indirect immunofluorescence assay 7 days after 6 weekly i.p. injections of 3×10^7 irradiated parasitized erythrocytes.

from Eqn 4 and 0·54 or 0·72 when calculated according to Eqn 5, from VBcs or VF_2 respectively. From their mean value we can estimate, according to Eqn 6 that about 6 (range 4–8) independent loci regulate the antibody responsiveness to f ag. of *S. typhimurium* in selection I. A possible interpretation of these findings is that among the 10 loci regulating responsiveness to SE, 6 operate also nonspecifically in the responsiveness to f ag. of *S. typhimurium*. It is worth mentioning that the quantitative responsiveness to f ag. of *S. typhimurium* in selection III is also regulated by about 6 independent loci (Table III).

Response to P. berghei *antigens* (*Heumann* et al., *1979*)
The comparison of the interline differences in responsiveness to *P. berghei* (Table V) and to the selection antigen indicates a non specific effect of 45%. According to Eqn 1, VE is 0·48. VA, calculated according to Eqn 5 from VBcs, is 0·37, which gives an n value equal to 3. We may therefore hypothesize that 3 genes among those which regulate antibody responsiveness to SE in selection II operate also for the control of *P. berghei* antibody synthesis.

Effect of the selection for antibody responsiveness on the other immunologic functions

The impact of the genetic differences between H and L lines on immunological responses other than antibody production is so far only known in selection I.

The results indicate similar potentialities in H and L mice for several T mediated reactions: skin graft rejection, graft versus host reaction, delayed type hypersensitivity and responses to the mitogenic effect of PHA (Biozzi *et al.*, 1975).

These data demonstrate the independence of the genetic control of humoral and cellular immunity, the implications of which have been discussed in the introduction.

Selective breeding for antibody responsiveness in guinea-pigs

This experiment is still incomplete since the results of 8 generations only are available. The model of selective breeding is similar to that used for selection I in mice. The antigens used were SE and chicken erythrocytes (CE) alternated at each generation (Ibanez *et al.*, 1980). The continuous normal frequency distribution of the phenotypes in the F_0 population and the progressive divergence of H and L lines indicate that the character is subject to polygenic regulation.

The constant increase of the cumulated R until F_8 means that the selection limit is not yet attained. The mean heritability of the character realized in the 8 generations is $0{\cdot}18 \pm 0{\cdot}04$, which is very similar to that observed in mice. The selective breeding will be continued until the selection limit. According to the data available, we provisionally estimate that the additive variance of the F_0 population is 0·41. Considering the RT at the 8th generation, we may calculate from Eqn 6 that about 3 independent loci are responsible for the interline difference at the present time. A similar estimate was obtained after 8 generations of selective breeding in mice (selection I).

In the guinea-pig selection, the nonspecific effect operated for the 3 unrelated antigens tested so far: f and s ags of *S. typhimurium* and human erythrocytes.

The remarkable similarity of the results obtained in mice and in guinea-pigs, particularly concerning the heritability value, suggests that the immunogenetic parameters defined by the method of bidirectional selective breeding may have a general significance.

Selective breeding for responsiveness of lymphocytes to phytohaemagglutinin (PHA)

The various tests for *in vivo* T cell mediated response are not quantitatively reliable enough to make sure that a genetic selection experiment can be successful. The *in vitro* blastogenic effect of PHA on T lymphocytes is a quantitative test for measuring the potentiality of these cells. The phenotypic character chosen for the selective breeding was therefore "quantitative response of lymph node cells to an optimal dose of PHA" measured by [^{3}H]-thymidine uptake after 2 days' culture *in vitro*. The results are expressed as the difference in counts per minute (ct/mt $\times$ 10^{-3}) between experimental and control cultures (Stiffel *et al.*, 1977). Since no sex effect was noticed, the means and the standard deviations were calculated from pooled data of both sexes.

Results of selection

The response to PHA in the F_0 constituted by 125 mice was 37 ± 12·8. The separation between the 2 lines was progressive and the selection limit was reached after 10 generations. The mean response was then 80·2 ± 28·4 in the H line (Hi/PHA), and 2·5 ± 3·8 in the L line (Lo/PHA), i.e. a 31-fold interline difference. The mean realized heritability was 0·24 ± 0·06. From the VA estimated in the F_0, the number of independent loci calculated from Eqn 6 was 19. The selective breeding had a clear asymmetrical effect. The response of Hi/PHA mice was twice that of F_0 whereas that of Lo/PHA mice was decreased by 15-fold. It should be noticed that in the 2 lines, the standard deviation is correlated with the mean level of the response. This correlation may be inherent in the method used for measuring the character investigated. However, the frequency distribution of individual phenotypes was normal in each population. This scale of measurements was therefore used for the genetic analysis.

TABLE VI

PHA responses in Hi/PHA, Lo/PHA and interline hybrids

	No. of mice	$[^3H]$-*thymidine uptake* $(ct/min \times 10^{-3})$[a] $\bar{x}$	*V*	
Hi/PHA	216	80·2	806·0	
Lo/PHA	215	2·5	14·4	VE = 420·5 (Eqn 1)
F_1	32	27·2	441·0	
BcH	27	39·5	767·0	VA = 71·7
				VD = 5·1
BcL	27	9·8	164·0	(Eqns 3 and 5)
	a = 38·8	d = −14·15		$\frac{d}{a} = -0{\cdot}36$

[a] Two days' culture of 4 × 10^5 lymph node cells in RPMI 1640 medium.

The results obtained in interline hybrids are reported in Table VI. The character "low responsiveness" was incompletely dominant in F_1 (36%).

From the estimates of the variance components indicated in that table, the number of loci calculated from Eqn 6 is 10. This figure is smaller than that reported above. A similar difference between the estimates of n, obtained from VA in F_0 and in interline hybrids, has been mentioned before in the results of the selections for antibody responsiveness. We may then hypothesize that responsiveness of lymph node cells to PHA is regulated by a number of independent loci between 10 and 19.

The selection was carried out for PHA responsiveness of lymph node cells. The interline difference was somewhat lower (5-fold) at the level of spleen cells. The responses of lymph node cells and spleen cells to another T mitogen, Concanavalin A, were similar to those obtained with PHA (Stiffel *et al.*, 1977, 1979). The tuberculin purified protein (PPD), a B mitogen, induced an equivalent proliferation of the spleen cells from the 2 lines. A small inter-line difference (2·5-fold) was observed when the spleen cells were stimulated by another B mitogen: *Escherichia coli* lipopolysaccharide (LPS). However, this is probably due to the activity of a subpopulation of T cells which influences the proliferation of B cells induced by LPS. These results demonstrate that T and B lymphocyte potentialities are subject to different genetic regulations.

Effect of the selection on immunological functions

The *in vitro* response of lymphocytes to mitogens is a rather artificial laboratory test. Nevertheless, it concerns an important cellular potentiality since Hi/PHA and Lo/PHA lines present a clear-cut difference in an *in vitro* test of immunological nature: the mixed lymphocyte reaction, and also differ for *in vivo* immunological phenomena such as graft versus host reaction and antibody responsiveness.

Mixed lymphocyte reaction (MLR)

The unidirectional MLR of Hi/PHA and Lo/PHA lymph node cells was investigated using irradiated lymphoid cells of 4 different inbred strains of mice as stimulator cells (Liacopoulos-Briot *et al.*, 1979).

The results show that the different allospecificites carried by the stimulator

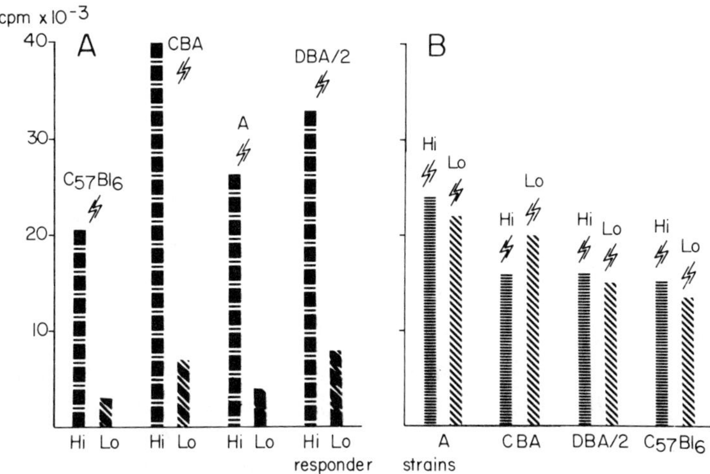

FIG. 3. *Mixed lymphocyte reaction. (A) [^3H]-thymidine uptake by Hi/PHA and Lo/PHA lymph node cells stimulated by irradiated spleen cells of 4 inbred strains of mice. (B) [^3H]-thymidine uptake by lymph node cells of the inbred strains of mice stimulated by irradiated spleen cells of Hi/PHA or Lo/PHA mice. (4 × 10^5 stimulator and 4 × 10^5 responder cells are cultivated for 3 days in RPMI 1640 medium supplemented with foetal calf serum (10%) and 2-ME (5 × 10^{-5}M). (From Liacopoulos-Briot* et al., *1979,* Cell Immunol. **44**, *29, by courtesy of Academic Press.)*

cells produced a markedly higher MLR in Hi/PHA than in Lo/PHA cells ($P < 0{\cdot}001$) (Fig. 3A). In contrast, a similar response was induced in the 4 inbred strains by the cells of the 2 selection lines, which indicates that the alloantigenicity of these cells was not modified by the selective breeding (Fig. 3B). These results show that the same group of genes regulates the intensity of T lymphocyte responsiveness to both PHA and alloantigens. The genes involved in this regulation are not implicated in the control of the expression of Ia antigens on lymphocytes.

Graft versus host reactivity (GVH)

The intensity of *in vivo* GVH reaction was measured by the proliferation of intravenously injected parental lymph node cells in the spleens of lethally irradiated F_1 hybrids. The results obtained in F_1 hybrids between Hi/PHA or Lo/PHA and CBA or DBA/2 strains are reported in Table VII.

The proliferative response of Hi/PHA lymphocytes is higher than that of Lo/PHA lymphocytes when stimulated by either CBA or DBA/2 alloantigens. On the contrary, Hi/PHA and Lo/PHA alloantigens produce a similar stimulation of CBA and DBA/2 lymph node cell proliferation. These results indicate that the same group of genes controlling the *in vitro* responsiveness to PHA also regulates the potentiality of T lymphocytes to mount a GVH reaction *in vivo* (Mouton *et al.*, 1980).

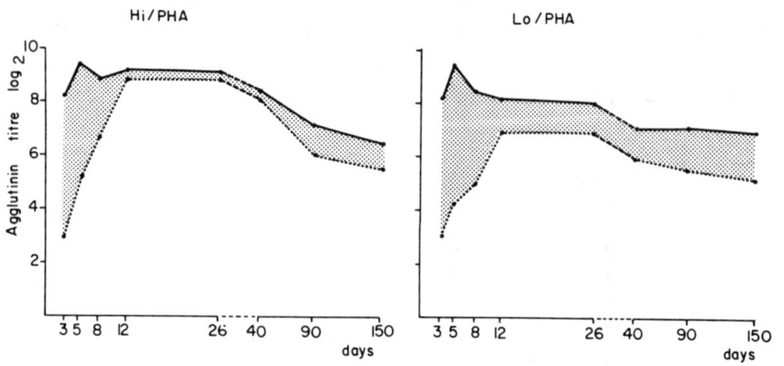

FIG. 4. *Kinetics of total (continuous line) and ME resistant (dotted line) agglutinin titres in Hi/PHA and Lo/PHA mice immunized with 2×10^8 SE i.v.*

Antibody response to a T-dependent antigen: SE

The kinetics of agglutinin response of Hi/PHA and Lo/PHA lines to an optimal immunization with SE show that only ME resistant antibodies are produced in Hi/PHA mice after the 12th day whereas an important synthesis of ME sensitive antibodies persists until the 150th day in Lo/PHA mice (Fig. 4). A possible explanation for these results is that the genes regulating T lymphocyte responsiveness to PHA may also control the activity of a T helper cell population involved in the switch between IgM and IgG antibody synthesis (Mouton *et al.*, 1980). The difference between Hi/PHA and Lo/PHA mice in the total antibody responses to SE is very small (2-fold) compared with the interline

TABLE VII

Induction of graft v. host reaction by Hi/PHA and Lo/PHA cells

Cell donors	Spleen incorporation[a] of $[^3H]$-thymidine ct/min $\times 10^{-3} \pm$ s.d.) in irradiated recipients[b]				
	$(Hi/PHA \times CBA)F_1$	$(Lo/PHA \times CBA)F_1$	p	$(Hi/PHA \times DBA/2)F_1$	$(Lo/PHA \times DBA/2)F_1$	p
Hi/PHA	235 ± 94 (22)[c]		} < 0.001	406 ± 153 (15)		} < 0.001
Lo/PHA		89 ± 58 (27)			116 ± 54 (15)	
CBA	213 ± 92 (12)	175 ± 75 (11)	n.s.			
DBA/2				385 ± 135 (9)	311 ± 120 (9)	n.s.

[a] Measured 4 days after i.v. injection of 5×10^6 lymph node cells.
[b] 900 rads on day −1.
[c] Number of mice.

difference observed in selection I carried out for responsiveness to this antigen (120-fold) (Fig. 2).

The independence of the genetic control of PHA responsiveness and of antibody production is therefore verified in both selective breedings, since, as mentioned before, PHA responsiveness is equivalent in the 2 lines of selection I.

Genetic regulation of the phagocytic activity of the reticulo-endothelial system (RES) macrophages

RES macrophages play an important role in various biological functions such as: immunoresponsiveness, nonspecific defence against infections and tumours, interferon production, lipid and iron metabolism, etc.

Macrophages are characterized by 2 distinct functions: powerful phagocytic activity and metabolism of the phagocytized material (bactericidal effect on living micro-organisms). These functions are subject to separate genetic regulation. It has been mentioned before that the selective breeding for antibody responsiveness (selection I) greatly modifies the rate of antigen metabolism in macrophages without altering their phagocytic activity.

The genetic study was carried out for phagocytic activity measured by the rate of blood clearance of colloidal carbon particles injected i.v. More than 95% of these injected particles are phagocytized by liver and spleen macrophages in contact with the circulating blood. The phagocytic activity is expressed by the phagocytic index K (Biozzi *et al*, 1953; Stiffel *et al.*, 1970a).

The comparison of the phagocytic index K in 10 inbred strains of mice shows that the intrastrain variability produced by environmental effects (30%) is smaller than the mean interstrain variability (87%). This function is therefore subject to genetic regulation. However, the interline differences are relatively small, which suggests that the basic phagocytic activity is a physiological homeostatic constant (Mouton *et al.*, 1976). Therefore no attempt was made to modify this basic activity by selective breeding.

The phagocytic activity of RES macrophages can be markedly stimulated in different ways.

The injection of a glyceryl trioleate (triolein) emulsion only stimulates the phagocytic activity without modifying the other functions in which the macrophages participate (antibody responsiveness and resistance to experimental infections).

The stimulation of RES macrophages by bacteria such as *Mycobacterium tuberculosis*, BCG strain (BCG) or *Corynebacterium parvum* (*C. parvum*), or bacterial products, had a more complex effect related to immunological phenomena: adjuvant effect on antibody responsiveness; induction of cell mediated immunity; and modification of the resistance to various experimental infections and tumours (reviewed in Stiffel *et al.*, 1970a).

The genetic regulation of the stimulation of the macrophage phagocytic activity produced by triolein and by BCG was investigated by the method of genetic selection described above.

•elective breeding for macrophage responsiveness to triolein

The phenotypic character was the phagocytic index K measured 48 h after i.v. injection of triolein, when the stimulation of the macrophages was maximal. In the F_0 the K × 10^3 value was 50 in males and 93 in females. This was an increase of about 5-fold compared with the basic K value. In both sexes a normal frequency distribution of the phenotypes was obtained when the K values were expressed as natural logarithms (ln (K × 10^3)). The results are given as the average of means ($\bar{x}$) and variances (V) measured separately in males and females in order to eliminate the sex effect. The value for F_0 is then 4·06 ± 0·57.

The selective breeding produced a progressive divergence between a line with high K response to triolein (KTH) and a line with low K response to triolein (KTL). The selection limit was reached after 21 consecutive generations of selection.

The response to selection, with a mean RG value of 0·06 resulted in a RT of 2, corresponding to a 7-fold interline difference in terms of K values. The mean heritability was 0·09, which gives a VA estimate in F_0 equal to 0·03. According to this VA value the number of independent loci is 16.

The effect of the selective breeding was quite strong. The KTL mice were almost unresponsive to triolein whereas the macrophage stimulation of KTH mice was 3-fold higher than that of normal random-bred mice (Mouton *et al.*, 1975).

The results in the homozygous generations of KTH and KTL mice (F_{21}–F_{41}) and in interline hybrids are shown in Table VIII. The response

TABLE VIII
Response to triolein in KTH, KTL and interline hybrids

	No. of mice	*Phagocytic index K* (Ln (K × 10^3))[a]		
		$\bar{x}$	*V*	
KTH	727	5·0	0·19	VE = 0·25 (Eqn. 1)
KTL	712	3·0	0·17	
F_1	76	2·8	0·38	
F_2	83	3·3	0·42	VA = 0·1, VD = 0·07 (Eqn. 5)
BcH	77	4·3	0·67	VA = 0·19, VD = 0·13 (Eqn. 5)
BcL	60	2·5	0·30	

$a = 1;\ d = -1{\cdot}2;\ \frac{d}{a} = -1{\cdot}2$

[a] Index K measured from the blood clearance of 8 mg/100 g of colloidal carbon 48 h after i.v. injection of 0·2 ml/20 g of a 10% triolein emulsion.

of F_1 hybrids shows a complete dominance or even a slight overdominance of the "low character" ($d/a = -1{\cdot}2$). Considering the VE value, the largest part of VF_2 (60%) is produced by environmental effects. The two VA evaluations obtained by Eqn 5 from VF_2 and VBcs would give, according to Eqn 6, an estimate of 3–5 independent loci. This is probably an underestimation of n, due to sampling errors, which also prevents the use of Eqn 4 to calculate VA.

As mentioned above, the effect of triolein is restricted to the stimulation of the phagocytic activity without modification of other macrophage functions. In fact the resistance to *Salmonella* infection is similar in both KTH and KTL lines infected, when stimulated by triolein.

The antibody response to SE was studied in KTH and KTL mice treated with triolein. It was only slightly higher in the KTH line (Mouton *et al.*, 1976). This confirms the independence of the phagocytic and metabolic activities of the macrophages, already demonstrated by the results of selection I.

Selective breeding for macrophage responsiveness to BCG

BCG and *C. parvum* are among the most powerful stimulants of the RES macrophages. Their effect on the phagocytic activity in random-bred mice and in inbred lines depends on the interaction of both genetic and environmental factors (Stiffel *et al.*, 1970b).

A bidirectional selective breeding was attempted for stimulation of the phagocytic activity by BCG. Two i.v. injections of heat-killed BCG (300 μg/mouse) were given 3 days apart. The phagocytic index K was measured 3 and 8 days later, during the period of the plateau response, and was expressed, as above, as ln ($K \times 10^3$).

The BCG treatment increased the K value by about 5-fold. In the F_0, K was $4{\cdot}8 \pm 0{\cdot}5$. A small sex effect in favour of female responsiveness was observed. Therefore the means ($\bar{x}$) and variances (V) were expressed as the average of the values obtained in both sexes.

Figure 5A shows the mean K values in 8 generations of the 2 lines referred to as K.BCG.H and K.BCG.L lines. A significant interline difference was observed in F_3 and persisted in all the successive generations but in this selection, unexpectedly, a strong and progressive depression of the macrophage responsiveness to BCG occurred in both lines. In the F_8 this depression, compared with the F_0 response, was about 70% in the K.BCG.H line and more than 80% in the K.BCG.L line. In fact, the F_8 K.BCG.L mice were completely unresponsive to BCG stimulation.

An attempt at genetic analysis of interline divergence is represented in Fig. 5B. The selection limit was reached after 3 generations with a mean realized heritability of 0·37. The RT was quite small: 0·51. It represents only about 25% of the macrophage stimulation produced by BCG in the F_0. Therefore the genetic effect was limited. The low value of the additive variance of the F_0 suggests that alleles at a single locus are affected by selective breeding.

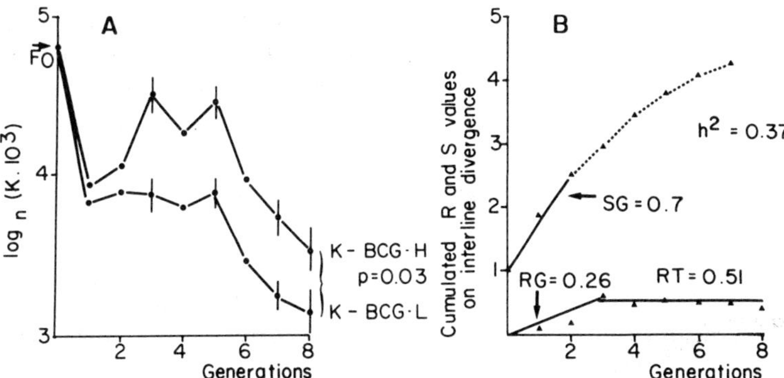

FIG. 5. *Selective breeding of mice for responsiveness to BCG stimulation. (A) Means of K values in 8 generations of K.BCG.H and K.BCG.L lines (± s.e.). (B) Cumulated values of R and S on interline divergence.*

The reason for the marked and progressive decrease of responsiveness to BCG affecting both lines throughout the selective breeding (Fig. 5A) is unknown. It may be a special sensitivity to the inbreeding depression resulting from the close colony reproduction in each line. A progressive rise of the inbreeding coefficient occurred even in the absence of brother–sister mating. This hypothesis is substantiated by the finding that the stimulation of the macrophage phagocytosis produced by BCG is higher in outbred mice than in inbred lines, some of which are very poorly responsive (Stiffel *et al.*, 1970b).

Another explanation for the depression observed in Fig. 5A may be that the repeated administration of BCG in consecutive generations resulted in the transmission of some maternal factors (antibodies ?) which interfered with the progeny's responses to BCG. Nevertheless, the depression is not restricted to the BCG induced stimulation since the phagocytic index K in the F_8 mice of both lines measured after the administration of *C. parvum* was also 4-fold lower than in random-bred mice. The peak K values after an i.v. injection of 500 μg of heat-killed *C. parvum* were 3·93 ± 0·4 in K.BCG.H line and 3·47 ± 0·4 in K.BCG.L line. The interline difference in the response to *C. parvum* was 0·46 ($p < 0{\cdot}01$), which is similar to that observed for BCG responsiveness, RT = 0.51 ± 0·008. If the depression effect is due to the passive transmission of maternal antibody to the progeny, then the antigenic substance responsible for macrophage stimulation would be the same in BCG and in *C. parvum*. Because of the depression in responsiveness to BCG, the selective breeding was interrupted at the F_8 generation.

Conclusion

The results presented demonstrate that the principal immunologic functions are subjected to independent polygenic regulation. The intensity of the response of each function can be drastically modified by bidirectional selective breeding. High and Low responder lines of animals homozygous for all the loci regulating each immunological function can be obtained. These lines are of paramount importance for the study of the genetic regulation of immunoresponsiveness and its role on the efficacy of anti-infectious immunity.

References

Biozzi, G., Benacerraf, B. and Halpern, B. N. (1953). *Br. J. Exp. Pathol.* **34**, 441.

Biozzi, G., Stiffel, C., Mouton, D., Bouthillier, Y. and Decreusefond, C. (1971). *In* "Progress in Immunology" (B. Amos, ed.) Vol. 1, pp. 529–545. Academic Press, New York.

Biozzi, G., Stiffel, C., Mouton, D. and Bouthillier, Y. (1975). *In* "Immunogenetics and Immunodeficiency" (B. Benacerraf, ed.) pp. 179–227. MTP Publishing Co, Lancaster.

Biozzi, G., Mouton, D., Sant'Anna, O. A., Passos, H. C., Gennari, M., Reis, M. H., Ferreira, V. C. A., Heumann, A. M., Bouthillier, Y., Ibanez, O. M., Stiffel, C. and Siqueira, M. (1979a). *Current Topics Microbiol. Immunol.* **85**, 31.

Biozzi, G., Mouton, D., Heumann, A. M., Bouthillier, Y., Stiffel, C. and Mevel, J. C. (1979b). *Immunology* **36**, 427.

Cavalli-Sforza, L. L. and Bodmer, W. F. (1971). "The Genetics of Human Populations". Freeman, San Francisco.

Colombani, M., Pla, M., Mouton, D. and Degos, L. (1979). *Immunogenetics* **8**, 237.

Falconer, D. S. (1960). "Introduction to Quantitative Genetics". Ronald Press, New York.

Feingold, N., Feingold, J., Mouton, D., Bouthillier, Y., Stiffel, C. and Biozzi, G. (1976). *Eur. J. Immunol.* **6**, 43.

Heumann, A. M. et Stiffel, C. (1978). *Ann. d'Immunol.* (*Inst. Pasteur*) **129C**, 13.

Heumann, A. M., Stiffel, C., Monjour, L., Bucci, A. and Biozzi, G. (1979). *Infect. Immun.* **24**, 829.

Howard, J. G., Courtenay, B. M. and Desaymard, C. (1974). *Eur. J. Immunol.* **4**, 453.

Ibanez, O. M., Reis, M. H., Gennari, M., Ferreira, V. C. A., Sant'Anna, O. A., Siqueira, M. and Biozzi, G. (1980). *Immunogenetics* **10**, 283.

Liacopoulos-Briot, M., Stiffel, C., Lambert, F. and Decreusefond, C. (1979). *Cellular Immunol.* **44**, 29.

Lieberman, R., Stiffel, C., Asofsky, R., Mouton, D., Biozzi, G. and Benacerraf, B. (1972) *J. Exp. Med.* **136**, 790.

Mouton, D., Bouthillier, Y., Feingold, N., Feingold, J., Decreusefond, C., Stiffel, C. and Biozzi, G. (1975). *J. Exp. Med.* **141**, 306.

Mouton, D., Bouthillier, Y., Heumann, A. M., Stiffel, C. and Biozzi, G. (1976). *In* "The RES System in Health and Disease: Functions and Characteristics" (S. M. Reichard, M. R. Escobar and H. Friedman, eds) pp. 225–236. Plenum, New York.

Mouton, D., Heumann, A. M., Bouthillier, Y., Mevel, J. C. and Biozzi, G. (1979). *Immunogenetics* **8**, 475.

Mouton, D., Stiffel, C. and Biozzi, G. (1980). *In* "Immunologic Defects in Laboratory Animals" (M. E. Gershwin and B. Merchant, eds) Plenum, New York.

Passos, H. C., Siqueira, M., Reis, M. H., Ferreira, V. C. A., Ibanez, O. M., Sant'Anna, O. A. and Biozzi, G. (1977). *J. Immunol.* **119**, 1439.

Sant'Anna, O. A., Bouthillier, Y., Siqueira, M. and Biozzi, G. (1979). *Immunology* **37**, 849.

Siqueira, M., Bandieri, A., Reis, M. H., Sant'Anna, O. A. and Biozzi, G. (1976). *Eur. J. Immunol.* **6**, 241.

Stiffel, C., Mouton, D. and Biozzi, G. (1970a). *In* "Mononuclear Phagocytes" (R. Van Furth, ed.) pp. 335–381. Blackwell, Oxford.

Stiffel, C., Mouton, D., Bouthillier, Y., Decreusefond, C. and Biozzi, G. (1970b). *J. RES Soc.* **7**, 280.

Stiffel, C., Liacopoulos-Briot, M., Decreusefond, C. and Lambert, F. (1977). *Eur. J. Immunol.* **7**, 291.

Stiffel, C., Liacopoulos-Briot, M., Decreusefond, C. and Lambert, F. (1979). *Ann. d'Immunologie* (*Inst. Pasteur*) **130C**, 841.

Wiener, E. and Bandieri, A. (1974). *Eur. J. Immunol.* **4**, 457.

25

The Role of Macrophages in Genetic Control of the Immune Response

ALAN S. ROSENTHAL, JAMES W. THOMAS, JOYCE SCHROER and J. THOMAS BLAKE

*Department of Immunology,
Merck Sharp & Dohme Research Laboratories,
Rahway, New Jersey, USA*

Macrophage function in antigen-specific T cell proliferation

Macrophages facilitate a variety of thymus-dependent immunological phenomena in man and experimental animals and are thus essential for development of cellular and humoral immunocompetence (Fig. 1). They serve at least four distinct, but yet interlocking functions in host defence. First, the

We would like to thank Mrs Lorri Caffrey for her skilful preparation of this paper.

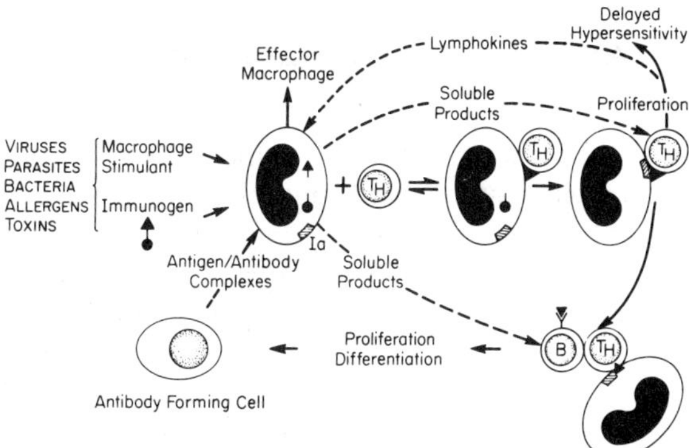

FIG. 1. *Macrophage regulation of immunity.*

induction of T lymphocyte proliferation requires their physical association with macrophages bearing antigen (Rosenthal *et al.*, 1978). Second, the macrophage is a principal site of immune response gene control (Rosenthal, 1978). Third, macrophages have a number of plasma membrane receptors, such as those for the Fc portion of immunoglobulin, which augment the killing and phagocytosis of infectious agents during secondary immune responses (Zuckerman and Douglas, 1979). Fourth, macrophages secrete a wide range of biologically active molecules which influence development of the afferent limb of the immune response as well as being directly responsible for many of the major clinical and pathological aspects of chronic allergic and inflammatory diseases (Davies and Bonney, 1979). This review will consider the role of the macrophage in antigen recognition by T lymphocytes as well as their function in immune response gene control.

Macrophages are required for *in vitro* induction in antigen-specific T cell proliferation as well as for mediator production by T lymphocytes. This is most easily seen in the lack of T cell proliferation in populations of lymphoid cells depleted of macrophages and by the restoration of proliferation by readdition of macrophage-rich adherent cells but not by lymphocytes, granulocytes, or fibroblasts (Rosenstreich and Rosenthal, 1974). While the precise molecular events are not defined it seems clear that recognition of soluble protein antigens by the T lymphocyte is usually proceeded by an initial uptake and processing of antigen by the macrophage (Waldron *et al.*, 1973). Macrophage function is not predicated upon or restricted by the immune state of the animal. Lastly, macrophages and lymphocytes must share genetic identity at some portion of the major histocompatibility complex (MHC) for successful detection of the antigenic signal borne by the macrophage (Rosenthal and Shevach, 1973).

The concepts presented in this brief report are principally derived from studies of inbred mice and strain 2 and 13 guinea-pigs. The general applicability of these biological observations in man are emerging (Bergholtz and Thorsky, 1977, 1978).

Antigen uptake by macrophages

It is important to develop an appreciation for the nature of the antigen uptake process and the physical state of macrophage-associated antigen (Table I). Uptake of protein antigens by macrophages is usually assessed in our laboratory both isotopically and by their capacity to activate primed T cell proliferation. Uptake occurs at 37°C via an initial binding step not requiring the expenditure of metabolic energy and is followed by a second temperature-dependent event (Waldron *et al.*, 1974). When this latter step is carried out in glucose-free medium, immunological activity, i.e. the ability to induce antigenic specific

TABLE I

Supernatants of peritoneal exudate cells enhance the response of immune T cell to DNP-OVA, but have little effect on response to GLT^{15}. Response of BALB/c lymphocytes primed in vivo *with 100 μg GLT^{15} and 10 μg DNP-OVA per mouse.*

Addition to culture	Antigen-specific lymphocyte proliferation DNP-OVA 200 μg/ml	GLT¹⁵ 200 μg/ml
	[a] ct/min ± s.e. ³H-TdR incorporation	
0	1·21 ± 0·3	0·04 ± 0·01
BALB PEC	31·92 ± 1·55	11·11 ± 2·84
B6 PEC	24·23 ± 4·31	0·24 ± 0·14
BALB supernatant	10·57 ± 1·19	0·03 ± 0·02
B6 supernatant	12·79 ± 5·17	0·10 ± 0·04

[a] mean ct/min ± s.e. for 3 experiments; ct/min is (Expt'l-Control) for each experiment. Naive mice are primed with antigen in CFA in the hind footpads and boosted with equivalent antigen in CFA 10–21 days later. 1–4 weeks after that, the popliteal and femoral lymph nodes are removed, teased, pressed through a 200 wire mesh screen and incubated on a nylon wool adherence column for 60 min. On elution, a T cell enriched, adherent cell depleted population of immune lymph node lymphocytes (LNL) is obtained. This population contains 90–95% T cells, 1–5% B cells, and 0·1–0·5% macrophages. The immune LNL are then incubated with or without antigen or reconstituting peritoneal exudate cells (PEC) (induced with sterile, mineral oil in non-immune donors) as a source of macrophage. Cultures are carried out in flat bottom microtitre plates with 2×10^5 LNL and 5×10^4 PEC per well in a volume of 200 μl of medium RPMI 1640 (Grand Island Biological Co., Grand Island, NY) supplemented with fresh L-glutamine (0·3 μg/ml), gentamicin (10 μg/ml), penicillin (200 units/ml), 2-mercaptoethanol ($2{\cdot}5 \times 10^{-5}$ M), 10 mM Hepes Buffer, and 7·5% foetal calf serum (FCS). The cultures were carried out at 37°C in humidified atmosphere of 5% CO_2 and 95% air for 96 h. 16–24 h prior to harvesting, 1 μCi of tritiated thymidine (6·7 Ci/mM, New England Nuclear Co., Boston, MA) was added per well. Tritiated thymidine incorporation was measured after harvesting by liquid scintillation spectrometry and results reported as mean ct/min ± s.e. of the mean for triplicate determinations or as ct/min (number of counts above control, e.g., Experimental (Ag)-Control (No Ag.)

proliferation, is reduced to the level seen when macrophages are exposed to antigen at either 4°C or at 37°C with sodium azide and 2-deoxyglucose, agents that inhibit aerobic and anaerobic metabolism respectively. It is of considerable interest that cytochalasin B, an agent which specifically disrupts contractile microfilament structure, does not affect uptake of immunologically relevant proteins.

Trypsinization of macrophages pulsed with antigen at 4°C (antigen restricted to the plasma membranes) removes most immunological activity without altering the ability of such macrophages to take up new antigens. If, however, trypsinization is progressively delayed by prior culture at 37°C, macrophages pulsed with antigens at 4°C become progressively resistant to the effects of trypsinization such that by 120 min the macrophage's immunological potential is not reduced. More surprisingly, antibody against antigens (as high as 0·5 mg/ml) does not affect the ability of antigen-pulsed macrophages to initiate T cell proliferation (Ellner and Rosenthal, 1975; Unanue *et al.*, 1969).

How do macrophages interact with lymphocytes?

Prior to proliferation, lymphocytes from an immune animal have been observed to cluster specifically around antigen-bearing macrophages (Lipsky and Rosenthal, 1973, 1975a). Instead, at least two types of physical interactions occur between macrophages and lymphocytes. The first is not dependent on the presence of antigen and is without immunologic commitment. This step requires active macrophage, but not lymphocyte, metabolism, divalent cations and a trypsin-sensitive macrophage site. This binding does not distinguish T or B lymphocytes and is reversible in such a way that, at any given time, binding represents an equilibrium between cellular association and dissociation (Lipsky and Rosenthal, 1973). When this step has brought specifically immune lymphocytes into apposition with antigen-bearing macrophages, a second type of binding results (Fig. 2). This latter phenomenon is dependent upon the presence of antigen and a sharing on lymphocyte and macrophage of histocompatability linked gene products. This association is not easily reversed and results in proliferation of the bound lymphocyte (Lipsky and Rosenthal, 1975a).

When viewed from the perspective of population dynamics, antigen-specific lymphocyte-macrophage interaction lasts longer (24–72 h) than that observed between T cells and macrophage in the absence of antigen (1–5 h) (Ben-Sasson *et al.*, 1978). In the mouse it is possible to demonstrate that macrophages serve a second critical immune function in expanding the clones of antigen-specific T cells. This latter influence does not depend on direct physical contact. Soluble "factors" factors produced by supernatants derived from guinea-pig peritoneal exudate cells can, under certain circumstances, replace intact macrophage in the lymph node lymphocyte assay (Rosenthal *et al.*, 1979; Rosenwasser and Rosenthal, 1978) for complex multideterminant soluble

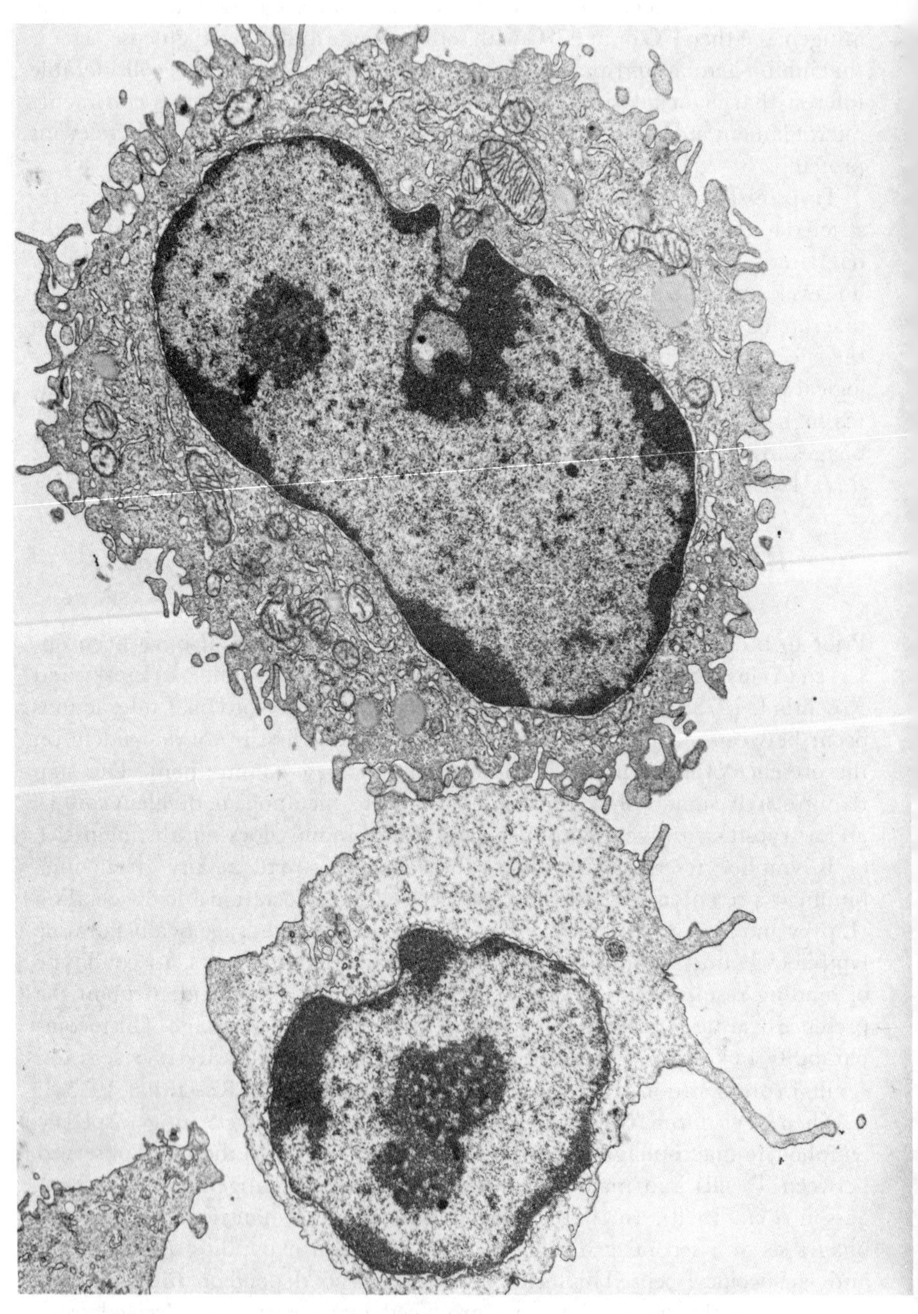

FIG. 2. *Electronmicrograph of an activated lymphocyte physically associated with an antigen-bearing macrophage.*

protein antigens like dinitrophenyl ovalbumin (DNP-OVA). When an antigen of restricted heterogeneity like the terpolymer L-glutamic acid, L-lysine, L-tyrosine (GLT) is used, intact macrophages are required and furthermore, the interaction only occurs between macrophage and primed lymphocytes having MHC identity. Table I demonstrates the difference in macrophage requirement for the T cell response to the antigens GLT and DNP-OVA.

Using peritoneal exudate T lymphocytes, Schwartz and his colleagues have mapped more precisely the macrophage–T cell interaction requirement to the *I-A* subregion of the MHC (Schwartz, *et al.*, 1978). Subsequent experiments examining the response to two antigens, the random terpolymer (L-glu^{55}-L-lys^{36}-L-phy^{9}) GLΦ and myoglobin, under dual *Ir* gene control (one gene each in *I-A* and *I-C* subregions), have revealed more about this *I* region requirement. For the GLΦ case, the antigen-presenting cells must come from animals possessing both genes (Schwartz *et al.*, 1979; Rosenwasser and Rosenthal, 1979). For myoglobin, macrophages obtained from animals having only *I-A* region identity mediate immune responses to the (1–32, 1–53 amino acid) fragment but frequently less well to the (1–55 amino acid) fragment of myoglobin, whereas macrophages from animals having only *I-C* region identity were capable of mediating immune responses only to the (1–55 amino acid) fragment (Richman *et al.*, 1980). Richman and coworkers speculated that independent dual *Ir* gene control might be mediated by macrophage-associated determinant selection as previously postulated (Rosenthal, 1978).

For other antigens under *Ir* gene control, soluble factors released by macrophages following incubation with antigen have been shown to allow helper T cells to stimulate B cells to make antibody in an H–2 restricted manner (Erb *et al.*, 1976a, b). The factor, called genetically related factor (GRF), is 50 000–60 000 daltons and reacts with anti-Ia sera. However, soluble macrophage products have not been found which elicit antigen-specific lymphocyte proliferation in the guinea-pig.

A linkage between physical and functional macrophage–lymphocyte interaction in the antigen recognition process is found by using cytochalasin B, a reagent that inhibits recognition of antigen-specific signals by T lymphocytes but does not affect mitogenic signals such as PHA. Cytochalasin B inhibit antigen-initiated lymphocyte proliferation and antigen-dependent lymphocyte–macrophage interaction when added immediately to culture, but was progressively less effective when added later in the culture period. This suggested that cytochalasin B acts selectively on an early event in antigen-specific proliferation. Since it neither interferes with uptake of antigen by macrophages nor inhibits PHA-induced proliferation, antigen recognition itself is disrupted, not the machinery of DNA synthesis. The effects of cytochalasin B are thus likely to result from its inhibition of the antigen-independent phase of macrophage–lymphocyte interaction (Lipsky and Rosenthal, 1975b).

Histocompatibility restriction of macrophage–T lymphocyte interaction

Antigens under control of *H*-linked genes and specific alloantisera that recognize cell-associated antigenic determinants of the major histocompatibility complex provide useful probes of the function and cellular location of MHC-linked products critical in the T lymphocyte antigen recognition process. Alloantisera block the antigen-specific T cell responses in a highly predictable manner (Eardley and Sercarz, 1976).

The requirement for at least some *I* region identity between macrophage and T cells for proliferation was paralleled by the ability of anti-Ia sera to block proliferation (Greineder *et al.*, 1976; Schwartz *et al.*, 1976a; Shevach and Rosenthal, 1973). Ia antigens have been demonstrated on the surface of some macrophage in the guinea-pig (10–20%) (Yamashita and Shevach, 1977) and mouse (8–15%) (Schwartz *et al.*, 1976b). The Ia-bearing macrophage subset thus appears to have enhanced antigen-presenting function since killing macrophages with anti-Ia sera and complement blocks the capacity of macrophage-rich populations to support a proliferative response to a soluble protein antigen (Schwartz *et al.*, 1978; Mottram and Miller, 1980) as well as *Listeria monocytogenes* (Farr *et al.*, 1979). The precise mechanisms by which macrophage-associated Ia molecules regulate immune responsiveness is not known. Our current appreciation of the central role of the macrophage in the regulation of the immune response suggests that the site for the inhibitory effect of the alloantiserum is on the macrophage itself and would be supported by blockade of the physical and/or functional interaction of the macrophage and T cell.

Not surprisingly, the site of alloantiserum blockade of functional macrophage–lymphocyte interaction can be examined directly by assessing the effect of alloantiserum on antigen-induced macrophage–lymphocyte physical interaction. Binding of lymph node cells by antigen-pulsed macrophages was determined after 20 h of culture. Anti-2 serum completely inhibited the binding of lymphocytes from strain 2 guinea-pigs to strain 2 macrophages pulsed antigen but not antigen-specific clustering of strain 13 macrophages and lymphocytes.

Immune response gene influences on macrophage–T lymphocyte interaction

An additional restriction on the interaction of antigen-pulsed macrophages with immune T cells was observed when macrophages obtained from a parental animal that lacked a given *Ir* gene were briefly exposed in a pulse-wash mode with an antigen controlled by that gene and then mixed with (nonresponder

× responder)F_1 T cells. Macrophages from nonimmunized strain 2 and (2 × 13) F_1 guinea-pigs pulsed with polymers of L-glutamic acid-1-lysine (an antigen, the response to which is controlled by a strain 2-linked *Ir* gene) activate immune F_1 T lymphocyte proliferation equally, while the magnitude of stimulation observed with strain 13 pulsed macrophages is approximately 10% of that seen when strain 2 or (2 × 13) F_1 macrophages are used (Shevach *et al.*, 1974). One explanation for the failure of the nonresponder macrophage to activate the (nonresponder × responder) F_1 T cell is an intrinsic defect in *Ir* gene product function in the nonresponder macrophage.

Determinant selection: immune response gene function at the level of the macrophage

We have proposed that during immunologically relevant macrophage–T lymphocyte interaction, the two cells come into close functional contact in areas of shared histocompatibility antigens. Thus, the *Ir* gene-controlled antigen recognition structures on the T cell are physically related to the sites for macrophage–T lymphocyte binding specified in the same haplotype (Shevach and Rosenthal, 1973).

Our study proposes a simple, and perhaps more unifying explanation of what an immune response gene "does". It states that a given macrophage's repertoire of *Ir* gene products function to specify what portions of a given polypeptide antigen is seen by the T cell. This can be tested by assessing the relationship of antigen structure, i.e. amino acid sequence, and conformation to macrophage function in T cell activation.

Synthetic polymers and peptides have provided information on the role of a few amino acids in determining the response to these antigens (Benacerraf and Dorf, 1976) and insight into the complexity of cellular interactions (Katz *et al.*, 1973). The inexact nature of the sequence and conformation of these polymers encouraged the study of highly defined, but often more complex protein antigens (Crumpton, 1974; DeWeck, 1974; Rechlin, 1975). Major conclusions drawn from those observations were, first, that the specificity of humoral and cellular responses can be spatially separated (Senyk *et al.*, 1971), individual determinants within the same molecule may be under the control of separate *Ir* genes (Schwartz *et al.*, 1978), and, lastly, that nonsequential amino acids may form conformational determinants for both antibody and T cells (Atassi, 1978; Schwartz *et al.*, 1979a, b). Studies on defined antigens and their peptide derivatives are powerful probes for dissecting the nature of the specificity of the *Ir* gene product as well as that of the T cell receptor and antibody. Table II summarizes the principal defined antigens available for immunological studies.

Species variants of insulin with limited amino acid differences were previously used in our own, as well as other, laboratories to map the intramolecular sights recognized by T and B cells from inbred strains of guinea-pigs

TABLE II

Defined protein antigen	*Species variants studied peptides studied*	*Modified, fragmented or synthetic peptides studied*	*Amino acid sequences*	*X-ray crystallography*	*MHC-linked* Ir *gene control*
Collagen	–	+	partial	–	+
α_1 chains			> 1000		
α_2					
Cytochrome	> 100	+	104	+	+
Ferrodoxin	+	–	49–97	+	?
Fibrinogen	+	+	49–68	–	+
A chains					
B					
β-Galactosidase	+	–	–	–	?
	mutants of *E. coli*				
Glucagon	–	+	29	–	?
	few exist				
Haemoglobin	+	+	141–146	+	?
α	many				
β					
Insulin		> 15	+	51	+
Lysozyme	+	+	129	+	+
Myelin basic protein	+	+	170	–	?
Myoglobin	+	+	153	+	+
Staphylococcus nuclease	–	+	104	+	+

(Barcinski and Rosenthal, 1977). Both the T cell proliferative and T helper responses were found to be under the control of *Ir* genes linked to the guinea-pig MHC (GPLA). Strain 2 guinea-pig T cells respond to a well defined area on the A chain of insulin (A8-A9-A10). In strain 13 guinea-pigs, the T cell response was not defined but was believed to be directed at some determinant(s) on the B chain of insulin. These *Ir* genes appear to operate at the level of the macrophage by a process of determinant selection (Rosenthal *et al.*, 1978). It was not clear whether antibody specificity was correspondingly directed against the same intramolecular regions as T cell responsiveness.

To establish the fine specificity of the determinants of this *Ir* gene-controlled response in strain 13 guinea-pigs, we have used synthetic peptide fragments of the insulin B chain. Multiple peptide sequences were used to map the minimal determinants required for activation of T cell proliferation and for expression of T helper cell activity.

T lymphocyte enriched peritoneal exudate lymphocytes (PELs) from strain 13 guinea-pigs immunized with pork insulin proliferate *in vitro* to the immunizing antigen as well as to sulphonated B chain, partially to oxidized B chain, and to some, but not all, synthetic fragments of the insulin B chain (Table III). As expected from previously published data (Barcinski and Rosenthal, 1977), strain 2 guinea-pigs which recognize the amino acid 8, 9, 10 of the A chain loop do not respond to insulin B chain or its fragments. The oxidized form of the B chain was less stimulatory than the sulphonated B chain, which was probably due to the performic acid oxidation procedure used to produce the former product. Of note is the ability of all fragments which contain the *N*-terminal 16 amino acids of the B chain to stimulate insulin-primed T cells. Hormonally inactive desoctapeptide insulin (DES) which has the 8 carboxy terminal amino acids removed is also able to stimulate DNA synthesis equal to the native molecule (data not shown). B chain fragments (1–8), (9–16), (17–30) and (22–30) do not activate insulin immune T cells. The inability to stimulate DNA synthesis was not due to toxicity or induction of suppression since co-culture or prepulsing of cells with nonstimulatory fragments failed to suppress the response to insulin, B chain, B(1–16) or PPD in culture (data not shown). Furthermore, molar equivalent dose-response curves showed the B chain fragment 1–16 was equal the native insulin at all concentrations tested.

Figure 3 shows the amino acid sequence of the important *N*-terminal amino acids of guinea-pig insulin compared to that of pork insulin. Since guinea-pig insulin has been previously shown not to be stimulatory (Barcinski and Rosenthal, 1977), 4 amino acid differences in this region could be of importance for T cell activation.

To further map the T cell response within this 16 amino acid region, additional peptides were synthesized representing B(1–10), B(1–13), B(5–13) and B(5–16). At the molar concentrations used above, a low level of T cell activation was noted; therefore, a several fold molar excess was required to elicit the response to these fragments. Table IV gives the moles of peptide

TABLE III

Proliferative response to insulin and synthetic B chain peptides by T lymphocytes from inbred strain 13 guinea-pigs immunized to pork insulin.

Antigen (*10µg/ml*)	*Lymphocyte DNA synthesis* ^{3}*H-thymidine incorporation* ($\triangle$ *ct/min* $\times$ *10*^{3})
Beef insulin	52·3 ± 1·5[a]
Insulin B chain (sulphonated)	57·1 ± 1·7
Insulin B chain (oxidized)	19·9 ± 0·4
B(1–8)[b]	2·6 ± 0·9
B(1–16)	51·3 ± 2·7
B(1–23)	60·0 ± 5·1
B(9–16)	1·2 ± 0·7
B(17–30)	1·7 ± 0·3
B(24–30)	1·1 ± 0·2

[a] Mean ± s.e. of 3–5 experiments.
[b] Amino acid sequence in relation to B chain (30 amino acids).

For the T cell proliferation assay, guinea-pigs were immunized with 100 µg of antigen in saline emulsified with an equal volume of complete Freund's adjuvant (CFA) containing 0·5 mg/ml of killed *Mycobacterium tuberculosis*, H37Ra (Difco). Peritoneal exudate cells (PECs) were obtained by lavaging the peritoneal cavity of immune guinea-pigs, 4 days after the injection of 25 ml of sterile oil (Marcol 52; Humble Oil and Refining Co., Houston, Texas). The PECs were washed twice in HBSS and divided into two fractions, one of which was treated with mitomycin C (40 µg/ml; Sigma Chemical Co., St Louis, Mo) for 60 min at 37°C at a concentration of 5–15 × 10^6 cells/ml. After 4 washes with HBSS, this cell population was used as a source of macrophages. In situations requiring pulsed macrophages, virgin guinea-pigs were used as the source of PECs that were subsequently incubated with antigen as previously described (Rosenstreich and Rosenthal, 1973). The second PEC fraction was used to obtain a population of highly enriched antigen-reactive T cells (PELs) after passage through a nylon wool adherence column (Lipsky *et al.*, 1976). This population was used to assess T cell proliferation by incorporation of radiolabelled thymidine into DNA. PELs resuspended in RPMI 1640 with 5% FCS were cultured in microtitre plates with round-bottom wells (Cooke Laboratory Products Div., Dynatech Laboratories Inc., Alexandria, Va) for 72 h in a 5% CO_2 humidified atmosphere at 37°C at a concentration of 1·2 × 10^6 PELs/ml and 0·3 × 10^6 PECs/ml in the presence of continuous antigen. Tritiated thymidine (6·7 Ci/m M; New England Nuclear Corp., Boston, Mass.) 1 µCi/well was added 18 h prior to termination. The cells were harvested onto glass filter paper by the use of a semiautomated microharvesting device. Tritiated thymidine incorporation was determined by liquid scintillation spectrometry and the results reported as number of counts above the control (ct/min) unless otherwise stated.

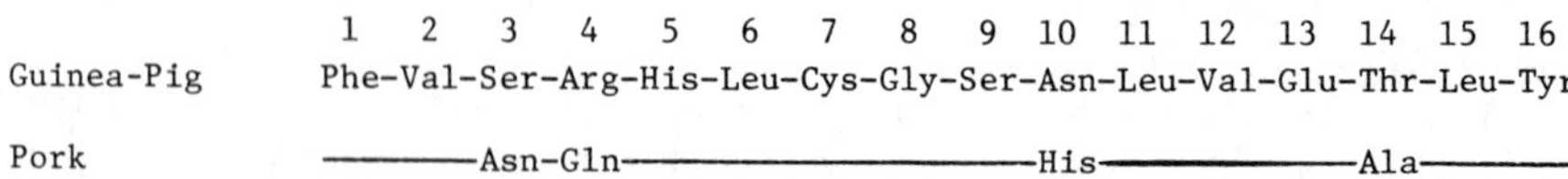

FIG. 3. *The amino acid sequence of the* N-*terminal 16 residues of guinea-pig insulin B chain is compared to that of pork insulin. Identities are shown by solid lines.*

TABLE IV

DNA synthesis can be induced in strain 13 guinea-pigs immune to insulin by molar excess of N-terminal peptides contained in the B(1–16) fragment (methods are described in Table III).

Antigen	*Peak ^{3}H-thymidine incorporation (Δ ct/min $\times 10^{-3}$)*	*Moles peptide/ moles insulin*	*% Stimulation*
Insulin	31·6 ± 0·4	—	—
B(1–16)	35·6 ± 2·0	1·0	100+
B(1–10)	17·2 ± 0·6	3·0	54
B(1–13)	15·9 ± 0·6	3·0	50
B(5–13)	8·1 ± 3·7	5·5	26
B(5–16)	29·3 ± 1·9	8·0	93

per mol of insulin required to induce the maximum DNA synthesis in insulin immune PELs. Peptides B(1–10), B(1–13) and B(5–13) are capable of inducing about half the amount of tritiated thymidine incorporation of insulin or B(1–16) when used in antigen excess. However, the fragment B(5–16) can produce 90% of the T cell activation seen with the immunizing native antigen. Maximum stimulation is attained at 200–250 μg protein. Costimulation of insulin immune T cells with multiple combinations of these peptides did not show any evidence of additive proliferation.

If the immune response to insulin requires recognition of "non-self" residues within the molecule, then only two residues appear to be critical for stimulation within the B(1–16) peptide. Accordingly, the relative contribution of residues 10 (histidine) and 14 (asparagine) were assessed for their importance in the activation of insulin immune T cells (Table V). Peptides either identical to the guinea-pig sequence ($Asn_{10} \rightarrow Thr_{14}$), or individually substituted residues,

TABLE V

Position 10 of insulin B chain is critical for T cell activation of insulin immune strain 13 guinea-pigs

Antigen (10μg/ml)	*Δ ct/min*
Beef insulin	63·4 ± 0·42[a]
B chain	50·5 ± 0·31
B(1–16)	54·4 ± 0·45
B(5–16)	41·0 ± 0·41
B(5–16) [Ala → Thr][b]	49·9 ± 0·35
B(5–16) [His → Asn][b]	3·2 ± 0·03
B(5–16) [Ala → Thr + His → Asn][b]	1·6 ± 0·02

[a] Mean ± s.e. of 2 experiments. For detailed methodology see Table III.
[b] Square brackets indicate substitution(s) made from original sequence of pork insulin towards sequence of guinea-pig insulin B chain fragment.

were assayed for stimulation of DNA synthesis in insulin immune PELs. Alteration of position 14 (Ala → Thr) does not alter the DNA synthetic response; however, change in position 10 (His → Asn) removes over 90% of the proliferative response. This single residue therefore appears critical for the T cell immune response to insulin in strain 13 guinea-pigs.

Since the specificity of the proliferating T cells appears to be the same for the B(1–16) fragment and the whole insulin molecule, a hapten-carrier system was employed to evaluate the specificity of T cell helper function in fragment immune guinea-pigs. Strain 13 guinea-pigs were primed with DNP-OVA i.p. and subsequently immunized with B(1–16), B chain, pork insulin or CFA alone as described in Methods. The titre of anti-DNP antibody was measured immediately before (day 0) and 8 days after boosting. The results shown indicate that animals immunized with insulin, B chain and B(1–16) were able to generate significant antihapten response to DNP-insulin (Fig. 4). Control animals did not show a significant rise in anti-DNP titres. These results indicate that T helper cells are primed by a fragment of the whole molecule and that this common determinant generates helper cell activity equivalent to that of intact native insulin. These experiments do not directly identify T helper and proliferating T cells to be the same clone rather than distinct subpopulations, but they do establish that the fine specificity of their antigen receptor is similarly constrained.

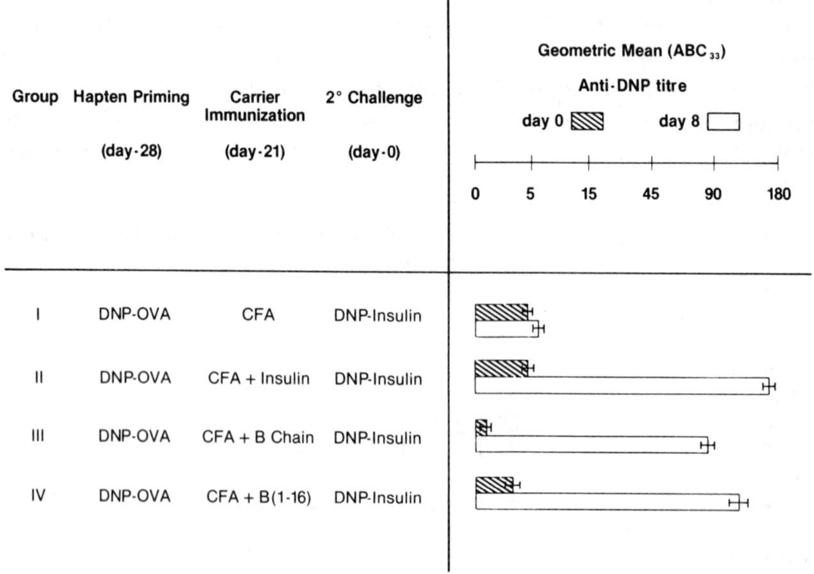

FIG. 4. *Determinant specificity of T helper function: evidence that insulin B chain peptides can generate T helper function in strain 13 guinea-pigs. Synthetic B chain and B(1–16) were able to prime T helper cells as efficiently as pork insulin, DNP-OVA-primed and DNP-pork insulin-boosted animals. The anti-DNP antibodies were obtained from strain 13 guinea-pig sera after an immunization schedule designed to access T helper function.*

One can next ask whether immune response genes operate via the presenting function of macrophages. F_1 (2 × 13) guinea-pigs were immunized either with pork insulin or the B(1–16) peptide. The PELs obtained from these animals were then stimulated in culture with antigen pulsed strain 2 or strain 13 mitomycin-treated macrophages (PECs). The results of several experiments are shown in Table VI. T cells from F_1 animals immunized with insulin

TABLE VI

Evidence that only strain 13 macrophages (MΦ) can present B(1-16) to F_1 (2 × 13) insulin or fragment immune T cells while both strain 2 and strain 13 macrophages can present insulin to insulin immune F_1 (2 × 13) T cells

	Stimulation (Δct/min) of F_1 (2 × 13) T cells immunized with:			
	B(1-16)		*Pork Insulin*	
Pulsed with:	*MΦ strain 2*	*MΦ strain 13*	*MΦ strain 2*	*MΦ strain 13*
B(1-16)	7·4 ± 0·6[a]	90·3 ± 6·0	3·5 ± 0·4	35·1 ± 1·1
Pork	3·5 ± 0·4	65·5 ± 4·4	29·6 ± 0·3	39·9 ± 1·2
PPD	39·2 ± 0·9	30·5 ± 4·5	37·3 ± 0·3	35·0 ± 1·0

[a] Mean ± s.e. of 3 experiments. Methods are as described in Table III.

demonstrate the ability of insulin or PPD pulsed macrophages from either strain 2 or strain 13 to induce DNA synthesis. The somewhat lower proliferative response seen with strain 2 macrophages is consistent with that seen in parental animals immunized with insulin (Barcinski and Rosenthal, 1977). However, the proliferative response to the B(1–16) fragment is seen only when antigen is presented on strain 13 macrophages. Strain 2 macrophages are unable to present the fragment to insulin immune T cells. On the left side of Table VI, we see a different pattern of response when F_1 animals are immunized with the B(1–16) peptide. Strain 2 macrophages, though able to present PPD quite well, are unable to activate T cells to respond to either insulin or B(1–16). Since the F_1 T cells can respond to both the A chain determinant of strain 2 T cells and the B(1–16) determinant of strain 13, the genetic restriction seen in the secondary proliferative response appears to depend upon the determinant(s) presented to the T cell. This strain-related determinant specificity of the response would suggest that *Ir* genes operate at the level of the macrophage as a function of antigen presentation.

Taking advantage of the single tyrosine in the B(1–16) peptide, we were able to analyse a number of guinea-pig sera for antibodies binding this fragment as well as B chain and insulin. The antibody binding of sera at the peak of the primary response (21 days after immunization), does not show determinant preference seen at the T cell level (Table VII). The results clearly show that both strain 2 and strain 13 guinea-pigs develop very high titre antibody against insulin when immunized with insulin in CFA. The ability of these sera to bind B chain are significantly less. These same individual sera bind radio-

TABLE VII

A comparison of strain 2 and strain 13 antibodies directed against insulin, B chain or B(1-16) fragment

Immunizing antigen and strain	Mean of ABC_{33} titres[a] of antibodies against: Insulin	B chain	B(1-16)
Insulin (strain 2)	4·37 ± 0·71	0·41 ± 0·39	< 0·1
Insulin (strain 13)	5·03 ± 0·12	0·57 ± 0·23	< 0·1
B chain (strain 13)	0·9 ± 0·30	2·74 ± 1·08	0·46 ± 0·41
B(1-16) (strain 13)	< 0·1[b]	< 0·1[b]	1·32 ± 0·52

[a] Expressed as log of mean titre ± S.D. of 3–6 animals per group.
[b] No detectable antibody titres, indicates ⩽ 3% binding above normal sera control. For detailed methodology, see Table III.

labelled B(1–16) peptide only slightly greater than control serum. When animals are immunized with B(1–16) or B chain, the antibody produced is capable of binding the immunizing antigen but no significant binding is detected against the parent molecule. These data indicate that the B cell product or antibody recognizes features different from the determinants "seen" by T cells and differs in that B cells but not T cells prefer the original tertiary structure of the immunizing antigen. These results cannot exclude the presence of a small subset of antibody with the same specificity as the T cell. The data do, however, emphasize that the dominance of restricted regions of the antigen for eliciting T cell responses differ from those at the level of antibody or the B cell.

Conclusions

Previous data, as well as the present ones, indicate that only limited molecular regions on a globular protein need be recognized for generation of cellular immunity and for generation of T helper cell activity. Denatured proteins can retain the ability to induce delayed hypersensitivity but loose antibody reactivity (Gell and Benacerraf, 1959) and retain their ability to elicit specific helper cells (Ishizaka, *et al.*, 1974). In our model antigen insulin, the peptide sequence of the first 16 amino acids of the insulin B chain contains, for the strain 13 guinea-pig, all of the immunogenic information present in the native molecule as reflected in the generation of T cell proliferation and in the expression of T cell helper activity. B(5–16) is as active as B(1–16) and contains all of the immunologically important determinants. Synthetic sequences of the region B(5–16) having the amino acid sequences present in guinea-pig insulin, or possessing only the B14 alanine of beef insulin, but not the histidine 10th position, are not stimulatory. Using the (1–16) peptide, this reactivity was found to be reciprocal in that either peptide or whole molecule could be used as the immunogen. These observations support the concept that T cell responses are specific for a primary amino acid sequence on the antigen, and also emphasize the restricted nature of the T cell recognition process.

Several smaller peptides from the same region were also found to stimulate T cell proliferation, albeit less effectively than B(1–16). All of the peptides which activate T cells contain a common amino acid variation at the 10th position. This histidine for aspargine exchange makes guinea-pig insulin unique among mammalian insulins, being unable to form hexamers with zinc (Blundell *et al.*, 1972). Using a computer-generated space-filling model developed by Richard Feldman of the NIH (American National Institute Health), we have located this residue as projecting from the planar surface of the molecule. The other amino acid exchange (14th residue) within the B(5–16) peptide is not available on the surface of the molecule. If one considers variations from "self" to be a key in the recognition process, then the B-10 position assumes a critical role for T cell activation. A single amino acid has recently been shown to be critical for immune response to another peptide, human fibrin peptide (Thomas *et al.*, 1979a, b). However, the failure of peptide B(9–16) to induce T cell proliferation emphasizes that the presence of this exchange alone is not sufficient for T cell activation. Moreover, a synthetic fragment consisting of B(1–4)-(9–16) also fails to activate insulin immune T cells, indicating that more than fragment size is important. Possibly another residue(s) important for *Ir* gene product interaction is contained within the 5–9 region. A requirement for recognition of two specificities—one for *Ir* and another T cell—within even such a limited peptide sequence as the 5–16th amino acid of the B chain is consistent with recent hypotheses for the mechanism of the *Ir* gene function (Benacerraf, 1978; Rosenthal, 1978).

While primary structure is of key importance in T cell activation, the role of conformation in orienting an amino acid sequence for recognition should not be overlooked. For example, the B(5–13) peptide is the smallest found to stimulate insulin immune T cells; however, slightly larger peptides B(1–13) and B(5–16) are more powerful stimulators of T cell proliferation. These additional residues may in some way sustain a propensity to reform the alpha helix found in this region of the native molecule (Blundell *et al.*, 1972). The decreased reactivity of the oxidized B chain may also reflect a loss or derangement of tertiary structure. Helical regions tend to be important sites of immunological determinants in at least two other proteins, nuclease (Sacks *et al.*, 1978) and cytochrome c (Corradin and Chiller, 1979). Though transient in solution, such conformation may be essential for activation on the cell surface. Reasonably, both recognition events taking place during antigen presentation and the physicochemical nature of the antigen are important in achieving maximum T cell activation. Such a mechanism could conformationally approximate two nonsequential amino acids (e.g. B–5 and B–10) to create a single topographical determinant for cytochrome c (Schwartz *et al.*, 1979a, b). Currently, we are attempting to resolve the extent to which recognition of specific residues and conformational integrity are necessary for T cell activation by the synthesis of pseudopeptide analogues.

The antibody specificity of the response to insulin and its fragments in inbred guinea-pigs does not reflect the same characteristics as that of the T cell. Using radiolabelled species variants of insulin and isoelectrically focused sera, determinant specific antibody spectrotypes could not be detected in strain 2 sera (Thomas *et al.*, 1980). In the present study employing radiolabelled fragment for which strain 13 T cells are highly specific, we could not detect significant binding in either strain 2 or strain 13 serum with high anti-insulin titres. Even though immunizing with the B(1–16) fragment will produce antibodies which bind the fragment, they do not appear to bind the native molecule. The determinants recognized by these antibodies are probably not available on the surface of the insulin molecule. These results may be somewhat analogous to the data obtained in mice hyperimmunized with nuclease in which the antibody titre in low responders reached the same level as seen in high responders. However, when these hyperimmune sera were examined for binding of the nuclear fragment (99–146), the pattern of response was similar to that noted in the primary (Sacks *et al.*, 1978) suggesting that the failure to find determinant restriction of antibody specificity in the guinea-pig is not due to the magnitude of the response in the primary. Thus, shared specificity between antibody and T cell could be present but not detectable because it represents such a small percent of the total anti-insulin response. This has been recently emphasized in H-2^b mice where hybridoma antibodies have been produced which bind the same A chain loop region seen by strain 2 guinea-pig T cells (Loblay *et al.*, 1980). More importantly, the fragment studied here is quite small in comparison to the nuclease fragment which is about the same size as the whole insulin molecule. Nonetheless, in our present studies of insulin where the T cell response is directed at a limited epitope, an antibody population with identical specificity to the T cell does not constitute a detectable portion of the antibody response.

The function of *Ir* genes has been closely associated with the Ia molecules on the surface of macrophages (Rosenthal and Shevach, 1973; Paul *et al.*, 1976) and B cells (Benacerraf, 1976). Since previous experiments indicate that antibody directed against these Ia molecules could block *in vitro* responses against the antigen but antibody against the native antigen could not (Shevach *et al.*, 1972; Ellner *et al.*, 1977). An antigen fragment has been shown to induce specific T cell function directed against the insulin molecule yet we have also shown that very high titre antisera cannot bind this same peptide. Taken together, one can propose that the failure of antibodies directed against the native molecule to block T cell activation is most easily explained by its failure to bind antigen fragment(s) generated during critical phase of induction of T cell reactivity.

Finally, we presented experiments in which parental macrophages bearing native antigen were used to activate F_1 T cells from animals immune to synthetic sequences of the B chain. They demonstrated that *Ir* gene products distinguish separate determinants within the same molecule and that the process of determinant selections operates at the macrophage level. If antigen metabolism alone were the mechanism of *Ir* gene function, F_1 T cells would be expected to respond to the fragment presented by either strain 2 and strain 13 macrophages. This was not the case; rather, the defect in strain 2 presentation appears to be a lack of a specific associative relationship between Ia and the restricted molecular region rather than inability to derive the appropriate degradative product.

Summary

Both T helper and proliferative responses can be induced by a polypeptide fragment representing a highly restricted region of the native molecule and that, as with the intact native insulin molecule, *Ir* gene control of the response to such fragments appears to reside at the level of the macrophage. Presentation of this processed antigen requires MHC restricted physical interaction between the fragment bearing macrophage and specific T cell. These data support the concept that a potential degradation product(s) of an antigen, in the form of a peptide, contains all of the necessary information for mediation of an *Ir* gene controlled T cell response to the native antigen. Studies of the binding of anti-insulin antibody to these fragments, as contrasted with their binding to native insulin, emphasizes that there is a differing pattern of determinant specificity which exists between B and T cells in response to antigens of defined structure.

References

Atassi, M. Z. (1978). *Immunochemistry* **15**, 909.

Barcinski, M. A. and Rosenthal, A. S. (1977). *J. Exp. Med.* **145**, 726.

Ben-Sasson, S. Z., Lipscomb, M. F., Tucker, T. and Uhl, J. W. (1978). *J. Immunol.* **120**, 1902.

Benacerraf, B. (1976). *In* "The Role of Products of the Histocompatibility Gene Complex in Immune Response" (D. H. Katz and B. Benacerraf, eds) p. 715. Academic Press, New York and London.

Benacerraf, B. (1978). *J. Immunol.* **120**, 1809.

Benacerraf, B. and Dorf, M. E. (1976). *Proc. Cold Spring Harbor Symp. Quant. Biol.* **41**, 65.

Bergholtz, B. O. and Thorsky, E. (1977). *Scand. J. Immunol.* **6**, 779.

Bergholtz, B. O. and Thorsky, E. (1978). *Scand. J. Immunol.* **8**, 63.

Blundell, T., Dodson, G., Hodgkin, D. and Mercela, D. (1972). *Adv. Protein. Chem.* **26**, 279.

Corradin, G., and Chiller, J. M. (1979). *J. Exp. Med.* **2**, 436.

Crumpton, M. J. (1974). *In* "The Antigens" (M. Sela, ed.) Vol. 2, p. 1. Academic Press, New York and London.

Davies, P. and Bonney, R. J. (1979). *J. Reticulo. Soc.* **26**, 37.

DeWeck, A. L. (1974). *In* "The Antigens" (M. Sela, ed.) Vol. 2, p. 142, Academic Press, New York and London.

Eardley, D. D. and Sercarz, E. E. (1976). *J. Immunol.* **116**, 600.

Effros, R. B., Doherty, P. C., Gerhard, W. and Bennink, J. (1977). *J. Exp. Med.* **145**, 557.
Ellner, J. J. and Rosenthal, A. S. (1975). *J. Immunol.* **114**, 1563.
Ellner, J. J., Lipsky, P. E. and Rosenthal, A. S. (1977). *J. Immunol.* **118**, 208.
Erb, P., Feldmann, M. and Hogg, N. (1976a). *Eur. J. Immunol.* **6**, 365.
Erb, P., Meier, B. and Feldmann, M. (1976b). *Nature* **263**, 601.
Farr, A. G., Kiely, J. M. and Unanue, E. R. (1979). *J. Immunol.* **122**, 2395.
Gell, P. G. H. and Benacerraf, B. (1959). *Immunology* **2**, 64.
Greineder, D. K., Shevach, E. M. and Rosenthal, A. S. (1976). *J. Immunol.* **117**, 1594.
Ishizaka, K., Kishimoto, T., Delespesse, G. and King, T. P. (1974). *J. Immunol.* **113**, 70.
Katz, D. H., Hamoaka, T., Dorf, M. E., Maurer, P. H. and Benacerraf, B. (1973). *J. Exp. Med.* **138**, 734.
Lipsky, P. E. and Rosenthal, A. S. (1973). *J. Exp. Med.* **138**, 900.
Lipsky, P. E. and Rosenthal, A. S. (1975a). *J. Exp. Med.* **141**, 138.
Lipsky, P. E. and Rosenthal, A. S. (1975b). *J. Immunol.* **115**, 440.
Lipsky, P. E., Ellner, J. J. and Rosenthal, A. S. (1976). *J. Immunol.* **116**, 876.
Loblay, R. H., Schroer, J. and Rosenthal, A. S. (1980). *In* "Macrophage Regulation of Immunity" (E. Unanue and A. S. Rosenthal, eds) pp. 87–94. Academic Press, New York and London.
Mottram, P. L. and Miller, J. F. A. P. (1980). *Eur. J. Immunol.* **10**, 165.
Paul, W. E., Shevach, E. M., Thomas, D. W., Pickerel, S. F. and Rosenthal, A. S. (1976). *Proc. Cold Spring Harbor Symp. Quant. Biol.* **41**, 571.
Rechlin, M. (1975). *Adv. Immunol.* **20**, 71.
Richman, L. K., Stober, W. and Berzofsky, J. A. (1980). *J. Immunol.* **124**, 619.
Rosenthal, A. S. (1978). *Immunol. Rev.* **40**, 136.
Rosenstreich, D. L. and Rosenthal, A. S. (1973). *J. Immunol.* **110**, 934.
Rosenstreich, D. L. and Rosenthal, A. S. (1974). *J. Immunol.* **112**, 1085.
Rosenthal, A. S. and Shevach, E. M. (1973). *J. Exp. Med.* **138**, 1194.
Rosenthal, A. S., Barcinski, M. A. and Blake, J. T. (1977). *Nature* **267**, 156.
Rosenthal, A. S., Barcinski, M. A. and Rosenwasser, L. J. (1978). *Fed. Proc.* **37**, 79.
Rosenthal, A. S., Thomas, J. W., Schroer, J., Yokomuro, K., Blake, J. T. and Rosenwasser, L. J. (1979). *In* "Recent Developments in Immunologic Tolerance and Macrophage Function" (P. Baram, C. W. Pierce and J. R. Battisto, eds) p. 57. Elsevier, North Holland.
Rosenwasser, L. J. and Rosenthal, A. S. (1978). *J. Immunol.* **120**, 1991.
Rosenwasser, L. J. and Rosenthal, A. S. (1979). *J. Immunol.* **123**, 1141.
Sacks, D. H., Berzofsky, J. A., Pisetsky, D. S. and Schwartz, R. H. (1978). *Springer Sem. Immunopathol.* **1**, 51.
Schwartz, R. H., David, C. S., Sachs, D. H., and Paul, W. E. (1976a). *J. Immunol.* **117**, 531.
Schwartz, R. H., Dickler, H. B., Sachs, D. J. and Schwartz, B. D. (1976b). *Scand. J. Immunol.* **5**, 731.
Schwartz, R. H., Yano, A. and Paul, W. E. (1978). *Immunol. Rev.* **40**, 153.
Schwartz, R. H., Solinger, A. M., Ultee, M. E., Margoliash, E., Yano, A., Stimpfling, J. H., Chen, C., Meryman, C. F., Maurer, P. H. and Paul, W. E. (1979a). ICN-UCLA Symposium, Keystone, Colorado.
Schwartz, R. H., Yano, A., Stimpfling, J. H. and Paul W. E. (1976b). *J. Exp. Med.* **149**, 40.
Senyk, G., Williams, E. B., Nitecki, D. E. and Goodman, J. W. (1971). *J. Exp. Med.* **133**, 1294.
Shevach, E. M. and Rosenthal, A. S. (1973). *J. Exp. Med.* **138**, 1213.
Shevach, E. M., Paul, W. E. and Green, I. (1972). *J. Exp. Med.* **136**, 1207.
Shevach, E. M., Green, I. and Paul, W. E. (1974). *J. Exp. Med.* **139**, 679.

Thomas, D. W., Meitz, S. K. and Wilner, G. D. (1979a). *J. Immunol.* **123**, 759.
Thomas, D. W., Meitz, S. K. and Wilner, G. D. (1979b). *J. Immunol.* **123**, 1299.
Thomas, D. W., Schroer, J. A., Danho, W., Bullesbach, E., Fohler, J. and Rosenthal. A. S. (1980). *In* "Macrophage Regulation of Immunity" (E. Unanue and A. S. Rosenthal, eds) pp. 3–14. Academic Press, New York and London.
Unanue, E. R., Cerottini, J. C. and Bedford, M. (1969). *Nature* **222**, 1193.
Waldron, J. A., Horn, R. G. and Rosenthal, A. S. (1973). *J. Immunol.* **111**, 58.
Waldron, J. A., Horn, R. G., and Rosenthal, A. S. (1974). *J. Immunol.* **112**, 746.
Yamashita, U. and Shevach, E. M. (1977). *J. Immunol.* **119**, 1584.
Zuckerman, S. H. and Douglas, S. D. (1979). *Ann. Rev. Microbiol.* **33**, 267.

26

Genetic Control of Idiotype Expression

DAVID H. SACHS

Transplantation Biology Section, Immunology Branch, National Cancer Institute, National Institutes of Health, Bethesda, Maryland, USA

Introduction

When regarded as an antigen, an immunoglobulin molecule possesses numerous determinants against which specific antibodies can be raised. The idiotype of an immunoglobulin can be defined as the set of antigenic determinants which distinguish it from all other immunoglobulins produced by the same animal. Such antigenic individuality was first demonstrated for myeloma antibodies (Slater *et al.*, 1955) and was later shown to apply to induced antibodies as well (Kunkel *et al.*, 1963; Oudin and Michel, 1963; Gell and Kelus, 1964). Subsequent analyses of the primary structure of immunoglobulin molecules suggested that such individuality ought to reflect structural properties of the variable regions of immunoglobulin heavy and/or light chains, and this prediction has indeed been verified for numerous idiotypic determinants (reviewed by Nisonoff *et al.*, 1975). In view of the large body of sequence data indicating that variable (V) region diversity is predominantly a function of the hypervariable (HV) segments of the V region (Wu and Kabat, 1970), it seems likely that idiotypic determinants should be a reflection of HV segment diversity, and for the purposes of this paper, we shall assume that this relationship exists.

The other major property of antibody molecules determined by the sequence of the HV segments is of course antigen binding activity. As shown schematically in Fig. 1, these two properties may or may not be related. If

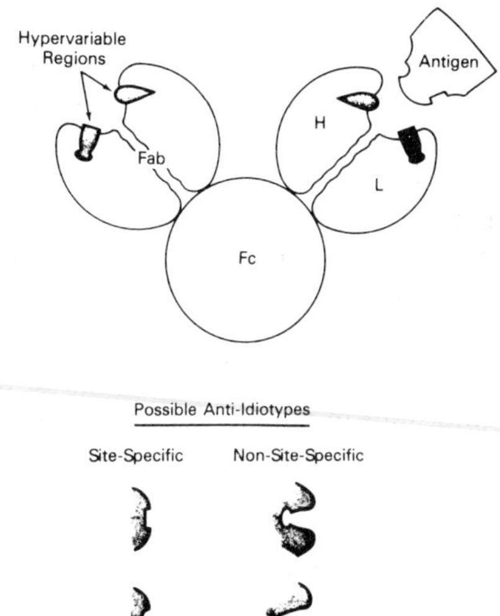

FIG. 1. *Schematic representation of an antibody molecule. Hypervariable regions of the heavy* (*H*) *and light* (*L*) *chains are seen to be responsible both for antigen complementarity and for idiotypic determinants both within and outside of the antigen binding site* (*site-specific and non-site-specific, respectively*).

an anti-idiotypic antibody reacts with a determinant within the binding site such that it interferes with antigen binding, such an anti-idiotype is said to be site-specific, or antigen-inhibitable. On the other hand, one can clearly envision unique structural determinants caused by the HV segment which should have no effect on antigen binding because, as illustrated in Fig. 1, they are not within the binding site. Antibodies can therefore bind to such idiotypic determinants independent of antigen binding. For simplicity Fig. 1 shows only 1 HV segment of each Ig chain, although there are in fact 3 such segments per chain, making the number of possible idiotypic determinants per antibody molecule quite large (Padlan, 1977).

Any one anti-idiotypic antibody does not react with the entire array of idiotypic determinants of an Ig molecule, but rather with a single determinant or "idiotope". The distinction between idiotypes and idiotopes is of more than just semantic importance. Most assays for idiotype measure only idiotope levels, since these assays generally involve dilution of the anti-idiotypic reagent to near the end of its binding curve, at which point inhibition by idiotype is of course most sensitive. At this point, however, only those idiotopes against which the highest titer of antibodies are present will be detected. Thus, the vast majority of studies of expression of idiotype are in fact studies of the expression of idiotopes.

Furthermore, since there is no *a priori* reason why a particular HV segment cannot be used in the construction of a large number of different binding sites, idiotopes may be shared by antibodies of very different specificities. Thus, in addition to the existence of non-site-specific idiotypic determinants, one might predict the presence of idiotypic determinants on Ig molecules which do not bind the antigen against which the original antibody was directed. This prediction has indeed been substantiated in several systems, as will be discussed further below.

It is thus clear that the detection of idiotype is very dependent on the kind of assay used. Most of the studies on genetic control of idiotype expression which we will discuss have employed antigen-binding assays, and therefore deal with site-specific idiotypes. However, it is worth keeping in mind that if, as has been suggested by Jerne (1974), idiotype–anti-idiotype interactions are of general significance in the physiologic regulation of immune responses, then it would seem most likely that such regulation would occur at the level of idiotope recognition rather than at the level of specific binding site recognition. Genetic control of idiotype expression by anti-idiotype would then involve regulation of sets of idiotope-bearing Ig molecules rather than only those with a given binding specificity.

In this chapter I shall attempt to catalogue many of the idiotypic determinants for which genetic control of expression has been studied, to examine several of the levels of genetic control which have been described, and to discuss some possible implications of the data examined. Although work relevant to the genetic control of idiotype expression has been reported in several species, I have confined the discussion here to work carried out in the mouse model. In addition, I have frequently chosen examples from our own work in the staphylococcal nuclease system, although other systems might have provided equally satisfactory examples. I apologize in advance for the incompleteness of this survey and hope that investigators in this rapidly expanding field will not be offended if I have inadvertently omitted mention of other relevant experimental findings.

Idiotypic markers

Anti-idiotypic reagents have been prepared against a large and rapidly increasing number of antibodies. Many of the early anti-idiotypes studied were prepared against antigen binding myeloma proteins which offered the obvious advantage of consisting of a single immunogen. Since normal antibody populations are generally heterogeneous, one might expect immunization against such induced antibody populations to lead either to a complex mixture of anti-idiotypes or, if no single antibody species were of sufficient immunogenic concentration, to no apparent anti-idiotypic activity at all. However, there have now been a large number of anti-idiotypes described against induced antibody populations. In order for such reagents to be produced it is probably necessary either for the humoral response to the antigen in question to be restricted in heterogeneity or for one or a few clones to be responsible for the majority of the antibody produced. Thus, in the phosphorylcholine (PC) system, only one major antibody population appears to be produced when normal BALB/c mice are immunized with PC, and this antibody shares idiotype with the myeloma protein TEPC 15 (Lieberman *et al.*, 1974). In the case of antiarsanyl (ARS) responses, the humoral antibody produced is more heterogeneous, but individual animals appear nevertheless to devote a substantial fraction of their total anti-ARS response to the production of the same restricted antibody population (Pawlak *et al.*, 1973).

The same is probably true for those protein antigens for which anti-idiotypes have been produced against normal antibody populations. Thus, for example, in the nuclease system (Sachs *et al.*, 1978), all animals of the prototype strain are found to produce substantial levels of the same idiotype-bearing antibodies when immunized with this antigen. In this case, it is clear that antibodies are produced against multiple antigenic determinants and that there is heterogeneity in the response to certain individual determinants as well. Nevertheless, restricted clonality of the response has been correlated with a particular isoelectric focusing pattern, or spectrotype of the induced antibodies (Miller and Sachs, in preparation). There are, of course, numerous antigens for which no characteristic idiotype has been obtained when purified antibodies have been used as immunogen, and presumably such antibody populations would not show restricted heterogeneity on isoelectric focusing.

With the recent advent of hybridoma technology (Köhler and Milstein, 1975), it has become possible to obtain virtually limitless amounts of monoclonal antibodies against a wide variety of antigens. Thus, anti-idiotypic antibodies against individual induced antibody molecules are now possible, permitting correlations between the idiotype markers thus observed and those observed for normal humoral responses. A prediction one might make is that for those responses for which production of anti-idiotypes has been possible using induced antibody populations, anti-idiotypes to hybridoma antibodies and to normal antibody populations will often crossreact, an example of which has already been reported (Marshak-Rothstein *et al.*, 1980). Conversely, those humoral responses which have not readily permitted production of anti-idiotype reagents may be quite heterogeneous, and therefore one might predict that anti-idiotypes to monoclonal antibodies would only infrequenly define idiotypes of the normal antibody population. In this regard, one series of antigens for which we have found it difficult to produce anti-idiotypes against normal humoral antibodies has been the H-2 antigens (Sachs, unpublished observations). Recently we have produced a series of anti-idiotypic reagents against anti-H-2K^k hybridoma antibodies and have found these to be unique, even with regard to examination of other hybridoma antibodies with apparently identical serologic specificity (Sachs *et al.*, 1980).

Idiotypic determinants of myeloma proteins have been classified as unique for the myeloma used for immunization (IdI) or cross-reactive with related antibodies (IdX) (Weigert and Riblet, 1978). In the case of normal antibody populations, Nisonoff has used the term cross-reactive idiotype (CRI) to describe idiotypic determinants which appear during the normal response to a particular antigen in many or all animals of a given inbred strain (Nisonoff *et al.*, 1977). Regardless of the source of the immunizing antibodies, only CRI determinants provide useful markers for studies of the genetic control of idiotype expression, since such studies depend on the detection of the idiotype markers among the progeny of appropriate crosses, and only markers with high levels of penetrance can be studied effectively. Many of the idiotypic markers for which such genetic mapping studies have been possible are summarized in Tables I and II.

Linkage between idiotype expression and Ig structural genes

Ig structural gene markers

In contrast to the idiotypic determinants discussed so far, there are another series of antigenic determinants of immunoglobulin chains which can be detected by immunization between different strains of inbred mice. Such determinants are called allotypes, and generally reflect polymorphism of amino acid sequence in the constant regions of the immunoglobulin chains. A large number of such allotypic markers have been identified and associated with most of the heavy chain classes (Lieberman, 1978). Any one strain inherits a set of these markers for each of the heavy chain classes, and by the most recent conventions, this set has been assigned a designation, such as Igh-C^a, in which Igh-C refers to the heavy chain constant region genes and the superscript *a* to the allele carried by a given strain (Green, 1979). Because no recombinants have yet been found between the allotypic markers of the various heavy chain classes within a given allelic set, the genes encoding these different heavy chain classes are thought to be very closely linked, and the entire complex is often referred to as the heavy chain allotype linkage group.

In contrast, although one might similarly expect to detect polymorphism of light chain constant regions by the use of allotypic reagents, no reliable markers of this type have yet been described for the κ chain constant region, despite the fact that greater than 95% of mouse Ig contains κ light chains. However, three other types of genetic markers for the detection of κ chain diversity have recently been described. The first is a peptide, called the I_B peptide, detected in tryptic digests of whole mouse κ chain preparations from

TABLE I
Cross-reactive idiotypes of monoclonal antibodies

Idiotype designation	*Antigen*	*Prototype antibody*	*Reference*
DEX	α-1,3 dextran	J558, M104, U102	Blomberg *et al.* (1972)
S117	A-CHO	S117	Berek *et al.* (1976)
UPC10	β-2,6 and β-2,1 polyfructans	UPC10, MOPC173	Bosma *et al.* (1977)
GAL	β-1,6 D-galactan	XRPC24	Mushinski and Potter (1977)
Inulin	β-2,1 fructans	E109	Lieberman *et al.* (1976)
TEPC15	Phosphorylcholine	T15, S63, H8	Lieberman *et al.* (1974)
460	DNP	MOPC460, MOPC315	Rosenstein *et al.* (1978)

TABLE II
Cross-reactive idiotypes of induced antibodies

Idiotype designation	*Antigen*	*Prototype strain*	*Reference*
ARS	*p*-azophenyl-arsonate	A/J	Pawlak *et al.* (1973)
A5A	A-CHO	A/J	Eichman (1973)
ACH_D	A-CHO	AKR	Krammer *et al.* (1978)
BGL	poly-G,L,Phe	B10.A(5R)	Kipps *et al.* (1977)
DEX	α-1,3 dextran	BALB/c	Riblet *et al.* (1975)
GA-1	poly-Glu,Ala,Tyr	D1.LP	Ju *et al.* (1979)
GAT	poly-Glu,Ala,Tyr	BALB/c	Thèze and Sommé (1979)
Inulin	polyfructosans	BALB/c	Lieberman *et al.* (1979)
Lysozyme	Hen egg white lysozyme	B10.A	Harvey *et al.* (1979)
M511	PC-KLH	BALB/c	Ruppert *et al.* (1980)
NASE A-E	Staphyloccal nuclease	A/J	Sachs *et al.* (1978)
NP^b	NP-BGG	C57BL/6	Karjalainen and Mäkelä (1978)
TGAL	poly-(T,G)--A--L	C3H.SW	Schwartz *et al.* (1978)
T15	R36A pneumo-cocci	BALB/c	Cosenza and Köhler (1972)

AKR, C58, RF and PL strains and not from numerous other strains tested (Edelman and Gottlieb, 1970). Sequence analyses have shown that the I_B peptide is derived from the V region of about 5% of the κ chains from positive strains. Presence of this peptide can thus be used as a marker for the presence of a framework (i.e., nonhypervariable) portion of the light chain variable region.

A second kind of marker recently described (Gibson, 1976; Claflin, 1976) is based on the pattern of bands obtained by isoelectric focusing of light chains. Characteristic differences in the presence or absence of certain bands in different inbred strains have been observed, and these differences appear also to constitute markers for the κ chain framework. The fact that no allotypic markers or structural variants have been noted for the κ chain constant region (Igk-C) probably indicates that there is very little diversity in the constant regions of available mouse strains (Weigert and Riblet, 1978). However, by analogy to the heavy chain allotype linkage group, these framework markers should nevertheless be satisfactory for the detection of linkage between Igk-C and idiotype expression.

Similarly, two other markers recently demonstrated to be linked to Igk-C are the Lyt-2 and Lyt-3 loci, loci which determine expression of the corresponding Lyt-2 and Lyt-3 antigens on subpopulations of T cells. Linkage between the Lyt-2,3 loci and Igk on chromosome 6 was first suggested by the finding that a congenic strain produced intentionally to introduce Lyt-2,3 antigens from AKR to the B6 background also carried the I_B peptide from the AKR strain (Gottlieb, 1974). This linkage has been confirmed by several other studies (summarized in Weigert and Riblet, 1978), and the Lyt-2,3 alleles can therefore now be used as markers for the κ chain locus, although the distance between these 2 loci has not yet been determined.

Heavy chain-linked idiotype markers

Most of the idiotype markers shown in Tables I and II have been demonstrated by classical genetic studies to be dependent upon loci linked to the heavy chain allotype linkage group. Three major methods for establishing such linkage have been used, and for several of the markers a combination of methods have established the linkage and provided mapping data by which relative distances between *Ig* genes determining these markers can be estimated.

The first method for establishing linkage is the use of classic backcross genetics. An example of the use of this methodology for establishment of linkage between nuclease idiotype markers and Igh-C allotype markers is shown in Table III (Fathman *et al.*, 1977). Idiotype in this system is defined by the inhibition of antibody-mediated inactivation of nuclease, and this inhibition has been shown by a variety of criteria to be binding-site related (Fathman and Sachs, 1976).

In the study shown in Table III, the characteristic A/J idiotype was examined by this method in a series of backcross progeny of the type (B10.A × A/J) backcrossed to B10.A. This particular backcross was chosen because the *H-2*^{a} haplotype is a high responder to nuclease, and therefore all of the progeny produced sufficient antinuclease antibodies to be informative. Since the B10.A strain does not express the A/J idiotype, one would expect this backcross to lead to segregation of those genes from A/J responsible for

TABLE III
Expression of A/J idiotype in (B10.A × A/J) × B10.A backcross progeny[a]

Animal No.	*Igh-C phenotype*	*Inhibition of inactivation (%)*	*Significance* (P < 0·05)
1	b/b	4.0	—
3	b/b	0·0	—
4	b/b	0·8	—
5	b/b	−2·4	—
7	b/b	1·9	—
9	b/b	2·4	—
12	b/b	0·3	—
14	b/b	27·1	+
15	b/b	42·3	+
17	b/b	−4·7	—
18	b/b	−0·9	—
19	b/b	−5·6	—
2	b/e	27·0	+
6	b/e	42·2	+
8	b/e	55·8	+
10	b/e	24·7	+
11	b/e	33·3	+
13	b/e	54·3	+
16	b/e	55·3	+

[a] From Fathman *et al.* (1977).

idiotype expression. Animals were typed by standard allotyping reagents in order to determine whether they were Igh-$C^{b/b}$ homozygotes or Igh-$C^{b/e}$ heterozygotes, and antinuclease antibodies from each individual animal were examined for inhibition of inactivation by the anti-A/J idiotype reagent. As can be seen in Table III, all animals which inherited the Igh-C^{e} allotype showed significant expression of the A/J idiotype, while 10 of 12 Igh-$C^{b/b}$ homozygotes did not show significant A/J idiotype expression. By X^2 analysis this data indicates highly significant linkage between genes coding for the A/J idiotype and those determining heavy chain allotype ($P < 0{\cdot}005$), and this is thus an example of the use of classic backcross genetics for establishing such linkage.

In addition to analysis of linkage, such backcross analyses also permit the identification of recombinant events between genetic markers. Thus, as also seen in Table III, 2 of the 12 Igh-$C^{b/b}$ homozygotes appeared to express significant amounts of the A/J idiotype, and this expression was verified by repeated analysis of these sera and by multiple bleedings. Thus, the possibility was raised that these 2 animals represented recombination events in which the genes responsible for idiotype expression from the Igh-C^{e} haplotype had recombined with genes responsible for the Igh-C^{b} allotype markers.

The obvious possible artifact of failure to detect the Igh-C^{e} allotype markers in these putative recombinant animals was shown to be very unlikely by the use of a much more sensitive haemagglutination inhibition assay for allotype (Pisetsky and Sachs, 1977). However, this high recombination frequency (about 10%) was still surprising, and therefore a much larger backcross analysis was performed. A total of 101 backcross animals of this type were examined. Among 36 Igh-C$^{b/e}$ heterozygotes, all were found to express significant amounts of the A/J idiotype. However, among 65 Igh-C$^{b/b}$ homozygotes, 7 putative recombinants expressing the A/J idiotype were detected (Pisetsky and Sachs, 1977). Thus a recombination frequency of nearly 10% was observed. In addition, of the ultimate test for true recombination is the examination of progeny of such putative recombinants, and this was also performed for the nuclease recombinants. Each putative recombinant was further backcrossed to B10.A and offspring were tested for the A/J idiotype. Approximately 50% of the offspring from each putative recombinant tested were found to express the A/J idiotype (Pisetsky and Sachs, 1977), thereby confirming that these animals did represent true recombination events. As will be discussed later, although these findings confirm the occurrence of recombination, they do not distinguish between recombination of a structural or a regulatory locus.

The second methodology commonly used to establish linkage involves the evaluation of responses in congenic strains. The production of Igh-C congenic lines is illustrated in Fig. 2, which shows schematically the production of the CB.20 line (Potter and Lieberman, 1967). Production of such lines involves crossing of two strains, in this case (BALB/c × C57BL), and successive backcrossing of the hybrid to the BALB/c partner. At each generation selection of appropriate offspring which have received the required Igh-C^{b} allele is performed by standard allotype testing, and after a given number of backcrosses (20 for the CB.20 line), the offspring are intercrossed and homozygotes selected. Such animals should contain all of the background genome of the BALB/c animal and differ only at the Igh-C locus and closely linked loci.

The use of such strains for establishment of linkage between markers is illustrated in Table IV. As seen in this table, the A5A idiotype marker is detectable in the A/J strain and in the C.Al-20 strain, but not in the BALB/c. Since the C.AL-20 strain represents a congenic line possessing the same heavy chain allotype linkage group as A/J, these data strongly suggest that expression of this marker is determined by an Igh-C-linked locus. Such linkage has also been demonstrated for this marker by classic backcross analysis (Pawlak *et al.*, 1973).

During the production of such congenic lines, there is of course the possibility for recombination to take place. Thus, it is conceivable that congenic lines possessing a given heavy chain allotype linkage group may in fact possess variable region markers from the congenic partner. Such recombination has indeed been demonstrated for the BAB-14, an animal similar to the CB.20, but possessing many idiotype markers from BALB/c (Eichmann, 1975).

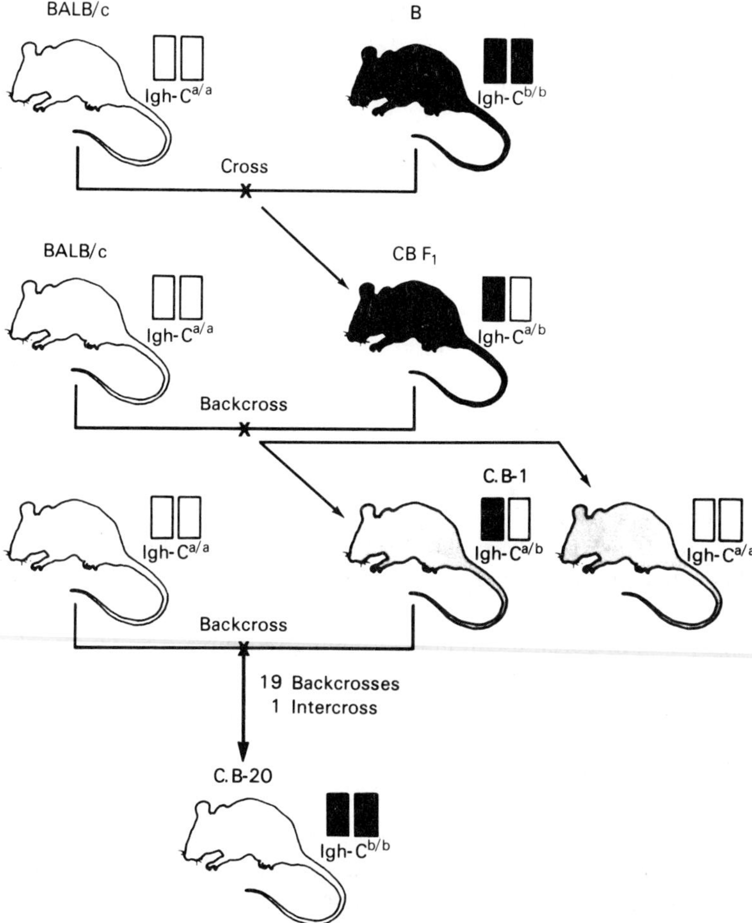

FIG. 2. *Schematic representation of the breeding scheme used to produce the C.B–20 allotype congenic line from BALB/c and C57BL parental lines (Potter and Lieberman, 1967).*

Other, less extensive recombination events may have occurred in other allotype congenic lines and not yet have been detected. Thus, failure to detect linkage by examination of congenic lines may not necessarily imply independence of the two markers, and a formal backcross analysis might be indicated.

The third methodology which has recently become increasingly important in the establishment of linkage and recombination frequencies involves the use of recombinant inbred lines (Bailey, 1971; Taylor *et al.*, 1975). These lines have been produced by crossing of 2 inbred lines, subsequent intercrossing of the F_1 progeny, and selection of breeding pairs among the F_2 progeny from which successive pedigreed inbreeding was then performed. This procedure leads to a scrambling of all of the genetic information in the original 2 lines, such that each recombinant inbred line obtained contains an in-

TABLE IV
Demonstration of Igh-C linkage by congenic lines[a]

	Strain				
Marker	*BALB/c* (*Igh-C^a*)	*C57BL* (*Igh-C^b*)	*A/J* (*Igh-C^e*)	*C.B-20* (*Igh-C^b*)	*C.AL-20* (*Igh-C^e*)
DEX	+	−	−	−	−
S117	+	−	−	−	−
ARS	−	−	+	−	+
A5A	−	−	+	−	+
BGL	−	+	−	+	−
NASE-C	−	+	−	+	−

[a] From Weigert and Riblet (1978).

dependent assortment of alleles at all segregating loci. Because the animals are sufficiently inbred, all loci of each line are theoretically homozygous, but the lines differ from each other for distinct segments of each chromosome. In addition to providing evidence for linkage between markers, these lines have also recently been useful in determining recombination frequencies between different markers and between idiotypes and heavy chain allotype markers (Weigert and Riblet, 1978).

Light chain-linked idiotype markers

Obviously, whenever a backcross analysis is performed, both heavy chain and light chain linkage groups should be segregating. Therefore, the fact that numerous idiotype markers have been determined to be linked to the Igh-C locus suggests either that idiotype expression is entirely dependent on the heavy chain, or that all mouse strains used in such backcross analyses can express the appropriate light chains to produce the idiotypic markers studied. Because there are numerous examples showing the contribution of light chain to idiotypic determinants, the former possibility would seem to be unlikely. In addition, Gottlieb and coworkers have made use of the linkage between Lyt-2, 3 markers and the κ chain locus to demonstrate that ARS idiotype marker expression is influenced by the Igk locus as well as by the Igh locus (Laskin *et al.*, 1977).

These workers noted that numerous previous studies involving backcrosses of idiotype positive and idiotype negative strains for examination of the ARS idiotype had never employed as the idiotype negative strain one of those 4 strains shown to express the I_B peptide (Gottlieb, 1974). They therefore examined a backcross between A/J and the PL/J strain, an idiotype negative strain which expresses the I_B peptide and is also different from A/J at the Lyt-3 locus, PL/J being Lyt-3·1, while A/J is Lyt-3·2. Among the progeny examined, there was a strong association between idiotype levels expressed and the Lyt-3 phenotype, high levels of idiotype being found only in Lyt-3 heterozygotes. Thus, in a case in which Igk polymorphism exists, linkage of idiotype expression to the Igk locus was detectable.

It seems likely, therefore, that light chain loci are involved in idiotype expression, but that the great similarity between light chain loci of all available inbred strains has made detection of light chain-linked idiotype markers difficult. Thus, in comparison to the corresponding heavy chain markers, there appears to be much less detectable polymorphism of both Igk-C and Igk-V markers.

Nature of genes controlling idiotype expression

Ig-linked genes

Using the methods described in the preceding section, several studies have now shown recombination between the expression of idiotype markers and Igh-C allotypic markers. In addition to the nuclease system described above, such classic recombination has also been observed for at least 12 other markers, with recombination frequencies ranging from 0·42% (V_{DEX}) to 3·8% (S117) (Weigert and Riblet, 1978). In several cases it has been possible to breed the recombinant animal, to select appropriate offspring inheriting the recombining chromosome, and to thus establish a new congenic heavy chain recombinant strain.

The most straightforward explanation for such apparent linkage between idiotype expression and Igh-C markers is undoubtedly that the idiotype markers represent structural V-region genes or HV regions of such genes, and that these elements are arrayed linearly along the chromosome bearing the Igh-C loci. In this case, the exceptionally high recombination frequency seen for some of the idiotypic markers would suggest either a very large chromosomal segment devoted to such V gene information, or some unusual property of this chromosomal region leading to a very high apparent recombination frequency. Recent studies of the molecular biology of immunoglobulin genes have shown the occurrence of gene rearrangements during the ontogeny of antibody producing cells (Tonegawa *et al.*, 1976). Such studies suggest that unorthodox joining mechanisms are indeed operative during the generation of immunoglobulin chains, and may therefore support the hypothesis that the linkage of idiotype expression to allotype markers is a function of structural genes. That is, absence of an idiotype in the population of antibodies elicited by a particular antigen would imply the absence of the corresponding V gene or HV segment in the structural gene repertoire. As such, one might hope to construct a linear map of idiotype markers which would reflect the linear order of the corresponding V genes on the immunoglobulin structural gene chromosomes. Early maps for such markers have already been constructed (Eichmann, 1973; Weigert and Riblet, 1978), although some inconsistencies still remain with regard to map distances.

Despite the plausibility of such a structural basis for control of idiotype expression, there is considerable evidence that idiotype expression is subject to both positive and negative regulation *in vivo*. For example, there is now evidence for several of the idiotype markers listed in Tables I and II, that *in vivo* administration of exogenous anti-idiotype can have a profound effect on idiotype expression upon subsequent challenge with antigen. In several cases such effects have been shown for expression of idiotypes for which Igh-C-linked control of expression has likewise been established. In both the ARS and TEPC 15 systems, for example, administration of exogenous anti-idiotype leads to failure of animals to produce the CRI upon subsequent challenge with antigen (Nisonoff *et al.*, 1977; Cosenza and Köhler, 1972). In the case of anti-ARS idiotype suppression, specific antibody is nevertheless produced, in quantity and affinity equivalent to that of unmanipulated animals. However, the CRI, which would ordinarily be a major component of the humoral response, has been found to be missing.

Even more striking evidence for regulation of idiotype expression is provided by the work of Cazenave and colleagues, who have been able to induce expression of an idiotype marker in a strain in which the corresponding V gene information should be missing according to a structural hypothesis for idiotype expression (Le Guern *et al.*, 1979). Thus, unlike BALB/c mice, DBA/2 mice ordinarily do not express the 460 idiotype (Ab1 in the Cazenave nomenclature) when immunized with DNP-ovalbumin. However, when DBA/2 animals were treated with anti-idiotype to 460 (Ab2), they uniformly began to produce 460 idiotype in their serum (Ab3), although this idiotype did not correlate with anti-DNP binding activity. When such Ab3 producing DBA/2 animals were then challenged with DNP-ovalbumin they began to produce anti-DNP antibodies bearing the 460 idiotype.

One explanation for these findings is that the nonantigen binding Ab3 molecules use the same hypervariable regions responsible for the 460 idiotopes (see Introduction), but not in the unique combination required for antigen binding activity. However, the unique combination may exist within this population and then be expanded upon subsequent challenge with antigen. We have recently obtained similar evidence for the induction of inappropriate idiotype expression in the nuclease system, using a series of non-site-specific idiotypic determinants (Sachs *et al.*, in preparation).

The mechanism by which idiotype is expressed after such *in vivo* treatment remains unclear, and the argument can be made that such induction of idiotype occurs via very different pathways than those involved in the normal immune response. However, the fact remains that those very strains which have been considered negative for certain idiotype markers in mapping and recombination studies can, under certain circumstances, produce those idiotype markers. Therefore, the possibility must be entertained that even in the unmanipulated animal, control mechanisms of a regulatory nature determine idiotype expression. In fact, one cannot yet rule out the possibility that all of the *Ig*-linked genes which have so far been mapped are in fact involved in regulating expression of *V* genes, perhaps at a level far removed from structural gene expression, such as at the level of intercellular network interactions (Jerne, 1974).

Non-*Ig*-linked loci

Given the relationship between idiotype expression and antibody activity discussed above, it is clear that any gene involved in the control of the immune response to a particular antigen must of necessity also exert some control on idiotype expression. Thus, there are a large number of immune response genes (*Ir* genes) which have been shown to control responsiveness of inbred strains of mice to a variety of antigens, and all of these genes should also be considered in the control of idiotype expression. The most widely studied *Ir* genes are those linked to the MHC, known as *Ir-1* (Benacerraf and McDevitt, 1972). However, numerous studies have also shown genetic control of immune responses linked neither to the MHC nor to the *Ig* structural gene loci (for review see Berzofsky, 1980).

Of necessity, such control of idiotype expression by non-Ig-linked genes must be on a regulatory rather than a structural basis. Thus, an *Ir* gene such as the H-2-linked *Ir* gene controlling responsiveness to the synthetic polypeptide TGAL determines the overall antibody production to TGAL among inbred mouse strains (McDevitt *et al.*, 1972). If one examines 2 H-2 congenic strains such as C3H (H-2^k) and C3H.SW (H-2^b) which differ only at H-2 and closely linked loci, the anti-TGAL idiotype level measured following immunization with TGAL is much higher in the C3H.SW responder strain than in the congenic partner (Schwartz *et al.*, 1978; Pincus *et al.*, 1978). Such control is, however, strictly quantitative, since the idiotype levels reflect the amount of anti-TGAL antibody produced.

On the other hand, *Ir* gene control can lead to control of idiotype expression even between strains both of which are responders. Thus, for example, in the antinuclease antibody response, it has been shown that H-2-linked *Ir* genes exert control on the relative amount of antibody produced against different antigenic determinants of the nuclease molecule (Berzofsky *et al.*, 1977). Thus, when hyperimmune sera from H-2^b (low responder) and H-2^a (high responder) congenic strains were examined, the ratio of antibodies to different determinants was significantly different (Table V). Clearly, if one were measuring the idiotype of antibodies against determinants in the region 99–149, it would appear that the H-2-linked *Ir* gene controlled the level of expression of such an idiotype despite the fact that the overall antinuclease responses of the strains is similar. Evidence has also been obtained in the nuclease system for the existence of at least one non-H-2-linked *Ir* gene which controls the overall hyperimmune level of antinuclease responses and which is responsible for the great difference in total antinuclease produced between

TABLE V

Concentrations of antibodies to subregions of nuclease in antinuclease sera[a]

Strain	*H-2* *haplotype*	*Antinuclease activity*[b] *(units/ml)*	*Antibody binding sites* (μ *M*)[c] *anti-(99-149)*	*anti-(1-126)*	*Ratio* *anti-(99-149)/anti-(1-126)*
B10	*b*	120	0·26 ± 0·03	1·2 ± 0·15	0·22
B10.A	*a*	113	0·71 ± 0·03	0·8 ± 0·12	0·89
A.BY	*b*	1200	2·55 ± 0·09	17·2 ± 0·36	0·15
A/J	*a*	920	5·75 ± 0·30	12·7 ± 0·55	0·45

[a] Hyperimmune pooled sera from each strain was assessed; data from Berzofsky *et al.* (1977)

[b] Measured as units of nuclease inhibited/ml serum.

[c] Measured by radioimmunoassay with ^{14}C-labelled fragments.

the A background animals and the B10 background animals, as seen in Table V (Pisetsky *et al.*, 1978). Again, such a gene must also be considered as regulating the idiotype levels of antibodies produced, although in this case Igh-C-linked loci are of much greater importance, as noted above.

It is important to note that in the case of such non-Ig-linked control of idiotype expression, low idiotype producing strains would nevertheless be expected to be capable of producing the relevant idiotopes. The reason for which such idiotopes are not produced is that the relevant antigenic determinant is recognized differentially by the strains compared. Thus, such control does not necessarily imply anything about the structure of the receptors involved. Although this caveat is easily accepted for immunoglobulin idiotypes, it is perhaps less obvious for T cell idiotypes, since the structure of the T cell receptor is not yet known. An example of such a dilemma can be seen in the recent studies of Krammer and Eichmann (1977), in which control of T cell receptor idiotypes by both *Igh-C*-linked and *MHC*-linked genes was reported. In this study, a backcross of (AKR × SJL)F_1 animals to the SJL parental was performed. Animals were divided into four groups, of the type: (1) H-2$^{s/s}$, Igh-C$^{b/b}$; (2) H-2$^{s/s}$, Igh-C$^{b/d}$; (3) H-2$^{s/k}$, Igh-C$^{b/b}$; (4) h-2$^{s/k}$, Igh-C$^{b/d}$. Lymph node T cells from each group were activated agains B6 stimulator cells in a mixed lymphocyte culture, and the resulting T cell blasts were tested for expression of a putative AKR anti-B6 receptor idiotype. Since only group 4 was found to be significantly positive for idiotype expression, the authors concluded that both *H-2*-linked and *Igh-C*-linked genes from the AKR parental (H-2$^{k/k}$, Igh-C$^{d/d}$) were required for idiotype expression. The authors were of course unable to distinguish between a regulatory influence of the *H-2*-linked genes or involvement of H-2 products in the T cell receptor. However, in view of both the differential response to different determinants discussed above for the antinuclease response, and the probable sharing of specificities between $H\text{-}2^k$ and $H\text{-}2^b$, it is worth considering that the response of an $H\text{-}2^{s/k}$ animal to $H\text{-}2^{b/b}$ might involve responses to different determinants than the response of $H\text{-}2^{s/s}$ to the same stimulator. Such non-*Ig*-linked control of idiotype expression could in fact constitute the regulatory mechanism explaining these results. Of course, direct involvement of H-2-linked products in the receptor is also a possible explanation, but would imply that idiotype expression by T cell receptors has a different structural basis than that of B cell receptors. In view of the high level of current interest in T cell receptors and their idiotypes, it is worth keeping in mind the possible regulatory influences of non-*Ig*-linked genes on idiotype expression.

Conclusions

We have examined several levels at which genetic control of idiotype expression may be exerted. Foremost is control by *Ig*-linked genes, the simplest explanation for which would probably involve a structural mechanism. By such an hypothesis, the genes controlling idiotype expression would be responsible for the primary sequence of a particular antibody heavy and/or light chain V region or the hypervariable segments thereof. However, we have also noted that there is considerable evidence of regulation of expression of idiotypes even in systems for which *Ig*-linked control of idiotype expression has been demonstrated. Therefore, the possibility that regulatory rather than structural genes are responsible for *Ig*-linked idiotype expression must still be entertained.

There is also now considerable genetic mapping data supporting a linear array of *Igh-C*-linked genes controlling expression of different specific idiotypes. Thus, if regulatory genes are in fact responsible for this level of control, these genes would appear nevertheless to behave as classic genetic units with respect to segregation and recombination. If regulation occurs at an intercellular level, such as via anti-idiotype receptors or suppressor cells, then these mechanisms must in turn be controlled by *Ig*-linked genes.

On the other hand, it seems clear that regulatory genes must be responsible for non-*Ig*-linked genetic control of idiotype expression. We have examined several mechanims by which such control could be manifested, and have noted the importance of considering such mechanisms in the interpretation of data concerning idiotype expression on T cell receptors.

Idiotype expression is presently a central theme in immunologic research. From a theoretical viewpoint, it seems possible that anti-idiotype–idiotype interactions may be important in regulation of immune response (i.e., the network theory), a topic which has been covered extensively in another symposium in this volume (Theme 2). In addition, understanding of the genetics of *Ig*-linked idiotype expression may help to unravel the mechanism by which diversity of immunoglobulin variable regions is generated. Idiotype markers also provide valuable tools for examining cellular interactions in the immune response, in particular for following the origin of specific cellular receptors.

From a more practical viewpoint, control of idiotype expression by means of exogenous anti-idiotype administration could provide a specific mode of immunotherapy. Since both augmentation and suppression of specific immune responses have been obtained by this means, one might envision the use of anti-idiotypes to increase responses to infectious agents or perhaps to tumour antigens, or to decrease responses of an autoimmune nature or to transplantation antigens for purposes of organ grafting. In any case, it seems likely that studies of the mechanisms by which idiotype expression is controlled will flourish over the next few years, and that many of the perplexing questions posed in this review will not long remain unanswered.

References

Bailey, D. W. (1971). *Transplantation* **11**, 325.

Benacerraf, B. and McDevitt, H. O. (1972). *Science* **175**, 273.

Berek, C., Taylor, B. A. and Eichmann, K. (1976). *J. Exp. Med.* **144**, 1164.

Berzofsky, J. A., Schechter, A. N., Shearer, G. M. and Sachs, D. H. (1977). *J. Exp. Med.* **145**, 123.

Berzofsky, J. A. (1980). *In* "Biological Regulation and Development" (R. F. Goldberger, ed.) Vol. 2. Plenum Press, New York. (In press.)

Blomberg, B., Geckeler, W. R. and Weigert, M. (1972). *Science* **177**, 178.

Bosma, M. J., DeWitt, C., Hausman, S. J., Marks, R. and Potter, M. (1977). *J. Exp. Med.* **146**, 1041.

Claflin, J. L. (1976). *Eur. J. Immunol.* **6**, 669.

Cosenza, H. and Köhler, H. (1972). *Proc. Natn. Acad. Sci. U.S.A.* **69**, 2701.

Edelman, G. M. and Gottlieb, P. D. (1970). *Proc. Natn. Acad. Sci. U.S.A.* **67**, 1192.

Eichmann, K. (1973). *J. Exp. Med.* **137**, 603.

Eichmann, K. (1975). *Immunogenetics* **2**, 491.

Fathman, C. G. and Sachs, D. H. (1976). *J. Immunol.* **116**, 959.

Fathman, C. G., Pisetsky, D. S. and Sachs, D. H. (1977). *J. Exp. Med.* **145**, 569.

Gell, P. G. H. and Kelus, A. S. (1964). *Nature, London* **201**, 687.

Gibson, D. (1976). *J. Exp. Med.* **144**, 298.

Gottlieb, P. D. (1974). *J. Exp. Med.* **140**, 1432.

Green, M. C. (1979). *Immunogenetics* **8**, 89.

Harvey, M. A., Adorini, L., Miller, A. and Sercarz, E. E. (1979). *Nature, London* **281**, 594.

Jerne, N. K. (1974). *Ann. Immunol., Paris* **125c**, 373.

Ju. S-T., Pierres, M., Germain, R. N., Benacerraf, B. and Dorf, M. E. (1979). *J. Immunol.* **123**, 2505.

Karjalainen, K. and Mäkelä, O. (1978). *Eur. J. Immunol.* **8**, 105.

Kipps, T. J., Benacerraf, B. and Dorf, M. E. (1977). *Eur. J. Immunol.* **7**, 865.

Köhler, G. and Milstein, C. (1975). *Nature, London* **256**, 495.

Krammer, P. H. and Eichmann, K. (1977). *Nature, London* **270**, 733.

Krammer, P., Taylor, B. A. and Eichmann, K. (1978). *Z. ImmunForsch. Immunobiol.* **154**, 284.

Kunkel, H. G., Mannik, M. and Williams, R. C. (1963). *Science* **140**, 1218.

Laskin, J. A., Gray, A., Nisonoff, A., Klinman, N. R., and Gottlieb, P. D. (1977). *Proc. Natn. Acad. Sci. U.S.A.* **74**, 4600.

Le Guern, C., Aissa, F. B., Juy, D., Mariamé, B., Buttin, G. and Cazenave, P-A. (1979). *Ann. Immunol., Paris* **130c**, 293.
Lieberman, R. (1978). *Immunopathology* **1**, 7.
Lieberman, R., Potter, M., Mushinski, E. B., Humphrey, W. Jr and Rudikoff, S. (1974). *J. Exp. Med.* **139**, 983.
Lieberman, R., Potter, M., Humphrey, W. Jr, Mushinski, E. B. and Vrana, M. (1975). *J. Exp. Med.* **142**, 106.
Lieberman, R., Potter, M., Humphrey, W. Jr and Chien, C. C. (1976). *J. Immunol.* **117**, 2105.
Lieberman, R., Bona, C., Chien, C. C., Stein, K. E. and Paul, W. E. (1979). *Ann. Immunol., Paris* **130**, 247.
McDevitt, H. O., Deak, B. D., Shreffler, D. C., Klein, J., Stimpfling, J. H. and Snell, G. D. (1972). *J. Exp. Med.* **135**, 1259.
Marshak-Rothstein, A., Siekevitz, M., Margolies, M. N., Mudgett-Hunter, M. and Gefter, M. L. (1980). *Proc. Natn. Acad. Sci. U.S.A.* **77**, 1120.
Mushinski, E. B. and Potter, M. (1977). *J. Immunol.* **119**, 1888.
Nisonoff, A., Hopper, J. E. and Springer, S. B. (1975). "The Antibody Molecule." Academic Press, New York.
Nisonoff, A., Ju, S-T. and Owen, F. L. (1977). *Immunological Rev.* **34**, 89.
Oudin, J. and Michel, M. (1963). *C. R. Acad. Sci., Paris* **257**, 805.
Padlan, E. A. (1977). *Proc. Natn. Acad. Sci. U.S.A.* **74**, 2551.
Pawlak, L. L., Mushinski, E. B., Nisonoff, A. and Potter, M. (1973). *J. Exp. Med.* **137**, 22.
Pincus, S. H., Sachs, D. H. and Dickler, H. B. (1978). *J. Immunol.* **121**, 1422.
Pisetsky, D. S. and Sachs, D. H. (1977). *J. Exp. Med.* **146**, 1603.
Pisetsky, D. S., Berzofsky, J. A. and Sachs, D. H. (1978). *J. Exp. Med.* **147**, 396.
Potter, M. and Lieberman, R. (1967). *Adv. Immunol.* **7**, 91.
Riblet, R., Blomberg, B., Weigert, M., Lieberman, R., Taylor, B. A. and Potter, M. (1975). *Eur. J. Immunol.* **5**, 775.
Rosenstein, R. W., Zeldis, J. B., Konigsberg, W. H. and Richards, F. F. (1978). *Mol. Immunol.* **16**, 361.
Ruppert, V. J., Williams, K. and Claflin, J. L. (1980). *J. Immunol.* **124**, 1068.
Sachs, D. H., Berzofsky, J. A., Pisetsky, D. S. and Schwartz, R. H. (1978). *Springer Semin. Immunopathol.* **1**, 51.
Sachs, D. H., Bluestone, J. A., Epstein, S. L. and Ozato, K. (1980). *Transplant. Proc.* (in press).
Schwartz, M., Lifshitz, R., Givol, D., Mozes, E. and Haimovich, J. (1978). *J. Immunol.* **121**, 421.
Slater, R. J., Ward, S. M. and Kunkel, H. G. (1955). *J. Exp. Med.* **101**, 85.
Taylor, B. A., Cherry, M., Bailey, D. W. and Shapiro, L. S. (1975). *Immunogenetics* **1**, 529.
Thèze, J. and Sommé, G. (1979). *Eur. J. Immunol.* **9**, 294.
Tonegawa, S., Hozumi, N., Matthyssens, G., and Schuller, R. (1976). *Cold Spring Harbor Symp. Quant. Biol.* **41**, 877.
Weigert, M. and Riblet, R. (1978). *Springer Semin. Immunopathol.* **1**, 133.
Wu, T. T. and Kabat, E. A. (1970). *J. Exp. Med.* **132**, 211.

Theme 7: Summary
Genetic Regulation of Immune Responsiveness

M. SELA

Department of Chemical Immunology, The Weizmann Institute of Science, Rehovot, Israel

Immunity is not inherited, but the susceptibility to lead to a good or poor immune response is definitely under strict genetic control, and is in most, but by no means all cases, linked to the major histocompatibility locus of the species. The initial observations, mainly from the laboratories of Benacerraf, of McDevitt and our own, were obtained thanks to the successful combined use of synthetic antigens (simple chemically) and inbred strains of mice and guinea-pigs (simple genetically).

This whole field of research started developing in the 1960s, with most of the crucial observations made in the second half of that decade, but the tremendous and amazing progress, with all its implications for our present-day understanding of immune phenomena was obtained in the last decade, in an almost exponential expansion. It is, therefore, not surprising that much of what we know today has been elucidated in the last 3 years, and many of the most interesting and as yet unanswered questions have been posed also only in the last few years. Thus, the summary of this theme can be only sketchy and selective.

Two genetic regions regulate immune responses. The major histocompatibility complex (MHC) and the immunoglobulin V_H genes. These genes and their products mediate such regulations by controlling essential cell interactions involving helper and suppressor T cells, and by determining the specificity of T lymphocyte clones stimulated by antigen.

The realization that the *Ir* genes are H-linked led to the identification of a new region of the MHC, the *I* region, where *Ir* genes map, and to the demonstration that this region codes for glycoprotein antigens, Ia molecules, expressed selectively on macrophages, B cells and activated T cells. It was then demonstrated that T cells are committed to MHC gene products and to T-dependent antigens concomitantly. Another important discovery was the critical role of antigen presentation by macrophages to stimulate T cells, and the contribution of Ia molecules to the specificity of helper T cells and delayed type hypersensitivity (DTH) T cells. The *I* region controls T–B cell interactions and is related also to macrophage-T cell interactions. One of the most recent events has been the discovery of T cell regulatory factors bearing I region controlled determinants.

As Benacerraf clearly exposed (Chapter 23), *Ir* genes are identical with Ia molecules because: (1) they map onto the same genetic region; (2) specific helper and DTH T cells bind antigen, and are stimulated only when antigen is presented in conjunction with the appropriate Ia molecule; (3) stimulation of these T cells by antigen on antigen-presenting cells is blocked by appropriately specific anti-Ia serum; (4) *Ir* gene complementation for responses to a synthetic polypeptide antigen composed of glutamic acid, lysine and phenylalanine, parallels clearly the complementation between *I–E* controlled

α chain and *I–A* controlled β chain; (5) the expression of Ia-7 specificity controlled by the *I–E* subregion correlates with the *Ir* α gene of the above mentioned antigen.

How do Ia molecules selectively and specifically restrict T cell responses? Two mechanisms can be evoked. In one, a specific interaction between Ia molecules and antigen is postulated to permit effective presentation of the complex. According to the other, during T cell differentiation in the thymus, individual clones are restricted to display receptors for certain antigens and certain Ia molecules selectively. Benacerraf (Chapter 23) favours the first hypothesis on the basis that the specificity of *Ir* genes does not match the specificity of T cell responses controlled by the genes.

Another topic discussed by him was the control of suppressor T cell responses specific for a hapten. I.v. administration of haptenated spleen cells induces suppressor T cells which are hapten specific, and possess both idiotypic and I–J determinants on their surface. From these cells a suppressor factor was obtained which induces a second set of suppressor T cells, which are anti-idiotypic. The first set of cells can be enriched on antigen-coated plates, whereas the second set can be enriched on idiotype-coated plates. Moreover, hapten-specific cells suppress immune induction, whereas anti-idiotypic cells suppress immune cells at the effector phase of the response. The antigen-specific suppressor factor is not MHC restricted but is functionally restricted by V_H genes. In contrast, the effector suppressor cells and the factor they produce are restricted in their activity by both V_H genes and *I* region genes. Benacerraf believes that allo-reactive cells arise as a consequence of the commitment of T cells to self-MHC antigens, and because of immunization with virally infected syngeneic cells. Indeed, immunization with Sendai virus on syngeneic cells stimulates cells that are concomitantly specific for Sendai on syngeneic cells and also for allogeneic cells.

Not all genetically controlled immune responses are linked to the major histocompatibility locus of the species. Some are linked to the allotype, to the coat colour, or to the X-chromosome. It appears that on the X-chromosome of mice, *Ir* genes, histocompatibility antigen loci, and loci controlling T and B lymphocyte surface antigens are to be found together. These associations are homologous to those of the MHC-complex on the 17th chromosome.

The workshop (5.6)* on this topic reached the conclusion that there is no definite example of multigenic immune response regulation excluding formally *H-2* linked control. Examples discussed included red blood cells, T-independent antigens, cellular membrane determinants and parasites. The non *H-2* linked genes have been tentatively mapped in the case of allotype linkage for antipig insulin response, Ea-4 linkage for anti-H-2 response, "d" coat colour linkage for anti*Brucella* response, and X-chromosome linkage for antilipopolysaccharide response. In the case of non *H-2* controlled anti-red blood cell response a defect was allocated to B cell.

David Sachs (Chapter 26) discussed the genetic control of idiotype expression. Foremost is the control by Ig-linked genes, the simplest explanation for which would involve a structural mechanism. By such a hypothesis, the genes controlling idiotype expression would be responsible for the primary sequence of a particular antibody heavy and/or light chain V region or the hypervariable segments thereof. However, there is considerable evidence for regulation of expression of idiotypes even in systems for which *Ig*-linked control of idiotype expression has been demonstrated. Therefore, the possibility that regulatory rather than structural genes are responsible for *Ig*-linked idiotype expression must still be entertained.

Understanding of the genetics of *Ig*-linked idiotype expression may help to unravel the mechanism by which diversity of immunoglobulin variable regions is generated. Sachs suggests that, from a more practical viewpoint, control of idiotype expression by means of exogenous anti-idiotype administration could provide a specific mode of immunotherapy. Since both augmentation and suppression of specific immune re-

* Reference numbers indicate Abstract numbers in: Abstracts 4th International Congress of Immunology, Paris, 1980.

sponses have been obtained by this means, one might envision the use of anti-idiotypes to increase responses to infectious agents or to tumour antigens, or to decrease responses of an autoimmune nature or to transplantation antigens for purposes of organ grafting.

Biozzi (Chapter 24) dealt with genetic selections for relevant immunological functions such as antibody response, macrophage activity and T cell response to phytohaemagglutinin. All these functions may be drastically modified by selective breeding for high and low responder lines of mice. The genetic regulation is under polygenic control. Individual phenotypes for each of the functions investigated are determined by the interaction of genetic and environmental factors, and each function has an independent genetic regulation.

High antibody responder mice are more resistant than low responders against the type of infection in which antibody plays a protective role, such as malaria, pneumococcus or trypanosomiasis. High macrophage activity lines of mice are more resistant than low activity lines against the types of infection in which macrophage function constitutes the principal protective mechanism (*Salmonella, Brucella, Yersinia, Leishmania*).

A workshop (5.5) on polygenic regulation of immune responsiveness discussed polygenic control in inbred strains of mice. In the F liver antigen system the dominance of nonresponsiveness is seen as a way of preventing autoimmunity. Studies were also reported in humans and guinea-pigs. Controversial results were discussed about delayed hypersensitivity and antibody affinity in high and low Biozzi mice.

Rosenthal (Chapter 25) discussed the role of macrophages in genetic control of immune response. T cell recognition of antigen requires an initial uptake of antigen by metabolically intact presenting cells of macrophage lineage. Presentation of antigen associated with macrophages is restricted by major histocompatibility complex in that only syngeneic or semisyngeneic presenting cells and T cells respond. When evaluating antigens of restricted heterogeneity, the response to which is controlled by *I* region-linked immune response genes, only macrophages of responder haplotype present antigen to F_1 responder by nonresponder T cells.

From studies with defined synthetic segments of insulin reacting with guinea-pig macrophages and T cells, Rosenthal concludes that MHC restriction and *Ir* restriction depend upon successful physical macrophage–lymphocyte interaction, and thus that macrophages represent a principal site of expression of *Ir* gene influence. He also suggests that the T cell does not recognize native determinants but rather interacts with selected molecular domains of processed antigen. Ia must represent at least in part cellular interaction structures. Additional associative interaction takes place between Ia and processed antigen. This process he calls "determinant selection".

The workshop on the role of macrophage Ia molecules in *Ir* gene control of specific immune responses (5.2) addressed itself to four questions. 1. Is there only one antigen-presenting cell or can more than one cell type present antigen? Everybody agreed that both macrophages and dendritic cells could function under some circumstances. 2. Do Ia-bearing molecules function in antigen presentation? The answer is that anti-Ia antibodies, including monoclonal reagents, inhibit T cell responses by reacting with Ia molecules on the antigen presenting cell and not on the T cell. The T cell receptor has a higher affinity for the antigen-Ia complex than for free antigen. 3. Do antigen-presenting cells process antigen? Here, there is no clear answer. The T cell certainly recognizes only a fragment of a protein antigen, while kinetic studies of antigen presentation suggest that 20 to 30 min are required for macrophages to effectively stimulate T cells, whereas antigen uptake takes only 5 min. And the last question, 4. What is the relationship between macrophage presentation and suppressor cell induction? There appear to be specific determinants which stimulate only suppressor cells, but no evidence was presented as to whether macrophages are involved in presentation of such determinants. Finally, interesting data was presented, supporting the notion that *Ir* gene products are the Ia-bearing molecules. It should be also mentioned that the isolation of antigen-Ia complexes, which can induce T cell functions both *in vitro* and *in vivo*, suggests that this complex is the biologically active component from macrophages involved in T cell stimulation.

The workshop on functions of *I* region genes in the regulation of immune responses (5.1) considered three main areas: *I* region control of restriction of lymphocyte interaction, *Ir* gene control of immune responsiveness, and cellular expression and serology of Ia antigens. Macrophages seem to have played a crucial role in most workshops as well as symposium lectures and this workshop expressed general agreement that helper and prolifering T lymphocytes display "restriction", defined as recognition of discreet *I* region determined "self" products, in their interaction with macrophages. This was supported by work with long-term lines and with cloned T cell populations. In addition, results were presented to further support the concept that the T lymphocyte *Ir* phenotype is determined by the *Ir* genotype of the developmental environment and the antigen presenting cells used in priming. Particularly, it was shown that this could be obtained in fully allogeneic chimaeras as well as in semiallogeneic ones previously used.

Is there a comparable restriction in the interaction of T and B lymphocytes? Or are all such restrictions artifacts due to the fact that the B cell population is usually the source of the antigen presenting cells? The restriction might depend on the state of differentiation of the B cell.

What is the significance of the finding that animals which are low responders to certain antigens may nonetheless develop T cells capable of responding to these antigens after priming with nonreactive antigens to which the animals are high-responders? This is a heteroclitic situation in which the *Ir* phenotype determines that two cross-reactive antigens behave such that the first one is a better immunogen and a better stimulant but that both probably use the same *Ir* determined system when the second one is an *Ir* controlled nonimmunogen.

How do *Ir* genes regulate the fine specificity and idiotype of the antibodies produced? It was suggested that the mechanism through which *Ir* genes determine expression of idiotypes on B cells might really reflect the fact that the receptor of the T cells for the antigen expresses that idiotype, and that anti-idiotype specific T cells (or antibodies) then lead to the preferential expression of idiotype in the pool of activated B cells.

Some mention during the workshop was made also of the genetic control of delayed type hypersensitivity responses (DTH). DTH response to the synthetic antigen (T,G)-A--L is genetically controlled in mice, like the humoral responses, and the gene regulating the responses is mapped in the *I–A* subregion of the *I* region in the *H-2* complex. Efficient DTH responses require T–T cell collaboration. The first cell is the (T,G)-A--L activated T cell which is of the Ly-1^+ type and is radioresistant, whereas the second cell is not stimulated by antigen and is radiosensitive and of Ly-$1,2,3^+$. Two types of non responders were found. In one type ($H\text{-}2^k$ haplotype) the defect is in their second cell, which is not triggered by the activated T cell and antigen to manifest the DTH response. In the other type ($H\text{-}2^s$ haplotype) the defect is expressed in both activation and manifestation steps of DTH, on the antigen presenting cell level.

The workshop on the genetic control of T cell suppression (5.3) focused on the contributory roles of either the major histocompatibility complex or the immunoglobulin/heavy chain complex set of genes in the induction of regulatory T cell subsets. The mixed leukocyte reaction may induce suppressor T cells which could dampen the antibody response to a T independent antigen. The impact of antigen density on the induction of MHC restricted suppressor T cells was also discussed. It is clear that the induction signals for suppression are influenced by genes of the major histocompatibility locus, the *Ig-h* locus, and possibly other unidentified regions. The sequence of events in the mouse includes the induction of idiotype bearing I^-J^+ T cells and the consequent generation of anti-idiotypic regulatory cells.

The workshop on antigen specific helper and suppressor factors bearing I region determinants (5.4) discussed helper factors from T cells, long-term cell lines and hybridomas. As a rule, these molecules bind antigen, bear V_H or idiotypic determinants shared with similar antibodies, lack Ig constant region determinants and possess Ia (I-A) coded determinants. Several molecules directly activate B cells together with antigen, whereas others require additional T cell function for activity. Similar molecules may be obtained from murine and human cells. Ly-1^+ cells produce these helper molecules.

Specific suppressor factors could also be obtained from T cells, long-term lines and hybridomas. These were similar to helper factors in constitution, and have a mol. wt of 50 000 to 70 000. In addition, most suppressor factors possess Ia (I-J) coded determinants, although one factor, specific for sheep red blood cells, lacked detectable H-2 specificities. One group found the factor to consist of two dissimilar chains, one binding the antigen and the other bearing Ia determinants, whereas others found only one chain possessing I-J and antigen-binding activity, though the function of this molecule is still undefined.

Heterogeneity of I-J determinants on suppressor factors was described, monoclonal anti-I-J antibodies have been produced, and heteroantisera specific for either all helper or all suppressor factors were described. An interesting workshop was devoted to the genetic regulation of immune responsiveness in innate resistance and the efficacy of prophylactic immunization against microbial and parasitic infections (5.7). Both innate susceptibility and efficacy of prophylactic immunization have been found to be under major genetic control, with a wide range of different microbial and parasitic infections. While these genes are predominantly non-H-2 linked in mice, one example of the converse discussed was the involvement of *MHC*-linked regulation of susceptibility to infection with a nematode (*Trichinella spiralis*). Even here, however, other genes are clearly involved. The extent of genetic association for different infections is largely undetermined. However, several loci have been clearly identified.

In addition to identification of susceptibility genes in inbred and congenic mice, considerable use has been made of the Biozzi high and low antibody responding lines of mice. Resistance to various infections is conferred either by high antibody responsiveness or by the macrophage hyperactivity of low responder animals which influences intracellular infections. The exceptional resistance of Biozzi low line (selection I) mice to *Salmonella typhimurium* was demonstrated to be due to genes distinct from the major *Ity* locus. One interesting example of genetic control in nonmurine species concerned the polymorphism of response to prophylactic immunization against an intestinal nematode in sheep.

While considerable progress is being made in the identification and mapping of genes controlling susceptibility to infection, we as yet know relatively little about the mechanisms whereby they exert their effects. Macrophages may be involved intrinsically or extrinsically. A role for NK cells in resistance to several haemotropic protozoa was proposed on the basis of correlative strain differences, but this awaits direct demonstration. Suppressor T cell involvement in susceptibility to human leprosy and murine *Leishmania tropica* infection is demonstrable, but it is not yet known whether these are primary genetic events.

Does a summary need another summary? I doubt it. But maybe it is worth emphasizing once again that the most important findings of the last few years include the realization of the importance of the thymic environment in determining responsiveness to antigen-self in chimaera experiments; the pinning down of macrophage, the antigen presenting cell, as site of *Ir* gene defect; as well as the expression of idiotypes on T cells and T cell factors.

Theme 8

The MHC and its Role in the Immune Defence

Presidents:
A. SVEJGAARD
L. DEGOS

Symposium Chairman:
W. F. BOOMER

27

The Role of H-2 *I* Region Genes in Regulation of the Immune Response

HUGH O. McDEVITT

Division of Immunology, Department of Medicine, Stanford University School of Medicine, Stanford, California USA

Introduction

During the last 12 years, research in a great many laboratories has produced evidence which gives the *I* region of the H-2 major histocompatibility system a major role in a very long list of immunologic functions (McDevitt and Benacerraf, 1969; Benacerraf and McDevitt, 1972; Klein, 1975; Möller, 1976; Katz and Benacerraf, 1976). A partial list of these functions is given in Table I.

This is an impressive array of functions to be attributed to a single and

TABLE I
Immunologic functions regulated by the H-2I region

1. Genetic control of the immune response (*Ir*) genes (McDevitt and Benacerraf, 1969; Benacerraf and McDevitt, 1972).
2. Genetic control of immune suppression (*Is*) genes (Katz and Benacerraf, 1976).
3. Interaction between T cells and B cells (Katz and Benacerraf, 1976).
4. Interaction between T cells and macrophages (Möller, 1978).
5. Stimulation of the MLR and GVH reactions (Klein, 1975).
6. One of several components of T cell derived helper and suppressor factors (Mozes *et al.*, 1975; Taniguchi and Takei, 1980).
7. Structural genes for the Ia antigens (Möller, 1976).

This work was supported in part by the following NIH grants: AI 07757; AI 11313; and AM 26908.

rather limited set of structural gene products. As will be discussed below, the Ia antigens which are readily detected on B cells and macrophages include 4 glycopeptides (2 of 34 000 mol. wt and 2 of 29 000 mol. wt) clearly encoded by the *I* region of the H-2 complex, as well as a fifth invariant glycopeptide which is associated in the cell with the other 4 glycopeptides, but is nonpolymorphic and therefore is not yet known to be encoded by the H-2 *I* region (Jones, 1977; Jones *et al.*, 1978, 1979). While there are other *I* region gene products expressed on T cells, including the *I-J* region gene products (Okumura *et al.*, 1976) and at least one *I-C* region gene product (Rich *et al.*, 1978), the relatively small number of gene products encoded by the *I* region naturally leads to the question of how these glycopeptides can control or at least influence all of the functions listed in Table I.

Major characteristic of H-2 linked immune response genes

For the purposes of this discussion, I will focus only on *Ir* genes and briefly review the major facts concerning them, since the other immunologic functions in Table I have been extensively reviewed in other chapters. There are 4 major characteristics of H-2 linked immune response genes which must be considered in any discussion of the mechanism by which *I* gene products mediate *Ir* gene functions.

First, the recognition process influenced by *Ir* genes is highly stereospecific and can readily discriminate a few or single amino acid differences in insulin (Rosenthal, 1978), lysozyme (Adorini *et al.*, 1979), and cytochrome *C* (Solinger *et al.*, 1979), as well as larger differences in random sequence synthetic polypeptides (McDevitt and Benacerraf, 1969; Benacerraf and McDevitt, 1972).

Second, *Ir* genes determine which antigenic determinants will elicit a cellular and humoral response, resulting in distinct H-2 linked differences in antibody specificity between 2 strains, both of which respond to the antigen in question. This was originally noted for branched multichain synthetic polypeptides (Mozes *et al.*, 1969) and has subsequently been demonstrated for several other antigens of more defined structure (Rosenthal, 1978; Adorini *et al.*, 1979; Solinger *et al.*, 1979).

Third, there is impressive evidence that the *I* region genotype of the antigen-presenting macrophage is one site of *Ir* gene action, and is the point at which the *I* region determines which antigenic determinants will elicit a specific T cell and B cell response (Rosenthal, 1978; Schwartz *et al.*, 1978).

Fourth, blocking studies with anti-Ia sera suggest that Ia antigens themselves are the *Ir* gene products, and are involved in the presentation of all antigens to T cells (Rosenthal, 1978; Schwartz *et al.*, 1978; Niederhuber, 1978; Hodes *et al.*, 1979). Indeed, a number of authors have advanced the concept that the Ia antigens are a type or class of antigen-specific receptor molecules (Benacerraf, Ch. 23, this vol; Rosenthal, Ch. 25, this vol; Snell, 1978).

We are thus presented with the following picture: 4 readily detected Ia molecules, and perhaps a few more which are not so readily detected, generate a receptor system of great specificity and great diversity—able to recognize specific antigenic determinants on insulin, cytochrome C, lysozyme, and indeed almost all T cell-dependent antigenic molecules. The present situation is analogous to that of the studies of Landsteiner in 1935, at which time a great deal was known about antigenic determinants which were recognized by antibody, and very little was known about the recognition molecules themselves (Landsteiner, 1936). In reviewing the available evidence, Landsteiner considered Erlich's side-chain theory (which postulated many different cells, each with a distinct receptor specific for a foreign toxin or antigen) as improbable, and embraced Pauling's later theory of a single receptor molecule which could be folded in a great many different ways to assume a great many different shapes (Landsteiner, 1936). It seems worth noting that further studies of the structure of antigens did not solve the problem of antibody specificity, and that we must be cautious in attributing such a great deal of specificity and such a variety of immunologic functions to a relatively small set of glycopeptides.

There are, of course, other possible mechanisms and at least 3 of these deserve careful consideration:

1. Ia molecules are a larger set than present evidence indicates, and combinatorial associations, regulatory polymorphisms, and the possibility that several different classes of Ia molecules may be involved in recognition of a single antigenic molecule, result in generation of hundreds or thousands of different Ia combinations which associate with antigens.
2. Ia antigens are enzymes which influence the presentation of antigen by enzymatic modification of the Ia-antigen complex (Parish *et al.*, 1978).
3. Ia antigens determine the T cell receptor repertoire by an unknown mechanism such as the type that has been postulated by Jerne and elaborated upon by Zinkernagel (Zinkernagel *et al.*, 1980).

To decide among these alternatives, we must have more information than is currently available. In particular, we need much more complete information on the following points:

1. The number of genes in the *I* region and the total number of *I* region gene products.
2. The nature of T cell receptors for Ia antigens and for foreign antigens, and the relation between the two.
3. The molecular nature of the association between Ia antigens and foreign antigens in the antigen-presenting macrophage.
4. The molecular nature of *I-A* and *I-J* gene products in T cell-derived helper and suppressor factors.

In the absence of this type of detailed information, we have no basis for making a decision among the various possibilities for the mechanism of *Ir* gene function. If Ia antigens are in fact a type of antigen-receptor molecule, then it seems apparent that there must be more of these gene products than we have yet detected. If, on the other hand, *I* region gene products act by modifying the Ia-antigen complex or by functioning as the basis for generation of a T cell receptor repertoire (in which self Ia antigens are either not recognized or not responded to, while altered self Ia antigens are recognized and responded to by the T cell repertoire) then it is not immediately apparent that the Ia antigens should be found in close association with foreign antigens in macrophages and with T cell-derived helper and suppressor factors. In both of the latter cases, it would seem that *I* region molecules might exert their affect without the necessity for continuous close association with foreign antigen molecules. Since this seems to be the case, it again raises the possibility that Ia antigens convey some type of specific receptor function.

Recent studies have indicated that Ia antigens do have multiple combinatorial associations as well as complex regulatory polymorphisms. These could lead to considerable molecular diversity, and the nature of these associations will be described briefly, since they have some bearing on the question of whether Ia antigens can function as specific receptor molecules. The underlying theme of these combinatorial associations is genic interaction, a phenomenon which is also prominent in many *I* region functions, and may be an integral mechanism for *Ir* gene regulation of the immune response.

At the functional level, interaction between the *I-A* and *I-E* regions is required to generate an immune response to some antigens, such as the terpolymer (Glu-Lys)Phe, which are under *H-2* linked *Ir* gene control. For (G,L)Phe, the $H\text{-}2^a$, $H\text{-}2^b$, and $H\text{-}2^k$ haplotypes are all nonresponders, while the F_1 between the $H\text{-}2^a$ and $H\text{-}2^b$ is a responder as is the recombinant B10.A(5R) which carries the $I\text{-}A^b$ and $I\text{-}E/C^k$ alleles [Benacerraf and Dorf, 1976]. The presence of the proper allele in the *I-A* and *I-E/C* regions, in either the *cis* or *trans* configuration, confers responsiveness to (G,L)Phe. Similar genic interaction has also been reported for immune suppression genes (Benacerraf and Dorf, 1976).

A similar phenomenon of gene interaction is encountered in the study of macrophage presentation of antigen to T cells in *in vitro* antigen-induced T cell proliferation, and in *in vitro* antibody producing systems (Schwartz *et al.*, 1978; Rosenthal, Ch. 25, this vol.; Hodes *et al.*, 1978). In both types of immune response, an adherent antigen-presenting cell, presumably a macrophage, is required for the response. Antisera against either the *I-A* or *I-E/C* region gene products will block antigen-induced T cell proliferation or eliminate the antigen-producing system (Benacerraf and Dorf, 1976; Hodes *et al.*, 1978). Mixing experiments indicate that the antigen-presenting macrophage must express both *I-A* and *I-E/C* region gene products in order to function effectively in antigen presentation. Thus, at the functional level, *Ir* gene controlled responses, in some cases, require the proper allele in the *I-A* and *I-E/C* regions, and the antigen-presenting macrophage must express both *I-A* and *I-E/C* region gene products. Neiderhuber (1978) has also presented evidence that *I-J* region gene products must be expressed in the antigen-presenting macrophage for an *in vitro* primary antibody response. This raises the possibility that for some antigen-presentation functions, the macrophage must express gene products of the *I-A*, *I-J*, and *I-E/C* regions in concert.

Recent studies by Jones *et al.* (1978) have shown that gene interaction also occurs in the formation of Ia antigen molecules on the cell surface, in this case on the surface of spleen B lymphocytes. Most gene interactions which have been detected to date involve gene products of the *A* and *E* subregions. These gene products are listed in Table II, which also indicates that distinct

TABLE II
I *region gene products*

Region	*Product*	*Mol. wt*	*Expression*
A	A_a	34 000	B cells, macrophages, activated T cells
A	A_b	28 000	B cells, macrophages, activated T cells
A	A_e	28 000	B cells, macrophages, activated T cells
E	E	34 000	B cells, macrophages, activated T cells
J	J_1(?)	—	Suppressor T cells
J	J_2(?)	—	Amplifier or helper T cells
J	J_3(?)	—	Macrophage
C	C	—	MLR suppressor T cell

I region gene products encoded by the *I-J* and *I-C* regions are selectively expressed on suppressor T cells, on an amplifier or helper T cell population, on macrophages, and for the *I-C* region gene products on the MLR suppressor T cell. The available evidence indicates that there are several distinct *I-J* region gene products (Taniguchi and Takei, 1980; Okumura *et al.*, 1976; Niederhuber, 1978; Murphy, pers. comm.). Because of the lack of detailed biochemical characterization of *J* and *C* region gene products, our attention must focus primarily on *A* and *E* region gene products.

Figure 1 is an autoradiography of a 2-dimensional gel electrophoresis of the *I* region gene products which are readily detected with anti-Ia sera. The gene products are labelled internally with ^{35}S-methionine and immunoprecipitated from detergent lysates of the *in vitro* labelled cell populations. More acidic molecules migrate to the right, more basic molecules migrate to the left, and the small "a" in the figure denotes actin which is mol. wt 44 000. Antisera directed to the *I-A* region precipitate 2 sets of polymorphic spots, denoted A_a and A_b, and an invariant polypeptide labelled I_i. It is not clear yet whether I_i is expressed on the cell surface, but A_a and A_b join together to make a 2-chain dimer on the B lymphocyte and presumably the macrophage surface.

Antisera to the *I-E/C* subregion of the *H-2* region immunoprecipitate a

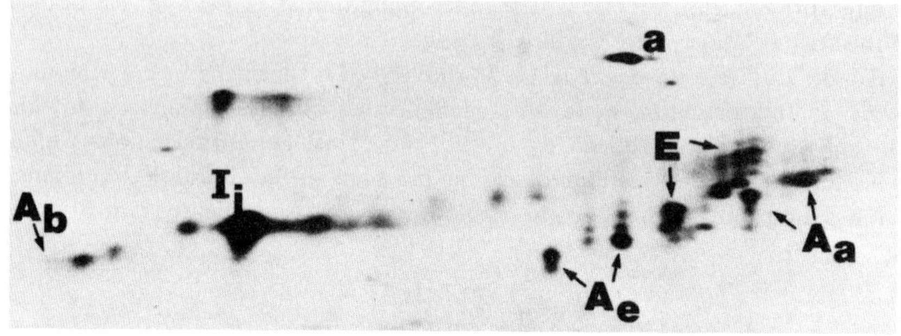

FIG. 1. *Mouse nonequilibrium pH gradient electrophoresis 2-dimensional gel Ia pattern ^{35}S-methionine labelled B10.D2 spleen extracts (d haplotype) immunoprecipitated with B10 anti-B10.D2 antiserum. A, actin, a 44 000 mol. wt protein nonspecifically precipitated in almost all immunoprecipitates and serving as a marker protein; A_a and A_b, acidic and basic polypeptide gene products precipitated by antisera specific for the* I-A *subregion of I; E and A_e, polypeptides precipitated by antisera specific for the* I-E *subregion. Polypeptide I_i is an invariant spot found in all Ia immunoprecipitates and is associated with several related polypeptides progressively more acidic and of slightly higher mol. wt. All of these spots are associated with the I_i spot and are found in all immunoprecipitates obtained with antisera against the whole* I *region, the* I-A *subregion, or the* I-E/C *segment. (I thank Patrica Jones for permission to reproduce this gel.)*

distinctly different set of polypeptides denoted as E and A_e, and also immunoprecipitate the I_i invariant polypeptide chain (it should be noted that the multiple forms of each of these 5 gene products can be shown to be due to glycosylation by both pulse-chain studies as well as the use of tunicamycin to inhibit glycosylation). A_e has been so designated because an extensive series of studies using several different recombinant *H-2* haplotypes have demonstrated conclusively that the 28 000 mol. wt chain in immunoprecipitates brought down by anti-I-E/C sera is encoded in the *A* subregion, but exists on the cell surface in combination or association with an *E* region encoded 34 000 mol. wt polypeptide (Jones *et al.*, 1978).

Despite the relatively small number of gene products of the *I* region which are found on macrophages and B lymphocytes, a series of different types of combinatorial associations has been demonstrated which by themselves add somewhat to the molecule diversity of Ia antigens, and in series could create considerable additional molecular diversity.

Jones *et al.* (1978) have shown that one gene product of the *I-A* region, A_e, and a gene product of the *I-E* region, E_a, form a 2-chain molecule on the cell surface. These studies also showed that this genic interaction could occur in both the *cis* configuration as is seen in the H-$2^{k,d,i^3,i^5}$, and in the *trans* configuration as shown in the (B10 × B10.A)F_1 (Table III). (B10 mice, which are *H-2*^{b}, synthesize A_e but do not glycosylate it or express it at the cell surface, presumably because of a failure to synthesize detectable amounts of the I-E/C_a polypeptide gene products.) In an F_1 between 2 strains carrying *H-2* haplotypes which express both A_e and E, there are 4 different possible molecular combinations which can be generated by combinatorial associations between the two different alleles of A_e and E_a.

Jones has also shown (Jones, pers. comm.) similar combinatorial associations between the A_a and A_b polypeptide gene products in appropriate F_1 combinations, so that in an F_1 carrying 2 different alleles of A_a and 2 alleles of A_b, a total of 4 different combinations can be generated by combinatorial associations. Thus, in appropriate F_1's, combinatorial associations between A_a and A_b, and between E and A_e, could generate 8 different Ia molecules on the cell surface. If the regulatory role of *I* region gene products is mediated by both the A_a and A_b dimer, as well as the E and A_e dimer, appropriate F_1's would generate 16 different combinations of the 4 polypeptide chains. If *I-J* region gene products are also required, a point which is controversial (Schwartz *et al.*, 1978; and Niederhuber, 1978), then the number of combinatorial associations of all 3 sets of molecules would be correspondingly increased.

TABLE III

Gene interaction in the formation of Ia antigens

Interacting gene products	Cis *interaction*	Trans *interaction*
$A_a : A_b$	+	+
$E : A_e$	+	+

Nevertheless, the maximum number of possible combinatorial associations of *I-A*, *I-J*, and *I-E/C* gene products for the known gene products of these regions would presumably not exceed 32–64 distinct molecular combinations. This is a rather small set of molecules to constitute an antigen-recognition system with the exquisite and relatively diverse recognition characteristics of the known *Ir* genes. This statement is based on the assumption that each of the Ia molecules interacts with antigen at only a restricted part of the topography of the Ia molecule, in a manner analogous to an antibody-combining site. On the other hand, if Ia molecules can interact with foreign antigens via multiple discrete sites on the surface of these Ia molecules, then a considerable degree of site diversity could be generated from the numbers of combinatorial associations described above. This statement is based on the demonstration by Fathman (Kimoto and Fathman, 1980) that mice heterozygous for *I* region genes demonstrate a marked increase in the number of T cell clones which recognize hybrid Ia antigen determinants and fail to react with either parent. However, the molecular mechanisms by which Ia molecules on the cell surface could interact with antigens at multiple sites on the Ia molecule itself, is completely unknown.

For this reason, one must entertain the possibility that there are considerably more *I* region gene products than have currently been detected. (One must also, of course, entertain the possibility that Ia antigens regulate immune responses by one of the other mechanisms listed above.) Several regulatory polymorphisms have been detected which result in marked alteration in the amount or form in which particular *I* region gene products are expressed. These regulatory polymorphisms are listed in Table IV.

TABLE IV
E *and* A_e *regulatory polymorphism*

Haplotype	A_e *Cytoplasm*	A_e *Surface*	*E Cytoplasm*	*E Surface*
k, d, r, p	+	+	+	+
b, s	+	−	−	−
f, q	−	−	−	−
ap5	−	−	+	−

As has been known for some time (Möller, 1976), the $H\text{-}2^b$ and $H\text{-}2^s$ haplotypes fail to synthesize detectable amounts of the E_α polypeptide chain. The study by Jones *et al.* (1978) showed that in these haplotypes the A_e gene product is synthesized in the cytoplasm, but is not glycosylated or expressed on the cell surface. Using this information, Jones was able to show that the $H\text{-}2^f$ and $H\text{-}2^q$ haplotypes, in addition to failing to synthesize detectable amounts of the E_α polypeptide chain, also apparently fail to synthesize a cytoplasmic precursor of the A_e polypeptide chain which is found in the $H\text{-}2^b$ and $H\text{-}2^s$ haplotypes. Murphy *et al.* (1980) in studying the $H\text{-}2^{ap5}$ haplotype carried by the A.TFR5 strain found that this strain synthesized only 5–10% of the normal levels of the E_α polypeptide chain. When this strain was crossed with strains capable of synthesizing A_e (e.g. $H\text{-}2^b$ or $H\text{-}2^s$ strains), then normal levels of the $I\text{-}E^k$ gene products encoded by the $H\text{-}2^{ap5}$ haplotype were synthesized and encoded by the $H\text{-}2^b$ or $H\text{-}2^s$ parental haplotypes. These regulatory polymorphisms are of great interest of themselves and presumably contribute to the diversity of *Ir* and Ia phenotypes, but their relevance here is to suggest that *I* region gene products known to be involved in macrophage antigen presentation can be expressed at levels at or below the level of detectability by present-day methods. This, of course, raises the possibility that other *I* region gene products exist which have not yet been detected, either because they do not induce alloantibodies, or because they are present in amounts too small for detection. This is analogous to the present state of affairs in biochemical detection of *I-J* and *I-C* region gene products in T cells and in macrophages.

A relatively small increase in the number of Ia molecules acting in concert (i.e. some representative of each type of Ia molecule is required for antigen recognition and *Ir* gene function), could lead to the generation of a very large number of different combinations, particularly in mice heterozygous for all or most *I* region loci. At the present time there is nothing to exclude this possibility. The fact that antisera to the *I-A* subregion alone, or monoclonal antibodies to Ia antigen, can block macrophage-antigen presentation simply indicates that these gene products are required for this function, but does not establish that they are the only such required gene products. It is quite possible that additional *I* region gene products are also involved in the generation of

Ir gene control recognition processes. The availability of strains carrying *I* region mutations or deletions would be of great help in further analysis of this system. However, the correlation of alteration or loss of a gene product with loss of a function only establishes the requirement for that gene product for the function, and does not establish that the gene product is sufficient for that function. A great deal more will have to be known about the molecular organization of the *I* region, the number of gene copies, and their diversity before we can assess the possible role of the Ia antigens as a true, if primitive, antigen-receptor system.

In summary, several tentative conclusions can be made:

1. Ia antigens appear to be the *Ir* gene products.
2. Combinatorial association as well as regulatory polymorphisms contribute to *I* region receptor diversity and genetic diversity.
3. The currently available number of *I* region gene products is a minimum estimate and is probably larger, although how much larger is a matter of conjecture.
4. If the number is large (e.g. 20–50 or more) these molecules may constitute in themselves a true antigen-recognition system.

References

Adorini, L., Harvey, M. A., Miller, A. and Sercarz, E. E. (1979). *J. Exp. Med.* **150**, 293.

Benacerraf, B. and Dorf, M. (1976). *In* "The Role of Products of the Histocompatibility Gene Complex in Immune Responses" (D. H. Katz and B. Benacerraf, eds) pp. 225–248. Academic Press, New York and London.

Benacerraf, B. and McDevitt, H. O. (1972). *Science* **175**, 273.

Hodes, R. J., Ahmann, G. B., Hathcock, K. S., Dickler, H. B. and Singer, A. (1978). *J. Immunol.* **121**, 1501.

Hodes, R. J., Hathcock, K. S. and Singer, A. (1979). *J. Immunol.* **123**, 2823.

Jerne, N. K. (1971). *Eur. J. Immunol.* **1**, 1.

Jones, P. (1977). *J. Exp. Med.* **146**, 1261.

Jones, P. P., Murphy, D. B. and McDevitt, H. O. (1978). *J. Exp. Med.* **148**, 925.

Jones, P. P., Murphy, D. B., Hewgill, D. and McDevitt, H. O. (1979). *Molec. Immunol.* **16**, 51.

Katz, D. H. and Benacerraf, B. (eds) (1976). "The Role of Products of the Histocompatibility Gene Complex in Immune Responses", Academic Press, New York and London.

Kimoto, M. and Fathman, C. G. (1980). *J. Exp. Med.* (in press).

Klein, J. (1975). "Biology of the Mouse Histocompatibility-2 Complex", Springer-Verlag, New York.

Landsteiner, K. (1936). "The Specificity of Serological Reactions," p. 148. Dover Publications, Inc., New York.

McDevitt, H. O. and Benacerraf, B. (1969). *Adv. Immunol.* **11**, 31.

Möller, G. (ed.) (1976). *Transpl. Rev.* **30**, (entire volume).

Möller, G. (ed.) (1978). *Immunol. Rev.* **40** (entire volume).

Mozes, E., McDevitt, H. O., Jaton, J-C. and Sela, M. (1969). *J. Exp. Med.* **130**, 493.

Mozes, E., Isac, R. and Taussig, M. J. (1975). *J. Exp. Med.* **141**, 703.

Murphy, D. B., Jones, P. P., Loken, M. R. and McDevitt, H. O. (1980). *Proc. Natn. Acad. Sci. U.S.A.* (in press).

Niederhuber, J. E. (1978). *Immunol. Rev.* **40**, 28.

Okumura, K., Herzenberg, L. A., Murphy, D. B., McDevitt, H. O. and Herzenberg, L. A. (1976). *J. Exp. Med.* **144**, 685.

Parish, C. R., Jackson, D. C. and McKenzie, I. F. C. (1978). *In* "Ir Genes and Ia Antigens" (H. O. McDevitt, ed.) pp. 243–254, Academic Press, New York and London.

Rich, S. S., Orson, F. M. and Rich, R. R. (1978). *In* "Ir Genes and Ia Antigens" (H. O. McDevitt, ed.) pp. 559–568, Academic Press, New York and London.

Rosenthal, A. S. (1978). *Immunol. Rev.* **40**, 136.

Schwartz, R. H., Yano, A. and Paul, W. E. (1978). *Immunol. Rev.* **40**, 153.

Snell, G. D. (1978). *Immunol. Rev.* **38**, 3.

Solinger, A. M., Ultee, M. E., Margoliash, E. and Schwartz, R. H. (1979). *J. Exp. Med.* **150**, 830.

Taniguchi, M. and Takei, I. (1980). *Nature* **283**, 227.

Zinkernagel, R. M., Althage, A., Waterfield, E., Kindred, B., Welsh, R. M., Callahan, G. and Pincetl, P. (1980). *J. Exp. Med.* **151**, 376.

28

The MHC and Immune Response in Man

J. DAUSSET and L. CONTU

Institut de Recherches sur Maladies du Sang, Hôpital Saint-Louis, Paris, France

Abbreviations

ADCC: antibody-dependent cell cytoxicity; DNP: dinitrophenyl; *EBV*: Epstein Barr virus; GLT: synthetic random terpolymer of L-glutamic acid–L-lysine–L-tyrosine; *HLA*: human leukocyte antigens (major histocompatibility complex in man); *H-2*: major histocompatibility complex in the mouse; *HSV*: Herpes simplex virus; *I* region: immune region; Ia: *I* region-associated antigens; *Ir*: immune response (gene); *Is*: immune suppressor (gene): *MHC*: major histocompatibility complex; MLR: mixed leukocyte reaction; NK cells: natural killer cells; PBL: peripheral blood lymphocytes; PPD: tuberculin purified protein derivative; RgV1: resistance Gross virus gene; RR: relative risk; SLE: systemic lupus erythematosus; SRBC: sheep red blood cells; TNP: trinitrophenyl; TT: tetanus toxoid; KLH: keyhole limpet haemocyanin.

Introduction

That the human *MHC* or *HLA* complex has a role in the immune response is highly probable, although this has not yet been demonstrated directly as it has been in mice (Benacerraf and McDevitt, 1972) and in monkeys (Dorf *et al.*, 1974). There are many reasons why such a demonstration is difficult:

(a) the number of "ethical" antigens is few, and it is very difficult to perform systematic and well-planned immunizations in man;

(b) the great heterogeneity of human populations and thus the extreme complexity of their genetical situations;

(c) our knowledge of the *HLA-D* region is very incomplete, lagging far behind that of the *I* region, its equivalent in mice.

Three approaches are nevertheless possible and have already been exploited:

(a) studies on true "experiments of Nature" represented by HLA associated or linked diseases, mostly those in which an immunological process is proven or suspected;

(b) searching for correlation between HLA antigens and various immunological parameters;

(c) *in vitro* mixing cell populations of two different individuals, looking for the restriction phenomenon in cell co-operation.

It must be recalled that *HLA* genes can be classified as follows (Klein, 1979). The first class of genes is the classical *HLA-A*, *-B*, *-C* genes. Both heavy and light chains of their products have marked homology with immunoglobulins. The second class of genes is the *Ia* equivalent: the DR genes. The third class of genes governs the factors of the complement pathway (C2, C4 and Bf).

However, the length of the HLA complex is such that it can contain several hundred genes, which for the time being are unknown.

HLA and the immunological process in pathology

Bacterial infections

HLA-associated diseases, true "experiments of Nature," are an invaluable source of information on the function of *HLA* complex genes. It is striking, however, that very few *infectious diseases* due to a well-defined nonviral microorganism have yet been found to be clearly associated with HLA. This almost negative finding is probably due to the multiplicity of antigenic determinants borne by germs and to the heterogeneity of the immune response of each individual which is probably polygenic—both non-*HLA* and *HLA*-linked genes being involved. However, in spite of this complexity there are some indications that during epidemics in the past, a part of the population—the most susceptible—was eliminated. For example, the B7 antigen has almost disappeared from a Dutch colony established in Surinam which was attacked by yellow fever and typhoid fever epidemics (De Vries and Van Rood, 1977).

It is important to point out that an association with HLA antigens can be detected in unrelated patients only when the susceptibility gene is in linkage disequilibrium with an *HLA* gene, giving a detectable product. In the case of nonpreferential association, only family studies allow detection of a linkage. This is probably the case in the tuberculoid form of leprosy which segregated in familes with *HLA* haplotypes (a different haplotype in each family) (De Vries *et al.*, 1976).

One of the mechanisms proposed to explain the HLA and disease association was that of mimicry between *HLA* gene products and bacterial antigens. Much work has been done on various streptococcus and staphylococcus protein fractions (Rapaport and Chase, 1965). Streptococcal M proteins inhibit some anti-HLA antisera, but not all of the same specificity (Hirata and Terasaki, 1970). Lipopolysaccharides from Gram-negative bacteria behave in the same way (Hirata *et al.*, 1973). Recently, a cross-reactivity between B27 lymphocytes and *Klebsiella aerogenes* was demonstrated (Ebringer, 1978; Welsh *et al.*, 1980). This cross-reactivity seems to be limited to B27 cells of AS patients. Extracts of culture *Klebsiella* K43 are able to transform a B27 normal lymphocyte into a reactive lymphocyte (Geczy *et al.*, 1980).

Viral infections

The only virus disease clearly associated with HLA (Bw35) is subacute thyroiditis (de Quervain disease) due to the Semliki forest virus. Certain other viral diseases have been said to be associated with HLA, such as paralytic polio, recurrent herpes labialis (Ryder *et al.*, 1979). In mice the *Rgv-1* gene is dominant, providing resistance to the leukaemic Gross virus. In man the absence of a gene of that type on both chromosomes should lead to a disease which appears to be recessive. A linkage with *HLA* is strongly suggested by the appearance of several cases among HLA identical siblings (Hors *et al.*, 1980). In each of these families a different haplotype was present.

Likewise a viral aetiology is suggested for juvenile insulin dependent diabetes. *Coxsackie B4* virus was cultivated from the pancreas of a child during the first acute phase of diabetes (Yoon *et al.*, 1979). Many other diseases associated with HLA are good candidates for a viral aetiology, as for example, multiple sclerosis. However the mechanism of this interaction and of the association with *HLA* genes is still obscure. Are the HLA products (or products of closely linked genes) serving as receptors? (Helenius *et al.*, 1978; Oldstone *et al.*, 1980). Is it an immune response gene defect against the virus itself or against a self-virus modified antigen leading to autoimmunization? Is it the interaction between HLA product and virus at the surface of the target cell which is lacking or abnormal, preventing the cell lysis? In brief, the search for an obvious association of linkage of *HLA* and infectious diseases of a known viral agent has until now been rather disappointing but most studies were carried out before the era of DR typing, and only a few familial studies have been done. A second examination would perhaps provide some surprises.

Parasitic infections

Diseases due to animal parasites have not until now received full attention regarding their association with HLA antigens.

The observation made in Sardinia that the frequencies of some *HLA* genes (*A1, B5, B17, Bw21*) and of the *A2, B17* haplotype differ between the populations living in lowland villages (where malaria was endemic) and in unexposed highland villages significantly more than the other "neutral" genetic markers, suggests the possibility that the *HLA* complex may play a role in susceptibility to malaria infection (Piazza *et al.*, 1973). A recent finding is a strong association between high serum antibodies to *Plasmodium falciparum* and some of the antigens quoted above (Osoba *et al.*, 1979).

In *Schistosoma mansoni* infection, the pathogenesis and the clinical evolution of disease have been shown to be due primarily to immune mechanisms. Hepatosplenomegaly, a major disease manifestation, has been found recently to be very strongly associated with HLA-A1 and B5 antigens in Egyptian children (Salam *et al.*, 1979). Of particular interest is the presence in the serum of patients of factors that specifically inhibit lymphocyte ability to respond *in vitro* to parasite antigens (Colley *et al.*, 1977) and the progressive specific loss of responsiveness to *Schistosoma* antigens by lymphocytes from patients in the chronic phase of infection. This loss seems to result from the appearance of specific suppressor cells (Ottesen, 1979). We shall see below that a dominant gene of low response against *Schistosomiasis japonicum* is *HLA*-linked.

Immunological abnormalities

We turn now to diseases due to an immunological abnormality such as allergic diseases, atopy, autoimmune diseases, immune deficiencies, complement factor defects, where some well-established facts have emerged. For example, many diseases classified among autoimmune diseases are associated in Caucasians with the Dw3/DR3 markers and most frequently with the haplotype *A1, Cw7, B8, Dw3, DR3.* However, not all autoimmune diseases are associated with the same HLA formula. And even in Caucasians an obviously autoimmune disease like Hashimoto disease seems to be associated with DR5 and, like Hydralazine-SLE, with DR4 (Table I). Other autoimmune diseases such as acquired haemolytic anaemia is apparently not HLA associated. The impression gained of the *A1, B8, Cw7, Dw3, DR3* haplotype is that it confers a general susceptibility to various autoimmune manifestations which probably occur because of other genes and environmental influence. In many of these DR3 associated diseases, a decrease of suppressor cells has been described (Balazs *et al.*, 1979; Zilko *et al.*, 1979; Bach, pers. comm.).

TABLE I
HLA-DR and diseases

	Antigen	*Relative risk*
Multiple sclerosis	DR2	4·1
Optic neuritis	DR2	2·4
Goodpasture syndrome	DR2	15·0
C2 deficiency	DR2	Linked to A25, B18
Dermatitis herpetiformis	DR3	15·4
Coeliac disease	DR3	10·8 (also DR7)
Sicca syndrome	DR3	9·7
Addison's disease	DR3	6·3
Graves' disease	DR3	3·0
Juvenile diabetes	DR3	5·6 (also DR4)
Myasthenia gravis	DR3	2·5
SLE	DR3	5·8
Idiopathic membranous nephropathy	DR3	12·0
Rheumatoid arthritis	DR4	4·2
Pemphigus	DR4	14·4
IgA nephropathy	DR4	4·0
Hydralazine-SLE	DR4	5·6
Hashimoto's disease[a]	DR5	3·2
Pernicous anaemia	DR5	5·4
Juvenile rheumatoid arthritis	DR5	5·2

[a] Mayr (pers. comm.). For references see Ryder *et al.*, 1979.

TABLE II
HLA and complement factors

C2, C4 total deficiencies
Recessive diseases linked to HLA
C2 mostly with A25, C2°, B18, Dw2, DR2 haplotype
C4 with different haplotypes

C4 partial deficiencies

C4	Fs°	BfF1	B18	DR3
C4	Fs°	Bfs	B15	DR4
C4	Sf°	Bfs	B8	DR3
C4	s°		B44	
C4	s°		Bw35	
C4	F_1[a]	Bfs	B17	DR7

[a] Haemolytically inactive.

The second well-documented fact is the frequent presence of the *C2°* and *C4°* deficiencies gene in the *HLA* complex. The disease appears only in homozygous individuals. Partial C4 deficiencies are borne by different *HLA* haplotypes (Table II) (Hauptman, 1979).

Some close relationships between HLA molecules at the cell surface and C

(Arnaiz-Villena *et al.*, 1975) and Fc receptors (Solheim *et al.*, 1976) have been published.

The correlations with immune deficiencies are confused but a peculiar abnormality has been observed in several cases of complex immune deficiencies, with partial defect of expression of the HLA-A, -B antigens (Schuurman *et al.*, 1979; Touraine *et al.*, 1980).

For the other immune disorders such as allergy, atopy, the data are not sufficiently well documented to be introduced as yet in this discussion. The reader can consult Marsh *et al.* (1979) and Dausset and Svejgaard (1977).

HLA correlations with immunological parameters

Humoral response

The first question which comes to mind obviously concerns the possible correlation between the production of a given antibody and the presence of a certain HLA antigen in the producer, by analogy with *Ir* dominant genes in mice.

The first studies were carried out on the anti-Rh immunization of Rh negative individuals. No correlation was found between antibody production to Rh antigens and HLA (Hors *et al.*, 1974; Petranyi *et al.*, 1975; Brain and Hammond, 1974; Van Rood *et al.*, 1975; Murray *et al.*, 1976). It is worth noting that about 40 to 50% of individuals, in spite of multiple transfusions (over 100) are apparently unable to develop anti-Rh or anti-HLA antibodies. They can be called nonresponders. Moreover it has been observed that often the same individuals develop both anti-Rh and anti-HLA antibodies (Salmon and Schwartz, 1960; Brain and Hammond, 1974). They can be called good responders. Until now no genetical marker has been found which might distinguish these two groups. However these data strongly suggest a genetical control of the humoral immune response in man, possibly due to the appearance of suppressor cells or factors (Sasportes *et al.*, 1978).

It has also been tempting to study in normal human beings the correlation between the appearance and titre of antibodies after clinical and routine vaccination and HLA. Several studies devoted to anti-influenza vaccination were unsuccessful (Sybesma *et al.*, 1973; Spencer *et al.*, 1976; McKenzie *et al.*, 1979). Likewise no correlation has been found with antidiphtheria toxoid (McMichael *et al.*, 1977a) or antiherpes virus antibodies (Henderson *et al.*, 1973). It is also worth mentioning the collaborative negative work done in Hungary studying several antigens such as polystaphylococcus, *B. pertussis* (Petranyi *et al.*, 1974a).

A systematic study has been done in normal human beings using immunization with an "ethical" antigen: the flagellin from *Salmonella Adelaide*. Allotypes Glm (1), Glm (17) and G3m (21) occurred more frequently among IgG antibody responders, and HLA-B12 occurred more frequently among IgM antibody responders. The effect of Gm phenotypes on the IgG antibody response was influenced by the HLA phenotypes and vice versa. Thus, among the G1m 1–2–3+) individuals the HLA-B8 were high responders while the HLA-B7 were low responders (Whittingham *et al.*, 1980).

In order to mimic as much as possible the situation in mice, Scher *et al.* (1975) used a synthetic antigen in humans, the GLT. They nevertheless failed to find a correlation with HLA.

In brief, it appears that until now, and in spite of several careful studies, it has been impossible to classify according to HLA the responders and the nonresponders on the bases of the humoral response against xeno- or allo-antibodies, even when using small doses of synthetic antigens. However it should be stressed again that all these studies were performed before the introduction of DR typing, and most of the time without family studies.

Other methods might also be useful. Comparison between monozygotic and dizygotic twins which in one instance gave inconsistent results (Haverkorn *et al.*, 1975) and above all family studies using lod score analysis, could be very fruitful.

When we look at autoantigens the situation is different. The most remarkable example is that of Caucasoid individuals B8, Dw3, DR3. They were found to be prone to develop many autoantibodies as antiacetylcholine-receptors in myasthenia gravis (Naeim *et al.*, 1978) or anti-B pancreatic islet cells in insulin-dependent juvenile diabetes (Nerup *et al.*, 1978). This particularity is not extended to all antigens, however, as was clearly shown by Scott *et al.* (1976).

Delayed hypersensitivity

Hopes have been pinned on another approach, that of a possible correlation with tests of delayed hypersensitivity. These studies, performed with various antigens, remain almost negative (Buckley *et al.*, 1973; Van Rood *et al.*, 1975; Morris *et al.*, 1977; Alföldy *et al.*, 1977).

Lymphocyte proliferation *in vitro*

Much more promising results were collected by seeking a correlation between HLA and proliferative response *in vitro* by sensitization to various antigens. The aim of this method was to detect high responders and low responders in a panel of unrelated individuals and/or in families. Some authors have found a high response against streptococcus antigen (group C) (SK/SD). Higher responders were most frequently B5 (Greenberg *et al.*, 1975). This result was not confirmed in Japan (Kawa *et al.*, 1978), but of course the genetical background was different. However, more recently, Greenberg *et al.* (1980) conducted accurate studies in 9 families. They found an elevated response against another purified group A streptococcus antigen inherited as a dominant character with an *HLA* haplotype, the haplotypes being different in each family.

Other authors have described a low response. The first clear-cut result was obtained in xeno-MLR between man and mouse. Cukrova *et al.* (1977) elegantly demonstrated that individuals A25, B18 and also Dw2 have a significantly low proliferative response against lymphocytes of 6 congenic mouse strains. It should be noted that the A25, B18, Dw2 haplotype frequently contains the C2° deficiency gene. The relationship between these two facts has not been clarified.

A completely independent and very encouraging result was observed in normal individuals after routine antivariola vaccination where Cw3 individuals responded significantly less in a proliferation *in vitro* test than all the other individuals (De Vries *et al.*, 1977).

A further indication of this trend, i.e. dominance of the low response over the high response, was also found by Sasazuki *et al.* (pers. comm.) studying 92 volunteers after a primary immunization with tetanus toxoid. The 78 high responders showed no association with any HLA specificity. However, of 14 low responders 57% were B5 positive compared with 28% high responders. Moreover 58% low responders bore Dw12 compared to 11% of high responders. It was a good demonstration of the existence of an *HLA*-linked gene inhibiting the proliferative response *in vitro*, i.e. an *Is* gene, in humans. Recently the same authors (Sasazuki *et al.*, 1980a) demonstrated that this *Is* gene located in the haplotype *A24, B52, Dw12, DR2* in Japanese people has a broad specificity since the low response was also observed against other antigens such as tetanus toxoid, *Candida*, *Trichuris vulpis* and *Schistosoma japonicum*.

Working on the same lines, Sasazuki *et al.* (1980) studied the proliferative response of 6 family members against membrane streptococcus A antigens (type 12, strain SS 95/12). The found a clear-cut linkage with *HLA* haplotypes, the haplotypes being different in each family. Likewise a low response to influenza A was found associated to Bw35 (Cunningham-Rundles *et al.*, 1979).

These observations taken together seem to indicate clearly that dominant Is genes are widely distributed both in Mongoloids and in Caucasoids. These findings are of high theoretical and practical importance since it is the first well-established relationship between HLA and an essential stage of the immune response against T dependent antigens.

Macrophage antigen degradation

It is known that the low and high responder Biozzi's mice differ by their speed of antigen degradation by macrophage. A slow degradation leads to a high antibody production (Biozzi *et al.*, 1979). In a human random population the degradation index has a bimodal distribution (Fig. 1). The low degraders are significantly associated with DR3. An interaction seems to exist with the *Gm* genes since all DR3 low degraders fell in the G1m (1–2–3+) phenotype (Legrand *et al.*, 1980).

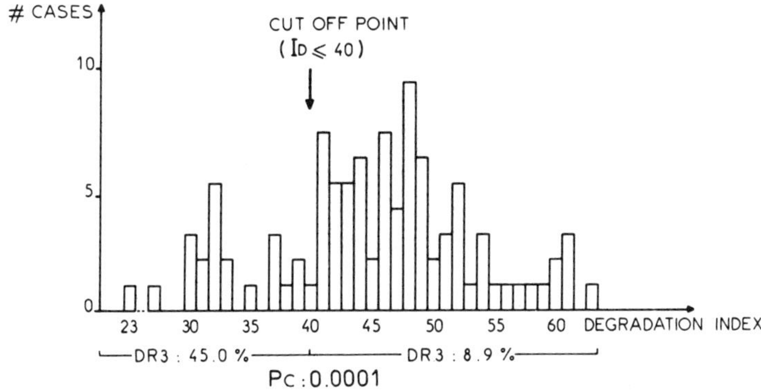

FIG. 1. *Distribution of degradation rate by macrophages and its correlation with HLA-DR3. 101 normal unrelated individuals tested for SRBC degradation by macrophages. The index of degradation (ID) gave a bimodal distribution (cut-off point at 40 ID). All the DR3 low degrader bear the Gm allotype (G1m (1–2–3+)* ($p < 0{\cdot}001$).

HLA restriction

The restriction phenomenon is probably the most convincing presently available argument for an intervention of *HLA* genes in the immune response. Identity at HLA products is apparently required so that cell–cell co-operation can occur at the different stages of the immune response.

Restriction during antigen presentation by macrophages

This point has been well established by Scandinavian teams (Hansen *et al.*, 1978; Hirschberg *et al.*, 1979), used PPD as the antigen of tuberculin PBL of positive individuals as the cells. Monocytes assimilated to macrophages were first pulsed with PPD and then added to PBL. Proliferation was only observed when the lymphocytes and monocytes shared an HLA-D/DR. Antigen (PPD) and D/DR determinants must be present on the same cell. Indeed a mixture of incompatible pulsed monocytes with compatible monocytes and lymphocytes will be inactive. The monocytes must be alive. When the responder is HLA-D/DR heterozygous as well as the monocyte donor, two populations of sensitized lymphocytes are present. These can be separated physically. Thus there is clonal expression. By an *in vivo* sensibilization, followed by an *in vitro* immunization, memory cells can be generated which only recognize PPD in the presence of monocytes bearing the HLA-D/DR of those which served for the first presentation of the antigen. The PPD response can be inhibited by antisera recognizing the shared DR.

Similar results have been obtained using the KLH (Rodney *et al.*, 1979) or the *herpes simplex virus* (HSV) as antigen. In this system, human epithelial Langerhans cells can replace the macrophage (Thorsby *et al.*, 1980).

The same conclusions have also been reached using tetanus toxoid as an antigen (Bright and Munro, 1980). It has also been shown that specific anti-DR blocked this reaction (Geha *et al.*, 1979). However, the restriction is not strict; certain cross-reactions have been observed between the HLA-determinants (Thorsby *et al.*, 1980).

Restriction during the help and suppressor phase of the proliferative response

Help

HLA-D/DR restriction has also been documented for the proliferative response against hapten modified cells. High responses require D/DR sharing between modified TNP cells and responding cells (Charmot and Mawas, 1979; Seldin *et al.*, 1979).

The role of macrophages has not been specifically studied here. Thus it is not known whether restriction is at the presentation or the T help level.

Suppression

A comprehensive picture is progressively emerging regarding T suppressor restriction during the allogenic proliferative reaction (MLR). Early observations were made on MLR inhibition specifically induced on some responding cells (Bean *et al.*, 1977; Thomsen *et al.*, 1978; Kristensen and Jorgensen, 1978). The story became clearer, however, when a multiparous Dw2 homozygous woman was shown to be unresponsive against her husband's lymphocytes Dw1, DR1, DR4 (Engleman *et al.*, 1978, 1979). this unresponsiveness was due to suppressor T cells. When added to a primary MLR they inhibited the proliferation, provided that the responding cells shared the Dw2 determinant with the wife. Further, only when the hysband's cells (or a few other stimulator cell types) were used, was the suppression detected. This suppression has been shown to be dependent on a soluble factor(s), released in the MLR supernate by the female cells. This factor is highly specific to the D product of the responder. Thus it acts in feedback on its own T cells and on any responding T cells sharing at least one D/DR specificity. Conversely the D specificity of the stimulator seems to be indifferent. It is assumed that there are two subsets of T cells, one secreting the factor, another accepting it.

Sasportes *et al.* (1978) were able to produce first suppressor cells and later a suppressor factor after twice allogeneic immunization *in vitro*. This factor is produced by T cells which are adherent to nylon and radioresistant. It acts in feedback on its own T cells and on certain others. Again, the factor has no specificity for the stimulating cell. It has been suggested by Sasportes *et al.* (1979) that this factor(s) is (are) responsible for the beneficial effect of pretransplantation transfusing. It could also be important in explaining foeto-maternal tolerance and could play a role in autoimmunity

Restriction during T–B co-operation for antibody production

Here the data are only preliminary. Two models of antibody formation were studied: antitetanus toxoid (Mudawwar *et al.*, 1978) and anti SRBC (Friedman *et al.*, 1980). In the first the helper factor carried both an idiotype antitetanus toxoid (or SRBC) or a DR determinant. In the second, the helper factor was produced in an allogeneic system. The treatment of the B stimulating cells by a monoclonal anti-DR abrogates the factor production. In both cases no restriction was documented.

Restriction during the lytic phase

This is probably the phase of the immune response where restriction is most evident. It has been shown in man with virus or hapten modified cells and as well with cells bearing the H–Y target.

The most frequently used virus was that of influenza (McMichael *et al.*, 1977b, 1978). Generally speaking, the sharing of at least one HLA-A or -B determinant between the T killer cells and target cells is required.

It has been established that the killing by T cells is virus specific. The target is self-specific and is most probably the A and B molecules themselves, as has been shown by population studies and by inhibition by monoclonal antibodies (Biddison and Shaw, 1979; Shaw *et al.*, 1980). The site where the virus interacts with the HLA molecule may be distinct from the serologically defined antigen. In this case, to which part of the HLA molecule is this restriction directed? Recently an A2 cell (M7) was found which was serologically indistinguishable from other A2 cells but nonetheless behaved differently: when in association with influenza virus it could not be killed by an immune anti-influenza T cell from an A2 individual (Biddison *et al.*, 1980a). Biochemically the A2 molecule of the M7 cells was slightly different from the others (Biddison *et al.*, 1980b). Thus the interaction between the virus and the A2 molecule apparently occurs at a specific site on the HLA molecule which is different from that which is serologically detected. It should be added that this A2 (M7) cell is killed by its own immunized T cells. These findings indicate that different HLA products may facilitate T cell responses to different pathogens which would result in an evolutionary advantage for HLA heterozygosity.

An important point is that there is no fixed hierarchy of the HLA antigens either with the same virus tested on different individuals or with different viruses tested against the same individuals (Shaw *et al.*, 1980).

The restriction rules nevertheless are not always followed. Lipinski *et al.* (1979) observed the appearance of T killer cells only in a small percentage of patients (mostly A1 positive) after infectious mononucleosis. The T killer cells act on any target regardless of HLA type. However, the HLA molecules seem to be necessary since the cell line EBV infected lacking HLA (Daudi) are not killed.

Experiments with measles virus (Ewan and Lachemann, 1977) and with vaccine virus (Perrin *et al.*, 1977) likewise did not show any HLA restriction.

Contradictory results have also been published as far as *hapten* modified target cells are concerned. The first study by Dickmeiss *et al.* (1977) using

DNP modified cells indicated the necessity of an HLA-A or/and B sharing between the killer cells and the target. Indeed subsequent studies on TNP modified cells (Charmot and Mawas, 1979) have not found the restriction. Thus it seems that the phenomenon is less specific in man than in experimental animals (Shaw and Shearer, 1978).

H-minor

Goulmy *et al.* (1979) described two cases of A2 positive women immunized after the rejection of a bone marrow graft for their male siblings HLA identical donors. Their T killer cells were acting almost exclusively against A2 male cells, i.e. against the H–Y minor histocompatibility antigen "in the context" of the A2 molecules. The same was observed for B7. Two T cell clones were demonstrated by differential absorption. It remains to be explained why only certain A or B products are involved in this type of reaction.

In brief, the restriction phenomenon as observed in man is the formal proof that class I and II HLA products are involved in the immune response. However many exceptions have been documented and could be due to technical difficulties in dissociating this phenomenon from other kinds of killing (NK, ADCC).

Discussion

From these data taken together we may speculate and try to visualize what the immune situation may be in humans. We shall do this in the light of the two genetic controls of the *Ir* described in animals. The first is antigen specific and governed by MHC linked *Ir* or *Is* genes. This is the Benacerraf and McDevitt model. The second is antigen nonspecific influencing the level of the humoral response. It is polygenic but with a main gene(s) MHC linked. This is the Biozzi model (Biozzi *et al.*, 1979).

We assume that the *H-2* complex, as was almost always the case until now, is a faithful homologue of *HLA*. In this case the *D* region would possess loci equivalent to *IA, IB, IJ, IE, IC* with their serologically defined alleles. In other words several allelic series like the present *DR* series should be postulated as well as *Ir* and *Is* genes.

In this case the involvement of HLA gene products would be extremely complicated and subtle, and for the time being impossible to imagine. They would intervene at each step of the immune response at the antigen presentation, at each co-operation between the different subsets of immune competent cells when a specifically HLA restricted message sent from an emitter cell to an acceptor cell and also at the target lytic phase. The mechanism applies both to immunity and tolerance.

With this extreme complexity and variety of possible intervention in mind, we shall discuss a general concept of the role of the HLA gene complex in the defence and homeostasy of the human organism and also of the human species.

According to this hypothesis HLA haplotypes are not merely a chance gathering of genes. They probably have been brought and maintained together by some selective advantage, which would be their common effective immunological performance against a particular type of aggression. It is known for example, that in Biozzi's low and high responder mice the $H\text{-}2^s$ (low) and $H\text{-}2^{dq}$ (high) haplotypes were selected for good or bad antibody production (Colombani *et al.* 1979). Some Ig allotypes were also selected (Lieberman *et al.*, 1972). Moreover synergy between *MHC* genes is known as in mice for the constitution of IA–IE hybrid molecules (Jones *et al.*, 1978; Lafuse *et al.*, 1980) and in man for the C2–C4 complement cascade. A 2-gene control of the responsiveness to some antigens and of the generation of antigen-specific suppression has been well documented (Dorf and Benacerraf, 1975; Benacerraf and Dorf, 1976).

Thus according to our hypothesis each *HLA* haplotype would bear a different genetic set of constellations of interacting genes, conferring a particular immune capacity sometimes beneficial, sometimes detrimental, according to the type of immunological challenge. We have already emphasized the peculiarities of the *A1, B5, DR3* haplotype. Another example is the *A3, B7, DR2* haplotype. Individuals with B7, (Dw2, DRw2) have been said to possess a higher delayed hypersensitivity (Persson *et al.*, 1975; Bertrams and Gruneklee, 1977) a low migration test against some viruses (Platz *et al.*, 1974) and a low natural killer response (Petranyi *et al.*, 1974b). Moreover a certain opposition seems to exist between B8, DR3 and B7, DR2 (Dausset, 1977) since B7, DR2 apparently protects against diseases associated with B8, DR3 (Ryder *et al.*, 1979).

However each individual possesses two such constellations of *HLA* genes. In the mouse, true complementation between the *H-2* haplotypes is well documented. Likewise the *HLA* haplotypes could act in interallelic or interloci complementation, conferring on the individual a *final* immune capacity sometimes beneficial, sometimes detrimental, according to the type of challenge.

An example of this complementary effect is observed in the CML killing of a child's lymphocytes while those of both parents were not killed (Schendel *et al.*, 1978).

At the level of a population, it can be assumed that this population includes high and low responders for each immunological trait. That is once again sometimes beneficial, sometimes detrimental, according to the type of aggression.

If the immune trait is polygenically controlled as in Biozzi's mice, the trait is distributed in the population in a Gaussian normal curve. During the epidemics in the past, for example, the most vulnerable individuals were negatively selected for their antibody response.

If an immune character is governed by one (or a major) dominant *HLA*-linked gene either of positive response or of active unresponsiveness, the distribution in the population will be altered and a bimodal distribution could appear, as in the case of *Schistosoma* lymphocyte proliferation or that of the macrophage degradation rate already quoted.

Finally one must emphasize the great importance for humanity of the unravelling of the subtle mechanisms of man's immunological defence. Thanks to the HLA markers, a great advance has been made in this direction.

An even better understanding of immune regulation will allow beneficial manipulations of the human immune system either for immunization for example as against tumour antigens, or for tolerance as in organ transplantation.

Summary

The role of the *HLA* complex in immune response is no longer an hypothesis. First of all, this role is suggested by:

(a) the obvious biochemical homology between the HLA and immunoglobulin for both light and heavy chains of class I products;

(b) the numerous associations or linkages between HLA antigens and diseases with immunological processes especially those with autoimmune manifestations;

(c) the correlation found between certain HLA antigens or haplotypes and some immunological parameters such as the lymphocyte proliferation *in vitro* governed by dominant genes of low or high response or as the antigen degradation by macrophages.

Secondly, the HLA role in the immune response is proven by the restriction phenomenon. Immune response requires an active co-operation between immune competent cells: apparently this co-operation is possible only if these cells recognize each other by identities for some HLA gene products of both class I or class II.

We can speculate that the *HLA* complex, like the *H-2* complex, possesses several polyallelic series, which intervene at the various steps of the immune response. Each *HLA* haplotype bears its own genetic profile of immune response capacity due to the whole of *Ir* and *Is* genes, acting synergistically. Each individual has their own immune capacity, thanks to a complementary effect between its two haplotypes, beyond other non-*HLA*-linked genes, and each population is balanced to cope with different types of aggression.

References

Alföldy, P., Gyodi, E., Dombi, E. and Toth, T. (1977). *Haematologica* **11**, 93–102.

Arnaiz-Villena, A. and Festenstein, H. (1975). *Nature* **258**, 732–734.

Balazs, Cs., Stenszky, V., Kozma, L., Szerze, P. and Leövey, A. (1979). *Transplant. Proc.* **11**, 1314.

Bean, M. A., Kodera, Y., Cummings, K. B. and Bloom, B. R. (1977). *J. Exp. Med.* **146**, 1455–1460.

Benacerraf, B. and Dorf, M. E. (1976). *Cold Spring Harbor Symp. Quant. Biol.* **41**, 455–465.

Benacerraf, B. and McDevitt, H. O. (1972). *Science* **175**, 273–279.
Bertrams, J. and Gruneklee, G. (1977). *Tissue Antigens* **10**, 273–277.
Biddison, W. E. and Shaw, S. (1979). *J. Immunol.* **122**, 1705–1709.
Biddison, W. E., Ward, F. F., Shearer, G. M. and Shaw, S. (1980a). *J. Immunol.* **124**, 548–552.
Biddison, W. E., Krangel, M. S., Strominger, J. L., Ward, F. E., Shearer, G. M. and Shaw, S. (1980b). *J. Exp. Med.* (in press).
Biozzi, G., Mouton, D., Sant'Anna, O. A., Passos, H. C., Gennari, M., Reis, M. H., Ferreira, V. C. A., Heumann, A. M., Bouthillier, Y., Ibanez, O. M., Stiffel, C and Siqueira, M. (1979). "Current Topics in Microbiology and Immunology" pp. 31–98. Springer-Verlag, Berlin.
Brain, P. and Hammond, M. G. (1974). *Eur. J. Immunol.* **4**, 223–225.
Bright, S. and Munro, A. (1980). IV Int. Congr. Immunol. Paris (Abstr.).
Buckley, C. E., Dorsey, F. C., Corley, R. B., Ralph, W. R., Woodbury, M. A. and Amos, D. B. (1973). *Proc. Natn. Acad. Sci. U.S.A.* **70**, 2157–2161.
Charmot, D. and Mawas, C. (1979). *Eur. J. Immunol.* **9**, 723–730.
Colley, D. G., Hieny, S. E., Bartholomew, R. K. and Cook, J. A. (1977). *Am. J. Trop. Med. Hyg.* **26**, 917–925.
Colombani, J. M., Pla, M., Mouton, D. and Degos, L. (1979). *Immunogenetics* **8**, 237–243.
Cukrova, V., Rychlikova, M. and Demant, P. (1977). *Immunogenetics* **4**, 531–540.
Cunningham-Rundles, S., Brown, A., Gross, D., Braun, D., Hansen, J. A., Good, R. A., Armstrong, D. and Dupont, B. (1979). *Transpl. Proc.* **11**, 1849–1852.
Dausset, J. and Svejgaard, A. (1977). "HLA and Disease". Munksgaard, Copenhagen.
Dausset, J. (1977). *In* "HLA and Disease" (J. Dausset and A. Svejgaard, eds) pp. 296–310. Munksgaard, Copenhagen.
De Vries, R. R. P., Lai A Fat, R. F. M., Nijenhuis, L. E. and Van Rood, J. J. (1976). *Lancet* **2**, 1328–1330.
De Vries, R. R. P. and Van Rood, J. J. (1977). "Histocompatibility Testing" (W. F. Bodmer, J. R. Batchelor, J. G. Bodmer, H. Festenstein and P. J. Morris, eds) p. 409. Munksgaard, Copenhagen.
De Vries, R. R. P., Kreeftenberg, H. G., Loggen, H. G. and Van Rood, J. J. (1977). *New Engl. J. Med.* **297**, 692–696.
Dickmeiss, E., Soeberg, B. and Svejgaard, A. (1977). *Nature* **270**, 526–528.
Dorf, M. E., Balner, H., de Groot, M. L. and Benacerraf, B. (1974). *Transpl. Proc.* **6**, 119–123.
Dorf, M. and Benacerraf, B. (1975). *Proc. Natn. Acad. Sci. U.S.A.* **72**, 3671–3675.
Ebringer, A. (1978). *New Sci.* **79**, 865–867.
Engleman, E. G., McMichael, A. J. and McDevitt, H. O. (1979). *J. Exp. Med.* **147**, 1037–1043.
Engleman, E. G., McMichael, A. J., Batey, M. E. and McDevitt, H. O. (1978). *J. Exp. Med.* **147**, 137–146.
Ewan, P. and Lachmann, P. (1977). *Clin. Exp. Immunol.* **30**, 22–31.
Friedman, S. M., Irigoyen, O. H., Gay, D. and Chess, L. (1980). *J. Immunol.* **124**, 2930–2935.
Geczy, A. F., Alexander, K. and Bashir, H. V. (1980). *Nature* **283**, 782–784.
Geha, R. S., Milgrom, H., Broff, M., Alpert, S., Martin, S. and Yunis, E. J. (1979). *Proc. Natn. Acad. Sci. U.S.A.* **76**, 4038–4041.
Goulmy, E. L. S., Hamilton, J. D. and Bradley, B. A. (1979). *J. Exp. Med.* **149**, 545–546.
Greenberg, L. J., Gray, E. D. and Yunis, E. J. (1975). *J. Exp. Med.* **141**, 935–943.
Greenberg, L. J., Ckopyk, R. L., Bradley, P. W. and Lalouel, J. M. (1980). *Immunogenetics* (in press).
Hansen, G. S., Rubin, B., Sorensen, S. F. and Svejgaard, A. (1978). *Eur. J. Immunol.* **8**, 520–525.

Hauptman, G. (1979). *Blood trans. Immunohematology* **22**, 587–614.
Haverkorn, M. J., Hofman, B., Masurel, N. and Van Rood, J. J. (1975). *Transplant. Rev.* **22**, 120–124.
Helenius, A., Morein, B., Fries, E., Simons, K., Robinson, P., Schirrmacher, V., Terhorst, C. and Strominger, J. (1978). *Proc. Natn. Acad. Sci. U.S.A.* **75**, 3846–3850.
Henderson, B. E., Dworsky, R., Menck, H., Alena, B., Kenle, W., Henle, G., and Terasaki, P. (1973). *J. Natu. Cancer Inst.* **51**, 1443–1447.
Hirata, A. A. and Terasaki, P. I. (1970). *Science* **168**, 1095–1096.
Hirata, A. A., McIntire, F. C., Terasaki, P. I. and Mittal, K. K. (1973). *Transplant* **15**, 441–445.
Hirschberg, H., Bergh, O. J., Thorsby, E. (1979). *J. Exp. Med.* **150**, 1271–1276.
Hors, J., Dausset, J., Gerbal, A., Salmon, C., Ropartz, C. and Lanset, S. (1974). *Haematologia* **8**, 217–221.
Hors, J., Steinberg, G., Andrieu, J. M., Jacquillat, C., Minev, M., Messerschmitt, J., Malinvaud, G., Fumeron, F., Dausset, J. and Barnard, J. (1980). *Eur. J. Cancer* **16**, 809–815.
Jones, P. P., Murphy, D. B. and McDevitt, H. (1978). *J. Exp. Med.* **148**, 925–939.
Kawa, A., Matsuyama, T., Fujii, H., Nakamura, S., Ogaki, S., Ode, H., Koreeda, N., Nomoto, K., Arima, N. and Kanehisa, Y. (1978). *Tissue Antigens* **12**, 236–237.
Klein, J. (1979). *Science* **203**, 516–521.
Kristensen, T. and Jorgensen, F. (1978). *Tissue Antigens* **11**, 443–448.
Lafuse, W. P., McCormick, J. F. and David, S. C. (1980). *J. Exp. Med.* **151**, 709–715.
Legrand, L., Hors, J. and Dausset, J. (1980). IV Int. Congr. Immunol. Paris (Abstr.).
Lieberman, R., Stiffel, C., Asofsky, R., Mouton, D., Biozzi, G. and Benacerraf, B. (1972). *J. Exp. Med.* **136**, 790–798.
Lipinski, M., Fridman, W. H., Tursz, T., Vincent, C., Pious, D. and Fellous, M. (1979). *J. Exp. Med.* **150**, 1310–1322.
Marsh, D. G., Chase, G. A., Freidhoff, L. R., Meyers, D. A. and Bias, W. B. (1979). *Proc. Natn. Acad. Sci. U.S.A.* **76**, 2903–2907.
Marsh, D. G., Hsu, S. H., Hussain, R., Meyers, D. A., Freidhoff, L. R. and Bias, W. (1980). *J. All. Clin. Immunol.* (in press).
McKenzie, S. S., Wetherall, J. D., Flower, R. L. P., Fimmel, P. J. and Dawkins, R. G. (1979). *Vox Sang.* **37**, 201–208.
McMichael, A. J., Sasazuki, T. and McDevitt, H. (1977a). *Transpl. Proc.* **9**, 191–194.
McMichael, A. J., Ting, A., Zweerink, H. J. and Askonas, B. A. (1977a). *Nature* **270**, 524–526.
McMichael, A. (1978). *J. Exp. Med.* **148**, 1458–1467.
McMichael, A. J., Pilck, J. R., Brodsky, F. M. and Parham, P. (1980). *J. Exp. Med.* (in press).
Morris, P. J., Vaugham, H., Tait, B. D. and Mackay, I. R. (1977). *Austr. N.Z.J. Med.* **7**, 616–624.
Mouzon A. de, Ohayon, E., Ducos, J., Hauptmann, G. (1979). *Lancet* **2**, 1364.
Mudawwar, F. B., Yunis, E. J. and Geha, R. S. (1978). *J. Exp. Med.* **148**, 1032–1043.
Murray, S., Dewar, P. J., Lee, E., McNay, R. A. and Collins, A. K. (1976). *Vox Sang.* **30**, 91–104.
Naeim, F., Keesey, J. C., Herrmann, C. Jr, Lindstrom, J., Zeller, E. and Walford, R. L. (1978). *Tissue Antigens* **12**, 381–386.
Nerup, J., Platz, P., Ryder, L. P., Thomsen, M. and Svejgaard, A. (1978). *Diabetes* **27**, 247–250.
Oldstone, M. B. A., Tishon, A., Dutks, F. J., Kennedy, S., Ian, T., Holland, J. J. and Lampert, P. W. (1980). *J. virol.* **34**, 256–265.
Osoba, D., Dick Heather, M., Voller, A., Goosen, T. J., Goosen, T., Draper, C. C. and de The G. (1979). *Immunogenetics* **8**, 323–338.
Ottesen, E. A. (1979). *J. Immunol.* **123**, 1639–1644.

Perrin, L. H., Zinkernagel, R. M. and Oldstone, M. B. A. (1977). *J. Exp. Med.* **146**, 949–969.

Persson, I., Ryder, L. P., Staub-Nielsen, L. and Svejgaard, A. (1975). *Tissue Antigens* **6**, 50–53.

Petranyi, G. G., Ivanyi, P. and Hollan, S. R. (1974a). *Vox sang.* **27**, 470–482.

Petranyi, G., Benczur, M., Onody, C. E. and Hollan, S. R. (1974b). *Lancet* **1**, 736.

Petranyi, G. G., Ivanyi, P. and Hollan, Z. (1975). *Folia Haemat.* **102**, 29–34.

Piazza, A., Belvedere, M. C., Bernoco, D., Conighi, C., Contu, L., Curtoni, E. S., Mattin, P. L., Mayrr, W., Richiardi, P., Scudeller, G. and Cepellini, R. (1973). *In* "Histocompatibility Testing," pp. 73–84. Williams and Wilkins, Baltimore.

Platz, P., Dupont, R., Fug, T., Ryder, L., Thomsen, M., Svejgaard, A. and Jersild, C. (1974). *Proc. Roy. Soc. Med.* **67**, 22–28.

Rapaport, F. T. and Chase, R. M. (1965). *Science* **145**, 407.

Rodey, G. E., Luehrman, L. K. and Thomas, D. W. (1979). *J. Immunol.* **123**, 2250–2254.

Ryder, L. P., Andersen, E. and Svejgaard, A. (1979). "HLA and Disease Registry", 3rd report, *Tissue Antigen.* Munksgaard, Copenhagen.

Salam, E. A., Ishaac, S. and Mahmoud, A. A. F. (1979). *J. Immunol.* **123**, 1829–1831.

Salmon, C., Schwartz, D. (1960). *Revue d'Hémat.* **2**, 162–173.

Sasazuki, T., Kohno, Y., Iwamoto, I., Tanimura, M. and Naito, S. (1978). *Nature* **272**, 359–361.

Sasazuki, T., Ihta, N., Hayase-Kaneoka, R. and Kojima, S. (1980a). *J. Exp. Med.* (in press).

Sasportes, M., Fradelizi, D. and Dausset, J. (1978). *Nature* **276**, 502–504.

Sasportes, M., Wollman, E., Cohen, D., Fradelizi, D., Carosella, E., Cathely, G. and Dausset, J. (1979). *C. R. Acad. Sci. Paris* **289**, 41–46.

Schendel, D. J., Wank, R. and Dupont, B. (1978). *Eur. J. Immunol.* **9**, 634–640.

Scher, I., Berning, A. K., Strong, D. M. and Green, I. (1975). *J. Immunol.* **115**, 36–40.

Schuurman, E. K. B., Van Rood, J. J., Vossen, J. M., Schellekens, P. T. A., Felkamp-Vroom, T. M., Doyer, E., Gmelig-Meyline, F. and Visser, H. K. (1979). *Clin. Immunol. Immunophath.* **14**, 418–434.

Scott, B. B., Cooks, E. M., Hambling, M. H. and Losowsky, M. S. (1976). *J. Immunogenetics* **3**, 185–189.

Seldin, M. F., Rich, R. R. and Dupont, B. (1979). *J. Immunol.* **122**, 1828–1833.

Shaw, S. and Shearer, G. M. (1978). *J. Immunol.* **121**, 290–299.

Shaw, S., Shearer, G. and Biddison, W. B. (1980). *J. Exp. Med.* **151**, 235–245.

Solheim, B. G., Thorsby, E. and Muller, E. (1976). *J. Exp. Med.* **143**, 1568–1573.

Spencer, M. J., Cherry, J. D. and Terasaki, P. I. (1976). *New Engl. J. Med.* **294**, 13–16.

Sybesma, J. P. H. B., Holtzer, J. D., Borat-Eilers, E., Moes, M. and Zegers, B. J. M. (1973). *Vox Sang.* **25**, 254–262.

Thomsen, M., Dickmeiss, E., Jakobsen, B. K., Platz, P., Ryder, L. P. and Svejgaard, A. (1978). *Tissue Antigens* **11**, 449–456.

Thorsby, E., Bergholtz, B. and Berle, E. (1980). *J. Exp. Med.* (in press).

Touraine, J. L., Betuel, M. and Philippe, N. (1980). *Blut* (in press).

Van Rood, J. J., Van Hooff, J. P. and Keuning, J. J. (1975). *Transplant. Rev.* **22**, 95–104.

Welsh, J., Avakian, H., Cowling, P., Ebringer, A., Wooley, P., Panay, G. and Ebringer, R. (1980). *Br. J. Exp. Path.* **61**, 85–91.

Whittingham, S., Mathews, J. D., Schanfield, M. S., Mathews, J. V., Tait, B. D., Morris, P. J. and Mackay, I. R. (1980). *Clin. Exp. Immunol.* **40**, 8–15.

Yoon, J. W., Austin, M., Onodera, T. and Notkins, A. L. (1979). *New Engl. J. Med.* **300**, 1173–1179.

Zilko, P. J., Dawkins, R. L., Holmes, K. and Witt, C. (1979). *Clin. Immunol. Immunol. Immunopath.* **14**, 418–434.

29

HLA and Disease

A. SVEJGAARD, N. MORLING, P. PLATZ, L. P. RYDER and M. THOMSEN

Tissue-Typing Laboratory of the Blood Grouping Department, State University Hospital of Copenhagen, Denmark

Introduction

Within the last decade, it has become clear that a variety of diseases occur preferentially in individuals who have inherited certain genetic factors controlled by the major histocompatibility complex (MHC) of man, i.e. the HLA system. The group of diseases which have been found to be associated with HLA factors span from clear-cut immunologic disorders (e.g. gluten hypersensitivity, myasthenia gravis, and systemic lupus erythematosus), via diseases suspect of autoimmune pathogenesis (e.g. insulin-dependent diabetes, thyreotoxicosis, and rheumatoid arthritis), over conditions of unknown etiology (e.g. multiple sclerosis and psoriasis vulgaris) to diseases without immunologic abnormalities (e.g. idiopathic haemochromatosis and congenital adrenal hyperplasia).

Abbreviations
AS: ankylosing spondylitis; C2: second component of complement; C4: fourth component of complement; *HLA*: the MHC of man; IDDM: insulin-dependent diabetes; *MHC*: major histocompatibility complex; 21-OH: 21-hydroxylase.

This study was aided by grants from the Danish Medical Research Council, the Medical Research Council of EEC, the Dagmar Marshall Foundation, and Gaardon's Fund.

The information inherent in these associations has considerable impact on our understanding of disease heterogeneity and the inheritance of disease susceptibility, and with the increasing knowledge of the biological function of the HLA system, the associations are likely to bring new clues to the etiologies and/or pathogenesis of these diseases. From a practical point of view, some associations are already now being used diagnostically, and it would appear that some have prognostic value.

The main impetus to this research was the discovery of Lilly *et al.* in 1964 that the susceptibility of mice to viral leukaemogenesis is largely controlled by the *MHC* (the H-2 system) of that species. The *HLA* system had hardly been recognized as the *MHC* of man before studies of HLA in malignancies were reported: Amiel (1967) found evidence that Hodgkin's disease may be associated with HLA, whereas Kourilsky *et al.* (1967) found no association between HLA and acute leukaemia. The first definite associations were not discovered until 1972 when the striking associations between HLA and psoriasis (Russell *et al.*, 1972) and coeliac disease (Falchuk *et al.*, 1972) were found. The following year the extraordinarily strong association between HLA-B27 and ankylosing spondylitis was discovered (Brewerton *et al.*, 1973; Schlosstein *et al.*, 1973), and at the same time it became clear that associations with HLA-D (MLC) factors in some cases may be stronger than those with the classical HLA-A and B antigens (Jersild *et al.*, 1973). When HLA-DR typing became possible and more widely used, the HLA-D associations were confirmed and new associations were found.

The purpose of this survey is to review our present knowledge about HLA and disease associations and to discuss how these associations can be used in diagnosis and prognosis and in studies of disease heterogeneity and genetics. Finally, the various mechanisms which can explain the associations are summarized. A general introduction to the HLA system has been given elsewhere (Svejgaard *et al.*, 1979).

The associations

Table I summarizes most of the associations which have been found between HLA and disease. The information has been extracted from the data in the HLA and Disease Registry in Copenhagen (Ryder *et al.*, 1979; Svejgaard and Ryder, in prep.). Numerous investigators have contributed to this information and it is obviously impossible to quote them all here. The diseases have arbitrarily been listed according to the HLA-A, B, C, and D/DR antigen(s) showing the strongest association with the disease in question; for simplicity we are not distinguishing between HLA-D and DR antigens in this report although there are occasional differences (Platz *et al.*, 1980). To save space, only data on Caucasians are shown. For each disease and each antigen, we have given the frequency of the antigen in patients and controls and the relative risk of the disease for individuals carrying that antigen. The relative

TABLE I
HLA associated disorders

Condition	*HLA*	*Frequency (%)* *Patients*	*Controls*	*Relative Risk*
Hodgkin's disease	A1	40	32·0	1·4
Idiopathic haemochromatosis	A3	76	28·2	8·2
	B14	16	3·8	4·7
Behçet's disease	B5	41	10·1	6·3
Congenital adrenal hyperplasia[a]	B47	9	·6	15·4
Ankylosing spondylitis	B27	90	9·4	87·4
Reiter's disease	B27	79	9·4	37·0
Acute anterior uveitis	B27	52	9·4	10·4
Subacute thyroiditis	B35	70	14·6	13·7
Psoriasis vulgaris	Cw6	87	33·1	13·3
Dermatitis herpetiformis	D/DR3	85	26·3	15·4
Coeliac disease	D/DR3	79	26·3	10·8
	D/DR7 also increased			
Sicca syndrome	D/DR3	78	26·3	9·7
Idiopathic Addison's disease	D/DR3	69	26·3	6·3
Graves' disease	D/DR3	57	26·3	3·7
Insulin-dependent diabetes[a]	D/DR3	56	28·2	3·3
	D/DR4	75	32·2	6·4
	D/DR2	10	30·5	·2
Myasthenia gravis[a]	D/DR3	50	28·2	2·5
	B8	47	24·6	2·7
S.L.E.[a]	D/DR3	70	28·2	5·8
Idiopathic membraneous nephropathy[a]	D/DR3	75	20·0	12·0
Multiple sclerosis	D/DR2	59	25·8	4·1
Optic neuritis	D/DR2	46	25·8	2·4
C2 deficiency	D/DR2			
	B18			
Goodpasture's syndrome[a]	D/DR2	88	32·0	15·9
Rheumatoid arthritis[a]	D/DR4	50	19·4	4·2
Pemphigus (Jews)[a]	D/DR4	87	32·1	14·4
IgA nephropathy[a]	D/DR4	49	19·5	4·0
Hydralazine-induced SLE[a]	D/DR4	73	32·7	5·6
Hashimoto's thyroiditis[a]	D/DR5	19	6·9	3·2
Pernicious anaemia[a]	D/DR5	25	5·8	5·4
Juvenile rheumatoid arthritis:				
pauciart[a]	D/DR5	50	16·2	5·2
all cases[a]	D/DRw8	23	7·5	3·6

The above information has been extracted from the HLA and Disease Registry in Copenhagen (Ryder *et al.*, 1979; Svejgaard and Ryder, in prep.). Studies indicated by [a] are referenced in Svejgaard *et al.* (1980a). Antigen frequencies refer mainly to a Danish population, but when only one or a few studies are available, the control frequencies published by these authors are given. for simplicity we have not here or in the text distinguished between HLA-D and DR antigens although there are occasional differences—for example, DR4 shows a stronger association with insulin-dependent diabetes than does Dw4.

risk indicates how many times more frequently a disease develops in individuals with the antigen as compared to the frequency of the disease in individuals not possessing this antigen. For example, it appears from Table I that idiopathic haemochromatosis occurs 8·2 times more frequently in HLA-A3-positive than in A3-negative individuals. A relative risk above one means a positive association while risks below one are seen for negative associations. The principles and methods for the calculations have been described elsewhere (Ryder *et al.*, 1979).

Diagnostic and prognostic value

When an HLA factor occurs with high frequency in patients with a given disease and with low frequency in the normal population, HLA typing may sometimes be useful as "diagnostic test". For example, typing for HLA-B27 may be considered a diagnostic test of ankylosing spondylitis with 10% "false negatives" (= the frequency of B27 in healthy individuals). It should be noted that the diagnostic value of HLA typing depends on the *a priori* probability of the disease based on clinical and other laboratory findings. Thus, HLA typing has its maximal value in early, unclear cases of suspected ankylosing spondylitis.

In congenital adrenal hyperplasia due to 21-hydroxylase (21-OH) deficiency, it is possible to HLA type foetal cells and thus make prenatal diagnosis of this disease in offspring of parents who have earlier given birth to a child with 21-OH deficiency: all offspring having the same HLA type as the affected sibling will have the abnormality. The same is true in idiopathic haemochromatosis, but antenatal diagnosis does not seem indicated. However, by HLA-typing the siblings of a patient with idiopathic haemochromatosis it is possible to predict which siblings will eventually develop this disease and thus depletion of the iron stores can be instituted before tissue damage develops. In such cases, HLA typing has prophylactic value.

In some cases, a disease seems to run a more severe course in patients having the disease associated HLA antigen than in patients without this antigen. For example, multiple sclerosis progresses more rapidly in D/DR2-positive than in D/DR2-negative patients, and there is a higher probability that thyreotoxocosis will relapse in D/DR3-positive than in D/DR3-negative patients with this disease. However, it is too early to judge whether this information is of practical prognostic value. Nevertheless, it may be anticipated that HLA typing may find its place in the evaluation of the prognosis for some of the diseases listed in Table I.

Genetics and heterogeneity of diseases

The relations between HLA and disease have contributed to genetics in two major ways: firstly, some genes have unexpectedly been mapped within or close to the HLA system, and secondly, information has been obtained about the inheritance of the susceptibility to a variety of diseases. In several cases, the associations have helped to detect heterogeneity within entities which by itself is important genetic information.

Idiopathic haemochromatosis and congenital adrenal hyperplasia due to 21-hydroxylase (21-OH) deficiency are two examples of unexpected mapping of disease genes within or close to *HLA*. Thanks to HLA studies (Kravitz *et al.*, 1979; Simon *et al.*, 1977) idiopathic haemochromatosis has now been established as a clear-cut recessive disorder closely linked to *HLA* because almost all affected sibpairs are HLA identical. Moreover, virtually all apparently healthy siblings HLA identical with an affected sib appear to have the biochemical abnormalities of this disease. The exact nature of the defect in idiopathic haemochromatosis is not known but seems to involve an increased iron absorption in the gut. Accordingly, it would appear that a gene influencing iron absorption is closely linked to *HLA*. The 21-OH deficiency is probably due to the lack of the enzyme, 21-OH, and because this deficiency has now been mapped inside the *HLA* system (Dupont, 1980), close to the *HLA-B* locus, it is likely that the gene coding for 21-OH belongs to the *HLA* system. The common, severe form of 21-OH deficiency is associated with the rare HLA-B47 antigen and it may be calculated that about half of all haplotypes carrying a *B47* gene also carries a 21-OH deficiency gene. Most recently, it has been found (Dupont, in press) that a mild form of 21-OH deficiency is associated with HLA-B14. Thus, there appears to be two different 21-OH deficiency genes within the HLA system.

Deficiency of C2 is particularly interesting from a genetic point of view because the C2 deficiency (C2°) gene occurs preferentially in a special haplotype: *HLA-A25,B18,Dw2*. It is possible that the *C2°* gene originally arose by a mutation on such a haplotype. On the basis of the present linkage disequilibrium between *A25* and *B18* in *C2°*-carrying haplotypes, it may be estimated that this mutation might have taken place almost 2000 years ago (Svejgaard and Ryder, 1979). Similar mutational events may also explain the associations between HLA on the one hand and idiopathic haemochromatosis and 21-OH deficiency on the other.

Ankylosing spondylitis was earlier considered a "polygenic" disorder (Carter, 1969), but the HLA studies show now that there is an *HLA* gene of "major effect" which confers dominant susceptibility to this disorder (Thomson and Bodmer, 1977). It remains to be established how often Reiter's disease and reactive arthropathies develop into ankylosing spondylitis, but it seems that these arthropathies have a more severe prognosis in B27-positive patients (Leirisalo *et al.*, 1980). Further genetic analyses of this disease spectrum are complicated by the observation that nonsymptomatic sacroiliitis is quite frequent in otherwise healthy B27-positive controls (Calin and Fries, 1975).

The first clear-cut separation of a disease into two subgroups by means of HLA was the observation that psoriasis vulgaris but not pustular psoriasis is

HLA associated (Svejgaard *et al.*, 1974) which confirmed earlier clinical distinction between these two types of psoriasis. Moreover, HLA studies even seem to indicate heterogeneity within psoriasis vulgaris because HLA is only associated with early onset and not with late onset psoriasis (Svejgaard *et al.*, 1974) and because the frequency of psoriasis among first degree relatives is higher when psoriasis patients carry the psoriasis-associated HLA antigens than when they do not (Svejgaard and Ryder, 1979). This latter observation also indicates that if there are unknown HLA factors involved in the development of psoriasis in patients lacking the known psoriasis-associated HLA factors, then these unknown factors have a smaller influence. As discussed elsewhere (Svejgaard *et al.*, 1975), the susceptibility to psoriasis conferred by HLA seems to be dominant.

The genetics of diabetes has long been an enigma. HLA studies showed first of all that only insulin-dependent diabetes mellitus (IDDM) is associated with HLA whereas noninsulin-dependent, maturity onset diabetes is not, which finally proved that these two disorders have different genetic backgrounds and should be treated separately in genetic analyses. The unravelling of the genetics of IDDM is probably one of the most fascinating topics of HLA and disease studies at the time of writing. During the 8th international histocompatibility workshop, a large number of IDDM patients from many parts of the world were HLA typed. The analyses of these data (Svejgaard *et al.*, 1980b) showed that IDDM is positively associated with HLA-DR4 in all three major ethnic groups (Negroid, Caucasian, and Mongoloid) with DR3 in most, and with DRw8 in some populations, while DR2 showed negative associations in all populations. The workshop IDDM study doubled the amount of available information on HLA-haplotype sharing among affected sibpairs, and the analysis of all these data showed clearly that the susceptibility to IDDM cannot be dominant (with incomplete penetrance). These studies also make a recessive model (with incomplete penetrance) unlikely because the frequency of the susceptibility gene compatible with the data would be so high that one would have to postulate a penetrance so low that it does not fit with the well-known frequency of IDDM among all siblings of IDDM propositi. Thus, the only "simple" model which has not been ruled out for the inheritance of the susceptibility to IDDM is the intermediate one according to which there is a gene dose effect which gives a higher penetrance in individuals homozygous for the susceptibility gene than in heterozygous individuals. However, there is some evidence against this model because the risk of IDDM seems to be higher for *HLA-DR3/4* heterozygotes than it is for *DR3/3* and *DR4/4* homozygotes. Moreover, the age-at-onset may be different for DR4-positive patients and DR4-negative ones which may indicate heterogeneity of IDDM. Nevertheless, these results were obtained by pooling data from different sources (Svejgaard *et al.*, 1980b) and they need confirmation in homogeneous populations. If true, they indicate that there are at least two different IDDM susceptibility genes within the *HLA* system—one associated with *DR3* and one with *DR4*.

The association between HLA and myasthenia gravis is most pronounced in the subgroup of patients with an early onset and without a thymoma. This type of myasthenia is most frequent in females and it is an old observation that such patients respond better to thymectomy than older patients with thymoma.

Two of the classical organspecific autoimmune disorders have only very recently been found to be HLA associated: Hashimoto's thyroiditis and pernicious anaemia. Both of these "thyreogastric" diseases have now been shown to be associated with HLA-D/DR5 (Farid, 1980; Thomsen *et al.*, 1980; Weissel *et al.*, in press) and strikingly not with D/DR3 which clearly separates them from the other organspecific autoimmune disorders.

Even when there is no association between HLA and a disease, it is sometimes possible to obtain information on disease heterogeneity by HLA studies. This has been illustrated by Pedersen *et al.* (1980) who found that there are two forms of dominant, hereditary cerebellar ataxia: one linked to HLA and the other not. This has now been confirmed (Morton *et al.*, 1980). Pedersen *et al.* (1980) even provided evidence that there is clinical differences between the two forms: while dementia and extrapyramidal signs were absent in the HLA-linked form, both of these were present in the non-HLA linked form.

Mechanisms

Apart from C2 deficiency and 21-OH deficiency, the mechanisms behind the HLA associations are largely unknown. In fact, we do not know whether the HLA factors now known to be associated with the diseases are causally involved or whether they are merely markers for as yet unknown factors occurring in linkage disequilibrium with the known ones. Sucn linkage disequilibrium is a fundamental characteristic of the HLA system: virtually every known HLA factor shows positive association with at least one other HLA factor controlled by a gene at a nearby locus, and it can be anticipated that this is true also for as yet unknown markers.

When attempts are made to hypothesize mechanisms behind the associations, one may consider what is known about the major histocompatibility complex (*MHC*) in man and other species (Svejgaard *et al.*, 1979; Klein, 1975). For example, it appears that both HLA-ABC and D/DR antigens are involved in thymus-dependent immunity: the ABC antigens on target cells are involved in the lysis by T effector lymphocytes of virus-infected or hapten-conjugated cells, while the D/DR antigens control the co-operations between macrophages, T helper lymphocytes, and B lymphocytes; the HLA-D/DR antigens may thus be identical with the immune response (Ir) determinants, and if they are not, the genes controlling them are at least believed to map very close to the Ir determinants and probably have a pronounced linkage disequilibrium with these. Even if the D/DR antigens are Ir determinants, it should be kept in mind that in mice there are several closely linked *Ir* loci within the *MHC* which also appears to contain immune suppressor (*Is*) genes. Accordingly, there is probably more than one *Ir* locus in *HLA*, too, and this system may also contain *Is* genes.

In addition to ABC and D/DR antigens, the *HLA* system also controls some components of the complement cascade: properdin factor Bf of the alternative and second (C2) and fourth (C4) component of the classical activation pathway. These three factors may not be the only enzymatic factors controlled by *HLA*: the gene controlling 21-OH probably also belongs to the *HLA* system. It may be worth noting that both the loci for HLA controlled complement factors and that for 21-OH deficiency have been mapped close to the *HLA-B* locus.

Finally, the *H-2* system of mice has been shown to influence a variety of quantitative traits, and it seem likely that the HLA system has more biological functions than those listed above.

With the above considerations in mind, it seems reasonable to assume that the pathogenesis in disorders "primarily" associated with HLA-D/DR antigens involve inadequate action of Ir or Is determinants some of which may be the D/DR antigens themselves. Diseases "primarily" associated with HLA-ABC factors may involve preferential restriction phenomena or molecular mimicry. However, both HLA-D/DR, B, and C associated disorders could also involve as yet unknown variants of HLA controlled complement components. In the following, we give some examples on how one might explain some of the associations, but we wish to stress that all of these examples are as yet only hypothetical.

Coeliac disease and perhaps dermatitis herpetiformis may represent involvement of an Ir determinant with specificity for a component in gluten, hypersensitivity to which causes coeliac disease. However, the situation is probably not so simple because coeliac disease is associated with both DR3 and 7 while dermatitis herpetiformis apparently is only associated with DR3.

An HLA-DR3 associated *Ir* gene could also be involved in most, if not all, of the other DR3 associated disorders, in which autoimmune antibodies are found. One problem here is that quite a number of different autoantibodies are involved, and if it is only one Ir determinant which is responsible for all the associations, it must be postulated that it has a rather broad specificity. It is perhaps more plausible that the hypothetical Ir determinant might have a more basic, general role for certain immune responses. Lack of a common *Is* determinant could also explain these associations. Conversely, there may be a cluster of DR3-associated Ir determinants with specificities towards various organs, but quite a number of genes must then be postulated. Each of these possibilities fit the observation that the different antibodies tend to occur together in the same patients and in their relatives. For several of these disorders, it is often assumed that they are triggered by environmental (infectious?) agents which could trigger the autoimmune process. The tissue specificity of an infecting virus could determine which organ becomes affected

The association of both pernicious anaemia and Hashimoto's thyroiditis with HLA-D/DR5 but not D/DR3 may indicate the action of another Ir determinant in these disorders.

Preferential HLA-ABC restriction in T lymphocyte mediated lysis of virus infected or hapten conjugated cells might explain the associations between HLA-B35 and subacute thyroiditis and between HLA-B5 and Behçet's disease. For example, the HLA-B35 antigen could be particularly effective in the presentation to T effector lymphocytes of a putative thyrotropic virus which may be the cause of this disease.

A case for molecular mimicry was made when Australian investigators (Seager *et al.*, 1979) observed that certain rabbit anti-*Klebsiella* antibodies lysed lymphocytes from HLA-B27 patients with ankylosing spondylitis (AS). However, it was clear from the beginning that this could not be simple molecular mimicry because these antibodies did not react with lymphocytes from B27-positive healthy individuals including relatives of patients with AS. More recently, the same group of investigators (Geczy *et al.*, 1980) found that a factor from the supernatant of *Klebsiella* cultures could "convert" B27 positive lymphocytes from healthy individuals to react with the rabbit anti-*Klebsiella* antibodies. Accordingly, it seems as if B27 positive lymphocytes have a certain affinity for a factor in *Klebsiella*, i.e. it could be a special case of preferential restriction. However, it is not readily understood how this phenomenon should lead to AS, and it is worth noting that a number of other micro-organisms seem to be responsible for various reactive arthropathies. This is particularly true of *Yersinia* infections which are occasionally followed by acute arthritis particularly in B27 positive individuals. It is possible that these reactive arthropathies are due to circulating immune complexes which are trapped in the capillaries of the joints. If this is true, it may be speculated that some variant of a complement component could be involved. This variant could be responsible for a poor phagocytosis of certain immune complexes and/or could give them a size which could lead them to be trapped in the capillaries in question. None of the presently known complement variants seem to fit this idea, but it should be kept in mind that these variants are detected by differences in electrophoretic behaviour and it is well-known that the majority of mutations (amino-acid substitutions) does not lead to changes in the electric charge of a protein. Recently, it has been found that one of the electrophoretic variants of C4 in some individuals in haemolytically inactive (Dupont and O'Neill, pers. comm.; DeMouzon and Hauptmann, pers. comm.). This variant is associated with HLA-Cw6 and HLA-B17, but the occurrence of this variant in psoriasis remains to be investigated. If it shows a "primary" association with psoriasis, it may again be speculated whether this disorder could be due to immune complexes.

At the time of writing, we consider the mechanisms discussed above (i.e. Ir and/or Is determinant involvement, preferential ABC restriction, and complement variation) the best candidates for most of the presently known HLA and disease associations. However, these mechanisms are unlikely to be involved in idiopathic haemochromatosis or 21-OH deficiency. As discussed elsewhere (Svejgaard and Ryder, 1976), it is possible that HLA factors may interfere with ligand-receptor interactions. It has also been suggested that some HLA factors may serve as receptors for virus but there is not much evidence supporting this assumption. Finally, the HLA-D/DR antigens are differentiation antigens and it may be speculated that other HLA antigens may control other cellular interactions which could lead to associations between HLA and various diseases. Obviously, the last word has not yet been said about HLA and disease and in particular not about the mechanisms underlying the associations.

References

Amiel, J. F. (1967). *In* "Histocompatibility Testing 1967" (E. S. Curtoni *et al.*, eds) pp. 79–81. Munksgaard, Copenhagen.

Brewerton, D. A., Caffrey, M., Hart, F. D., James, D. C. O., Nicholls, A. and Sturrock, R. D. (1973). *Lancet* **i**, 904.

Calin, A. and Fries, J. F. (1975). *New Engl. J. Med.* **293**, 835.

Carter, C. O. (1969). *Br. Med. Bull.* **25**, 52.

Dupont, B. (1980). *In* "Histocompatibility Testing 1980" (P. I. Terasaki, ed.). University of California, Los Angeles (in press).

Falchuk, Z. M., Rogentine, G. N. and Strober, W. (1972). *J. Clin. Invest.* **51**, 1602.

Farid, N. (1980). Data submitted to the HLA and Disease Registry.

Geczy, A. F., Alexander, K. and Bashir, H. V. (1980). *Nature* **283**, 782.

Jersild, C., Fog, T., Hansen, G. S., Thomsen, M., Svejgaard, A. and Dupont, B. (1973). *Lancet* **ii**, 1221.

Kidd, K. K., Bernoco, D., Carbonara, A. O., Daneo, V., Steiger, U. and Ceppellini, R. (1978). *In* "HLA and Disease" (J. Dausset and A. Svejgaard, eds) pp. 72–80. Munksgaard, Copenhagen.

Klein, J. (1975). "Biology of the Mouse Histocompatibility-2 Complex" Springer-Verlag, New York.

Kourilsky, F. M., Dausset, J., Feingold, N., Dupuey, J. M. and Bernard, J. (1967). Proceedings 1st International Congress Transplantation, Paris, 1967, pp. 515–521. Munksgaard, Copenhagen.

Kravitz, K., Skolnick, M., Cannings, C., Carmelli, D., Baty, B., Amos, B., Johnson, A., Mendell, N., Edwards, C. and Cartwright, G. (1979). *Am. J. Hum. Genet.* **31**, 601.

Leirisalo, M., Skylv, G., Kousa, M., Voipio-Pulkki, L-M., Hvidman, L., Darm-Nielsen, E., Nissislä, M. and Laitinen, O. (1980). Data submitted to the HLA and Disease Registry.

Lilly, F., Boyse, E. A. and Old, L. J. (1964). *Lancet* **ii**, 1207.

Morton, N. E., Lalouel, J-M., Jackson, J. F., Currier, R. E. and Yee, S. Data submitted to the HLA and Disease Registry.

Pedersen, L., Platz, P., Ryder, L. P., Lamm, L. U. and Dissing, J. (1980). *Human Genetics* **54**, 371.

Platz, P., Jakobsen, B. K., Morling, N., Ryder, L. P., Svejgaard, A., *et. al.*, (1980). in prep.

Russell, T. J., Schultes, L. M. and Kuban, D. J. (1972). *New Engl. J. Med.* **287**, 738.

Ryder, L. P., Andersen, E. and Svejgaard, A. (1979). "HLA and Disease Registry. Third Report". Munksgaard, Copenhagen.

Schlosstein, L., Terasaki, P. I., Bluestone, R. and Pearson, C. M. (1973). *New Engl. J. Med.* **288**, 704.

Seager, K., Bashir, H. V., Geczy, A. F., Edmonds, J. and Vere-Tyndall, A. de (1979). *Nature* **277**, 68.

Simon, M., Bourel, M., Genetet, B. and Fauchet, R. (1977). *New Engl. J. Med.* **297**, 1017.

Svejgaard, A. and Ryder, L. P. (1976). *Lancet* **ii**, 547.

Svejgaard, A. and Ryder, L. P. (1979). *In* "Genetic Analysis of Common Diseases: Applications to Predictive Factors in Coronary Disease" (C. Sing and M. Skolnick, eds) pp. 523–543. Alan R. Liss, New York.

Svejgaard, A. and Ryder, L. P. (1980). Fourth Report from the HLA and Disease Registry (in prep).

Svejgaard, A., Staub Nielsen, L., Svejgaard, E., Kissmeyer-Nielsen, F., Hjortshøj, A. and Zachariae, H. (1974). *Br. J. Derm.* **91**, 145.

Svejgaard, A., Platz, P., Ryder, L. P., Staub Nielsen, L. and Thomsen, M. (1975). HL-A and disease associations—a survey. *Transplant. Rev.* **22**, 3.

Svejgaard, A., Hauge, M., Jersild, C., Platz, P., Ryder, L. P., Staub Nielsen, L. and Thomsen, M. (1979). *In* "Monographs in Human Genetics" (2nd edn) (L. Beckman *et al.*, eds) Vol. 7. S. Karger, Basel.

Svejgaard, A., Morling, N., Platz, P., Ryder, L. P. and Thomsen, M. (1980a). *Transplant. Proc.* (in press).

Svejgaard, A., Platz, P. and Ryder, L. P. (1980b). *In* "Histocompatibility Testing 1980" (P. I. Terasaki, ed.). University of California, Los Angeles (in press).

Thomsen, M., Ryder, L. P., Svejgaard, A. and Gimsing, P. (1980). *In* "Genetics and Heterogeneity of Common Gastrointestinal Disorders" Academic Press, New York and London.

Thomson, G. and Bodmer, W. F. (1977). *In* "HLA and Disease" (J. Dausset and A. Svejgaard, eds) pp. 84–93. Munksgaard, Copenhagen.

Weissel, M., Hofer, R., Zasmeta, H. and Mayr, W. R. (in press). *Tissue Antigens.*

30

Structure of Products of the Major Histocompatibility Complex in Man and Mouse

JACK L. STROMINGER

The Biological Laboratories, Harvard University, Cambridge, Massachusetts, USA

This chapter will summarize available data on the structure of products of the major histocompatibility complex and several related topics. My laboratory work has focused on products of the human *HLA-A*, *-B*, *-C*, and *-DR* genes. These genes correspond to the murine *H-2K*, *H-2D*, *H-2L* and *Ia* genes respectively—the products of which have been studied extensively by others. The studies of the murine antigens will be described here principally when they contribute additional information. A more comprehensive review can be found elsewhere (Strominger *et al.*, 1980). These genes are all very polymorphic, for example, in the range of 25 alleles known at the *HLA-A* and *-B* loci and more than 200 at each of the *H-2K* and *-D* loci in feral mouse populations. A most interesting question is the location of regions of amino acid diversity within these molecules which reflect the genetic polymorphism and how these diversity regions relate to the natural functions of these molecules. Evolutionary pressure related to the biological functions leads to the polymorphism and, therefore, the regions of diversity must pinpoint functionally important regions of these molecules.

This research was supported in part by National Institute of Health Grant AI 10736. Research contributions by Harry T. Orr were supported in part by the Leukemia Society of America Fellowship.

HLA-A, -B and -C antigens

The complete structure of a papain-solubilized human histocompatibility antigen, HLA-B7 was reported during 1979 (Orr *et al.*, 1979a, b, c; Lopez *et al.*, 1979). A schemic depiction of the structure of the HLA-A and -B antigens is shown in Fig. 1. They are composed of 2 chains: the large glycoprotein subunit has a size of 44 000 daltons on SDS-PAGE (but in fact is closer to 41 000 daltons by sequence analysis) and traverses the cell membrane; the small, noncovalently associated subunit, β_2-microglobulin, has a size of 11 500 daltons. The large chain can be divided into 5 regions:

1. an *N*-terminal region of about 13 500 daltons which bears the single glycan moiety of the molecule but has no disulphides;
2. a 2nd region of about 10 500 daltons which has an internal disulphide bridge;
3. a 3rd region which also is about 10 500 daltons and has an internal disulphide bridge, (the first 3 regions are outside the cell membrane);

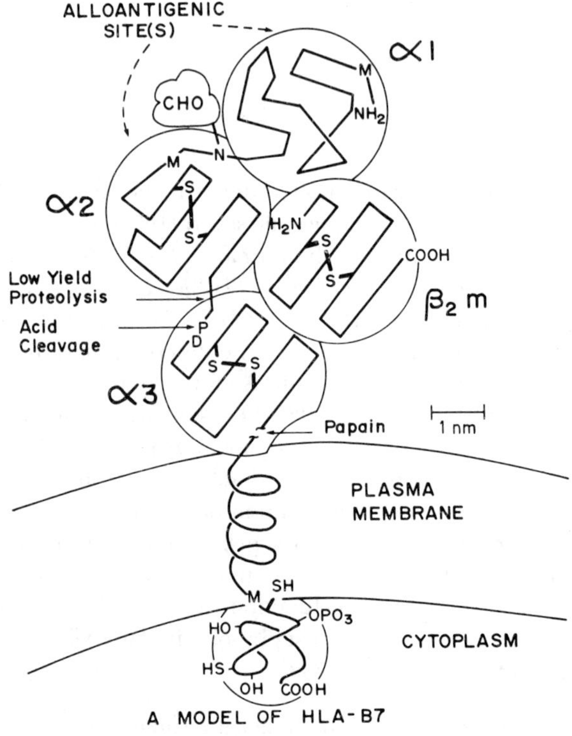

FIG. 1. *Schematic representation of the structure of an HLA-A or -B antigen.*

4. a 4th region of about 3000 daltons which is the hydrophobic, intramembranous portion of the molecule, and then finally,
5. a small hydrophilic region of about 3500 daltons which is intracytoplasmic and may play some role in the function of these antigens, perhaps by interaction with cytoskeletal elements.

β_2-Microglobulin is attached noncovalently to the large extramembranous region of the molecule.

All 3 extracellular regions (called α_1, α_2, and α_3) are probably folded into domains with a β-pleated sheet structure, as is β_2-microglobulin. However, the manner in which β_2-microglobulin is associated with the putative domains of the heavy chain of the molecule is not known. One of the most interesting and unresolved questions about the structure is the role of β_2-microglobulin. It has been suggested that this small subunit locks the molecule (in particular, the α_1 domain which has no internal disulphides) in a conformation which is alloantigenically active. There appear to be multiple sites which contribute to the diversity and hence to the alloantigenicity of these molecules. At least 2 of these sites are located in α_1 and α_2. Finally, a phosphate residue occurs on a serine residue of the small, internal region (Pober *et al.*, 1978); is it metabolically active and may play a role in the functioning of these molecules.

The large extracellular region is solubilized by papain removing the hydrophilic, intracellular piece, and the hydrophobic, intramembranous piece. Two important features occur in the sequence of the intracellular region. One is a clustering of dibasic amino acids near the membrane interface, that may serve to position the molecule in the membrane. The other is the very large number of serine and threonine residues, approximately a third of the residues. One or more of these serines carry a phosphate group. The intramembranous piece is essentially a copolymer of a few hydrophobic amino acids and its sequence is the only uncertain feature of the structure of the molecule. It is very difficult to get very accurate sequence for a structure in which individual amino acids are repetitive.

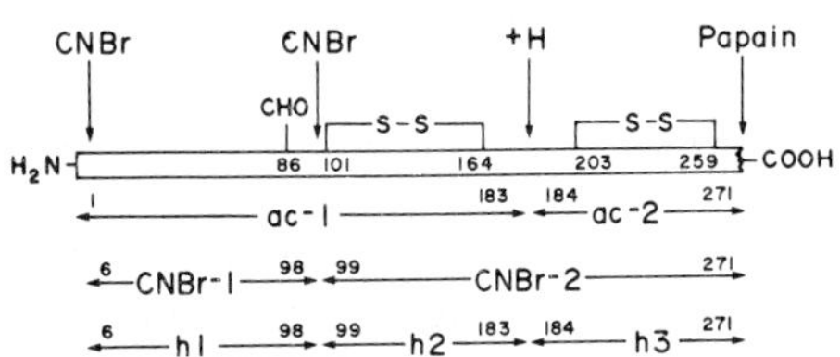

FIG. 2. *Fragmentation of HLA-B7.*

In order to work out its complete amino acid sequence, fragmentations of the papain-solubilized molecule had to be carried out first. In the case of HLA-B7 antigens, the fragmentations used were formic acid cleavage and CNBr cleavage which fortuitously gave fragments h_1, h_2, and h_3, corresponding approximately to α_1, α_2, and α_3, the 3 regions of the molecule (Fig. 2).

Subsequent tryptic and chymotryptic digestions yielded the peptides from which the complete sequence of HLA-B7 was elucidated.

In addition, 97% of the sequence of HLA-A2 has now been worked out (Orr, in prep.) as has the complete sequence of H-2K^b (Martinka *et al.*, 1980). Comparisons of the structures of 3 complete molecules, 2 from man and 1 from the mouse, reveal several interesting features. The sequence homology between HLA-A2 and HLA-B7 is in the range of 80–85% (Fig. 3). Even though these molecules are encoded a great distance apart (in terms of map units) on the 6th chromosome, they nevertheless have very strong sequence homology, and therefore must have arisen by gene duplication. The homology of the murine antigen to the human antigens is in the range of 70–75%, again a high degree of homology. These molecules have not diverged very greatly since the separation of the species. However, since HLA-A and -B antigens

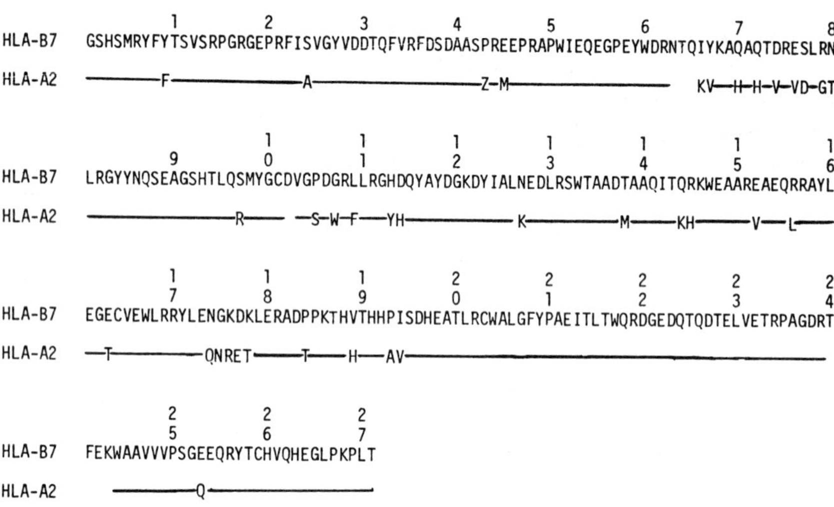

FIG. 3. *Complete amino acid sequence of papain-solubilized HLA-B7 and its comparison with 97% of the sequence of HLA-A2.*

are more homologous to each other than H-2K^b, the gene duplication yielding the multiple loci must have occurred after the mouse-human speciation. Comparing the HLA-A2 and HLA-B7 sequences (Fig. 3), substitutions between these A and B locus antigens occur throughout the molecules. However, 3 regions occur in which there is a clustering of differences, 1 in α_1 (residues 65–80) and 2 in α_2 (residues 105–115 and 174–178). The sequence homology drops to 50% or less in these regions while it is greater than 90% throughout the rest of the molecules. Comparing the mouse H-2K^b antigen (Martinka *et al.*, 1980) with HLA-B7, a cluster of differences is found in the region of residues 61–82 (Fig. 4). The differences at residues 105–115 are not as striking in terms of forming a cluster.

The 3rd region of diversity is found between the 2 disulphide loops. A

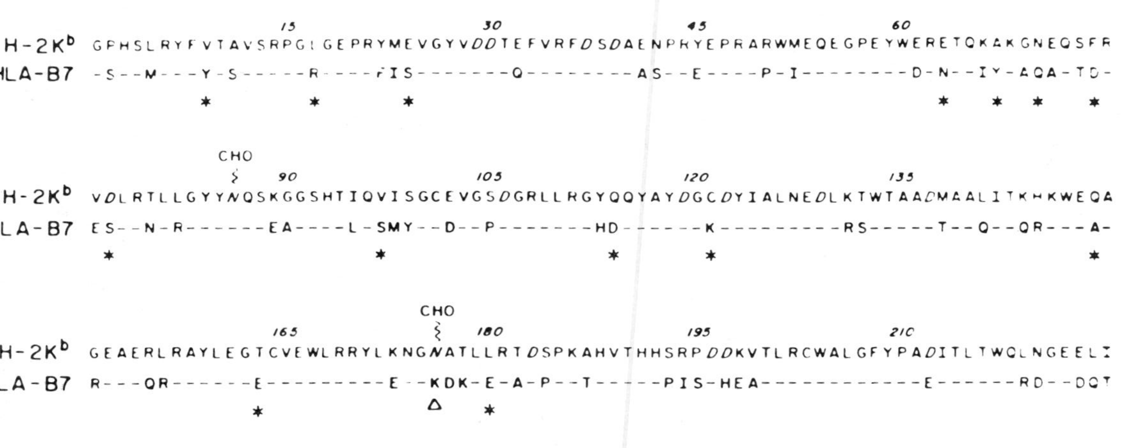

FIG. 4. *Complete amino acid sequence of papain-solubilized H-2K^b and its comparison in the HLA-B7* (8).

stretch of 5 residues from residue 174 to 178 is completely different in HLA-A2 and HLA-B7, in fact, the largest contiguous stretch of sequence difference between these molecules. Comparing H-2K^b and HLA-B7, there are 14 differences in 27 residues between positions 173–199. This diversity region has a number of interesting features. The murine histocompatibility antigen contains 2 glycan residues, one at position 86, as in the HLA-A and -B antigens, and the other at position 176. The homologous location of these 2 carbohydrates within α_1 and α_2 in H-2K^b further strengthens the homology relationship between α_1 and α_2 (see below). Position 176 is, however, not glycosylated in HLA-B7, -A2, or apparently in any other HLA molecules. The asparagine in this position in the H-2 antigens is replaced by another residue in all of the HLA antigens studied. Another interesting feature of this region is that the acid cleavage site Asp$_{183}$-Pro$_{184}$ is not found in HLA-A2, HLA-A28, nor in any of the H-2 antigens so far studied. All of these regions of sequence diversity may play some role in the formation of the alloantigenic determinants. It is possible that the differences in the region 173–199 represent species specific and/or isotypic differences, rather than allospecific differences. This possibility is supported by the fact that so far no mutations in this region have been found in the H-2 mutant mice (see below).

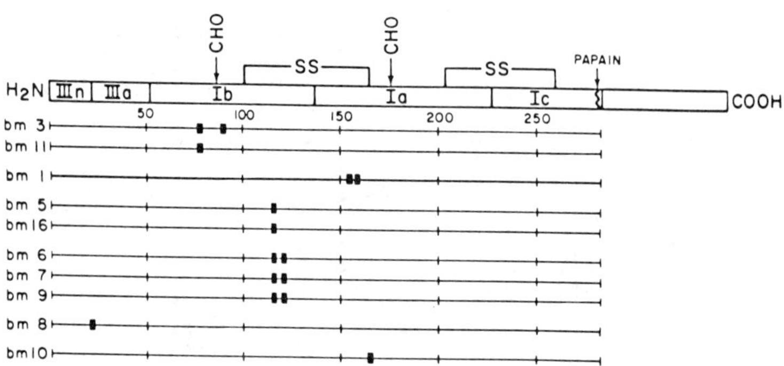

FIG.5. *Location of mutations in H-2K^b molecules of mutant mice* (9).

In the mouse, a large number of mutants of H-2K^b were identified by the rejection of skin grafts by litter mates (Nairn *et al.*, 1980). These mutants retained serological allospecificity but lost recognition by cytotoxic T cells (CTLs). Since T cell killing is also allospecific, there must be at least 2 regions of diversity. Tryptic peptide maps have localized these mutations in 4 regions (Fig. 5). Two of these regions correspond to the regions of amino acid diversity (residues 65–80 and 105–120). One mutant has an alteration at residue 23, a residue which, interestingly, is different in the 3 antigens sequenced. Two mutations at residue 155–156 have been detected. There are, therefore, at least 4 regions where a change in structure can lead to a change in function of these molecules. It remains to be determined, of course, whether these are really the functional regions or whether in some cases a change in structure might lead to a conformational change at a distant position.

Within the past year, an HLA-A2 variant has been detected in the human population (Biddison *et al.*, 1980). It was detected during a study in 15 subjects of the killing of influenza virus infected B lymphocytes by HLA-A2-restricted influenza directed cytotoxic T cells. In one individual the serological type was indistinguishable from other HLA-A2. It was only in this subject that the influenza virus infected cells were not killed by the CTL. In addition, his cells were not killed by HLA-A2-directed allospecific CTLs, nor could they stimulate the production of such CTLs. A study of his HLA-A2 antigen revealed that it had a unique heavy chain which, by isoelectric focusing (IEF), differs by a single charge from other HLA-A2 heavy chains. The location of the change(s) in the variant remains to be established, but these experiments point to a method for detecting variant molecules in the human population.

Another important feature of the structural data is the fact that α_3 is virtually completely conserved. One possible difference was found between HLA-A2 and HLA-B7 in this region, at residue 253. As this is an acid–amide difference it is possible that this difference is due to an error in the HLA-B7 sequence. It is noteworthy that no duplicate amino acids were detected in this region in sequencing a mixture of allospecificities obtained from pooled human blood lymphocytes (Trägårdh *et al.*, 1979). In fact, the sequence of the principal amino acid residue at each position in this pooled material differed at only 12 residues from HLA-B7 (Trägårdh *et al.*, 1980).

The amino acid sequence of papain solubilized HLA-A28 is about 40% completed (Orr, in prep.) and it is very interesting because only a few scattered differences have been found between HLA-A28 and HLA-A2 (3 differences in 101 residues sequenced). These 2 allospecificities cross-react serologically. When the sequence of HLA-A28 is completed, the differences from HLA-A2 may also help to point to a region of the molecule which is serologically important.

Earlier studies had revealed a number of similarities between histocompatibility antigens and immunoglobulins, a point of considerable evolutionary interest in view of the possible role of histocompatibility antigens as cell-bound defence molecules and of immunoglobulins as circulating defence molecules. Once the complete sequence of HLA-B7 was available, it was possible to compare its sequence to all sequenced proteins using a computer program designed to detect evolutionary relationships. Only the region of the second disulphide loop (α_3) showed significant sequence homology to other proteins. It had a highly significant sequence homology to immunoglobulin C region domains, with particular conservation around the regions of the 2 cysteines. From the α_3 sequence, it has been predicted that this region folds into a "sandwich" of 2 β-pleated sheets in a manner similar to that of immunoglobulin domains. By circular dichroism, it has been determined that HLA antigens contain a high percentage of β structure.

In contrast, α_1 and α_2 have only general features which suggest immunoglobulin-like structures but they have no statistically significant homology to any sequenced proteins including V or C region immunoglobulin domains, e.g. α_2 has a disulphide loop within the range of sizes of V region loops. α_1 and α_2 do have some sequence homology to each other, suggesting that they arose from a common ancestral gene, but neither region has significant homology to α_3. α_1 and α_2 are the regions which are presumed to contain the functionally important portions of the molecule. Presumably considerable evolutionary pressure has been placed on these regions, and if indeed they arose from the same ancestral genes as did the α_3 regions and the immunoglobulin domains, then they have diverged sufficiently far so that evidence of homology is no longer apparent from the amino acid sequence.

More precise information about the structure of these molecules can, of course, be obtained from their crystal structure. Towards this end HLA-A2, -A28 and -B7 have recently been crystallized (Bjorkman *et al.*, in prep.). The best crystals were obtained from HLA-A2. They were of sufficient size to yield a diffraction pattern with resolution beyond 0·3 nm. Within the next 3 or 4 years it may be possible to elucidate the crystal structure of an HLA antigen.

Much less information is presently available about the products of the HLA-C and H-2L genes. These molecules are also composed of polypeptide chains of 44 000 and 12 000 daltons. *N*-terminal sequencing and tryptic peptide mapping of the H-2L molecules established that they are indeed products of a separate gene from H-2K and H-2D (Coligan *et al.*, 1980). In the case of HLA-C, only serological data and independent capping support the idea that the HLA-C antigen is clearly a distinct gene product. The amount of the HLA-C antigen on the surface of the cell appears to be much smaller than the amount of HLA-A and -B antigen, thus making its isolation for structural studies considerably more difficult.

Biosynthetic studies of HLA-A and -B antigens and of the H-2K and -D antigens are of considerable interest in view of the prominence of these proteins as intrinsic membrane proteins (Ploegh *et al.*, 1979; Krangel *et al.*, 1979; Doberstein *et al.*, 1979). In addition these studies have provided the reagents and potential for cloning the respective cDNAs. If successful and because of the relative rapidity of DNA sequencing compared to protein sequencing, they will provide tools for the isolation of many additional clones for the very rapid accumulation of sequence information from a larger number of alleles. Such clones would also provide the tools for undertaking a study of the genomic organization of the regions in the major histocompatibility complex which encode these genes. Studies of this kind have been initiated in several laboratories, including our own, and rapid progress in the next few years is anticipated.

These purified antigens can also be employed in functional studies. Of course, the most interesting aspect of function is the recognition of allogeneic histocompatibility antigens by cytotoxic T lymphocytes (CTLs). Earlier purified HLA-A and -B antigens incorporated into liposomes were utilized in a secondary response to generate allospecific xenogeneic CTLs (Englehard *et al.*, 1978). Most recently a human cytotoxic T lymphocyte line which is specific for one of the histocompatibility antigens, HLA-B7, has been developed (Reiss *et al.*, 1980). This line was developed from a mixed lymphocyte culture using as the stimulator the standard lymphoblastoid cell line JY (HLA-A2, B7 homozygous) and as the responder the peripheral lymphocytes from an HLA-$A2^+$, $-B7^-$ individual. This T cell line required T cell growth factor for outgrowth and maintenance in culture (TCGF) and for its cytolytic activity periodic stimulation with the stimulating antigen. At an effector to target ratio of 0·08 to 1, it killed targets bearing HLA-B7 to 30%. Cytotoxic T lymphocyte lines which recognize other HLA allospecificities or which recognize HY in an HLA-A2 restricted system have also been developed and clones (Goulmy *et al.*, 1980; Charmot *et al.*, 1980). The availability of these lines together with the availability of purified HLA antigen should make it possible in the next few years to understand an important and long standing problem in immunology, the nature of the T cell receptor and its interaction with foreign histocompatibility antigens. It may be noteworthy, therefore, that a heteroantiserum prepared against the HLA-B7-directed CTL line and absorbed extensively with B lymphoblastoid cell lines immunoprecipitated only 2 polypeptides from membranes of this line with sizes of 78 000 and 33 000 daltons (Reiss *et al.*, 1980). Earlier data employing anti-idiotypic serum had suggested that the murine T cell receptor carried a V regions idiotype and might have a size of about 70 000 daltons (Binz and Wigzell, 1977). Similar techniques have recently extended these data to both human and marmoset cells (Lea *et al.*, 1979; Marchalonis *et al.*, 1980).

HLA-DR antigens

Like the HLA-A and -B antigens, HLA-DR antigens also contain 2 polypeptide chains. These two chains of 34 000 (α) and 29 000 (β) daltons are in an extremely tightly linked noncovalent complex and both chains span the membrane, but only the heavy (α) chain, is phosphorylated (Kaufman and Strominger, 1979). The heavy chain also contains 2 glycan moieties (a complex and a high mannose oligosaccharide) while the light chain (β) contains only 1, a complex oligosaccharide (Shackelford, in prep.). The difference in apparent mol. wt of the 2 chains on SDS-PAGE is largely due to the difference in glycosylation. Only *N*-terminal sequencing has been carried out so far. Although the chains have no apparent sequence homology to each other at the *N*-terminus, they appear to share a number of gross structural features. The sites of papain proteolysis in the native molecule are similar in both chains and separate analogous regions. The distribution of the methionines is also similar in the 2 chains, and the cysteines and carbohydrate are found in the analogous CNBr fragments (Fig. 6). *N*-terminal sequence analysis has shown that all of the HLA-DR antigens so far isolated have sequence homology to the murine I-E/C antigen, that is, the α-chain of HLA-DR has *N*-terminal

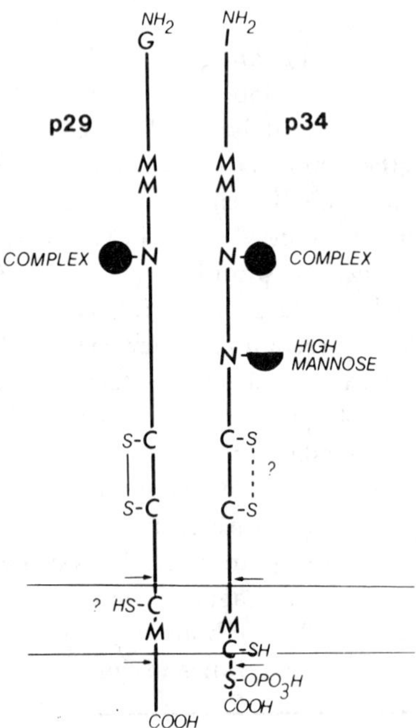

FIG. 6. *Schematic representation of the structure of an HLA-DR antigen.*

sequence homology to the α-chain of murine I-E/C, and similarly the β-chain of HLA-DR has sequence homology to the β-chain of murine I-E/C. Most of the available data indicate that it is the light chain of the HLA-DR (and I-E/C) antigens which is polymorphic (Shackelford and Strominger, 1980; Kaufman *et al.*, 1980). Tryptic peptide mapping has indicated that the light chains of different HLA-DR specificities differ from each other while no tryptic peptide differences were found in the tryptic peptide maps of the HLA-DR heavy chains (Silver and Ferrone, 1979; Kaubman *et al.*, 1980). Similarly, 2 dimensional gel analysis (SDS-PAGE and isoelectric focusing) of the HLA-DR antigens from a number of homozygous typing cells led to the same conclusion (Shackelford and Strominger, 1980). The heavy chains are more acidic and the IEF patterns of the heavy chains of different HLA-DR specificities are virtually identical. By contrast, a number of different patterns can be seen in the IEF patterns of the HLA-DR light chain. One other important feature is the occurrence of a 3rd chain called M1 (for middle band) which is co-precipitated with all the HLA-DR antigens examined and which does not vary in mol. wt or isoelectric point. It is analogous to the invariant spot immunoprecipitated along with the murine Ia antigens (Jones *et al.*, 1979).

The complexity of the band patterns seen in the IEF pattern suggested that some of the variability might be due to glycosylation differences. However, even after treatment of cells with tunicamycin, under which circumstances HLA-DR antigens lacking *N*-linked glycans are synthesized, the light chains from different HLA-DR specificities still showed different IEF patterns (Shackelford and Strominger, 1980). HLA-DRw1 and 2, -DRw3 and 6, and -DRw4, 5 and 7 appear to be closely related chemically. These similarities correspond to known cross-reaction patterns among the HLA-DR antigens. Interestingly, each HLA-DR specificity appeared to contain 2 different light chains. Similarly, although in the case of the heavy chain the IEF patterns of all of the HLA-DR specificities were identical, again apparently 2 different heavy chains were present. It is not presently known whether the occurrence of these 2 chains is due to a real biological phenomenon or might be attributed to some chemical artifact during the isolation of these materials.

Finally, 2 monoclonal antibodies, L203 and L227, which recognize monomorphic determinants on HLA-DR antigens (i.e. they react with antigens of all known HLA-DR specificities) have recently been described (Lampson and Levy, 1980). These antibodies precipitated 2 different sets of Ia-like molecules. These observations with the Raji cell line (HLA-DRw3,6) have been confirmed and, moreover, it has been shown that the light chains precipitated by the L203 and L227 monoclonal antibodies have different IEF patterns (Shackelford *et al.*, in prep.). There is also some evidence that the heavy chains recognized by these 2 monoclonal antibodies may not be identical. Since Raji is a HLA-DR heterozygous cell line, the experiments were repeated with WT46 and Arnt, both DRw6 homozygous cell lines (Fig. 7). Again 2 light chains were observed, one of which was only recognized by L203 and the other was recognized by both monoclonal antibodies. In addition L227 appears to recognize precursors of the DR heavy and light chains, not seen by L203. In addition, preclearing experiments were carried out in which one monoclonal antibody was used to preclear followed by immunoprecipitation with the second. Again, it was apparent that these 2 monoclonal antibodies recognize independent sets of molecules. Moreover, M1, the invariant molecule, was largely associated with the population of molecules precipitated by the monoclonal antibody L227 (Fig. 7). Thus chemical data are accumulating to support the idea derived from careful analysis of alloantisera that the HLA-DR antigen preparations contain several sets of molecules which may be the products of separate genetic loci.

This idea, is, of course, in accord with the fact that at least 2 subregions encoding molecules of this type are found in the *Ia* region of the mouse (*I-A* and *I-E/C*). Both the A_α and A_β chains are encoded in the *I-A* subregion and both of these chains are polymorphic. In addition, the *I-A* subregion encodes E_β, the polymorphic chain of the I-E/C antigens. The E_α chain, which shows only very limited sequence variability, is encoded in the *I-E/C* subregion. The entire system in mice is made more complex by the recent observations that trans gene complementation can occur so that 4 types of I-E/C molecules can occur in outbred mice ($E_{\alpha1}E_{\beta1}$, $E_{\alpha2}E_{\beta2}$, $E_{\alpha1}E_{\beta2}$, and $E_{\alpha2}E_{\beta1}$). In the human HLA-DR antigens, only the polymorphic chain, β, is certainly encoded in the major histocompatibility complex, but by analogy with the mouse, it seems likely that the HLA-DR α-chain is also encoded in this region.

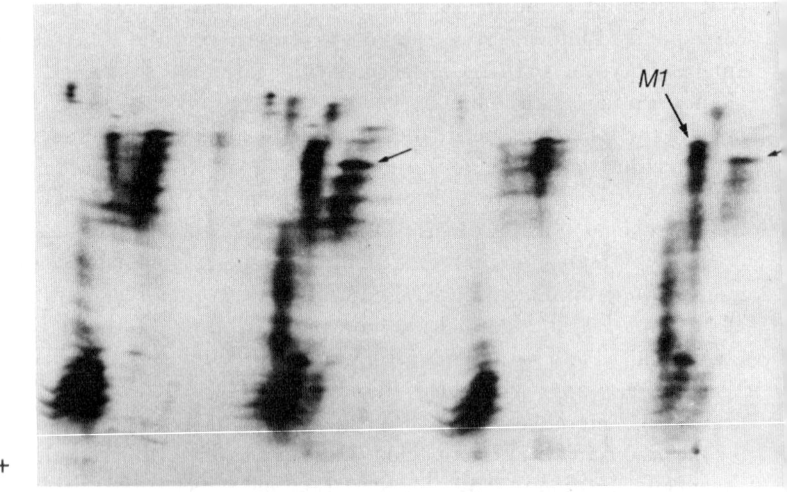

FIG. 7. *Analysis of WT46 with monoclonal antibodies (32). The cell line WT46 was labelled for 4 h with [^{35}S]-methionine and the antigens were extracted with NP-40. The extract was aliquoted and precipitated with L227 or with L203. Each aliquot was reprecipitated with the same antibody and then each precleared extract was then treated with the reciprocal monoclonal antibody. The immunoprecipitates were analysed by 2-dimensional gel electrophoresis (SDS-PAGE followed by IEF) as described in reference 27. The brackets at the bottom indicate the placement of the SDS gel pieces on the IEF gel at the anode. The pieces are oriented with MW decreasing from left to right. The arrow indicated the presumed precursor of 1 of the 2 light chains.*

Thus, the studies of the structure of HLA-DR and I-A or I-E/C molecules have lagged considerably behind the studies of HLA-A and -B and of H-2K and -D antigens. Similarly, studies of biosynthesis with a view to cloning genes of the HLA-DR chains (Korman *et al.*, 1980) and studies of function using the purified HLA-DR antigens (Engelhard *et al.*, 1980) have been initiated but have not progressed as far as the corresponding studies of the HLA-A and -B antigens.

In summary, then, since the time of the 3rd International Congress of Immunology in Sidney, Australia, in 1977 there has been an explosion of information about the structure of the human HLA-A and -B antigens and the corresponding murine H-2K and D antigen. Similar studies of HLA-DR antigens and of murine Ia antigens (I-A and I-E/C) have commenced. It seems possible that gene cloning will be accomplished before the next International Congress and will lead to a very rapid accumulation of primary sequence information. It will also make possible an examination of the organization of these genes in the major histocompatibility complex. Purified antigens, the structural information obtained about them and studies of mutant antigens are being used to approach a precise definition of the function of these extraordinarily polymorphic and interesting cell surface molecules.

References

Biddison, W. E., Krangel, M. S., Strominger, J. L., Ward, F. E., Shearer, G. M. and Shaw, S. (1980). *Human Immunol.* (in press).

Binz, H. and Wigzell, H. (1977). *Cont. Top. Immunobiol.* **7**, 113.

Bjorkman, P., Strominger, J. L. and Wiley, D. C. (in prep).

Charmot, D., Malissen, B., Chiotto, M. and Mawas, C. (1980). *Tiss. Antigens* (in press).

Coligan, J. E., Kent, T. J., Nairn, R., Nathenson, S. G., Sachs, D. H. and Hanson, T. H. (1980). *Proc. Natn. Acad. Sci. U.S.A.* **77**, 1134.

Doberstein, B., Garoff, H., Warren, G. and Robinson, P. J. (1979). *Cell* **17**, 759.

Engelhard, V. H., Kaufman, J. F., Strominger, J. L. and Burakoff, S. J. (1980). *J. Exp. Med.* (in press).

Engelhard, V. H., Strominger, J. L., Mescher, M. and Burakoff, S. J. (1978). *Proc. Natl. Acad. Sci. U.S.A.* **75**, 5688.

Goulmy, E., Blokland, E., Charmot, D., Malissen, B. and Mawas, C. (1980). *J. Exp. Med.* (in press).

Jones, P. P., Murphy, D. B., Hewgill, D. and McDevitt, H. O. (1979). *Mol. Immunol.* **16**, 51.

Kaufman, J. F. and Strominger, J. L. (1979). *Proc. Natn. Acad. Sci. U.S.A.* **76**, 6304.

Kaufman, J. F., Andersen, R. L. and Strominger, J. L. (1980). *J. Exp. Med.* (in press).

Korman, A. J., Ploegh, H. L., Kaufman, J. F., Owen, M. J. and Strominger, J. L. (1980). *J. Exp. Med.* (in press).

Krangel, M. S., Orr, H. T. and Strominger, J. L. (1979). *Cell* **18**, 979.

Lampson, L. and Levy, R. (1980). *J. Immunol.* **125**, 293.

Lea, T., Forre, O. T., Michaelsen, T. E. and Natvig, J. B. (1979). *J. Immunol.* **122**, 2413.

Lopez de Castro, J. A., Orr, H. T., Robb, R. J., Kostyk, T. G., Mann, D. L. and Strominger, J. L. (1979). *Biochemistry* **18**, 5704.

Marchalonis, J. J., Warr, G. W., Rodwell, J. D. and Karush, F. (1980). *Proc. Natn. Acad. Sci. U.S.A.* **77**, 3625.

Martinka, J. M., Uehara, H., Ewenstein, B. M., Kindt, T. J., Coligan, J. E. and Nathenson, S. G. (1980). *Biochemistry* (in press).

Nairn, R., Yamoga, K. and Nathenson, S. G. (1980). *Am. Rev. Genetics* (in press).

Orr, H. T. (in prep.).

Orr, H. T., Lancet, D., Robb, R. J., Lopez de Castro, J. A. and Strominger, J. L. (1979a). *Nature* **282**, 266.

Orr, H. T., Lopez de Castro, J. A., Parham, P., Ploegh, H. L. and Strominger, J. L. (1979b). *Proc. Natn. Acad. Sci. U.S.A.* **76**, 4395.

Orr, H. T., Lopez de Castro, J. A., Lancet, D. and Strominger, J. L. (1979c). *Biochemistry* **18**, 5711.

Ploegh, H. L., Cannon, L. E. and Strominger, J. L. (1979). *Proc. Natn. Acad. Sci. U.S.A.* **76**, 2273.

Pober, J. S., Guild, B. C. and Strominger, J. L. (1978). *Proc. Natn. Acad. Sci. U.S.A.* **75**, 6002.

Reiss, C. S., Hemler, M. E., Engelhard, V. H., Meir, J. W., Strominger, J. L. and Burakoff, S. J. (1980). *Proc. Natn. Acad. Sci. U.S.A.* (in press).

Shackelford, D. (in prep.).

Shackelford, D. A. and Strominger, J. L. (1980). *J. Exp. Med.* **151**, 144.

Shackelford, D., Lampson, L. and Strominger, J. L. (in prep.).
Silver, J. and Ferrone, S. (1979). *Nature* (*Lond.*) **279**, 436.
Strominger, J. L., Engelhard, V. H., Fuks, A., Guild, B. C., Hyafil, F., Kaufman, J. F., Korman, A. J., Kostyk, T. G., Krangel, M. S., Lancet, D., Lopez de Castro, J. A., Mann, D. L., Orr, H. T., Parham, P. R., Parker, K. C., Ploegh, H. L., Pober, J. S., Robb, R. J. and Shackelford, D. A. (1980). *In* "The Role of the Major Histocompatibility Complex in Immunobiology?" (B. Benaceraf and M. E. Dorf, eds) Garland Press, New York (in press).
Trägårdh, L., Rask, L., Wiman, K., Fohlman, J. and Peterson, P. A. (1979). *Proc. Natn. Acad. Sci. U.S.A.* **76**, 5829.
Trägårdh, L., Rask, L., Wiman, K., Fohlman, J. and Peterson, P. A. (1980). *Proc. Natn. Acad. Sci. U.S.A.* **77**, 1129.

Theme 8: Summary

The MHC and its Role in the Immune Defence

WALTER F. BODMER

Imperial Cancer Research Fund, London

The similarities between the major histocompatibility systems of man, *HLA* and of the mouse, *H-2*, both at the genetic level and in terms of the structures of their products has, if anything, increased as our knowledge of their complexity has progressed. There are gaps in both species for example the lack of a human equivalent for *Q* and *TL*, and the lack of evidence so far for C2 and factor B in the *H-2* region. However, only *H-2K* and *HLA-A* remain truly out of line. Flaherty *et al.* (8.1.10),* have found a new allele for Qa-1 and emphasise the increasing complexity of the *Q* region but also its close relationship with *TL* and *H-2K* and *D*. As knowledge of other species' major histocompatibility systems, such as in the rat, syrian hamster, Rhesus monkey and chicken increases, so does, on the whole, their similarity with *HLA* and *H-2*. However, the apparent lack of polymorphism for class 1 determinants (HLA-ABC and H-2KD equivalents) in the Syrian hamster is a surprise (8.1.09). Wild mouse populations show extraordinary variability for H-2 just like their human counterparts.

Fascinating data on structural comparisons for the class 1 products are now available through the extensive amino acid sequence data in the mouse from Nathenson's laboratory and in man from Strominger and his colleagues, as summarized in Chapter 30. Domains of the HLA-ABC and H-2KDL products are clearly defined and major structural homologies are evident with respect to, for example, the position of disulphide loops, hydrophobic regions and "variable" regions. Cross-reactive products, such as A2 and A28, show the expected close similarity, while locus and allele differences remain surprisingly large. Now that crystals of the HLA-A2 molecule have been obtained, the 3-dimensional structure of these products may soon be established. This should answer important questions for example about the position on the molecules of the serological determinants and the nature of their interactions with $\beta2$ microglobulin. The homology of the third outer domain nearest the cell surface with the IgG heavy chain constant region domains is tantalizing. Rather than implying variability with respect to recognition this, perhaps, emphasizes the possibility of analogies with complement, since it is to that region of immunoglobulin that complement binds. Or is there a better analogy with the Fc receptor?

The domain structure of the class 1 products, including the limited homology between the first and second domains, emphasizes the possibility of a complex organization of regions at the DNA level as discussed by Demant (8.1.07) for the polymorphic variants common to H-2K, D and L and by Bodmer for the monomorphic HLA-ABC determinants detected by monoclonal antibodies. The data on H-2L mutants and their relationship to the H-2D mutants (8.2.28), can be interpreted in terms of a

* Reference numbers indicate Abstract numbers in: Abstracts 4th International Congress of Immunology, Paris, 1980.

common region for the class 1 products coded by the same DNA region. Will the different protein domains delineated by the amino acid sequence data have their corresponding DNA regions and how will these relate to the different types of specific or private and cross-reacting or public determinants?

Work on the structure of the Ia and HLA-DR determinants is progressing. There is still, however, argument about the number of gene products and their chain composition. In the mouse the distinction between the I-E/C and I-A products is clear, but there is a suggestion that there may be more than one type of I-E/C product (8.1.26). The invariant spot with an intermediate mol. wt of about 30 000, first found in the mouse by Jones and McDevitt, is now also seen in man in many laboratories, but its relationship in both species to the Ia products is controversial. Its structure appears to be different from the so far recognized 33 000 mol. wt, (8.2.21,22,37) α chains, which leads to the suggestion that the chain plays some functional role in its association with the other Ia chains, perhaps with respect to intracellular transport. It is, however, puzzling that this chain though glycosylated appears not to be expressed on the cell surface. Another possibility suggested by de Kretser, Bodmer and coworkers, is that the 30κ chain seen inside the cell may be processed into another 33κ, α chain on the cell surface. Data from several laboratories (Strominger, Bodmer, Crumpton, Acolla, 8.1.01, Fellous, 8.1.1, Peterson, 8.2.17,.37) suggest that there are two 28κ, β chains associated with the HLA-DR products. The different polymorphic β chains may share monomorphic and cross-reactive determinants, contributing to the present confusion concerning the number of loci detected by HLA-DR serology. If each β chain associates with a specific α chain, then the differences between these α chains may explain apparent α chain polymorphism and remain consistant with the possibility that the structural genes for the α chains may not be in the HLA or *H-2* regions. The genetic control in these regions may be for which of a set of alternative chains coded for elsewhere in the genome is expressed. The mouse Ia α chain recombinant described by Rose and Cullen (8.2.27), may help to answer this question. Specific chain combinations can explain the intriguing complementation for expression of Ia products described by Freed *et al.* (8.2.09), but minimize the possibilities for generating Ia variability by chain combination, as suggested by McDevitt in Chapter 27. Only Goyert and Silver (8.2.10), showed evidence suggesting clearly the existence of an I-A equivalent in man though the SB system described by Shaw *et al.* (8.6.13), using primed lymphocyte testing, seems another plausible candidate for a human I-A equivalent and further studies with monoclonal antibodies, including especially cross-species testing (8.1.27), may soon help to provide an answer. The persistent reports from Parrish and colleagues (8.2.25), of possible carbohydrate differences contributing to polymorphism, need to be evaluated in relation to variation in carbohydrate side chains, which has been described for other products, including HLA-DR on melanomas by Strominger. Such variation could make a limited contribution to the polymorphic differences and indeed exists between human and mouse class 1 products. But the same sugar differences are likely to be found on glycoproteins and glycolipids, so that any claims for their functional significance and the relation of glycolipids and glycosyl transferases to the *H-2* and *HLA* regions must be treated with considerable caution.

Monoclonal antibodies are making a major contribution to this, as to other fields, for example in the definition of determinants, purification of products (for example, H-2, 8.2.23) and through blocking in functional studies. Cross-blocking studies using monoclonal antibodies may define molecular domains by a form of complementation analysis (8.1.20, 8.2.13). Care is needed in such studies to control for the problems of affinity and antibody concentration. Occasional enhancement of the reactivity of one antibody by another (8.1.20) suggests subtle conformational effects, on antibody reactivity.

The close association between determinants identified by cellular techniques and those defined serologically, together with the effects of blocking by monoclonal antibodies, clearly indicate that the known serological products are the basis for at least some of the cellular reactions. The discrepancy between serology and cellular typing, for example, using CML targets to detect subvariants of HLA-B12 (8.1.18), is not unexpected and reflects the different recognition properties of the two assays. One must surely expect that eventually all the cellular products will be detectable serologically even if the actual determinants involved in the cellular reactions are different from those detected by the antibodies. Association due to linkage disequilibrium is at its most exteme for determinants on the same product coded for by different DNA regions of the same gene. Cloning of T cells will help to clarify these problems (8.6.10), and together with the identification of suppressor T cells in man (8.6.02) will help in the identification of the human equivalent of the mouse I-J product as well as in the characterization of human helper and suppressor (8.6.12) factors.

The contribution of cloned T cells to the delineation of specificities recognized by cellular interactions is illustrated strikingly by the data of Fathman and his colleagues (11.2.10). They have shown that it is possible to obtain cloned T cells which react with heteropolymeric products made up of chains from the *Ia* region. These clones recognize specific combinations of chains and so provide an explanation for "heterozygote" determinants.

The role of HLA-ABC products in T cell immune recognition and killing is clearly established in many systems. Differences in flu related killing associated with different allelic determinants have been described by Biddison *et al.* (8.4.01) and McMichael and his colleagues, who also show suggestive evidence for the role of such differences in the protective effects of different alleles against flu. Varying effects of HLA-ABC polymorphic differences on T cell recognition as observed in the EBV system (Workshop 9.2) may simply reflect differences in the extent to which polymorphic differences interfere with the proper functional interaction between the T cell receptor and its target antigen. This association may be refined as the maturity of an immune response develops, and so lead to an increase in the observed effects of HLA-ABC polymorphic restriction during the progress of a T cell immune response.

Changes in H-2 and HLA expression on tumours, especially loss of the determinants, may reflect selection during tumour progression for escape from T cell immunity. Acquisition of new determinants must, it seems, now be treated with some caution in the light of the possibility of contamination between cultures (8.1.32, .23). The so called "bare" lymphocyte syndrome in which HLA-ABC and β_2m are not expressed on the surface of lymphocytes throws a fascinating light on the functional importance of these determinants for the immune system (Van Rood, Touraine *et al.* 8.5.67). Individuals with this syndrome have severe immune deficiency and synthesize no antibody. The deficiency is not linked to HLA and appears to involve a specific control of the expression of $\beta 2$ microglobulin during the maturation of lymphocytes. Van Rood suggests that the major deficiency is in the proper homing of lymphocytes to the lymphoid organs. Perhaps analogous phenomena are associated with the absence of these determinants from certain tumours favouring, for example, the possibilities for metastasis.

Lymphocyte proliferation, whether in mixed lymphocyte cultures (8.6.01), or in the context of antigen specific stimulation (8.4.02, 8.4.08 and 8.4.15) seems to be dependent on HLA-DR. Perhaps HLA-DR can also serve as a basis for T cell cytotoxicity with appropriate targets (8.4.10). The presence of HLA-DR products on, and their synthesis by, activated T cells is now very clear (8.2.01, also Charron and McDevitt, Strominger and Kunkel), though the functional significance of this is not obvious. Does the fact that activated T cells bind externally added Ia reflect the presence of specific receptors for particular factors? The presence of HLA-DR on melanomas (Strominger, Pollack *et al.*, 8.1.30) is intriguing. It is another warning to be careful in the interpretation of apparent tumour specific antigens, and also poses the question as to a possible role for these products in nonimmune functions.

If the gene for 21 hydroxylase deficiency is really in the *HLA* region then this poses yet another puzzle for nonimmune, and indeed perhaps nonsurface related, functions controlled by the *MHC*. The population associations of the 21 hydroxylase mutations with certain HLA alleles (8.5.49), though statistically significant, may simply reflect founder effects and not have any functional significant comparable to other linkage disequilibria observed within the *HLA* region.

The abundant evidence for immune response genes in the mouse is slowly finding its parallel in man as, for example, in the case of *HLA* linked control of proliferation stimulation by streptoccoccal cell wall products (8.4.13). The wide variety of diseases connected with autoimmune involvement which are associated with DR3 (and B8) suggests the possibility of a generalized immune response difference associated with these alleles. This is further supported by the general allergy response differences reported by Marsh *et al.* (8.4.09). The observation by Legrand *et al.* (8.4.06) of differences in the rate of macrophage degradation of antibody coated sheep red blood cells as a function of HLA-DR3, paralleling the differences between Biozzi's high and low responder mice, provides one possible mechanism for such general immune response differences. This contrasts with the specificity of the immune response differences associated with allelic variation as emphasized by McDevitt in the symposium. Perhaps allelic variation associated with differential efficiency in antigen presentation or cellular immune attack is enough to account for the observed apparently specific immune response differences. In that case we do not need to search for a variability generating mechanism in the *HLA-DR* and *H-2-I* regions but may be left once again with a complement function analogy.

The many earlier suggestions and expectations of a role for Gm differences in immune response are supported by Wittingham *et al*'s further data on antibody response to Flagellin and associations with chronic active hepatitis (8.4.17), by the role of Gm differences in macrophage degradation of sheep red cells (8.4.06) as well as by Sasazuki's striking and succinct observation of HLA and Gm identity amongst sibs with Graves disease.

Most HLA and disease associations still lack detailed functional explanations but manv do provide valuable data for diagnosis, prognosis and nosology as summarized by Dausset (Chapter 28) and Svejgaard (Chapter 29) in the symposium. There are still apparently unresolved statistical problems connected with the estimation of gene frequencies and increased linkage disequilibrium in patient populations. The evidence that, even for the apparently recessive mechanisms such as in juvenile onset insulin dependent diabetes, there is some effect of heterozygosity for the relevant HLA genes, *DR3* and *DR4*, is now fairly strong. The association of DR3 with coeliac disease is well established and appears to be with *DR3/DR3* homozygotes. The association of DR7, with coeliac disease, but only in *DR3/DR7* heterozygotes, is an intriguing new observation (8.5.03,.09,.07). In families with multiple cases of rheumatoid arthritis there is a strikingly high frequency of DR4 80% or more (8.5.31), as also observed by J. G. Bodmer and colleagues in other cases involving severe rheumatoid arthritis. It is reassuring to see the first example of an HLA association involving an autoimmune disease, namely that, with Systemic Lupus Erythematosis described by McDevitt, Bodmer, Walford and their colleagues in 1971, now being confirmed both with respect to DR4, reflecting the B15 association and DR3 reflecting a B8 association. Interesting new, or comparatively new, associations involve the pauciarticular form of Juvenile Rheumatoid arthritis with DR5 (8.5.64), many studies on IgA nephropathy associated with Bw35 and possibly DR4 (8.5.21, .26, .35, .36), and Behçet's disease associated with B5 in both Turkey and Greece (8.5.52, .46).

In the search for the mechanism underlying the association between ankylosing spondylitis and B27, while the data on cross-reactions involving *Klebsiella* seem very questionable (8.5.04, 8.5.71) and associations of other antigens with AS in B27 negative individuals lack conviction, the association with a cross-reactive determinant (8.5.43) is intriguing. So also are the possibilities of chemotactic factors associated with reactive arthritis (8.5.53) and the role of immune complexes suggested by Svejgaard in Chapter 29. Variations in complement levels with HLA, especially an apparently clear cut variation in C3 level with DR2 ranging from high in *DR2/DR2* homozygotes through medium in heterozygotes and low in other genotypes, are reminiscent of the initial observations of Demant and his colleagues on complement level variation controlled by H-2 differences (8.5.73). More relevant perhaps for function are the suggested variations in natural killer activity and response to, as well as production of, interferon described by Petranyi and Bloom and their colleagues (11.5.04,.22). It remains to be seen whether these are a product of the disease state or are functions controlled in some way by the HLA region.

The influence of HLA matching on kidney transplant survival remains significant, though much less than might have been hoped for (8.3.14). Cross-matching for HLA antibodies remains, however, important and it is clear that to assess the clinical significance of the presence of antibodies after transplantation, their specificities need to be carefully analysed. Thus, several groups have defined antibodies following transplantation, which react specifically with monocytes and also possibly with certain epithelial tissues (8.3.04,05,07,10). Particularly intriguing are the differences, found by Baldwin and his colleagues (8.3.04), between maternal antisera, with or without platelet absorbtion, and monoclonal antibodies using immunofluorescence on kidney sections. The major challenge for bone marrow grafts, done mainly between HLA identical sibs, is to remove the cells which are responsible for the graft versus host disease. Thierfelder and his colleagues have made a promising start using treatment of the bone marrow with appropriate antisera (8.3.19). There is still, however, doubt as to whether it is killer or suppressor T cells that are involved (8.3.20) and there are interesting suggestions for an important role for natural killer cells (8.3.06).

Many questions concerning the nature of the major histocompatibility genetic regions will only be answered through knowledge of their DNA sequence. The first steps towards this have been taken by many laboratories and have led to interesting information concerning the biosynthesis of the HLA-ABC and DR products and their H-2 equivalents (8.2.16,17,26,29,33). The products are synthesized, as expected for membrane proteins, on the endoplasmic reticulum, have signal sequences and are appropriately glycosylated as they pass to the surface of the cell. Data from the laboratories of Strominger, Bodmer and Peterson (8.2.29) using the Daudi cell line, which lacks HLA-ABC and β2 microglobulin on the cell surface and is in fact a mutant for production of β2 microglobulin, show the important role for β_2m in controlling the final processing of the HLA-ABC products and through this their expression on the cell surface. Many laboratories have DNA clones but none have yet reported their clear cut identification as being derived from HLA or H-2. However, the DNA sequences will surely be accumulated very rapidly.

Based on the recombination fraction within the *HLA* and *H-2* regions, and on the proportion of the DNA from a gene cluster which one might expect to code for protein as indicated for example, from data on the haemoglobins, it is likely that there are as many as 100 peptide products of the HLA region with the approximate size of the HLA-A, B, and C products. Clearly, much still remains to be uncovered in this fascinating genetic region. The rate of advance in the analysis of protein products, and of the RNA and DNA from which they are derived has been, and will continue to be, considerable. We must wait with bated breath for new developments to answer our questions about the region during the coming 3 years, before the next international congress.

Theme 9

Viral Immunity—T Killer Cells (including Alloreactivity)

Presidents:
R. M. ZINKERNAGEL
J. P. LEVY

Symposium Chairman:
K. T. BRUNNER

31

Surveillance of Self: CMI to Virally Modified Cell Surface Defined Operationally by the MHC

P. C. DOHERTY

The Wistar Institute, Philadelphia, USA

Introduction

The cell-mediated immune (CMI) response in virus infections is concerned essentially with eliminating virally modified cells (Zinkernagel and Doherty, 1979). The cells in question may be sited in solid tissues, such as liver (Blanden, 1974), or at mucosal barriers like the respiratory epithelium (Yap *et al.*, 1978). The same general principles seem to apply in each case. The thymus derived lymphocytes (T cells) cannot be shown to recognize virus unless it is presented in association with major histocompatibility complex (MHC) glycoproteins, the structures that we have thought of for many years as transplantation antigens.

The central biological function of these MHC antigens is apparently to focus self-monitoring effector T cells onto virally modified cell surface. The glycoproteins which were historically thought to define "foreignness" are now known to play a key role in maintaining the functional integrity of self. The specificity of any T cell response is determined both by the invading virus and by the self MHC antigens encountered during stimulation. Nonself is thus always defined within the context of self.

The MHC-restriction phenomenon

The MHC of the different species is described at length in other chapters of this volume. Genetic mapping experiments with *H-2* recombinant mice have shown operationally that T cell specificity for virally modified cells is restricted to *H-2K* or *H-2D* compatible interactions (Table I). A variety of experimental

TABLE I
Cytotoxic T cell activity is restricted to H-2K or H-2D compatible interactions

Immune T cells		*Lysis of virus-infected targets*[a]						
Mouse strain	H-2 type K I-A D	*B10* bbb	*B10.Br* kkk	*B10.D2* ddd	*B10.A(2R)* kkb	*B10.A(5R)* bbd	*B10.S* sss	*B6.H2*^{bm1} bm1, bb
B10	*bbb*	+	–	–	+	+	–	+
B10.Br	*kkk*	–	+	–	+	–	–	–
B10.D2	*ddd*	–	–	+	–	+	–	–
B10.A(5R)	*bbd*	+	–	+	–	+	–	–
B10.A(4R)	*kkb*	–	+	–	+	–	–	–
bm1	*bm1, bb*	+	–	–	–	–	–	+
A.TL	*skd*	–	–	+	–	+	+	–

[a] Lysis is seen whenever the T cells and the targets share one allele at either *H-2K* or *H-2D*. The presence of only a common *I*-region allele does not lead to cytotoxicity. The B10.A(4R) mouse is a low-responder to virus presented in association with *H-2D*^{b}. The H-2K^{bm1} and H-2K^{b} antigens are serologically very similar and differ by only one or two amino acids, but there is complete discrimination between these two H-2 glycoproteins by virus-immune CTL. The experimental evidence for this table is reviewed by Zinkernagel and Doherty, 1979.

approaches have been used to demonstrate that different sets (or clones) of virus-immune T cells are associated with each allele at the *H-2K* or *H-2D* locus, the first of these studies being summarized in Table II.

The phenomenon of *H-2K* and *H-2D* restriction is now established for all virus systems that have been examined in depth in the mouse, being defined at the level of cytotoxicity *in vitro* and inflammatory process and virus elimination *in vivo* (Table III). A comparable restriction to HLA-A and HLA-B compatible interactions has also been clearly demonstrated for secondary cytotoxic cell responses to influenza A virus and Epstein–Barr virus-modified cells in man (Table III). The need to focus effector T cells onto virally modified cell surface rather than free virus particles (which can be eliminated by

TABLE II

Different T cell specificities are associated with each H-2K *or* H-2D *allele: Stimulation of (bbb × ddd)F_1 lymphocyte populations in irradiated, virus-infected recipients*

	Lysis of virus-infected targets					
Irradiated recipient[a]	bbb	ddd	kkd	ddd	ddb	bbd
bbb	+	−	−	−	+	+
ddd	−	+	+	+	+	+
ddb	+	+	−	+	+	−
bbd	+	+	+	+	−	+

[a] The recipient mice are irradiated (850 rad), injected with virus and cells and spleen cells are assayed after a further 6 or 7 days (Zinkernagel and Doherty, 1975).

circulating antibody and macrophages) presumably applies to all mammals and, perhaps, to birds (Wainberg *et al.*, 1974).

Fine specificity of the virus-immune T cell response

Virus-immune effector T cells show extraordinary specificity for self *H-2* determinants. A change of two amino acids between the mutant $H\text{-}2K^{bml}$ and wild-type $H\text{-}2K^{b}$ glycoproteins (Nathenson *et al.*, 1980) leads to a complete divergence of effector T cell function (Tables I and IV). Differences between these two H-2 antigens can also be detected by alloreactive T cells (Sherman, 1980), though there is a great deal of cross-reactivity in the overall alloimmune response to $H\text{-}2K^{bml}$. The self-restricted, virus immune T cell response thus seems to show more precise discrimination than is found for alloreactivity.

While virus-immune effector T cells demonstrate a greater capacity to differentiate between mutant and wild-type *H-2* glycoproteins than is readily found by serological means (alloimmune sera do not discriminate readily between $H\text{-}2K^{b}$ and $H\text{-}2K^{bml}$, the converse seems to be true for specificity for viral components (Table V). Influenza A virus haemagglutinin (HA) glycoproteins, which do not cross-react at all when examined serologically, are apparently recognized by effector T cells generated as a result of exposure to any influenza A virus. Massive, secondary cytotoxic T cell responses are seen when mice primed with one influenza A virus are challenged with a second, serologically different influenza A virus. The same phenomenon has been shown for man, the mouse and the rat (Table V). The spectrum of cross-reactivity does not, however, extend to the closely related influenza B viruses.

There is thus a temptation to argue that the potential receptor repertoire specific for self MHC glycoproteins is much more stringently constrained than that for alloantigen or for virus. This may simply reflect the functional need to ensure self-tolerance in the face of a biological mechanism which requires

TABLE III

Association of the MHC with CMI in virus infections

Virus	*Classification*	*Phenomenon*[a]	*Species*	*MHC region*	*Reference*[b]
Lymphocytic choriomeningitis	Arenavirus	CMC	Mouse	*H-2K-D*	Blanden *et al.* (1975)
		Inflammation	Mouse	*H-2K-D*	Doherty *et al.* (1976a)
		Clearance	Mouse	*H-2K-D*	Zinkernagel and Welsh (1976)
		DTH	Mouse	*H-2K-D*	Zinkernagel (1976c)
		CMC	Rat	*AgB*	Zinkernagel *et al.* (1977)
Ectromelia	Poxvirus	CMC	Mouse	*H-2K-D*	Blanden *et al.* (1975)
		Clearance	Mouse	*H-2K-D*	Kees and Blanden (1976)
Vaccinia	Poxvirus	CMC	Mouse	*H-2K-D*	Koszinowski and Ertl (1975)
		CMC	Rat	*AgB*	Zinkernagel *et al.* (1977)
Sendai	Paramyxovirus	CMC	Mouse	*H-2K-D*	Doherty and Zinkernagel (1976)
Influenza	Orthomyxovirus	CMC	Mouse	*H-2K-D*	Yap and Ada (1977)
		CMC	Rat	*AgB*	Marshak *et al.* (1977)
		CMC	Man	*HLA*	McMichael *et al.* (1977)
		Clearance	Mouse	*H-2K-D*	Yap *et al.* (1978)
		DTH	Mouse	*H-2I*	Leung *et al* (1980)
Coxsackie	Enterovirus	CMC	Mouse	*H-2*	Wong *et al.* (1977)
Rabies	Rhabdovirus	CMC	Mouse	*H-2K-D*	Wiktor *et al.* (1977)
Vesicular stomatitis virus	Rhabdovirus	CMC	Mouse	*H-2K-D*	Hale *et al.* (1978) Zinkernagel *et al.* (1978c)
Reovirus I and II	Reovirus	CMC	Mouse	*H-2K-D*	Finberg *et al.* (1979)
		DTH	Mouse	*H-2K/I-A,D*	Weiner *et al.* (1980)
Herpes simplex	Herpesvirus	CMC	Mouse	*H-2K-D*	Pfizenmaier *et al.* (1977)
Epstein Barr virus	Herpesvirus	CMC	Man	*HLA*	Rickinson *et al.* (1980)

[a] CMC, cell-mediated cytotoxicity; Inflammation, cell concentration in cerebrospinal fluid; Clearance, elimination of virus or bacteria by cell transfer into infected recipients; DTH, delayed-type hypersensitivity measured by footpad swelling. [b] The reference given is to the first paper published on the topic. Many of these results have been confirmed by others.

TABLE IV

Major findings that have contributed to the analysis of H-2 restriction of virus-immune T cells

Experiment	Reference
1. H-2 homology is required between T cell and target	Zinkernagel and Doherty (1974)
2. Mapping of phenomenon to H-2K and H-2D	Blanden *et al.* (1975)
3. Different T cell specificities are associated with H-2K and H-2D	Zinkernagel and Doherty (1975)
4. Discrimination at the level of a point mutation in $H\text{-}2K^b$	Zinkernagel (1976a) Blanden *et al.* (1976)
5. T cells (A) developing in thymus of an $F_1(A \times B)$ radiation chimaera interact with H-2 different (B) virus-infected cells	Pfizenmaier *et al.* (1976) Zinkernagel (1976a)
6. The capacity to recognize virus in association with a particular *H-2K* or *H-2D* allele may be dictated by radiation-resistant cells in thymus	Zinkernagel *et al.* (1978)[a]
7. Mature T cells (A) depleted of alloreactivity for B may be induced to recognize B virus-infected cells	Doherty and Bennink (1979)

[a] This is an extremely important set of findings, which has stimulated an immense amount of debate and research. However, the interpretation is still controversial, and the experimental system may be much more complex than was originally envisaged.

TABLE V

T cell specificity for viral antigens

Experimental system	Reference
1. The T cell response overall is cross-reactive for all influenza A viruses, but not for influenza B viruses. This has been shown for man, the mouse and the rat.	Effros *et al.* (1977) Doherty *et al.* (1977) Zweerink *et al.* (1977) McMichael *et al.* (1977) Marshak *et al.* (1977) Biddison *et al.* (1979)
2. The T cells that cross-react for different influenza A viruses recognize targets modified by exposure to liposomes containing the viral haemagglutinin antigen	Koszinowski *et al.* (1980)
3. T cells distinguish between the haemagglutinins of type I and type II reoviruses	Finberg *et al.* (1979)
4. T cell cross-reactivity for targets infected with the Sindbis, Bebaru and Semliki Forest α-viruses	Mullbacher *et al.* (1979)
5. Cross-reactive recognition of targets expressing the G protein of the Indiana and New Jersey strains of vesicular stomatitis virus	Rosenthal and Zinkernagel (1980)

that T cells monitor the integrity of cell-surface in the context of self MHC components (Doherty and Bennink, 1980a). The possibility of autoreactivity may be minimized by ensuring that surveillance of self is limited to a particular active site (defined by the $H\text{-}2^{bml}$ mutation on the H-2 molecule). Obviously, the same constraint need not apply for recognition of either a novel virus glycoprotein, or an alloantigen. The T cell may be able to focus onto any newly encountered determinant expressed on either structure.

The analogy between cell-mediated immunity and graft rejection

The possibility that rejection of virally modified self cells is comparable to allograft rejection was first raised by the experiments of Holterman and Majde (1969), and was given a biological basis by the discovery (and subsequent analysis, Tables III and IV) of the MHC-restriction phenomenon (Zinkernagel and Doherty, 1974, 1979). How is a self cell made to seem "allogeneic" as a result of infection with a virus?

Two possible mechanisms have been discussed at length (Zinkernagel and Doherty, 1974; Doherty *et al.*, 1976b; Zinkernagel and Doherty, 1979). One idea is that the T cell expresses two separate, but in some way linked, receptors that interact with distinct virus and MHC determinants on the surface of the target cell. The broad alternative is that a complex of viral and H-2 antigens is recognized by a single T cell receptor. Evidence is now accumulating that viral and H-2 glycoproteins may associate on cell membrane, and that T cell recognition is optimal when these two components are in close proximity (Tables VI and VII). This does not neccessarily mean that the "one receptor" argument is correct, though it does seem to fit best with models which propose the operation of a single, high-affinity recognition unit. The binding site of such a recognition unit might well be comprised of 2 separately encoded elements, specific for MHC and viral determinants respectively. Ultimately, the problem will only be solved by direct genetic and molecular characterization of the T cell receptors.

The realization that self-monitoring T cells must, before evidence of either binding or of function can be detected, focus onto MHC antigens also provides an explanantion for the existence of alloreactivity. The fact that virus-immune T cells seem to be restricted (Table IV) by the so-called "private" H-2 specificities, while alloreactivity is also associated with the "public" determinants, indicates that the lytic function of T cells is mediated via high affinity binding to any part of the MHC glycoprotein. The limitation to a particular site on the self H-2 antigen presumably reflects the operation of physiological mechanisms concerned with the maintenance of self-tolerance (Doherty and Bennink, 1980a).

Alloreactivity may thus be considered to reflect cross-reactive recognition of foreign H-2 determinants by a single T cell receptor which is normally

TABLE VI

Evidence that viral and H2- glycoproteins may associate on cell membrane

Phenomenon	Reference
1. Cocapping of retrovirus and H-2 glycoprotein	Schrader *et al.* (1975) Zarling *et al.* (1978)
2. Secreted Friend virus containing H-2 glycoprotein of the responder, but not of the nonresponder, H-2 type	Bubbers *et al.* (1977)
3. Cocapping of vaccinia virus and H-2 glycoprotein	Senik *et al.* (1979)
4. CTL interact with cell surfaces modified by exposure to liposomes containing both viral and H-2 glycoproteins, but this is not seen following treatment with separate liposomes incorporating comparable amounts of viral and H-2 antigens respectively	Finberg *et al.* (1978a) Loh *et al.* (1979) Hale *et al.* (1980)
5. Sequential immunoprecipitation indicates that from 10–30% of vesicular virus G protein and the H-$2K^k$ molecule are complexed	Hale (1980)
6. Coprecipitation of retrovirus gp71 and H-2^k antigens under conditions of gentle detergent solubilization	Honeycutt and Gooding (1980)

TABLE VII

Blocking of virus-immune T cells with monoclonal antibodies

Phenomenon	Reference
1. A monoclonal antibody to an H-2 molecule blocks influenza virus-specific but not Bebaru virus-specific CTL	Blanden *et al.* (1979)
2. Monoclonal antibodies to influenza virus HA blocks subtypespecific but not cross-reactive CTL[a]	Effros *et al.* (1979)
3. One monoclonal antibody to the viral HA molecule blocks influenza-immune CTL function associated with H-$2D^d$ but not H-$2K^d$	Frankel *et al.* (1979)
4. A mixture of monoclonal antibodies to the H-2 and viral HA molecules blocks all influenza-immune CTL activity	Askonas and Webster (1980)
5. Dosing mice with monoclonal antibody at 3 h after administration of influenza virus blocks generation of the subtypespecific CTL preferentially	Greenspan and Doherty (1980)

CTL: cytotoxic T lymphocyte. [a]Subtypespecific: specific for a particular viral HA type. Cross-reactive: recognizing cells infected with all influenza viruses.

specific for either virus, or for a complex of viral and self MHC glycoproteins. The latter idea is readily accommodated by the one receptor hypothesis, while proponents of the two receptor model may argue that alloantigen is recognized by the receptor for virus alone (Langman, 1978): alloreactivity is thus considered to operate via a one receptor mode and self-monitoring via a two receptor mode. Some evidence is available that T cells which normally interact with modified self cell surface may also be alloreactive (Finberg *et al.*, 1978b; Boehmer *et al.*, 1979; R. Schwartz, pers. comm.).

The fact that alloreactivity now seems to be a biological irrelevancy, while elimination of virally modified self cells is obviously central to survival, does not necessarily mean that the latter preceded the former in a phylogenetic sense. Prevention of mutual parasitism seems to be of vital importance to the well-being of more primitive life forms (Burnet, 1972; Borysenko, 1976; Hildemann, 1979). The cell-mediated immune system may well have evolved from mechanisms concerned with recognition of foreign components and macro-organisms of the same, or different, species.

Role of the thymus in cell-mediated immunity

Much of the analysis of the MHC-restricted phenomenon (Table IV) has been concerned with determining whether or not T cells of one H-2 type (A) can be induced to respond to virus presented in the context of another H-2 antigen (B). The question has obvious implication for understanding the nature of the T cell repertoire (Doherty *et al.*, 1976b; Zinkernagel and Doherty, 1979). Such experiments are only possible if the T cells of type A which are alloreactive for B can first be removed. This may be achieved by inducing either or state of developmental tolerance (radiation chimaeras, allophenic mice) or acute tolerance (negative selection).

Experiments with $A \rightarrow (A \times B)\ F_1$ radiation chimaeras (irradiated $(A \times B)$ F_1 mice are reconstituted with bone marrow cells of type A) have been interpreted as indicating that A, T cells which develop in an $(A \times B)F_1$ environment may be induced to respond to B+ virus when primed with virus presented on $(A \times B)F_1$ stimulator cells. However it is not yet clear whether these A, T cells can always respond to B+ virus following sensitization in irradiated recipients of type B (Zinkernagel *et al.*, 1980, Doherty and Bennink, 1980b).

The acute removal of A, T cells which are alloreactive for B (negative selection by filtration through irradiated mice or by adsorption on monolayers) sometimes leads to the emergence of T cell clones which are capable of responding to B+ virus (Doherty and Bennink, 1979a, b; Stockinger *et al.*, 1980). However this is not invariably the case (Bennink and Doherty, 1978a). The problem with the negative selection approach is that there is always the possibility that the procedure used to remove the alloreactive precursors may also eliminate clones of A, T cells which have low affinity for B, but high affinity for B+ virus.

The most interesting and controversial finding, which is presumably reviewed elsewhere in these proceedings by Zinkernagel and others is that T cells from an $((A \times B)F_1 \rightarrow A)$ radiation chimaera can only be induced to respond to virus presented in the context of A and not of B. The restriction to A is considered to reflect the interaction of the developing thymocytes with radiation-resistant cells of type A (nurse cells?, see Wekerle and Ketelsen, 1979) that are encountered on the thymic stroma of the A recipient. The phenomenon could reflect either positive selection of T cell precursors which are potentially reactive to virus presented in the context of A (Zinkernagel, 1978; Bevan and Fink, 1978), or deletion of thymocytes which have even minimal affinity for B (Doherty and Bennink, 1979b, 1980a). Other experiments have, however, thrown doubt on the idea that the spectrum of the T cell precursor repertoire is totally determined by the thymus (Kindred, 1978; Zinkernagel *et al.*, 1980). What is the relative importance of intrathymic and postthymic maturation pathways?

TABLE VIII

Loss of thymic function in $(BalB/_6\ nu/nu \rightarrow (C_3H \times DBA/2\ F_1)$ *bone marrow chimaeras*[a]

Days after reconstitution[a]	*% specific* ^{51}*Cr release* *L cells kk* *Vacc*	*N*	*KHTGSV db* *Vacc*	*N*	*MC57G bb* *Vacc*	*N*
28	43	2	24	0	5	1
35	64	5	11	11	14	10
50	11	7	12	19	5	8

[a] From Doherty and Bennink (1980b). [b] Thymus cells were stimulated with virus for 6 days on 850 rad $(kk \times dd)F_1$ receipients.

The development of T cell competence on the part of thymocytes can be studied directly by examining the responder potential of adoptively transferred thymus cells in irradiated, virus-infected recipients. Functional precursors are first detected at 3 or 4 weeks after administration of bone marrow (Bennink and Doherty, unpublished data). However the capacity of thymocytes to develop into virus-immune cytotoxic T cells may be lost within 50 to 60 days of reconstituting the recipients (Table VIII). Other evidence (Doherty and Bennink, 1980b) indicates that this apparent "loss" of thymic function in an $(A \rightarrow (A \times B)F_1)$ chimaera may be accompanied by the transient appearance of T cells which are alloreactive for B and, perhaps, followed by the long-term production of suppressor T cells which inhibit this potential autoreactivity.

The continued analysis of thymic function is thus concerned with the roles that the organ plays in the evolution of MHC-restricted T cell function, on the one hand, and the maintenance of self-tolerance on the other (Doherty and Bennink, 1980a). This is likely to prove one of the more interesting areas of immunobiology over the next 3 or 4 years.

Polymorphism and the organization of the major histocompatibility complex

The realization that T cells can respond only to virus presented in association with MHC antigens (Zinkernagel and Doherty, 1974, 1979) has given us a biological reason (Doherty and Zinkernagel, 1975) for the extreme genetic polymorphism associated with *H-2K* and *H-2D* in the mouse, and HLA-A and HLA-B in man (Amos *et al.*, 1972; Bodmer, 1972; Burnet, 1972). The fact that T cells make little, if any, response to viruses presented in association with some H-2 glycoproteins (Table IX) reflects an underlying evolutionary need to ensure that the species as a whole does not fail to respond to a particular, novel pathogen. Furthermore, different groups (or demes) within a population may be undergoing positive selection for MHC genes that are associated with high responsiveness to virulent viruses operating within a particular ecological niche. It is interesting that the H-2 types found in most laboratory mice, which are presumably of temperate climate origin (Morse, 1978), are associated with nonresponsiveness to the essentially tropical, mosquito-borne alphaviruses (Table IX). The need for a balanced interaction between potentially lethal

TABLE IX
Defective virus-immune CTL responses are seen in the context of some H-2 *alleles*

Virus	*Group*	H-2 *allele*	*Reference*
Friend	retrovirus	K^d, D^d	Blank *et al.* (1976)
murine sarcoma	retrovirus	K^b, D^d	Gomard *et al.* (1977)
influenza A	myxovirus	K^b	Doherty *et al.* (1978)
Sendai	paramyxovirus	D^k	Zinkernagel *et al.* (1978b)
vaccinia	poxvirus	D^k	Zinkernagel *et al.* (1978b)
Sindbis, Bebaru Semliki Forest	α-viruses	all except D^k	Mullbacher and Blanden (1979)
SV40	papovavirus	K^d, D^k, K^q	Pfizenmaier *et al.* (1980)

viruses and the hosts that maintain them has been discussed previously in greater detail (Doherty, 1979).

The other line of defence that the individual possesses against failure to respond to a particular virus rests in the fact that the functions associated with *H-2K* and *H-2D* (or HLA-A and HLA-B) are apparently identical. Absence of any virus-immune T cell response in the context of glycoproteins encoded at both *H-2K* and *H-2D* seems to be fairly uncommon (Table IX). The existence of two such loci may reflect a duplication at some time during evolution. If so, virus infections may have exerted a strong selective pressure favouring the retention of such a duplication. Either the duplication arose before speciation to mouse and man, or we are considering an example of convergent evolution.

The fact that the MHC is inherited as integral unit may reflect long-term, successful interactions between T cell subsets associated with the different loci. The significance (or otherwise) of H-2I-restricted T cell help in the generation of the virus-immune cytotoxic T cell response is far from clear (Zinkernagel, 1978; Bennink and Doherty, 1978b; Ashman and Mullbacher, 1979). Is the lytic function of the T cell mediated via a complement-like molecule? C4 is encoded at H-2S. There may also be phenomenological associations between strong T cell responses restricted to (for instance) $H\text{-}2K^k$ and weaker responses mapping to $H\text{-}2D^b$ (Table X). Analysis to date (Table X) has not clarified whether this reflects a form of suppression, or some other MHC-related interaction.

Virus infections tend to kill young animals that have not yet reached reproductive age. The selective pressures exerted by viruses on contemporary man are probably minimal, though the potential for catastrophic pandemics still exists from pathogens like the Lassa fever virus. Our present spectrum of HLA types may reflect the influence of many pathogenic viruses, such as smallpox, during the middle ages, and influenza in the second decade of this century.

TABLE X

The T cell response to $H\text{-}2D^b$-vaccinia virus

	Virus-specific CTL activity		
T cell populations[a]	K^b	K^k	D^b
bbb	+	−	+
kkb	−	+	−
qkb	−	−	+
$(kkb \times bbb)F_1$	+	+	−
$(kkd \times bbb)F_1$	+	+	−
$(kkd \times bbb)F_1 \rightarrow$ 850 rad bbb[b]	+	−	+
$\searrow$ 850 rad kkb	−	+	−
$[(kkk \times bbb)F_1 \rightarrow bbb]$ chimaera	+	−	+
$[(kkk \times bbb)F_1 \rightarrow kkb]$ chimaera	−	+	−
[c]$kkb_{-bbb} \rightarrow$ 850 rad bbb	−	−	+
[c]$bbb_{-kkb} \rightarrow$ 850 rad kkb	−	+	+
[c]$bbb_{-kkb} + (kkb \times bbb)F_1 \rightarrow$ 850 rad kkb	−	+	+

[a] The *H-2K*, *I-A* and *H-2D* alleles are given. [b] The 850 rad recipients were irradiated one day, injected with virus and cells on the next day and spleen cells were taken for assay after a further 6 days. [c] The T cell populations were filtered through (−, = negative selection) irradiated (950 rad) recipients, and then stimulated with virus in a further set of irradiated recipients. From Zinkernagel *et al.* (1978b, d); Doherty *et al* (1978); Bennink and Doherty (1979); Doherty and Bennink (1979b).

Summary

Cell-mediated immunity (CMI) in virus infections reflects the surveillance of cell surface by immune thymus derived lymphocytes (T cells). The T cells which function to eliminate virus *in vivo* are apparently the same as those that mediate cytotoxicity *in vitro*. These cytotoxic T lymphocytes show two orders of specificity: for the virus in question and for self major histocompatibility complex (MHC) glycoproteins. The need to interact with MHC antigens serves to focus the effector T cell onto virally modified cell membranes, rather than onto free virus particles. The balance between potential responsiveness and self-tolerance that must be achieved to ensure that T cells operate to eliminate virus-infected, but not normal, self cells is probably a major function of the thymus. The fact that CMI always operates within the context of one or another MHC glycoprotein provides a biological basis for the extreme polymorphism of the MHC genes. Some MHC alleles are associated with absence of response to a particular virus. The existence of many alternative MHC genes ensures that nonresponsiveness to a novel pathogen will not be general throughout the species. Both the evolution of MHC-restricted cytotoxic T cell function and the present spectrum of *H-2* and HLA genes probably reflect selective pressures exerted by virus infections.

References

Amos, D. B., Bodmer, W. F., Ceppellini, R., Condliffe, P. G., Dausset, J., Fahey, J. L., Goodman, H. C., Klein, G., Klein, J., Lilly, F., Mann, D. L., McDevitt, H., Nathenson, S., Palm, J., Reisfeld, R. A., Rogentine, G. N., Sanderson, A. R., Shreffler, D. C., Simonsen, M. and Van Rood, J. J. (1972). *Fed. Pro.* **31**, 1087.

Ashman, R. B. and Mullbacher, A. (1979). *J. Exp. Med.* **150**, 1277.

Askonas, B. A. and Webster, R. G. (1980). *Eur. J. Immunol.* **10**, 151.

Bennink, J. R. and Doherty, P. C. (1978a). *J. Exp. Med.* **148**, 128.

Bennink, J. R. and Doherty, P. C. (1978b). *Nature Lond.* **276**, 829.

Bennink, J. R. and Doherty, P. C. (1979). *Proc. Natn. Acad. Sci. U.S.A.* **76**, 3482.

Bevan, M. J. and Fink, P. J. (1978). *Immunol. Rev.* **42**, 4.

Biddison, W. E., Shaw, S. and Nelson, D. (1979). *J. Immunol.* **122**, 660.

Blanden, R. V. (1975). *Transplant. Rev.* **19**, 56.

Blanden, R. V., Doherty, P. C., Dunlop, M. B. C., Gardner, I. D., Zinkernagel, R. M. and David, C. S. (1974). *Nature Lond.* **254**, 269.

Blanden, R. V., Dunlop, M. B. C., Doherty, P. C., Kohn, H. I. and McKenzie, I. F. C. (1976). *Immunogenetics* **3**, 541.

Blanden, R. V., Mullbacher, A. and Ashman, R. B. (1979). *J. Exp. Med.* **150**, 166.

Blank, K. J., Freedman, H. A. and Lilly, F. (1976). *Nature Lond.* **260**, 250.

Bodmer, W. F. (1972). *Nature Lond.* **237**, 139.

Boehmer, H. von, Hengartner, H., Nabholz, M., Lernhardt, W., Schreir, M. H. and Haas, W. (1979). *Eur. J. Immunol.* **9**, 592.

Borysenko, M. (1976). *Immunogenetics* **3**, 305.

Bubbers, E. J., Chen, S. and Lilly, F. (1978). *J. Exp. Med.* **147**, 340.

Burnet, F. M. (1972). *Nature Lond.* **245**, 359.

Doherty, P. C. (1980). *In* "Strategies of Immune Regulation." (A. Cunningham and E. Sercarz, eds). Academic Press, New York and London (in press).

Doherty, P. C. and Bennink, J. R. (1979a). *J. Exp. Med.* **149**, 150.

Doherty, P. C. and Bennink, J. R. (1979b). *J. Exp. Med.* **150**, 1187.

Doherty, P. C. and Bennink, J. R. (1980a). *Scand. J. Immunol.* (in press).

Doherty, P. C. and Bennink, J. R. (1980b). Manuscript submitted for publication.

Doherty, P. C. and Zinkernagel, R. M. (1975). *Lancet* **ii**, 1406.

Doherty, P. C. and Zinkernagel, R. M. (1976). *Immunology* **31**, 27.

Doherty, P. C., Dunlop, M. B. C., Parish, C. R. and Zinkernagel, R. M. (1976a). *J. Immunol.* **117**, 187.

Doherty, P. C., Gotze, D., Trinchieri, G. and Zinkernagel, R. M. (1976b). *Immunogenetics* **3**, 517.

Doherty, P. C., Effros, R. B. and Bennink, J. (1977). *Proc. Natn. Acad. Sci. U.S.A.* **74**, 1209.

Doherty, P. C., Biddison, W. E., Bennink, J. R. and Knowles, B. B. (1978). *J. Exp. Med.* **148**, 534.

Effros, R. B., Doherty, P. C., Gerhard, W. and Bennink, J. (1977). *J. Exp. Med.* **145**, 557.

Effros, R. B., Frankel, M. E., Doherty, P. C. and Gerhard, W. (1977). *J. Immunol.* **123**, 1343.

Finberg, R., Mescher, M. and Burakoff, S. J. (1978a). *J. Exp. Med.* **148**, 1620.

Finberg, R., Burakoff, S., Cantor, H. and Benacerraf, B. (1978b). *Proc. Natn. Acad. Sci. U.S.A.* **75**, 5145.

Finberg, R., Weiner, H. L., Fields, B. N., Benacerraf, B. and Burakoff, S. J., (1979). *Proc. Natn. Acad. Sci. U.S.A.* **76**, 442.

Frankel, M. E., Effros, R. B., Doherty, P. C. and Gerhard, W. (1979). *J. Immunol.* **123**, 2438.

Gomard, E., Duprez, V., Reme, T., Colombani, M. J. and Levy, J. P. (1977). *J. Exp. Med.* **146**, 909.

Greenspan, N. and Doherty, P. C. (1980). Manuscript submitted for publication.

Hale, A. H. (1980). *Immunogenetics* **10**, 469.

Hale, V. H., Witte, O. N., Baltimore, D. and Eisen, H. N. (1978). *Proc. Natn. Acad. Sci. U.S.A.* **75**, 970.

Hale, A. H., Ruebush, M. J. and Harris, D. T. (1980). *J. Immunol.* **125**, 428.

Hildemann, W. H. (1979). *Transplantation* **27**, 1.

Holterman, O. A. and Majde, J. A. (1969). *Nature Lond.* **233**, 624.

Honeycutt, P. J. and Gooding, L. R. (1980). *Eur. J. Immunol.* **10**, 363.

Kees, U. and Blanden, R. V. (1976). *J. Exp. Med.* **143**, 450.

Kindred, B. (1978). *Immunol. Rev.* **42**, 60.

Koszinowski, U. and Ertl, H. (1975). *Nature Lond.* **255**, 552.

Koszinowski, U. H., Allen, H., Gething, M. J., Waterfield, M. D. and Klenk, H. D. (1980). *J. Exp. Med.* **151**, 945.

Langman, R. E. (1978). *Rev. Physiol. Bioch. Pharmacol.* **81**, 1.

Leung, K. N., Ada, G. L. and McKenzie, I. F. (1980). *J. Exp. Med.* **151**, 815.

Loh, D., Ross, A. H., Hale, A. H., Baltimore, D. and Eisen, H. N. (1979). *J. Exp. Med.* **150**, 1067.

McMichael, A. J., Ting, A., Zweerink, H. J. and Askonas, B. A. (1977). *Nature Lond.* **270**, 524.

Marshak, A., Doherty, P. C. and Wilson, D. B. (1977). *J. Exp. Med.* **146**, 1773.

Morse, H. C. III (1978). "Origins of Inbred Mice." Academic Press, New York and London.

Mullbacher, A. and Blanden, R. V. (1979). *Immunogenetics* **7**, 551.

Mullbacher, A., Marshall, I. D. and Blanden, R. V. (1979). *Scand. J. Immunol.* **10**, 291.

Nathenson, S. G., Ewenstein, B. W., Marinho, J. M., Nairn, R., Nisizawa, T., Uehara, H. and Yamaga, K. (1980). *J. Supramol. Struct. Suppl.* **4**, 121.

Pfizenmaier, K., Starzinski-Powitz, A., Rodt, H., Rollinghoff, M. and Wagner, H. (1976). *J. Exp. Med.* **143**, 999.

Pfizenmaier, K., Jung, H., Starzinski-Powitz, A., Rollonghoff, M. and Wagner, H. (1977). *J. Immunol.* **119**, 939.

Pfizenmaier, K., Pan, S. H. and Knowles, B. B. (1980). *J. Immunol.* **123**, 1888.

Rickinson, A. B., Wallace, M. E. and Epstein, M. A. (1980). *Nature Lond.* **282**, 865.

Rosenthal, K. L. and Zinkernagel, R. M. (1980). *J. Immunol.* **124**, 2301.

Schrader, J. W., Cunningham, B. A. and Edelman, G. M. (1975). *Proc. Natn. Acad. Sci. U.S.A.* **72**, 5066.

Senik, A., Demant, P. and Neauported-Sautes, C. (1979). *J. Immunol.* **122**, 1461.

Sherman, L. A. (1980). *J. Exp. Med.* **151**, 1386.

Stockinger, H., Pfizenmaier, K., Rollinghoff, M. and Wagner, H. (1980). Manuscript submitted for publication.

Wainberg, M. A., Markson, Y., Weiss, D. W. and Doljanski, F. (1974). *Proc. Natn. Acad. Sci. U.S.A.* **71**, 3565.

Weiner, H. L., Greene, M. I. and Fields, B. N. (1980). *J. Immunol.* (in press).

Wekerle, H. and Ketelsen, U. P. (1980). *Nature Lond.* **283**, 402.

Wiktor, T. J., Doherty, P. C. and Koprowski, H. (1977). *Proc. Natn. Acad. Sci. U.S.A.* **74**, 334.

Wong, C. Y., Woodruff, J. J. and Woodruff, J. F. (1977). *J. Immunol.* **118**, 1165.

Yap, K. L. and Ada, G. L. (1977). *Immunology* **32**, 151.

Yap, K. L., Ada, G. L. and McKenzie, I. F. C. (1978). *Nature Lond.* **273**, 238.

Zarling, D. A., Keshet, I., Watson, A. and Bach, F. (1978). *Scand. J. Immunol.* **8**, 497.

Zinkernagel, R. M. (1976a). *J. Exp. Med.* **143**, 437.

Zinkernagel, R. M. (1976b). *Nature Lond.* **261**, 139.

Zinkernagel, R. M. (1976c). *J. Exp. Med.* **144**, 776.

Zinkernagel, R. M. (1978). *Immunol. Rev.* **42**, 202.

Zinkernagel, R. M. and Doherty, P. C. (1974). *Nature Lond.* **248**, 701.

Zinkernagel, R. M. and Doherty, P. C. (1975). *J. Exp. Med.* **141**, 1427.

Zinkernagel, R. M. and Doherty, P. C. (1979). *Advances Immunol.* **27**, 51.

Zinkernagel, R. M. and Welsh, R. M. (1976). *J. Immunol.* **117**, 1495.

Zinkernagel, R. M., Althage, A. and Jensen, F. C. (1977). *J. Immunol.* **119**, 1242.

Zinkernagel, R. M., Callahan, G. N., Althage, A., Cooper, J., Klein, P. A. and Klein, J. (1978a). *J. Exp. Med.* **147**, 882.

Zinkernagel, R. M., Althage, A., Cooper, S., Kreeb, G., Klein, P. A., Sefton, B., Flaherty, L., Stimplfling, J., Shreffler, D. and Klein, J. (1978b). *J. Exp. Med.* **148**, 592.

Zinkernagel, R. M., Althage, A. and Holland, J. J. (1978c). *J. Immunol.* **121**, 748.

Zinkernagel, R. M., Althage, A., Cooper, S., Callahan, G. N. and Klein, J. (1978d). *J. Exp. Med.* **148**, 805.

Zinkernagel, R. M., Althage, A., Waterfield, E., Kindred, B., Welsh, R. M., Callahan, G. and Pincetl, P. (1980). *J. Exp. Med.* **151**, 376.

Zweerink, H. J., Courtneidge, S. A., Skehel, J. J., Crumpton, M. J. and Askonas, B. A. (1977). *Nature Lond.* **267**, 354.

32

Interaction of Viruses and Lymphocytes in Evolution, Differentiation and Oncogenesis

SUSUMO OHNO, TAKESHI MATSUNAGA, JOERG THOMAS EPPLEN and TOYOHARU HOZUMI

Division of Biology, City of Hope Research Institute, Duarte, California, USA

Abbrevations

β_2m: $\beta_2$microglobulin; C: immunoglobulin constant region; DNP: dinitrophenol; H: immunoglobulin heavy chains or immunoglobuin heavy chain hinge region coding sequence; HyL: hydrophobic leader coding sequence; J: immunoglobulin junction coding sequence; KLH: keyhole limpet haemocyanine; L: immunoglobulin light chain; MHC: major histocompatibility complex; MuLV: murine leukaemia virus; NIP: 4-hydroxy-5-iodo-3-nitrophenacetyl; NP: 4-hydroxy-3-nitrophenacetyl; V: immunoglobulin variable region.

Curse of Prometheus laid upon the immune system

Upon wresting the control of the earth from the Titans, Zeus assigned the task of creating living creatures to two Titan brothers who had sided with him in the epic battle just concluded. Because Epimetheus, who had been endowed only with hindsight, had the first hand in this creation, all the good attributes were exhausted in the creation of other animals. Thus, man was made naked and weak. Prometheus took pity on this miscreation and gave man intelligence for the eventual use of fire. Upon the completion of their task, Zeus punished not Epimetheus but Prometheus for the impertinence of his foresight. The moral of this Greek myth is very profound, for the Darwinian model of evolution by natural selection is a strictly Epimethean model, where foresight is the forbidden fruit.

Foresight imposed *status quo* on variable region genes

As a difference of several orders of magnitude exists between the generation time of parasitic viruses and bacteria and that of vertebrate hosts, in an evolutionary race for adaptive changes one invariably expects these parasites to gain the upper hand. The antiviral antibody selected on the basis of its past merit would be useless against a new mutant strain of that virus. Thus, we come to realize that unlike all other biological systems, the immune system had to acquire Promethean foresight. Indeed, in recent years the immune system has demonstrated ample capacity to deal with all sorts of odd, man-made nonbiological molecules that are the products of post-World War II synthetic chemistry. One can be reasonably certain that this biological world had not experienced most of these man-made molecules until the present day. It follows then that the ability to generate antibodies directed against those odd molecules was conferred to the mammalian genome by apparent foresight (Cohn, 1968; Ohno, 1979). Promethean foresight of the immune system depends upon its ability to generate randomly a very large variety of antigen-binding sites specified by a large number of V genes; the extent of contribution by somatic mutations determining the total number of V genes in the mammalian genome. As the expression of each antigen-binding site by lymphocytes is made clonal, nearly every individual comes to possess a variety of minority clones that, by chance, happen to express antigen-binding sites directed against antigens not yet in existence.

The curse of Prometheus is found in the *status quo* imposed upon V genes of the immune system. In the past, black plagues and smallpox epidemics ravaged the Eurasian continent. Yet these great epidemics should have exerted

This work was supported by NIH grants No. 1 RO1 AG00042 and No. 1 RO1 AI15620 and by the Wakunaga Pharmaceutical Company, Ltd. J.T.E. is a recipient of Fellowship grant No. Ep712, from the Deutsche Forschungs Gemeinschaft.

no selective pressure upon variable region genes of the human genome, for the simple reason that the ability to generate antigen-binding sites directed against *Pasteurella pestis* and *Variola major* was made inherent in nearly all human individuals long before their encounter with those virulent pathogens. While it is true that during the first encounter with a new virulent pathogen, individuals who happened to be endowed with the greatest number of relevant clones enjoy a decisive selective advantage, this cannot be a stable inheritable characteristic. Unequal crossing-overs constantly occurring among numerous V genes would equalize the above kind of advantages and disadvantages in relatively short order (Ohta, 1980).

Since V genes of the mammalian immune system placed upon the Promethean pedestal are beyond the reach of natural selection, autoimmune diseases, no matter how severe, should not cause the elimination of antiself V genes from the genome. This, then, is the curse of Prometheus laid upon the immune system for the impertinence of its foresight. Were it not in the nature of V genes to endow nearly every individual with relevant clones directed against any pathogen as well as against any self antigen, subsequent development of helper and suppressor T cells would have been superfluous, for helper T cells regulate the speed of expansion of pre-existing clones against pathogens, whereas suppressor T cells prevent the expansion of antiself clones already in existence.

Viruses attempt to disguise their antigens as the host's selves, the host counters by polymorphism of MHC antigens

Development of the Promethean immune system that can keep up with rapid adaptive changes of viruses and bacteria must have forced these parasites to exercise the one remaining option in escaping from immunological persecution by the host. The sound strategy devised was to disguise their antigens as components of the host. Although smallpox epidemics should have exerted no appreciable influence upon V genes of the human genome, as already noted, those unfortunate individuals whose blood group and/or other plasma membrane antigens too closely resembled relevant antigens of *Variola major* must have been selectively eliminated by such epidemics. This tells us that natural selection by favouring genetic polymorphism of host plasma membrane antigens succeeded in placing the Promethean immune system under its surveillance, albeit indirectly. Since the list of pathogens is endless, the best that each species can hope for by generating genetic polymorphism of plasma membrane antigens is survival of the majority of a population after periodical encounters with various virulent pathogens. Extraordinarily extensive genetic polymorphism of MHC antigens observed in all mammalian species studied, as well as the invariable presence of duplicated gene loci (e.g. *H-2D*, *H-2K*, *Ia-1* to *Ia-5* of the mouse) in the MHC region of the mammalian genome then indicates that these MHC antigens are the principal tool with which the host immune system attempts to distinguish disguised selves of pathogens from true selves.

T cell receptors recognize alien antigens in association with MHC antigens

After every conceivable experiment has been done and all the possible alternatives have been explored, one finds that the original article on the subject said it all. We found this to be true of the X inactivation mechanism that operates in mammalian females (Lyon, 1961). Our feeling is that the same is also going to be the case with MHC restrictions in the cell-mediated immune system (Zinkernagel and Doherty, 1974). The original interpretation was that cytoxoic T cells do not recognize viral antigens *per se* on the infected target plasma membrane, but specific perturbations of self MHC antigens caused by their association with viral antigens; the "altered self" phenomenon. It has been proposed that much of the germ line V genes of the immune system are directed against all the allelic MHC antigens of the species (Jerne, 1971). If, by viral pertubations, self MHC antigens come to resemble allo-MHC antigens specified by other MHC alleles, infected individuals can readily mobilize anti-allo-MHC V genes in their genome for the persecution of the virus. Thus, the above noted view on the germ line V genes and the original "altered self" concept are quite complementary. Viewed in this light, violent graft rejections caused by MHC incompatibilities are but inadvertent consequences of the immune system's choice of MHC antigens as the principal tool of discrimination between viral disguised pseudoselves and true selves.

The nature of self-restricting antigens

The other side of the "altered self" concept is that when confronted with virally infected, allo-MHC targets, the host cell mediated immune systems choose to ignore viral antigens and exclusively react against allo-MHC antigens. While the above may not hold true in every instance, it does reveal the immune system's preoccupation with the recognition of MHC antigens. In a sense, MHC antigens are self restricting, but there are other reported instances of similarly self-restricting antigens.

Early preimplantation mouse embryos are thought to be H-2 antigen (−), and so presumably are embryonal carcinoma cells. It has been shown that cytotoxic T cells can be raised against such H-2 antigen (−) embryonal carcinoma cells and that their cytotoxicity towards other embryonal carcinoma cells and spermatogonia is restricted not with regard to H-2 but with regard to F9 antigen (Wagner *et al.*, 1978). In a similar vein, it has been the experience of many that cytotoxic T cells directed against H-2Qa antigens (Flaherty,

1978) are self restricted. We also expect the cell mediated immune response against Tla antigens of the mouse to be self restricting (Forman, 1979). This self restriction was also observed on one of the "differentiation antigens" as defined by Cantor and Boyse (1977). When female mice of H-Y nonresponder H-2^k haplotype were immunized against purified testicular Sertoli cells from syngeneic males, anti-SG cytotoxic T cells were generated. These T cells lysed only testicular Sertoli cells and ovarian granulosa cells of the mouse, but of divergent H-2 haplotypes (Ciccarese and Ohno, 1978).

It will be of extreme interest if in the future it is shown that the common denominator of all self-restricting plasma membrane antigens is their use of β_2m or β_2m-like polypeptide as a subunit, as ubiquitously expressed MHC antigens indeed do.

Polymorphic MHC antigens show differential associative affinities towards the same alien antigens

In order to significantly alter the configuration of self MHC antigens, viral antigens as well as H-Y and other minor histocompatibility antigens must engage in intimate association with each other at one time or another in the life cycle of cells. We can think of only two reasons for such an invariable association. It should be noted that the two are not mutually exclusive:

(1) β_2m-MHC antigen dimers serve as the plasma membrane anchorage sites of testis-organizing H-Y antigen and other organogenesis-directing plasma membrane antigens. Indeed, in the absence of its proposed anchorage sites, Daudi β_2m (−), HLA (−) human male Burkitt lymphoma cells failed to maintain H-Y antigen on their plasma membrane (Beutler *et al.*, 1978; Fellous *et al.*, 1978). Instead Daudi cells excreted H-Y antigen to the culture medium (Nagai *et al.*, 1979). Accordingly, viruses found it to their advantage to displace these functionally important host antigens with their own (Ohno, 1977).

(2) β_2m-MHC antigen dimers function as the vehicle of transport towards the plasma membrane for those antigens, which would otherwise remain in the cellular interior because their messenger RNAs, are translated by free ribosomes. This would apply to those viral antigens that are found as much in the cellular interior as on the plasma membrane. Conversely, some of the antigen equipped with HyL, therefore, whose messenger RNAs are translated by membrane-bound ribosomes, may be kept on the plasma membrane by β_2m-MHC antigen dimers instead of being excreted. With regard to H-Y antigen, the findings already noted on Daudi cells can also be used to support the above hypothesis. If self MHC antigens can receive lasting imprints of alien antigens during their association in the cellular interior, the continued association after their emergence on the plasma membrane appears irrelevant. Yet it appears that if given a choice, T cell receptors invariably recognize that MHC antigen which remains in closest association with an alien antigen on the

target plasma membrane. It may be that the persistent association is a reflection of a profound alteration inflicted on that MHC antigen.

Indeed, on the plasma membrane of F_1 $H\text{-}2^b/H\text{-}2^d$ mouse cells, Friend MuLV antigen preferentially remains in association with $H\text{-}2D^b$ (Bubbers and Lilly, 1977), and it is this (MuLV + altered $H\text{-}2D^b$) antigen complex which is recognized by cytotoxic T cell receptors (Blanks and Lilly, 1977). Along a similar vein, it has been shown that in the presence of testosterone, H-Y antigen on the plasma membrane of male $H\text{-}2^b$ mice associates with $H\text{-}2D^b$ but not with $H\text{-}2K^b$ (Flaherty *et al.*, 1979). Not surprisingly, in the presence of $H\text{-}2D^b$ antigen, anti-H-Y T cell receptors ignore all other H-2 antigens and recognize the (H-Y + altered $H\text{-}2D^b$) antigen complex (Simpson and Gordon, 1977).

Confusion between altered self-MHC and unaltered self- or allo-MHC

Inasmuch as MHC antigens as one class of molecules must be endowed with a finite number of conformational alternatives and most of these alternatives must be manifesting themselves in the form of allelic MHC antigens in a polymorphic population, it is really no surprise if one allelic MHC antigen altered by an alien antigen comes to resemble another allelic MHC antigen in the unaltered state. Indeed when anti-H-Y cytotoxic T cells derived from female $H\text{-}2^b$ mice were cloned and then propagated, aside from lysing male $H\text{-}2^b$ cells that were their intended target, they also indiscriminately lysed male and female cells alike that carried $H\text{-}2D^d$ antigen (von Boemer *et al.*, 1979). It would appear that the (H-Y + altered $H\text{-}2D^b$) antigen complex comes to resemble unaltered $H\text{-}2D^d$ antigen, as schematically illustrated in Fig. 1. Inasmuch as nature does not practice the transplantation of allografts, the above confusion is of no consequence.

The fact that anti-(H-Y + altered $H\text{-}2D^b$) cytotoxic T cells made no apparent distinction between male and female $H\text{-}2D^d$ cells offered as their targets indicated that either H-Y antigen does not associate with $H\text{-}2D^d$, or by association, $H\text{-}2D^d$ antigen alters but a very little. Indeed female mice of the $H\text{-}2^d$ haplotype have long been known as poor responders against H-Y antigen. As shown in Fig. 1, when anti-H-Y female cytotoxic T cells that preferentially recognized the (H-Y + $H\text{-}2K^d$) antigen complex were raised *in vitro*, they lysed nearly half as much self ($H\text{-}2^d$ female cells) as their intended $H\text{-}2^d$ male target (Matsunaga and Ohno, 1980). It would appear that by association, H-Y antigen altered $H\text{-}2K^d$ just enough to provoke an anti-H-Y response, but not enough to prevent the cytotoxic T cell receptor from confusing unaltered $H\text{-}2K^d$ and/or $H\text{-}2D^d$ antigens with the (H-Y + $H\text{-}2K^d$) antigen complex. *In vitro*, the role of suppressor T cells might be to prevent such a self destructive cell mediated immune response.

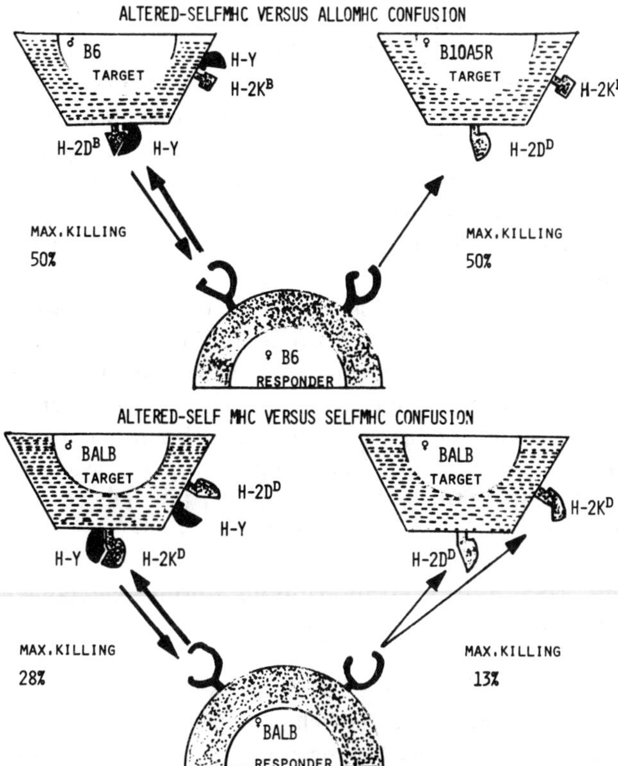

FIG. 1. *Anti-H-Y cytotoxic T cells of the mouse confuse altered self H-2 antigens with unaltered allo- or self-H-2 antigens; the cause of autoimmune response?* Top: *Anti-H-Y cytotoxic female $H\text{-}2^b$ T cells confuse (H-Y + altered $H\text{-}2D^b$) antigen complexes with unaltered allo-$H\text{-}2D^d$, thus, indiscriminately lysing male and female $H\text{-}2D^d$ cells alike presented as the targets.* Bottom: In vitro *raised anti-H-Y cytotoxic T cells of $H\text{-}2^d$ female mice have difficulty in distinguishing (H-Y + altered $H\text{-}2K^d$) antigen complexes from unaltered $H\text{-}2D^d$ and/or $H\text{-}2K^d$ antigens of the self, thus, lysing nearly half as much female $H\text{-}2^d$ cells (self) as their proper male target.*

Differential use of the same V_H gene by T cell receptors and immunoglobulin heavy chains

Provided that the same pool of V genes contribute the antigen binding sites to T cell receptors as well as immunoglobulins, the T cell receptor's inclination to recognize the (alien + altered self MHC) antigen complex on the target plasma membrane should also be reflected in humoral antibodies directed against the same plasma membrane antigen. Indeed, starting with the original findings by Binz and Wigzell as well as by Rajewsky and Eichmann, increasing evidence indicates that T cell receptors derive their antigen binding sites from V_H genes, while receiving no contribution from V_L genes. One of the more convincing demonstrations of the above utilized V_HIg-1b genetic marker which is a V_H allotype of the mouse. The anti-NP hapten humoral antibody of the $V_{\lambda L}V_HNP^b$ composition exhibits a unique heteroclicity in that this antibody raised against NP demonstrates a far greater binding affinity to a related hapten NIP than to NP itself. Anti-NP T cell receptors of the same mouse also exhibit the same heteroclicity towards NIP, thus, suggesting their antigen binding sites to have been specified by the V_HNP^b allelic gene (Cramer *et al.*, 1979). The above finding, however, created one unresolved dilemma. In the case of anti-NP humoral antibodies, the heteroclicity towards NIP is the unique property of $V_{\lambda L}V_HNP^b$ and not of $V_{\kappa L}NP^b$. How V_HNP^b alone of the T cell receptor without help from $V_{\lambda L}$ can express this heteroclicity? At any rate, the antigen binding specificity is not often, if ever, demonstrable in V_H monomers. Here we show that the pretranscriptional coding sequence fusion mechanism that unites one of the numerous Vs with the C, even if indirectly in the B cell nucleus, can also unite two or more V_H coding sequences in tandem in the T cell nucleus. We thus suggest that the antigen binding sites of T cell receptors are furnished by two V_H coding sequences fused in tandem. We acknowledge here that the possibility of $V_H + V_H$ fusion dawned on us during our conversation with Dr Melvin Cohn.

$V_L + J_L$ and $V_H + D_H + J_H$ pretranscriptional fusion mechanisms for immunoglobulin subunits

In the mammalian genome, three unlinked clusters of genes specify Ig κ-class L chains, λ-class L chains and several classes of H chains. Furthermore, within each cluster, numerous V genes are separated by a million or more base pairs from a small number of C genes. Thus, it was earlier realized that in order to specify each Ig transcript containing one each of V and C coding sequences, one of the numerous Vs must somehow be brought to the proximity of the C. In the case of κ-class light chains, the above essential has recently been shown to be accomplished by a pretranscriptional coding sequence fusion between one of the Vs and one of the several short J coding sequences (Sakano *et al.*, 1979; Seidman *et al.*, 1979). Since these five or so short Js are likely to be tandem duplicates of HyL of the C when the C was specifying an independent $\beta_2$microglobulin-like peptide (Ohno, 1980), a cluster of them accompany the C. Accordingly, a single V + J coding sequence fusion event causes that V + J, remaining unattached Js and the C coding sequences to be included in the same transcript; subsequent removal of intervening sequences producing mature Ig κL messenger RNA. When one each of the Vs and Js are brought together by a pretranscriptional fusion enzyme of enzymes, the cardinal fusion signal sequence $\frac{\text{CCACAGTG}}{\text{GGTGTCAC}}$ immediately downstream from the V coding sequence and its complementary fusion signal $\frac{\text{CACTGTGG}}{\text{GTGACACC}}$ immediately

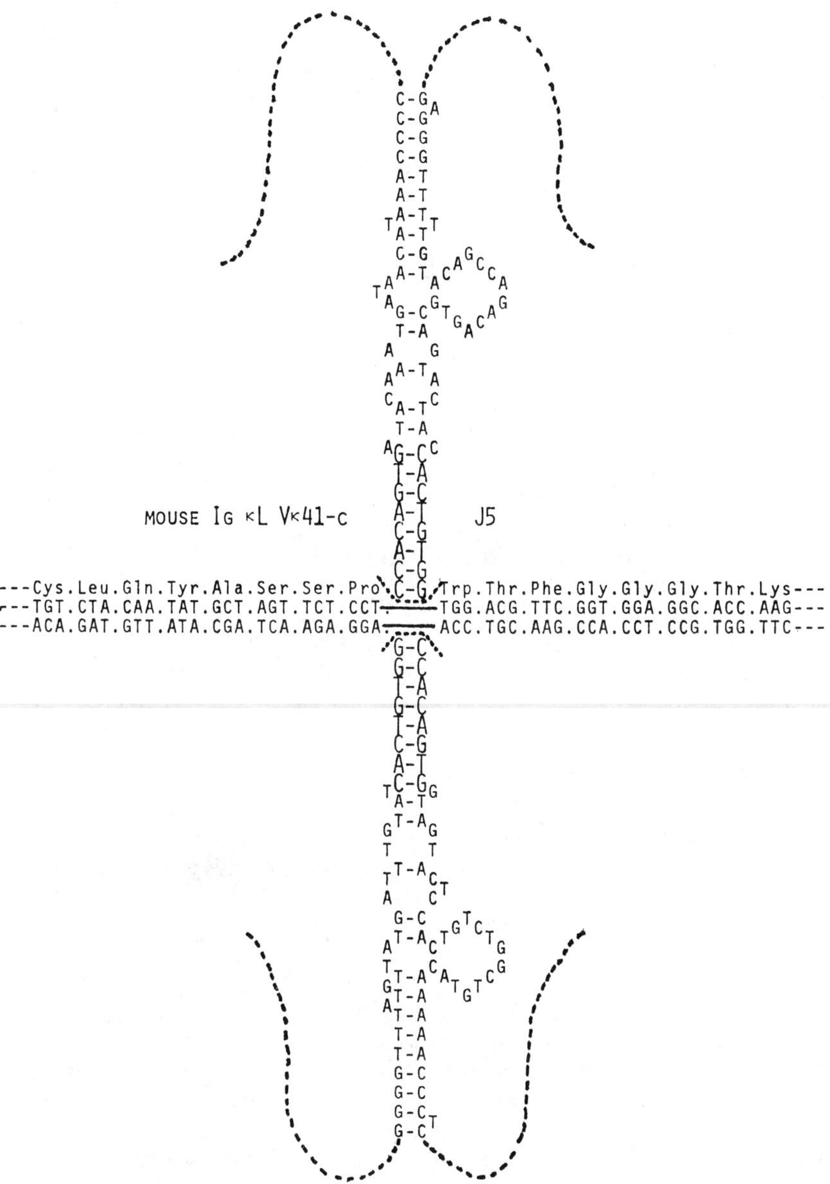

FIG. 2. *The cardinal fusion signal sequence* $\frac{CCACAGTG}{GGTGTCAC}$ *attached to Vκ41-c coding sequence of the mouse and its complementary fusion partner signal* $\frac{CACTGTGG}{GTGACACC}$ *adorning Jκ5 in the coupled, ready-to-be-fused configuration. In the actual fusion of Vκ41c and J5, the complementarity between the above noted 8-base-long signal sequences is reinforced by additional complementary sequences. Among them,* $\frac{CATAAACC}{GTATTTGG}$ *on the V side and* $\frac{GGTTTATG}{CCAAATAC}$ *on the J side seemed to have been conserved reasonably well.*

upstream from the J coding sequence, initiate extensive sideways base pairing between them to form the cross-configuration at the V and J coding sequence junction on DNA. The resulting V + J coding sequence fusion presumably discards a million or more base pairs of DNA (Fig. 2).

However, the finding represented in Fig. 2 has not revealed the all-important V + J pretranscriptional fusion mechanism in its entirety, for there remain two unresolved questions. First of all, unless a V + J coding sequence fusion happened to involve the last J nearest to the C, a transcript would have to contain a number of unattached J coding sequences situated between the fused (V + J) and the C. Since each J is equipped with its own upstream

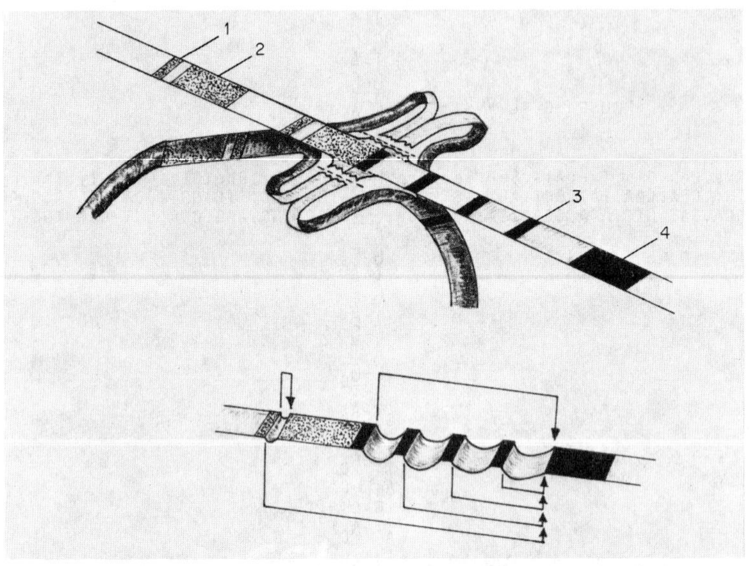

FIG. 3. *A pretranscriptional V + J coding sequence fusion event occurring in the gene cluster for mouse Ig κL and the consequent production of transcripts containing one fused V + J, three unattached J's and one C coding sequences are schematically illustrated. 1, hydrophobic leader sequence; 2, variable region coding sequence; 3, junction coding sequence; 4, constant region coding sequence.*

Top: *Because the cardinal fusion signal sequence* $\frac{CCACAGTG}{GGTGTCAC}$ *resides immediately downstream of each Vκ coding sequence, while its complementary partner signal* $\frac{CACTGTGG}{GTGACACC}$ *adorns each Jκ, any combination of Vκ and Jκ can be brought together by the enzyme that recognizes the above pair of signals. The sideways pairing initiated by the pair produces the cross-figuration at the Vκ + Jκ coding sequence junction. The resulting V + J fusion eliminates a very long stretch of DNA; longer than one million base pairs containing varying numbers of V's and J's.* Bottom: *The RNA transcript of the above rearranged DNA segment. For it to become mature cytoplasmic messenger RNA for Ig κL, only two proper pairs of splicing signals should be recognized as indicated by 2 arrows above the transcript. The presence of three unattached J's, however, creates the possibility of 4 different types of illicit splicing as indicated by arrows below the transcript.*

splicing signal, splicing with the C during the processing of that nuclear transcript is more likely to involve one of the unattached Js than the fused V + J, thus resulting in the formation of nonsense messenger RNA. The pretranscriptional fusion mechanism has to contain a built-in safeguard against the inadvertent splicing noted above (Fig. 3). In each of the three chromosomes carrying Ig genes, a large subcluster of numerous V genes and a small subcluster made of several Js and one or more Cs is separated by a million or more base pairs of void as already noted; roughly a genetic distance of one cross-over unit. When viewed in the light of immense distance, the fusion signal sequence barely 40 or so base pairs long loses its impressiveness. In order for the fusion enzyme in the B cell nucleus to be able to recognize one V and one J separated by such an immense distance, each V and each J must be endowed with additional, more conspicuous characteristics to make their positions known.

In Fig. 4, the solutions to both questions are shown using J-1, J-2 and J-5 coding sequence of mouse κL as examples. It should be noted that each J coding sequence is an imperfect palindrome, internal base sequence complementarity extending to adjacent noncoding sequences. Accordingly, even in germ line DNA, each J should be obvious because it assumes a small cross-configuration (Fig. 4).

It is of interest to note here that the cardinal 8-base-long pretranscriptional fusion signal sequence CCACAGTG directly attached to Vκ41-c of Fig. 2 represents the core of the prototype 14-base-long splicing signal sequence *CCC ACA.G*/G*U* GAG AG from which all the upstream as well as downstream splicing signals have been derived (Ohno, 1980). It would appear that the pretranscriptional coding sequence fusion mechanism for the formation of Ig transcripts evolved from the ubiquitous posttranscriptional splicing mechanism that removed intervening sequences from nuclear transcripts of many genes. It follows then that the 8-base-long downstream fusion signal attached to each J being complementary to the above noted CCACAGTG is also largely complementary to that Js own upstream splicing signal located at the other end because of the latter's derivation from the prototype CCC ACA.G/*GU GAG AG* (intervening sequence bases in italics). Accordingly, each unattached J in Ig transcripts, by assuming a hairpin loop configuration, manages to hide its upstream splicing signal by base pairing; e.g., the upstream splicing signal CUG AAA.C/*Gu AAG UA* of unattached J-1 in Fig. 4 is base paired with a sequence centred by the complementary fusion signal CACUGUGG. The above then is a safeguard against inadvertent splicing involving unattached Js and the C. Naturally, the pretranscriptional fusion with V discards the fusion signal sequence from J, and by so doing renders its upstream splicing signal accessible to the splicing enzyme, thus, ensuring the representation of one each of V, J and C coding sequences in contiguity in mature cytoplasmic messenger RNA.

The situation is a little different in an IgH chain gene cluster, for it was found that antiphosphorylcholine V_Hs used by certain mouse myeloma antibodies first fuse with very short D coding sequences which are good

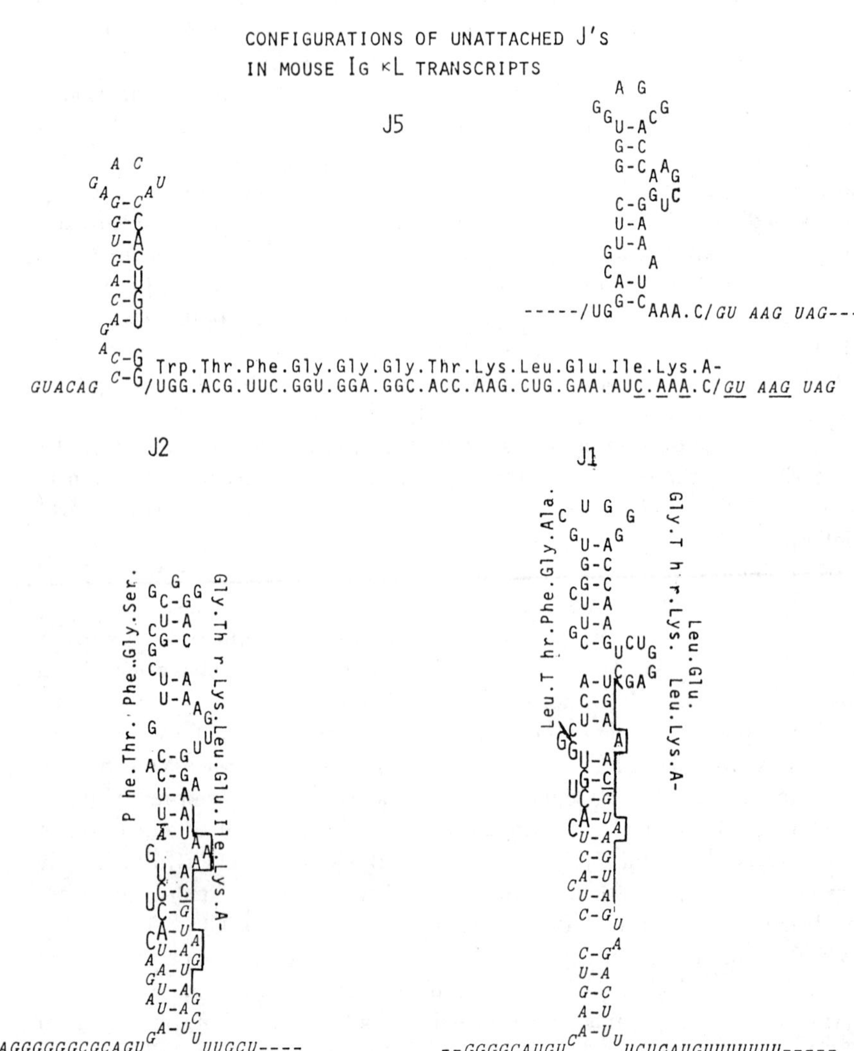

FIG. 4. *Hairpin loop configurations of unattached J5, J2, and J1 in mouse Ig κL transcripts. All J coding sequences including JH's are imperfect palindromes. Only in J5 does the complementary fusion partner signal CACUGUGG form another hairpin loop with its immediate upstream bases, thus, leaving the AAA.C/*GU AAG UA *portion of the J5's upstream splicing signal sequence accessible to the splicing enzyme. The above apparently reflects the terminal position of J5. Being farthest away from the Cκ, J5 would never be transcribed without the prior fusion with V. In unattached J2 as well as J1, the AAA.C/*GU AAG UA *portion of their upstream splicing signals is made inaccessible to the splicing enzyme, because of base pairing.*

only for 5 amino acid residues, and only then does $(V_H + D_H)$ fuse with the J_H (Early *et al.*, 1980). Interestingly, each D_H coding sequence such as $\frac{\text{Tyr.Tyr.Gly.Ser.T}}{\text{TAC.TAC.GGT.AGT.A}}$ is a nearly perfect palindrome. Furthermore, it is equipped with the downstream fusion signal sequence at one end for the fusion with V_H, and the upstream fusion signal at the other end for the fusion with J_H, and the two partner fusion signals are naturally complementary to each other. It follows then that in the germ line DNA, each D_H stands out as conspicuously as each J by assuming the configuration of a small cross. Each V_L or V_H coding sequence in the germ-line DNA can also signal its presence to the fusion enzyme by the possession of two crosses, the second being larger than the first, for we found that the first and second hypervariable regions are invariably included in independent pseudo-palindrome sequences. This point is illustrated in the first and second hypervariable regions of V_HM141 (Sakano *et al.*, 1980) in Fig. 5.

$V_H + V_H$ pretranscriptional fusion for T cell receptors

If this insertion of an extra step represented by D_H in the pretranscriptional coding sequence fusion mechanism of IgH chains is universal in spite of the fact that D_H may contribute as little as 1 or as many as 14 amino acid residues to IgH chains (Sakano *et al.*, 1980), it must mean that this extra step in the B cell nucleus acts as an irreversible commitment towards Ig heavy chain formation.

What occurs in the nuclei of killer, helper and suppressor T cells? We have noted that the 42 base-pair-long sequence made of the last 31 base pairs of the intervening sequence after HyL, and the first 11 base pairs of the V_HM603 coding sequence are largely complementary to the upstream fusion signal of V_HS107 (Early *et al.*, 1980). Thus, the enzyme that causes the pretranscriptional fusion of V_H and D_H has an apparent potential to fuse V_HS107 and V_HM603 in tandem; both V_H being directed against phosphorylcholine. However, in view of the very early ontogenic separation of the T cell lineage from the B cell lineage (Cantor and Boyse, 1977), we feel that the pretranscriptional fusion enzyme that causes $V_H + D_H + J_H$ as well as $V_L + J_L$ coding sequence fusion in the B cell nucleus can not be utilized by the T cell nucleus for tandem $V_H + V_H$ fusions. It is necessary for the latter to recognize a related but different set of fusion signal base sequences. We found such downstream fusion signals residing within the first two-thirds of the intervening sequence that follows HyL of V_HM141 (Sakano *et al.*, 1980). The postulated fusion between V_HM141 and V_HS107 is illustrated in Fig. 6.

It should be recalled that $V_L + J_L$ (Fig. 2) and presumably also $V_H + D_H$ and then $(V_H + D_H) + J_H$ coding sequence fusions in B cell nuclei depend upon the complementarity between the two sets of fusion signal sequences; that between the cardinal $\frac{\text{CCACAGTG}}{\text{GGTGTCAC}}$ and $\frac{\text{CACTGTGG}}{\text{GTGACACC}}$ or their immedi-

VHM141

HYPERVARIABLE I HYPERVARIABLE II

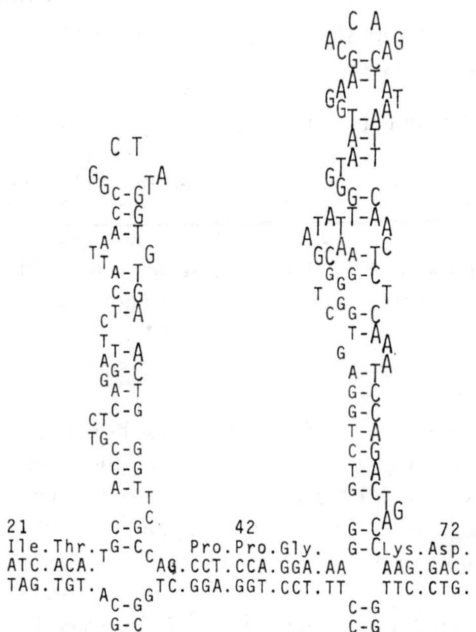

FIG. 5. *Contrary to certain previous claims, the first and second hypervariable regions residing within each V_L and V_H coding sequence do not show sufficient internal base sequence complementarity within themselves. But each is invariable included in a longer palindrome sequence. This point is illustrated on V_HM141. Accordingly, the enzyme responsible for pretranscriptional fusion shall have no difficulty in recognizing individual V's, D's and J's on the germ line DNA. Bases of first and second hypervariable regions are shown in larger capital letters. While the first specifies only 5 amino acid residues, the second specifies 19. Naturally, their inclusions in palindrome hairpin loops might account for selectively high mutational base substitutions, deletions, and insertions affecting these regions; not only first and second hypervariable regions within each V, but also individual D's and J's (Fig. 4) that constitute the third hypervariable region of antigen binding sites.*

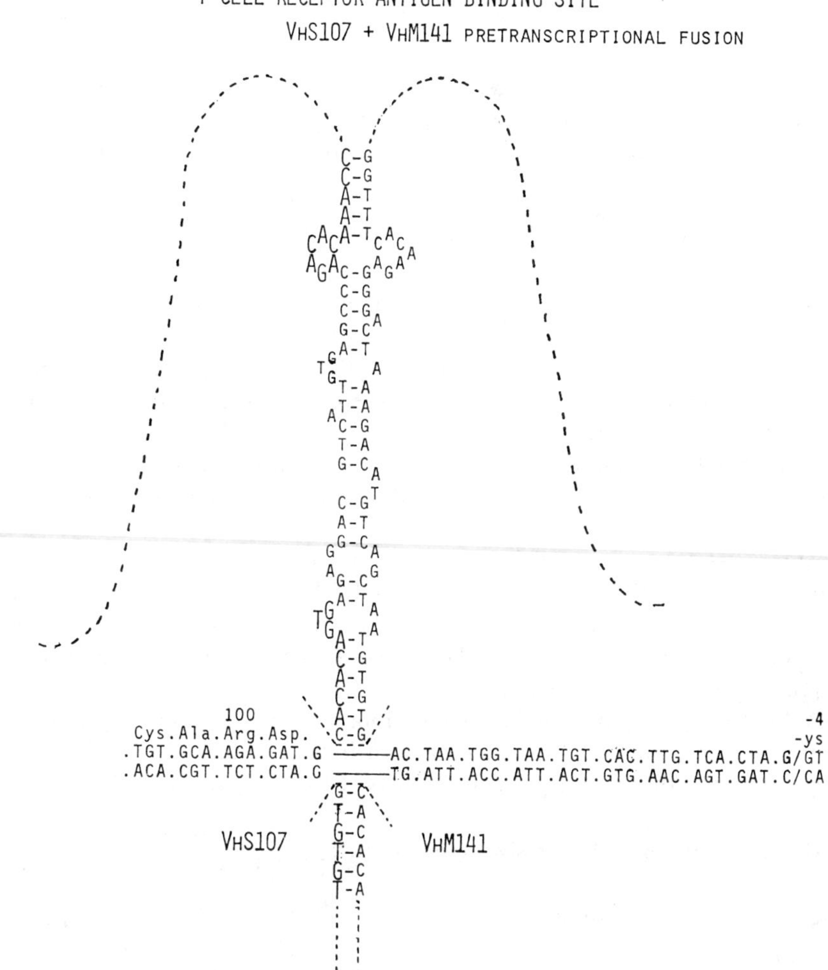

FIG. 6. *The feasibility of the* $V_H + V_H$ *pretranscriptional coding sequence fusion in the T cell nucleus is illustrated choosing* V_H*S107* (*Early* et al., *1980*) *and* V_H*M141* (*Sakano* et al., *1980*) *as upstream and downstream fusion partners. Both of the two conserved upstream fusion signal sequences for* $V_H + D_H$ *fusion residing immediately adjacent to* V_H*S107 coding sequence are shown in larger capital letters. When the extensive sideways base pairing of this figure is compared with that shown in Fig. 2, a strong measure of support is found for our notion that* $V_H + V_H$ *fusions in T cell nuclei and* $V_L + J_L$ *as well as* $V_H + D_H + J_H$ *fusions in B cell nuclei are catalysed by two different enzymes that recognize pairs of related but slightly different fusion signal base sequences.*

ate derivative, supplemented by that between $\frac{\text{ACAAAAACC}}{\text{TGTTTTTGG}}$ and $\frac{\text{GGTTTTTGT}}{\text{CCAAAAACA}}$ or their immediate derivatives (Sakano *et al.*, 1979, 1980; Early *et al.*, 1980). Figure 6 suggests that for proposed tandem $V_H + V_H$ coding sequence fusions in T cell nuclei, only specific portions of the above noted pair of upstream fusion signals are utilized for the side-wise base pairing; the complementarity between $\frac{\text{CACACA}}{\text{GTGTGT}}$ and $\frac{\text{TGTGTG}}{\text{ACACAC}}$ is supplemented by that between $\frac{\text{AAACC}}{\text{TTTGG}}$ and $\frac{\text{GGTTT}}{\text{CCAAA}}$. The differential use of fusion signal base sequences would insure that $V_H + D_H$ and then $(V_H + D_H) + J_H$ coding sequence fusions can occur only in B cell nuclei, whereas $V_H + V_H$ fusions can take place only in T cell nuclei.

By having two or more V_Hs fused in tandem as their antigen binding site, the antigen discriminating power of T cell receptors is elevated to the equivalent of at least Ig LH dimers (Fig. 7).

Anti-KLH receptors excreted by suppressor T cells of H-2^b mice have been shown to contain the KLH binding site and I-J^b antigenic determinants in unseparable coupling; their combined molecular weight being in the range of 50 000 (Taniguchi *et al.*, 1979). The above appears to limit the number of V_Hs involved in tandem fusion to two (Fig. 7).

After the $V_H + D_H$ pretranscriptional fusion in the B cell nucleus, V_HS107 contributes the amino acid sequence down in Asp of the 101st position to IgH chains. In the transcript of the fused V_HS107 + V_HM141 of Fig. 8, one finds the upstream splicing signal sequence $\frac{\text{T-yr. T-yr. C-y-}}{\text{U.UA U.AC U.G}/\textit{U GCA AG}}$ within the V_HS107 coding sequence; the first of the two Tyrs of the above occupying 93rd position (bases of an intervening sequence in italics). Since the absence of *G* at the head of the intervening half of the above upstream signal has to be compensated by an addition of an extra *G* at the intervening sequence end of its partner downstream splicing signal (Ohno, 1980), the regular downstream splicing signal $\frac{\text{-ys. Ile. Le}}{\textit{UCA CUA G}/\text{GU. AUC. CU}}$ of V_HM141 for the removal of its intervening sequence should now be read as $\frac{\text{-s. Ile. Le}}{\textit{UCA CUA GG}/\text{U. AUC. CU}}$. Accordingly, the processing of the (V_HS107 + V_HM141) transcript by T cells should unite the two V_H coding sequences at

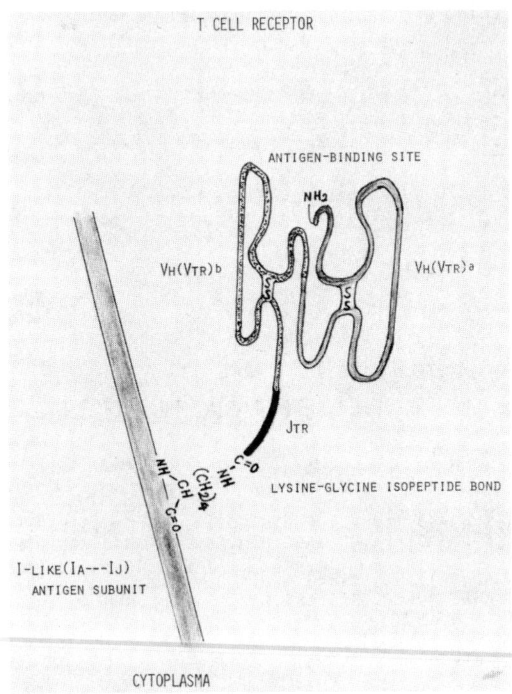

FIG. 7. *The schematic illustration of T cell receptors as we conceive them. This scheme is heavily influenced by the finding of Tada's group on anti-KLH suppressor T cell receptors. Its antigen binding site is furnished by two V_H's directed against the same antigen in tandem fusion. The possible source of J_{TR} carboxyl terminal amino acid sequence is shown in Fig. 8. We believe that J_{TR} and one or the other subunit of I-J and other I-like antigens are linked together by the isopeptide bond; here shown as glycine-lysine.*

the junction $\begin{matrix}\text{Tyr. Try. Cy-s. Ile. Le}\\ \text{UAU.UAC.CG/U.AUC.CU}\end{matrix}$ (Fig. 8). Since V_HM141 is involved as a downstream partner of this $V_H + V_H$ fusion, the translation of V_HM141 coding sequence can continue beyond Ser of the 97th position until the chain terminating codon is encountered which is not yet evident in the sequence data presented by Sakano *et al.* (1980), thus, gaining at least 30 additional amino acid residues (Fig. 8). In schematic drawings of Fig. 7, the amino acid sequence beyond the 97th Ser of V_HM141 is identified as J_{TR}, since the $(V_H + V_H)$ antigen binding site of T cell receptor is thought to bind to one of the two subunits of I-J and other I-like MHC antigens via J_{TR} (Fig. 7).

In view of the unseparable coupling between the antigen binding site and I-J antigenic determinants observed in anti-KLH suppressor T cell receptors (Taniguchi *et al.*, 1979), we propose the isopeptide linkage between the antigen binding site furnished by two tandemly fused V_Hs and a subunit of I-like MHC antigen; e.g., nuclear protein ubiquitin and histone H-2A are linked

SPLICING OF (V_HS107 + V_HM141) TRANSCRIPT

```
 97      VHS107
--T-yr.T-yr.C-y -s.Ala.Asp.
--U.AU U.AC U.G/ U GCA AGA [UGA] CUA [AUG] GUA AUG UCA CUU

 G UC A CU A G G/U.AUC.CUU.UCC.CAG.------------------
                -s.Ile.Leu.Ser.Gln.------------------
                  -3         1

                VHM141
```

JTR OF (V_HS107 + V_HM141)

T CELL RECEPTOR ANTIGEN BINDING SITE

```
            97
--TYR.CYS.ALA.SER.Asp.Thr.Val.Arg.Glu.Val.Gln.Cys.Glu.Pro.Ala.Gln.Ile.
--UAC.UGU.GCC.AGA.GAC.ACA.GUG.AGG.GAA.GUC.CAA.UGU.GAG.CCU.GCA.CAA.AUA.

  Pro.Leu.Cys.Arg.Asp.His.Asn.Gln.Gln.Gly.Ala.Val.Arg.Thr.Gln.Gly.Leu.
  CCU.CUC.UGC.AGG.GAU.CAC.AAC.CAG.CAG.GGG.GCG.GUG.AGG.ACC.CAA.GGA.CUU

(the sequence data end)
```

FIG. 8. *A possible manner of processing the fused $V_H + V_H$ transcript and subsequent translation of its processed cytoplasmic messenger RNA to yield T cell receptor antigen binding sites are illustrated using the fused $V_HS107 + V_HM141$ as an example.* Top: *The removal of a newly created intervening sequence from the fused $V_HS107 + V_HM141$ transcript. Bases of an intervening sequence are shown in italics and the precise positions of a pair of intervening-coding boundaries are indicated by slashes. The rules that enable us to identify each pair of splice sites in all transcripts have been described in detail elsewhere (Ohno, 1980).* Bottom: *The continuous translation of the processed messenger RNA adds 30 extra amino acid residues to the carboxyl terminus of the fused $V_HS107 + V_HM141$ polypeptide beyond Ser of the 97th position (199th in the fused antigen binding site) of V_HM141. The presence of a chain terminating codon is not yet in evidence in the sequence data (Sakano* et al., *1980).*

by a lysine-glycine isopeptide bond (Fig. 7). It must be this linkage with I-like antigen subunit that anchors T cell receptors to the plasma membrane. The second alternative origin of J_{TR} is the constant coding sequence reserved only for T cell receptors; the pretranscriptional fusion between 2 V_Hs being followed by a second fusion between (fused $V_H + V_H$) and one of the D_Hs. According to this view, D_Hs are duplicates of the hydrophobic leader of the T cell-specific C. Thus, each T cell receptor transcript should contain (fused $V_H + V_H + D_H$), a number of unattached D_Hs and the C. Evidence suggesting the existence of such J_{TR} (C) which is class-specific for receptors of suppressor and killer T cells has been presented (Owen *et al.*, 1979).

On target plasma membrane, humoral antibodies also see alien antigens in association with MHC antigens

Although the antigen binding sites of T cell receptors as well as IgH chains are apparently derived from the same pool of V_H genes, it is worth remembering that a given antigen, as a rule, provokes multiclonal responses from B cells, thus revealing the luxury of multiple choices among V_H genes. Furthermore, receptors of helper and suppressor T cells that regulate B cell responses do not recognize alien antigens in association with H-2D and H-2K antigens as do cytotoxic T cells but in association with I-A to I-J antigens in the case of mice. Although H-2D, H-2K and I-A to I-J antigens are specified by the same gene complex, there exists no further similarity between these two classes of antigens. Another difference between the antigen binding sites of humoral antibodies and that of T cell receptors lies in the fact that that of the former is represented by $V_L + V_H$ combinations while the T cell receptor antigen binding sites are furnished by two tandemly furnished V_Hs according to our view. In spite of all these differences noted above, the fact remains, nevertheless, that so long as alien antigens remain in almost invariable association with one or the other of MHC antigens on the target plasma membrane, humoral antibodies should also recognize not alien antigens alone, but antigen complexes formed between alien antigens and altered self MHC antigens.

Evidence in favour of the above has been slowly accumulating. A certain class of anti-H-2^b antibodies raised in MuLV (−) B10A (H-$2D^d$H-$2K^k$) mice against MuLV (+) B10 (H-$2D^b$H-$2K^b$) cells lysed both MuLV (+) and MuLV (−) B10 cells presented as targets. Furthermore, the cytotoxicity of this antibody towards the former can be absorbed out by the latter as expected of anti-H-2^b antibody. In addition, however, this antibody lysed MuLV (+) but not MuLV (−) selves/B10A cells (Ivani *et al.*, 1980). One plausible explanation is that this class was not a real anti-H-2^b antibody, and instead the antibody was directed against (MuLV + altered H-$2D^b$) and/or (MuLV + altered H-$2K^b$) antigen complexes, and that the overall conformation of one or the other of the above two complexes became sufficiently similar to (MuLV + altered H-$2D^d$) and/or (MuLV + altered H-$2K^k$) antigen complexes.

Certain humoral H-Y antibodies appear to recognize less H-Y antigen itself and more of the altered MHC antigens, whereas the converse may be true of other H-Y antibodies. A good example of the former is found in human H-Y antibody reported by Goulmy *et al.* (1977). Of male and female human cells of various HLA haplotypes offered as its cytotoxic targets, this antibody lysed only male human cells carrying HLA-A2 antigenic determinants. Yet, this was not anti-HLA-A2 antibody, for it did not lyse HLA-A2 female cells. Furthermore, even absorption of this antibody was possible only by human male HLA-A2 cells. By contrast, mouse H-Y antibody customarily raised in

H-2^b female mice apparently represent the latter, for its male specific cytotoxicity can be readily extinguished by absorption with male cells of any mammalian species (Wachtel *et al.*, 1975). However, the cytotoxicity of this antibody towards appropriate male mouse targets (spermatozoa and epidermal cells) demonstrates very pronounced H-2 dependence; male cells of H-2^b and H-2^d haplotypes are susceptible to lysis, while those of H-2^k are resistant; a recombinant haplotype H-2^a(H-$2D^d$H-$2K^k$) exhibiting intermediate susceptibility (Scheid *et al.*, 1972). Thus, it would appear that even mouse H-Y antibody does recognize (H-Y + altered H-2) antigen complexes. We have already noted that anti-H-Y cytotoxic T cell receptors raised in H-2^b female mice preferentially recognize (H-Y + H-$2D^b$) antigen complex. The reason that this receptor recognizes more H-$2D^b$ than H-Y may be found in the manner of association; H-Y not covering up most H-$2D^b$ antigenic determinants. We believe that homoral H-Y antibody raised in the same female mouse preferentially recognize (H-Y + H-$2K^b$) antigen complex in which much of the H-$2K^b$ antigenic determinants are made inaccessible by association with H-Y. None the less, even the above H-Y antibody appears to confuse the (H-Y + altered H-$2K^b$) antigen complex with unaltered H-$2K^k$. The above noted mouse H-Y antibody can be IgM or IgG, and the antibody of both classes demonstrate nearly the identical cytotoxic potency towards the appropriate male targets; the maximal 60% killing of H-2^b or H-2^d male epidermal cells until 1/8th dilution. Yet, the male specific cytotoxicity of IgM H-Y antibody can be absorbed out with only 1/12th as many male cells as the number required for the absorption of IgG antibody: $0{\cdot}32 \times 10^6$ male mouse spleen cells/μl against $4{\cdot}0 \times 10^6$ male cells/μl. As shown in Fig. 9, we have found that the male specific cytotoxicity of IgM H-Y antibody can be greatly reduced by absorption with a very large number ($3{\cdot}0 \times 10^6$ spleen cells/μl) of female mouse cells of either H-$2D^k$H-$2K^k$(C3H) or H-$2D^b$H-$2K^k$-(B10A2R) haplotypes, while the same number of H-2^b(B6) or H-2^d(BALB) female cells did not show an appreciable absorption. The above suggested the cross-reactivity between the (H-Y + altered H-$2K^b$) antigen complex and unaltered H-$2K^k$ antigen. Since the comparable experiment on IgG H-Y antibody would have required the use of $37{\cdot}0 \times 10^6$ female H-$2K^k$ cells/μl, the experiment proved impractical.

Summary

In order to cope with rapid mutation rates of parasitic viruses and bacteria, the mammalian immune system violated the Epimethean rule of evolution and acquired Promethean foresight. V genes in the mammalian genome, by random mutations and reassembly, generate a very large number of antigen binding sites; many of which are directed against antigens not yet in existence. As the penalty for the above audacity, status quo prevails among the V genes, as to their antigen binding capacities. Consequently, everlasting contests

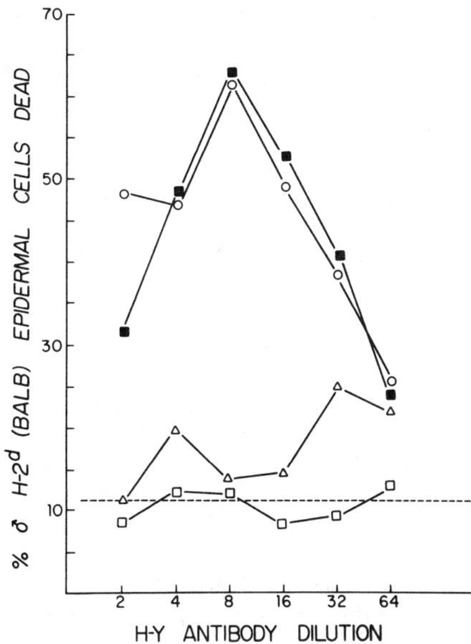

FIG. 9. *One example showing that mouse H-Y antibody of the IgM class raised in* $H\text{-}2^b$ *females may confuse unaltered* $H\text{-}2K^K$ *antigen with* ($H\text{-}Y$ + *altered* $H\text{-}2K^b$ *and/or* $H\text{-}Y + H\text{-}2D^b$) *antigen complexes. The male specific cytotoxicity of this antibody titrated on male* $H\text{-}2^d$ (*BALB*) *epidermal cells was completely absorbed out by as little as* $0{\cdot}32 \times 10^6$ *male* $H\text{-}2^d$ (*BALB*), $H\text{-}2^b$ (*B6*) *as well as* $H\text{-}2^k$ (*C3H*) *spleen cells/μl of antibody, whereas as many as* $3{\cdot}6 \times 10^6$ *female spleen cells of* $H\text{-}2^d$ *as well as* $H\text{-}2^b$ *haplotypes totally failed to absorb. However, the same number of female cells of* $H\text{-}2^k$ *as well as recombinant* $H\text{-}2D^bH\text{-}2K^k$ (*B1OA2R*) *haplotype/μl nearly absorbed out the male specific cytotoxicity of this antibody.* ■: *unabsorbed H-Y antibody;* □: *absorbed with* $0{\cdot}5 \times 10^6$ *male* $H\text{-}2^d$ *spleen cells/μl;* ○: *absorbed with* $3{\cdot}6 \times 10^6$ *female* $H\text{-}2^d$ *spleen cells/μl.* △: *absorbed with* $3{\cdot}22 \times 10^6$ *female* $H\text{-}2^k$ *spleen cells/μl.*

between parasitic viruses and the host immune system involve the former's attempts to disguise their antigens as selves of the host and the host's attempts to distinguish these viral pseudoselves from true selves. The host utilizes extensively polymorphic MHC antigens as the principal tool for pseudoself v. true self distinction. The key for generation of diverse humoral antibodies is found in the $V_L + J_L$ or $V_H + J_H$ pretranscriptional fusion mechanism. We propose that the key for generation of diverse T cell receptors is found in $V_H + V_H$ pretranscriptional coding sequence fusion.

References

Beutler, B., Nagai, Y., Ohno, S., Klein, G. and Shapiro, I. (1978). *Cell* **13**, 509–513.
Blanks, K. J. and Lilly, F. (1977). *Nature* **269**, 808–809.
von Boehmer, H., Hengartner, H., Nabholz, M., Lernhardt, W., Schreier, M. H. and Haas, W. (1979). *Eur. J. Immunol.* **9**, 592–597.
Bubbers, J. E. and Lilly, F. (1977). *Nature* **266**, 458–459.

Cantor, H. and Boyse, E. A. (1977). *Immunol. Rev.* **33**, 105–124.
Ciccarese, S. and Ohno, S. (1978). *Cell* **13**, 643–650.
Cohn, M. (1968). *In* "Nucleic Acids in Immunology". Springer-Verlag, Berlin, Heidelberg and New York.
Cramer, M., Krawinkel, U., Melchers, I., Imanishi-Kari, T., Ben-Neriah, Y., Givol, D. and Rajewsky, K. (1979). *Eur. J. Immunol.* **9**, 332–338.
Early, P. Huang, H., Davis, M., Calame, K. and Hood, L. (1980). *Cell* **19**, 981–992.
Fellous, M., Gunther, E., Kemler, R., Wiels, J., Berger, R., Guenet, J. L., Jakob, H. and Jacob, F. (1978). *J. Exp. Med.* **148**, 58–70.
Flaherty, L. (1978). *In* "Workshop on the Origin of Inbred Strains of Mice". Academic Press, New York and London.
Flaherty, L., Zimmerman, B. and Wachtel, S. S. (1979). *J. Exp. Med.* **150**, 1020–1027.
Forman, J. (1979). *J. Immunol.* **123**, 2451–2455.
Goulmy, E., Bradley, B. A., van Leeuwen, A., Lansberg, Q., Munro, A., Termijtelen, A. and van Rood, J. T. (1977). *Tissue Antigens* **10**, 248.
Ivani, P., Melief, J. M., van Mourik, P. Vlug, A. and de Greeve, P. (1980). *Nature* **282**, 843–845.
Jerne, N. K. (1971). *Eur. J. Immunol.* **1**, 1–9.
Lyon, M. F. (1961). *Nature* **190**, 372–373.
Matsunaga, T. and Ohno, S. (1980). *Transplantation* (in press).
Nagai, Y., Ciccarese, S. and Ohno, S. (1979). *Differentiation* **13**, 155–164.
Ohno, S. (1977). *Immunol. Rev.* **33**, 60–69.
Ohno, S. (1979). *Perspec. Biol. Med.* **19**, 527–532.
Ohno, S. (1980). *Differentiation* **17**, 1–15.
Ohta, T. (1980). Population Genetics of Multigene Families. Springer-Verlag, Berlin, Heidelberg and New York.
Owen, F. L., Finnegan, A., Gates, E. R. and Gottlieb, P. D. (1979). *Eur. J. Immunol.* **9**, 948–955.
Sakano, H., Huppi, K., Heinrich, G. and Tonegawa, S. (1979). *Nature* **280**, 288–294.
Sakano, H., Maki, H., Kurosawa, Y., Roeder, W. and Tonegawa, S. (1980). *Nature* (in press).
Scheid, M., Boyse, E. A., Carswell, E. A. and Old, L. J. (1972). *J. Exp. Med.* **135**, 938–955.
Seidman, J. G., Max, E. E. and Leder, P. (1979). *Nature* **280**, 370–375.
Simpson, E. and Gordon, R. D. (1977). *Immunol. Rev.* **35**, 59–75.
Taniguchi, M., Saito, T. and Tada, T. (1979). *Nature* **278**, 255–258.
Wachtel, S. S., Koo, G. C. and Boyse, E. A. (1975). *Nature* **254**, 270–272.
Wagner, H., Starzinski-Powitz, A., Rollinghoff, M., Goldstein, P. and Jakob, H. (1978). *J. Exp. Med.* **147**, 251–264.
Zinkernagel, R. M. and Doherty, P. D. (1974). *Nature* **251**, 547–549.

33

Action of Antibody and Complement in Regulating Virus Infection

MICHAEL B. A. OLDSTONE, J. G. P. SISSONS and ROBERT S. FUJINAMI

Department of Immunopathology, Scripps Clinic and Research Foundation, La Jolla, California, USA

Much of the work described in this review was done in collaboration with several investigators at Scripps Clinic and Research Foundation. From the authors' laboratory, special recognition is given to P. Lampert and A. Tishon. The long association with N. Cooper of the Department of Molecular Immunology regarding the complement aspects of this work is acknowledged. In addition, the author thanks H. Müller-Eberhard and R. Schreiber for making the isolated components of the complement system available.

This is Publication No. 2197 from the Department of Immunopathology, Scripps Clinic and Research Foundation, La Jolla, California 92037, USA. This research was supported by U.S.P.H.S. grants AI-09484, AI-07007, NS-12428 and NS-14068.

Introduction

During infection viruses provide a supply of macromolecular antigens which in most, if not all, instances elicit a host immune response. The interrelationship between virus antigens expressed on infectious virions or on the surface of infected cells and the immune response leads to immunopathologic injury. Depending on the type of cell(s) infected (neurones, oligodendrocytes, myocardial cells, lymphocytes or fibroblasts), the numbers of cells involved and the intensity of the immune response, the end result may be stopping the spread of virus infection and clearance of a nidus of infected cells leading to immunity or severe tissue injury. During acute viral infection the imbalance between the immune response and virus replication in target cells causes either termination of disease or death of the host. By comparison the time-scale is lengthened and both a continuous host immune response against the virus and ongoing viral replication occurs in chronic virus infections. In addition, by a variety of mechanisms, infected cells may evade the host's immune response, thus allowing continuous virus replication, persistence of virus and chronic or degenerative disorders.

Viruses are obligate intracellular pathogens and their efficient elimination from a host requires that continuing intracellular virus replication be prevented. The major way of achieving this is by destruction of virus infected cells by a number of immunological mechanisms. These include antibody independent and antibody dependent cell mediated cytotoxicity against virus infected target cells as well as the action of antibody and complement. This chapter is concerned with those effects of the immune response on virus infected cells and on infectious virions which are medicated by antibody and complement.

Antibody and complement acting jointly can destroy virus infected cells prior to the release of infectious virus progeny. Further, infectious virus units released into the fluid phase can be neutralized directly by antibody, while complement by a variety of mechanisms can both enhance and accelerate destruction of the infectious virion–antibody complex. These interactions on virus infected cells and virions can be studied *in vitro* and there is reason for thinking that these activities may also be important *in vivo*. Spread of virus infection occurs principally by three mechanisms. First, virus budding from the plasma membrane is released into the fluid phase. Such infectious virions can then be transported to areas where they adsorb to and infect other permissive cells. The second mechanism is the spread of virus into adjacent cells via cytoplasmic bridges. In this manner infectious virions are protected from hostile immune reagents present in the fluid phase. The third mechanism of spread is whereby infectious virus nucleic acid becomes integrated into the host's genetic material and is passed from mother to daughter cells during cell division. Regardless of the mechanism of virus spread, for the immune

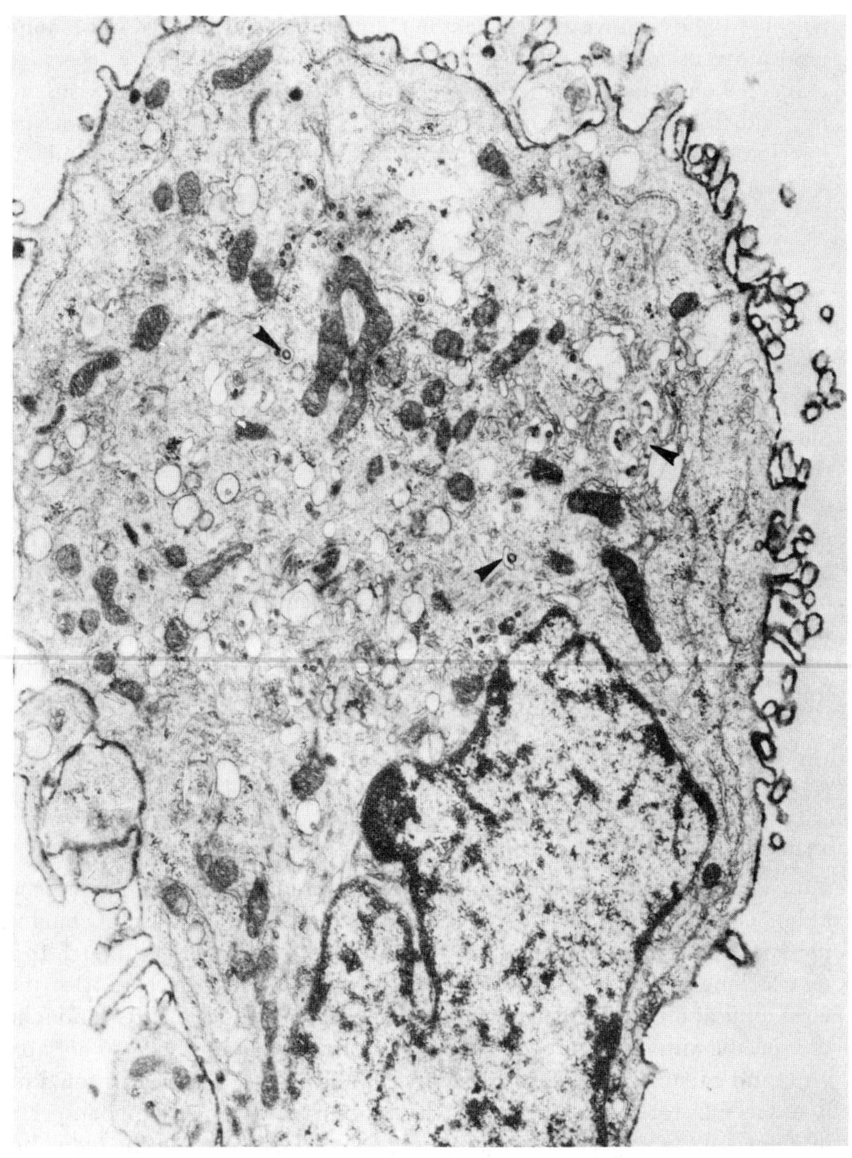

FIG. 1. *Expression of viral antigens on the cell's surface in the absence of virus budding from the plasma membrane. Murine primary neuronal cells were infected with mouse hepatitis virus (MHV), a positive strand RNA virus that does not bud from the plasma membrane but exits from cytoplasmic vesicles. The photomicrograph shows expression of MHV antigens on the surface of infected cells prior to the release of infectious virus. Cell stained with monospecific antibody to MHV conjugated to peroxidase. Arrows point to virions. Picture courtesy of Drs R. Knobler and M. Dubois-Dalq.*

response to be effective and efficient in eliminating virus infected cells, unique viral antigens must be expressed on the cell's surface which are recognized and acted on. This frequently occurs even in infected cells in which virus does not bud from the plasma membrane (Fig. 1). Immune destruction of virus infected cells prior to the assembly and release of infectious virions eliminates a factory of continuing virus production.

Lysis of virus infected cells

It is clear from work done over the last 2 to 3 decades that specific antibody and complement can lyse virus infected cells (reviewed: Wiktor *et al.*, 1968; Brier *et al.*, 1971; Rawls and Tompkins, 1975; Oldstone and Lampert, 1979; Sissons and Oldstone, 1980). However, much of the work on antibody and complement lysis of virus infected cells has been done with heterologous systems of virus infected cells, antibody and complement. Such systems frequently contain cross-reactive and natural antibodies to cell surface antigens and makes any critical assessment of the role of complement and/or antibody difficult (see Sissons and Oldstone, 1980). For this reason it is imperative to use a homologous or autologous system. In this chapter, study of human system, either homologous or autologous, is used in order that extrapolations from lessons learned *in vitro* can be made to *in vivo* probabilities.

Action of antibody

Specificity

The absolute specificity of antiviral antibody for lysis of virus infected cells is quite clear. For example, virus infected cells can only be lysed in the presence of IgG containing antibody to the infecting virus. Hence, neither IgG binding nor specific immune lysis occurs with uninfected cell targets. Although fresh sera lacking antibody to a given virus cannot lyse cells infected with that virus, lytic ability is attained upon the addition of monospecific IgG containing the specific antiviral antibody. Further, serum having antibody to only one virus and capable of mediating lysis of cells infected with that virus could not lyse cells infected with other viruses. Lysis occurred when either monospecific immune IgG to a specific virus was added to the sera or when the individual lacking antibodies to a particular virus was vaccinated with that virus and his sera assayed at least 6 days later (see Table 1). In the latter case the association of immune specific lysis was accompanied by specific binding of IgG to the target cell expressing the appropriate virus antigens on its surface. These various observations are summarized in Table I and described in detail by Perrin *et al.* (1976).

Antibody responses to viral antigens during infection follows a sequence similar to that observed with nonviral antigens. IgM antibody usually reaches maximal titres at 3 to 4 weeks after exposure to virus and then falls to low

TABLE I

Specificity of antiviral antibody in lysis of virus infected target cells

Serum source	History (previous exposure) HSV blisters	Measles	Mumps	Treatment used	Human target cells infected with (viruses): Herpes simplex I IgG binding	Herpes simplex I Immune Lysis (%)	Measles IgG binding	Measles Immune lysis (%)	Mumps IgG binding	Mumps Immune Lysis (%)
A	Yes	Yes	No	None	+	> 90	+	> 90	Nil	< 5
A	Yes	Yes	No	Add mumps IgG	+	> 90	+	> 90	+	> 90
A	Yes	Yes	Yes	Mumps vaccination serum tested 14 days later	+	> 90	+	> 90	+	> 90
B	No	No	No	None	Nil [a]	< 7	Nil	< 5	Nil	< 5
B	No	No	No	Add measles IgG	Nil	< 7	+	> 90	Nil	< 5
B	No	Yes	No	Measles vaccination serum tested day 14	Nil	< 7	+	> 90	Nil	< 5
B	No	Yes	Yes	Mumps vaccination serum tested day 14	Nil	< 7	+	> 90	+	> 90

[a] Nil: not detectable.

Details as to binding assay and test for specific immune lysis given in Perrin *et al.* (1976).

or undetectable levels. Titres of IgG antibody rise in parallel to IgM but in contrast to the decay in IgM titres persist for years. We have studied the generation of specific cytotoxic antibody(s) in 3 individuals during the course of mumps virus vaccination, 5 individuals during the course of measles virus vaccination and in 2 individuals during acute measles virus infection. Sera obtained from these persons prior to vaccination or infection with a specific virus uniformly showed neither the presence of binding nor lytic antibody to that particular virus. Following vaccination or infection lytic antibody was detected as early as 6 days and usually peaked by 10 to 14 days. In several individuals tested, serum obtained 3 days after vaccination had no cytolytic activity. It is likely that antibody to viral glycoproteins expressed on the surfaces of infected cells are important in immune lysis. This is clearly so in lysis of measles virus infected cells where antibody directed against the viral haemagglutinin or against the viral haemolysin (fusion protein), the only two glycopeptides of measles virus, have been shown to be involved (Sissons *et al.*, 1979). Many viral antigens are thymus dependent (Burns *et al.*, 1975). Currently there is little information about antibody subclass response to specific viral polypeptides (i.e., IgG1, IgG2, IgG3 or IgG4). In this regard restriction of an antibody response to a unique subclass would be of interest and likely of biological importance as certain subclasses fail to fix complement or fix it poorly, while other subclasses have other differing properties (reviewed by Spiegelberg, 1974). It is of interest that unique restrictions when they do occur have been found with responses to carbohydrate antigens (Spiegelberg, 1974).

Requirement for divalent antibody

Several studies have focused upon whether the entire igG molecule or one of its fragments is needed for complement dependent lysis of virus infected cells. In experiments with measles virus, herpes simplex virus or mumps virus infected human cells, it was found that the Fab′2 piece of IgG antibody to these various viruses was as efficient in lysing virus infected cells as was the total IgG (Joseph *et al.*, 1975; Perrin *et al.*, 1976). Recently it has been possible to study lysis of virus infected cells using purified antiviral IgG, the isolated purified components of the complement system and virus infected cells (Sissons *et al.*, 1980a, b). The results of these studies are shown in Figs 2 and 3. Despite the binding of equivalent amounts of IgG, its Fab′2 or Fab′ fragments to the surface of a virus infected cell per given amount of protein offered, dose related lysis was found only with IgG and its Fab′2 fragment but not with comparable amounts of Fab′ (Fig. 2). Binding of 4×10^7 molecules of Fab′2 or $6{\cdot}5 \times 10^7$ molecules of IgG antibody per cell, roughly equivalent amounts of IgG or Fab′2, was required for lysis of 50% of measles virus infected cells in the presence of isolated complement show that the inability of Fab′ to initiate lysis did not result from its failure to bind to virus antigens on the cell's surface, and that complement dependent immune lysis of virus infected cells can occur in the absence of the Fc portion of the IgG molecule. Further, these studies strongly suggested that the alternative complement pathway and

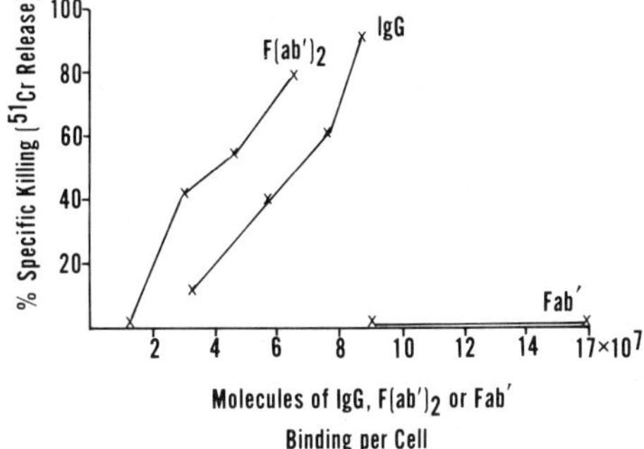

FIG. 2. *Lysis of measles virus infected HeLa cells requires the whole IgG or its Fab'2 fragment (containing antibody to measles virus). Despite the inability of Fab' fragment to induce lysis it bound to infected cells as equivalently as whole IgG or the Fab'2 piece. See Sissions* et al., *1979 for experimental details. Similar results were obtained with immune lysis of cells infected with herpes simplex type 1 virus (see Perrin* et al., *1976). Complement sources used were either the individual purified components (Sissons* et al., *1979) or fresh human serum devoid of measles or herpes simplex virus antibodies (Perrin* et al., *1976).*

not the classical complement pathway was involved in lysis of virus infected cells (Joseph *et al.*, 1975). C1, the first component of complement, reacts with the Fc portion of antibody formed in the immune complex. This binding is to the C1q subunit. Thereafter, C4 and C2 components of the classical complement pathway become activated. The fact that the Fc portion of immune IgG is not needed for lysis of virus infected cells in the homologous and autologous human models studied indicates that activation of the classical complement pathway is not necessary for lysis. The suggestion is that the functional integrity of the alternative complement pathway is required. The evidence for the above and the role of these two pathways in lysis of virus infected cells are discussed below.

Action of complement

Essential requirement of the alternative pathway

The complement system consists of over 20 immunochemically distinct serum proteins capable of interacting with each other, with antibody and with cell membranes. These interactions lead to several biologic sequelae including the lysis of virus infected cells. There are two principal pathways by which complement is activated. The classical pathway is activated when IgG, principally subclasses 1 and 3, or IgM antibody complexed with antigen, reacts with the first component of complement, C1. Reaction occurs by a binding site on the Fc fragment of IgG with the C1q component of the C1 macromolecule. By this means C1 is activated and subsequently cleaves C4 and C2 which forms the classical pathway C3 cleaving enzyme C42 . The alternative pathway of complement activation provides a distinct means whereby C3 can be cleaved. In this pathway complement components are activated indepen-

TABLE II

Requirement of a functional alternative complement pathway for ant

Treatment of complement	Per cent of virus infected cell lysis observed Measles (Edmonston strain)						
	HeLa	*HEp-2*	*Lymphoblastoid WI-L2*	*Raji*	*8866*	*Glia (339 MG)*	*Neuroblastoma (IMR-32)*
Whole serum fresh	>90	>90	>90	>90	>90	>90	>90
Whole serum heated 50 °C/20 min	<10	<10	<10	<10	<10	<10	<10
Block classical pathway							
C2 genetically deficient sera	>90	>90	>90	ND	ND	ND	ND
C2 removed	>90	>90	>90	>90	>90	>90	>90
C4 removed	>90	>90	>90	>90	>90	>90	>90
Block alternative pathway							
Factor B removed	<10	<10	<10	<10	<10	<10	<10
Factor D removed	<10	ND	ND	ND	ND	ND	ND
Properdin removed	2	ND	ND	ND	ND	ND	ND
Reconstitution of the alternative pathway							
Add Factor B back to factor B depleted serum	>90	>90	>90	>90	>90	>90	>90
Add Factor D back to factor D depleted serum	>90	ND	ND	ND	ND	ND	ND
Add properdin back to properdin depleted serum	>90	ND	ND	ND	ND	ND	ND
Use of purified components of the alternative pathway (C3, B, D, P, β1H, C3bINA)* and C5, C6, C7, C8, C9**	>90	ND	ND	ND	ND	ND	ND

dent of antibody and of C1, C4 and C2 (reviewed Müller-Eberhard and Schreiber, 1980). Six plasma proteins interact in the alternative pathway of complement activation. These are C3 itself; factor B, a 93 000 mol. wt glycoprotein; factor D, a 24 000 mol. wt serine protease; properdin, a 224 000 mol. wt protein; β1H, a 150 000 mol. wt protein; and C3b inactivator (C3b INA), an 88 000 mol. wt protein. β1H and C3b INA together inactivate C3B. Currently it is believed that a continuous low grade conversion of C3 to its major active fragment, C3b, occurs in plasma. Normally this C3b in the fluid phase, or on surfaces, is rapidly inactivated by the two control proteins, β1H and C3b INA acting in sequence. However, on surfaces of known activators of the pathway, such as yeast cell walls and certain types of Gram-negative bacteria, C3b deposited from the fluid phase is protected from the action of β1H and C3b INA. This protected C3b then binds factor B which is cleaved

To determine the participation of the two complement pathways in IgG antiviral dependent lysis of virus infected cells, specific complement components were immunochemically removed: C4, C2, factor B, facter D, properdin or serum genetically deficient in C2 was used. In reconstitution studies, physiological amounts of specific reagents were added to depleted serum.

TABLE II *continued*

dependent lysis of human cells infected with a variety of RNA and DNA viruses

	Measles (M-VAC strain)	*Measles (Schwartz strain)*	*SSPE-Halle strain*	*Influ. A⁰*		*Mumps*		*HSV-I*	*HSV-II*
Autologous fibroblasts	*HeLa*	*HeLa*	*HeLa*	*Conjunctivia*	*HE_{p-2}*	*Autologous fibroblasts*	*HeLa*	*Autologous fibroblasts*	*HeLa*
85	>90	>90	>90	81	88	80	>90	85	89
<10	<10	<10	<10	<10	<10	<10	<10	<10	<10
ND	>90	>90	>90	ND	81	ND	>90	84	ND
>90	>90	>90	>90	ND	ND	ND	ND	ND	ND
>90	>90	>90	>90	78	75	80	82	85	87
<10	<10	<10	<10	<10	<10	<10	<10	<10	<10
ND	ND	ND	ND	ND	ND	ND	ND	ND	ND
ND	ND	ND	ND	ND	ND	ND	ND	ND	ND
88	>90	>90	>90	82	76	84	>90	85	>90
ND	ND	ND	ND	ND	ND	ND	ND	ND	ND
ND	ND	ND	ND	ND	ND	ND	ND	ND	ND
ND	ND	ND	ND	ND	ND	ND	ND	ND	ND

by factor D, giving the alternative pathway C3 cleaving enzyme $\overline{\text{C3bBb}}$. Properdin (P) binds to this enzyme and retards its otherwise rapid intrinsic decay. Hence, the alternative pathway is a positive feedback system in that C3b is both a product of the reaction and a constituent of the C3 cleaving enzyme. In addition, the pathway can be activated as an amplification loop whenever C3b is generated following C3 cleavage by the classical pathway. Following C3 cleavage by either pathway, C5 is cleaved and then sequential nonenzymatic binding of C6 through C9 results in assembly of the membrane attack complex, C5b9, which is inserted into the lipid bilayer of membranes, creating a permeability defect which allows osmotic lysis to occur. A description of current knowledge in the human complement system is given in this volume by Müller-Eberhard (1980).

A detailed analysis of the participation of various human complement

ND: Not done. These experiments were done with Luc Perrin, Patrick Sissons, Robert Schreiber and Neil Cooper. The components of the alternative complement pathway* and membrane attack system** were a gift from Hans Müller-Eberhard. For experimental details see Joseph *et al.* (1975), Perrin *et al* (1976), Sissons *et al.* (1979), Sissons *et al.* (1980).

components in lysing a variety of human cell lines infected with a spectrum of viruses has been made (Joseph *et al.*, 1975; Perrin *et al.*, 1976; Sissons *et al.*, 1979; Sissons *et al.*, 1980a, b). The data which is summarized in Tables I and II indicates that both specific antibody for the relevant virus and the components of the alternative pathway of complement activation are needed for lysis. The evidence for the alternative pathway of complement activation occurs from experiments showing lysis of virus infected cells in sera depleted of C4 or C2. The absence of C4 or C2 abrogates classical pathway activation and yet lysis of virus infected cells occurs as efficiently as lysis in whole serum (Fig. 3). In addition, the dependence of lysis on antibody and the alternative pathway, but not the classical pathway, of complement activation was also observed using serum depleted of complement components by affinity chromatography or employing genetically deficient C2 sera (Table II). Finally, and most convincingly, it has recently been shown that immune lysis of virus infected cells occurs with specific IgG and the isolated purified components of the alternative pathway (Fig. 3). Thus, using HeLa cells infected with measles virus as a model, lysis was mediated by antibody and a mixture composed of purified proteins of the alternative pathway of activation (C3, factor B and D, P, β1H, C3b INA) and membrane attack complex (C5 through C9) of complement. It was also found that properdin, which is known not to be required for the initial activation of the alternative pathway, was nevertheless necessary for lysis of virus infected cells (Sissons *et al.*, 1980a, b), which contrasts with its unessential role in lysing nonnucleated cells such as erythrocytes.

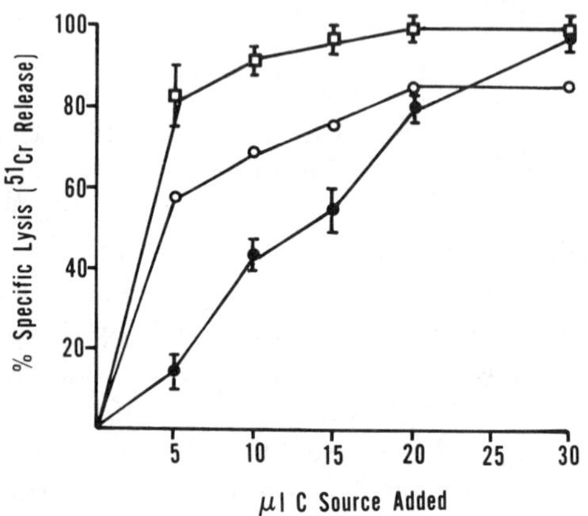

FIG. 3. *Evidence for the requirement of the alternative pathway in lysing measles virus infected cells in the presence of antiviral antibody. Dose related lysis of measles virus infected HeLa cells coated with human IgG antibody to measles virus and the following human complement source:* □ *whole serum;* ● *serum depleted of C4;* ○ *purified complement components: C3, B, D, P, β1H, C3bINA, C5, C6, C7, C8, C9. When whole serum was heated at 56°C for 30 min or when B or P were left out of the complement component mix, less than 5% lysis occurred. Each point represents the mean of duplicate assay ± 1 s.e. For experimental details see Sissons* et al., *1979.*

The alternative pathway dependence for lysis of virus infected cells by human antibody and complement is well established. Nevertheless, the classical pathway is activated on the surface of antibody-coated infected cells, despite the inability of the classical pathway to cause lysis. Perrin *et al.* (1976) noted that C4 bound to the plasma membranes of HeLa cells infected with and expressing measles virus antigens on their surface when fresh serum or factor B depleted serum containing antimeasles virus antibodies was used. This finding was supported by parallel studies showing some consumption of the early components of the classical pathway. The inability of the classical pathway to lyse virus infected cells may reflect the fact that the amplifying effect of the alternative pathway is always required for lysis of such nucleated cells or that the classical pathway may be partially blocked. The binding of various components of the alternative complement pathway to the surfaces of virus infected cells after these cells were sensitized with antiviral antibody was shown by immunofluorescence and immunoelectron microscopy (using monospecific antibodies to the various purified complement components—Perrin *et al.*,1976; Oldstone and Lampert, 1979).

While the alternative complement pathway is responsible for lysis of a variety of human cell lines infected with viruses in the presence of human serum containing specific antiviral antibodies (Table II, reviewed by Oldstone and Lampert, 1979), both the classical and the alternative complement pathway have been implicated in lysis of a variety of virus infected cells in heterologous model systems (Ehrnst, 1978; Hicks *et al.*, 1976; reviewed Oldstone and Lampert, 1979). For example, mixing primate cells infected with measles virus, human, or rabbit antibodies against measles virus and rabbit or guinea-pig complement source, Hicks *et al.* (1976) and Ehrnst (1978) noted that both complement pathways were involved in the lysis of measles virus infected targets, but each pathway could function independently. These results were confirmed in our laboratory and the mechanism studied. Using two rabbit sera containing antibodies to measles virus and acting as their own complement source, we noted that both lysed measles virus infected HeLa cells by the alternative and by the classical complement pathway. However, when the sera were extensively absorbed against uninfected HeLa cells to remove cross-reacting antibodies to HeLa cell surface determinants, lysis of virus infected cells no longer proceeded by the classical pathway, but was restricted to the alternative complement pathway. This and other results had pointed to the difficulty in using heterologous systems if one wishes to sort out mechanisms of antibody and complement lysis of virus infected cells (reviewed Oldstone and Lampert, 1979).

Molecular mechanism of lysis

Membranes activate complement independent of antibody but antibody is required for lysis

The observation that lysis of virus infected cells required both antibody and the alternative complement pathway initially seemed contradictory, particularly as initiation of alternative pathway by other activators (yeast cell walls, certain bacteria or their products, red blood cells, etc.) occurs independently of antibody (reviewed Müller-Eberhard and Schreiber, 1980). It is now clear that infected cells can activate the alternative complement pathway independent of antibody. However, these cells do not lyse unless antibody is present. This was shown by the ability of measles virus infected HeLa cells to activate the alternative pathway in a system composed only of purified C3, Factors B and D, P, β1H and C3b INA (Sissons *et al.*, 1980b). Hence, mixing these purified complement components with HeLa cells acutely infected with measles virus in the total absence of antibody, there was a progressive uptake of ^{125}I labelled C3b onto the cell's surface. This C3b uptake was blocked by EDTA and was not shown by uninfected cells (Fig. 4). When antiviral IgG

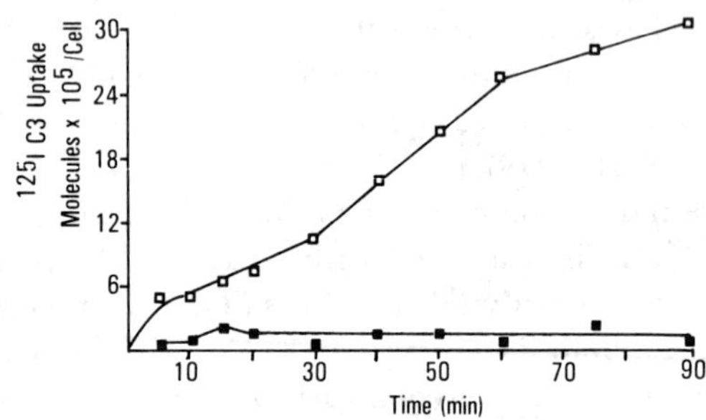

FIG. 4. *C3 (C3b) is bound to the surfaces of virus infected cells in the absence of antiviral antibody. The uptake of ^{125}I C3 onto measles virus infected HeLa cells (□) and uninfected HeLa cells (■) in the presence of purified C3, Factors B and D, β1H, C3b INA and P and 0·01* M *EDTA. See Sissons* et al. *(1980b) for experimental details.*

was bound to the cell surface, the rate of C3 uptake occurred more rapidly (Fig. 5). The ability to activate the alternative pathway as evidenced by ^{125}I labelled C3 uptake directly paralleled the expression of viral glycopeptides on the cell's surface. Lysis occurred only after the addition of divalent antibody in the presence of a complement source. Experimentally, despite the binding of C3b to the cell's surface in the absence of antibody, such cells cultured for 24 h in human serum devoid of antibodies to measles virus did not demonstrate significant lysis over the spontaneous ^{51}Cr released from uninfected control cells or infected cells inoculated in heat inactivated serum.

The question then arises why, if virus infected cells can activate the alternative pathway alone, is antibody required for lysis? The evidence indicates that virus infected cells are relatively weak activators of the alternative pathway and that antibody to the virus enhances the deposition of C3b on the cell surface. This occurs probably by increasing the number of C3b binding sites and also perhaps by antibody protecting bound C3b from C3b INA and β1H. Our findings with virus infected cells have recently been extended by other investigators to the activation of the alternative pathway by zymosan and certain erythrocytes (Moore *et al.*, 1980; Schenkein and Ruddy, 1980), where it was found that C3b deposition, which occurred independent of antibody, was enhanced in the presence of IgG.

Regarding the divalent antibody requirement, it has been conclusively shown in the lysis of virus infected cells that a large amount of antibodies (at least 5×10^6 IgG molecules must bind per infected cell for lysis to occur and that Fab′2 fragments are as effective as whole IgG, while Fab′ is almost totally ineffective) (Perrin *et al.*, 1976; Sissons *et al.*, 1980a). The precise mechanism whereby divalent antibody is required is unclear. However, it is tempting to hypothesize that divalent antibody clusters or groups membrane bound C3b, perhaps protecting the C3b from its inactivating enzymes. Experiments in which cell membrane fluidity was limited showed that lysis occurred in the absence of capping (Perrin *et al.*, 1976; Sissons *et al.*, 1979). Hence the

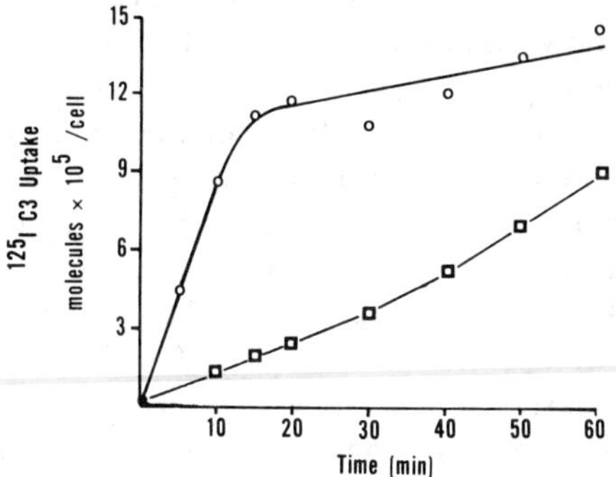

FIG. 5. *Antimeasles virus IgG enhances the uptake of C3 (C3b) onto virus infected cells. The uptake of ^{125}I C3 onto measles virus infected HeLa cells coated with IgG (○) in the presence of purified C3, Factors B and D, β1H, C3b INA and P; onto measles virus infected HeLa cells in the absence of IgG (□) in the presence of purified C3, Factors B and D, β1H, C3b INA and P. See Sissons* et al. *(1980b) for experimental details.*

two unanswered questions regarding mechanism of lysis of virus infected cells by antibody and complement are first the precise role played by divalent antibody and second, the nature of the virus induced changes in the cell membrane that allows activation of the alternative pathway.

Generality and implications of antibody and alternative complement pathway mediated lysis of virus infected cells

The lysis of virus infected cells by antibody and the alternative complement pathway is a general phenomenon. Table II shows that a variety of RNA and DNA viruses infecting several different human cell lines are lysed by these means. In addition to the DNA viruses of herpes simplex virus 1 and 2 shown, there is evidence that cytomegalovirus is lysed by a similar mechanism. In addition to lysis of cells infected with measles virus of the Edmonton strain, cells infected with M-VAC, Schwartz, SSPE-Halle strains of measles virus, and parainfluenza viruses are also lysed by antiviral antibody and the alternative pathway components (Oldstone and Lampert, 1979). The fact that multiple human cells of wide backgrounds (epithelial, lymphoid, neural, glial, autologous fibroblasts) infected with viruses are lysed by antiviral antibody and a functional alternative pathway further indicates the generality of these findings and suggests its potential biological importance *in vivo*.

The biological implications of these findings are several. First, the observation that virus infected cells themselves actually activate the alternative pathway independent of antibody suggests that the alternative pathway of complement activation may be a means of early nonspecific host defence against a wide range of invading micro-organisms. In this regard it is of interest that certain Gram-negative bacteria and parasites can also activate the alternative pathway directly. At present there is little evidence to assess the importance of this mechanism in man *in vivo*. It is possible, however, that the deposition of C3b on virus infected cells could render them, early in infection, susceptible to attack by neutrophils and macrophages, cells which bear C3b receptors. The second implication is based on the finding that the lytic activity of complement found in fresh serum is absent in other body fluids like cerebral spinal fluid and thoracic duct fluid. In addition, the functional activity of the alternative complement pathway is labile when compared to the classical pathway as a 1:4 dilution of fresh serum usually abrogates lysis dependent on the alternative complement pathway by 50% or more, whereas a 1:50 or greater dilution of fresh serum is needed to cause a 50% reduction in lysis by the classical pathway. The second implication is that patients with genetic or acquired deficiencies for complement components of the alternative pathway may not handle acute virus infections as well as individuals with normal complement pathways and hence may have a higher incidence of latent and/or overt virus infections. At present deficiencies of the alternative pathway protein (factors B and D, P) have not yet been described. This may be partly due to the conventional screening method used for total haemolytic complement in serum which only assesses integrity of the classical and not the alternative pathway. In man, distinct genetic deficiency states have been described for complement components of the classical pathway of activation (C1r, C1s, C4 and C2) as well as deficiencies of C3 and terminal components (C5 through C9). These genetically deficient patients are usually homozygous for a null gene and there is a complete absence of the individual component, with heterozygotes having half normal levels. Deficiencies of C1, C4 and C2 are associated with a high incidence of rheumatic or immune complex diseases similar to systemic lupus erythematosus. Patients with total deficiency of C3 have frequent recurrent bacterial infections while those with deficiencies in the terminal components have a high incidence of chronic neisseria infection. At present there is no firm evidence to suggest that patients with complement deficiencies are especially prone to virus infections; however, the numbers of cases are relatively small and more clinical observations are needed. The fact that the alternative pathway lytic activity for infected cells can be almost abrogated in 1:4 diluted serum and is negligible in cerebral spinal and thoracic duct fluids suggests that thirdly, antibody may act against virus infected cells in the absence of an effective complement effector system. As discussed below (next section), antibody in the absence of complement can initiate the persistence of virus in infected cells. By antibody stripping viral antigens off the plasma membranes, these cells retain viral genetic information and persist in the face of a hostile immune environment (cytotoxic lymphocytes, antibody and complement). The fourth implication is that the virus–antibody complexes formed on the plasma membranes can be shed in the fluid phase and serve as a source of phlogogenic immune complexes (see below, Fig. 6). Trapping of these circulating complexes leads to immune complex disease of renal glomeruli, blood vessels and the choroid plexus (reviewed Oldstone, 1975).

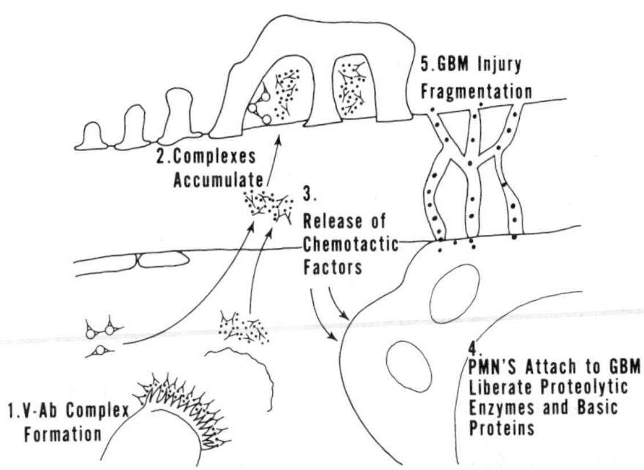

FIG. 6. *A schematic drawing hypothesizing the formation of virus–antibody immune complexes in the fluid phase, subsequent trapping in tissues and immune complex injury* in vivo. *Note the formation of immune complexes by shedding of plasma membrane bound virus–antibody complex from infected cells and by the interaction of antibody and virions or viral antigens in the fluid phase.*

The fate of virus–antibody plasma membrane bound immune complexes have been studied in depth using measles virus infected cells (Joseph and Oldstone, 1974, 1975; Lampert *et al.*, 1975; Perrin and Oldstone, 1977; Fujinami and Oldstone, 1979, 1980). Under physiologic conditions, virus–antibody complexes precipitate, patch and aggregate on the plasma membrane with the immune complex subsequently relocating to a polar region on the cell's surface. Capping of virus–antibody complexes on the plasma membrane, first described in detail for measles virus, has now been noted for a wide variety of other RNA and DNA viruses infecting multiple cell lines. Once formed, the majority (>85%) of the measles virus–antibody immune complexes are shed from the cell's surface and only infrequently internalized by cell ingestion (Lampert *et al.*, 1975; Perrin and Oldstone, 1977). In contrast to the shedding of the majority of membrane bound measles virus–antibody immune complexes from the cell's surface, Ig-anti Ig complexes and cell surface antigen–antibody to cell surface antigen complexes were predominantly internalized and degraded with lesser amounts of complexes ($<33\%$) shed into culture fluids.

Immune complex disease occurs in most, if not all, virus infections in which there is ongoing viral replication and a continuing host immune response (reviewed Oldstone, 1975). Immunopathologic studies indicate this to be a common pathogenic mechanism for human nephritides and arteritis and choroid plexus disease. The shedding of virus–antibody complexes from the plasma membrane of virus infected cells may be an importance source of these complexes.

Escape of virus infected cells from immune lysis

Antibody induced antigenic modulation and resultant virus persistence

Overview of phenomena and parameters involved

Expression of viral antigens on the surfaces of infected cells can be altered in a variety of ways (see review Oldstone and Lampert, 1979), one way being by the action of specific antiviral antibody. The loss of a specific antigen on the surface of cells cultured in the presence of specific antibody was first observed by Boyse, Old and associates (1963, 1965, 1967) and termed antigenic modulation. These investigators noted that the phenotype expression of TL antigen on normal thymus cells (TL^+) was suppressed by TL antibodies both *in vivo* and *in vitro*. Subsequently, a variety of virus infected cells were shown to have similar effects. This occurred with several retroviruses (Aoki and Johnson, 1972; Ioachim and Sabbath, 1979; Genovesi *et al.*, 1977; Doig and Chesebro, 1978; Calafat *et al.*, 1976) and measles virus infected cells (Joseph and Oldstone, 1975; Fujinami and Oldstone, 1979, 1980).

Antibody induced antigenic modulation is dependent on active metabolism of affected cells. In addition, a virus infection is required in which the virus *per se* does not significantly shut off host protein synthesis. For example, infection of permissive cells with measles virus causes cytopathology due to plasma membrane fusion and resultant plasma membrane dysfunction. Measles virus does not shut off the cells' protein synthesis. When measles virus infected cells are cultured in the presence of antibodies, viral antigens responsible for cell–cell fusion (haemolysin, i.e. fusion protein) are removed from the cell's surface, minimizing fusion and allowing cell survival and virus persistence.

Modulation continues as long as sufficient antibody remains in the culture fluids to bind to and strip viral antigens from the cell's surface. Once the initial phase has begun, cells can be cultured in serum containing antibodies and a functional lytic complement source. The end result is that the amount of viral antigen expressed on the cell's surface diminishes to a level that is insufficient for immune mediated lysis. Infected cells cultured in the presence of antibody grow at a rate similar to uninfected cells. When antibody is removed the cells re-express antigens on their surface and reclaim their sensitivity to immune lysis. In some systems (i.e., measles virus infected HeLa cells) viral antigens return rapidly to the cell's surface when antibody is removed after 3 or 4 days of exposure to antibody. In contrast, the longer the cells are cultured in antibody (>5 days), the longer the time needed to re-express measles virus antigen after antibody has been removed (Joseph and Oldstone, 1975). Studies with the TL system have indicated that modulation did not require the whole Ig molecule, but that Fab fragment by itself was sufficient to induce modulation and that the modulating activity was enhanced by complement (see review by Stackpole *et al.*, 1978).

Mechanism of virus persistence in human chronic measles virus infection (*SSPE*) In man many naturally occurring infections are associated with virus persistence in the presence of a specific antiviral antibody response. Examples include persisting infection with herpes simplex virus, cytomegalovirus, hepatitis B virus and measles virus infection. In humans, measles virus infection follows an acute self-limiting course as the patient mounts an immune response which clears the virus from his tissues. Convalescence is associated with low titres of antibody to measles virus and immune lymphocytes that remain throughout life. In contrast to this usual situation is chronic measles virus infection, called subacute sclerosing panencephalitis (SSPE). SSPE is associated with measles virus persistence and abnormally high titres of antimeasles virus antibodies in body fluids and serum; yet the complement system is functionally active and cytotoxic immune lymphocytes are present in peripheral blood (ter Meulen *et al.*, 1972; Joseph *et al.*, 1975; Perrin *et al.*, 1977; Kreth *et al.*, 1979).

To explain the event seen in SSPE, we have suggested that antibody to measles virus modulates or strips viral antigens off surfaces of virus infected cells (Joseph and Oldstone, 1975; Fujinami and Oldstone, 1980). This is based on experimental evidence that specific measles virus antibodies added to cultured infected cells modulate viral antigens from the cell's surface, causing these cells to express less viral antigens and thereby avoid immune lysis by both humoral or cell mediated mechanisms. Further, during antibody induced antigenic modulation, the numbers of nucleocapsids accumulated inside the cell dramatically increase and they are positioned in a random arrangement. This *in vitro* picture parallels the distribution of nucleocapsids seen in cells obtained by biopsy from patients with SSPE (Iwasaki and Koprowski, 1974).

Molecular events accompanying antibody induced modulation of measles virus infected cells have been recently uncovered (Fujinami and Oldstone, 1979, 1980). It was noted that viral polypeptides on the cell's surface as well as viral polypeptides inside the cell were altered. While the stripping of the measles virus surface glycoproteins was expected, the alterations in viral polypeptides expressed only inside the cell was not. The polypeptides altered inside of infected cells were the P (a phosphoprotein with molecular weight of 70 000) and M or matrix protein (molecular weight of 36 000). Using isotope labelling and quantitative studies, it was found that ^{35}S and ^{32}P labelled residues of

P protein were decreased by 80% or more, while the M protein showed significantly increased incorporation of ^{32}P during modulation. It is interesting to speculate that changes in the phosphorylation of M protein might alter nucleocapsid recognition and alignment of the plasma membrane, thereby inhibiting viral maturation, all consequences noted in cells chronically infected with measles virus. P protein complexes with the nucleocapsid and L protein of measles virus to form the replicative complex. Hence, P protein may be a rate limiting protein in the regulation of measles virus synthesis. The loss of the fusion protein from the surface of virus infected cells has a known biological consequence. This is the prevention of cell–cell fusion. Cell fusion ordinarily results in giant cell and syncytia formation leading to cell death. Cells lacking fusion protein molecules on their surfaces are relatively normal in cytomorphology, retain viral genetic information and survive for prolonged times in culture.

While the biological consequences of the aberrations in P and M polypeptides during antibody induced modulation of measles virus infected cells are unclear, it is clear that antibody induced modulation is specific, as the aberrations in measles virus polypeptides are associated only with antibodies binding to measles virus antigens on the cell's surface and not to antibody binding to nonviral structural antigens expressed on the cell's surface. Hence, perturbation of membranes of infected cells, *per se*, is not associated with the molecular events occurring during antibody induced antigenic modulation.

The biological importance of antibody induced antigenic modulation is that it provides a mechanism whereby cells infected with certain viruses can reduce the expression of viral antigens on their surfaces, maintain viral genetic information and escape immunologic surveillance. It is clear from several *in vitro* models with a variety of viruses that modulation takes place under physiologic conditions (multivalent antibody and 37°C). Further, there are several systems in which antibody induced antigenic modulation can be shown *in vivo*. The initiation of antibody induced antigenic modulation can occur via two mechanisms. First, cells found in areas having low or inefficient complement systems can react with antibody made externally or produced *in situ* by plasma cells. For example, we have studied paired serum and cerebral spinal fluid from 2 patients with SSPE. Either the serum or cerebral spinal fluid independently was able to strip measles virus antigens from the surface of infected HeLa cells. However, lysis only occurred with serum as the cerebral spinal fluid, although containing high titres of cytotolic antibodies to measles virus, lacked an effective complement system. A second factor favouring antibody induced modulation over antibody and complement mediated lysis is that 50-fold less antibody is needed for modulation of measles virus antigens than is required for lysis of measles virus infected cells. Thus, quantitatively the local production of antibody by plasma cells favours modulation over immune lysis. Once virus persistence is initiated by antibody, persistence can be maintained by several mechanisms, the most likely being the generation of virus mutants by infected cells.

Action and mechanism of complement inactivation of virus–antibody immune complexes

Antibody may neutralize virus infectivity in several ways, although in the presence of complement, neutralization is frequently more efficient. There are a number of possible mechanisms whereby complement plays a role. First, complement and antibody may aggregate virus particles, thereby both preventing their adsorption to cells and reducing the net number of infectious particles. This effect has been observed with several viruses including herpes simplex, polyoma and rabies virus. In these studies of agglutination of virus by antibody and complement, the early components of the classical pathway are required (reviewed Oldstone, 1975; Cooper and Welsh, 1979). The features of this reaction are electron micrographic evidence of agglutination and sucrose gradient evidence of the formation of heavy aggregates (Fig. 7). A second and less common mechanism of neutralization of virus with antibody and complement occurs by blanketing or covering individual viral particles. In this instance, virions initially mixed with antibody are covered by complement without the formation of aggregates (Fig. 7). This event is observed under stringent experimental conditions with infectious bronchitis virus and herpes simplex virus and requires the early components of the classical complement system. Like aggregation, blanketing (covering) achieves neutralization by covering virion attachment sites. Blanketing is segregated from aggregation

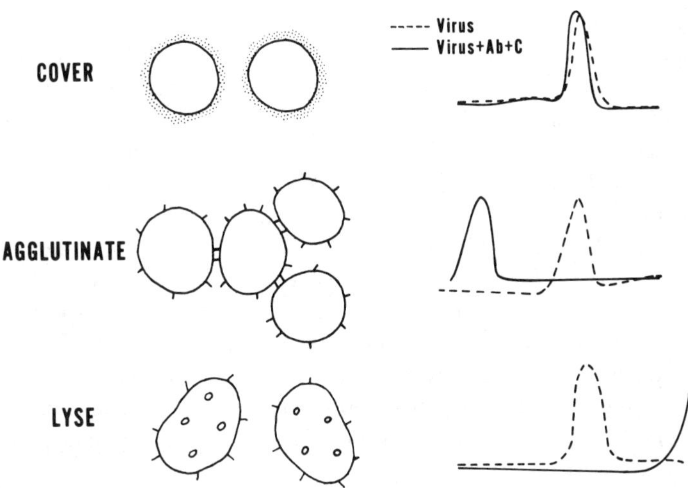

FIG. 7. *A schematic drawing showing the electron micrographic and sucrose density gradient (following fate of virus nucleic acid) evidence for differences between formed virion–antibody–complement complexes. Viral neutralization occurs via the three mechanisms of covering (blanketing), aggregating or lysing. Reproduced from Oldstone (1975) with permission from S. Karger AG, Basel.*

on the basis of electron microscopic and density gradient studies (Fig. 7). Although not as yet reported, it is possible that a virus not permissive for a specific cell that bears a C3 (C3b or C3d) receptor may now infect that cell owing to the attachment of C3 on its virion surface. A third mechanism whereby antibody and complement neutralize viruses is by lysis of virions (Fig. 7). Immune lysis of virions occurs with those viruses containing lipid moieties in their membranes and requires the participation of antibody and the terminal or membrane complement components (C5–C9). Similar to studies of lysis of red blood cells, lysed virions show distinctive ultrastructure pits or craters of 8–10 nm in diameter (Fig. 7). Immune lysis of virions has been demonstrated with a variety of viruses in the herpes, corona, arena, paramyxo and myxovirus groups. In addition to the distinctive electron micrographic pictures of pits or craters found on the surfaces of virions or of disrupted virus particles (Fig. 8), density gradient analysis shows the release of viral nucleic acid from the virion (Fig. 7). A fourth mechanism whereby complement deposited on antibody coated virus particles may cause neutralization is by the opsonization of these aggregates by phagocytic cells bearing C3b receptors. The neutralization of viruses by antibody and complement, the physiochemical, morphological and biological consequences have been reviewed (see Oldstone, 1975; Cooper and Welsh, 1979). Some viruses may be neutralized by complement in the absence of antibody. For details the reader is referred to a recent review by Cooper and Welsh (1979).

Conclusion

Evidence for the human system shows that virus infected cells are lysed by antibody and complement *in vitro*, and that this lysis is dependent on a functional alternative complement pathway and specific antiviral antibody. Virus infected cells themselves activate the alternative pathway independent of antibody, but divalent IgG antibody is a necessary requirement for lysis. Immune lysis of virus infected cells occurs with a variety of different cell types infected by a wide spectrum of both DNA and RNA viruses. These observations strengthen the likelihood that antibody and complement mediated lysis of virus infected cells is an important mechanism in preventing the spread of virus infections *in vivo*. Once the infected cell is lysed, the infectious virions released can be neutralized by antibody in the fluid phase. The neutralization of virus particles by antibody is enhanced by complement and occurs by several mechanisms including blanketing or covering of virions, aggregation of virions, lysis of virions or preparing virions for phagocytic cells that bear C3b receptors.

Although virus–antibody–complement union affords a host protection in terms of removal of virus infected cells and neutralization and clearing of unwanted infectious agents, the same union affords the host the hazard of immunopathologic disease. First, destruction of a large number and/or critical

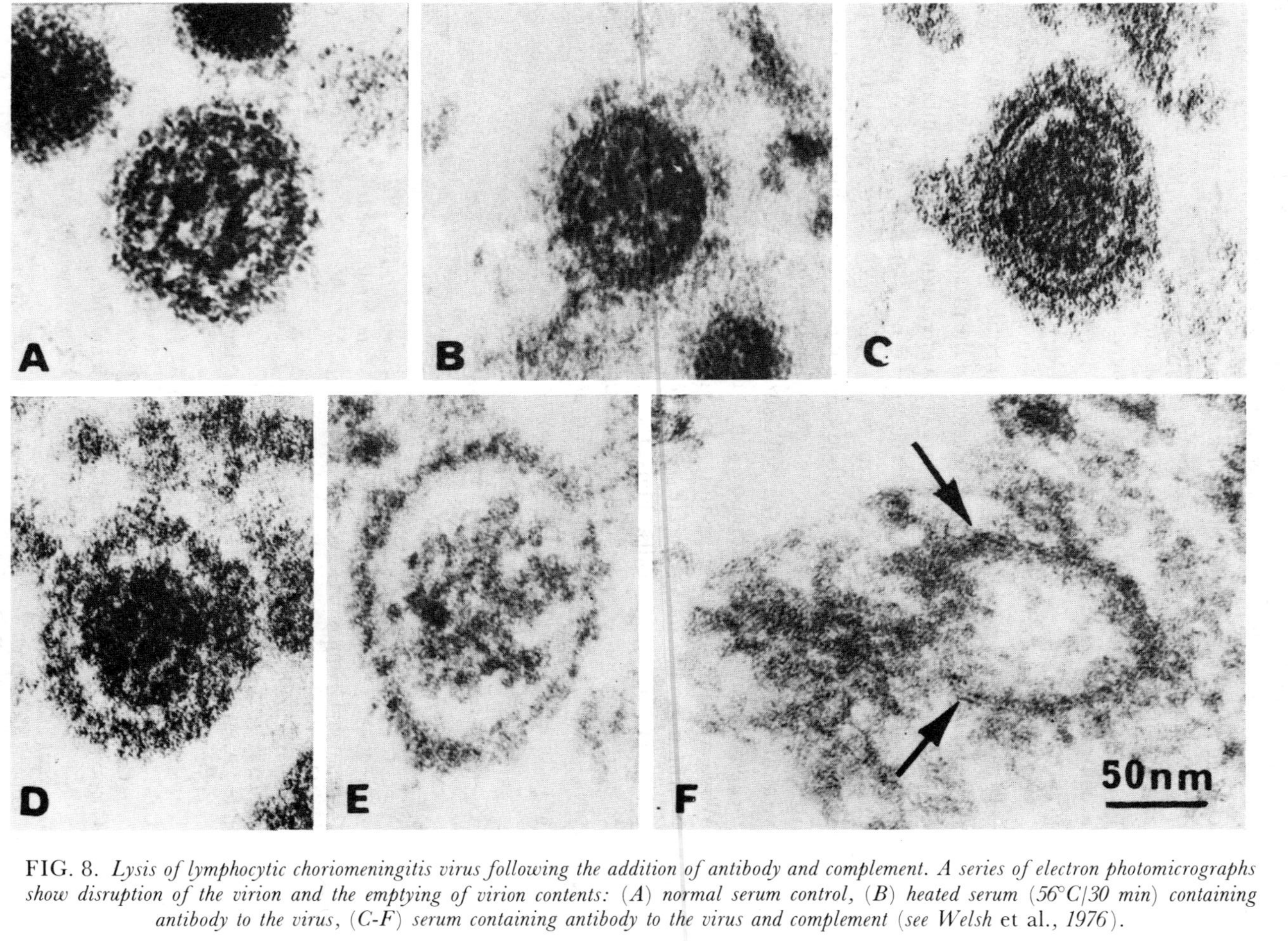

FIG. 8. *Lysis of lymphocytic choriomeningitis virus following the addition of antibody and complement. A series of electron photomicrographs show disruption of the virion and the emptying of virion contents:* (*A*) *normal serum control,* (*B*) *heated serum* (*56°C/30 min*) *containing antibody to the virus,* (*C-F*) *serum containing antibody to the virus and complement* (*see Welsh* et al., *1976*).

cells in the body can lead to immunopathologic mediated injury and severe disease. Second, virus–antibody immune complexes can be formed and shed into fluid phase. The trapping of such complexes in glomeruli, vessels and choroid plexus can lead to the well-known manifestations of immune complex disease. Factors affecting the amount of virus carried, the magnitude of the antiviral immune response and the presence and functional ability of the complement system are likely to be of prime importance in determining the accompanying tissue injury, virus clearance and perhaps the initiation of virus persistence.

Antibody induced redistribution of viral antigens on the surfaces of infected cells leads to aggregation, capping and/or modulation. Evidence indicates that the regulation of viral antigens expressed on the plasma membranes of infected cells is specific and that antibody may provide a signal to the membrane that specifically alters viral coded events occurring inside the cell. Antibody induced modulation of viral antigens occurs *in vitro* and *in vivo* and can be shown to be a source of shedding virus–antibody immune complexes into the fluid phase. In addition, antibody-induced antigenic modulation reduces the number of viral antigens expressed on the cell's surface and allows the infected cell to escape immune lysis by antibody and complement or cytotoxic lymphocytes. While avoiding immune assault, such infected cells maintain viral genetic information and may generate a series of mutants that further allows virus persistence in infected cells. Thus, the end result of a virus infection relates to a combination of specific characteristics of a virus, the cells in which the virus replicates, and the function and activity of the host's immune system, as modified by several host effector systems.

References

Aoki, T. and Johnson, P. A. (1972). *J. Natn. Cancer Inst.* **183**, 192.

Boyse, E. A., Old, L. J. and Stockert, E. (1965). *In* "Immunopathology, IVth International Symposium" (P. Grabar and P. A. Miescher, eds), p. 23. Schwabe and Co., Basel.

Boyse, E. A., Old, L. J. and Luell, S. (1963). *J. Natn. Cancer Inst.* **31**, 987.

Boyse, E. A., Stockert, E. and Old, L. J. (1967). *Proc. Natn. Acad. Sci. U.S.A.* **58**, 954.

Brier, A. M., Wohlenberg, C., Rosenthal, J., Mage, M. and Notkins, A. L. (1971). *Proc. Natn. Acad. Sci. U.S.A.* **68**, 3073.

Burns, W. H., Billings, L. C. and Notkins, A. L. (1975). *Nature* **256**, 654.

Calafat, J., Von Blitterswijk, W. J., Verbeet, M. and Hageman, P. C. (1976). *J. Natn. Cancer Inst.* **56**, 1019.

Cooper, N. R. (1980). *In* "Basic and Clinical Immunology" (3rd edn) (H. H. Fudenberg, D. P. Stites, J. L. Caldwell and J. V. Wells, eds). Lange Medical Publications, San Francisco (in press).

Cooper, N. R. and Welsh, R. M., Jr. (1979). *In* "Springer Seminars in Immunopathology" (P. Miescher and H. J. Müller-Ebergard, eds) Vol. 2 (No. 3), pp. 285–310. Springer-Verlag, New York.

Doig, D. and Chesebro, B. (1978). *J. Exp. Med.* **148**, 1109.

Ehrnst, A. (1978). *J. Immunol.* **121**, 1206.

Fujinami, R. S. and Oldstone, M. B. A. (1979). *Nature* **279**, 529.
Fujinami, R. S. and Oldstone, M. B. A. (1980). *J. Immunol.* **125**, 78.
Genovesi, E. V., Marx, P. A. and Wheelock, E. F. (1977). *J. Exp. Med.* **146**, 520.
Hicks, J. T., Klutch, M. J., Albrecht, P. and Frank, M. M. (1976). *J. Immunol.* **117**, 208.
Ioachim, H. L. and Sabbath, M. (1979). *J. Natn. Cancer Inst.* **62**, 169.
Iwasaki, Y. and Koprowski, H. (1974). *Lab. Invest.* **31**, 187.
Joseph, B. S. and Oldstone, M. B. A. (1974). *J. Immunol.* **113**, 1205.
Joseph, B. S. and Oldstone, M. B. A. (1975). *J. Exp. Med.* **142**, 864.
Joseph, B. S., Cooper, N. R. and Oldstone, M. B. A. (1975). *J. Exp. Med.* **141**, 761.
Kreth, H. W., ter Meulen, V. and Eckert, G. (1979). *Med. Microbiol. Immunol.* **165**, 203.
Lampert, P. W., Joseph, B. S. and Oldstone, M. B. A. (1975). *J. Virol.* **15**, 1248.
ter Meulen, V., Katz, M. and Muller, D. (1972). *Current Topics Microbiol Immunol.* **57**, 1.
Moore, F. D., Fearon, D. T. and Austen, K. F. (1980). *Fed. Proc.* **39**, 1058 (Abstr.).
Müller-Eberhard, H. J. (1980). *In* "Immunology, 1980" (M. Fougereau, ed.). Academic Press, New York (in press).
Müller-Eberhard, H. J. and Schreiber, R. (1980). *Adv. Immunol.* **29**, 1.
Old, L. J., Stockert, E., Boyse, E. A. and Kim, J. H. (1968). *J. Exp. Med.* **127**, 523.
Oldstone, M. B. A. (1975). *In* "Progress in Medical Virology" (J. L. Melnick, ed.) Vol. 19, pp. 84–119. Karger, Basel.
Oldstone, M. B. A. and Lampert, P. W. (1979). *Springer Sem. Immunopathol.* **2**, 261.
Perrin, L. H. and Oldstone, M. B. A. (1977). *J. Immunol.* **118**, 316.
Perrin, L. H., Joseph, B. S., Cooper, N. R. and Oldstone, M. B. A. (1976). *J. Exp. Med.* **143**, 1027.
Perrin, L. H., Tishon, A. and Oldstone, M. B. A. (1977). *J. Immunol.* **118**, 282.
Rawls, W. and Tompkins, W. (1975). *In* "Viral Immunology and Immunopathology" (A. Notkins, ed.) p. 99. Academic Press, New York.
Schenkein, H. A. and Ruddy, S. (1980). *Fed. Proc.* **39**, 1059 (Abstr.).
Sissons, J. G. P. and Oldstone, M. B. A. (1980). *Adv. Immunol.* **29** (in press).
Sissons, J. G. P., Schreiber, R. D., Perrin, L. H., Cooper, N. R., Oldstone, M. B. A. and Müller-Eberhard, H. J. (1979). *J. Exp. Med.* **150**, 445.
Sissons, J. G. P., Cooper, N. R. and Oldstone, M. B. A. (1980a). *J. Immunol.* **123**, 2144.
Sissons, J. G. P., Oldstone, M. B. A. and Schreiber, R. D. (1980b). *Proc. Natn. Acad. Sci. U.S.A.* **77**, 559.
Spiegelberg, H. L. (1974). *Adv. Immunol.* **19**, 259.
Stackpole, C. W., Jacobson, J. B. and Lardis, M. P. (1978). *J. Exp. Med.* **140**, 939.
Welsh, R. M., Lampert, P. W., Burner, P. A. and Oldstone, M. B. A. (1976). *Virology* **73**, 59.
Wiktor, T. J., Kuwert, D. and Koprowski, H. (1968). *J. Immunol.* **101**, 1271.

34

Clonal Analysis of Cytolytic T Lymphocytes and their Precursors

J.-C. CEROTTINI

Unit of Human Cancer Immunology, Ledwig Institute for Cancer Research, Lausanne, Switzerland

Introduction

Although considerable progress in our understanding of T cell responses has been made over the last 10 years, it is evident that such studies have been severely limited by the lack of assay systems allowing the quantitation of effector T cells and their immediate precursors and/or the analysis of their fine specificity. In view of these limitations, considerable efforts have recently been devoted to the development of techniques that allow studies of individual T cell clones rather than heterogeneous cell populations. In contrast to effector cells involved in helper, suppressive or delayed hypersensitivity activities, cytolytic T lymphocytes (CTL) express a specific function that can be measured directly in a short-term quantitative assay (^{51}Cr release assay). It is therefore not too surprising that initial attempts to isolate functional T cell

Abbreviations

CTL: cytolytic T lymphocyte; TCGF: T cell growth factor; CTL-P: cytolytic T lymphocyte precursor; MCL: mixed leukocyte culture; MoLV: Moloney leukaemia virus.

clones have concentrated on the establishment of permanent CTL lines. Later, a similar approach has been applied to the isolation of homogeneous populations of helper and suppressor lymphocytes.

Early attempts to establish CTL lines involved repeated stimulation *in vitro* of alloreactive CTL populations with appropriate stimulator cells. With one exception (Dennert, 1979), these studies showed that the cell populations, although retaining specific proliferative activity, lost their lytic capacity after several months in culture. In contrast, CTL populations cultured in media supplemented with T cell growth factor(s) (TCGF) present in supernatant from concanavalin A stimulated spleen cells were found to undergo continuous proliferation without losing lytic activity (Gillis and Smith, 1977). Based on these findings, a general procedure was developed in which cell populations were first enriched for CTL of a given specificity by repeated stimulation with antigen, then maintained in continuous proliferation in the presence of TCGF and finally cloned by either limiting dilution or in soft agar (always in the presence of TCGF) (for a more detailed discussion of this procedure, see Nabholz *et al.*, 1980). By using this approach, it has been possible to isolate clonal CTL lines from different origins and with different specificities. Some of these lines have been maintained in continuous proliferation for several years and therefore appear to have an unlimited lifespan. Although such clones are useful tools for biochemical or somatic cell genetic studies, they appear to be derived from a small proportion of CTL which are selected for during culture in TCGF-containing medium. Therefore, these clones are not likely to represent the whole repertoire of CTL present in the initial cell populations. Moreover, this approach does not allow any quantitation of the number of CTL precursors (CTL-P) reactive to a given antigen.

Recently, limiting dilution microculture systems have been developed that allow direct measurement of CTL-P frequencies (Skinner and Marbrook, 1976; Fischer-Lindahl and Wilson, 1977; Teh *et al.*, 1977b; Ryser and MacDonald, 1979a). In addition, by using similar microculture systems, it has been possible to obtain large numbers of individual CTL clones which subsequently could be expanded and maintained in culture for several months. The aim of this chapter is to summarize the basic features of limiting dilution microculture systems, and their application to the determination of CTL-P frequencies and to the analysis of specificity, phenotype stability and Lyt phenotype of CTL clones. For further discussion of this topic, the reader is referred to a recent review article (MacDonald *et al.*, 1980).

Limiting dilution microculture systems

It is well documented that the immediate precursors of CTL are small, inactive lymphocytes which undergo extensive proliferation and differentiation upon antigenic stimulation. Therefore, a CTL-P, although it has no lytic activity, can be detected through the ability of its clonal progeny to lyse appropriate target cells. In the various limiting dilution microculture systems developed for the measurement of CTL-P frequencies, the same basic approach has been taken: large numbers of cultures are set up containing decreasing numbers of responder lymphocytes (including CTL-P) and a fixed number of antigen-bearing stimulator cells. In theory, detection of CTL activity after antigenic stimulation indicates that the culture tested contains at least one CTL-P reactive to the antigen used. When the number of CTL-P per culture becomes limiting, some cultures contain no CTL-P and, thus, are negative when assayed for CTL activity after appropriate antigenic stimulation.

As pointed out by Miller *et al.* (1977), limiting dilution assays to measure CTL-P frequency for various antigens should meet the following conditions (a) the CTL-P must be the only limiting cell type in the suspension being diluted; (b) the culture conditions must be such that a single CTL-P can produce viable progeny upon specific antigenic stimulation; and (c) the assay for CTL must be sufficiently sensitive to detect the progeny of a single CTL-P.

Recent developments in tissue methodology indicate that the above conditions can be met provided optimal concentrations of stimulating cells, accessory cells and serum are used (Miller *et al.*, 1977; Ryser and MacDonald, 1979a). In addition, maximal sensitivity of the culture system is dependent on the presence of nonspecific factors including TCGF (since the topic of T cell stimulating growth factors is outside the scope of this chapter, the interested reader is referred to Volume 51 of Immunological Reviews). Whether these factors are responsible for the activation of greater number of CTL-P or simply increase clone size (and therefore detection efficiency) has yet to be determined. Whatever the mechanism of action might be, it is evident that the presence of these factors in the limiting dilution microculture system eliminated the possible requirement of alloreactive helper T cells for CTL induction.

The basis of the limiting dilution assay developed in our laboratory is to culture various limiting numbers of responder lymphocytes in the presence of an excess of irradiated antigen-bearing stimulator cells and an optimal concentration of secondary mixed leukocyte culture supernatant as a source of TCGF. In studies of alloreactive CTL-P, spleen cells or tumour cells bearing the appropriate alloantigens have been used as a source of stimulator cells. Virally infected spleen cells or virally induced tumour cells have been used as stimulator cells in studies dealing with CTL-P reactive against virus associated surface antigens in syngeneic systems. With syngeneic tumour cells, addition of irradiated syngeneic spleen cells as a source of accessory cells was found to give optimal results (Brunner *et al.*, 1980). After 7 days of culture, individual microcultures are assayed for lytic activity against appropriate ^{51}Cr-labelled target cells, and the percentage of positive (cytolytic) microcultures is determined for each responder cell dose. Since a positive response can result indistinguishably from the presence of any number of CTL-P whereas a negative response can result only from the absence of CTL-P, the zero-order term of the Poisson equation is used to describe the relation between the number of cells tested per culture and the percentage of nonresponding cultures per group (for discussion of this concept, see Miller *et al.*, 1977). Therefore, if the frequency of CTL-P in a given population is represented by f, then the percentage of nonresponding cultures (y) is related to the number of responding cells per culture (x) according to the equation $\ln y = fx + \ln a$, where a is the y-intercept, theoretically equal to 100%. Practically, experimental x- and y-values are fitted to the Poisson equation by the least-squares method or, better still, by the method of chi-squared minimization or log likelihood maximization.

It should be noted that, even if it is established that CTL-P are the only limiting cell type under the conditions employed in a given assay, the frequency estimates obtained are minimal estimates since the efficiency of detection of these precursors cannot be assessed with certainty. Moreover, comparison between the frequencies of CTL-P that have been obtained by various groups in similar antigenic combinations indicates that the plating efficiency can vary considerably according to the culture conditions used.

Frequencies of CTL precursors

Minimal estimates of the frequency of CTL-P directed against a variety of antigens have been obtained recently. Thus, the mean frequency of CTL-P in C57BL/6 (H-2^b) spleen reactive against DBA/2 (H-2^d) alloantigens was found to be 1 in 400 (MacDonald *et al.*, 1980). Interestingly, the mean-frequency measured in a congenic H-2^b anti-H-2^d situation was not very different (1:737). Moreover, in two series of recombinant strains (H-2^b anti-H-2^d and H-2^b anti-H-2^a), it appeared that similar frequencies (approximately equal to 50% of the frequency directed against the whole determinant haplotype) of CTL-P were reactive with K and D end determinants. Unexpectedly, the mean CTL-P frequency in C57BL/6 spleen against three independently derived K^b mutants was found to be within the range of frequencies (between 1:772 and 1:1165) observed in entirely H-2 incompatible combinations (Widmer and MacDonald, 1980).

Tissue distribution analysis in C57BL/6 mice of the frequency of anti-DBA/2 CTL-P indicated a higher frequency in lymph node (1:68) and in peripheral blood (1:180) lymphocytes than in spleen. In the thymus, the frequency was lower (1:1634) than in the spleen, but increased 17-fold (to 1:96) after treatment with hydrocortisone *in vivo* (Taswell *et al.*, 1979). In bone marrow, the frequency observed (1:2131) could be interpreted as a contamination of bone marrow cell suspensions by peripheral blood.

A recent study by Maryanski *et al.* (1980b) showed that frequency determinations were feasible even when such frequencies were very low, e.g. in spleens of congenitally athymic (nu/nu) C57BL/6 mice. Minimal estimates of the frequency of anti-DBA/2 CTL-P ranged from 1:12 400 to 1:159 000 in unseparated nude spleen cell suspensions. However, the determinations were not always statistically acceptable, possibly due to the large number of cells cultured. Better results were obtained with nylon wool nonadherent nude spleen cells. Therefore, when CTL-P frequencies are relatively low, prior enrichment of CTL-P by negative or positive selection procedures might improve the accuracy of the limiting dilution assay. This consideration should be kept in mind when frequencies of CTL-P directed against antigens other than major histocompatibility antigens are determined. In the few systems studied so far, it appears that the frequency of CTL-P is much lower than that of anti-H-2 CTL-P, ranging from approximately 1 in 10^4 in an oncornavirus-induced lymphoma system (Brunner *et al.*, 1980) or in a chemically-modified syngeneic spleen cell system (Fischer-Lindahl and Wilson, 1977; Ching and Marbrook, 1979) to $\leqslant 1$ in 10^5 in a male H-Y antigenic system (MacDonald *et al.*, 1980) or in an influenza virus-infected cell system (Komatsu *et al.*, 1978).

The search for qualitative and quantitative effects of specific immunization on CTL responses has been the subject of many investigations in the past. The concept that memory existed at the level of CTL responses was first suggested by the observation that mice preimmunized with allogeneic tumour cells developed, after challenge with the same tumour cells, a response with accelerated kinetics and higher peak levels of cytolytic activity. Subsequent studies showed that the expression of memory after *in vitro* secondary antigenic stimulation was even greater than after *in vivo* challenge. Indeed, most of the recent studies dealing with the generation of CTL directed against nonmajor histocompatibility antigens have relied on the combination of *in vivo* primary immunization and *in vitro* secondary stimulation. Although the cellular basis for anamnestic CTL responses remains to be clarified, it appears that it involves an increased number of CTL-P. By using limiting dilution assay systems for CTL-P frequency, direct evidence has been provided that immunization *in vivo* may be accompanied by a selective increase in CTL-P directed against the immunizing antigen. This increase ranged from 2·6-fold in an allogeneic system (Ryser and MacDonald, 1979b) to 10- to 30-fold in two syngeneic systems (MacDonald *et al.*, 1980). Other studies indicated that the frequency of CTL-P dramatically increased following antigenic stimulation *in vitro*. Using C57BL/6 spleen cells as a source of responder cells, Maryanski *et al.* (1980a) found that the frequency of anti-DBA/2 CTL-P was 1:5 in mixed leukocyte culture (MLC) populations that had been stimulated with irradiated DBA/2 spleen cells for 5 days. When the MLC cells were separated on the basis of size, it was observed that the CTL-P frequency was as high as 1:2 in the large sized cell fraction as compared to 1:200 in the small lymphocyte fraction. Quantitative comparison of CTL-P (as measured by limiting dilution assay) and CTL (as measured by ^{51}Cr release assay) in these separated populations revealed a striking degree of correlation. Thus, it appears very likely that the operationally defined CTL-P in day 5 MLC populations were indeed mature CTL. High CTL-P frequencies were also observed in long-term MLC populations, i.e. at a time when CTL had reverted into small lymphocytes devoid of lytic activity (Ryser and MacDonald, 1979b). Taken together with other studies

(Teh *et al.*, 1977a), these results indicate that limiting dilution microculture systems can detect cells of the CTL lineage irrespective of whether or not they express cytolytic function, i.e. they detect the original CTL-P, CTL and memory CTL-P derived from CTL.

Lyt phenotype of CTL precursors and their clonal progeny

Many studies have recently been devoted to the characterization of the Lyt phenotype of CTL-P in various antigenic systems. Originally, as a result of the work of Cantor and Boyse (1975, 1976), it became widely accepted that alloreactive CTL-P expressed the Lyt-$1^-2^+3^+$ phenotype whereas H-2-restricted CTL-P were confined within the Lyt-$1^+2^+3^+$ subset. Recently, however, it was suggested that there were two subsets of alloreactive CTL-P, one expressing the Lyt-$1^+2^+3^+$ phenotype and the other the Lyt-$1^-2^+3^+$ phenotype, and that activation and/or proliferation of one or the other subset depended on the additional activation of Lyt-$1^+2^-3^-$ helper cells (Alter and Bach, 1979; Wettstein *et al.*, 1979). More recently, evidence was presented that both alloreactive and H-2 restricted (unprimed) CTL-P were Lyt-$1^+2^+3^+$ (Simon and Abenhardt, 1980; Nakayama *et al.*, 1980).

It should be pointed out that these results were obtained by stimulating *in vitro* (under mass culture conditions) various T cell subpopulations negatively selected for by treatment with anti-Lyt antisera plus complement. Such studies suffer from several important limitations in interpretation. In the first place, precursor assays done under normal mass culture conditions are complicated by the possible dependence of CTL induction on other cell types and/or soluble factors. More importantly, even under optimal culture conditions, any quantitative interpretation of such assays depends on the unproven assumption that there exists a linear relationship between the number of CTL-P in a given lymphoid cell population and the lytic activity displayed by this population after appropriate antigenic stimulation.

In view of these limitations, a more direct approach has recently been used whereby the frequency of CTL-P directed against whole H-2 haplotype differences and against H-2 mutant alloantigens was determined before and after treatment with appropriate anti-Lyt antisera plus complement (MacDonald *et al.*, 1980; Cerottini and MacDonald, 1980). In both systems, the absolute number of CTL-P was reduced by 90% and 98% by treatment with anti-Lyt-1 and anti-Lyt-2 alloantisera, respectively, in the presence of complement. These results thus demonstrate that most, if not all, alloreactive CTL-P express the Lyt-$1^+2^+3^+$ phenotype. In this respect, there appears to be no difference between CTL-P directed against independently derived H-2 haplotypes and those reactive against mutant alloantigens.

These results are consistent with recent quantitative immunofluorescence studies of the Lyt phenotype of peripheral T cells (Ledbetter and Herzenberg, 1979). As assessed by flow microfluorometry, it is now evident that most, if not all, peripheral T cells express the Lyt-1 antigen, whereas only 30% of these cells express the Lyt-2 antigen. This implies that peripheral T cells can be divided into 2 subclasses only, namely Lyt-1^+2^- and Lyt-1^+2^+, instead of 3 as originally proposed on the basis of antibody cytotoxicity studies (Cantor and Boyse, 1975). The most likely explanation for the discrepancy in these results is that T cells, though expressing the Lyt-1 antigen, vary in their susceptibility to lysis by anti-Lyt-1 serum plus complement. In the experiments mentioned above, the CTL-P frequency in the cell population remaining after treatment with anti-Lyt-1 serum plus complement was only 2- to 3-fold lower than that in untreated cells (Cerottini and MacDonald, 1980). However, by taking into account both the frequency and the number of cells lysed by anti-Lyt-1 plus complement (approximately 75% of the nylon wool purified spleen cells used in these experiments), it became evident that 90 out of 100 CTL-P had been eliminated by this treatment.

It should be pointed out that the same considerations apply to the Lyt phenotype of CTL. In contrast to the widely-held view that CTL express the Lyt-$1^-2^+3^+$ phenotype, recent studies came to the conclusion that some, if not all, CTL are Lyt-$1^+2^+3^+$ (Nakayama *et al.*, 1979; Wettstein *et al.*, 1979). Quantitative immunofluorescence studies performed on MLC populations clearly indicated that essentially all the cells in the large sized fraction (containing the CTL) expressed the Lyt-1 antigen (Cerottini and MacDonald, 1980). Furthermore, recent studies in our laboratory showed that CTL clones directed against alloantigens or virus-associated antigens all expressed the Lyt-1^+2^+ phenotype as assessed by flow microfluorometry.

Taken together, these results strongly suggest that CTL-P, irrespective of their specificity, exhibit the Lyt-$1^+2^+3^+$ phenotype and differentiate into Lyt-$1^+2^+3^+$ progeny CTL. Interestingly, it appears that there exists in addition a distinct population of alloreactive precursor cells which express the Lyt-1^+2^- phenotype and differentiate into Lyt-1^+2^- effector cells able to mediate lectin-dependent non-specific lysis, although they appear not to be directly cytotoxic (Cerottini and MacDonald, 1980). The antigenic specificity of these effector cells has yet to be determined, but preliminary results indicate that alloantigens other than those encoded by the K/D regions of the major histocompatibility complex may be involved.

Specificity analysis of CTL clones

Until recently, conclusions regarding CTL specificity have been based on the study of CTL populations. Considerable information has been gained by using various approaches, including genetic analysis of CTL-mediated lysis, depletion of effector cells by absorption on target cells, and inhibition by unlabelled target cell or antibodies. However, it is clear that definitive analysis of CTL specificity can only be provided by studies at the single cell level rather than at the population level. For example, while the phenomenon of H-2 restriction has been documented in many syngeneic CTL systems, it has often been observed that this restriction is not complete, since some degree of cytolysis also occurs against H-2-incompatible target cells (especially when strong responses are elicited). When measured at the population level, this cross-reactivity can be explained by (a) a homogeneous population of CTL reacting with both syngeneic and (to a much lesser extent) allogeneic target cells, (b) a heterogeneous population of CTL with some effector cells reacting only with syngeneic target cells, and other effector cells reacting with both syngeneic and allogeneic target cells with the same efficiency, or (c) a more complex combination of both of these possibilities. Although attempts have been made to investigate cross-reactivity by unlabelled target cell inhibition of the lytic activity displayed by CTL populations, this method cannot accurately distinguish between these possibilities. Furthermore, the methods available for detecting individual effector cells are not easily amenable to the study of CTL specificity. Therefore, recent approaches have concentrated on the specificity analysis of CTL clones generated under limiting dilution conditions.

In early studies, CTL clones have been generated directly from (unprimed) CTL-P using the limiting dilution microculture systems described above. The number of responder cells per culture has to be selected in such a way that the frequency of cytolytically positive microcultures is low, thus ensuring a high probability that CTL contained in individual cultures are derived from single CTL-P. Under optimal culture conditions, the size of the clones is sufficient to allow assays against 2 (sometimes even up to 4) different target cells. Using this approach, Teh *et al.* (1978) demonstrated that approximately 4% of H-2^k anti-H-2^b CTL clones were also reactive with H-2^d target cells. Direct evidence was also provided for the existence of CTL cross-reacting with TNP-modified syngeneic and allogeneic target cells (Teh, 1979). In a recent study (Brunner *et al.*, 1980), the clonal progeny of individual CTL-P reacting against Moloney leukaemia virus (MoLV)-associated antigens were tested for cytolytic activity against syngeneic and allogeneic MoLV-induced tumour cells. Of a total of 576 microcultures set up with 200 C57BL/6 regressor spleen cells, 198 (35%) were cytolytically positive, and of these, 145 (73% of all positive cultures) lysed only syngeneic target cells. In addition, 13 cultures (7% of all positive cultures) were identified clearly as containing CTL with similar lytic activity against both syngeneic and allogeneic target cells. In all these studies, however, no attempt was made to ascertain the monoclonality of the CTL obtained under limiting dilution conditions.

A slightly modified approach has recently been developed in order to increase the probability that CTL are monoclonal even at a relatively high percentage of positive cultures (Taswell *et al.*, 1980). Based on the observation that the frequency of operationally defined CTL-P dramatically increases after *in vitro* stimulation of responder cell populations with appropriate stimulating cells in mass culture, very small numbers (between 1 and 5 cells per microculture) of such *in vitro* stimulated cell populations are cultured in the presence of the relevant antigen-bearing cells, accessory cells (whenever needed) and a source of TCGF. Under optimal conditions, positive microcultures contain approximately 5×10^4 cells on average on day 7. This estimated clone size corresponds to approximately 16 divisions with a doubling time of 11 h for the 7 day culture period. Such putative clones can be expanded readily, subcloned by limiting dilution and maintained in culture for extended periods of time under appropriate culture conditions (Taswell *et al.*, 1980; Weiss *et al.*, 1980).

This approach was used in a recent study of cross-reactivity of alloreactive CTL (Taswell *et al.*, 1980). Using two different target cells, a total of 287 positive microcultures were analysed for specific, heteroclitic and cross-reactive lysis. The overall phenotype distribution was found to be 81% specific, 11% heteroclitic and 8% cross-reactive. Moreover, 22 clones could be subcloned and in virtually every case the subclones retained the specificity phenotype of the original clone from which they were derived.

A similar approach was used by Weiss *et al* (1980) to further document the specificity pattern of C57BL/6 CTL clones directed against MoLV-derived tumour cells. Using 4 target cell types, 3 specificity patterns were observed, one reactive with the syngeneic MoLV-derived tumour only, one cross-reactive with an allogeneic MoLV-derived tumour, and one cross-reactive with normal allogeneic cells. Subclones derived from 14 clones exhibited a high degree of stability in terms of lytic activity and specificity over a 4 month period of observation.

Taken together, these results indicate that CTL generated against a given set of antigens may express distinct specificities. In view of the large number of homogeneous CTL populations which can be derived by the method described above, it now appears feasible to investigate the repertoire of CTL specific for a particular antigen by testing the lytic activity of expanded clones on a panel of target cells. The recent study of Sherman (1980) suggests that such a repertoire may be very diverse. By examining the reactivity pattern of B10.D2 anti-H-2K^d CTL clones on a panel of 7 different H-2K^d mutants, a minimum of 23 distinct specificities could be defined. It is thus conceivable that the size of the CTL repertoire may approach the size of the B cell repertoire. However, many more studies using the experimental approach described in this chapter are needed to resolve this important question.

References

Alter, B. J. and Bach, F. H. (1979). *Scand. J. Immunol.* **10**, 87.
Brunner, K. I., MacDonald, H. R. and Cerottini, J.-C. (1980). *J. Immunol.* **124**, 1627.
Cantor, H. and Boyse, E. A. (1975). *J. Exp. Med.* **141**, 1390.
Cantor, H. and Boyse, E. A. (1976). *Cold Spring Harbor Symp. Quant. Biol.* **41**, 23.
Cerottini, J.-C. and MacDonald, H. R. (1980) (manuscript submitted).
Ching, M. L. and Marbrook, J. (1979). *Eur. J. Immunol.* **9**, 22.
Dennert, G. (1979). *Nature* **277**, 476.
Fischer-Lindahl, K. and Wilson, D. B. (1977). *J. Exp. Med.* **145**, 508.

Gillis, S. and Smith, K. A. (1977). *Nature* **268**, 154.

Komatsu, J., Nawa, J., Bellamy, A. R. and Marbrook, J. (1978). *Nature* **274**, 802.

Ledbetter, J. A. and Herzenberg, L. A. (1979). *Immunological Rev.* **47**, 63.

MacDonald, H. R., Cerottini, J.-C., Ryser, J.-E., Maryanski, J. L., Taswell, C., Widmer, M. B. and Brunner, K. T. (1980). *Immunological Rev.* **51**, 93.

Maryanski, J. L., MacDonald, H. R. and Cerottini, J.-C. (1980a). *J. Immunol.* **124**, 42.

Maryanski, J. L., MacDonald, H. R., Sordat, B. and Cerottini, J.-C. (1980b) (manuscript submitted).

Miller, R. G., Teh, H.-S., Harley, E. and Philipps, R. A. (1977). *Immunological Rev.* **35**, 38.

Nabholz, M., Conzelmann, A., Acuto, O., North, M., Haas, W., Pohlit, H., von Boehmer, H., Hengartner, H., Mach, J.-P., Engers, H. and Johnson, J. P. (1980). *Immunological Rev.* **51**, 125.

Nakayama, E., Shiku, H., Stockert, E., Oettgen, H. F. and Old, L. J. (1979). *Proc. Natn. Acad. Sci. U.S.A.* **76**, 1977.

Nakayama, E., Dippold, W., Shiku, H., Oettgen, H. F. and Old, L. J. (1980). *Proc. Natn. Acad. Sci. U.S.A.* **77**, 2890.

Ryser, J.-E. and MacDonald, H. R. (1979a). *J. Immunol.* **122**, 1691.

Ryser, J.-C. and MacDonald, H. R. (1979b). *J. Immunol.* **123**, 128.

Sherman, L. A. (1980). *J. Exp. Med.* **151**, 1386.

Simon, M. M. and Abenhardt, B. (1980). *Eur. J. Immunol.* **10**, 334.

Skinner, M. A. and Marbrook, J. (1976). *J. Exp. Med.* **143**, 1562.

Taswell, C., MacDonald, H. R. and Cerottini, J.-C. (1979). *Thymus* **1**, 119.

Taswell, C., MacDonald, H. R. and Cerottini, J.-C. (1980). *J. Exp. Med.* **151**, 1372.

Teh, H.-S. (1979). *Immunogenetics* **8**, 99.

Teh, H.-S., Philipps, R. A. and Miller, R. G. (1977a). *J. Exp. Med.* **146**, 1280.

Teh, H.-S., Harley, E., Philipps, R. A. and Miller, R. G. (1977b). *J. Immunol.* **118**, 1049.

Teh, H.-S., Philipps, R. A. and Miller, R. G. (1978). *J. Immunol.* **120**, 425.

Weiss, A., Brunner, K. T., MacDonald, H. R. and Cerottini, J.-C. (1980) (manuscript submitted).

Wettstein, P. J., Bailey, D. W., Moorbraaten, L. E., Klein, J. and Frelinger, J. A. (1979). *Proc. Natn. Acad. Sci. U.S.A.* **76**, 3455.

Widmer, M. B. and MacDonald, H. R. (1980). *J. Immunol.* **124**, 48.

Theme 9: Summary
Viral Immunity—T Killer Cells

HILARY KOPROWSKI

The Wistar Institute, Philadelphia, Pennsylvania, USA

In the past several decades, viral immunology has been limited principally to the study of the capacity of the host to produce antibodies against viral antigens. As to the role of cell-mediated immune (CMI) responses in virus infections, a number of published studies reported results that were wrong either because the experimental tools used were inadequate or because conceptual approaches were lacking. This state of affairs was modified by the adoptive transfer experiments of Mackaness, Blanden and colleagues and drastically changed by Zinkernagel and Doherty's discovery (in 1974) of the major histocompatibility complex (MHC) restriction of virus-immune T cells. The latter finding once again gave viral immunology respectable status within the immunology community; more important, the world of infectious disease once again became interesting to those concerned with a basic understanding of the immune response.

Analysis of the MHC restriction phenomenon

MHC restriction of virus-immune T cells in the mouse had clearly been accepted by the time of the 1977 Sydney meeting. There were reports at this stage that virus-immune T cell functions in the rat were restricted by the RT1 complex, and the first account of McMichael's studies of influenza viruses in man indicated that HLA restriction also occurred in human lymphocyte populations. The generalization cannot yet be made with absolute certainty that HLA restriction applies for all virus-immune T cell responses in man. However, evidence has been provided by Epstein, Pope and Sugamura *et al.* (9.8.19)* that memory lymphocyte populations circulating in the blood of people who have been exposed to the Epstein–Barr virus are, on secondary stimulation *in vitro*, only able to mediate lysis of HLA-identical virally modified target cells. Furthermore, Moss *et al.* (9.2.14) have shown that this virus-immune T cell effector function is blocked by the incorporation into the assay system of antibodies directed against the HLA antigens of the target cell. As with the influenza-specific cytotoxic T cell response studied by McMichael and Gotch (9.2.13) and Lucas *et al.* (9.2.12) T cell recognition is restricted to HLA-A and HLA-B compatible interactions. The fact that the DR antigens (in the *I* region) do not seem to be involved also parallels findings for the mouse model.

Even so, HLA restriction has not yet been demonstrated for all the viruses that have

* Reference numbers indicate Abstract numbers in: Abstracts 4th International Congress of Immunology, Paris, 1980.

I wish to thank Peter Doherty and Rolf Zinkernagel for their helpful advice and Martha Courant for her editorial assistance.

received a reasonable amount of attention. For instance, Lucas *et al* (9.2.12) have been able to show autologous preference in the measles virus model but have not yet been able to confirm absolute HLA restriction of effector T cell function. The specificity of the H-2 restriction phenomenon in the murine virus-immune T cell response has also come under increasing scrutiny. The results of experiments by Ertl indicate that there may be cross-reactivity between H-2^b and H-2^d in the secondary influenza-immune T cell response. A claim of this type obviously needs to be analysed rigorously at a clonal level. There has also been further investigation of the question of whether T cells of one H-2 type can be induced to respond to virus-infected stimulator cells of another H-2 type. The results of Zinkernagel's experiments (Chapter 18) with the $F_1 \rightarrow$parent radiation chimaeras have been interpreted to mean that, in a $(P_1 \times P_2)$ $F_1 \rightarrow P_1$ chimaera, T cell recognition is totally channelled towards responsiveness in the context of P_1. The other possibility is that there exists a specific deletion of that T cell repertoire which has to do with P_2. The *in vivo* negative selection experiments of Bennink and Doherty (9.2.01) indicate that P_1 T cells acutely depleted of allo-reactivity of P_2 could be sensitized to P_2 + virus, at least in some situations. Further evidence of widespread cross-reactivity of this type has been provided by the studies of Stockinger *et al.* (9.2.19) in which the investigators claim that, following removal of alloreactive precursors by adsorption onto appropriate monolayers, T cells of one H-2 type can be acutely sensitized by exposure to virus-infected stimulator cells of any other H-2 type. This observation should either become part of the established dogma or be refuted within the next 4 years. The possibility that T cells express at least 2 receptors with different specificity characteristics will be less likely if it is shown that lymphocytes respond to virus-infected cells expressing other H-2 antigens in an H-2-restricted way. At present, the question as to whether or not the virus-immune T cell repertoire is rigorously restricted to self is completely open.

Obviously, thorough studies of the properties of cloned T cell lines should be made for further analysis of the T cell repertoire. It would be a good step forward if the various alloreactive T cell clones now available could be tested for cytotoxicity on various virus-infected target cells, particularly since clones of Pfizenmaier *et al.* (9.2.15) which are specific for herpes virus presented in association with H-$2D^k$, are also cytotoxic for normal cells that bear the H-$2D^d$ alloantigen.

Inflammation and susceptibility in virus infections

The idea that rejection of virally modified self cells is essentially analogous to allo-reactivity has been supported by a number of *in vivo* experiments. For instance, the cell transfer experiments of Leung and Ada show that the effector T cells responsible for the elimination of influenza virus-modified lung cells are restricted to H-2K and H-2D and are of the Ly-23^+ phenotype. Although delayed hypersensitivity cells (which are Ly-1^+ and H-2 (I-A)-restricted) can be shown to operate when tested in a footpad assay system, these cells do not seem to be involved in eliminating virally modified cells. The analysis of cell-mediated immunity in the context of the MHC restriction phenomenon has provided clear answers about the nature of the triggering and effector events in virus elimination.

A detailed understanding of the overall inflammatory process, however, will require further studies of the type described by Mokhtarian *et al.* (9.7.20) concerning the role of lymphokines and other possible effector populations that operate in concert with, or following recruitment by invading T cells. It should also be remembered that, although T cell function is MHC-restricted, many factors involved in susceptibility to virus infection have no obvious relationship to the strong transplantation systems. The studies of Chalmer (9.1.01) on murine cytomegalovirus infection indicate that the susceptibility of mice to lethal infection with this virus is influenced by both H-2 and non-H-2 linked genes. The earlier studies of Mims, Koprowski, Bang and others, which show that resistance to viruses resides in cell populations such as the macrophage and reflects the extent of virus growth, are still valid when the nature of host resistance to viruses is considered. The MHC restriction phenomenon is concerned essentially with defining the nature of T cell recognition.

The fine specificity of T cells

The question of T cell specificity for MHC antigens has been approached mainly by the use of H-2 mutant mice. These experiments have shown considerable precision in the specificity of recognition. However, studies of T cell specificity for viral glycoprotein have revealed a much broader range of cross-reactivity than would have been expected from the serological analysis of viral constituents. The broad cross-reactivity of the influenza-immune T cell response for all A virus subtypes (described for the mouse before the 1977 Meeting) has now been demonstrated in man both by McMichael's laboratory (9.2.13), and by Lucas *et al.* (9.2.12). Furthermore, Rosenthal and Zinkernagel (9.2.17) have shown that vesicular stomatitis virus-immune T cells cross-react with serologically unidentical virus subtypes. However, this should not be taken as an indication that the T cell receptor is less specific than the immunoglobulin molecule. Experiments with influenza A viruses have shown clearly that what is being studied is polyclonal responses, which no doubt include lymphocytes with a number of different specificities. The extreme precision for H-2 antigens shown by the experiments with H-2 mutants probably reflects the need to maintain self-tolerance to all except the active site, which seems to be involved in T cell recognition (and which is equivalent to the H-2 private specificity). Such tolerance for viral glycoproteins or for other histocompatibility antigens (alloantigens) is apparently unnecessary and presumably accounts for the less precise response of the alloreactive and virus-specific T cells as compared with the H-2 restricted self-monitoring function.

The nature of cell-surface changes recognized by virus-immune T cells

The question of how viruses modify the cell in a way that can be recognized by the effector T cell has received considerable attention both from virologists, who have suddenly become interested in immunology, and from immunologists, who are now returning to the study of infectious disease. Doherty and Zinkernagel's hypothesis that virus-immune T cells are specific for some form of complex between the virus and the MHC antigens is supported by the studies of Hammerling *et al.* (9.2.07), which show that the adenovirus type 2 early membrane glycoprotein is bound to rat transplantation antigens on a virus-transformed cell line. Additional support for the idea that the viral and H-2 glycoproteins must be in close proximity is provided by numerous experiments in which T cell recognition is restricted to an H-2 antigen incorporated into the same liposome as viral antigens and integrated into the cell membrane. These observations have been reported for Sendai and pox viruses, which have fusion capacity; other viruses probably replicate within the cells, but this replication may simply reflect the need for presentation of a suitable antigen at the plasma membrane. The possible importance of virus carbohydrate is suggested by the studies of Forman and colleagues (9.2.04) in which tunicamycin treatment was shown to modify T cell recognition of vesicular stomatitis virus target cells. The role of carbohydrates is of interest, especially when one considers the experiments of Sandrin, McKenzie, Higgins and Parish (8.1.34), which indicate that the Ia antigen is of a dual carbohydrate and protein nature.

The general conclusion that can be drawn is that liposome technology offers the most powerful approach available for the analysis of the nature of the viral antigens recognized by cytotoxic T cells. The recent demonstration that T cell recognition can be blocked by monoclonal antibodies directed against influenza A virus glycoproteins offers another possible method for the dissection of T cell specificity patterns. However, such antibody blocking experiments also indicate that the inhibition may be steric and not the result of actual binding to the site recognized by the cell. For instance, Greenspan, Gerhard and Doherty(pers. commun.) have shown that cytotoxic T cells, generated following immunization with a mutant influenza A virus that was selected in the presence of a particular monoclonal antibody, are prevented from interacting with target cells infected with the wild type virus by incorporation of that particular antibody into the assay system.

Immunopathology and immunosuppression

Of course, not all problems in biology can be solved by convenient *in vitro* assays that happen to work to the advantage of the investigator. Tremendous problems remain in the understanding of virus diseases, of which one of the most interesting is human hepatitis. Results from Dwyer's laboratory (9.6.07) at Yale indicate that the majority of the inflammatory cells in the livers of people with hepatitis are T cells and suggest that the cell-mediating liver injury is of thymus-derived lineage. It is also interesting that a very severe liver lesion can be produced by the transferral of virus-immune T cells into mice infected with hepatotropic lymphocytic choriomeningitis virus. Other groups are also attempting to determine the status of T cells in patients with hepatitis. There is documentation for the existence in chronic hepatitis of serum inhibitors of T cell proliferation, shown by Ramić *et al.* (9.6.11), and of suppressor T cells, shown by de Moura *et al.* (9.6.04). The experiments of Levo *et al.* (9.6.06) further indicate that the cellular immune function in carriers of hepatitis B is confined to the T cell compartment.

The phenomenon of immune suppression as the result of virus infection has been recognized for some time. Chaturvedi and Mather (9.7.04) and Semenov *et al.* (9.7.30) have presented evidence that infection with flaviviruses results in the development of autoreactive T cell subsets. Such phenomenon are of obvious interest for an analysis of the possibility that virus triggers autoimmune processes in diseases such as multiple sclerosis. These effects may not be mediated solely by effector T cells. Recent studies by Stevens (pers. comm.) in the Marek's disease system indicate that infection with this virus results in the generation of antibody populations that bind to normal peripheral myelin. There are other mechanisms of virus-induced immunosuppression, including direct effects of viruses on the T cells and the possible development of suppressor T cells in a mouse tumour virus system.

The presence of sensitized lymphocytes at the time of infection with respiratory syncytial virus (RSV), an infant disease, may be protective, but the studies of Welliver *et al.* (9.7.32) indicate that cell-mediated immunity developing in the face of infection with RSV may also constitute part of the pathological process. This is hardly surprising, as any process that results in widespread cell death will obviously have pathological consequences, particularly in the case of nonlytic viruses such as lymphocytic choriomeningitis virus.

It should also be recognized that, although much current research is obsessed with the CMI response, the part played by other facets of the host response still requires an immense amount of investigation. The detailed studies of Oldstone and colleagues with the complement system serve to highlight the complexity of these phenomena. We must eventually develop an overview of virus pathogenesis that incorporates CMI, antibody-mediated effects, complement and interferon in the context of the physiological and genetic characteristics of the host.

General discussion

Clearly, a new golden age of viral immunology has begun. The recognition of the MHC restriction phenomenon and the availability of monoclonal antibodies to viruses and of nucleic acid sequencing techniques offers the possibility of an understanding in the near future of the mechanisms underlying viral pathogenicity in animals. The molecular basis of events in the intact organism, as well as in the isolated tissue culture cell, should soon be understood, and there is good chance now that the complex jigsaw puzzle that constitutes the host–virus interaction will be put together.

It is important that the momentum gained over the past 5 or 6 years in the analysis of immune responses in virus diseases not be lost. The continued interest of immunologists in infectious disease processes can be assured, in part, by the availability of funding. However, the best minds will pursue this topic only if its potential for major advances in biological understanding continues to be recognized. The virologist must impress upon immunologists that only the surface has been scratched. The problems of viral persistence and pathogenesis and the analysis of such questions in the context of immune response should constitute one of the major areas of growth in immunobiology within the next 10 years. Old questions of microbiology can now be addressed with the best available immunobiological techniques. There are many exciting new roads to be taken.

As a result of the availability of monoclonal antibodies, novel manipulations of host–parasite interactions are now possible. Our own studies with influenza viruses and with rabies virus have indicated the possibility of many promising new means for the analysis of regulation and effector function and of the overall immune response. The development of better vaccination procedures and improved methods for treatment is only one consequence that is likely to result from this approach. The continued analysis of these practical questions in the context of viral pathogenesis and immune response is the approach most likely to lead to further breakthroughs of ultimately clinical importance. Moreover, the possibility should be recognized that monoclonal antibodies may prove to be therapeutically significant in many otherwise intractable infectious processes.

Much of the interest of basic immunologists in virus infections is presently directed towards the analysis of the virus-immune cytotoxic T cell response. However, this is only one part of the answer, and we should like to persuade immunologists to remain in the field of infectious disease even after these problems are solved. As far as T cell functions are concerned, the major question now seems to concern the relative roles of the thymic and extrathymic environments in determining the spectrum of T cell restriction. Answers may come from the rigorous analysis of specificity profiles shown by T cell clones and from further detailed studies of the nature of regulation in the virus-immune T cell response. Radiation chimaeras are now known to be a much more complex experimental model than originally thought. Recently, both Singer and Doherty (pers. comm.) have shown that the restricting function of the thymus seems to be lost between 50 and 60 days after irradiation. It is not clear whether the restricting element in the thymus is no longer functional or whether suppressor T cell subsets have evolved. The problem is further confused by the results of Singer, which indicate that the cells in the thymus 14 days after reconstitution of the chimaeras are mainly of host origin. There is a tendency among many workers in the field to consider the radiation chimaera too complex for analysis. However, it seems that the experimental advantages of being able to mix cells of various histocompatibility types should counterbalance these arguments. Careful analysis of radiation chimaeras may reveal much about the evolution of T cell responsiveness.

Another area of major significance concerns molecular events on the surface of the virus-infected target cell. Experiments with liposomes are providing a great deal of fascinating information. The demonstration by Koszinowski and colleagues (9.2.09) that the cross-reactive T cells resulting from immunization with influenza A viruses recognize viral haemagglutinin antigen in liposomes incorporated into the cell surface may provide a solution to this problem. The major histocompatibility complex antigen may constitute a rosetta stone for a hitherto unknown cell surface language, as suggested by Eisen (pers. comm.) which may be unravelled by this approach. Perhaps the people working in this area should be considered the new anatomists of Immunology.

The recent studies of DNA sequencing of immunoglobulin genes should have convinced even the most steadfast cellular immunologist that molecular biology has something to offer the field. The monoclonal antibody technology developed by Gerhard and colleagues for the influenza A viruses is rapidly leading to an understanding of the nature, variation and structure of the viral haemagglutinin antigen. The efforts of the influenza research community to analyse these mutant viruses by nucleic acid and protein sequencing and by crystallographic techniques should greatly increase our knowledge of viral glycoproteins and, indeed, of all glycoproteins expressed on the surface of virus-infected cells. Finally, the fact remains that some viruses do incorporate nucleic acid sequences of their hosts, and these virus "variants" may have a selective advantage in replication over viruses that do not incorporate such sequences. If these variants express antigenic determinants coded by the host sequences, the fun of studying viral immunology will extend to the next International Congress of Immunology and possibly to many Congresses thereafter.

Theme 10

Tumour Immunology

Presidents:
G. KLEIN
J. C. SALOMON

Symposium Chairman:
G. MATHÉ

35

Present Concepts in Immune Surveillance

N. A. MITCHISON and L. J. KINLEN

Imperial Cancer Research Fund Tumour Immunology Unit, University College, London and Imperial Cancer Research Fund Cancer Epidemiology and Clinical Trials Unit (University of Oxford), Radcliffe Infirmary, Oxford, UK

Introduction

The hypothesis of immune surveillance proposes that a high proportion of early cancers are eliminated by the immune system, and therefore predicts that individuals under immunosuppression, whether congenital or acquired should display a high incidence of cancer. In the course of 19 years that have passed since it was first proposed, this hypothesis has become untenable in any general sense. It was proposed at a time when T cells had no known function other than to reject allografts. Now that we understand quite well what the proper functions of these cells are, the hypothesis has become redundant from a theoretical standpoint. More seriously, observations made on immunosuppressed mice and men offer little support: "Approximately, 6900 nudes were observed in the 7-year period 1969–1975 . . . spontaneous malignant tumours were not observed in any animal." (Rygaard and Povlsen, 1976.)

Even if a failure as a broad generalization, immune surveillance survives happily in more limited applications. This chapter traces three particular ideas: natural killing, surveillance of lymphoma and of u.v.-induced cancer of skin, and the role of viral antigens. At the end we shall ask how far these local surveillance effects can be generalized.

Natural killing

The concept of a natural killer (NK) cell was introduced 5 years ago in order to account for the ability of lymphocytes from normal individuals to kill tumour cells *in vitro*. The cell has subsequently become defined by the group of properties outlined in Fig. 1 (Cantor *et al.*, 1979; Herberman *et al.*, 1979;

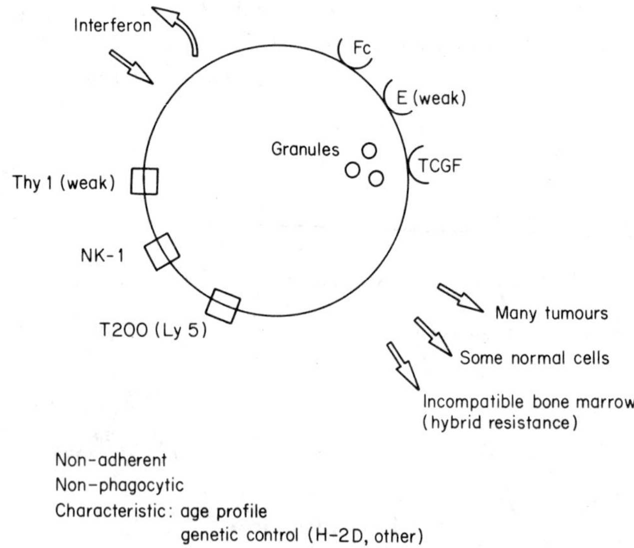

FIG. 1. *The NK cell.*

Kiessling and Wigzell, 1979). It possesses Fc receptors; these can be blocked by aggregated immunoglobulins without interfering with the ability to kill, thus distinguishing the NK cell from the killer (K) cell which mediates antibody dependent cell cytotoxicity (ADCC). A weak receptor for sheep erythrocytes is present in human NK cells, which enable these cells to be rosetted under favourable conditions. The Thy-1 antigen is present on mouse NK cells, also in a weak form which enables these cells to be killed under favourable conditions, e.g. with certain monoclonal anti-Thy-1 antibodies. Some, but perhaps not all, NK cells multiply in response to T cell growth factor. These three characteristics indicate that NK cells belong to the T cell lineage, perhaps at an early stage of differentiation. NK-1 and T200 (Ly-5) are other markers which have been identified in the mouse; T200 is present on other lymphocytes as well. Characteristic granules are present in the cytoplasm of human NK cells.

Both in man and the mouse NK cells are activated by interferon, at least in part because this agent induces the differentiation of cells with NK activity from inactive precursors. NK cells are nonadherent and nonphagocytic. They have a characteristic age profile, being present in small numbers in rodents up to the age of weaning, then rising sharply, to fall slowly in old age. NK activity is under genetic control, with a major gene control at or close to H-2D and multiple minor controls elsewhere.

Many, but not all, tumours are killed by NK cells. So also are a limited range of normal cells, particularly stem cells from thymus and bone marrow. An important finding, which links NK activity to a well-established form of *in vivo* cytotoxicity, is that hybrid resistance to parental bone marrow (the Hh phenomenon) is mediated by NK cells (Cudkowicz and Hochman, 1979). This linkage was based originally on the parallel genetics observed in the two systems (Harmon *et al.*, 1977), and is now supported by other evidence.

Nude mice are rich in NK cells, so that the low incidence of tumours in this type of animal raises no difficulties for surveillance mediated by these cells. However, because most but not all of the evidence for antitumour activity has been obtained *in vitro*, the question remains as to whether NK cells do in fact operate surveillance. It was important therefore to find a genetic lesion for NK cells comparable to the genetic lesion which the nude mouse provides for T cells. This has now been done, in the form of beige mice (Roder and Duwe, 1979) and the similar (but rare) Chediak–Higashi syndrome in man (Roder *et al.*, 1980). Beige mice are partially but not completely deficient in NK cells; unfortunately the difference from normal mice declines with age (Herberman *et al.*, 1979).

Thus far little information is available concerning the susceptibility of beige mice to cancer. Young beige mice do not display increased susceptibility to chemical carcinogens (Salomon, 1980). On the other hand a small colony of aged beige mice have exhibited a high incidence of lymphoma, as shown in Table I (Loutit *et al.*, 1980). The question must be considered to be still open; beige mice can expect to have a hard time in cancer laboratories for the next few years.

TABLE I
Lymphomas in aged beige mice

C3H × 101.bg/bg (15–18 months)
11/40 lymphomas

Loutit *et al.* (1980).

Surveillance of lymphoma and of skin cancer

A considerable body of evidence concerning surveillance in man is accumulating, mainly from the excellent kidney transplant registries. These provide a unique source of information concerning the incidence of cancer under conditions of immunosuppression. Some recent analyses are illustrated in Tables II–IV, which permit several conclusions to be drawn (Hoover and Fraumeni, 1973; Kinlen *et al.*, 1979).

TABLE II
Non-Hodgkin's lymphoma in transplant recipients

Years after transplantation	*Observed*	*Expected*
<2	19	0·26
2–3	6	0·16
≥4	9	0·16

$n = 3823$
UK and Australasia: Kinlen *et al.* (1979)

(a) There is no sign that Hodgkin's lymphoma is under immune surveillance. This is contrary to what might have been expected from the association of this disease with HLA, the only known example of this type of association with cancer (Greene *et al.*, 1979).
(b) Non-Hodgkin's lymphoma has a marked increased incidence and an early onset. This is a highly particular form of cancer, and even among this group of lymphomas the disease which occurs among transplant recipients has a special pathology and pattern of distribution. This suggests that an oncogenic virus may be involved, a matter to which we shall return in the third part of this chapter.

TABLE III
Skin cancer in transplant recipients

	Ob.	*Exp.*
Skin and lip cancers (USA)	21	4·99–16·17[a]
Squamous cell carcinoma (UK)	3	0·13[b]
Other cancers (UK + Australasia) (excluding skin cancer and non-Hodgkin's lymphoma)	30	17·79[b]

[a] Hoover and Fraumeni (1973)
[b] Kinlen *et al.* (1979)

TABLE IV

Squamous cell carcinoma in transplant recipients (Australasia)

Age	*Rate*[a] ♂	*Rate*[a] ♀
14–24	3	0
–34	13	6
–44	16	15
–54	40	19
–64	24	19

[a] per 1000 yearly; 5834 person-years.
Kinlen *et al.* (1979).

(c) The risk of skin cancer is markedly increased, but this is confined to squamous cell carcinoma, leaving basal cell carcinoma largely unaffected. The rate for squamous cell carcinoma in Australasia is so high that over 50% of men and 35% of women would develop the disease by 55 years of age if they were to behave like the immunosuppressed recipients. Other cancer incidences do not rise, except those of mesenchymal origin. Ultra-violet light is strongly implicated as a causal agent. The squamous cell carcinomas occur almost entirely in those parts of the body exposed to sunlight, and further analysis provides evidence of a positive interaction between immunosuppression and u.v. exposure (Hoover and Kinlen, 1980).

(d) The incidence of squamous cell carcinoma is higher among males than females. This observation is in accordance with the hypothesis of X-linked recessive immune deficiency genes introduced in connection with Duncan's syndrome, as discussed below.

The human data suggest that u.v.-induced squamous cell carcinoma may be exceptionally strongly antigenic, and may normally be kept under control by that part of the immune system which is susceptible to immunosuppression of the type applied to transplant recipients. This conclusion parallels to a remarkable extent that drawn from a fine series of studies of u.v.-induced tumours in mice, illustrated in Fig. 2. Careful comparisons have been made of the effects of various forms of immunosuppression on chemical and u.v. carcinogenesis in mice. These show, for u.v. induction only, a shorter latent period in mice exposed to antilymphocyte globulin; to a lesser extent, this applies to other immunosuppressive agents (Daynes *et al.*, 1979).

Ultra-violet skin tumours of mice belong to the narrow category of tumours which are so strongly antigenic that they cannot normally be transplanted into normal syngeneic hosts (Kripke, 1974). They carry individual-specific tumour antigens which elicit strong cytotoxic cell responses. It was natural to inquire how such tumours came to develop in their autochthonous hosts. It turns out that treatment with u.v. light elicits the formation of a population of suppressor T cells, which develop prior to the occurrence of overt tumours. These T_S cells are specific, in the sense that they act only upon u.v.-induced

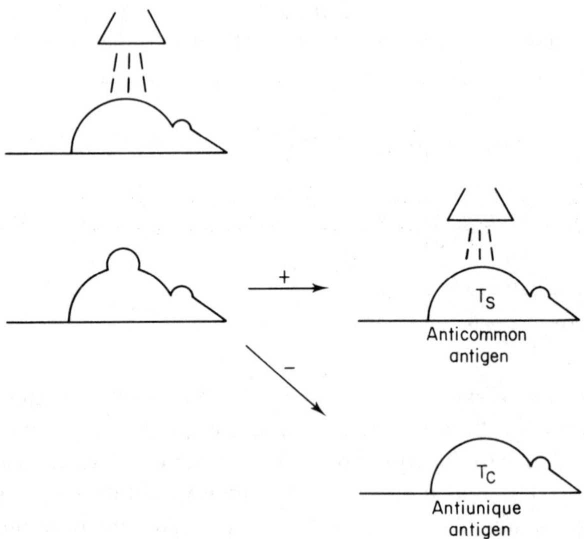

FIG. 2. *Ultra-violet tumours.*

tumours and not upon other immune responses; they do not, however, discriminate between one u.v. tumour and another (Fisher and Kripke, 1978). Presumably either they develop as multiple sets of T_S cells in parallel, each specific for a single TSTA; or alternatively, they recognize a common suppressor determinant shared between different u.v. tumours. The second alternative is the more attractive, not only because of the difficulty with numbers that the first alternative encounters, but also because instances are known in basic immunology of a suppressor determinant affecting separate but adjacent helper determinants (Sercarz *et al.*, 1978). These T_S cells are active *in vivo* in cell transfer tests, and in tests *in vitro*, but it is not yet known whether they are fully responsible for the growth of autochthonous tumours.

This remarkable situation has inspired further study of the impact of u.v. irradiation on the immune system. The outcome, together with that of older

TABLE V
Ultra-violet-induced defects in immunoreactivity
(other than with tumours)

1	No local GVH
2	DNCB atopy
3	Langerhans cells absent
4	TNP-spleen adherent cells induce suppression, not DTH
5	Spleen adherent cells do not present GAT

(1) Kripke (1977), (2) Haniszko, Suskind (1963), (3) Toews *et al.* (1980), (4) Greene *et al.* (1979), (5) Letvin *et al.* (1980).

work, is summarized in Table V (Haniszko and Suskind, 1963; Kripke, 1977; Letvin *et al.*, 1977; Greene *et al.*, 1979; Toews *et al.*, 1980). Evidently there is a gross impairment of immune function associated with the loss of antigen-presenting cells from the epidermia, which results eventually in a generalized abnormality of antigen presentation. This in turn favours the development of suppressive immune responses. This conclusion is reminiscent of the effects of "macrophage" depletion on the *in vitro* immune response, which is known to favour activation of suppressor T cells (Feldmann and Kontiainen, 1976). There is other evidence of a link between Langerhans cells of epidermis and spleen adherent cells of the type illustrated in Fig. 3; for references see Mitchison, 1979, 1980. The consequences of u.v. treatment of skin clearly favour some kind of traffic of antigen-presenting cells from skin to internal lymphoid organs.

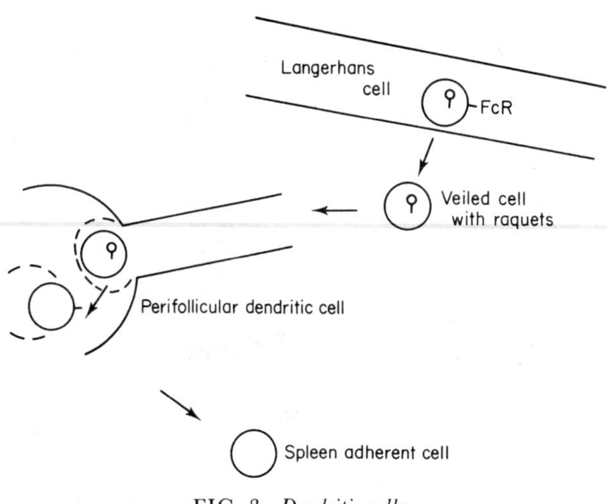

FIG. 3. *Dendritic cells.*

Viral antigens and immune surveillance

Current ideas about the nature of the viral antigens involved in oncogenesis are summarized in Fig. 4. The two proteins most closely connected with malignant transformation are the DNA-associated 53K host protein, and the P60 viral protein associated with the inner side of the cell membrane (Purchio *et al.*, 1978). The distribution between host- and virus-coded proteins is somewhat nominal, as "host" proteins may well be encoded by endogenous viral genes and "viral" genes may have been picked up from hosts in the past. 53K host proteins have been found in association with the SV40 virus-coded DNA-binding T proteins (Lane and Crawford, 1979); within chemically-induced tumours (Deleo *et al.*, 1979); and as part of the Epstein–Barr virus (EBV) nuclear antigen (EBNA) (Luka *et al.*, 1980). In the first and second instances the 53K proteins are now known to be serologically closely related (Lane and Crawford, 1979). There will be more of a problem with EBNA, because this antigen is so poorly immunogenic in animals. Perhaps one of the other herpes viruses may provide better material for serological analysis; the monoclonal antibody approach would seem logical (Howes *et al.*, 1979).

The point which is most relevant here is that neither of the candidate transformation-specific proteins are accessible to the immune system from outside the cell, and cannot therefore be involved in immune surveillance. The only possible exception is the *sarc* gene-product in avian cells; there is limited and controversial evidence that this may be accessible to antibody from outside.

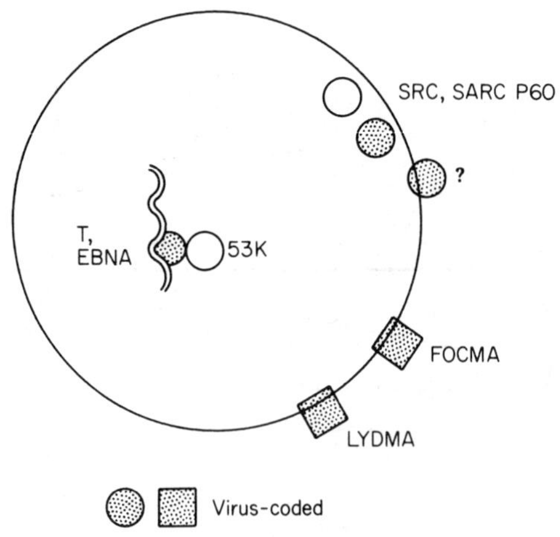

FIG. 4. *Virus-related antigens.*

Viral antigens which are better candidates for immune surveillance are shown in the little square boxes in Fig. 4. Feline oncornavirus membrane antigen (FOCMA) (Essex *et al.*, 1979) and EBV lymphocyte-determined membrane antigen (LYDMA) (Klein, 1978) are accessible (by definition) to the surveillance system. Neither of these are tumour-antigens in the same sense as the candidate transformation-antigens mentioned above; they are present rather in the virus-infected premalignant cell (although FOCMA is still referred to as a "tumour-specific antigen"). One could illustrate the way surveillance may operate on this type of antigen perfectly well from cat data, but perhaps the most dramatic example is provided by the impact of EBV on immunosuppressed humans.

Duncan's syndrome is an X-linked recessive lymphoproliferative condition (Purtilo *et al.*, 1977). What appears to happen is that an X-chromosome transmits an immune response defect. Males who inherit the chromosome cannot resist EBV virus infection in the normal way (the virus normally produces symptomless infection in infants or infectious mononucleosis in adolescents). Instead, they either succumb to uncontrolled proliferation of their infected B lymphocytes with symptoms such as rupture of the spleen; or they develop tumours of B lymphocyte origin. Apparently the uncontrolled cellular proliferation favours mutation (in a general sense, probably involving chromosomal rearrangements) to malignancy. Thus, in this instance immune surveillance clearly operates on premalignant cells.

One further point is worth making. Duncan's syndrome provides a dramatic example of the damaging effect of X-linked recessive gene(s) on the workings of the immune system. One may well guess that every single gene may effect something as complex as the immune system. If so, and if in accordance with genetic theory most rare genes are recessive, males will be immunologically less fit than females as a rule. It has been argued that the sex incidence of childhood leukaemias fit this expectation (Purtilo, 1979), a suggestion which of course assumes that this form of cancer is under immune surveillance. The sex incidence of squamous carcinoma, as shown in Table IV, evidently fits this expectation.

Conclusion

We have chosen 3 examples of immune surveillance in operation: lymphomas in old beige mice, squamous carcinoma in immunosuppressed transplant recipients, and B cell tumours in Duncan's syndrome. All of these represent instances of the kind of data which can be collected from examining genetic or acquired lesions in the immune system. The question is whether this kind of information applies to other forms of cancer which develop in normal individuals.

Rather than generalize from insufficient information, let us make two predictions. One is that the tremendous effort now going into interferon clinical trials will tell us the truth about NK cells. We need to know whether NK cells are activated strongly in a way which can be related to any antitumour effect of the agent. The second is that if squamous carcinoma is the tip of an immunological iceberg, then manipulation of the T cell system should have some impact on other forms of cancer. Manoeuvres of intervention have certainly been under discussion for long enough.

References

* Cantor, H., Kasai, M., Shen, F. W., Leclerc, J. C. and Glimcher, L. (1979). *Immunol. Rev.* **44**, 3.

Cudkowicz, G. and Hochman, P. S. (1979). *Immunol. Rev.* **44**, 13.

Daynes, R. A., Harris, C. C., Connor, R. J., and Eichwald, E. J. (1979). *J. Natn. Cancer Inst.* **62**, 1075.

* Supplemented by personal communication from senior author.

Deleo, A. B., Jay, G., Appella, E., Dubois, G. C., Law, L. W., and Old, L. J. (1979). *Proc. Natn. Acad. Sci. U.S.A.* **76**, 2420.

Essex, M., Grant, C. K., Sliski, A. J. and Hardy, W. D. (1979). *In* "Antiviral Mechanisms in the Control of Neoplasia" (P. Chandron, ed.), p. 427. Plenum Press, New York.

Feldmann, M. and Kontiainen, S. (1976). *Eur. J. Immunol.* **6**, 302.

Fisher, M. S. and Kripke, M. L. (1978). *J. Immunol.* **121**, 1139.

Greene, M. H., McKeen, E. A., Li, F. P., Blattner, W. A. and Fraumeni, J. F. (1979). *Int. J. Cancer* **23**, 777.

Greene, M. I., Sy, M. S., Kripke, M. and Benacerraf, B. (1979). *Proc. Natn. Acad. Sci. U.S.A.* **76**, 6591.

Haniszko, J. and Suskind, R. R. (1963). *J. Invest. Dermatol.* **40**, 183.

Harmon, R. C., Clark, E. A., O'Toole, C. and Wicker, L. S. (1977). *Immunogenetics* **4**, 601.

* Herberman, R. B., Djeu, J. Y., Kay, D., Ortaldo, J. R., Riccardi, C., Bonnard, G. D., Holden, H. T., Fagnan, R., Santoni, A. and Puccetti, P. (1979). *Immunol. Rev.* **44**, 43.

Hoover, R. and Fraumeni, J. F. (1973). *Lancet* **1**, 55.

Hoover, R. and Kinlen, L. (1980). In prep.

Howes, E. L., Clark, E. A., Smith, E. and Mitchison, N. A. (1979). *J. Gen. Virol.* **44**, 81.

* Kiessling, R. and Wigzell, H. (1979). *Immunol. Rev.* **44**, 165.

Kinlen, L. J., Sheil, A. G. R., Peto, J. and Doll, R. (1979). *Brit. Med. J.* **2**, 1461.

* Klein, G. (1978). *IARC Sci. Publ.* (24, Pt. 2), 815.

Kripke, M. L. (1974). *J. Natn. Cancer Inst.* **53**, 1333.

Kripke, M. L. (1977). *J. Reticuloendothelial. Soc.* **22**, 217.

* Lane, D. P. and Crawford, L. V. (1979). *Nature* **278**, 261.

Letvin, N. L., Greene, M. I. and Benacerraf, B. (1977). *Proc. Natn. Acad. Sci. U.S.A.* **77**, 2881.

Loutit, J. F., Townsend, K. M. S. and Knowles, J. F. (1980). *Nature* **285**, 66.

Luka, J., Jornvall, H. and Klein, G. (1980). *J. Virol.* (in press).

Mitchison, N. A. (1979). *Clin. Exp. Dermatol.* **4**, 489.

Mitchison, N. A. (1980). *In* "Regulatory T Lymphocytes" (B. Pernis and H. J. Vogel, eds) (in press).

* Purchio, A. F., Erikson, E., Brugge, J. S. and Erikson, R. L. (1978). *Proc. Natn. Acad. Sci. U.S.A.* **75**, 1567.

Purtilo, D. T. (1979). *Lancet* **1**, 327.

Purtilo, D. T., Deflorio, D., Hutt, L. M., Bhawan, J., Yang, J. P. S., Otto, R. and Edwards, W. (1977). *New Engl. J. Med.* **297**, 1077.

Roder, R. J. and Duwe, A. (1979). *Nature* **278**, 451.

Roder, J., Haliotis, T., Klein, M., Korec, S., Jett, J. R., Ortaldo, J., Herberman, R. B., Katz, P. and Fauci, A. S. (1980). *Nature* **284**, 553.

Rygaard, J. and Povlsen, C. O. (1976). *Transp. Rev.* **28**, 41.

Salomon, J. C. (1980). Pers. comm.

Sercarz, E. E., Yowell, R. L., Turkin, D., Miller, A., Araneo, B. A. and Adorini, L. (1978). *Immunol. Rev.* **39**, 108.

Toews, G. B., Bergstresser, P. R. and Streilein, J. W. (1980). *J. Immunol.* **124**, 445.

* Supplemented by personal communication from senior author.

36

Immunostimulation of Tumour Growth

R. T. PREHN and H. C. OUTZEN

The Jackson Laboratory, Bar Harbor, Maine, USA

Introduction

The idea that one of us has been forwarding for nearly 10 years (Prehn, 1971; Prehn and Lappé, 1971), namely that an active immune response may aid and abet tumour growth directly, rather than by suppression of an otherwise antitumour portion of the immune reaction, has not been widely accepted. This lack of acceptance, despite a considerable amount of experimental data congenial with such an idea, is probably due, in part, to the widespread perception that an immune reaction is basically a defence reaction; thus, teleologically, there is no obvious evolutionary rationale for an immune reaction that would stimulate the growth of target tumour cells. This widespread perception is, in our opinion, not justified. In this chapter we will present some of the reasons for believing that an immune reaction can be, and often is, a direct cause of hyperplasia, and some speculations concerning the mechanisms by which an immune reaction could be directly stimulatory to tumour growth.

Supported by: CD 32 (Am. Cancer Soc.), CA 20920 (NIH) and CA 24901 (NIH).

It is customary to approach the study of the role of immunity in tumour growth by analogy with the role of immunity in resistance to viral, bacterial, or parasitical infections. Although there are similarities, the analogies with cancer can easily be exaggerated. All of these foreign invaders have evolved over many aeons and evolution has fitted each of them with various strategies for evading host immunity, and host immunity, in these systems, is usually clearly defensive. The strategies differ markedly from organism to organism and probably little can be learned from them about the mechanisms that might apply to a deviant clone of cells derived from the host itself. The cancer cell evolves only within the short span of the duration of the disease in a single animal and does not, except in the possible cases of some viral tumours, or long transplanted tumours, accumulate adaptive mechanisms over many generations. It therefore seems more reasonable to find models for tumour cell regulation in the regulation of normal cells; tumour cells and normal cells are very similar, especially as compared with the vast differences between a parasite and a cancer. The regulation of normal growth should thus have much in common with the defences against neoplasia.

It seems doubtful if such an important issue as growth regulation would have been left, by evolution, entirely to one mechanism, although seemingly there must be a final common pathway. Rather, there are probably numerous interlocking and redundant regulatory devices; we postulate that the immune reaction is one of these. The immune mechanism itself probably evolved from some more primitive mechanism involved in normal growth control, and still manifests this growth regulatory function in relation to such things as wound healing and neoplasia.

Immunostimulation of normal tissues

The evidence that the immune system is involved in the regulation of non-neoplastic growth, including growth promotion, is extensive. The most striking observation is that non-neoplastic hyperplasia is quite regularly associated with leukocytic infiltrates—lymphoid cells, plasma cells, and macrophages (Prehn and Lappé, 1971; Prehn, 1977a). To the pathologist, this association is as common as "bread and butter." In at least one case the lymphoid cell reaction in a tick bite was described as so extensive as to mimic lymphoma while, at the same site, the epithelial hyperplasia was so severe that epithelial carcinoma was suspected (Allen, 1948). That such associations are probably aetiological, with the infiltrate producing the hyperplasia, is suggested by those experimental systems in which alloimmunity results in hyperplasia. For example, skin grafting across a very weak histocompatibility barrier in rabbits produced a chronic acanthosis and epithelial hyperplasia in the graft (Chai, 1980). Even when skin was grafted across a greater barrier, in which rejection of the graft occurred, the rejection was preceeded by an acute wave of mitotic activity (Lambert and Frank, 1966). In these cases, the immune reaction clearly was the cause of the hyperplasia. Numerous other examples in which an immune reaction appears to have produced hyperplasia in normal tissues have been documented (Prehn and Lappé, 1971; Prehn, 1977a).

It should be noted that in the allograft system it is very difficult to ascribe the epithelial proliferation to a blockage or suppression of an otherwise inhibitory immune reaction. In order to account for the allograft proliferation on the basis of suppressor cell activity, one would have to postulate that autografts are prevented from undergoing chronic hyperplasia by an immune response—a response which is only suppressed when the tissue is allografted!

If one admits, therefore, that immunity can directly stimulate a normal tissue allograft to undergo hyperplasia, can one then surround a tumour with lymphoid cells and be confident that they are not stimulating tumour growth? By analogy with the allograft, a weak or incipient immune reaction would be stimulatory to the target, but a greater reaction would be cytotoxic. Thus, when we find suppressor cells in tumour systems, they may well be reducing the immune response to a tumour-stimulatory range rather than simply removing an inhibition to tumour growth.

Immunostimulation of transplanted tumours

Since, by analogy with normal tissue allografts, it appears that a weak immune reaction may be stimulatory, but a strong reaction may be cytotoxic, it will be necessary to titrate the immune response in a variety of tumour systems before the general picture of the role of immunity in tumour growth can be perceived. This was first done with modified Winn tests, in the case of transplanted, 3-methylcholanthrene induced, syngeneic sarcomas; tumour cell aliquots were mixed with varying numbers of specifically immune or non-immune spleen cells and the mixtures inoculated subcutaneously into immuno-crippled recipient mice. Low ratios of immune spleen cells to tumour cells (i.e., 1 : 1) resulted in better tumour growth than did greater or lesser ratios of spleen cells, and also better growth than did the same low ratios of non-immune spleen cells. Evidence of specificity was obtained, but large ratios of nonimmune spleen cells were often very stimulatory to tumour growth (Prehn, 1972).

Thus, the data of these first experiments conformed with the expectations of the immunostimulation theory. A weak immune response, as represented by low proportions of immune spleen cells, stimulated tumour growth. Comparable data have been reported from experiments with transplanted tumours in completely *in vitro* systems (Prehn, 1976) and when the leukocytes tested were those actually separated from a tumour mass (Blazar *et al.*, 1978). Many other investigators have presented similar data (see Prehn, 1977a).

Although in the modified Winn test experiments the recipient animals had been immunocrippled to eliminate a host contribution to the reaction, some host immune capacity probably survived. Perhaps small numbers of spleen cells, in co-operation with the tumour, gave rise to suppressors which interfered with the immune response and so abrogated immune surveillance. Such an explanation could be invoked even in the case of the *in vitro* experiments, albeit with somewhat more difficulty. However, it cannot be invoked in *in vitro* experiments in which the target cells were stimulated by low concentrations of antibody with no immune cells in the system (Shearer, 1973; Heidrick *et al.*, 1978). It is also our belief that, in view of the precedent set by the normal tissue allografts, abrogation of surveillance, even if suppressor cells are present, is an unlikely explanation. A direct stimulation of tumour growth, in analogy with the presumably direct production of hyperplasia in the allografts, seems a far simpler hypothesis. The role of suppressor cells, if present, would then be to adjust the level of immunity to the stimulatory range.

Immunostimulation of oncogenesis

Although the titration of the immune response, *vis-à-vis* transplanted tumours, gave results, both *in vivo* and *in vitro*, in conformity with the expectations of the immunostimulation hypothesis, data obtained from the study of transplanted tumours may be misleading. However, the hypothesis has now been tested in several systems of oncogenesis. In the first study of this type, mice were again immunocrippled by adult thymectomy and sublethal irradiation. They were then immunologically restored to varying degrees by giving, intravenously, varying numbers of normal syngeneic spleen cells. Immediately after receiving the spleen cells the animals were challenged by subcutaneous 3-methylcholanthrene.

The results were exactly parallel to those obtained with the modified Winn tests. Those animals that had been partially restored with small numbers of normal, syngeneic spleen cells were more susceptible to oncogenesis than were those that had been either maximally restored or than were those that had not been restored at all. This effect was probably immunological because of the facts that the phenomenon disappeared when the concentration of oncogen was very low (yielding relatively nonimmunogeneic tumours) (Prehn, 1975), when bone marrow cells were substituted for the spleen cells, or when the spleen cells had been heavily irradiated. Of course, no test for specificity could be done in this type of oncogenesis experiment. These experiments have been repeated several times (Prehn, 1977b). Essentially similar results have been obtained by titration of the immune capacity in several other systems: in nude mice, in a skin papilloma system, and when titration was done directly with varying dosages of X-ray (Outzen, 1978, 1980). Most recently it has been shown, by titration of anti-skin autoantibody, that such antibody in low titre, but not in high, promotes papilloma formation in response to a hydrocarbon oncogen (Ryan *et al.*, 1980).

It thus seems clear that there exists a rather general phenomenon, both *in vitro* and *in vivo*, both with transplanted tumours and with oncogenesis: when the putative immune response is titrated, tumour growth is favoured by low to intermediate levels of the immune capacity. On the other hand, a normal or near normal level of immunity paradoxically produces a result similar to that produced by little or no immunity, a fact which may explain why severe immunocrippling so often fails to increase, or to decrease, the incidence of neoplasia (Weston, 1973). The analogies with the results of normal tissue allografting across barriers of varying degrees, from none (autograft) to great, seem nearly perfect.

Possible mechanisms

The spleen cells used in our laboratories for titration are obviously a complex mixture of a variety of cell types, and we have, as yet, made no attempt to fractionate this "black box" to see which cell or combination of cells might be stimulatory. We were more concerned with trying to titrate the total response in all its complexity. However, others have made some beginnings in this analysis and have reported that some cell types are more effective than others (Umiel and Trainin, 1974; Norburg, 1977; Small, 1977). Despite this, our own bias is to believe that the phenomenon is basically quantitative and to predict that any sufficiently active immune effector—be it antibody, lymphoid cells, or macrophages—will exhibit the same general phenomenon. We have already mentioned that antibody can do it (Shearer, 1973; Heidrick *et al.*, 1978), there is a suggestion that lymphotoxin is stimulatory to targets when titrated to very great dilutions (Kolb and Granger, 1970), macrophages can be stimulatory (Evans, 1978; Mantovani, 1978), and Salmon has shown a similar quantitative curve in connection with nonspecific stimulation of tumour growth by macrophages (Salmon, 1980). There is also evidence that NK cells can stimulate tumour cell growth under certain conditions (Kristensen, 1979).

The fact that immunostimulation of tumour growth usually seems to be dependent upon an intermediate ratio of effector to target is reminiscent of the precipitin reaction and the prozone phenomenon (Kabat and Mayer, 1964). It suggests, perhaps, that immunostimulation of tumour is based upon a somewhat analogous mechanism. The argument against a mere abrogation of a surveillance mechanism has already been discussed, and the very chronic nature of the hyperplasia in the skin allograft system, already cited, argues against a compensatory hyperplasia.

It is now becoming increasingly clear that the local clustering of cell surface receptors is an important molecular event in a number of physiological processes involving transmembrane signalling and cell activation. This clustering of receptors appears to be effected by cross-linking produced by the binding of a multivalent ligand to the receptors. Examples occur in the degranulation and desensitization of mast cells and basophils (Segal *et al.*, 1977; Dembo *et al.*, 1979), in the activation and inhibition of lymphocytes (Dintzis *et al.*,

1976; Pike and Nossal, 1979) and in the activity of peptide hormones such as insulin and epidermal growth factor (Kahn *et al.*, 1978; Schechter *et al.*, 1979). Inasmuch as normal and tumour tissues should share many regulatory devices, it will be our thesis that such clustering of surface receptors is also important in regulating tumour growth and that the immune mechanism affects tumour growth, at least in part, by modifying the degree of cross-linking of certain receptors on the tumour cell surface.

In the situations in which the cross-linking of surface receptors is the molecular signal to the cell, the degree of cross-linking is not linearly related to the concentration of the reacting ligand. The cross-linking curves, in relation to ligand concentration, have distinct maxima, much as a precipitation reaction shows a prozone, with maximum precipitation occurring at a narrow optimum ratio of antigen to antibody. In the case of histamine release from basophils, for example, it is clear that the maximal release coincides with the maximal cross-linking obtainable by a multivalent antigen, but the maximal cross-linking, in turn, coincides with an *intermediate* concentration of the cross-linking antigen (Dembo *et al.*, 1979; Perelson and De Lisi, 1980).

Not only is there a distinct optimal concentration of most ligands for the production of maximal cross-linking, but there may also be an optimal degree of cross-linking for the production of a maximal functional effect on the cell. In the case of the activation of the B cell by a T-independent antigen, a sufficient increase in the number of reactive sites on the polymeric antigen may increase the cross-linkage on the cell surface past the point of maximal activation. With sufficient cross-linking the cell apparently becomes unresponsive or tolerant (Feldmann, 1972; Weigel *et al.*, 1980). The concentration of cross-linking ligand that will produce maximal target cell activation apparently varies from tissue to tissue; tumour has been reported to be more sensitive than is the corresponding normal tissue (Chen *et al.*, 1977).

From the foregoing, we postulate that some degree of cross-linking of specific growth regulatory receptors coincides quite generally with cellular activation and differentiation and/or mitotic stimulation. The degree of surface cross-linkage on resting normal cells could be either too high or too low to stimulate (or to permit) hyperplastic growth. By analogy with slime moulds, which may secrete a specific surface "cement", the regulatory cross-linking molecules may be secreted, at least in part, by the cells themselves, and might be considered chalones (Muller and Gerisch, 1978). Perhaps these postulated growth regulating moieties, secreted by the cells themselves, are the tumour growth factors of the type described by Todaro (1979).

Given the above, it follows that, if the effector moieties of an immune response were similar or identical, in specificity, to the moieties that normally cross-link cell surfaces, the immune response could competitively either augment or decrease the degree of cross-linkage. The result would depend in part upon the valency of the immune moiety as well as its concentration *vis-à-vis* the "normal" cross-linking agents. Alternatively, an immune reaction directed against receptors unrelated to those normally involved in growth regulation, might alter the cross-linkage of the latter by steric interference with the physiological cross-linking moieties.

The above speculations serve merely to demonstrate that one can easily conceive of mechanisms by which immunity could stimulate as well as inhibit target cells; those based upon a modification of surface cross-linking seem particularly appealing, but the details cannot yet be more than guessed at.

Conclusions

In summary, the evidence that a modest level of immune reactivity contributes to tumour growth is strong and pervasive. If immunity plays a role in stimulating hyperplasia among non-neoplastic tissues, there is no reason to suppose that it does not do the same for tumour. Reasonable mechanisms to account for the phenomenon can be proposed. Furthermore, the hypothesis can be easily reconciled with observations that leukocytic infiltrates in tumours are often associated with a relatively good prognosis (Prehn, 1977a).

We presume that the successful tumour has, probably through a process of selection, adjusted its antigenicity so that, in the context of the rest of its growth characteristics and the reaction pattern of the particular host, the immune reaction is usually in a stimulatory range. The hypothesis thus accounts for the otherwise perplexing tendency of transplanted tumours to remain immunogenic through many transplant generations despite their immunogenic heterogenicity (Prehn, 1970); there may be positive selection by the immune reaction. If this is so, it suggests that manipulation of host immunity in either direction, i.e. either *to increase or to decrease the reaction*, may often inhibit the tumour and be of benefit to the patient. The clinician probably need not be concerned over the possibility that a chemotherapeutic agent might interfere with an immune reaction against the tumour; the chances are that such interference, regardless of its nature, may well be therapeutic.

References

Allen, A. C. (1948). *Am. J. Pathol.* **24**, 367.

Blazar, B. A. *et al.* (1978). *J. Immunol.* **120**, 1887.

Chai, C. K. (1980). *Transplantation* (submitted).

Chen, H. W. *et al.* (1977). *Exp. Cell Res.* **109**, 253.

Dembo, M. *et al.* (1979). *J. Immunol.* **122**, 518.

Dintzis, H. M. *et al.* (1976). *Proc. Natn. Acad. Sci. U.S.A.* **73**, 3671.

Evans, R. (1978). *Br. J. Cancer* **37**, 1086.

Feldmann, M. (1972). *J. Exp. Med.* **135**, 735.

Heidrick, M. L. *et al.* (1978). *J. Natn. Cancer Inst.* **60**, 1419.

Kabat, E. A. and Mayer, M. M. (1964). *In* "Experimental Immunochemistry" (2nd edn) (Charles C. Thomas, ed.). Springfield.

Kahn, C. R. *et al.* (1978). *Proc. Natn. Acad. Sci. U.S.A.* **75**, 4209.

Kolb, W. P. and Granger, G. A. (1970). *Cell Immunol.* **1**, 122.

Kristensen, E. (1979). *Proc. Soc. Exp. Biol. Med.* **162**, 467.
Lambert, P. B. and Frank, H. A. (1966). *Transplantation* **4**, 159.
Mantovani, A. (1978). *Int. J. Cancer* **22**, 741.
Muller, K. and Gerisch, G. (1978). *Nature* **274**, 445.
Norburg, K. C. (1977). *Cancer Res.* **37**, 1408.
Outzen, H. C. (1978). *In* "Proceedings of the Symposium on the Use of Athymice (Nude) Mice in Cancer Research" (D. Houchens and A. Overjera, eds), pp. 93–99. Gustav Fisher, New York.
Outzen, H. C. (1980). *Int. J. Cancer* (in press).
Perelson, A. S. and De Lisi, C. (1980). *Math. Biosciences* **48**, 71.
Pike, B. L. and Nossal G. J. V. (1979). *Eur. J. Immunol.* **9**, 708.
Prehn, L. M. (1976). *J. Nat. Cancer Inst.* **56**, 833.
Prehn, R. T. (1970). *J. Nat. Cancer Inst.* **45**, 1039.
Prehn, R. T. (1971). *J. Reticuloendothelial Soc.* **10**, 1.
Prehn, R. T. (1972). *Science* **176**, 170.
Prehn, R. T. (1975). *J. Nat. Cancer Inst.* **55**, 189.
Prehn, R. T. (1977a). *J. Nat. Cancer Inst.* **59**, 1043.
Prehn, R. T. (1977b). *Int. J. Cancer* **20**, 918.
Prehn, R. T. and Lappé, M. (1971). *Transplant. Rev.* **7**, 26.
Ryan, W. L. *et al.* (1980). *Proc. Soc. Exp. Biol. Med.* **163**, 212.
Salmon, S. E. (1980). *Lancet* (submitted).
Schecter, Y. *et al.* (1979). *Nature* **278**, 835.
Segal, D. M. *et al.* (1977). *Proc. Natn. Acad. Sci. U.S.A.* **74**, 2993.
Shearer, W. T. (1973). *Science* **182**, 1357.
Small, M. (1977). *J. Immunol.* **118**, 1517.
Todaro, G. (1979). *Cold Spring Harbor Symp. Quant. Biol.* **6**, 113.
Umiel, T. and Trainin, N. (1974). *Transplantation* **18**, 244.
Weigel, F. W. *et al.* (1980). *J. Theoret. Biol.* (submitted).
Weston, B. J. (1973). *Contemp. Topics Immunobiol.* **2**, 237.

37

The Antigens of Chemically Induced Tumours

E. S. LENNOX

MRC Laboratory of Molecular Biology, University Medical School, Cambridge, England

Introduction

Among the antigens of chemically induced rodent tumours it is those detected in transplantation assays that attract so much attention because of their apparently wide diversity. In addition these tumours, particularly the sarcomas, are easy to transplant and easy to grow in tissue culture they are much studied.

On the whole not much progress has been made in finding the molecular basis for this diversity, mainly because sera with specificities corresponding to those of the tumour-specific transplantation antigens (TSTA) have not been generally available. With only the cumbersome transplantation assay to follow the purification from tumour cells of material with transplantation activity, progress has been slow. This is sure to change with the use of monoclonal technology. This chapter reviews the problem of these diverse antigens, indicates what progress has been made by monoclonal antibody analysis and

Abbreviations
MCA = methylcholanthrene; NG = nitrosoguanine; TSTA = tumour specific transplantation antigen; MuLV = murine leukaemia virus; A-MuLV = Abelson virus; SV 40 = Simian virus 40; GP-70 = envelope glycoprotein of retraviruses, mol. wt 70 000; p30 = core protein or retraviruses, mol. wt 30 000.

I thank Dr R. C. Nowinski for generously making his monoclonal antibodies available to me and Ms L. Croft for essential, expert assistance.

suggests that these antigens are recombinant envelope glycoproteins, GP-70, of rodent leukaemia viruses.

Diversity of transplantation antigens

How diverse are the transplantation antigens of the chemically induced tumours? There is an impression that the number of possible antigens is very large because cross-reaction is seldom reported. In the most extensive study reported, Basombrio (1970) reported that among 25 independent tumours from the same inbred strain of mice, there were no reproducible cross-reactions. Ten of these had been tested in pair by pair combinations and the other 15 had been tested in combinations against single tumours. Weak cross-reactions were found, but could not be easily reproduced or assigned to cross-reacting pairs. Cross-reactions have been reported from time to time with several tumours, but they are never emphasized.

In a careful study of the question of cross-reactions Leffell and Coggin (1977) showed that two independent tumours induced by methylcholanthrene (MCA) in BALB/c mice could cross-react or not depending on details of immunization and challenge, but these same conditions did not lead to cross-reaction with a syngeneic SV-40 induced sarcoma. In addition, Economou *et al.* (1977) demonstrated common as well as unique tumour rejection antigens in a group of methylcholanthrene induced squamous cell carcinomas.

The diversity of TSTA might have been due to an underlying diversity of antigens in an already heterogeneous population of cells that are the carcinogen sensitive targets. That this is not the case has been shown by experiments of Basombrio and Prehn (1972) and Embleton and Heidelberger (1972) using cloned lines of cells grown *in vitro* as targets for tumour induction by MCA. In each case tumours with individual TSTA were induced. Although some cross-reaction was observed, it was clear that not all TSTA diversity could be explained by the pre-existing antigenic heterogeneity of the cells susceptible to tumour induction.

Since the collection of noncross-reacting TSTA seems large, there have been many attempts to associate them with another diverse collection of transplantation antigens—those of the major histocompatibility complex. Not only do biochemical properties distinguish them from H-2 antigens (Natori *et al.*, 1977; Sikora *et al.*, 1979) but no linkage has been shown between the genes for H-2 and TSTA (Klein and Klein, 1975). Occasionally some MCA sarcomas display MHC antigens which seem inappropriate to the genotype of the animal in which the tumour has been induced (Schirrmacher *et al.*, 1980; Law *et al.*, 1980). While this is a phenomena that requires explaining, it cannot be the common source of diverse TSTA for even in one of the best documented cases of "inappropriate H-2" it was also shown that the TSTA was not this antigen (Parmiani, 1980).

Attempts to make the antisera so necessary to molecular characterization of TSTA have been on the whole disappointing because usually the sera do not reflect the specificities of the TSTA. There have been exceptions. Parker and Rosenberg (1977) had some success in producing an antiserum against one tumour that had specific antibodies not cross-reacting with the other. The reverse was not accomplished and no biochemical analysis was done with this serum. Brown *et al.* (1978) with a set of 10 BALB/c MCA induced sarcomas prepared several syngeneic antisera and tested them against all 10 tumours. There were extensive cross-reactions which they attempted to correlate with expression by these tumours of protein components of the murine leukaemia viruses (MuLV).

With specific goat antisera, they assayed the core protein p30 and the envelope protein GP-70 in extracts of all of these tumours. They concluded the following.

(a) Each tumour had a unique TSTA but not all tumours express MuLV components.

(b) Tumours that do not express MuLV p30 or GP-70 do not elicit formation of antitumour or antiviral antibodies in the syngeneic immunizations. Tumours that do express GP-70 usually elicit antibody formation but these sera are negative on cells that do not express GP-70.

(c) Primary tumours rarely express MuLV but do so after subsequent, repeated passage in syngeneic mice.

(d) The viruses thus expressed after passage are comprised of antigenically distinct ones. For example, one of the early passage tumours reacted with the goat anti-GP-70 but not with the syngeneic antisera prepared against other tumours.

(e) In sum, syngeneic anti-MCA tumour sera are likely anti-MuLV.

Incidentally, it was with two of this set of tumours that Leffell and Coggin (1977) showed transplantation cross-reaction depending on details of immunization and challenge.

De Leo *et al.* (1977, 1978) also analysed a set of BALB/c MCA induced sarcomas for a wide variety of surface antigens, in an attempt to distinguish them from the distinct TSTAs. Among others antisera that detect MuLV antigens were used: goat anti-Rauscher p30; goat anti-Rauscher GP-70, rat anti-G_{ix} (a GP-70 specificity) and mouse anti-GSCA (gross cell surface antigen).

Three main points emerge from their experiments:

(a) The presence or absence of TSTA could not be correlated with MuLV antigens. The results with the tumour Meth A, which was available in two forms, were particularly striking as a derivative that grows in the ascites, Meth A(a), as well as the original one that grows as a solid tumour, Meth A(s). While Meth A(s) had no detectable MuLV antigens, Meth A(s) was positive for all assayed. None the less Meth A(a) and Meth A(s) have the same TSTA.

(b) A specific antiserum prepared against Meth A(a) was cytotoxic for Meth A(a) cells and its activity could be absorbed by Meth A(a) or

Meth A(s) cells passaged *in vivo* or *in vitro* but by no other normal cells, foetal cells or cells of any other of a large collection of sarcomas and lymphoid tumours.

(c) A similar specific antiserum could be made against CMS4 another BALB/c MC sarcoma, also $MuLV^-$.

Thus the experiments of De Leo *et al.* (1977, 1978) and Brown *et al.* (1977) tend to dissociate TSTA and MuLV components and on the whole identify MuLV specific antibodies in syngeneic antisera as a nuisance, in the way of the research for TSTA specific antibodies.

Later experiments with the Meth A specific antiserum by De Leo *et al.* (1979) showed its reactivity with a protein of mol. wt 53 000 (p53) in the extracts of a wide variety of transformed cells, even though they did not seem to share the cytotoxic specificities defined by the anti-Meth A serum. This makes it possible that p53 reacts with another antibody in this serum.

Against this background, the coming of the monoclonal technology was a fresh approach. There are, so far as I know, two published works on analysing antigens of MCA induced sarcomas: Simrell and Klein (1979) and Lennox *et al.* (1980).

In their experiments Simrell and Klein did many fusions using the spleens of C57/B16 mice bearing syngeneic tumours or immunized with them. Monoclonal antibodies (McAb) from cloned spleen-myeloma hybrid lines were analysed in detail against a large collection of MCA tumours and MuLV virus preparations. Two of their McAbs, in addition to reacting with the immunizing tumour, also reacted with several virus preparations including one from the tumour itself. One McAb reacted strongly with the immunizing tumour, did not react with the virus preparations tested but cross-reacted to varying degrees with some of a large collection of other sarcomas. Thus no strictly tumour-specific McAbs were found, but the last mentioned was much more discriminating than was the serum of the mouse from which the spleen cells were taken for the fusion.

In my own laboratory we have done many immunizations with a series of B10 MCA sarcomas attempting to find sera with tumour specificity after suitable absorptions. By and large this has not succeeded but with one tumour, B10/MC6A, a syngeneic serum was raised that showed some specificity for this tumour. When the spleen of this mouse was used for fusion, 7 stable doubly cloned antibody forming lines were isolated by screening on the immunizing tumour. Five showed tumour specificity and 2 cross-reacted widely (Lennox *et al.*, 1980). Several "specific" clones were intensively studied (Cohn, J., Lowe, T. and Lennox, E., unpublished data). The properties of one in particular A1/4B1.7.10 are described here. Its binding properties to a wide variety of normal tissues and tumours, including other B10 MCA induced sarcomas is shown in Table I. It is the rarity of its cross-reaction that tempts us to think this McAb recognizes the TSTA. When, however, the assay of 4B1 binding is made more sensitive by increasing the number of target cells and as well as the amount of second antibody used in the indirect binding

TABLE I

Binding of the "specific" McAb A1/4B1.7.10 to tumours and normal cell targets

Target	Description	Number tested	Binding
Sarcomas			
B10/MC6A	Immunizing tumour	1	+ + +
B10/MC·	Independent tumours	5	–
(B10BR × B10D2)/MC·	Independent tumours	2	–
(B10 × BALB/c)/MC·	Independent tumours	2	–
B10/MC·	Independent tumours	2	+
Lymphomas			
From: B10, BALB/c, BALB/B, B6 and AKR mice	Virus induced	6	–
Embryonic tumours			
Teratocarcinoma	Non differentiating	3	–
PSA5E	Endoderm derivative	1	–
Normal tissue culture cells			
B10 fibroblasts	Primary—from embryos	3	–
BALB/c fibroblasts	Line—from embryos	1	–
BALB/c not fibroblast	Line—from liver	1	–
Normal tissue			
B10 mice, from heart, kidney, liver, lung, muscle	Trypsinized	–	–
B10, BALB/c, AKR mice, thymus cells		–	–
B10 liver, brain, testes	Homogenized	–	–

Data from Cohn, J., Low, T., and Lennox, E. (unpublished data).
Binding measured in an indirect assay using ^{125}I-Rabbit Fab$_2$ anti mouse Ig.
+ + + ≈ 10 times background in a standard assay
+ ≈ 2–4 times background in a standard assay
– ⩽ 2 times background in a standard assay

assay, then cross-reaction is seen with 3 tumours B10/MC6B, B10/MC4 and B10/MC9.

To widen the search for cross-reaction with our specific McAbs we began a collaboration with Drs P. Patek, J. Collins and M. Cohn at the Salk Institute, San Diego, who had induced a large collection of BALB/c tumours. In order to study the stages in tumour induction, with and without the pressure of the immune system, they had prepared a large number of transformed cell lines (Patek *et al.*, 1978). These had been induced *in vitro* from a cloned BALB/c normal embryo fibroblast line (BALB/c N) and a cloned normal BALB/c liver cell line (BNL) using various transforming agents including chemical carcinogens as well as viruses. Transformants selected by clonal growth in agarose—

BALB/c N and BNL do not grow in agarose—were cloned again and kept as cell lines which were passed either in thymectomized, X-irradiated, foetal liver reconstituted mice or normal mice. We then tested a large number of these lines for the A1/4B1 antigen (Lennox, Patek, Collins and Cohn, unpublished data).

Several points emerge from this (Table II).

TABLE II
A1/4B1 antigen on in vitro *transformed BALB/c lines*[a]

Normal line	*Transforming agent*[b]	*Number of independent transformed lines tested*	*Passed in mice*[c]	*A1/4B1*[d] *binding*
BALB/c-N	MCA	2	No	–
Embryo fibroblast			Yes (1)	–
			(7)	+ to + + +
	SV40	3	No	–
			Yes (1)	+
	A-MuLV	1	No	–
			Yes (1)	–
	NG	1	No	–
			Yes	N.T.
BNL				
Normal BALB/c liver	MCA	3	No	–
			Yes (3)	–
	NG	1	No	–
	SV40	1	No	–
			Yes (3)	–
			(1)	+ + +

[a] Data from Patek, P., Collins, J., Cohn, M. and Lennox, E. (unpublished data).
[b] MCA = methylcholanthrene (or epoxide); SV40 = Simian virus 40; A-MuLV = Abelson virus; NG = nitrosoguanine.
[c] Numbers in parentheses are the total number of independent lines tested from all the transformants, each derived after separate passage in mice.
[d] Binding assay and scoring described in Table I.

(a) The untransformed lines are A1/4B1 negative.
(b) All the transformed lines that have not been passed in animals are A1/4B1 negative whether transformed by Abelson MuLV, SV40, MCA or NG (nitrosoguanine). Ten independent transformed lines were tested.
(c) Several of the transformed lines after passage through animals became 4B1 positive. This included derivatives of MCA transformants and SV40 transformants.

While we do not have a precise measure for the frequency of appearance of a line that is $4B1^+$ after passage in animals of a $4B1^-$ transformant, our analysis shows it not to be infrequent. It is also clear that both $4B1^-$ and

$4B1^+$ lines arise from the same $4B1^-$ transformant when lines passed through different animals are compared. Moreover, the appearance of 4B1 antigen did not depend on whether the cells were passed in immune competent or immune deficient animals.

In a very sketchy experiment in $(B10XBALB/c)F_1$ mice (Lowe, T. and Lennox, E., unpublished data), we assayed whether one of the $4B1^+$ BALB/c lines shared a transplantation antigen with B10/MC6A. In our standard transplantation assay, animals are immunized by 3 injections of 10^7 irradiated cells, then challenged with a single dose of just enough live cells to ensure tumour growth in all the immunized animals (usually about 10^5 cells). Protection was shown both ways, that is 6A immunized mice were protected against 6A and the BALB/c $4B1^+$ tumour and vice versa. Clearly this experiment is incomplete for specificity of protection was not tested. We are doing more complete experiments to determine whether there is a correlation between the presence of the 4B1 antigen and the specific TSTA of B10/MC6A. Until that is done any attempt to relate one to the other remains speculative.

Naturally, the appearance of the 4B1 antigen in this way on the BALB/c tumours invites speculation that it is MuLV related. Fortunately, at this time, we began a collaboration with Dr P. Klein of the University of Florida, Gainesville. He had made McAbs against a C57/B16 tumour (Simrell and Klein, 1979), had found two monoclonals that reacted with MuLV and was analysing the viral specificities of these McAbs attempting to correlate these specificities with those of the anti MuLV McAbs of Lostram *et al.* (1979), who had prepared several McAbs against envelope proteins of MuLV and had screened them against a large panel of MuLV and nonmurine retroviruses. On the basis of their reactions with viruses of this panel several of their monoclonals were shown to react with a GP-70 molecule and to fall into three patterns of reactivity which they label $GP\text{-}70^a$, $GP\text{-}70^b$, $GP\text{-}70^c$ (Stone and Nowinski, 1980).

To summarize, both in Klein's laboratory and ours, we have shown a correspondence between the antigens recognized by antibody 16-B7 (anti-$GP\text{-}70^a$) and 4B1 in the following ways.

(a) On several cell lines and on isolated virus, 4B1 and 16-B7 mutually compete for binding.

(b) 4B1 binding occurs on several of Klein's B6 tumour lines. When it does it correlates with 16-B7 binding.

(c) The BALB/c *in vitro* transformed lines which are positive for 4B1 are also positive for 16-B7.

Finally, we succeeded in isolating (Evan, G., unpublished data) the 4B1 binding protein from ^{125}I labelled cells from 6A and from one of the BALB/c sarcomas that is $4B1^+$. In both cases a protein of about 70K, running at the same position in acrylamide gels as in those bound by 16-B7, was found.

Conclusion

All these experiments suggest strongly that A1/4B1, the "specific" monoclonal is recognizing a determinant on a GP-70 molecule. Since the 4B1 antigen had seemed so discriminatory among the B10 sarcomas and was a candidate for the specific TSTA (Lennox *et al.*, 1980) where does its identification as a GP-70 determinant leave the problem of the molecular nature of TSTA?

There are two clear choices. One is to argue that since the 4B1 antigen turns up on a GP-70, it cannot be identifying a TSTA, for several laboratories have evidence against this correspondence. Both Brown *et al.* (1977) and De Leo *et al.*, (1977, 1978) have clearly shown that sarcomas that are GP-70 (and other MuLV proteins) negative by assay with several xenogeneic antisera do have TSTA. De Leo *et al.* (1977) even showed that $MuLV^+$ and $MuLV^-$ variants of the same tumour did not differ in TSTA. Moreover, since we eventually found cross-reactions of 4B1 with some BALB/c and B6 sarcomas, as well as among the B10 sarcomas, one could argue that it does not show the specificity expected of TSTA.

The other choice is to emphasize the many reasons to believe that the TSTA specificity might be borne on GP-70 molecules. Murine tumour cells certainly do express a wide variety of retroviruses and recombination among them yields a variety of recombinant GP-70 (Elder *et al.*, 1977; Haas and Patch, 1980).

To map TSTA specificities onto GP-70 specificities requires an explanation of the results of Brown *et al.* (1977) and De Leo *et al.* (1977, 1978), which make this mapping unlikely. We would have to assume, for example, that, contrary to our expectations, the xenosera against MuLV components are not universal in detecting all MuLV and that the $TSTA^+$ $MuLV^-$ tumours are wrongly characterized with regard to their MuLV status. We would also have to explain the serological cross-reaction of the tumours with monoclonal antibodies even though they are all supposed to have noncross-reacting TSTAs. This might be done by assuming either that the sera are less discriminating than the T cells responsible for tumour rejection via TSTA or by assuming that TSTAs are made up of ensembles of antigenic determinants from independent or associating molecules. We would also be forced to take the reports of cross-reacting TSTAs more seriously.

The possibility that TSTA diversity might arise from MuLV polymorphism is not a new one, of course, and was indeed suggested by De Leo *et al.* (1977). I am simply drawing attention to some new reasons for taking this possibility seriously.

In further support of this possibility I present the following, admittedly weak, evidence.

(a) The best characterized TSTA (Natori *et al.*, 1978) from the BALB/c sarcoma Meth A is a protein of mol. wt about 70 000, that does not bind to a lentil lectin column.

(b) The transplantation antigen of B10/MC6A was identified (Sikora *et al.*, 1979) as a molecule that is lentil lectin nonbinding and wheat germ agglutinin (WGA) binding.

(c) The GP-70 molecules of B10/MC6A are mainly WGA binding (Evan, G., unpublished data).

We are presently attempting by suitable transplantation experiments to test further this possible correspondence between specificities on GP-70 molecules and those of the tumour-specific transplantation antigens of the chemically induced sarcomas.

References

Basombrio, M. A. (1970). *Int. J. Cancer* **10**, 1.

Basombrio, M. A. and Prehn, R. T. (1972). *Int. J. Cancer* **10**, 1.

Brown, J. P., Klitzman, J. M., Hellström, I., Nowinski, R. C. and Hellström, K. E. (1978). *Proc. Natn. Acad. Sci. U.S.A.* **75**, 955.

De Leo, A. B., Shiku, H., Takahashi, T., John, M. and Old, L. J. (1977). *J. Exp. Med.* **146**, 720.

De Leo, A. B., Shiku, H., Takahashi, T. and Old, L. J. (1978). *In* "Biological Markers of Neoplasia: Basic and Applied Aspects" (R. W. Ruddon, ed.), pp. 25–34. Elsevier North-Holland, Inc.

Economou, G. C., Takeichi, N. and Boone, C. W. (1977). *Cancer Res.* **37**, 37.

Elder, J. H., Gautsch, J. W., Jensen, F. C., Lerner, R. A., Hartley, J. W. and Rowe, W. D. (1977). *Proc. Natn. Acad. Sci. U.S.A.* **74**, 4676.

Embleton, M. J. and Heidelberger, C. (1972). *Int. J. Cancer* **9**, 8.

Haas, M. and Patch, V. (1980). *J. Exp. Med.* **151**, 1321.

Klein, G. and Klein, E. (1975). *Int. J. Cancer* **15**, 879.

Law, L. W., Du Bois, G. C., Rogers, M. J., Appella, E., Pierotti, M. A. and Parmiani, G. (1980). *Transplant Proc.* **12**, 46.

Leffell, M. S. and Coggin, J. H. (1977). *Cancer Res.* **37**, 4112.

Lennox, E., Cohn, J. and Lowe, T. (1980). *Transplant. Proc.* **12**, 95.

Lostrom, M. E., Stone, M. R., Tam, M., Burnette, W. N., Pinter, A. and Nowinski, R. C. (1979). *Virology* **98**, 336.

Natori, T., Law, L. W. and Appella, E. (1977). *Cancer Res.* **37**, 3406.

Natori, T., Law, L. W. and Appella, E. (1978). *Cancer Res.* **38**, 359.

Parmiani, G. (1980). *Transplant Proc.* **12**, 50.

Parker, G. A. and Rosenberg, S. A. (1977). *J. Natn. Cancer Inst.* **58**, 1303.

Patek, P. Q., Collins, J. L. and Cohn, M. (1978). *Nature* **276**, 510.

Schirrmacher, V., Garrido, F., Hübsch, D., Garcia-Olivares, E. and Koszinowski, U. (1980). *Transplant. Proc.* **12**, 32.

Sikora, K., Koch, G., Brenner, S. and Lennox, E. (1979). *Br. J. Cancer* **40**, 8.

Simrell, C. R. and Klein, P. A. (1979). *J. Immunol.* **123**, 2386.

Stone, M. R. and Nowinski, R. C. (1980). *Virology* **100**, 370.

38

Immunology of DNA Virus-induced Tumours

YOSHIAKI ITO

Recombinant DNA Research Unit, National Institute of Allergy and Infectious Diseases, National Institutes of Health, Bethesda, Maryland, USA

Introduction

It had been demonstrated by Prehn and Main (1957) and Klein *et al.* (1960) that there was an antigen specific to the individual tumour and different from those shared by tumour and normal cells which was responsible for the rejection of a transplant of the tumour. These antigens are usually called tumour-specific transplantation antigens (TSTA). In early 1960s, it was established that animals immunized by polyoma virus or simian virus 40 (SV40) or by cells transformed by these viruses developed the immunity against the growth of transplanted tumour cells induced by respective viruses (Sjögren *et al.*, 1961;

I am grateful to Drs George Klein and Chungming Chang for their valuable discussions and to Dr Malcolm A. Martin for his continuous encouragement and support.

Habel, 1961; Defendi, 1963; Deichman and Kluchareva, 1964; Khere *et al.*, 1963; Koch and Sabin, 1963). The choice of these tumour viruses to study TSTA was based on this specificity of immune response induced in animals and antigens in tumour cells. This has led to the speculation that a virus coded protein(s) may be present on the surface of tumour cells induced by the viruses (Allison, 1980; Tevethia, 1980).

The search for these putative virus-coded proteins induced by DNA tumour viruses has long been fruitless. Recently, rapid progress has been made on the elucidation of the regions in virus genomes which are involved in the oncogenesis by these viruses. In the cases of polyoma virus, SV40, human papovavirus BKV, and some strains of human adenoviruses, nucleotide sequences of the entire genomes or those portions of the genomes have been determined and the proteins encoded in the segments of the genomes have been identified. A great deal of information has been accumulating as to how these virus-coded proteins might be involved in the process of tumour formation (reviewed in the books edited by Klein, 1980; Tooze, 1980).

There have been interesting observations in different fields of DNA tumour virology in relation to TSTA. For example, it has been reported that one of the early proteins of adenovirus type 2, 19K cell surface glycoprotein, is tightly associated with major histocompatibility antigens of rat cells transformed by the virus (Kvist *et al.*, 1978). Using adenovirus 12, Shiroki and coworkers (1979) have demonstrated that only a portion of the transforming gene is required to induce TSTA. In the case of Epstein–Barr virus, one of the early antigens, LyDMA, has been found in the plasma membrane (Svedmyr and Jondal, 1975). However, significance of these observations and understanding of the phenomena in molecular terms seem to require some more time.

As a tumour virologist, it seems most appropriate to focus my discussion entirely on polyoma virus and SV40 in this occasion for two reasons. One is that molecular biology of these two closely related but distinctly different viruses is nearly completely understood now and it is possible to discuss which of the virus-coded proteins might act as TSTA. Substantial work to correlate SV40-coded protein to TSTA has been done the results of which will almost certainly be unapplicable to the polyoma virus system. Secondly, of all the transforming proteins induced by DNA tumour viruses, a protein designated as middle-sized T antigen of polyoma virus has been attracting attention from tumour immunologists, since the protein believed to be essential in inducing tumours has been found to be associated with the plasma membrane. In addition, intriguing observations have recently been made on the structural arrangement of the protein with respect to the plasma membrane.

Organization of the genomes of polyoma virus and SV40

The genomes of polyoma virus (mouse virus) and SV40 (monkey virus) which contain approximately 5300 base pairs share strong nucleotide sequence homology suggesting that they may have evolved from a common ancestor (Soeda *et al.*, 1980). Approximately half of the circular genomes of these viruses (early regions) contains the genetic information required to induce tumours in susceptible rodents. In spite of the close relationship, there is a very important difference in the early regions of the two viruses: polyoma virus codes for an extra early protein, middle-sized T antigen (ca 55 000 mol. wt), in addition to large (ca 90 000–100 000 mol. wt) and small T antigens (ca 17 000–22 000 mol. wt) which are shared by these viruses (Ito, 1980). These early proteins or T (tumour) antigens are encoded in the genomes in an overlapping manner and the expression of each protein is accomplished

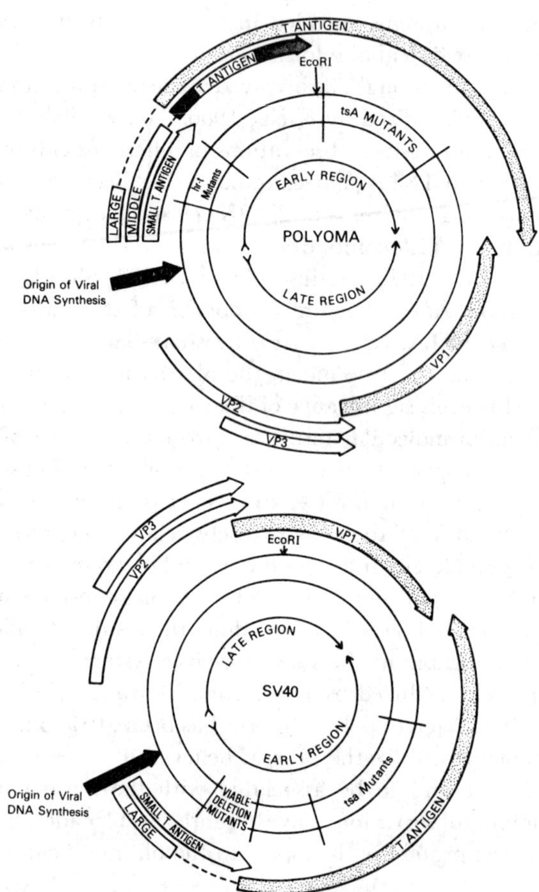

FIG. 1. *Organization of the genomes of polyoma virus and SV40. The restriction enzyme* Eco*RI cuts DNAs of both polyoma virus and SV40 once. The recognition site of the enzyme is taken as a reference point as map unit 0 in both cases. The circular maps of the genomes of the viruses are divided into 100 map units clockwise from 0 to 100 (polyoma virus) or 0 to 1·0 (SV40). The drawing is provided by courtesy of Dr Malcolm A. Martin, NIH, USA.*

by alternative RNA splicing. In particular, the carboxyterminal half of middle-sized T antigen (approximately 30 000 mol. wt) is encoded in the same DNA segment where a part of large T antigen is also encoded in a different reading frame (Fig. 1). There is no such segment of DNA in SV40 genome which has such a long open reading frame in two different frames. By lining up the homologous regions of the genomes of two viruses, it could be shown that the region of polyoma virus genome where two long open reading frames are located is indeed unique to polyoma virus. It appears that this segment of DNA in polyoma virus genome is "inserted" during the course of evolution (Soeda *et al.*, 1980).

The following may be my biased view; but until we find it otherwise, it helps to see similarities and differences of the two viruses clearly: polyoma virus probably has all the genetic functions which SV40 has and, in addition, it has middle-sized T antigen function which may be acquired by the virus after these two viruses had separated evolutionally.

Possible roles of each of the T antigen species in oncogenesis

SV40 is a monkey virus and grows in cultured monkey cells. SV40 or cells transformed *in vitro* by the virus induce tumours in the hamster and also in the mouse after lengthy tissue culture passages.

It is currently believed that the entire early region of the genome of the virus is required for the oncogenesis by the virus. Therefore, large T antigen is essential. The cells transformed by the mutant viruses lacking the ability to induce small T antigen can induce tumours under some conditions. Therefore, the role of small T antigen is less clear. There has been a suggestion that small T antigen might act like a tumour promoter (Seiff and Martin, 1980). So far as is known, all the tumour cells induced by SV40 have large T antigen. Most of large T antigen is present in the nuclei of tumour cells. Nuclear fluorescence staining obtained using anti-T serum from tumour-bearing animals is considered to be due to the presence of large T antigen which is a major antigen. Small T antigen is believed to be in the cytoplasm. Large T antigen binds to DNA specifically and nonspecifically and is involved in the initiation of viral DNA replication, control of the early RNA transcription, and induction of host cell DNA synthesis in infected cells.

Natural host for polyoma virus is mouse. The virus grows in cultured mouse cells. The virus induces tumours in the mouse, hamster, and rat when it is inoculated to young animals. Quite contrary to SV40, only about half of the early region of polyoma virus genome which encodes middle and small T antigens is required for the induction and the maintenance of the oncogenesis (Chowdhury *et al.*, 1980; Hassell *et al.*, 1980; Novak *et al.*, 1980). The DNA fragment capable of inducing small T antigen is not oncogenic (Chowdhury *et al.*, 1980). Middle and small T antigens are always present in tumour cells (except for the cases described below). Polyoma virus middle T antigen is associated with the plasma membrane of transformed mouse cells and has associated tyrosine phosphorylating protein kinase activity. The degree of the kinase activity and the rate of tumour growth appears to have direct correlation (Smith *et al.*, 1979; Ito *et al.*, 1980).

Is large T antigen of SV40 TSTA?

Tumours induced by polyoma virus or SV40 usually contain new antigen which can be recognized specifically by the sera from animals bearing these tumours. The antigen, designated as tumour (T) antigen, was originally demonstrated by complement-fixation test and is now known to be composed of a collection of components containing largely viral early proteins (Fig. 1). As summarized earlier, these tumour cells also contain new virus-specific antigen detected by the transplantation rejection test (TSTA). TSTA could be examined from two different stand points: one is to examine TSTA as an immunogen which induces in the animals an immune response specific to the virus and the other is to examine TSTA as an immunosensitive antigen present presumably on the surface of the tumour cells which responds to the specific immunity induced in the animals.

Substantial amounts of work have been done to try to find out the origin of SV40-specific TSTA. Specific immunity can be induced in animals by inoculating them with live SV40. Inactivated virus does not induce this immunity. Non-defective adenoviruses containing varying lengths of SV40 DNA inserted in the genome have been useful in specifying the region of the SV40 genome responsible for inducing the TSTA. While the hybrid virus containing 43% of the SV40 DNA (Ad2$^+$ND4) (mainly the early region from 11 to 54 map units, see Fig. 1) induces nuclear T antigen and TSTA, the ones containing either 32% of the SV40 genome (Ad2$^+$ND2) (from 11 to 44 map units) or 18% (Ad2$^+$ND1) (from 11 to 28 map units) induce TSTA but not nuclear T antigen (Lewis and Rowe, 1973; Jay *et al.*, 1978). Figure 1 shows that there is only one protein, large T antigen, known to be encoded in the region of the genome. Specific immune response could be induced by inoculating animals with virus-free transformed cells (usually X-irradiated before inoculation). By fractionating these cells, it has been shown that nuclear fractions contain most of the immunogenic activity (Anderson *et al.*, 1977a; Rogers *et al.*, 1977). Early proteins of SV40 can be obtained also from monkey cells in which SV40 is undergoing productive infection. These cells have also been shown to have immunogenic activity. A class of temperature-sensitive mutants, ts-A, which have mutations in A gene, induce thermolabile large T antigen. Using these mutants, it has been shown that the activity to induce TSTA is under A gene control (Anderson *et al.*, 1977b; Chang *et al.*, 1977a; Tevethia and Tevethia, 1977). The anti-T serum from tumour-bearing animals has been shown to immunoprecipitate both T antigens and the immunogenic activity. It has also been shown that SV40 T antigen and immunogenic TSTA copurify under various conditions (Chang *et al.*, 1979). Also it has been shown that both bind to DNA (Chang *et al.*, 1977b). Finally, purified large T antigen from transformed human cells (Chang *et al.*, 1979) or SV40-like protein containing a large part of SV40 large T antigen from the carboxyterminal end and some adenovirus-coded polypeptide at the amino-terminal region and shown to have all the known function of SV40 large T antigen (Tjian, 1978) have been shown to be a potent immunogen. 0·6 μg or 0·25 μg, respectively, of these purified proteins induced effective immune response in the animals (Chang *et al.*, 1979; Tevethia and Tjian, 1979). Taking all these together, it can be said that large T antigen of SV40 possesses the antigenic determinants to induce specific transplantation immunity in animals. At least some of these antigenic determinants seem to be located within the polypeptide chain of approximately 28 000 daltons in size from the extreme carboxy-terminal end of large T antigen (Jay *et al.*, 1978). It is not clear whether other parts of the molecule also have these determinants or whether any other protein also has immunogenic activity.

It is generally assumed that the surface of SV40-induced tumour cells has immunosensitive SV40-specific antigen. Characterization of this presumed cell surface protein is not as advanced as characterization of the immunogenic TSTA. Two SV40-coded proteins (56K and 42K) which share tryptic peptides with SV40 large T antigen induced in infected HeLa cells by Ad2$^+$ND2 were reported to be stably associated with the plasmal membrane (Deppert and Walter, 1976). Also, 28K protein induced by Ad2$^+$ND1 in KB cells was found in the plasma membrane fraction (Jay *et al.*, 1978). Soule and Butel (1979) and Soule *et al.* (1980) have fractionated SV40 transformed hamster and mouse cells and SV40 infected monkey cells and found that small fractions of large T antigen was present in the surface membrane fractions of these cells in addition to the nuclear fractions which contain a major part of the molecules. These results are certainly consistent with the view that the major nonvirion antigen, large T antigen, present in SV40-induced tumour cells may be immunosensitive as well as immunogenic TSTA.

Since large T antigen is a nuclear protein and has a DNA binding activity, the question remains as to why some fraction of large T antigen should be present in the plasma membrane. It has been suggested that there might be a subpopulation of large T antigen which has an affinity for cell membrane. They can be either a product of novel mRNA formed by rare splicing event (Berg, 1979) or a differently modified subpopulation of otherwise authentic large T antigen. There is little experimental evidence for any of these two at this moment. There is also a suggestion that large T antigen may be present in the plasma membrane accidentally without any significant role (Martin, 1980).

Structural and functional organization of middle-sized T antigen of polyoma virus with respect to plasma membrane

As mentioned earlier, large T antigen is often absent from polyoma virus-transformed cells. Therefore, large T antigen cannot be considered to act as TSTA universally in polyoma virus system. An obvious alternative candidate would be middle-sized T antigen. Since polyoma virus-coded middle-sized T antigen was found relatively recently, experiments to correlate the protein to TSTA have not been done yet. However, molecular characterization of the protein has been revealing intriguing properties of the protein which are relevant to TSTA.

Extraction of middle-sized T antigen of polyoma virus depends on the presence of detergent in the extraction buffer. When subcellular fractions were examined, the protein was found predominantly in plasma membrane fraction (about 85%) compared with cytoplasmic soluble fraction, endoplasmic reticulum fraction, and mitochondrial fraction (Ito *et al.*, 1977; Ito, 1979). It was not clear how much of the protein was present in nuclear membrane. The protein, however, could not be digested with trypsin from the outside of the cells. Also, attempts to demonstrate the immunofluorescene on the surface of cells using anti-T serum have been unsuccessful. On the other hand, amino acid sequence for middle-sized T antigen deduced from the nucleotide sequence for middle-sized T antigen predicted that the carboxyterminal region of the protein had a row of 22 hydrophobic amino acids flanked by hydrophilic ones and of 6 amino acids present after the hydrophobic cluster until predicted carboxyterminal end, 2 were Arginine and one was Lysine (Fig. 2) (Soeda *et al.*, 1979). This type of amino acid arrangements has been known recently to be characteristic to transmembrane proteins. From these, it has been postulated that the protein is probably inserted in the plasma membrane at the carboxy-terminal region and only a small part of the molecule from the carboxyterminal end is exposed to the outside of the cells. The rest of the molecule appears to be present inside of the plasma membrane (Ito and Spurr, 1979), since the amino-terminal half of the middle-sized T antigen is essentially the same as small T antigen and there is no evidence that small T antigen is associated with plasma membrane (Ito, 1979). This structural arrangement seems to be very similar to those of transforming proteins of several retroviruses such as $p60^{src}$ of avian sarcoma virus and p120 of Abelson murine leukaemia virus which share a variety of characteristics with middle T antigen: they are considered to be essential for oncogenesis and they have associated protein kinases which phosphorylate tyrosine residue (Eckhart *et al.*, 1979; Hunter *et al.*, 1980; Witte *et al.*, 1980). There is no evidence of glycosylation.

To further characterize middle-sized T antigen in plasma membrane, we have started to examine the structural arrangement of middle-sized T antigen with respect to plasma membrane using the outside-out and inside-out plasma

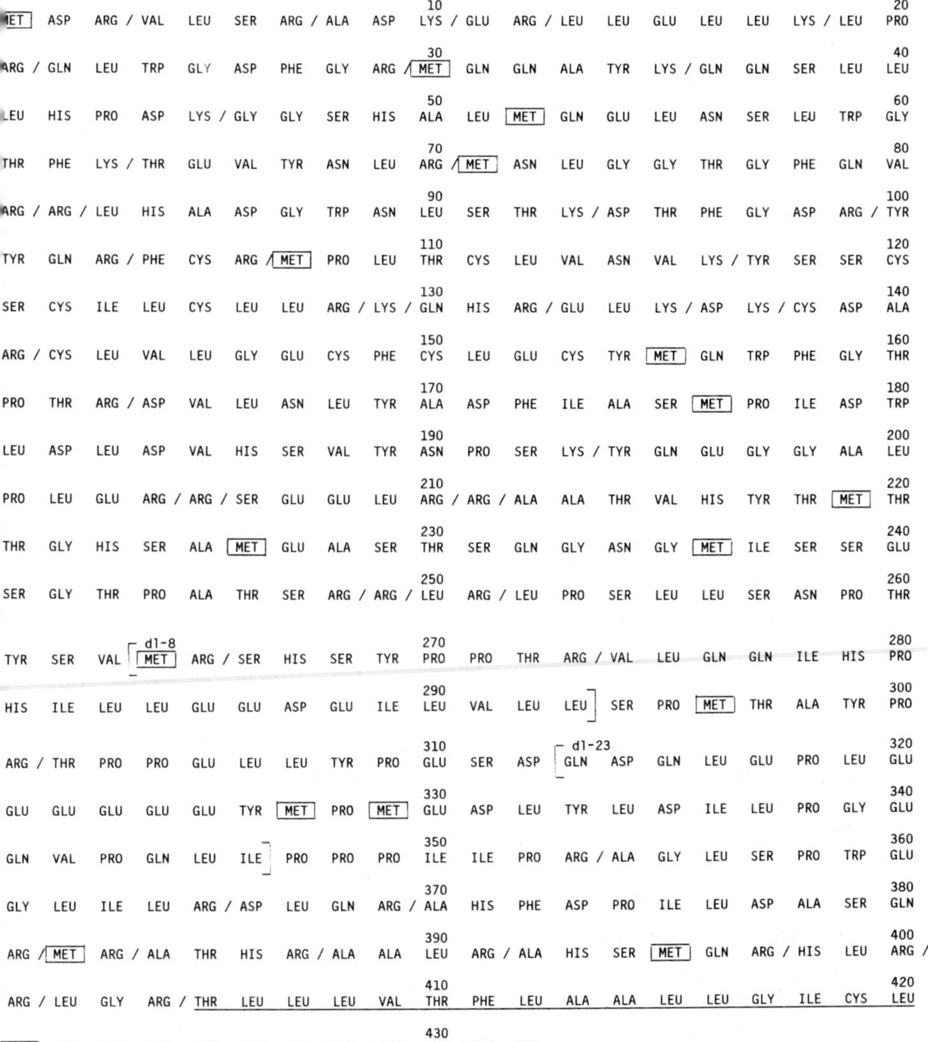

FIG. 2. *Postulated protein sequence of polyoma virus middle T antigen* (*Soeda* et al., *1979*).

membrane vesicles (Steck and Kant, 1974) made from polyoma virus transformed mouse cells in collaboration with S. E. Light and F. Hirata, NIH, USA. We have found recently, to our surprise, that middle-sized T antigen can be phosphorylated almost exclusively, on the surface of outside-out membrane vesicles but not on the inside-out ones. This indicates that phosphorylation of middle-sized T antigen should occur on the surface of intact cells. Indeed, we can now demonstrate that on the surface of live cells suspended in physiological saline, incorporation of ^{32}P into middle T antigen from γ-

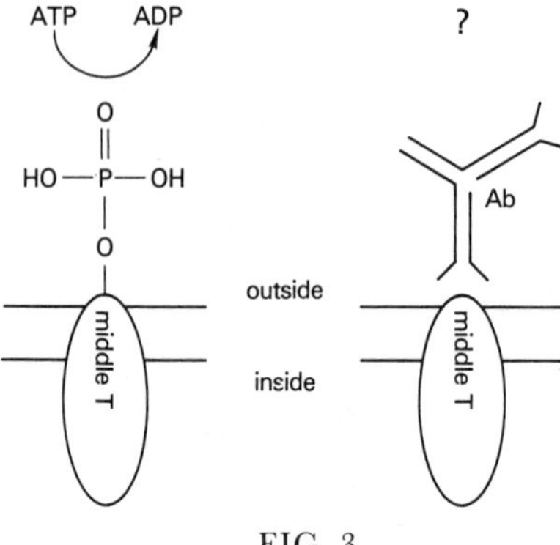

FIG. 3.

^{32}P-ATP occurs (manuscript in preparation). Current working hypothesis is illustrated in Fig. 3.

The localization of the site of phosphorylation of middle T antigen on the outside surface of the cells would have wide biological implications. As described above, middle-sized T antigen appears to be primarily important in inducing tumours and protein kinase activity associated to the protein appears to be the primary function of the protein for tumour growth. Then the significance of the phosphorylation of middle-sized T antigen (either by autophosphorylation or phosphorylation by other protein) or phosphorylation of some cellular protein by middle-sized T antigen needs to be considered in relation to cell surface components. From an immunological point of view, the first most important point to note would be the fact that the portion of the molecule is exposed to the outside of the cells. This would open the possibility that middle T antigen might serve as a TSTA. Then we need to know whether or not there is any immune response directed against the portion of the molecule which is located outside of the cells. Now that we know middle T antigen to be a transmembrane protein, specific effort will be made to obtain such evidence. One obvious possibility in doing so would be to make use of phosphorylation reaction for the detection of the antibodies; i.e., it would be rapid, sensitive, and accurate to test possible inhibitory activity present in sera against phosphorylation reaction. We have begun this approach in collaboration with George Klein's laboratory in the Karolinska Institute in Sweden.

If such antisera were available, it would be extremely intriguing to test whether or not they would interfere with tumour growth, since phosphorylation of or by middle-sized T antigen appears to have close relationship with the rate of tumour growth.

In any event, the polyoma virus-mouse system seems to offer a very interesting biological system to study oncogenesis by the virus and immune response of the host animals to it, since the mouse is the natural host for polyoma virus, the most important virus-coded protein for the oncogenesis is associated with plasma membrane, and probably the most important part of the molecule is exposed to the outside of the cells ready to interact with the host immune system.

Virus-coded and host cell-coded

One apparently disturbing observation in attempting to correlate middle-sized T antigen to TSTA is as follows: polyoma virus-induced mouse tumour cells passaged through animals for many years are free of any of the T antigen species, although freshly induced tumour cells do contain middle and small T antigens (G. Klein, personal communication and Y. Ito, unpublished observation). Yet, both tumour cells freshly induced and those passaged for a long period exhibit polyoma virus-specific TSTA (G. Klein, personal communication). This might indicate that middle-sized T antigen is not TSTA or at least middle-sized T antigen does not play a central role in TSTA. However, recent progress in tumour virology enabled us to offer an alternative, exciting explanation. As discussed above, the DNA segment which encodes the main part of the unique region of middle-sized T antigen appears to be "inserted" during the evolution of the virus. This inserted DNA segment must have come from mouse DNA from the region where "cellular middle-sized T antigen" is encoded. In many cases of transforming proteins of retroviruses, it has been established that there are cell-coded counterparts in their host cells which are very similar in character including the immunogenicity to those coded by the viruses. As mentioned above, middle-sized T antigen shares many characteristics with those transforming proteins of retroviruses. Presence of cellular proteins related to virus-coded proteins is not confined to the retrovirus system. Recently, Lane (1980) has isolated monoclonal antibodies against SV40 large T antigen which cross reacts with cellular protein of 68 000 mol. wt. It is likely that this 68K protein is cellular equivalent of large T antigen presumably required for cellular DNA replication. There is no reason to assume that there would be no cellular middle-sized T antigen in mouse cells.

If we accept that the existence of "cellular middle-sized T antigen" is highly probable, it is not difficult to imagine that in cells passaged through animals for many years, cellular middle-sized T antigen or similar protein might have taken over virus-coded middle-sized T antigen since virus-coded proteins may be too strongly antigenic. Cells containing such virus-coded proteins probably have selective disadvantage. It has been shown in the case of SV40 that highly tumorigenic spontaneously transformed mouse cells become less tumorigenic after transformation of these cells by SV40 (Mora *et al.*, 1977).

Summary and Conclusion

Two closely related but distinctly different papovaviruses, polyoma virus and SV40, were compared with respect to TSTA. SV40 codes for two transforming proteins, large and small T antigens. Polyoma virus codes for middle-sized T antigen in addition to large and small T antigens. In the case of SV40, large T antigen has a primary role in inducing oncogenesis. Purified large T antigen of SV40 is a potent immunogen against tumour cell challenge. Presence of large T antigen in cell surface membrane has been reported. In the case of polyoma virus, large T antigen is missing in many tumour cells. Instead, middle and small T antigens are universally present. Middle-sized T antigen is primarily responsible for inducing phenotype of tumour cells and has associated protein kinase activity. Middle-sized T antigen is a transmembrane protein located in the plasma membrane of transformed mouse cells. Recently it has been observed that the phosophorylation of middle-sized T antigen occurs on the surface of intact live cells. It is currently being investigated whether or not there is any antibodies capable of blocking phosphorylation of middle-sized T antigen on the cell surface. Polyoma virus-induced tumours kept in animals for many years do not have a detectable amount of T antigens but exhibit polyoma virus-specific TSTA. Possible explanation for this observation is discussed.

References

Allison, A. C. (1980). *In* "Viral Oncology" (G. Klein, ed.), pp. 481–487. Raven Press, New York.

Anderson, J. L., Martin, R. G., Chang, C. and Mora, P. T. (1977a). *Virology* **76**, 154.

Anderson, J. N., Martin, R. G., Chang, C., Mora, P. T. and Livingston, D. M. (1977b). *Virology* **76**, 420.

Berg, P. (1979). *Cold Spring Harbor Symp. Quant. Biol.* **44** (in press).

Chang, C., Anderson, J. L., Martin, R. G. and Mora, P. T. (1977a). *J. Virol.* **22**, 281.

Chang, C., Luborsky, S. W. and Mora, P. T. (1977b). *Nature* **269**, 438.

Chang, C., Martin, R. G., Livingston, D. M., Luborsky, S. W., Hu, C. P. and Mora, P. T. (1979). *J. Virol.* **29**, 69.

Chowdhury, K., Light, S., Garon, C. F., Ito, Y. and Israel, M. A. (1980). *J. Virol.* (in press).

Defendi, V. (1963). *Proc. Soc. Exp. Biol. Med.* **113**, 12.

Deichman, G. I. and Kluchareva, T. E. (1964). *Virology* **24**, 133.

Deppert, W. and Pates, R. (1979). *Nature* **277**, 523.

Deppert, W. and Walter, G. (1976). *Proc. Natn. Acad. Sci. U.S.A.* **73**, 2505.

Eckhart, W., Hutchinson, M. A. and Hunter, T. (1979). *Cell* **18**, 925.

Girardi, A. J. and Defendi, V. (1970). *Virology* **42**, 688.

Habel, K. (1961). *Proc. Soc. Exp. Biol. NY* **106**, 722.

Hassell, J. A., Topp, W. C., Rifkin, D. B. and Moreau, P. E. (1980). *Proc. Natn. Acad. Sci. U.S.A.* (in press).

Hunter, T. and Sefton, B. M. (1980). *Proc. Natn. Acad. Sci. U.S.A.* **77**, 1311.

Ito, Y. (1979). *Virology* **98**, 261.

Ito, Y. (1980). *In* "Viral Oncology" (G. Klein, ed.), pp. 447–480. Raven Press, New York.

Ito, Y. and Spurr, N. (1979). *Cold Spring Harbor Symp. Quant. Biol.* **44** (in press).

Ito, Y., Brocklehurst, J. R. and Dulbecco, R. (1977). *Proc. Natn. Acad. Sci. U.S.A.* **74**, 4666.

Ito, Y., Spurr, N. and Griffin, B. E. (1980). *J. Virol.* **35**, 219.

Jay, G., Jay, F. T., Chang, C., Friedman, R. M. and Levine, A. S. (1978). *Proc. Natn. Acad. Sci. U.S.A.* **75**, 3055.

Khera, K. S., Ashkenazi, A., Rapp, F. and Melnick, J. L. (1963). *J. Immunol.* **91**, 604.

Klein, G. (1980). "Viral Oncology." Raven Press, New York.

Klein, G., Sjögren, O., Klein, E. and Hellström, K. E. (1960). *Cancer Res.* **20**, 1561.

Koch, M. A. and Sabin, A. B. (1963). *Proc. Soc. Exp. Biol. Med.* **113**, 4.

Kvist, S., Ostberg, L., Persson, H., Philipson, L. and Peterson, P. A. (1978). *Proc. Natn. Acad. Sci. U.S.A.* **75**, 5674.

Lane, D. (1980). *Nature* (in press).

Lewis, A. M., Jr. and Rowe, W. P. (1973). *J. Virol.* **12**, 836.

Martin, R. G. (1980). *Adv. Cancer Res* (in press).

Mora, P. T., Change, C., Couvillion, L., Kuster, J. M. and McFarland, V. W. (1977). *Nature* **269**, 36.

Novak, U., Dilworth, S. M. and Griffin, B. E. (1980). *Proc. Natn. Acad. Sci. U.S.A.* **77**, 3278.

Prehn, R. T. and Main, J. M. (1957). *J. Natn. Cancer Inst.* **18**, 769.

Pretell, J., Greenfield, R. S. and Tevethia, S. S. (1979). *Virology* **97**, 32.

Rapp. F., Tevethia, S. S. and Melnick, J. L. (1966). *J. Natn. Cancer Inst.* **36**, 707.

Rogers, M. J., Law, L. W. and Appella, E. (1977). *J. Natn. Cancer Inst.* **59**, 1291.

Schaffhausen, B. S. and Benjamin, T. L. (1979). *Cell* **18**, 935.

Seif, R. and Martin, R. G. (1979). *J. Virol.* **32**, 979.

Shiroki, K., Shimojo, H., Maeta, Y. and Hamada, C. (1979). *Virology* **99**, 188.

Sjögren, H. O., Hellström, I. and Klein, G. (1961). *Cancer Res.* **21**, 329.

Smith, A. E., Fried, M., Griffin, B. E. and Smith, R. (1979). *Cell* **18**, 915.

Soule, H. R. and Butel, J. S. (1979). *J. Virol.* **30**, 523.

Soule, H. R., Lanford, R. E. and Butel, J. S. (1980). *J. Virol.* **33**, 887.

Soeda, E., Arrand, J. R., Smolar, N. and Griffin, B. E. (1979). *Cell* **17**, 357.

Soeda, E., Maruyama, T., Arrand, J. R. and Griffin, B. E. (1980). *Nature* **285**, 165.

Steck, T. L. and Kant, J. A. (1974). *In* "Methods in Enzymology" (S. Fleischer and L. Packer, eds), Vol. 31, pp. 172–180. Academic Press, New York and London.

Svedmyr, E. and Jondal, M. (1975). *Proc. Natn. Acad. Sci. U.S.A.* **72**, 1622.

Tevethia, S. S. (1980). *In* "Viral Oncology" (G. Klein, ed.), pp. 581–601. Raven Press, New York.

Tevethia, M. J. and Tevethia, S. S. (1976). *Virology* **69**, 474.

Tevethia, M. J. and Tevethia, S. S. (1977). *Virology* **81**, 212.

Tevethia, S. S., Tjian, R., unpublished observation, referred in a review by Tevethia, S. S. (1980). *In* "Viral Oncology" (G. Klein, ed.), pp. 581–601. Raven Press, New York.

Tjian, R. (1978). *Cell* **13**, 165.

Tooze, J. (1980). "Molecular Biology of DNA Tumour Viruses." Cold Spring Harbor Laboratory.

Witte, O. N., Dasgupta, A. and Baltimore, D. (1980). *Nature* **283**, 826.

Theme 10: Summary
Tumour Immunology

GEORGE KLEIN

Department of Tumour Biology, Karolinska Institute, Stockholm, Sweden

Immune surveillance (IS)

The central problem of this area, immune surveillance (IS) continued to be discussed in the somewhat simplistic terms that have become endemic in the area. It is still asked whether IS exists or not, implying that if it exists, it has to play a role for all tumours and all species. A built-in generalization of this type would appear as utterly unrealistic in all other areas of immunology. It is also often said that the "classical" theory of IS implies that it has to be mediated by T cells. While some modern reformulators of the theory, Burnet in particular, may have implied this, one can hardly speak of the original IS theory, except in direct reference to the originator, Paul Ehrlich.

Ehrlich made two statements: (a) neoplastic cells arise in normal tissues at an enormous frequency and (b) they are continuously eliminated by IS.

With regard to (a), Ehrlich was clearly wrong. In particular, he could not suspect the existence of many nonimmunological mechanisms that counteract neoplastic transformation. The multiple tumours of the xeroderma patients represent one example of what happens when a certain type of DNA repair is put out of function. He was also unaware of the vast influence of the cell genotype on the likelihood of neoplastic transformation, and of the multistep nature of progression. As to (b), Ehrlich did not—and could not—postulate any specific effector, nor is there any reason to single out T cells as the only potentially respectable mediator.

Many of the workshop papers showed an increasing awareness of the multifaceted nature of IS and the vast diversification of its mediators. Broadly speaking, the known biological systems show a clear polarization between two extremes:

A. *Naturally occurring, ubiquitous oncogenic viruses* have selected their host species for a highly effective and, sometimes completely watertight surveillance, directed *not* against the virus as such, but against some virally induced membrane change on the transformed cell. Polyoma in mice, EBV in man, *H. saimiri* in the squirrel monkey and (at a somewhat lower efficiency) FeLV-induced cat leukaemia can be quoted as examples. None of these systems has been analysed in detail for immunological mediation, but it may be expected (as also supported by the fragmentary evidence that is available) that selection has fixed multiple effector mechanisms, all directed against very few and perhaps only a single target site. One may refer to these as "*rejection geared systems*". Under these circumstances, tumour development is a biological accident of heavy, polyvalently acting immunosuppression.

B. *Spontaneous tumours* arise through a slow process of multistep progression, as a rule. In the course of progression, they are selected for nonimmunogenicity, i.e. an inability to provoke a rejection response on the genetic background of their own host. The mechanism for this absence of rejection, e.g. lack of antigenicity, suppression, enhancement, or a whole variety of other, experimentally demonstrated escapes is not known in detail for *any* spontaneous tumour, nor does it have to be unique or general. Unlike the situation described under A above, the host is not selected for IS, partly because there is no single transformation associated target to focus on, and partly because the majority of the tumours in this category occur after the reproductive age.

The chemically induced tumours show a wide range of behaviours between A and B above. They can approach both extremes and there are many intermediates. Most laboratory systems are highly artificial in using large doses of known carcinogens. They often cause polyclonal tumours (exemplified by Abstract 10.1.44)* that can hardly be regarded as being representative for naturally occurring tumours induced by environmental agents. The relatively strong immunogenicity of some tumours in this category may merely reflect the massiveness of the induction event and the rapid growth rate of some clones, obviating the need for the gradual, slow immunoselective modification at the level of the nascent tumour cell. This is well in line with the established fact that certain chemically induced tumours with relatively short latency periods tend to be more immunogenic than tumours that arise after a long latency.

A highly interesting special case is represented by the u.v.-induced skin tumours in mice. While strongly antigenic, these tumours are not rejected by u.v.-irradiated autochthonous or syngeneic hosts, due to a powerful suppression: u.v.-irradiation of the skin can generate the same suppression, in the absence of any tumours. Suppression can be transferred adoptively with T cells. It may be surmised that the system is *suppression geared*, in order to prevent the rejection of u.v.-irradiated ("mutagenized") normal skin. Interestingly, the suppressor cells prevent the rejection of u.v.-induced skin carcinomas in a group specific fashion, in spite of the antigenic individuality of these tumours. As Mitchison has pointed out (Chapter 35), this is reminiscent of other systems where the specific targets of the helper and the suppressor T cells are different on the same molecule, with Sercarz' lysozyme studies as the outstanding example.

In conclusion, IS cannot be discussed in all-or-none terms, either in relation to tumours in general, or in relation to one specific type of effector. As so beautifully exemplified by the immunology of parasitic diseases, the actual outcome of the immune response must be viewed in relation to the earlier selective history of the specific host-target combination.

Nature of the antigenic targets

Among the virus induced tumours, polyoma is still one of the most interesting systems, particularly now that the total base sequence of the viral DNA is known. The early region of the viral genome is utilized with an almost incredible economy. It codes for at least 3 antigenic products, totalling 170K in mol. wt. All 3 are the products of a single messenger corresponding to a 100K protein, if read in a single frame. Due to splicing and partial frameshifts, as explained in Chapter 38 by Ito, the synthesis of the 3 antigenic products, large, middle and small T, is now understood. There is not much (if anything) left to code for TSTA, the surveillance target, however. Ito has therefore argued that TSTA should be sought among the known antigenic products of the early region. Middle T antigen is the most likely candidate, due to its membrane localization. Ito showed, for the first time, that a small part of middle T is exposed on the outer cell surface and not only on the inner side of the membrane, as previously thought. Middle T is presently also the main candidate for the transforming function, as suggested by the analysis of transforming and nontransforming mutants. Since it is also a phosphorylated component, the possible analogies with the *sarc* protein are intriguing. Conceptually, it would make good sense if the mouse would have focused its surveillance on a regular, transformation associated change. However, different

* Reference numbers indicate Abstract numbers in: Abstracts 4th International Congress of Immunology, Paris, 1980.

results were reported by Barra *et al.* (10.1.03). By immunoprecipitation of labelled membrane components with the sera of rejector animals, they have identified a 37K product that was present in middle T negative cells and could induce a rejection reaction against polyoma tumours.

In the SV40 system, there is no middle T. Large T has been shown to induce rejection reactions in previous experiments. This makes good sense, since SV40 is a monkey virus. It induces highly antigenic tumours in the mouse that can only be transplanted to immunosuppressed recipients, as a rule. Clearly, this is an artificial system, compared to polyoma. Schmidt-Ullrich and Wallach (10.1.49) reported on the presence of a membrane associated, host cell modified large T antigen that could serve as the rejection target.

Monoclonal antibodies are now available against SV40 large T antigen, as mentioned by Ito. Unlike the exquisite specificity of the tumour-bearing animal serum against the T antigen carried in syngeneic tumour cells, the xenogeneic monoclonals cross-react with a cellular protein. While the nature of this protein and its relationship to large T antigen is interesting in itself, this finding illustrates a continuously recurring dilemma with the monoclonal antibodies. With a few notable exceptions, they are produced in foreign species. Perhaps we should recall the early days of tumour serology when it was all done across species barriers. While informative, it was hampered by frequent cross-reactions with normal cellular components. Many of these cross-reactions disappeared when syngeneic or autologous sera came into general use. Thus, while it must be acknowledged that the monoclonals clearly represent a great advance in this area as well, it must be remembered that xenogeneic monoclonals may not have the same distinctive ability between self and nonself as antibodies of the same species.

Mitchison (Chapter 35) pointed out that IS against virally transformed cells may frequently act on preneoplastic, rather than on fully autonomous tumour cells. This is reasonable and certainly true for the EBV-system. Haran-Ghera's findings (10.1.23) suggest that it is probably true for "spontaneous" AKR leukaemia. It might be possibly true for FeLV induced cat leukaemia, but it is probably not true for polyoma where viral oncogenesis appears to act more directly.

For the oncorna virus systems, Alaba and Law (10.1.01) found no relationship between the rejection-inducing TSTA and known viral proteins. In the Rous-system, Comoglio *et al.* (10.1.14) found a close association between *sarc* p60 and a host gene product, identified both by antisera and by monoclonal antibodies. The feline oncorna virus determined membrane antigen, FOCMA, is also a compounded host/viral component, and of particular interest because it serves as the target for natural surveillance. Chen *et al.* reported that there are two distinct forms of FOCMA, associated with virally transformed leukaemia and sarcoma cells, respectively (10.1.13). They differ from each other and from all known viral proteins.

In the EBV-system, LYDMA, the lymphocyte defined membrane antigen, is still identified by CMI reactions, particularly by the powerful HLA-restricted EBV specific memory T cells, present in the peripheral blood of healthy EBV-seropositives. Two different monoclonal antibodies were reported, directed against membrane antigens on EBV-carrying lymphoid lines. Both of them were interesting, but none of them necessarily identify LYDMA. The antibody reported by Thorley-Lawson (10.8.21) reacts preferentially with lymphoblastoid cell lines of normal origin, while the antibody of Wiels *et al.* (19.2.21) reacts against Burkitt lymphoma (BL) lines, but not lymphoblastoid lines (LCL) of normal origin. Since LCL and BL lines have quite different phenotypes, this is not surprising in itself. It will be of great interest to explore the nature of the reactive target structures and their possible relationship (if any) to EBV and to LYDMA.

If virus transformed, preneoplastic or potentially neoplastic cells represent the most likely targets for immune surveillance, it follows that tumours that appear in an increased frequency in immunosuppressed patients are the most likely sources of viruses involved in the aetiology of human tumours. This prediction is largely fulfilled by the findings of Purtilo *et al.* (9.7.25), showing that XLP, the X-linked lymphoproliferative syndrome that appears in multiple immunodeficient patients, is an EBV-associated (i.e. EBV-DNA carrying) lymphoproliferative disease. It appears to represent a clinically malignant variety of a normally self-limiting lymphoproliferative disease, mononucleosis. It is very different from Burkitt's lymphoma, a monoclonal tumour that is characterized not only by the presence of the viral genome, but also by a regular cytogenetic change. There are also data to indicate that at least some of the fatal lymphoproliferative lesions that arise in immunosuppressed renal transplant patients may have a similar (EBV)-aetiology.

As Mitchison pointed out, skin carcinoma is the second tumour form that shows a dramatic increase in immunosuppressed patients. The possibility of a viral aetiology must be considered here as well—u.v. (sunlight)—induction of highly antigenic, malignant epithelial cells is a conceivable alternative.

Concerning *TSTA-type antigens associated with chemically induced tumours*, Lennox reported further results (Chapter 37) obtained with his monoclonal antibodies, directed against two murine methylcholanthrene-sarcomas. In contrast to what has previously appeared, this antigen may be a highly variable form of C-virus determined gp 70 after all. The high variability, by mutation and by recombination, of the *env* gene product of the mouse oncorna virus systems may provide, at least theoretically, a basis for generating the necessary diversity. The evidence is not yet conclusive, however. The rat may provide a good species for comparison, since it is not infested with the same vast diversity of oncorna viruses as the mouse.

Lennox also showed, in agreement, with other reports, that the MC-TSTA is not related to H-2, biologically or biochemically.

In the *human tumour* area, important new data are being derived from the use of monoclonal antibodies. Several groups (10.1.24, 10.1.26, 10.1.28) described monoclonal antibodies that were specific for or at least highly reactive with human melanomas. It is still not clear whether the various antibodies identify qualitative or merely quantitative antigenic differences between melanoma and normal tissue. Nevertheless, the exchange of reagents and the increasing biochemical characterization of the target sites augurs well for rapid advances. On other human tumours, it was of particular interest to hear the report of Edgington and Leung (10.1.17) on an apparently tumour specific monoclonal antibody, reacting with a 53K membrane glycoprotein in human breast carcinoma.

There were a large number of papers that cannot be detailed here, on the incipient characterization of various tumour associated antigens, tissue or cell specific markers and oncofoetal antigens.

Effector mechanisms

Perhaps due to the disappointment with T cells as an all-encompassing surveillance mechanism, there was an enormous upsurge of interest in natural killer (NK) cells. When the pendulum has come back to equilibrium, it will probably turn out that NK cells represent one of several types of effectors that can act against some tumour cells. The involvement of the interferon (IF) system in triggering NK-cytotoxicity strengthens the suspicion that NK-cells may act as a "first line of defence" against virally infected targets. Bloom *et al.* and Blazar *et al.*, have previously shown this in a variety of virus systems. Here, Dubey *et al.* (10.8.05) have shown that feline sarcoma virus infection increases the NK sensitivity of human lymphoma lines. The NK-sensitivity of uninfected human and murine tumour cells provides a more erratic pattern. There are some regularities: certain types of tumours, e.g. T cell lymphomas, tend to show a high degree of NK-sensitivity. The work of the Stutman group (11.4.15,

11.4.43) has shown that there are different populations of naturally cytotoxic cells, with different genetic and age related distributions, that kill different types of tumours preferentially.

One of the foremost questions concerns the *in vivo* relevance of NK cells—most experiments have been carried out on *in vitro* systems. A new powerful tool has been introduced when John Roder described the selective NK-deficiency of the beige mouse. He now describes a similar NK-defect in the corresponding human disease (Chediak-Higashi Syndrome, 11.5.13). The report of Kärre *et al.* (10.2.17) showed that the beige mice are not only NK-deficient in the usual *in vitro* cytolytic test, but are also more susceptible to the *in vivo* growth of small inocula from NK-sensitive tumour lines than their immunologically normal syngeneic counterparts. This still does not tell us whether NK-cells are involved in protection against primary oncogenesis, but the presently ongoing tumour induction experiments in many laboratories will certainly give some hints. They will still have to be considered as hints, because the lysosomal defect of the beige mouse may affect oncogenesis at a nonimmunological level. It is therefore still important to test this question by alternative methods in parallel. H-2 and non-H-2 congenic mice differing in their NK activity provide another, independent alternative.

Many other reports testified of a diversification of the relevant effectors. Finlay-Jones *et al.* (10.7.09) reported on the role of both T cells and macrophages in the concomitant immunity of mice against a MC-sarcoma. A number of reports dealt with tumour infiltrating lymphocytes. The presence and activity of NK cells was quite controversial, but some workers, like Flannery *et al.* (10.2.08) found them present and active in chemically induced solid rat tumours. McKhann *et al.* (10.2.27) found a difference in effector preference, depending on the cell dose. While large cell doses from a MC-sarcoma could only be killed by the T cells of preimmunized mice, small cell numbers were effectively dealt with by a naturally occurring non-T effector.

In vitro tests may not always provide information on the relevant *in vivo* effector cells. This is exemplified by the report of Katacka *et al.* (10.2.18), finding no detectable killer T cells against antigenic guinea-pig tumours, in spite of positive Winn and blastogenesis tests.

It is often assumed that allograft killing of tumour cells must be necessarily mediated by T effectors. However, the report of Dan Cohen *et al.* (10.2.03), dealing with the transmissible canine venereal sarcoma, the only known naturally occurring tumour system propagated by cell transplantation showed that this allograft can induce a rejection response in resistant hosts that is mainly due to ADCC and monocytes. It is quite likely that the relative resistance of this tumour cell to cytotoxic T cells is partly or fully responsible for its ability to grow in allogeneic hosts.

Suppressors

The current tendency to attribute the absence of expected immunological reactivities to suppressors is a new occupational hazard in the field of tumour immunology. Reports indicating that not all forms of nonreactivity are due to suppressors are therefore of interest. Blank and Pincus (10.7.04) found that the nonresponsiveness of neonatally Gross-virus infected mice to their leukaemia cells is not due to suppressors, but to the clonal deletion of reactive T cells. The u.v.-skin carcinoma system continues to provide an outstanding case for suppressor mediation, as already mentioned. Fisher (10.3.13) showed that the situation is actually more complex, however, u.v.-irradiation was found to produce an X-ray resistant modification of the host that prevented rejection.

In a MC-sarcoma, Yamagishi *et al.* (10.1.56) reported the successful separation of an immunizing and an enhancing fraction by IEF. Both resistance and enhancement were adoptively transferable. Quite similar findings were made by Fujimoto and Yamanchi on a different tumour/mouse system (10.3.14). Their data also indicated that soluble antigens, shed from the tumour cell surface may be particularly active in inducing suppression.

A long-standing puzzle of tumour immunology, the "sneaking through" phenomenon, i.e. the ability of small tumour cell doses to grow in hosts that are perfectly capable to reject larger cell doses. The experiments of Gatenby and Creswick suggest that sneaking through can be attributed to suppressor T cells (10.3.15). Gabizon and Trainin (10.7.10) found that normal T cells can enhance a syngeneic T lymphoma—is this akin to the immunostimulation phenomenon of Prehn (Chapter 36)?

Naor *et al.* (10.7.23) reported a curious modulation in a Moloney-lymphoma, reproducible at will by back and forth passage between the mouse and the tissue culture bottle. While in *in vivo* form generated suppression, the *in vitro* form induced rejection. Both states were perfectly reversible. They used the YAC lymphoma, i.e. the prototype of the NK sensitive tumour cell. Is it conceivable that the *in vivo* form acts to suppress the NK-effector? The supprimability of the NK cell was actually demonstrated by Santoni *et al.* (10.7.26), in another system. Suppression could be attributed to activated macrophages.

Yefenof and Kedar (10.7.34) found an interesting difference between radiation induced and radiation leukaemia virus induced T cell lymphomas in the C57Bl mouse. Only the virus, not the radiation induced form was capable of generating cytotoxic lymphocytes and *also* suppressor cells—the radiation induced form generated neither. Ménard and Colnaghi (10.7.21) found that the level of natural antibodies against certain murine lymphoma cells was subject to T suppressor control in an unresponsive strain of mice.

Other escapes

Dormancy of tumour cells *in vivo* is one of the most striking features of certain human and animal neoplasms. Yet, its mechanisms are entirely unknown. If the tumour cells are antigenic and are presumably kept under control by immunological mechanisms, why are they not eliminated? The examples of polyoma in mice and EBV-transformed cells in man document the existence of an effective immune surveillance that protects the host against the uncontrolled proliferation of the transformed cells but falls short of complete elimination. Is antigenic modulation responsible? Only one paper dealt with this subject, using a model system. Weinhold and Wheelock (10.1.55) described a temporary, reversible modulation that could be attributed to a T cell mediated mechanism. Modulative (reversible) decreases in the sensitivity of tumour cells to *in vivo* rejection or to cytotoxic lymphocytes *in vitro* was also reported by Ioachim *et al.* (10.3.19) and by Palmer *et al.* (10.3.29) in different systems.

Only one paper dealt with cell cycle dependent variations in cytotoxic sensitivity to antibody and complement (10.3.27). Interestingly, the resistant phase of the cell cycle was different for different cell lines.

Stable antigenic losses were reported by Bosslet and Schirrmacher (10.3.04). A rejection-inducing tumour associated antigen could no longer be demonstrated in a spleen metastasizing variant of a chemically induced mouse lymphoma. The loss was stable in tissue culture. A different, although possibly related phenomenon was reported by de Baetselier *et al.* (10.3.09) showing a difference in the H-2 expression of metastatic and nonmetastatic sublines of the same original tumour.

A few reports dealt with the relationship between cell surfaces and rejectability. Churchill and Cameron (10.2.02) found a certain relationship between surface sialic acid content and tumour susceptibility to macrophage cytotoxicity. This represents an interesting contrast to earlier reports suggesting increased rejectability of cells deprived of surface sialic acid.

Immune complexes have often been implicated in the blocking of cell-mediated immunity. Carpentier *et al.* (10.3.06) reported considerable differences between metastatic and localized human breast carcinomas. Immune complexes dominated in the former, but it is not clear whether this represents a cause or a consequence of the biological difference. There is still no information on the postulated tumour relatedness —or otherwise—of the antigen component in this or any other immune complexes demonstrated in the sera of tumour patients. An immunochemical method that may permit such an analysis was reported by Gilead *et al.* (15.7.15).

We did not hear much about antibody induced enhancement, still a valid and powerful mechanism of tumour cell escape in experimental systems. However, several papers showed an increased immunoglobulin fixation on the surfaces of progressively growing human or animal tumours or, in some cases, metastatic or nonmetastatic tumours. There was no information on the specificity of the eluted antibodies, although they may represent an important tool to gain information on relevant tumour-associated antigens. In some cases they may be even more informative than monoclonal antibodies produced in foreign species.

Attempts to overcome immune unresponsiveness

Immune unresponsiveness to certain antigens, encountered on a given genetic background, is not a new problem in immunology. Modification of the antigen or coupling to well recognized antigens are some of the possibilities to overcome it. A variety of promising experiments have been presented along these and similar lines.

The Bach group (10.8.16) have supplied further evidence on the generation of cell-mediated immune responses against syngeneic murine leukaemia cells, following stimulation with a pool of allogeneic normal cells. On a human leukaemia system, analogous results were obtained by Gangal *et al.* (10.2.10). They showed that allogeneic stimuli can induce cytotoxicity against autochthonous leukaemia cells.

Kobayashi's group (10.4.11, 10.4.15) supplied further evidence on the efficiency of the "viral xenogenization" technique, to increase the immunogenicity of weakly antigenic tumours. Boon *et al.* (10.4.04) showed that highly antigenic variants could be treated by mutagenizing a low antigenic teratoma. The variants were capable of immunizing syngeneic hosts against the original tumour. Fioretti *et al* (10.4.10) showed that drug modified tumour cells can generate cytotoxic lymphocytes capable of inhibiting the original, unmodified tumour.

Somatic hybrids could also be used for similar purposes. Immunization with allogeneic hybrids has led to protection against weakly antigenic, syngeneic methylcholanthrene induced sarcoma cells (10.2.32). Interestingly, better effects were obtained in the Winn test than in the usual *in vivo* immunization/challenge experiments. The latter was attributed to the generation of suppressor cells. Baumal and Marks (10.4.02) reported that immunization with a hybridoma can protect against the weakly antigenic myeloma parent.

Clinical and experimental immunotherapy

Most experiments were concerned with nonspecific adjuvant therapy although some dealt with specific approaches. Of particular interest was the report of Grant and Norouba (10.8.07), showing regression of feline sarcoma virus induced solid tumours in 18 of 19 cases, after passive administration of anti-FOCMA antibodies. None of the untreated controls regressed spontaneously. Regression was maintained in spite of the fact that some of the regressor cats remained viremic. This raises some new questions about the role of cytotoxic antibodies, alone or in combination with an ADCC effect, against solid tumours. Monoclonal antibodies, directed against T cell associated differentiation antigens, were found to have a certain therapeutic effect in the study of Kirch and Hammerling (10.5.41).

The group of Rapp *et al.* (10.5.07) have applied their previous experimental system, based on the intralesional administration of BCG, combined with a cell wall preparation, to human head and neck carcinomas. They report encouraging but statistically not yet significant effects on survival. Intralesional injection of BCG into human lung tumours was found to induce functionally active T cells locally by Golub *et al.* (10.5.25). The effectiveness of PPD coupled tumour cells, in inducing rejection reactions against a syngeneic, noncoupled tumour in the presence of PPD reactive T cells, an approach pioneered by Lachmann, was supported by the report of Hamaoka *et al.* (10.5.28). The combination of nonspecific (BCG) and specific (tumour cell derived) immunotherapy gave encouraging results in the hands of Hanna *et al.*, in an experimental system (10.5.30).

Epilogue

In his article in "Immunology Today", distributed to all Congress participants, Gustav Nossal asks whether Tumour Immunology (Mr TI) is a terminal patient or still curable. Surely, this must be a case of mistaken identities. TI is not a patient at all. He is still a youngster who had a very complicated childhood. He was born like the hero of the Finnish national epos, Kalevala, the great poet Vejnemöjnen, after an immensely prolonged pregnancy. Vejnemöjnen was 600 years old at birth—TI was not quite that old but like V, he was regarded old and wise already in the cradle. Expectations were therefore enormous. He was pressured, pushed and pulled in all directions. Oscillations of great praise and even greater blame arrested his development. He became like little Oskar in the Tin Drum of Günther Grass. Sometimes he would scream at the top of his shrill voice so that all windows would break. At other time he would just sit, sullen, sour, and silent. He failed to grow normally.

What will happen next? Returning to an idyllic childhood on the quiet French countryside, under the tender loving care of an affectionate family is, by now, clearly out of the question. Let us hope that TI will go on to develop like a French intellectual of the postwar generation. Emerging from many intellectual and emotional conflicts, he will settle down to a more reflective existence. He will not forget his cultural heritage, but he will find practical solutions to seemingly impossible problems. Like our French intellectual friends of the postwar generation did when they arranged this marvellous Congress.

Theme 11

Natural Immunity and Macrophages

Presidents:
B. R. BLOOM
G. CUDKOWICZ
P. H. LAGRANGE

Symposium Chairman:
D. S. NELSON

39

Natural Cell-mediated Cytotoxicity

R. B. HERBERMAN, T. TIMONEN, J. R. ORTALDO, G. D. BONNARD and E. GORELIK

National Cancer Institute, Bethesda, Maryland, USA

Introduction

The phenomenon of cytotoxicity of tumour cells and of cultured cell lines derived from tumours by lymphocytrs of many normal individuals first became

Abbreviations
NK cell, natural killer cell; NC cell, natural cytotoxic cell; ADCC, antibody-dependent cell-mediated cytotoxicity; E rosettes, rosettes with sheep erythrocytes; $Fc_\gamma R$, receptors, receptors for the Fc portion of IgG; LGL, large granular lymphocytes; ly, conventional lymphocytes; T_G cells, T cells with $Fc_\gamma R$; IFN, interferon; BCG, bacillus Calmette-Guerin; poly I:C, poly inosinic: poly cytidylic acid; CTC, cultured T cells.

recognized during the course of studies attempting to examine specific cytotoxic activity of lymphocytes of tumour-bearing individuals against their own tumours or against tumours of the same histologic or aetiologic type. It was initially assumed in those studies that lymphoid cells from normal individuals would be unreactive and thus would serve as good baseline controls for comparison. However, it gradually became apparent that lymphocytes of some normal controls were actually more cytotoxic against some target cells than were the tumour-bearing individuals under study. Many investigators first attributed this anomalous control reactivity to a variety of *in vitro* artifacts (see discussion in Herberman and Gaylord, 1973), but it has subsequently been reasonably well established that much or all of this was due to natural cytotoxic cells. These findings have necessitated a re-evaluation of supposed disease-related cytotoxic reactivity of cancer patients, with a need to discriminate clearly between the activity of NK cells and of more specific immune effector cells (Herberman and Oldham, 1975).

The most extensively studied and characterized natural effector cell in man and rodents has come to be called a natural killer (NK) cell. This chapter will summarize the existing information with an emphasis on recent findings from our laboratory. It should be noted, however, that other types of natural effector cells have been found and these may also have important *in vivo* roles. Other natural effector cells include: (a) natural cytotoxic (NC) cells (Stutman *et al.*, 1980) in mice, that react primarily against monolayer cultures of solid tumour cells; (b) macrophages or monocytes from normal individuals, that may show considerable cytotoxic activity against tumour target cells in 48–72 h assays (Keller, 1980; Mantovani *et al.*, 1980); (c) K cells and macrophages or monocytes that can interact with natural antibodies to tumour cells, and thereby mediate antibody-dependent cell-mediated cytotoxicity (ADCC); and (d) granulocytes from normal individuals, that have been found to have cytostatic activity against a wide range of tumour target cells (Korec, 1980). For more details on NK cells and information on other aspects of natural cell-mediated immunity, the reader might consult recent reviews (e.g. Herberman and Holden, 1978; Herberman *et al.*, 1979a) and a new comprehensive book on this subject (Herberman, 1980).

Characteristics of NK cells

NK cells have generally been found to be nonadherent and nonphagocytic and therefore are considered to be a subpopulation of lymphocytes and not macrophages or monocytes. On the basis of initial cell separation studies, NK cells appeared to be null cells, i.e. lacking characteristic markers of either T cells or B cells. They clearly appear to be distinct from mature T cells, since high levels of NK activity have been found in nude or neonatally thymectomized mice. However, by using more sensitive techniques, evidence has accumulated for some association of NK cells with the T cell lineage. There have also been some suggestions that NK cells may be promonocytes (for detailed discussion, see Herberman, 1980).

Expression of T cell associated markers

In mice and humans, NK cells have been found to have several markers that suggest some relationship to T cells, possibly being early prethymic cells of the T cell lineage (summarized in Herberman, 1980). Each of these markers has been detected on at least a portion of NK cells and appears to be strongly associated with peripheral T cells. By using optimal conditions for the formation of rosettes with sheep erythrocytes (E rosette), 50–80% of human NK cells were found to have low affinity receptors for E (West *et al.*, 1977). As a further recent indication that human NK cells reside in the T cell lineage, treatment with specific anti-T cell sera plus complement caused virtual elimination of cytotoxic activity (Kaplan and Callewaert, 1978). In mice, it has been shown that treatment with high concentrations of anti-Thy-1 plus complement, or repeated treatments, eliminated most NK activity (Mattes *et al.*, 1979). In addition, it has been possible to select positively for a portion of NK cells from nude or conventional mice, using a monoclonal anti-Thy-1 antibody and the fluorescence activated cell sorter (Mattes *et al.*, 1979). Similarly, Koo and Hatzfeld (1980) have reported that monoclonal antibodies to Ly-1 can react with about 25% of mouse NK cells. Thus, it appears that at least some human and mouse NK cells have characteristic markers of the T cell lineage.

Expression of Fc_γ receptors and relationship to K cells

Another surface marker on NK cells is the $Fc_\gamma R$ (receptor for Fc portion of IgG). $Fc_\gamma R$ are readily detected on human NK cells and methods which deplete $Fc_\gamma R^+$ cells result in virtual elimination of NK activity. In mice and rats, NK cells initially appeared to lack $Fc_\gamma R$. However, when more sensitive depletion procedures were used, more than half of the NK lytic units were removed (Herberman *et al.*, 1977a; Oehler *et al.*, 1978a). The finding of $Fc_\gamma R$ on NK cells of each of the species studied raised questions about the relationship between NK cells and K cells mediating ADCC. One possible explanation for NK activity is that it is produced by K cells, which are "armed" with *in vivo* bound natural antibodies (Koide and Takasugi, 1977), or which react against target cells that become coated with antibodies secreted during the *in vitro* assay (Troye *et al.*, 1977). However, extensive studies in our laboratory and in some others have failed to confirm that IgG is involved in natural cell-mediated cytotoxicity (Herberman, 1980). Despite this, the NK and K cells appear to be in the same subpopulation of lymphocytes and share many characteristics. On the basis of experiments in which some target cells sensitive to NK activity were able to inhibit ADCC, it appears that NK and ADCC activities may be mediated by the same cells. It may be that the same cell can produce cytotoxic effects either by interaction with antibody-coated target cells via its $Fc_{\gamma}R$ or with some target cells via separate "NK receptors".

Expression of markers restricted to NK cells

In almost all studies of NK cells, the effector cells have been defined by their functional characteristics. However, for detailed studies of this population, it would be very helpful to identify markers that are restricted to, or are at least highly associated with, NK cells. In the mouse, several recent studies have described NK cell-associated surface antigens. If one or more of these antigens can be documented to be completely restricted to NK cells and their immediate precursors, we would have a powerful tool for enumerating and isolating them. NK 1·1 (Glimcher *et al.*, 1977), a similar NK alloantigen described by Burton (1980), and Qa-4 and Qa-5 (Koo and Hatzfeld, 1980) have thus far only been demonstrated on NK cells. Treatment of mouse spleen cells with antisera to these markers have been useful for almost complete depletion, or enrichment, of NK cells. In contrast, these reagents have not affected cytotoxic T cells or the few other functional or morphological cell types examined. However, it still needs to be documented that only NK cells, and interferon-inducible pre-NK cells, have these markers.

Ly-5 antigen appears to be present on most, or all mouse NK cells and thereby has been a useful marker for some detailed studies of differentiation of effector cells (Bloom *et al.*, 1980). However, this marker does not appear to be particularly selective for NK cells, being expressed on some cells of most types with haematopoietic origin (Scheid and Triglia, 1979). Also, since most investigators have found that anti-Ly-5 without complement can inhibit NK activity, it seems unlikely that this marker will be of use for positive selection of NK cells.

Antibodies to the cell surface ganglioside, asialo GM1, at low concentrations appear to be quite selective for mouse NK cells (Kasai *et al.*, 1980; Durdik *et al.*, 1980; Gidlund *et al.*, 1980). However, this marker is not entirely restricted to NK cells, since higher concentrations of antibody also inhibit cytotoxic T cells (Gidlund *et al.*, 1980).

Large granular lymphocytes

Although several of the above markers on mouse NK cells appear quite promising for selective depletion of cytotoxic activity, none has yet been shown to provide the basis for purification of NK cells. In contrast, some recent findings with human and rat NK cells have indicated that isolation of this effector cell population can be achieved. Timonen *et al.* (1979) found that the majority of human lymphocytes binding to NK-sensitive target cells and thereby forming conjugates were large lymphocytes with an indented nucleus and prominent azurophilic granules in the cytoplasm (large granular lymphocytes, LGL). It has been possible to enrich for LGL on discontinuous Percoll density gradients (Saksela and Timonen, 1980) and we have recently used this procedure to better characterize human NK cells (Herberman *et al.*, 1980b). Most of the NK and also ADCC activity has been found in the fractions with 75–85% LGL, whereas these fractions contained only 10–20% of the input peripheral blood lymphocytes (Fig. 1). In contrast, the fractions containing most of the small-medium lymphocytes have been virtually devoid of NK or ADCC activity. Thus, this procedure consistently results in at least 5-fold enrichment of NK and ADCC activities. The possibility that the LGL are responsible for the cytotoxic activity has been supported by observations that about 50% of the LGL can form conjugates with K-562 (a highly

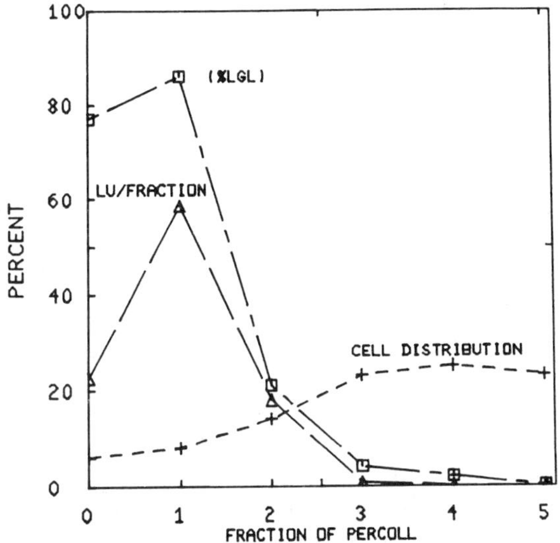

FIG. 1. *Separation of human peripheral blood nonadherent mononuclear cells on discontinuous Percoll density gradient. Distribution among the fractions of cells, LGL and NK activity (as LU/fraction) are shown.*

NK-sensitive target) or antibody-coated target cells and that most of these conjugate-forming LGL have the capacity to kill the attached target cells. Furthermore, almost all LGL were found to contain $Fc_{\gamma}R$, as measured by adherence to monolayers of immune complexes (Herberman *et al.*, 1980b). The combination of Percoll gradient centrifugation and monolayer adsorption procedures has yielded fractions containing 90% LGL and most of the NK activity of the input population.

LGL could also be discriminated from other lymphocytes by rosetting with E (Table I). About 50% of the LGL had low affinity E receptors, forming rosettes at 4° but not at 29°, and the remainder lacked detectable receptors. In contrast, most other nylon-nonadherent lymphocytes (ly) had high affinity E receptors, rosetting at 29° as well as at 4°. This has provided the basis for an alternative procedure for further purification of NK cells (Timonen *et al.*,

1980). Removal of high affinity E rosette forming cells from the LGL-containing Percoll fractions resulted in a subpopulation highly enriched for LGL and NK activity. Even with rosetting at 4°, 33% or less of the LGL-formed rosettes stable enough to result in their sedimentation into pellets upon Ficoll-Hypaque centrifugation.

TABLE I

Receptors for sheep erythrocytes and Fc_γ on LGL and on other lymphocytes

		% *E rosette-forming cells*			
Fraction	% *LGL*	*LGL, 4°*	*LGL, 29°*	*LY, 4°*	*LY, 29°*
Unseparated	14	57	10	95	84
$Fc_\gamma R+$	42	53	15	81	76
$Fc_\gamma R-$	1	—	—	97	89

These studies on separation of lymphocytes have also defined two morphologically distinct subpopulations of cells with $Fc_\gamma R$ and E receptors (and thus T_G cells). This was accompanied by a functional division, with only the T_G cells with LGL morphology having NK and ADCC activities. It will now be important to determine the distribution between the two cell types of other immune functions that have been associated with T_G cells, particularly suppressor activity.

Rat NK cells in spleen and peripheral blood also appear to be LGL and can be enriched by a procedure similar to that used for human cells (Reynolds *et al.*, 1980). In contrast, LGL have not been detectable in mouse spleens or peripheral blood and the mouse NK cell has not yet been found to have any special morphological features that would distinguish it from other lymphocytes.

Specificity of NK cells

An important issue to be considered is the specificity of natural cytotoxicity. Most of the early studies of rodent NK cells utilized leukaemia or lymphoma target cells and it was initially thought that only these cells were sensitive to NK activity. However, many of the initial observations on human NK were made with monolayer cell lines derived from carcinomas. Such data would suggest that NK cells might actually have a wide range of reactivity. This has been confirmed by extensive studies of the susceptibility of a wide variety of cells to NK activity (Herberman and Ortoldo, 1980). Some sarcomas and carcinomas have been found to be sensitive to NK activity, including some human primary tumours and cell lines. *In vitro* cell lines of tumours have usually been more susceptible to lysis by NK cells, but some *in vivo* tumour cells have also been susceptible. Although it initially appeared that NK reactivity was restricted to target cells of the same species, mouse and rat NK cells have been found to have activity against some human cell lines (Haller *et al.*, 1977). Reactivity of human NK cells against rodent target cells appears to occur less frequently. NK activity has also been shown not to be restricted to tumour cells, with some types of normal cells having some sensitivity to lysis (Herberman and Ortaldo, 1980; Nunn *et al.*, 1977).

Given this rather wide spectrum of reactivity for NK cells, the question then arises as to whether a single NK receptor reacts rather indiscriminately against all of the susceptible target cells or whether there is a variety of NK receptors with specificity for an array of possible antigens on target cells. There are several lines of evidence to support the latter possibility of recognition by NK cells of at least several broad antigenic specificities. Many of the data in this regard were obtained by the cold target inhibition assay. This assay consists of addition of various unlabelled target cells to the mixture of effector cells and ^{51}Cr-labelled target cells. Cells which can interact with the same NK cells mediating lysis of the labelled target cells will completely inhibit ^{51}Cr release. When different labelled target cells are used in such studies, varying patterns of inhibition are seen. Some cells which can strongly inhibit lysis of one target have little or no inhibitory activity for other target cells. In addition, there are some major differences in the reactivity of NK cells from different mouse strains against some target cells but not against others. Also, in view of the strong parallels between mouse NK cells and the cells mediating *in vivo* bone marrow resistance (Kiessling *et al.*, 1977), it seems likely that NK cells can specifically recognize the genetically determined Hh histocompatibility antigens.

More direct evidence for heterogeneity among NK cells in their ability to recognize various target cells has come from studies with human NK cells after selective adsorption of confluent monolayers of target cells, using a recently developed technique (Landazuri *et al.*, 1979). PBL from normal human donors were incubated on monolayers of 5 different NK-susceptible cell lines and the nonadherent cells were then tested for residual cytotoxicity against each of the targets (Herberman and Ortaldo, 1980). We found that virtually all reactivity could be removed against each of the adsorbing cell lines, but with 5 of the donors the selectively adsorbed cells still had considerable reactivity against one or more of the other target cells. These data appear to demonstrate that NK cells can recognize a variety of specificities on target cells and, furthermore, that recognition structure on NK cells are clonally distributed.

Factors affecting levels of NK and K cell activities

In mice and rats, the levels of NK and K cell activities follow a characteristic age-related pattern. Reactivity first appears at 3–4 weeks of age, reaches peak levels between 5 and 10 weeks of age, and then declines to low levels thereafter.

There are also considerable differences in levels of activity among various strains (Herberman, 1980). In man, NK activity is not so clearly age-related, with activity being found even in some cord blood samples. However, normal human donors do vary considerably in their levels of reactivity and some of this has been shown to be influenced by the HLA phenotype (Santoli *et al.*, 1976). It has been of considerable interest to determine the mechanisms responsible for the age-related and genetic differences and whether environmental factors may influence this activity. Some clues were initially obtained by observations that inoculation of mice with a variety of viruses, immune adjuvants such as BCG or *Corynebacterium parvum*, or tumour cells susceptible to NK activity, could induce a rapid and strong augmentation of reactivity (Herberman *et al.*, 1977b; Wolfe *et al.*, 1976). The finding that rat NK activity could be strongly boosted by poly I:C (Oehler *et al.*, 1978b), a potent interferon inducer, raised the possibility that interferon might play a central role in activating NK cells.

Augmentation of NK activity by interferon (IFN)

A variety of IFN-inducers has been found to augment NK activity in mice and inoculation of IFN itself led to boosting of activity within 3 h (Djeu *et al.*, 1979; Gidlund *et al.*, 1978). Incubation of mouse spleen cells with poly I:C or with IFN also has resulted in appreciable increases in NK activity. Similar observations have been made with human NK and K cells (Trinchieri and Santoli, 1978; Herberman *et al.*, 1978, 1979a, b). Administration of poly I:C to some patients resulted in increased levels of cytotoxicity after 2 days. Incubation of human peripheral blood lymphocytes with 3 different IFN preparations for 1 h or 18 h caused increased NK and K cell activities with most donors. The mediation of these effects by IFN has been supported in both mouse and human studies by demonstration that anti-IFN antibodies could eliminate the boosting effects by either the IFN preparations or poly I:C (Djeu *et al.*, 1979). In addition, in the human studies, high concentrations of the anti-IFN antibodies have caused the levels of NK and ADCC activities to decrease below spontaneous levels. Such data have suggested that IFN may be important in the spontaneous activation of these effector cells, or at least in the maintenance of their activities.

During the course of the above studies, there remained some concern as to whether IFN was indeed the molecule responsible for augmenting cytotoxic activity, since the antiviral substance in all the preparations was actually less than 1–10% of the total protein. To determine more definitely the role of IFN, we have recently had the opportunity to perform experiments with pure human leukocyte IFN (Rubinstein *et al.*, 1979). Incubation of human lymphocytes with this homogeneous protein for 1 h at 37°C resulted in substantial augmentation of NK activity, thus confirming the role of IFN in positive regulation of NK activity (Herberman *et al.*, 1980a).

The ability to separate LGL from conventional lymphocytes on Percoll gradients and to measure binding of lymphoid cells to NK-susceptible targets has allowed detailed examination of the interaction between effector cells and targets and of the mechanisms for augmentation of NK activity by IFN. One series of issues was whether only LGL formed conjugates with K562 and whether only this subpopulation could be activated for NK activity by IFN. There have been several previous indications for pre-NK cells that can be induced by IFN (e.g. Oehler *et al.*, 1978b; Bloom *et al.*, 1980) and these precursors may have some characteristics that differ from those associated with spontaneously active NK cells. Therefore, Percoll separated fractions of LGL and of conventional lymphocytes, with or without pretreatment by IFN, were tested for conjugate formation with K562 (Fig. 2). In addition to considerable

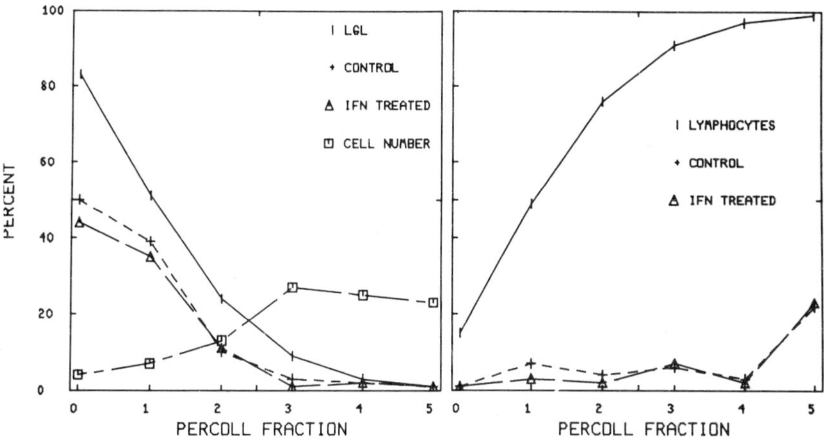

FIG. 2. *Conjugate formation of Percoll separated cells, at 1 : 1 ratio, with K562. Left: distribution of total cells, LGL and conjugate-forming LGL (with or without pretreatment with IFN). Right: distribution of total conventional lymphocytes and of those forming conjugates (with of without pretreatment with IFN).*

conjugate formation by LGL, some conventional lymphocytes (fraction 5) also formed conjugates. However, this was not unaccompanied by any detectable cytotoxic activity, even after pretreatment with IFN. These data indicate that both active NK cells and IFN-inducible precursors are LGL and that the conventional lymphocytes forming conjugates with K562 cells are not directly related to NK cells.

Another important question has been the mechanism for augmentation of NK activity by IFN. IFN was found substantially to increase the reactivity of LGL as well as unseparated lymphoid cells (Fig. 3), indicating that IFN can act directly on NK cells and cause augmentation of activity, without the need for accessory cells. Measurements of the kinetics of cytotoxicity also indicated that augmentation by IFN could be detected during the first hour of the assay. However, such cytotoxicity experiments failed to provide insight into which step or steps in the cytotoxic process were affected by IFN. Three

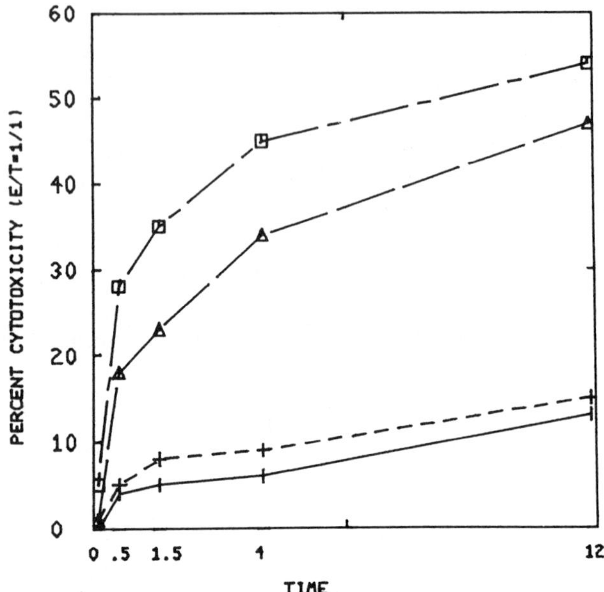

FIG. 3. *Kinetics of cytotoxicity of nonadherent human mononuclear cells, untreated* (*I*) *or pretreated for 1 h with 1000 U IFN* (+); *and of Percoll LGL fractions, untreated* (△) *or IFN-pretreated* (□).

main possibilities were considered: (a) induction on pre-NK cells of receptors for recognition of NK-susceptible targets; (b) triggering of the lytic machinery of conjugate-forming inactive NK cells; and (c) augmentation of the activity of already active NK cells. Measurement of conjugate formation by LGL provided a means to examine the first possibility directly. The treatment of LGL with IFN did not increase the proportion of cells forming conjugates with K562 (Fig. 2), indicating that the augmenting effects of IFN are beyond the induction of recognition receptors on LGL. To examine which of the other possibilities for IFN action were involved, we have performed experiments with the single cell agarose assay, developed by Grimm and Bonavida (1979). This method allows one to determine directly the proportion of conjugate-forming cells that produce lysis of their attached targets. During the first 4 h of the interaction between LGL and K562 (Fig. 4), both the rate of lysis and the proportion of active conjugate-forming cells were higher for the IFN-treated cells. However, with further incubation, the proportion of targets lysed by the untreated effectors approached or sometimes equalled that affected by the IFN-treated LGL. These data imply that IFN acts mainly to accelerate the rate of lysis by already active NK cells. However, since contact with target cells can induce LGL to produce IFN (Saksela *et al.*, 1980), the possibility remains that the late rise in the proportion of active NK cells in the control group was due to activation by the endogenously produced IFN. Another important point to note from the data in Fig. 4 is that a high proportion of

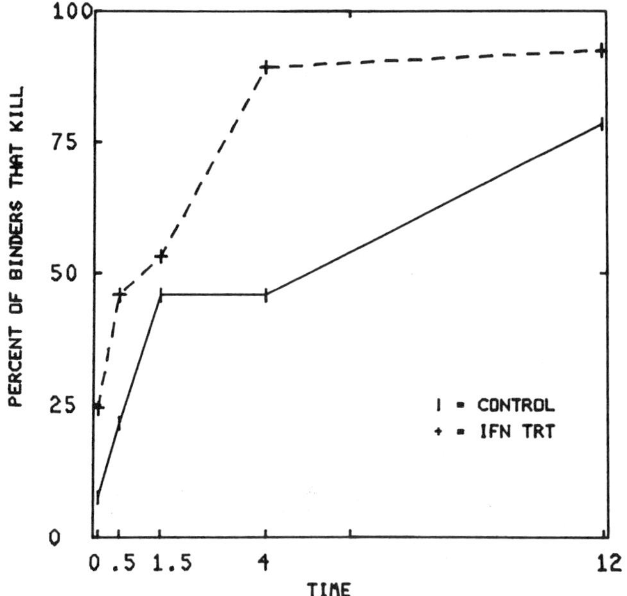

FIG. 4. *Kinetics of cytotoxicity in single cell agarose assay of untreated and IFN-treated Percoll separated LGL. The proportion of LGL forming conjugate with K562 (binders) that caused lysis of their attached targets at various times is shown.*

conjugate-forming LGL, often greater than 90%, have the ability to act as NK cells. Thus, not only are virtually all NK cells in the LGL population, but a substantial proportion of LGL (about 50%) can act as NK cells against one sensitive target cell. It remains to be determined whether many of the LGL that fail to bind and lyse K562 have reactivity against other NK-sensitive target cells. The results described above for the monolayer adsorption experiments suggest that this may indeed be the case.

Genetic regulation of NK activity

A most intriguing finding concerning the genetic regulation of mouse NK activity was reported by Roder and Duwe (1979), which indicated that the *beige* point mutation was associated with a selective and severe deficiency in NK activity. We have subsequently found that beige mice have some residual NK activity at levels similar to those of low NK strains, and IFN treatments of spleen cells from beige mice produce some augmentation of activity (Brunda *et al.*, 1980). Although the beige mutation does not result in complete loss in NK activity, the selective deficit associated with this gene may provide an important clue to the mechanisms involved in this form of cell-mediated cytotoxicity. Since the beige mutation in mice produces abnormalities analogous to the human Chediak-Higashi syndrome, we have recently studied two such patients, in collaboration with Drs John Roder and Anthony Fauci

(Roder *et al.*, 1980). These patients had markedly depressed NK activity when tested in a 4-h assay against the highly NK-susceptible target cell line K562, and they had a comparable depression in ADCC activity. As with beige mice, this deficit was also seen after pretreatment of the cells with IFN, or when tested in a longer term assay. However, the patients with Chediak-Higashi syndrome appeared to have a more profound defect in NK reactivity than the beige mice and it is intriguing to note that this syndrome has been associated with a high incidence of lymphoproliferative disease (Dent *et al.*, 1966). An important clue to the nature of the defective NK activity in the Chediak-Higashi patients has come from the observation that preincubation of lymphocytes with the cyclic nucleotide, guanosine monophosphate, caused an increase in reactivity to normal levels (Katz *et al.*, 1980).

Cytotoxicity by cultured T cells

A major limitation for detailed analysis of the characteristics and specificity of NK cells is that these cells only represent a small portion of the lymphoid cells in the blood or spleen (probably less than 1–2%). Even with the development of satisfactory isolation procedures, like the methods for enrichment of LGL, the low yield of cells imposes serious restrictions on the studies that can be performed. It would therefore be highly desirable to be able to propagate NK cells and expand them to large numbers. A further potential advantage in the growth of NK cells would be the ability to directly test our hypothesis of polyclonality of NK cells, with differing specificities.

During the past few years, it has become possible to propagate human or mouse T cells in the presence of T cell growth factor (Morgan *et al.*, 1976). Cultured T cells (CTC) from normal human donors were found to have considerable cytotoxic activity against a wide array of target cells (Alvarez *et al.*, 1978; Bonnard *et al.*, 1978; Schendel *et al.*, 1980). Since K562 was one of the target cells that were susceptible to lysis by CTC, we have investigated

TABLE II
Cytotoxicity by cultured T cells from human PBL

	Target cells			
			Mouse lymphoma	
Conditions	*K562*	*Alloblast*	*+Antibody*	*+PHA*
CTC above	+	+	+	+
+ protein A	=	=	↓	
+ IFN	↑	=	↑	↑
+ cold targets	↓	↓		
	only by homologous targets			

the possibility that at least some of the cytotoxicity was due to propagation of NK cells. In detailed studies on the nature of cytotoxicity by human CTC, we have obtained indications for 4 separate types of activity (Ortaldo *et al.*, 1980; Ortaldo, 1980), that are summarized in Table II: (a) cytotoxicity against K562 target cells; (b) cytotoxicity against allogeneic but not autologous or histocompatible mitogen-induced lymphoblasts; (c) ADCC against antibody-coated mouse lymphoma cells: and (d) lectin-induced cytotoxicity against the mouse lymphoma cells. The cytotoxicity against K562 and the alloblasts was distinguishable by the augmentation of only the former activity by pretreatment of CTC with IFN. Furthermore, in cold target inhibition experiments, unlabelled K562 could strongly inhibit lysis of ^{51}Cr-labelled K562, but did not appreciably affect lysis of labelled alloblasts. Conversely, unlabelled alloblasts only inhibited the lysis of labelled alloblasts. It seems likely that the activity against alloblasts was due to polyclonally activated cytotoxic T cells (Schendel *et al.*, 1980) and that the effectors for K562 were of a different nature and specificity. The possibility that the anti-K562 activity was due to NK cells was supported by the parallel findings of reactivity against antibody-coated targets. This appeared to be true ADCC by K cells since addition of protein A selectively blocked this reaction, as was previously demonstrated for ADCC (Kay *et al.*, 1979). The fourth type of cytotoxicity, in the presence of PHA, resulted in substratial cytotoxicity against the ordinarily resistant mouse lymphoma target cell.

The finding of apparent NK activity in CTC was encouraging and was consistent with our hypothesis of the T cell lineage of NK cells. However, the heterogeneity of effector cells in CTC interfered with the possible use of such cells for detailed studies of NK cells. To circumvent this heterogeneity, we have attempted to initiate cultures from Percoll-separated fractions of lymphocytes from normal human donors. The LGL-containing fractions (0 and 1), as well as the fractions with conventional lymphocytes (4 and 5), have proliferated in the presence of T cell growth factor. The CTC from fractions 0–1 maintained substantial levels of IFN-augmentable cytotoxic activity against K562 and antibody-coated target cells. In contrast, the CTC from the fractions containing conventional lymphocytes had little or no activity against these targets., even after pretreatment with IFN. Thus it appears promising that selected effector cell populations can be expanded by this procedure. We have recently initiated cultures from LGL-enriched fractions, further purified by removal of high affinity E-rosette forming cells. After 7–14 days, almost all of the cells in the cultures had the morphology of LGL. Studies are now in progress to evaluate the cytotoxicity of these cultures and to obtain clones of growing LGL.

In other laboratories, a few clones of mouse CTC, with cell surface characteristics of NK cells, have already been obtained (Dennert, 1980; H. Cantor, pers. comm.). The clones from the two laboratories differed in specificity, supporting the concept of heterogeneity of NK cells. Clones of mouse and human CTC have also been obtained in our laboratory (E. Kedar and N.

Navarro, unpub. observations) and intensive effeorts are now being made to characterize the phenotype and specificity of these cells. Hopefully, we will soon have documentation of proliferating cloned populations of NK cells that should be invaluable for analysis of the specificity of these effector cells and the nature of their interaction with target cells.

in vivo role of NK cells

The most important practical issue to be settled is the role of NK cells *in vivo*. There is increasing evidence that NK cells may play an important role in resistance against tumour growth and also in rejection of bone marrow transplants (summarized by Herberman and Holden, 1979).

Rapid *in vivo* clearance of radiolabelled tumour cells

To obtain more direct information about the role of NK cells in rapid *in vivo* elimination of tumour cells, we have recently examined the correlation between levels of NK activity and the ability of mice to destroy intravenously inoculated tumours that were prelabelled with ^{125}I-iododeoxyuridine (Riccardi *et al.*, 1979, 1980b, c). In young mice of strains with high NK activity, there was a greater decrease in recovery of radioactivity when measured in various organs at 2–4 h after inoculation than was seen in strains with low NK activity. Of the various organs examined, the degree of *in vivo* clearance of tumour cells from the lungs correlated best with levels of NK activity in the spleen. Recovery of radioactivity from the lungs of young mice with intermediate to high levels of NK activity was several fold less than that seen in strains with low NK activity. Such findings led to the prediction that NK cells could be isolated from the lungs, and indeed it has been possible to detect effector cells with the characteristics of NK cells in cell suspensions prepared by mincing of lung tissues (Puccetti *et al.*, 1980). The levels of NK activity detected in the lungs have been similar to those in the spleen and thus have also correlated well with the degree of *in vivo* clearance from the lungs. This occurrence of NK reactivity in the lungs and the ability to rapidly eliminate tumour cells from this organ raise the interesting possibility that NK cells may play a particularly important role in resistance against metastatic spread of tumours.

In parallel with the decline of NK activity in mice after 10–12 weeks of age, *in vivo* clearance of intravenously inoculated tumour cells was also found to decrease (Riccardi *et al.*, 1979, 1980b, d). Furthermore, a variety of treatments of mice that produced augmented or decreased *in vitro* reactivity also resulted in similar shifts in *in vivo* reactivity. Thus, this *in vivo* assay has correlated very well with NK cell reactivity against a variety of established tumour cell lines.

As further confirmation of the role of NK cells play in the resistance to growth of NK-susceptible transplantable tumours, transfer of NK cells into mice with cyclophosphamide-induced depression of NK activity was shown significantly to restore both *in vivo* and NK reactivities (Riccardi *et al.*, 1980a). The effectiveness of the transfer correlated with the levels of NK activity of donor cells in a variety of situations: (a) NK-reactive spleen cells were able to transfer reactivity whereas NK-unreactive thymus cells were ineffective; (b) spleen cells from young mice of high NK strains were considerably more effective than cells from older mice or from strains with low NK activity; (c) the cells responsible for transfer had the characteristics of NK cells, being nonadherent, nonphagocytic and lacking easily detectable Thy-1 antigen; and (d) cells from donors with drug-induced depression of NK activity were unable to transfer reactivity. These results extend the recent findings of Hanna and Fidler (1980), who showed the transfer of NK-reactive spleen cells to cyclophosphamide-treated mice could decrease the number of metastases developing in the lungs after challenge with NK-susceptible solid tumour cells.

In vivo reactivity against normal cells

It has been shown that NK cells can also lyse some normal cells such as subpopulations of bone marrow and thymus cells (Nunn *et al.*, 1977; Welsh *et al.*, 1979; Hansson *et al.*, 1979). To determine whether natural reactivity against normal cells could also occur *in vivo*, we have tested both *in vivo* and *in vitro* reactivities of normal mice against bone marrow cells and foetal fibroblasts (Riccardi *et al.*, 1980c). As with tumour targets, young mice of high NK strains rapidly eliminated a higher proportion of these normal cells than did older mice or those of a low NK strain. Furthermore, both *in vivo* and *in vitro* reactivities against these targets were modulated in parallel by NK-augmenting or depressing treatments.

Role of NK cells against primary tumours

It will be particularly important now to obtain information about the possible *in vivo* role of NK cells in resistance against primary tumours. The original formulations of the theory of immune surveillance focused on the central role of the immune response as a natural defence against neoplasia. Only more recently has the theory been modified to stress the relationship of thymus-dependent immunity to immune surveillance. It has been this modification of the theory which has aroused a series of criticisms of the concept of immune surveillance, and which even led to a counter theory of immune stimulation. Much attention has been directed towards two apparent contradictions to the theory of immune surveillance, the relatively low incidence of tumours in nude mice and the failure of some tumours to develop in thymectomized mice. Although these data do challenge the modified concept of immune surveillance, in which thymus-dependent immunological reactions are required for effective anti-tumour resistance, they do not really bear on the basic theory itself. The discovery that nude mice and neonatally thymectomized mice and rats have high levels of NK and ADCC activities, potentially very effective alternative mechanisms for immune surveillance, provides a good explanation for most of the available *in vivo* data.

The available information on the incidence of tumours in immunodeficient or immunosuppressed humans has also engendered controversy regarding the role of immune surveillance. With some forms of depressed immunity, the incidence of some types of tumours, especially those of the reticuloendothelial system, has been clearly increased. However, in other diseases associated with immune depression, e.g. leprosy, an increased incidence of cancer has not been noted. This variable association of immune depression with elevated tumour incidence might be related to different effects of disease or immunosuppressive regimens on NK and ADCC activities and other possible defence mechanisms. It will be very important to evaluate carefully the levels of these effector functions in the various conditions, to determine whether any correlate with the incidence of tumours in these patients.

One prediction of the immune surveillance hypothesis is that chemical carcinogens would cause depressed immune function, thereby impairing the ability of the host to reject the transformed cells. This postulate has been examined by many investigators in regard to the possible role of mature T cells and humoral immunity, and conflicting results have been obtained. In contrast, there is little information available on the effects of chemical carcinogens on NK cells. We have recently performed studies to determine the effects of urethane on NK activity (Gorelik and Herberman, 1980). A/J mice, which are sensitive to the carcinogenic effects of urethane, showed depressed and *in vivo* reactivity at 7 days after treatment and later developed multiple lung adenomas (Table III). In contrast, the NK and *in vivo* reactivities

TABLE III

Correlation between carcinogenesis and depression of NK activity by urethane

Mice	*Urethane treatment*[a]	*Spleen NK activity $LU_{10/10^7}$ cells*	*CPM $^{125}IUdR$ recovered from at 3 h*	*Average number lung adenomas at 3 months*
A/J	–	1·5	6800	0
A/J	+	0·01	21300	13·2
C57BL/6	–	5·9	2700	0
C57BL/6	+	5·1	2900	0·2

[a] Urethane (1 mg/g body weight) IP and NK and ^{125}IUdR assays after 7 days, using YAC-1 target cells.

of C57BL/6 mice, which are resistant to urethane carcinogenesis, were virtually unaffected by this treatment. Thus, carcinogenicity of urethane correlated with its ability to depress NK activity and this effect on host resistance may contribute to the development of neoplastic lesions.

The other principal challenge to the concept of immune surveillance has been that, in contrast to the antigenicity of virus-induced tumours, spontaneous tumours frequently lack detectable antigenicity and therefore might not be susceptible to control by the immune system. Much has been made of the findings that tumours arising *in vitro* are not more antigenic than those arising *in vivo* where the immune system might have been expected to select for tumours with weak or absent tumour-associated antigens. However, almost all of the negative evidence has been obtained by procedures designed to detect transplantation resistance and other immune responses which have generally been associated with immune T cell activity. If, as suggested here, there is a role for NK and K cells in immune surveillance, then the question of antigenicity and resistance to tumour growth needs to be asked by protocols designed to detect this function as well as that of immune T cell-mediated cytotoxicity.

References

Alvarez, J. M., de Landazuri, M. O., Bonnard, G. D. and Herberman, R. B. (1978). *J. Immunol.* **121**, 1270.

Bloom, B. R., Minato, N., Neighbor, A., Reid, L. and Marcus, D. (1980). *In* "Natural Cell-Mediated Immunity Against Tumors" (R. B. Herberman, ed.). Academic Press, New York and London (in press).

Bonnard, G. D., Schendel, D. J., West, W. H., Alvarez, J. M., Maca, R. D., Yasaka, K., Fine, R. K., Herberman, R. B., de Landazuri, M. O. and Morgan, D. A. (1978). *In* "Human Lymphocyte Differentiation: Its Application to Human Cancer" (B. Serrou and C. Rosenfeld, eds), pp. 319–326. Elsevier/North Holland Biomedical Press, Amsterdam.

Brunda, M. J., Holden, H. T. and Herberman, R. B. (1980). *In* "Natural Cell-Mediated Immunity Against Tumors" (R. B. Herberman, ed.). Academic Press, New York and London (in press).

Burton, R. C. (1980). *In* "Natural Cell-Mediated Immunity Against Tumors" (R. B. Herberman, ed.). Academic Press, New York and London (in press).

Dennert, G. (1980). Submitted for publication.

Dent, P. B., Fish, L. A., White, J. F. and Good, R. A. (1966). *Lab. Invest.* **15**, 1634.

Djeu, J. Y., Heinbaugh, J. A., Holden, H. T. and Herberman, R. B. (1979). *J. Immunol.* **122**, 175.

Durdik, J. M., Beck, B. N. and Henney, C. S. (1980). *In* "Natural Cell-Mediated Immunity Against Tumors" (R. B. Herberman, ed.). Academic Press, New York and London (in press).

Gidlund, M., Örn, A., Wigzell, H., Senik, A. and Gresser, I. (1978). *Nature* **223**, 259.

Gidlund, M., Haller, O., Örn, A., Ojo, E., Stern, P. and Wigzell, H. (1980). *In* "Natural Cell-Mediated Immunity Against Tumors" (R. B. Herberman, ed.). Academic Press, New York and London (in press).

Glimcher, L., Shen, F. W. and Cantor, H. (1977). *J. Exp. Med.* **145**, 1.

Gorelik, E. and Herberman, R. B. (1980). Submitted for publication.

Grimm, E. and Bonavida, B. (1979). *J. Immunol.* **123**, 2861.

Haller, O., Kiessling, R., Örn, A., Kärre, K., Nilsson, K. and Wigzell, H. (1977). *Int. J. Cancer* **20**, 93.

Hanna, N. and Fidler, I. J. (1980). *J. Natn. Cancer Inst.* (in press).

Hansson, M., Kärre, K., Kiessling, R., Roder, J., Andersson, B. and Häyry, P. (1979). *J. Immunol.* **123**, 765.

Herberman, R. B. (ed.) (1980). "Natural Cell-Mediated Immunity Against Tumors." Academic Press, New York and London (in press).
Herberman, R. B. and Gaylord, C. E. (eds) (1973). Conference and Workshop on Cellular Immune Reactions to Human Tumor—Associated Antigens. Natl. Cancer Inst. Monogr. No. 37, p. 1.
Herberman, R. B. and Holden, H. T. (1978). *Adv. Cancer Res.* **27**, 305.
Herberman, R. B. and Holden, H. T. (1979). *J. Natn. Cancer Inst.* **62**, 441.
Herberman, R. B. and Oldham, R. K. (1975). *J. Natn. Cancer Inst.* **55**, 749.
Herberman, R. B. and Ortaldo, J. R. (1980). *In* "Natural Cell-Mediated Immunity Against Tumors" (R. B. Herberman, ed.). Academic Press, New York and London (in press).
Herberman, R. B., Bartram, S., Haskill, J. S., Nunn, M., Holden, H. T. and West, W. H. (1977a). *J. Immunol.* **119**, 322.
Herbermann, R. B., Nunn, M. E., Holden, H. T., Staal, S. and Djeu, J. Y. (1977b). *Int. J. Cancer* **19**, 555.
Herberman, R. B., Djeu, J. Y., Ortaldo, J. R., Holden, H. T., West, W. H. and Bonnard, G. D. (1978). *Cancer Treat. Rep.* **62**, 1893.
Herberman, R. B., Djeu, J. Y., Kay, H. D., Ortaldo, J. R., Riccardi, C., Bonnard, G. D., Holden, H. T., Fagnani, R., Santoni, A. and Puccetti, P. (1979a). *Immunol. Rev.* **44**, 43.
Herberman, R. B., Ortaldo, J. R. and Bonnard, G. D. (1979b). *Nature* **277**, 221.
Herberman, R. B., Ortaldo, J. R., Djeu, J. Y., Holden, H. T., Jett, J., Lang, N. P. and Pestka, S. (1980a). *Ann. N.Y. Acad. Sci.* (in press).
Herberman, R. B., Timonen, T., Reynolds, C. and Ortaldo, J. R. (1980b). *In* "Natural Cell-Mediated Immunity Against Tumors" (R. B. Herberman, ed.). Academic Press, New York and London (in press).
Kaplan, J. and Callewaert, D. M. (1978). *J. Natn. Cancer Inst.* **60**, 961.
Kasai, M., Iwamori, M., Nagai, Y., Okumua, K. and Tada, T. (1980). *Eur. J. Immunol.* **10**, 175.
Katz, P., Roder, J., Herberman, R. B. and Fauci, A. S. (1980). *Clin. Res.* (in press).
Kay, H. D., Bonnard, G. D. and Herberman, R. B. (1979). *J. Immunol.* **122**, 675.
Keller, R. (1980). *In* "Natural Cell-Mediated Immunity Against Tumors" (R. B. Herberman, ed.). Academic Press, New York and London (in press).
Kiessling, R., Hochman, P. S., Haller, O., Shearer, G. M., Wigzell, H. and Cudkowicz, G. (1977). *Eur. J. Immunol.* **7**, 655.
Koide, Y. and Takasugi, M. (1977). *J. Natn. Cancer Inst.* **59**, 1099.
Koo, G. C. and Hatzfeld, A. (1980). *In* "Natural Cell-Mediated Immunity Against Tumors" (R. B. Herberman, ed.). Academic Press, New York and London (in press).
Korec, S. (1980). *In* "Natural Cell-Mediated Immunity Against Tumors" (R. B. Herberman, ed.). Academic Press, New York and London (in press).
Landazuri, M. O., Silva, A., Alvarez, J. and Herberman, R. B. (1979). *J. Immunol.* **123**, 252.
Mantovani, A., Peri, G., Polentarutti, N., Allavena, P., Bordignon, C., Sessa, C. and Mangioni, C. (1980). *In* "Natural Cell-Mediated Immunity Against Tumors" (R. B. Herberman, ed.). Academic Press, New York and London (in press).
Mattes, M. J., Sharrow, S. O., Herberman, R. B. and Holden, H. T. (1979). *J. Immunol.* **123**, 2851.
Morgan, D. A., Ruscetti, F. W. and Gallo, R. C. (1976). *Science* **193**, 1007.
Nunn, M. E., Herberman, R. B. and Holden, H. T. (1977). *Int. J. Cancer* **20**, 381.
Oehler, J. R., Lindsay, L. R., Nunn, M. E. and Herberman, R. B. (1978a). *Int. J. Cancer* **21**, 204.
Oehler, J. R., Lindsay, L. R., Nunn, M. E., Holden, H. T. and Herberman, R. B. (1978b). *Int. J. Cancer* **21**, 210.

Ortaldo, J. R. (1980). Submitted for publication.
Ortaldo, J. R., Timonen, T. and Bonnard, G. D. (1980). *Proc. Int. Symp. Cultured T Cells* (in press).
Puccetti, P., Santoni, A., Riccardi, C. and Herberman, R. B. (1980). *Int. J. Cancer* **25**, 153.
Reynolds, C. W., Timonen, T. and Herberman, R. B. (1980). Submitted for publication.
Riccardi, C., Puccetti, P., Santoni, A. and Herberman, R. B. (1979). *J. Natn. Cancer Inst.* **63**, 1041.
Riccardi, C., Barlozarri, T., Santoni, A., Herberman, R. B. and Cesarini, C. (1980a). Submitted for publication.
Riccardi, C., Santoni, A., Barlozzari, T. and Herberman, R. B. (1980b). *In* "Natural Cell-Mediated Immunity Against Tumors" (R. B. Herberman, ed.). Academic Press, New York and London (in press).
Riccardi, C., Santoni, A., Barlozzari, R. and Herberman, R. B. (1980c). Submitted for publication.
Riccardi, C., Santoni, A., Barlozzari, T., Puccetti, P. and Herberman, R. B. (1980d). *Int. J. Cancer* **25**, 475.
Roder, J. and Duwe, A. (1979). *Nature* **278**, 451.
Roder, J. C., Haliotis, T., Klein, M., Korec, S., Jett, J. R., Ortaldo, J., Herberman, R. B., Katz, P. and Fauci, A. S. (1980). *Nature* **284**, 553.
Rubinstein, M., Rubinstein, S., Familletti, P. C., Miller, R. S., Waldman, A. A. and Pestka, S. (1979). *Proc. Natn. Acad. Sci. U.S.A.* **76**, 640.
Saksela, E. and Timonen, T. (1980). *In* "Natural Cell-Mediated Immunity Against Tumors" (R. B. Herberman, ed.). Academic Press, New York and London (in press).
Saksela, E., Timonen, T., Virtanen, I. and Cantell, K. (1980). *In* "Natural Cell-Mediated Immunity Against Tumors" (R. B. Herberman, ed.). Academic Press, New York and London (in press).
Santoli, D., Trinchieri, G., Zmijewski, C. M. and Koprowski, H. (1976). *J. Immunol.* **117**, 765.
Scheid, M. P. and Triglia, D. (1979). *Immunogenetics* **9**, 423.
Schendel, D. J., Wank, R. and Bonnard, G. D. (1980). *Scand. J. Immunol.* (in press).
Stutman, O., Figarella, E. F., Paige, C. J. and Lattime, E. C. (1980). *In* "Natural Cell-Mediated Immunity Against Tumors" (R. B. Herberman, ed.). Academic Press, New York and London (in press).
Timonen, T., Saksela, E., Ranki, A. and Häyry, P. (1979). *Cell. Immunol.* **48**, 133.
Timonen, T., Ortaldo, J. R. and Herberman, R. B. (1980). Submitted for publication.
Trinchieri, G. and Santoli, D. (1978). *J. Exp. Med.* **147**, 1314.
Troye, M., Perlmann, P., Pape, G. R., Spiegelberg, H. L., Näslund, I. and Gidlöf, A. (1977). *J. Immunol.* **119**, 1061.
Welsh, R. M., Zinkernagel, R. M. and Hallenbeck, L. (1979). *J. Immunol.* **122**, 475.
West, W. H., Cannon, G. B., Kay, H. D., Bonnard, G. D. and Herberman, R. B. (1977). *J. Immunol.* **118**, 355.
Wolfe, S. A., Tracey, D. E. and Henney, C. S. (1976). *Nature* **262**, 584.

40

Interferon and the Immune System*

ION GRESSER

Institut de Recherches Scientifiques sur le Cancer,
Villejuif, Fance

Introduction

Interferon(s)† are proteins produced by animal cells, infected by viruses. Interferon can also be induced in the animal by a wide variety of substances, both natural and synthetic, and in cultures of lymphoid cells by mitogens or allogeneic cells. Virus induced interferon is called type 1 interferon [or interferon subclass α and β in the new nomenclature]. The interferon induced in lymphoid cells by some mitogens or allogeneic cells is called type 2 [or γ interferon] and can be distinguished from virus induced interferons by several criteria. To my knowledge the biologic effects obtained with type 1 interferon have also been obtained with type 2 interferon in so far as they have been

* Work cited in this text was aided by grants from the CNRS, DRET (contract 78–34–210), INSERM (ATP 59.78.91/3; 58.78.90/18), DGRST (contract 79.7.0205).
† Although there are several types of interferon distinguishable by certain physicochemical characteristics, they all exhibit common biologic effects, and thus for simplicity I will refer to interferons as "interferon" in the singular.

looked for. There are several reports suggesting however that some of the effects of type 2 interferon especially those on the immune system are more pronounced (antiviral unit for antiviral unit) than those seen with type1 interferon. If these preliminary findings are confirmed it may suggest that interferons may have different biologic functions. However, since type 2 interferon preparations are at present approximately 1000–10 000-fold less pure than type 1 interferon it is impossible to determine whether type 2 interferon is intrinsically more or less potent than type 1 interferon in a given system. Type 2 interferon preparations are contaminated with lymphokines which may affect its activity.

I will refer therefore to work done with virus induced interferon for 2 reasons. First, most of the work on the interaction of interferon with the immune system has been done with mouse or human virus induced interferon preparations. Secondly, these interferons have been purified to homogeneity, and it is now generally accepted that the biologic effects described are due to interferon. Some of these preparations can be diluted 100 000 000-fold and still inhibit the multiplication of a virus—or inhibit the multiplication of cells in culture. The specific activity of mouse interferon is about 10^9 biologic units/mg protein and it acts on cells *in vitro* at concentrations in the range of 3×10^{-14} M, or in other words, the equivalent of 1·0 pg/ml.

Interferon inhibits the intracellular multiplication of DNA and RNA containing viruses. It does not neutralize or combine with the virus outside of the cell: the antiviral effect is mediated by the cell. However, it turns out that interferon is *not* exclusively an antiviral substance—it also affects the division and the biologic activity of a wide variety of cells—including cells of the immune system. Thus, the antiviral effect of interferon is only one manifestation

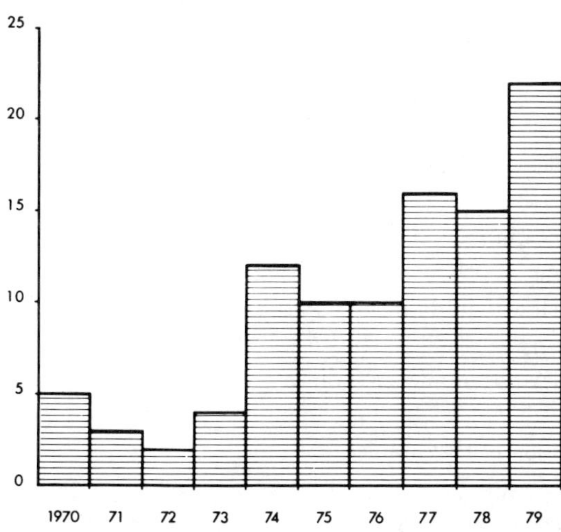

FIG. 1. *Number of articles/year on interferon in 3 journals of Immunology.*

of its effect on cells. Appreciation of the fact that interferon can interact with the immune system has been gradual. Figure 1 illustrates the progressive awareness that interferon has something to do with the immune system as exemplified by the increase in the number of articles dealing with interferon in 3 international journals of immunology between 1970 and 1979.

TABLE I

Effects of interferon on immune system (in vitro)

Cell multiplication
Inhibits mitogen or MLR induced lymphocyte proliferation

Antibody formation[a]
Inhibits but can *enhance*

Lymphocyte cytotoxicity
Enhances functions of differentiated effector cells: sensitized T NK[a] and K cells

Macrophage activity
Enchances phagocytosis, tumour cell killing

Surface antigens
Enhances expression of β2 microglobulin, H-2[a], HLA, Fc_γ receptors[a], concanavalin receptors, antigen receptors for synthetic polypeptides

Production or release of specific substances
Enhances cGMP[a], histamine

[a] Confirmed with EP interferon.

TABLE II

Effects of interferon on immune system (in vivo)

Cell multiplication
Inhibits multiplication of allogeneic lymphocytes in mice

Antibody formation
Inhibits or *enhances* in mice

Lymphocyte cytotoxicity
Enhances NK cell activity in mouse[a] and man

Macrophage activity
Enhances phagocytosis in mice, clearance

Surface antigens
Enhances expression of H-2 in mice

Delayed-type hypersensitivity[a]
Inhibits or *enhances* in mice depending on time of administration

[a] Confirmed with EP interferon.

I want first to list and describe some of the effects of mouse or human interferon preparations on the immune system (Tables I and II). Although the effects of interferon on various components of the immune system may be of interest *per se*, I think it is worthwhile to bear in mind, that significant amounts of interferon have with a few exceptions been detected only following virus infections. Interferon is an integral part of the host defence to viral infection. I believe a good working hypothesis at the outset would be to consider that the effects of interferon on the immune system also play a beneficial role in host defence against virus infection.

Most of these effects were obtained with partially purified interferon preparations but in some instances the biologic effects have been confirmed using electrophoretically pure (EP) mouse interferon.

Effect of interferon

Cell multiplication

Purified mouse and human interferon inhibit the multiplication of both normal and tumour cells *in vitro* and *in vivo*. It is not surprising therefore that interferon can also inhibit DNA synthesis in suspensions of mouse or human T or B lymphocytes stimulated by mitogens, some antigens or allogeneic lymphocytes. Treatment of mice with interferon or interferon inducers also results in an inhibition of the multiplication of transferred allogeneic donor lymphocytes (Table III).

TABLE III

Effect of exogenous interferon or interferon inducers on the generation of cytotoxic lymphocytes following transfer of C57BL/6 spleen cells into irradiated DBA/2 mice

No. of CB57BL/6 spleen cells injected	*Treatment of irradiated DBA/2 mice*	*Average no. of cells recovered from recipient spleens*	*% Specific lysis of DBA/2 target cells by transferred spleen cells Lymphocyte to target cell ratio*			*No. of lytic units present in recipient spleens*
			30 : 1	*10 : 1*	*3 : 1*	
3×10^6	None	$3·9 \times 10^6$	36	22	10	5·2
3×10^6	Control preparation	$3·4 \times 10^6$	36	21	9	4·5
3×10^6	Mouse interferon	$0·6 \times 10^6$	—	2·5	2·7	<0·1
10×10^6	None	$7·0 \times 10^6$	58	32		28
10×10^6	Control preparation	$5·5 \times 10^6$	43	25	NT	14
10×10^6	NDV	$0·4 \times 10^6$	2	0		<0·1
10×10^6	None	$7·3 \times 10^6$	42	29	17	22
10×10^6	Poly I·C + 1 h	$1·7 \times 10^6$	1	1	2	<0·4

Data taken from Cerottini *et al.* (1973). *Nature* **242**, 152–153.

Antibody formation

Interferon can inhibit or enhance the primary antibody response *in vitro*. Although the amount of interferon and several other experimental conditions are important factors—in our experience, the time of interferon addition was of prime importance. Thus, when interferon was added before or in the hours following addition of SRBC in a Mishell-Dutton type culture, a clear cut inhibitory effect on the number of PFC was observed. From the use of mosaic cell cultures, it seems that the effect is primarily on B lymphocytes rather than on T lymphocytes or macrophages.

When interferon was added several days *after* addition of antigen and shortly prior to assay, an increase in the number of PFC was observed (Table IV).

TABLE IV
Effect of partially purified mouse interferon added to spleen cell cultures during the terminal phase of antibody synthesis

	PFC/culture tested at 96 h after addition of SRBC	
	Exp. 1	*Exp. 2*
Control	3·620	1·436
Interferon added		
at 72 h	3·810	1·930
at 80 h	5·124	3·133
at 92 h	5·495	4·015

Data from Gisler *et al.* (1974). *J. Immunol.* **113**, 438–444.

In adult mice, inhibitory and enhancing effects on the response to T dependent and independent antigens have been reported. In our experiments with adult mice, only enhancement of antibody formation to SRBC has been observed. This was especially clear cut when interferon was administered several days after inoculation of antigen.

Lymphocyte cytotoxicity

Interferon also enhances the function of differentiated effector cells. Thus, it enhances the cytotoxicity of sensitized T lymphocytes and NK and K cells. The enhancing effect is observed within several hours and requires protein synthesis. Likewise, in mice and in man inoculation of interferon results in a rapid and significant increase in NK cell activity. Several interferon inducers also enhance the cytotoxicity of NK cells in mice and this effect can be abolished by injecting potent antimouse interferon antibody to neutralize the endogenous interferon.

Interferon acts directly on these cells. There is no good evidence for the production of a second effector substance. I believe it is still a matter of controversy whether interferon acts by increasing the lytic efficacy of individual NK cells or by recruitment of other cells or by inducing differentiation of a pre-NK cell.

Macrophage activity

Interferon affects the morphology and function of macrophages. It enhances phagocytosis of colloidal carbon particles as well as IgG-coated erythrocytes. Interferon renders macrophages cytotoxic for tumour cells, although the specificity of this effect is still controversial.

Surface antigens

As shown in Table I the expression of several surface antigens is increased by interferon treatment. The mechanism of this effect is unknown. My feeling is that it probably represents increased antigen synthesis, rather than an "unmasking" of surface antigens, or an accumulation of antigen because of decreased shedding.

There appears to be a differential effect of interferon on the expression of several surface antigens. Although interferon markedly enhances the expression of H-2 and HLA antigens, $\beta 2$ microglobulin and Fcγ receptors, it does not increase or increases to a much lesser extent the expression of Thy-1, Ia or DR antigens. It is not at all clear at present whether this differential effect is of biologic significance or merely reflects differences in the rate of "turnover" of different antigens.

Interferon enhances the expression of Fcγ receptors on lymphoid cells *in vitro* and possibly also *in vivo*.

Production or release of specific substances

Although interferon inhibits cell division, it can inhibit or enhance the synthesis of a variety of enzymes or important biologic mediators such as cGMP, histamine and prostaglandins. It is evident that a number of these mediators are also important in the modulation of the immune response.

Delayed hypersensitivity

Interferon can prolong skin allograft survival across the H-2 barrier in mice. Interferon has been shown to inhibit sensitization in mice to SRBC, or NDV when administered before injection of antigen. Interferon can also inhibit the response in mice previously sensitized to SRBC, NDV or picryl chloride when administered *prior to* challenge. The timing of interferon is crucial. When interferon was administered to mice *after* inoculation of antigen, it either had no effect or increased the expression of DTH. Furthermore, the sensitivity to this enhancing effect of interferon was strain dependent.

Conclusions

There are several ways of looking at the effect of interferon on the immune system. First let us consider its role in the course of viral infection. Significant levels of interferon appear *after* the virus has already multiplied to fairly high titres. In terms of timing, interferon is present therefore *after* the animal has been exposed to a certain antigenic mass. How is interferon of benefit to the viral infected host? Figure 2 attempts to co-ordinate the various experimental findings I have just enumerated with some sort of hypothesis as to the mode

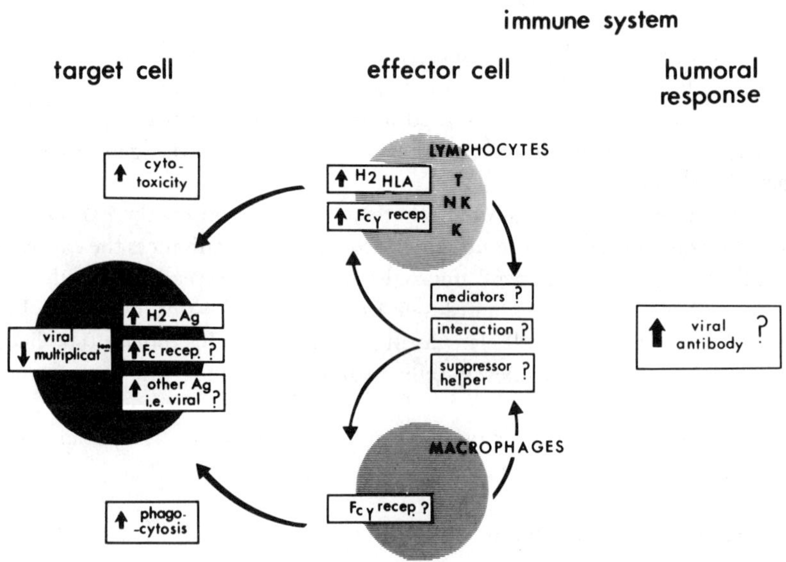

FIG. 2. *Effect of interferon in viral infection.*

of action of interferon in viral disease. There are first the effects of interferon on susceptible target cells, and then the effects of interferon on cellular and possibly humoral defence mechanisms. As for the target cells—interferon clearly inhibits viral multiplication. The importance to the host of this effect can easily be demonstrated by injecting mice with a virus and a potent antibody to interferon. The anti-interferon antibody neutralizes the endogenous interferon and the virus multiplies rapidly to very high titres with disastrous consequences for the host. In some experimental systems inoculation of anti-interferon antibody transformed an inapparent viral infection in a genetically resistant mouse into a fulminant lethal disease.

But what about the effects of interferon on the immune system? When one considers the ensemble of experimental findings, it is quite striking that the predominant effect appears to be one of *enhancement* rather than inhibition—enhancement of a variety of differentiated cell activities. Interferon enhances the cytotoxicity of sensitized T lymphocytes, NK and K cells, and the phagocytic activity of macrophages. These cells probably play a role in eliminating virus infected cells.

Interferon enhances the expression of some surface antigens both on potential target and effector cells (Fig. 2). Is the enhancement of the expression of histocompatibility antigens by interferon of importance for the host? Virus-sensitized T lymphocytes seem to play a beneficial role in viral infections by lysing virus-infected cells. Histocompatibility are considered important in the *in vitro* recognition and lysis of virus-infected cells by sensitized T cells both in murine and human systems. It may be important then that interferon not only enhances the cytotoxicity of sensitized T cells but also enhances the expression of those antigens (H-2 and HLA) that seem so necessary for recognition and effective T lymphocyte killing of virus-infected cells.

What about the interferon induced increase in Fcγ receptors? It has been shown that viral infection (herpes virus and cytomegaloviruses, for example) can result in an increase in Fc receptors, and immunoglobulin binding to these receptors leads in turn to inhibition of virus multiplication. Perhaps in some instances, it is the interferon resulting from local or systemic viral infection that is responsible for the increase in Fc receptors on target cells. Furthermore, the increase in the expression of Fcγ receptors on effector cells may play a role in the enhanced cytotoxicity of sensitized T lymphocytes, NK and K cells and the enhanced phagocytic activity of macrophages.

Does interferon enhance or inhibit the interaction between different lymphocyte or macrophage populations? For example, it is possible that some inhibitory effects may actually be due to the stimulation of suppressor cell activity. Little work has been done in this area to date.

As I have stated above, interferon enhanced the primary antibody response to SRBC in mice. It is possible that interferon might enhance production of antiviral antibody. To my knowledge, this point has not been investigated.

To what extent do the inhibitory effects of interferon on cell division play a role in the regulation of the immune response? There is no question that *in vivo* interferon can inhibit both tumour and normal cell division. In fact when given in large amounts to neonatal mice and rats, interferon markedly inhibits their growth and maturation. It is possible therefore that interferon is one of the factors that limits clonal expansion of lymphocytes, by inhibiting sensitization of uncommitted lymphocytes or by inhibiting the multiplication of lymphocytes already sensitized.

Lastly, interferon may have other effects of a more general nature—effects on temperature, and on the function of the endocrine or nervous systems which may influence the immune or non specific host defence mechanisms. For example, patients injected with both leukocyte and fibroblast interferon preparations become febrile. I think that there is a good possibility that this febrile response is due to interferon itself and not to contaminating pyrogens.

We know that an elevated temperature inhibits the multiplication of many different viruses and there is data suggesting that the effects of interferon on viral and cell multiplication are also more pronounced at raised temperatures.

Aside from the intrinsic interest in understanding how interferon may act as part of the host defence in viral infections, interferon may possibly be used in normal or immunosuppressed patients as antiviral prophylaxis or as an antitumour substance in patients with neoplastic disease. I would suggest that interferon may possibly be used one day in patients with immunologic disorders.

For these reasons the effects of interferon on the immune system will have to be carefully investigated. Interferon is one of the most potent biologic substances known, and as with all such substances they may under some conditions prove injurious. Treatment of newborn mice for 1 week with interferon can result in stunted growth, liver necrosis and death. Surviving mice develop a glomerulonephritis. Treatment of NZB/W mice with interferon exacerbates disease and shortens the survival time. Interferon has been detected in the blood of patients with severe systemic lupus erythematosis. It is not known whether this interferon is of benefit or harm to the patient.

There is one last point that may have some relevance for immunologists interested in mediators—interleukins, etc.—and it brings me back to my introductory remarks.

In the interferon field we started with a substance that was defined in terms of a given biologic activity. Other biologic effects were described, but it was only after purification was achieved, that one could state with conviction that:

(1) Interferon exerts different biologic effects and can affect the immune system in different ways.

I would suggest that:

(2) Other mediators now defined in terms of a given biologic activity may also exert several different biologic effects. Different biologic effects do not necessarily mean different substances.

We are only beginning to delineate some of the effects of mediators such as interferon on the immune system. We are at the level of phenomenology. We have not begun to explore mechanisms of action. I believe that there is an exciting future in the investigation of interferon and similar mediators—not only because of their role as intercellular messengers—but also because of their potential clinical usefulness in a wide variety of diseases of man.

References

De Maeyer, E. (1978). *Bull. Inst. Pasteur* **76**, 303.

De Maeyer, E. and De Maeyer-Guignard, J. (1979). *In* "Comprehensive Virology" (H. Fraenkel-Conrat and R. R. Wagner, eds) Vol. 15, pp. 205–284. Plenum Publishing, New York.

Epstein, L. B. (1977). *In* "Interferons and their Actions" (W. E. Stewart II, ed.) pp. 91–132. CRC Press, Cleveland.

Gresser, I. (1977). *Cell. Immunol.* **34**, 406.
Gresser, I. and Tovey, M. G. (1978). *Biochim. Biophys. Acta* **516**, 231.
Johnson, H. M. and Baron, S. (1976). *CRC Crit. Rev. Biochem.* **9**, 203.
Stewart II, W. E. (1979). *In* "The Interferon System". Springer-Verlag, Wien and New York.

41

Cytocidal Mechanisms of Phagocytic Cells

S. J. KLEBANOFF

Department of Medicine, University of Washington, Seattle, Washington, USA

Introduction

The professional phagocytes—neutrophils, eosinophils, and the cells of the mononuclear phagocyte system—are by definition cells which are particularly adept at the ingestion of foreign particles. When these particles are invading micro-organisms, phagocytosis serves to isolate the invaders in an intracellular vacuole, where the micro-organism is exposed to a variety of antimicrobial systems from which few survive. These same toxic systems may, under certain conditions, be released into the extracellular fluid where they can attack normal or malignant cells or parasites too large to be ingested.

A classification of the cidal systems of phagocytes is shown in Table I (for review see Klebanoff, 1975, 1980; Klebanoff and Clark, 1978). It is convenient to divide them initially into those which require oxygen and those which operate in its absence based on the inhibition but not loss of activity on the exposure of intact leukocytes to an atmosphere of nitrogen. It should be emphasized that the presence of antimicrobial activity under hypoxic conditions does not necessarily indicate that an oxygen-independent system is responsible for the death of the organisms under aerobic conditions; only that

TABLE I
Toxic systems of phagocytic leukocytes

Oxygen-dependent
Peroxidase-mediated
Peroxidase-independent
Superoxide anion
Hydrogen peroxide
Hydroxyl radical
Singlet oxygen
Oxygen-independent
Acid
Lysozyme
Lactoferrin
Acid and neutral hydrolases
Cationic proteins

antimicrobial systems are present which can kill the organism when oxygen is removed. This may be a back-up system not ordinarily needed. Nevertheless, toxic activity under hypoxic conditions, as well as the isolation of antimicrobial and cytotoxic agents from leukocytes which operate in the absence of oxygen, indicate the presence of oxygen-independent systems in leukocytes and it can be presumed that they contribute to the toxic activity of the cell. Further evidence for the presence of oxygen-dependent toxic systems in leukocytes is the demonstration of a killing defect in cells from patients with chronic granulomatous disease (CGD), a condition in which the leukocytes lack the phagocytosis-induced respiratory burst.

The oxygen-dependent toxic systems of phagocytes can be divided into those which are dependent on peroxidase (or possibly another haemprotein) and those which are operative in its absence. All phagocytic leukocytes respond to perturbation of the plasma membrane with a burst of oxygen consumption. This plasma membrane disturbance is generally a prelude to phagocytosis but need not be so. Leukocytes exposed to an antigen-antibody complex on a nonphagocytosable surface respond to it as it would to an appropriately opsonized particle. In addition there are a number of soluble agents which can react with cell surface components to initiate the respiratory burst. The oxygen consumed is converted to a number of highly reactive products: the superoxide anion (O_2^-); hydrogen peroxide (H_2O_2); hydroxyl radicals ($OH\cdot$); and possibly singlet oxygen ($^1O_2$). In recent years, there has been considerable interest in the role of these products of oxygen reduction and excitation in the toxic activity of phagocytes, with H_2O_2 being effective both in the presence and absence of peroxidase.

The oxygen-independent toxic agents in phagocytes include the fall in pH in the phagosome (and also presumably in pockets formed between adherent phagocytes and targets too large to be ingested), and a number of toxic agents released either into the phagosome or extracellularly. The membrane of the cytoplasmic granules fuses with that of the phagosome or the cell surface, the fused membranes rupture and the granule contents are discharged. The potentially toxic agents released in this way include lysozyme, lactoferrin, acid hydrolases, neutral proteases and a number of strongly basic proteins.

Oxygen-dependent toxic systems

Peroxidase-dependent toxic systems

Neutrophil

The peroxidase-mediated toxic system of phagocytes has been best studied in the neutrophil. The neutrophil peroxidase (myeloperoxidase, MPO) is present in exceptionally high concentration in the azurophil (or primary) granules of the resting neutrophil. Azurophil granule formation is limited to the promyelocyte stage of neutrophil development, and it is during this period that MPO is synthesized on cellular ribosomes and delivered via the endoplasmic reticulum and Golgi vesicles to the developing granules. Azurophil granule formation and MPO synthesis ceases at the termination of the promyelocyte stage. In the mature neutrophil, the peroxidase-positive azurophil granules are mixed with a second population of granules which are formed during the myelocyte stage of neutrophil development; these specific (or secondary) granules do not contain peroxidase (see Bainton *et al.*, 1971 for a more detailed description of the development of human neutrophils).

Myeloperoxidase, H_2O_2 and a halide form a very powerful toxic system (Klebanoff, 1967, 1968). Of the halides, chloride is effective at concentrations present within the neutrophil. Iodide is considerably more potent than chloride on a molar basis; however, its concentration in leukocytes is low and its contribution to the total halide pool thus may be small. The thyroid hormones thyroxine and tri-iodothyronine can replace iodide in the cell-free peroxidase system, presumably due to their deiodination (Klebanoff, 1967). Bromide ions (Klebanoff, 1968) and, under limited conditions of concentration, thiocyanate ions (Klebanoff and Clark, 1978) can also meet the halide requirement of the cell-free myeloperoxidase-mediated system.

The peroxidase combines with its substrate, H_2O_2, to form an enzyme–substrate complex (or complexes) which oxidizes the halide to form an agent or agents with potent toxic properties. With chloride as the halide, it is probable that hypochlorous acid (HOCl) is the primary oxidant formed (Agner, 1972; Harrison and Schultz, 1976) but chlorine (Cl_2) and the chloridinium ion (Cl^+) also may be produced. The oxidants formed from iodide may include iodine (I_2), iodinium ion (I^+) and hypoiodous acid (HOI) and comparable species may result from the oxidation of bromide or thiocyanate ions. Hypothiocyanate ion has been detected as a product of the lactoperoxidase—H_2O_2—thiocyanate system (Hoogendoorn *et al.*, 1977; Aune and Thomas, 1977). A well-described mechanism for the formation of singlet oxygen is the interaction of hypochlorite and H_2O_2 (Kasha and Khan, 1970) as follows:

$$H_2O_2 + OCl^- \rightarrow {}^1O_2 + H_2O + Cl^-$$

raising the possibility that hypohalites generated by the peroxidase system may yield singlet oxygen, a potentially toxic agent. Evidence has been presented which is compatible with the generation of $^1O_2$ by the peroxidase system (Rosen and Klebanoff, 1977; Piatt and O'Brien, 1979); however, these data are subject to alternate interpretations (Held and Hurst, 1978; Harrison *et al.*, 1978) and thus the formation of $^1O_2$ by the peroxidase system has not been definitely demonstrated.

It is probable that the highly reactive products of the peroxidase system attack the cell surface; 2 modes of attack have been proposed: halogenation and oxidation. When iodide is the halide employed, iodination of cell components occurs (Klebanoff, 1967) and the bound iodine can be demonstrated by autoradiographic techniques on the surface of the organism (Klebanoff, 1970b). Bromination (Klebanoff, unpublished data) and chlorination (Zgliczyński and Stelmaszyńska, 1975; Stelmaszyńska and Zgliczyński, 1978; Thomas, 1979; Selvaraj *et al.*, 1980) have also been observed and the substitution of a halide for hydrogen may contribute to the cell death. The products formed by the peroxidase system are powerful oxidants and oxidant damage to the cell would be expected. Sulphydryl oxidation (Thomas and Aune, 1977, 1978), lipid peroxidation (Buege and Aust, 1976), the oxidative cleavage of peptides (Alexander, 1974; Selvaraj *et al.*, 1974) and the oxidative deamination and decarboxylation of amino acids with the formation of aldehydes (Sbarra *et al.*, 1977) have been reported. The transport of metabolites across the cell membrane appears to be affected by these chemical changes. Thus, the uptake of lysine-^{14}C by *Lactobacillus acidophilus* is prevented by the MPO–H_2O_2–iodide system and, if this system is added following 60 min of lysine uptake, rapid discharge of the amino acid occurs (Klebanoff and Clark, 1978).

The MPO–H_2O_2–halide system has potent bactericidal activity against a variety of Gram-positive and Gram-negative organisms (Klebanoff, 1967, 1968; McRipley and Sbarra, 1967); it is also toxic to fungi (Lehrer, 1969; Klebanoff, 1970a; Lehrer and Jan, 1970; Diamond *et al.*, 1972; Howard, 1973), viruses (Belding *et al.*, 1970) and mycoplasma (Jacobs *et al.*, 1972) and to certain mammalian cells. The latter include spermatozoa (Smith and Klebanoff, 1970), erythrocytes (Klebanoff and Clark, 1975), leukocytes (Clark and Klebanoff, 1977a), platelets (Clark and Klebanoff, 1979b) and tumour cells (Clark *et al.*, 1975). This system also can inactivate certain soluble mediators, e.g. the chemotactic factors C5a and formylmethionyl-leucyl-phenylalanine (Clark and Klebanoff, 1979c) and α1 proteinase inhibitor (α1 antitrypsin) (Matheson *et al.*, 1979). Inactivation appears to result from the oxidation of the methionine residues of the mediators (Matheson *et al.*, 1979; Clark *et al.*, 1980).

In the intact cell, MPO released into the phagosome (or extracellular fluid) by the degranulation process reacts with H_2O_2 generated by the respiratory burst (or by certain ingested organisms) and a halide (largely chloride and/or iodide) to destroy ingested organisms, adjacent cells or soluble systems. The primary function of the neutrophil is the phagocytosis and destruction of micro-organisms and evidence suggesting the involvement of the peroxidase system in this antimicrobial activity has been reviewed (Klebanoff, 1975; Klebanoff and Clark, 1978). It is our view that many, perhaps most, ingested organisms are killed by the MPO–H_2O_2–halide system. It appears to be the predominant antimicrobial system during the early postphagocytic period and it would be anticipated that most organisms would not survive its action. Those that do are subject to attack by a variety of other antimicrobial systems. When MPO is absent as in hereditary MPO deficiency, these nonperoxidase systems combine with other host defence mechanisms to keep most patients in good health. Neutrophils from patients with hereditary MPO deficiency have a major candidacidal defect and their bactericidal activity is characterized by a lag period following which the organisms are killed (Lehrer and Cline, 1969; Lehrer *et al.*, 1969). Since MPO deficiency is the only recognized molecular lesion in these cells it can be assumed that the microbicidal defect is due to the absence of MPO.

There is strong evidence from *in vivo* models that neutrophils can, under certain conditions, damage adjacent tissues; the role of the peroxidase system in this extracellular toxicity, however, is not known. Appropriately stimulated intact neutrophils are toxic to adjacent cells *in vitro* and in some instances this toxicity appears to be mediated at least in part by the peroxidase system. Thus human neutrophils stimulated by phagocytosis (Clark and Klebanoff, 1975), concanavalin A (Clark and Klebanoff, 1979a), or phorbol myristate acetate (Clark, 1979; Jong and Klebanoff, 1980) can release the components of the peroxidase system (MPO, H_2O_2) into the extracellular fluid where they react with a halide to kill adjacent tumour cells. In contrast, we have been unable to detect peroxidase involvement in the toxic effect of neutrophils on tumour cells in the presence of antitumour cell antibody (Clark and Klebanoff, 1977b).

Mononuclear phagocytes

Mononuclear phagocytes are a continuum of cells which begin in the bone marrow as stem cells; promonocytes develop into monocytes which pass into the bloodstream where they circulate until they enter the extravascular tissue where they develop into macrophages. The peroxidases of the mononuclear phagocytes (for review see Klebanoff and Hamon, 1975; Klebanoff, 1980) are classified in Table II.

Granule peroxidase. A peroxidase is present in cytoplasmic granules of the blood monocyte of most species; the rabbit is an exception (Nichols *et al.*, 1971). The enzyme is formed and packaged in the bone marrow promonocyte where the enzyme can also be detected in the endoplasmic reticulum. The granule peroxidase also can be detected in mononuclear phagocytes which have recently left the bloodstream (Van Furth *et al.*, 1970; Daems *et al.*, 1973;

TABLE II
Peroxidase activity of mononuclear phagocytes

Granule peroxidase (myeloperoxidase)
Peroxidase present in the endoplasmic reticulum
Immature phagocytes (myeloperoxidase)
Mature phagocytes
Endocytosed peroxidase
Phagocytosis
Pinocytosis
Catalase

Simmons and Karnovsky, 1973) and can be found in the phagosomes of these cells (Daems *et al.*, 1973); however, as the macrophage matures, the granule peroxidase is generally lost. The granule peroxidase of the blood monocyte appears to be identical to that of the neutrophil (i.e. myeloperoxidase); peroxidase is absent from both cell types in hereditary MPO deficiency (Grignaschi *et al.*, 1963) suggesting that they are coded by the same gene and purified monocyte and neutrophil peroxidase have similar chemical and functional characteristics (Bos *et al.*, 1978). There is some evidence which suggests that the granule peroxidase contributes to the antimicrobial activity of the monocyte. Thus the monocytes of patients with hereditary MPO deficiency have a candidacidal defect and the peroxidase inhibitors azide, cyanide and sulphadiazine inhibit the fungicidal activity of normal, but not MPO-deficient monocytes (Lehrer, 1975).

Peroxidase of the endoplasmic reticulum. The peroxidase present in the endoplasmic reticulum of immature mononuclear phagocytes disappears at the termination of the promonocyte stage. However, some mature resident macrophages contain cytochemically identifiable peroxidase in the endoplasmic reticulum (see Klebanoff, 1980). Further, blood monocytes or macrophages which do not ordinarily contain peroxidase in this location may develop peroxidase activity in the rough endoplasmic reticulum and nuclear envelope following adherence of the cells to a surface *in vitro* (Bodel *et al.*, 1977, 1978). This peroxidase appears to differ from that of monocyte (and neutrophil) granules as it has been detected in the endoplasmic reticulum of adherent monocytes from a patient with hereditary MPO deficiency (Bainton, per. comm.). The peroxidase of the endoplasmic reticulum is not packaged into granules, nor is it released into the phagosome (Daems *et al.*, 1973). Its role in extracellular cytotoxicity, if any, is unknown.

Endocytosed peroxidase. Peroxidase in the extracellular fluid may be taken up by mononuclear phagocytes either as a constituent of a particle (phagocytosis) or in soluble (pinocytosis) and the cell could theoretically utilize this peroxidase to kill ingested organisms. We have recently found that eosinophil peroxidase (EPO), which is a strongly positive protein, forms a firm complex with staphylococci and the organisms coated with peroxidase are readily killed on the addition of H_2O_2 and a halide (Ramsey and Klebanoff, 1980). There was significantly increased killing of the staph-EPO complex as compared to control staphylococci by rabbit blood monocytes and alveolar macrophages (which do not contain granule peroxidase), and azide, a peroxidase inhibitor, inhibited the killing of staph-EPO but did not affect the killing of control staphylococci. This suggests that peroxidase bound to micro-organisms can react with H_2O_2 generated by the mononuclear phagocyte to kill the organism on which it is located.

Catalase. Catalase is present in very high concentration in rabbit alveolar macrophages (Gee *et al.*, 1970) and is discharged in part into the phagosome (Stossel *et al.*, 1972). Although catalase generally catalyses the degradation of H_2O_2 to oxygen and water, it is capable of peroxidatic reactions, (i.e. the oxidation of a number of other compounds by H_2O_2) when the H_2O_2 is maintained at low steady-state concentrations. Thus, catalase can react with H_2O_2 (generated by the glucose oxidase system) and iodide at pH 4·5 to form a microbicidal system toxic to bacteria (Klebanoff, 1969), fungi (Klebanoff, 1969) and viruses (Klebanoff and Hamon, 1975), and a granule preparation from rabbit alveolar macrophages was found to have bactericidal properties (Paul *et al.*, 1973) similar to those of catalase. These findings raise the possibility that the catalase of alveolar macrophages may be microbicidal *in situ*. However, direct evidence for such a microbicidal effect has not been found. No decrease in bactericidal activity was detected in rabbit alveolar macrophages in which catalase activity was decreased to 25% and 50% of normal by treatment with aminotriazole (Klebanoff and Hamon, 1975) and ethanol (Gee *et al.*, 1974) respectively, nor was bactericidal activity inhibited in another study by the addition of the catalase-inhibitors aminotriazole or nitrite (Bigger *et al.*, 1976). Thus catalase is either uninvolved in the bactericidal activity of rabbit alveolar macrophages or is present in considerable excess. Certain other mononuclear phagocytes, e.g. mouse peritoneal macrophages, have very low levels of catalase (Simmons and Karnovsky, 1973) arguing against the involvement of catalase in the batericidal activity of these cells.

Eosinophil

When blood smears are stained for peroxidase, the eosinophil stands out as the most heavily stained cell. As in the neutrophil (and monocyte), the peroxidase of the eosinophil is limited to cytoplasmic granules; it is seen in the matrix of the specific granules surrounding the central crystalline core and, as in the neutrophil and monocyte, is formed and packaged in the bone marrow during the progranulocyte stage (Bainton and Farquhar, 1970). The eosinophil peroxidase (EPO) differs both genetically and in its structure and properties from the neutrophil peroxidase. Thus patients with hereditary MPO deficiency lack peroxidase in neutrophils and monocytes but contain normal amounts in eosinphils (Grignaschi *et al.*, 1963) suggesting that the 2 enzymes are coded by different genes. Purified guinea-pig EPO and MPO differ immunologically and in their absorption spectrum, electrophoretic mobility, chromatographic behaviour, subunit structure and haem prosthetic group (Desser *et al.*, 1972). EPO and MPO also differ in the rate at which particular electron donors are oxidized and in their response to inhibitors (Migler and DeChatelet, 1978).

EPO, like MPO, has potent microbicidal activity (Lehrer, 1969; Migler *et al.*, 1978; Jong *et al.*, 1980) and is toxic to mammalian tumour cells (Jong and Klebanoff, 1980) and the schistosomula of *Schistosoma mansoni* (Jong *et al.*, 1979), when combined with H_2O_2 and a halide. In some studies, chloride was ineffective as the halide (Lehrer, 1969; Migler *et al.*, 1978) whereas in others (Jong *et al.*, 1980; Jong and Klebanoff, 1980) chloride could meet the halide requirement under certain experimental conditions (high EPO concentration, low pH). The EPO–H_2O_2-halide system was found to have a dual effect on mast cells: at relatively low concentrations of EPO, specific secretion occurred as indicated by ultrastructural evidence and by the release of histamine without concomitant lactic acid dehydrogenase (LDH) release, whereas when the EPO concentration was raised, lysis of the mast cells occurred with release of both histamine and LDH and with ultrastructural evidence of cell damage (Henderson *et al.*, 1980b).

EPO is a strongly basic protein which binds avidly to the surface of mast cell granules to form a complex with retention of peroxidatic activity (Henderson *et al.*, 1980a). Granules that had been depleted of histamine and other loosely bound mediators by suspension in 0·1 M phosphate buffer pH 7·0, bound a considerably greater proportion of the added EPO than did granules which retained their histamine content due to suspension in water. The mast cell granule–EPO complex retained peroxidatic activity; indeed, the complex had significantly greater iodinating and bactericidal activity than did the free enzyme when standardized to the same guaiacol units of peroxidase activity. The mast cell granule–EPO complex when combined with H_2O_2 and iodide also was more effective than was EPO in the stimulation of mast cell secretion (Henderson *et al.*, 1980b).

Basophil and mast cell

Basophils have been found by cytochemical techniques to contain peroxidase in their granules (Ackerman and Clark, 1971; Bentfeld *et al.*, 1977) and recently rat peritoneal mast cell granules have been shown to contain a small amount of peroxidatic activity (Henderson and Kaliner, 1978). Mast cell granules can catalyse the iodination reaction and has bactericidal activity when combined with H_2O_2 and iodide, although these activities are considerably potentiated by the binding of EPO to the mast cell granule surface (Henderson *et al.*, 1980a).

Oxygen-dependent but peroxidase-independent toxic systems

Peroxidase-independent toxic systems are clearly present in phagocytes (see above); however, some of these systems remain dependent on oxygen. Products of the respiratory burst are released either into the phagosome or extracellularly where they appear to contribute to the toxic activity of the phagocyte. They include the superoxide anion, hydrogen peroxide, hydroxyl radicals and possibly singlet oxygen.

Superoxide anion

Oxygen is initially reduced to its 1 electron reduction product, the superoxide anion. Superoxide anion production by neutrophils (Babior *et al.*, 1973), eosinophils (Tauber *et al.*, 1976; Klebanoff *et al.*, 1977; DeChatelet *et al.*, 1977) and some mononuclear phagocytes (see Klebanoff, 1980) has been reported, although production by the latter is variable as might be expected from the heterogenous nature of the cell population. The superoxide anion is both an oxidant and a reductant; however, it oxidizes and reduces a limited number of substances and there is little evidence to suggest that these direct actions of O_2^- are cytotoxic (see Fee and Valentine, 1977). Rather, it is probable that O_2^- exerts its toxicity through the products which it forms, namely H_2O_2, OH· and possibly $^1O_2$.

Hydrogen peroxide

The 2 electron reduction product of oxygen is hydrogen peroxide. It can be formed either directly from oxygen by divalent reduction or via the intermediate formation of the superoxide anion. For example, glucose oxidase appears to form H_2O_2 directly from oxygen (Massey *et al.*, 1969; Stankovich *et al.*, 1978) whereas xanthine oxidase forms H_2O_2, in part at least, from superoxide (Fridovich, 1970). It is possible for superoxide to be formed within the crevice of an enzyme molecule, or as an enzyme–superoxide complex, which is unavailable to the proteins for its assay, with dismutation occurring prior to release or diffusion into the surrounding medium. Nevertheless, even under these conditions, H_2O_2 would be the species available for reaction with adjacent cells or soluble substances. H_2O_2 generation by neutrophils (Iyer *et al.*, 1961), eosinophils (Baehner and Johnston, 1971; Mickenberg *et al.*, 1972; Klebanoff *et al.*, 1977) and mononuclear phagocytes (see Klebanoff, 1980) has been clearly demonstrated.

It is assumed that in the leukocyte, H_2O_2 is formed largely by the dismutation of the superoxide anion. This can occur spontaneously or be catalysed by the enzyme superoxide dismutase (see Fridovich, 1976). Spontaneous dismutation occurs most readily at pH 4·8 (the pKa of the dissociation: $HO_2^{\cdot} \leftrightharpoons O_2^- + H^+$) where the rate constant is $8{\cdot}5 \times 10^7$/MS (Behar *et al.*, 1970). At this pH, the protonated and nonprotonated forms of the radical are present in equal concentrations with the dismutation occurring as follows:

$$HO_2^{\cdot} + O_2^- + H^+ \rightarrow O_2 + H_2O_2$$

The rate constant decreases when the pH is lowered and $HO_2^{\cdot}$ predominates or when the pH is increased and O_2^- predominates. The rate constant at neutral pH is $4{\cdot}5 \times 10^5$/MS and it is probable that at very high pH or in aprotic environments where O_2^- is the sole species, spontaneous dismutation does not occur (Bielski and Allen, 1977). Superoxide dismutase catalyses the dismutation reaction over a wide pH range (rate constant $1{\cdot}9 \times 10^9$/MS, pH 5·0 to 9·5) (Rabini *et al.*, 1972); however, the difference in rate as compared to spontaneous dismutation is particularly significant at neutral or alkaline pH where spontaneous dismutation is relatively slow. Since the pH within the phagocytic vacuole and presumably also in the pocket between adherent leukocytes and target cells is acid, spontaneous dismutation would be expected to be rapid. Superoxide dismutase has not been detected in the extracellular or phagosome fluid; however, it may be a component of the target cell or micro-organism.

The involvement of H_2O_2 as a required component of the peroxidase-mediated microbicidal and cytotoxic system of phagocytes is considered above. H_2O_2 is also toxic non-enzymatically at relatively high concentration, and this nonenzymatic toxicity is increased by certain low mol. wt agents, e.g. ascorbic acid and iodide (see Klebanoff and Hamon, 1975). H_2O_2 has been found to be responsible for the toxic activity of phagocytes under certain experimental conditions *in vitro*. Thus, H_2O_2 has been implicated as the toxic species in the killing of the newborn larvae of *Trichinella spiralis* by human neutrophils and eosinophils (Bass and Szejda, 1979a, b) and in the toxic effect of macrophages on tumour cells (Nathan *et al.*, 1979a, b). Peroxidase was not required in these studies. the killing of intracellular trypomastigotes of *Trypanosoma cruzi* by mouse peritoneal macrophages correlated well with the formation of H_2O_2 by these cells (Nathan *et al.*, 1979c) and H_2O_2 appears to be partially responsible for the macrophage-induced suppression of lymphocyte proliferation (Metzger *et al.*, 1980). In another study (Lemarbre *et al.*, 1980) H_2O_2 was implicated in human pulmonary macrophage cytocidal activity against fibroblasts but not against tumour cells. These findings point to H_2O_2 as a toxic product of phagocytes which can be effective in the absence of peroxidase against certain targets.

Hydroxyl radicals

The further reduction of H_2O_2 results in the formation of the highly reactive hydroxyl radical. Haber and Weiss (1934) proposed the reduction of H_2O_2 by O_2^- (or its protonated form $HO_2^{\cdot}$) and this reaction

$$H_2O_2 + O_2^- \rightarrow O_2 + OH^- + OH\cdot$$

has become known as the Haber–Weiss reaction. It is now clear that the direct interaction of H_2O_2 and O_2^- to form OH· is too slow to be of major biological significance (see Fee and Valentine, 1977; Weinstein and Bielski, 1979). Rather, it is believed to be catalysed by a trace metal such as iron which is alternately oxidized by H_2O_2 and reduced by O_2^- with the overall reaction being the Haber–Weiss reaction (McCord and Day, 1978; Halliwell, 1978) as follows:

$$\begin{aligned} &H_2O_2 + Fe^{2+} \rightarrow Fe^{3+} + OH^- + OH\cdot \\ &O_2^- + Fe^{3+} \rightarrow Fe^{2+} + O_2 \\ \hline &H_2O_2 + O_2^- \rightarrow O_2 + OH^- + OH\cdot \end{aligned}$$

This catalytic activity of iron is increased by the chelating agent EDTA but is inhibited by certain other chelating agents, e.g. diethylenetriamine penta-acetic acid (DTPA) or desferrioxamine (McCord and Day, 1978; Halliwell, 1978). Inhibition of a reaction by superoxide dismutase, catalase and OH· scavengers such as mannitol or ethanol has been employed as evidence for a requirement for OH· formed by the metal-catalysed Haber–Weiss reaction (Beauchamp and Fridovich, 1970).

Since both H_2O_2 and O_2^- are generated by phagocytes, it might be anticipated that their interaction in a metal-catalysed Haber-Weiss reaction would result in the generation of OH·. Direct measurement of OH· formation by phagocytes has been attempted. Certain thioethers, namely methional and 2 keto-4-methylthiobutyric acid (KMB) are converted by one electron oxidants to the redical cation which degrades to release ethylene, which can be measured by gas chromatography. Hydroxyl radicals are among the one electron oxidants capable of this reaction (Beauchamp and Fridovich, 1970). Phagocytosis by neutrophils (Tauber and Babior, 1977; Klebanoff and Rosen, 1978; Weiss *et al.*, 1978a) or some mononuclear phagocytes (Weiss *et al.*, 1977; Drath *et al.*, 1979) is associated with the formation of ethylene from methional or KMB raising the possibility that this reaction can be employed as a measure of OH· formation by phagocytes. However, ethylene formation by neutrophils is largely dependent on myeloperoxidase; it is less than 10% of normal when leukocytes from patients with hereditary MPO deficiency are employed (Klebanoff and Rosen, 1978) which is in sharp contrast to the increased respiratory burst activity of these cells (Klebanoff and Pincus, 1971; Klebanoff and Hamon, 1972; Rosen and Klebanoff, 1976). Since the formation of OH· by MPO has not been demonstrated, this raises the possibility that ethylene formation by neutrophils is initiated largely by oxidants other than OH·. The residual ethylene formation by MPO-deficient neutrophils and that of mononuclear phagocytes which lack peroxidase may, however, be due to the OH· generated by these cells. Methane formation from dimethyl sulphoxide (DMSO) also has been employed as a chemical measure of OH· formation by phagocytes (Repine *et al.*, 1979).

An additional method which has been employed for the detection of OH· formation by phagocytes is electron spin resonance spectroscopy (ESR) using the spin trap 5,5-dimethyl-1-pyrroline-*N*-oxide (DMPO). DMPO reacts with OH· to form a characteristic ESR spectrum and this spectrum is observed when neutrophils ingest particles in the presence of DMPO (Green *et al.*, 1979; Rosen and Klebanoff, 1979). In contrast to ethylene formation, DMPO/OH· adduct formation, like the respiratory burst, is increased when MPO-deficient leukocytes are used (Rosen and Klebanoff, 1979). It should be emphasized, however, that DMPO also can form a radical adduct with O_2^- (or $HO_2^·$) and this DMPO/OOH· adduct may decompose to the OH· adduct (Rosen and Klebanoff, 1979; Finkelstein *et al.*, 1979).

The involvement of OH· in the microbicidal activity of neutrophils was proposed by Johnston *et al.* (1975) based on the inhibition of bacterial killing by superoxide dismutase or catalase bound to latex beads and by certain OH· scavengers. Further, both H_2O_2 and O_2^- appeared to be required for the killing of *Toxoplasma gondii* by macrophages, suggesting the possible involvement of OH· (Murray and Cohn, 1979; Murray *et al.*, 1979). These findings, together with the highly reactive nature of hydroxyl radicals and their probable formation in phagocytes, point to a role for OH· or "a strongly oxidizing OH·—analogous complex" (Bors *et al.*, 1979) in the toxic activity of phagocytes.

Singlet oxygen

Molecular oxygen contains 2 unpaired valence electrons with spins in the same direction. Singlet oxygen is an excited state of oxygen which is formed when an absorption of energy shifts one of the unpaired electrons to an orbital of higher energy with an inversion of spin (see Wasserman and Murray, 1979). There are 2 forms of singlet oxygen: delta singlet oxygen in which the newly paired electrons occupy the same orbital, and sigma singlet oxygen in which the electrons, now of opposite spin, occupy different orbitals. Singlet oxygen can dissipate its excess energy by the emission of light, and interest in the possible formation of singlet oxygen by phagocytes stemmed from the finding that light was emitted by stimulated phagocytes (Allen *et al.*, 1972). However, chemiluminescence *per se* is not a measure of singlet oxygen formation; it indicates the formation of an excited state with spectral analysis required to identify the nature of the excited species. Analyses to date have not revealed the characteristic spectrum of singlet oxygen decay but rather broad peak activity (Cheson *et al.*, 1976; Andersen *et al.*, 1977). Singlet oxygen, as well as other products of the respiratory burst, would be expected to react with cell or particle components to form excited products and it is presumably the decay of these secondary excitations which is responsible for the light emission.

The chemical reactivity of $^1O_2$ in aqueous solution is due largely, if not entirely, to the delta form due to its relatively long lifetime (2 μs in water) and its electronic configuration. Singlet oxygen is a strong electrophile which reacts with compounds in areas of high electron density to form characteristic, often oxygenated, products. That reactions of this sort on the surface of cells can be toxic is suggested by the photodynamic action of dyes. Certain dyes in the presence of light and oxygen are toxic to cells and one of the mechanisms proposed for this photodynamic action is the excitation of oxygen by the light-sensitized dye with the formation of $^1O_2$, which reacts with cell surface component to produce damage. Evidence for the formation of $^1O_2$ by stimulated phagocytes would be: (1) the demonstration of the characteristic emission spectrum of $^1O_2$ decay; (2) the detection of a specific $^1O_2$ product on incubation of phagocytes with an appropriate substrate; and (3) the inhibition of phagocytic cell function by $^1O_2$ quenchers and its potentiation by D_2O, an agent which increases the lifetime of $^1O_2$ in solution. Demonstration of $^1O_2$ is complicated by its short lifetime and by the lack of specificity of some of the procedures outlined above. Despite considerable effort, its formation by phagocytes has yet to be definitively demonstrated. Nevertheless, interest in its generation by phagocytes remains, based on the possibility of its formation by the peroxidase-mediated cytotoxic system (see above) and from the superoxide anion by one of a number of reactions (see Klebanoff, 1980). Although this and other indirect evidence (Krinsky, 1974) is suggestive, definitive proof of $^1O_2$ involvement in the toxic activity of phagocytes is lacking.

Oxygen-independent toxic systems

A variety of toxic systems which do not require oxygen are present in phagocytes (Table I). They have been reviewed previously by the author (Klebanoff, 1975; Klebanoff and Hamon, 1975; Klebanoff and Clark, 1978) and the description here will be limited largely to recent studies.

Interest in the role of the iron-binding protein lactoferrin in the toxic activity of phagocytes stemmed from the observation that this substance has bacteriostatic properties when not fully saturated with iron, presumably due to the chelation of iron required for the growth of the organisms. This antimicrobial activity of lactoferrin is weak as compared to that of other antimicrobial systems of phagocytes. More recently, iron has been proposed as a potential catalyst of the Haber–Weiss reaction and thus of OH· formation (see above). Lactoferrin thus may theoretically stimulate OH· formation by providing iron in an active form or inhibit it by the removal of iron from solution as an inactive chelate. Future studies are required to establish a role for lactoferrin in the control of OH· formation.

There is considerable literature on the presence and properties of cationic proteins in neutrophil granules (Klebanoff and Clark, 1978; Olsson and Venge, 1980). These proteins are toxic to micro-organisms (Odeberg and Olsson, 1975; Lehrer *et al.*, 1975; Modrzakowski *et al.*, 1979) and tumour cells (Clark *et al.*, 1976). An important recent development is the isolation of a cationic protein from rabbit and human polymorphonuclear leukocytes with potent bactericidal activity against certain Gram-negative bacterial species (Weiss *et al.*, 1978b; Elsbach *et al.*, 1979). The factor binds to the bacterial outer membrane and increases its permeability, and the extent of the damage is related to the bacterial lipopolysaccharide chain length (Weiss *et al.*, 1980). Eosinophil granules also contain a strongly cationic protein (major basic protein, MBP) in high concentration (Gleich *et al.*, 1973, 1974). MBP is toxic to the schistosomula of *Schistosoma mansoni* (Butterworth *et al.*, 1979), the newborn larvae of *Trichinella spiralis* (Wassom and Gleich, 1979), guinea-pig tracheal mucosa (Frigas *et al.*, 1980) as well as a number of other cell types (Gleich *et al.*, 1979), and presumably contributes to the toxic activity of eosinophils *in situ*.

Summary

A variety of toxic systems are present in phagocytes, some dependent on oxygen and others effective in its absence. Together they destroy most ingested organisms; they also can be released into the extracellular fluid and damage adjacent cells. The toxic systems differ quantitatively, and, to some degree qualitatively, among phagocytes and synergism among antimicrobial systems has been reported. For example, the neutrophil elastase has been reported to potentiate the antimicrobial activity of the MPO-mediated system and of neutrophil-derived cationic proteins (Odeberg and Olsson, 1976) and the fall in pH within the phagosome or between phagocyte and extracellular target would be expected to influence the toxic activity of peroxidases and cationic proteins. There appears to be a considerable excess in killing capacity in most instances, both as a result of the multiple killing mechanisms available in each phagocyte and the variety of phagocytes. The total armamentarium is impressive and certainly essential to the host defence.

References

Ackerman, G. A. and Clark, M. A. (1971). *Acta Haematol.* **45**, 280–284.

Agner, K. (1972). *In* "Structure and Function of Oxidation-Reduction Enzymes" (A. Akeson and A. Ehrenberg, eds), Vol. 18, pp. 329–335. Pergamon Press, New York.

Alexander, N. M. (1974). *J. Biol. Chem.* **249**, 1946–1952.

Allen, R. C., Stjernholm, R. L. and Steele, R. H. (1972). *Biochem. Biophys. Res. Commun.* **47**, 679–684.

Andersen, B. R., Brendzel, A. M. and Lint, T. F. (1977). *Infect. Immun.* **17**, 62–66.

Aune, T. M. and Thomas, E. L. (1977). *Eur. J. Biochem.* **80**, 209–214.

Babior, B. M., Kipnes, R. S. and Curnutte, J. T. (1973). *J. Clin. Invest.* **52**, 741–744.

Baehner, R. L. and Johnston, R. B. Jr (1971). *Br. J. Haematol.* **20**, 277–285.

Bainton, D. F. and Farquhar, M. G. (1970). *J. Cell. Biol.* **45**, 54–73.

Bainton, D. F., Ullyot, J. L. and Farquhar, M. G. (1971). *J. Exp. Med.* **134**, 907–934.

Bass, D. A. and Szejda, P. (1979a). *J. Clin. Invest.* **64**, 1415–1422.

Bass, D. A. and Szejda, P. (1979b). *J. Clin. Invest.* **64**, 1558–1564.

Beauchamp, C. and Fridovich, I. (1970). *J. Biol. Chem.* **245**, 4641–4646.

Behar, D., Czapski, G., Rabani, J., Dorfman, L. M. and Schwarz, H. A. (1970). *J. Phys. Chem.* **74**, 3209–3213.

Belding, M. E., Klebanoff, S. J. and Ray, C. G. (1970). *Science* **167**, 195–196.

Bentfeld, M. E., Nichols, B. A. and Bainton, D. F. (1977). *Anat. Rec.* **187**, 219–240.

Bielski, B. H. J. and Allen, A. O. (1977). *J. Phys. Chem.* **81**, 1048–1050.

Biggar, W. D., Buron, S. and Holmes, B. (1976). *Infect. Immun.* **14**, 6–10.

Bodel, P. T., Nichols, B. A. and Bainton, D. F. (1977). *J. Exp. Med.* **145**, 264–274.

Bodel, P. T., Nichols, B. A. and Bainton, D. F. (1978). *Am. J. Path.* **91**, 107–117.

Bors, W., Michel, C. and Saran, M. (1979). *Eur. J. Biochem.* **95**, 621–627.

Bos, A., Wever, R. and Roos, D. (1978). *Biochim. Biophys. Acta.* **525**, 37–44.

Buege, J. E. and Aust, S. D. (1976). *Biochim. Biophys. Acta.* **444**, 192–201.

Butterworth, A. E., Wassom, D. L., Gleich, G. J., Loegering, D. A. and David, J. R. (1979). *J. Immunol.* **122**, 221–229.

Cheson, B. D., Christensen, R. L., Sperling, R., Kohler, B. E. and Babior, B. M. (1976). *J. Clin. Invest.* **58**, 789–796.
Clark, R. A. (1979). *Clin. Res.* **27**, 290A.
Clark, R. A. and Klebanoff, S. J. (1975). *J. Exp. Med.* **141**, 1442–1447.
Clark, R. A. and Klebanoff, S. J. (1977a). *Blood* **50**, 65–70.
Clark, R. A. and Klebanoff, S. J. (1977b). *J. Immunol.* **119**, 1413–1418.
Clark, R. A. and Klebanoff, S. J. (1979a). *J. Immunol.* **122**, 2605–2610.
Clark, R. A. and Klebanoff, S. J. (1979b). *J. Clin. Invest.* **63**, 177–183.
Clark, R. A. and Klebanoff, S. J. (1979c). *J. Clin. Invest.* **64**, 913–920.
Clark, R. A., Klebanoff, S. J., Einstein, A. B. and Fefer, A. (1975). *Blood* **45**, 161–170.
Clark, R. A., Olsson, I. and Klebanoff, S. J. (1976). *J. Cell Biol.* **70**, 719–723.
Clark, R. A., Szot, S., Venkatasubramanian, K. and Schiffman, E. (1980). *J. Immunol.* **124**, 2020–2026.
Daems, W. Th., Poelmann, R. E. and Brederoo, P. (1973). *J. Histochem. Cytochem.* **21**, 93–95.
DeChatelet, L. R., Shirley, P. S., McPhail, L. C., Huntley, C. C., Muss, H. B. and Bass, D. A. (1977). *Blood* **50**, 525–535.
Desser, R. K., Himmerlhoch, S. R., Evans, W. H., Januska, M., Mage, M. and Shelton, E. (1972). *Arch. Biochem. Biophys.* **148**, 452–465.
Diamond, R. D., Root, R. K. and Bennett, J. E. (1972). *J. Infect. Dis.* **125**, 367–376.
Drath, D. B., Karnovsky, M. L. and Huber, G. L. (1979). *J. Appl. Physiol.* **46**, 136–140.
Elsbach, P., Weiss, J., Franson, R. C., Beckerdite-Quagliata, S., Schneider, A. and Harris, L. (1979). *J. Biol. Chem.* **254**, 11 000–11 009.
Fee, J. A. and Valentine, J. S. (1977). *In* "Superoxide and Superoxide Dismutases" (A. M. Michelson, J. M. McCord and I. Fridovich, eds), pp. 19–60. Academic Press, New York.
Finkelstein, E., Rosen, G. M., Rauckman, E. J. and Paxton, J. (1979). *Mol. Pharmacol.* **16**, 676–685.
Fridovich, I. (1970). *J. Biol. Chem.* **245**, 4053–4057.
Fridovich, I. (1976). *In* "Free Radicals in Biology" (W. A. Pryor, ed.), Vol. 1, pp. 277–299. Academic Press, New York.
Frigas, E., Loegering, D. A. and Gleich, G. J. (1980). *Lab. Invest.* **42**, 35–43.
van Furth, R., Hirsch, J. G. and Fedorko, M. E. (1970). *J. Exp. Med.* **132**, 794–812.
Gee, J. B. L., Vassallo, C. L., Bell, P., Kaskin, J., Basford, R. E. and Field, J. B. (1970). *J. Clin. Invest.* **49**, 1280–1287.
Gee, J. B. L., Kaskin, J., Duncombe, M. P. and Vassallo, C. L. (1974). *J. Reticuloend. Soc.* **15**, 61–68.
Gleich, G. J., Loegering, D. A. and Maldonado, J. E. (1973). *J. Exp. Med.* **137**, 1459–1471.
Gleich, G. J., Loegering, D. A., Kueppers, F., Bajaj, S. P. and Mann, K. G. (1974). *J. Exp. Med.* **140**, 313–332.
Gleich, G. J., Frigas, E., Loegering, D. A., Wassom, D. L. and Steinmuller, D. (1979). *J. Immunol.* **123**, 2925–2927.
Green, M. R., Hill, H. A. O., Okolow-Zubkowska, M. J. and Segal, A. W. (1979). *FEBS Lett.* **100**, 23–26.
Grignaschi, V. I., Sperperato, A. M., Etcheverry, M. J. and Macario, A. J. L. (1963). *Rev. Asoc. Méd. Argent.* **77**, 218–221.
Haber, F. and Weiss, J. (1934). *Proc. R. Soc. Lond. A* **147**, 332–351.
Halliwell, B. (1978). *FEBS Lett.* **92**, 321–326.
Harrison, J. E. and Schultz, J. (1976). *J. Biol. Chem.* **251**, 1371–1374.
Harrison, J. E., Watson, B. D. and Schultz, J. (1978). *FEBS Lett.* **92**, 327–332.
Held, A. M. and Hurst, J. K. (1978). *Biochem. Biophys. Res. Commun.* **81**, 878–885.
Henderson, W. R. and Kaliner, M. (1978). *J. Clin. Invest.* **61**, 187–196.

Henderson, W. R., Jong, E. C. and Klebanoff, S. J. (1980a). *J. Immunol.* **124**, 1383–1388.

Henderson, W. R., Chi, E. Y. and Klebanoff, S. J. (1980b). *J. Exp. Med.* (in press).

Hoogendoorn, H., Piessens, J. P., Scholtes, W. and Stoddard, L. A. (1977). *Caries Res.* **11**, 77–84.

Howard, D. H. (1973). *Infect. Immun.* **8**, 412–419.

Iyer, G. Y. N., Islam, D. M. F. and Quastel, J. H. (1961). *Nature* **192**, 535–541.

Jacobs, A. A., Low, I. E., Paul, B. B., Strauss, R. R. and Sbarra, A. J. (1972). *Infect. Immun.* **5**, 127–131.

Johnston, R. B. Jr, Keele, B. B. Jr, Misra, H. P., Lehmeyer, J. E., Webb, L. S., Baehner, R. L. and Rajagopalan, K. V. (1975). *J. Clin. Invest.* **55**, 1357–1372.

Jong, E. C. and Klebanoff, S. J. (1980). *J. Immunol.* **124**, 1949–1953.

Jong, E. C., Mahmoud, A. A. F. and Klebanoff, S. J. (1979). *Clin. Res.* **27**, 479A.

Jong, E. C., Henderson, W. R. and Klebanoff, S. J. (1980). *J. Immunol.* **124**, 1378–1382.

Kasha, M. and Khan, A. U. (1970). *Ann. N.Y. Acad. Sci.* **171**, 5–23.

Klebanoff, S. J. (1967). *J. Exp. Med.* **126**, 1063–1078.

Klebanoff, S. J. (1968). *J. Bact.* **95**, 2131–2138.

Klebanoff, S. J. (1969). *Proc. Soc. Exp. Biol. Med.* **132**, 571–574.

Klebanoff, S. J. (1970a). *Science* **169**, 1095–1097.

Klebanoff, S. J. (1970b). *In* "Biochemistry of the Phagocytic Process" (J. Schultz, ed.), pp. 89–110. North-Holland, Amsterdam.

Klebanoff, S. J. (1975). *Semin Hemat.* **12**, 117–142.

Klebanoff, S. J. (1980). *In* "Mononuclear Phagocytes: Functional Aspects" (R. vanFurth, ed.), pp. 1105–1137. Martinus Nijhoff, The Hague.

Klebanoff, S. J. and Clark, R. A. (1975). *Blood* **45**, 699–707.

Klebanoff, S. J. and Clark, R. A. (1978). *In* "The Neutrophil: Function and Clinical Disorders". North-Holland, Amsterdam.

Klebanoff, S. J. and Hamon, C. B. (1972). *J. Reticuloend. Soc.* **12**, 170–196.

Klebanoff, S. J. and Hamon, C. B. (1975). *In* "Mononuclear Phagocytes in Immunity, Infection and Pathology" (R. vanFurth, ed.), pp. 507–531. Blackwell Scientific, Oxford.

Klebanoff, S. J. and Pincus, S. H. (1971). *J. Clin. Invest.* **50**, 2226–2229.

Klebanoff, S. J. and Rosen, H. (1978). *J. Exp. Med.* **148**, 490–506.

Klebanoff, S. J., Durack, D. T., Rosen, H. and Clark, R. A. (1977). *Infect. Immun.* **17**, 167–173.

Krinsky, N. I. (1974). *Science* **186**, 363–365.

Lehrer, R. I. (1969). *J. Bact.* **99**, 361–365.

Lehrer, R. I. (1975). *J. Clin. Invest.* **55**, 338–346.

Lehrer, R. I. and Cline, M. J. (1969). *J. Clin. Invest.* **48**, 1478–1488.

Lehrer, R. I. and Jan, R. G. (1970). *Infect. Immun.* **1**, 345–350.

Lehrer, R. I., Hanifin, J. and Cline, M. J. (1969). *Nature* **223**, 78–79.

Lehrer, R. I., Ladra, K. M. and Hake, R. B. (1975). *Infect. Immun.* **11**, 1226–1234.

Lemarbre, P., Hoidal, J., Vesella, R. and Rinehart, J. (1980). *Blood* **55**, 612–617.

Massey, V., Strickland, S., Mayhew, S. G., Howell, L. G., Engel, P. C., Matthews, R. G., Schuman, M. and Sullivan, P. A. (1969). *Biochem. Biophys. Res. Commun.* **36**, 891–897.

Matheson, N. R., Wong, P. S. and Travis, J. (1979). *Biochem. Biophys. Res. Commun.* **88**, 402–409.

McCord, J. M. and Day, E. D. Jr (1978). *FEBS Lett.* **86**, 139–142.

McRipley, R. J. and Sbarra, A. J. (1967). *J. Bact.* **94**, 1425–1430.

Metzger, Z., Hoffeld, J. T. and Oppenheim, J. J. (1980). *J. Immunol.* **124**, 983–988.

Mickenberg, I. D., Root, R. K. and Wolff, S. M. (1972). *Blood* **39**, 67–80.

Migler, R. and DeChatelet, L. R. (1978). *Biochem. Med.* **19**, 16–26.

Migler, R., DeChatelet, L. R. and Bass, D. A. (1978). *Blood* **51**, 445–456.

Modrzakowski, M. C., Cooney, M. H., Martin, L. E. and Spitznagel, J. K. (1979). *Infect. Immun.* **23**, 587–591.
Murray, H. W. and Cohn, Z. A. (1979). *J. Exp. Med.* **150**, 938–949.
Murray, H. W., Juangbhanich, C. W., Nathan, C. F. and Cohn, Z. A. (1979). *J. Exp. Med.* **150**, 950–964.
Nathan, C. F., Brukner, L. H., Silverstein, S. C. and Cohn, Z. A. (1979a). *J. Exp. Med.* **149**, 84–99.
Nathan, C. F., Silverstein, S. C., Brukner, L. H. and Cohn, Z. A. (1979b). *J. Exp. Med.* **149**, 100–113.
Nathan, C. F., Nogueira, N., Juangbhanich, C., Ellis, J. and Cohn, Z. A. (1979c). *J. Exp. Med.* **149**, 1056–1068.
Nichols, B. A., Bainton, D. F. and Farquhar, M. G. (1971). *J. Cell. Biol.* **50**, 498–515.
Odeberg, H. and Olsson, I. (1975). *J. Clin. Invest.* **56**, 1118–1124.
Odeberg, H. and Olsson, I. (1976). *Infect. Immun.* **14**, 1276–1283.
Olsson, I. and Venge, P. (1980). *Allergy* **35**, 1–13.
Paul, B. B., Strauss, R. R., Selvaraj, R. J. and Sbarra, A. J. (1973). *Science* **181**, 849–850.
Piatt, J. F. and O'Brien, P. J. (1979). *Eur. J. Biochem.* **93**, 323–332.
Rabani, J., Klug, D. and Fridovich, I. (1972). *Israel J. Chem.* **10**, 1095–1106.
Ramsey, P. G. and Klebanoff, S. J. (1980). *Clin. Res.* **28**, 513A.
Repine, J. E., Eaton, J. W., Anders, M. W., Hoidal, J. R. and Fox, R. B. (1979). *J. Clin. Invest.* **64**, 1642–1651.
Rosen, H. and Klebanoff, S. J. (1976). *J. Clin. Invest.* **58**, 50–60.
Rosen, H. and Klebanoff, S. J. (1977). *J. Biol. Chem.* **252**, 4803–4810.
Rosen, H. and Klebanoff, S. J. (1979). *J. Clin. Invest.* **64**, 1725–1729.
Sbarra, A. J., Selvaraj, R. J., Paul, B. B., Mitchell, G. W. Jr and Louis, F. (1977). *In* "Movement, Metabolism and Bactericidal Mechanisms of Phagocytes" (F. Rossi, P. L. Patriarca and D. Romeo, eds), pp. 295–304. Piccin Medical Books, Padua.
Selvaraj, R. J., Paul, B. B., Strauss, R. R., Jacobs, A. A. and Sbarra, A. J. (1974). *Infect. Immun.* **9**, 255–260.
Selvaraj, R. J., Zgliczyński, J. M., Paul, B. B. and Sbarra, A. J. (1980). *J. Reticuloend. Soc.* **27**, 31–38.
Simmons, S. R. and Karnovsky, M. L. (1973). *J. Exp. Med.* **138**, 44–63.
Smith, D. C. and Klebanoff, S. J. (1970). *Biol. Reprod.* **3**, 229–235.
Stankovich, M. T., Schopfer, L. M. and Massey, V. (1978). *J. Biol. Chem.* **253**, 4971–4979.
Stelmaszyńska, T. and Zgliczyński, J. M. (1978). *Eur. J. Biochem.* **92**, 301–308.
Stossel, T. P., Mason, R. J., Pollard, T. D. and Vaughan, M. (1972). *J. Clin. Invest.* **51**, 604–614.
Tauber, A. I. and Babior, B. M. (1977). *J. Clin. Invest.* **60**, 374–379.
Tauber, A. I., Goetzl, E. J. and Babior, B. M. (1976). *Blood* **48**, 968.
Thomas, E. L. (1979). *Infect. Immun.* **23**, 522–531.
Thomas, E. L. and Aune, T. M. (1977). *Biochemistry* **16**, 3581–3586.
Thomas, E. L. and Aune, T. M. (1978). *Antimicrob. Agents Chemother.* **13**, 1006–1010.
Wasserman, H. H. and Murray, R. W. (eds) (1979). "Singlet Oxygen". Academic Press, New York.
Wassom, D. L. and Gleich, G. J. (1979). *Am. J. Trop. Med. Hyg.* **28**, 860–863.
Weinstein, J. and Bielski, B. H. J. (1979). *J. Am. Chem. Soc.* **101**, 58–62.
Weiss, S. J., King, G. W. and LoBuglio, A. F. (1977). *J. Clin. Invest.* **60**, 370–373.
Weiss, S. J., Rustagi, P. K. and LoBuglio, A. F. (1978a). *J. Exp. Med.* **147**, 316–323.
Weiss, J., Elsbach, P., Olsson, I. and Odeberg, H. (1978b). *J. Biol. Chem.* **253**, 2664–2672.
Weiss, J., Beckerdite-Quagliata, S. and Elsbach, P. (1980). *J. Clin. Invest.* **65**, 619–628.
Zgliczyński, J. M. and Stelmaszyńska, T. (1975). *Eur. J. Biochem.* **56**, 157–162.

42

Inflammation and Natural Immunity

ROBERT M. FAUVE

Unité d'Immunophysiologie cellulaire,
Institut Pasteur, Paris, France

Introduction

In order to persist and multiply in a given host, pathogens must overcome, first, the natural mechanisms of resistance, and later on, the specific effectors elicited by the antigenic determinants of invaders. In both steps, a complex system allows an increased number of effectors at the site of pathogens: inflammation.

As reviewed by Metchnikoff (1901), it has been known for nearly a century that an inflammation induced at the site of infection is able to increase strikingly the resistance of the host. Since we are dealing with natural immunity, we shall not examine in this review the induction of inflammation following the interaction between antigens and humoral or cellular effectors of specific

The work mentioned in this review was supported by grants from INSERM, DGRST, DRET, CNAM and the Ligue Nationale Française contre le Cancer. The secretarial help of C. Maczuka in the preparation of the manuscript is gratefully acknowledged.

immunity. We shall focus only on the different mechanisms explaining how an inflammatory reaction can increase natural immunity. Furthermore, it will be shown that some pathogens exhibit anti-inflammatory effects and that a local inflammation is of importance for the remote control of host resistance against pathogens.

Inflammation

The inflammatory process is one of the oldest phylogenic mechanisms of resistance since the first reaction of defence in primitive metazoa is the mobilization of amoebocytes at the site of aggression (Metchnikoff, 1892). Originally defined by this term because of the local warmth occurring at the site of injury, inflammation represents the host's responses to insults through various neurologic, vascular, humoral and cellular factors. The interrelationships of these factors can be summarized in a cascade of events that constitute the inflammatory process which were recently reviewed by Lepow and Ward (1972), Rocha e Silva and Garcia-Leme (1972), Zweifach *et al.* (1974),

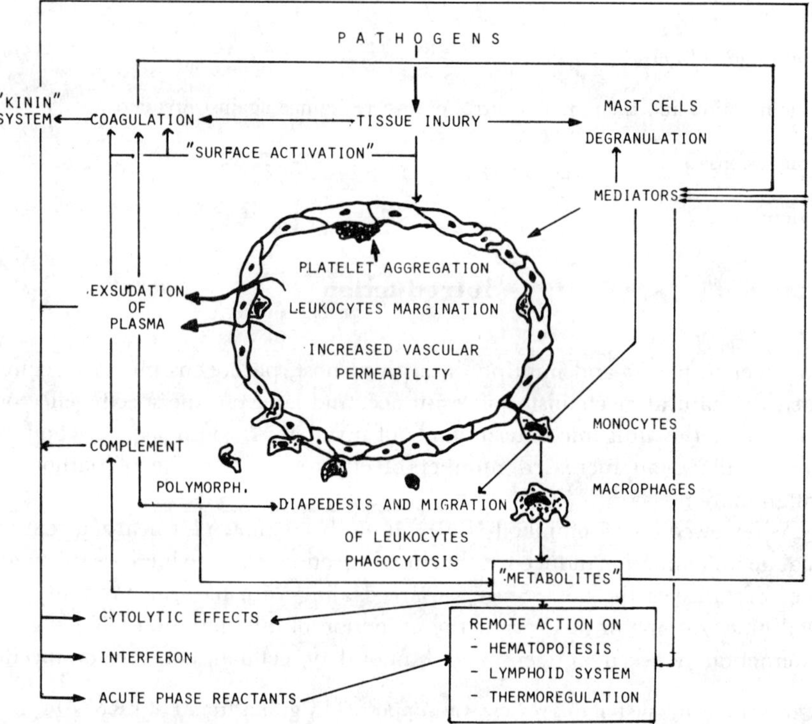

FIG. 1. *Diagram of the inflammatory reaction.*

Wilkinson (1974), Ryan and Majno (1977), Vane and Fereira (1978) and Movat (1979).

As shown in Fig. 1, a tissue injury induced by trauma, burn, radiation, different substances or pathogens is followed immediately by mast cell degranulation and liberation of some mediators. These mediators and some products resulting from "surface activation" induce vasodilatation which is followed rapidly by increased vascular permeability, platelet aggregation, and leukocyte migration. This increased vascular permeability allows the exudation of plasma with all the "participants" of the coagulation, fibrinolytic, and complement systems. In the same tissue, an increase in humoral factors such as circulating interferon, acute reactants and other substances with cytocidal properties is found at the site of inflammation. Platelet aggregation and leukocyte margination are followed by leukocyte diapedesis and migration through the basal membrane of the vessels. Once in the extravascular space, the movement of leukocytes towards injured cells, irritants or pathogens is controlled by chemotactic factors. Within the extravascular space, leukocytes release metabolic products or lyse, and thus release enzymes and mediators. These, in addition to some coagulation and complement factors, will contribute to increase locally the inflammatory process. Among leukocytes, monocytes are transformed into macrophages. The products of macrophage metabolism reinforce the inflammatory reaction. Macrophages with polymorphonuclear leukocytes will ingest and kill some pathogens. The accumulation at the site of the inflammatory focus of serum components and their split products, tissue debris, and mediators of inflammation, induces an alteration in the lymphatic system and the introduction in the circulation of substances that will act, at a distance, on the thermoregulation centre, haematopoietic tissue, and cells in which are synthesized acute phase reactants. Among these acute phase reactants are substances able: (1) to counteract the toxic effects of products resulting from the local tissue injury; (2) to damage pathogens; and (3) to increase the resistance of the host against the pathogen at a distance from the site of inflammation. Later, if the causal agent is not easily resorbed, the transition from acute to chronic inflammation is observed, as seen for instance with some adjuvants.

We shall now briefly examine the different systems involved during the inflammatory process and it will be shown that they can contribute to the natural resistance of the host against pathogens.

The coagulation system

As summarized in Fig. 2, plasma coagulates following a tissue injury induced in a nonsensitized host by different substances and pathogens or even by only a surgical trauma. As with the complement, the clotting mechanism occurs by two pathways; the intrinsic and the extrinsic pathway. As reviewed in the above-mentioned references on inflammation and in a recent book by Ogston and Bennet (1977), the extrinsic pathway starts with tissue thromboplastin,

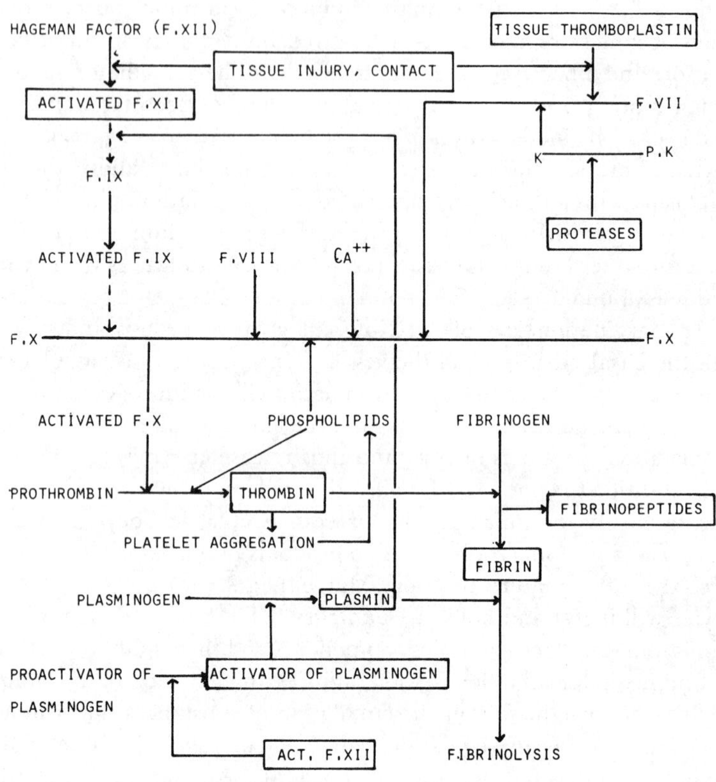

FIG. 2. *Diagram of the coagulation system.*

a poorly defined substance, which acts on factor VII. Factor VII can be also activated following contact with kallikrein (K) resulting from the action of proteases on prekallikrein (PK). Following these interactions factor X is activated.

The same activation of factor X occurs following the intrinsic pathway. Here again, tissue injury or contact with different substances are able to activate Hageman factor (FXII). This activated FXII will induce a cascade of factor activation, and following these interactions, FX is activated. The activation of FX leads to the transformation of prothrombin into thrombin, which induces not only platelet aggregation but also the transformation of fibrinogen to fibrin. Later on, the proactivator of fibrin in the presence of activated FXII transforms the proactivator of plasminogen into the activator of plasminogen, which transforms plasminogen in plasmin. Plasmin is able to split activated FXII and has a lytic action on fibrin. Furthermore, as demonstrated by Maillard and Favreau (1977), plasmin could increase the number of plaque-forming cells against T independent antigen, even with spleen cells depleted in T cells or macrophages. As will be seen later, some of these factors have an important function in complement and kinin systems. It is also known that fibrinopeptides are chemotactic for leukocytes and that fibrin helps phagocytic cells to move and ingest particles in inflammatory foci. The same kind of "catalytic" factors are produced following the activation of the complement.

The complement system

From the contributions of workers reviewed in the above-mentioned references, and more precisely by Vogt (1974), Müller-Eberhard (1975), and Hügli and Müller-Eberhard (1978), the activation of the complement system can be summarized as in Fig. 3. It is well known that the activation of the complement by the classical pathway starts with the activation of C_1 following its interaction with antigen–antibody complexes. More recently it has been shown that an

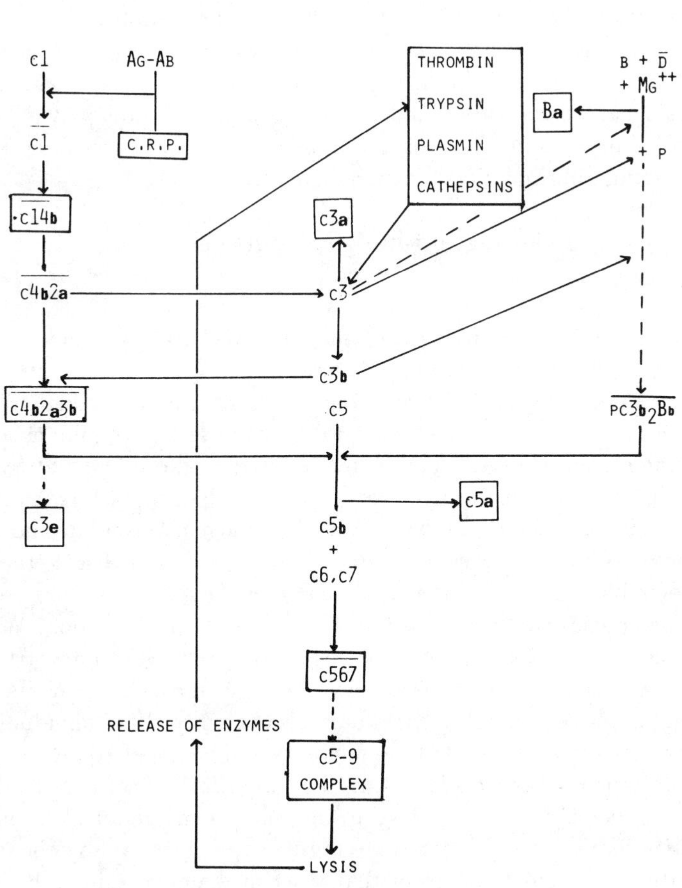

FIG. 3. *Diagram of the complement system.*

acute phase reactant, C reactive protein (CRP), is able also to activate C1. Following the work of Gotschlich and Edelman (1967), Volanakis and Kaplan (1971, 1974), Osmand *et al.* (1975), Siegel *et al.* (1975), Claus *et al.* (1977), CRP was shown to initiate the primary complement cascade upon interaction with C-polysaccharide or polycations following the activation of macromolecular C1. The binding specificity of CRP is related to the phosphocholine groups of C-polysaccharide. These findings are important since, at least in some experimental conditions, the classical pathway can be activated in the absence of antibodies.

The initial reactions of the alternative pathway occur when substances such as certain microbial polysaccharides interact with properdin (P), factor B, Factor $\overline{\text{D}}$ and C3 to achieve initial C3 cleavage. It is noteworthy that recently virus infected cells, bacteria and parasites (*Schistosoma mansoni*) were shown to induce this cleavage from both the classical and alternative pathways. Activating sequences interact with factors B and $\overline{\text{D}}$ to form the amplification C3 convertase. During these reactions, two products are released: C3a and C3e. Later, following the activation of C5, C5a and the complex $\overline{\text{C567}}$, among other products, are released. Finally, the complex C5-9 is involved in the lysis of cells. Following this lysis, some enzymes are released which are able to split C3 (trypsin, cathepsins, etc.). Some of these products not only play an important role in the inflammatory process, but also interact with other systems such as clotting, fibrinolytic and kinin systems.

Interactions between clotting, fibrinolytic, complement and kinin systems

As shown in Fig. 4, plasmin can split activated FXII, C1, C3 and transform prekallikrein in kallikrein. Plasmin can also split bradykinin from kininogens. Two other important links between these systems are kallikrein and FXII which interact to trigger the clotting and the kinin system. Again, as a result of these interactions, several factors are released in the inflammatory focus and, as we will see later, play a key role: complement factors, proteases, kallikrein and bradykinin, activators of plasminogen, thrombin and Hageman's factor (FXII). In fact, following the purification of FXII, the great number of publications on the biological activities of FXII and its split products lead to the conclusion that FXII is a key factor in inflammation. With all due respect to the work done in this area of research, it is noteworthy that M. Hageman, whose plasma was deficient in the factor which bears its name, died from pulmonary embolism. It should also be noted that individuals with the same deficiency show no bleeding tendency and no impaired inflammatory responses. As pointed out by Ryan and Majno (1977), these facts lead us to conclude "either that bradykinin is an insignificant mediator in human inflammation, that kinin activation (like clotting activation) can somehow occur *in vitro* without Hageman factor, or that other mediators can in such circumstances take over and compensate for the role of kinins". One has indeed to

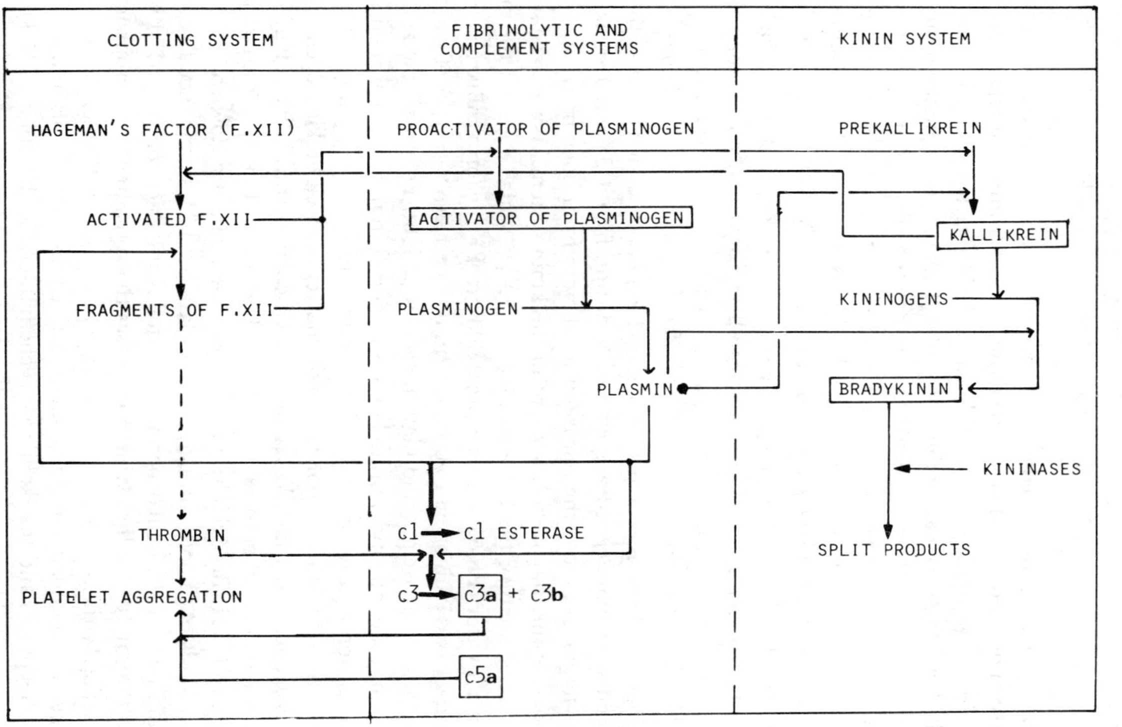

FIG. 4. *Interactions between the clotting, fibrinolytic and complement systems.*

be cautious when one considers all the products which are thought to trigger off and to sustain inflammatory reactions: they are called endogenous mediators.

Endogenous mediators

In contrast with exogenous mediators such as some bacterial products or other chemicals, endogenous mediators are those derived from the injured tissue.

Following *coagulation*, fibrinopeptides and fibrin degradation products are released. *Fibrinopeptides* can induce vascular leakage, are chemotactic for neutrophils and have been reported to enhance the effect of bradykinin.

Following the *activation of complement*, C1 4b is involved in immune adherence and viral neutralization. The complex C4b2a3b is considered to help immune adherence, to enhance phagocytosis and to stimulate lymphokine production. C5a, Ba, and C567 are chemotactic for phagocytic cells and both C5a and C3a are able to increase capillary permeabillty. For instance in human skin the minimum concentration which causes a wheal and erythema reaction is 2×10^{-12} M for C3a and 1×10^{-15} M for C5a. In addition to its chemotactic effect, C567 has been reported to enhance lymphocytotoxicity. Recently, a low molecular weight acidic fragment of C3, distant from C3a and designated C3e, was found to induce the release of leukocytes from bone marrow.

Bradykinin is the major effector agent of the kinin system. As we have seen (Fig. 4), a fragment of the Hageman factor (FXII) which is called the prekallikrein activator (PKA) activates prekallikrein (PK) to form kallikrein (K). Kallikrein cleaves kininogens to produce kinin. There are two types of kininogens: low molecular weight and high molecular weight. Following the action of kallikrein, a nonapeptide, bradykinin is removed from kininogen resulting in the formation of a heavy and a light chain held together by a disulphide bond. At the same time, from the high molecular weight kininogen, two fragments are formed which have transient vascular permeability enhancing activity. Another effect of these fragments is their ability to inhibit the contact activation of FXII. Bradykinin, in very low doses, causes a slow contraction of certain kinds of smooth muscle *in vitro*, dilatation of systemic blood vessels *in vivo*, and increased vascular permeability following injection. *In vitro*, it was observed that at 10^{-8} M, bradykinin increases the spreading of macrophages. In connection with the kinin system, it has been reported that kallikrein and plasminogen activator have chemotactic activity for neutrophils and mononuclear phagocytes and that kallikrein is chemotactic for basophils. The kinin system is controlled by the action of kallikrein antagonists in blood and tissues. Another modulator of the kinin system is the C1 esterase inhibitor which not only acts on the C1 component of the complement but which is also able to inhibit the effects of activated FXII, of kallikrein and plasmin. Bradykinin is quickly broken down by kininases present in plasma and tissues into inactive peptides.

Mediators released from tissues comprise the vasoactive amines, acidic lipids, lysosomal components, endopyrogens, substance P, neurotensin, tuftsin, and cyclic AMP.

The vasoactive amines are histamine and 5-hydroxy tryptamine or serotonin. Histamine and 5HT are found in the granules of mast cells and basophils, and in platelets. As we have seen, mechanical trauma, irradiation, heat, some venoms, toxins, surfactants, histamine liberators such as compound 48/80, ATP and some cationic proteins, are able to degranulate mast cells and to allow the release of histamine. Other agents are also able to trigger the platelet release reaction (platelet activating factor, enzymes such as trombin, trypsin, etc.). At the same time, other potential inflammatory mediators are derived or, as quoted by Ryan and Majno (1977), presumed to be derived from mast cells: eosinophil chemotactic factor, prostaglandins, slow reacting substances.

Slowly reacting substances and prostaglandins are acidic lipids which have been reported to induce arteriolar dilatation, pain, and fever. Among the many reports on prostaglandins (PG), it has been found that some of these compounds potentiate the plasma exudation induced by histamine and bradykinin and that PGE1, for instance, stimulates the intracellular accumulation of cyclic AMP (cAMP). It was found following such an accumulation that PGs are not only mediators of inflammation, but also modulators. For example, the increased content of cAMP could lead to decreased phagocytic activity. The recent finding that aspirin-like drugs and glucocorticoids are able respectively to inhibit the synthesis and the release of PGs is indirect proof that these compounds are important participants in the inflammatory reaction.

Lysosomal components are cationic proteins, and acid and neutral proteases. They are not only key factors in the inflammatory process, but some of these products are toxic for pathogens.

Other products of cell origin, *endopyrogens*, are proteins released from leukocytes (mostly from monocytes or macrophages). These products exert their effects by a central action on the hypothalamus. At this level, there are indications that prostaglandins may act as local neurohumoral transmitters. It has been shown that fever has a favourable effect against some viral and bacterial infections.

Substances P and neurotensin have kinin-like properties.

Tuftsin is a tetrapeptide fragment of immunoglobulin which is present in inflammatory foci. It has been reported that this peptide increases the phagocytic activity of polymorphonuclear leukocytes and macrophages. Furthermore, Tzehoval *et al.* (1978) have recently shown that tuftsin is able to increase the antigen specific, macrophage-dependent education of T lymphocytes.

All the systems and the mediators involved in inflammation are elements of a tangled web and some of the systems which were briefly summarized are quite well known (e.g. the alternate pathway of complement) in some species but not in others. Despite this complexity, it is clear that we have today enough elements to explain why inflammation is a cornerstone of natural resistance against pathogens.

Increased resistance against pathogens in inflammatory foci

As shown in Fig. 5, many factors illustrate how and why inflammation is so important in natural resistance against invaders. Acidic pH and hyperthermia are known to impede the survival of many pathogens. Following the activation of the complement, in addition to the lytic complex C5-9, other compounds such as C14b, C3a and C5a are known to increase the efficiency of the local mechanisms of resistance (viral neutralization, phagocytosis). Lysozymes have a minor lytic effect on virulent bacteria. In contrast, interferon was reported to act, not only against viruses, but also through indirect mechanisms on bacteria and malignant cells. Among cationic proteins, β-lysin has antibacterial effects. This thermostable cationic protein (mol. wt = 6000)

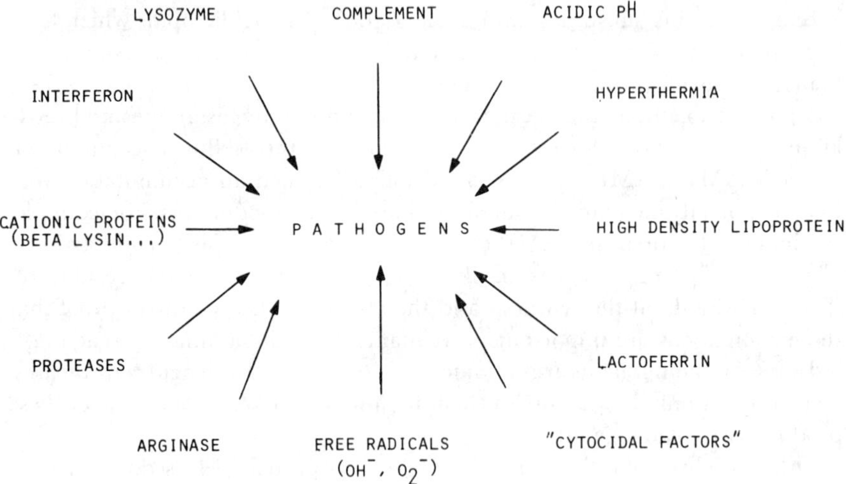

FIG. 5. *Inflammatory byproducts involved in host resistance against invaders.*

present in platelets and in body fluids is able, following its contact with the cell membrane, to kill bacteria within minutes (Donaldson and Tew, 1977). The same is true with some proteases. Arginase, whose synthesis and release were discovered recently in activated macrophages, may explain killing of schistosomula of *Schistosoma mansoni* (Olds *et al.*, 1980) and the killing of some malignant cells (Curie, 1978). As a consequence of the phagocytic process, free radicals OH^- and O_2^- are released in the vicinity of phagocytic cells and their effects on different pathogens, either bacteria, parasites or malignant cells, have been demonstrated (Jong *et al.*, 1979; Mantovani *et al.*, 1979; Murray and Cohn, 1979; Weiss *et al.*, 1980). Another substance which can be released by polymorphonuclear leukocytes is lactoferrin. As reviewed by Humbert *et al.* (1975) and Klebanoff and Clark (1978), lactoferrin is an iron binding protein present in the granules of PMN leukocytes which, when not fully saturated with iron, inhibits bacterial growth by binding the iron required as an essential microbial nutrient. Therefore lactoferrin is a bacteriostatic product. As quoted in general reviews on inflammation, many cytocidal factors have been described. Among them a trypanocidal factor has been found recently in normal serum by Rifkin (1978). Following the fractionation and the purification of serum lipoproteins, a trypanocidal activity was recovered in the high density lipoprotein (HDL) fraction. The identification of the trypanocidal factor as HDL was confirmed by the finding that serum from patients with a severe deficiency of HDL had no trypanocidal activity. Following the intravenous injection of HDL in mice infected with *Trypanozoma brucei* three days previously, the number of trypanosomes in the blood was strikingly decreased 24 hours after treatment.

All these factors allow one to understand the many weapons that pathogens have to face when they ingraft in a nonsensitized host. In addition to these effectors of natural resistance, other substances arrive at the vicinity of pathogens in the inflammatory focus: the acute phase reactants.

Acute phase reactants

Acute phase proteins or acute phase reactants (APR) are seric proteins whose concentration in blood is increased following and during the inflammatory process. They are considered in the general reviews mentioned previously and more precisely by Kof (1974).

The alpha 1 glycoprotein (AGP) very often called orosomucoid is an acidic protein. Its physical and chemical properties have been defined but its biological function is not completely known. It was shown that AGP inhibits thromboplastin and binds with progesterone and vitamin B_{12}. More recently, Chiu *et al.* (1977) have found that AGP *in vitro* decreases the blastogenesis induced by concanavalin A, pokeweed mitogen and PHA. A decreased mixed lymphocyte response was also observed.

The α-1 antitrypsin does not only bind to trypsin but also with some neutral proteases such as those from leukocytic origins.

Ceruloplasmin, an oxidase allows the binding of ferrous ions to apotransferrin. It was emphasized recently by Goldstein *et al.* (1979) that ceruloplasmin can act as a scavenger of superoxide anion radicals. Thus, ceruloplasmin can modulate the effects of these radicals in the inflammatory focus where it has been found that neutrophil-generated superoxide reacts with an extracellular precursor to generate a substance chemotactic for neutrophils (Petrone *et al.*, 1980).

Fibrinogen and haptoglobin have been found in the past to enhance the uptake of particles by phagocytic cells.

Complement components are also increased following and during inflammation. Among many reports, it was found by Schutte *et al.* (1974) that following surgery or in patients with active inflammatory diseases, properdin factor B (C3PA) and C1s levels showed the most dramatic changes. To a lesser extent, C1q, C4, C3 and C5 levels were also increased.

Besides transferrin, 3 other APR (CRP, α-2 macroglobulin and CSF) have great importance during inflammatory reactions. We have previously mentioned the importance of CRP in the classical pathway of the complement. As quoted by Mortensen (1979), CRP: (1) promotes C-dependent reactions of adherence and phagocytosis involving the macrophage Fc receptors; (2) suppresses platelet aggregation; (3) inhibits the lymphokine production; and (4) decreases the mixed lymphocyte proliferation following the binding of CRP to human and murine T lymphocytes. More recently, Mortensen (1979) has shown that this APR mediates the suppression of antibody induction to T dependent antigens by interacting with T cells and generating a suppressive T cell population.

As we have seen, high proteolytic activities can be demonstrated in an inflammatory focus and, as reviewed recently by Bata *et al.* (1979), lymphocyte responses can be modulated by protease–antiprotease interplay. Among these antiproteases (α–1 antitrypsin, antithrombin, interalpha trypsin inhibitor, antichymotrypsin and the inactivator of $C\bar{1}$ esterase), α-2 macroglobulin (α2M) has received special consideration. This macroglobulin, present in plasma in high concentration, is produced mostly by mononuclear phagocytic cells, as shown by Hovi *et al.* (1977). Except for the paradoxical activation of human leukocyte elastase by human α2M reported by Twumasi *et al.* (1977), this high molecular weight APR has polyvalent affinities and binds to many proteases. It was shown *in vitro* that α2M has inhibitory effects on the lymphocyte proliferative responses induced not only by lectins but also in mixed lymphocyte culture. Furthermore, it has been found *in vitro* that α2M decreases the antibody dependent and the PHA induced cytotoxicities. The precise mechanisms of these inhibitory effects are still unknown for some of these effects. Nevertheless, it seems reasonable to presume that α2M either at the site of inflammation or at a distance may modulate the lymphocyte responses.

Another acute phase reactant, the colony stimulating factor (CSF), is a protein involved in the regulation of haematopoiesis. More precisely, added to bone marrow cell *in vitro*, it stimulates the growth of granulocyte–macrophage colonies. CSF, which can be produced by macrophages, among other cells, has not only an effect on haematopoietic tissue but also on the natural resistance of the host. It was indeed shown by Handman and Burgess (1979) that pure CSF obtained from mouse lung conditioned medium is able to stimulate *in vitro* the *Leishmania tropica* killing by macrophages. When macrophages were incubated with CSF before infection with *L. tropica*, the uptake and the killing of parasites were increased. In contrast with normal macrophages in which *L. tropica* was found to survive unharmed and to multiply, when CSF was added to infected macrophages, an increased number of dead parasites was observed. This finding is of great importance since CSF is also considered as one lymphokine. Therefore, CSF is another example of a key factor of host resistance which can be induced following an antigen dependent reaction or following a "nonspecific" inflammation.

As we have seen, an inflammatory reaction not only allows locally a better phagocytosis, but also the release of harmful products against pathogens. How can such pathogens survive and multiply despite such a hostile environment? It is well known that some pathogens like virulent *Salmonella*, or *Mycobacterium tuberculosis* for instance are unharmed by the local acid pH and the proteolytic enzymes and that, although they are engulfed by phagocytic cells, they do multiply in macrophages. Other escape mechanisms have been described. Antigenic mimicry is a recent exciting explanation to account for the escape mechanisms of *Schistosoma mansoni*, for instance. Furthermore, since most pathogens, in the broadest sense of the term (viruses, bacteria, parasites, malignant cells), once established in a nonsensitized host are able to induce a tissue injury, one wonders why in many cases no inflammation is observed. This lack of inflammation in the vicinity of the pathogen may explain, at least in part, how some pathogens can repel the specific effectors of immunity, i.e. an immunorepulsion.

Immunorepulsion

In contrast with immunodepression or immunosuppression which act on systemic immunity, immunorepulsion is effective only in the vicinity of pathogens. As demonstrated by Fauve *et al.* (1974), malignant cells are able to repel macrophages. From the last review on this subject (James, 1977) and from more recent works (Razvorotnew *et al.*, 1977; Rabatic *et al.*, 1977; Johnson *et al.*, 1978; Stahl *et al.*, 1978; Cheung *et al.*, 1979), the existence of factor(s) has been reported in tumours or in the supernatant of cultured malignant cells. These factors are able to explain, at least in part, how malignant cells can impede the host resistance. Working with different tumours, these workers have isolated factors of molecular weight between 1000 and 12 000. Injected in mice or guinea-pigs, it was found that these malignant cell factors (MCF) decrease (1) the influx of polymorphonuclear leukocytes and macrophages in tissues injected with phlogogens; (2) the macrophage mediated resistance to *Listeria monocytogenes* infection; (3) the delayed hypersensitivity against sheep red blood cells; and (4) the host resistance when malignant cells and one of the described factors are injected in the same site in mice. *In vitro*, it has been found that MCF are able to decrease (1) the spreading and the chemotaxis of macrophages; and (2) the tumoricidal activity of macrophages induced by lipopolysaccharide. The precise nature of these factors is still not known. No precision is given concerning their mechanism of action. Nevertheless, according to recent findings (Fauve and Hevin, 1977; Stahl *et al.*, 1978), it was found, in contrast with bradykinin which is able to increase the spreading of murine macrophages, that MCF decreases the spreading of these cells. Furthermore, the effect of bradykinin can be inhibited if macrophages are incubated first with MCF, and the spreading inhibition of MCF is lost if macrophages are incubated first with bradykinin. These results suggest, but do not prove, that MCF competes with bradykinin for the same receptors. Concerning the key role of kinins in the inflammatory reaction, these preliminary findings may explain, at least in part, the decreased cellular infiltration in the vicinity of highly invasive malignant cells. Other pathogens are also able to behave as "immunorepellents". As reviewed by Fauve (1976), bacteria and parasites are also able to repel the effectors of the host resistance. Virulent bacteria such as *Staphylococcus aureus*, *Pseudomonas aeruginosa*, *Bordetella pertussis*, are able to decrease the inflammation at the site of injection and to impede the functions of phagocytic cells. Factors extracted from these bacteria were found to act on the Hageman's factor–kinin pathway or to act directly on phagocytes. Although no substances have been extracted from parasites until now, it is evident that such a local anti-inflammatory effect does exist with parasites. For instance, in the early stage of invasion of the liver by *Entamoeba histolytica* parenchymal cells are destroyed. Despite this injury, which is known in the liver to mobilize leukocytes quickly, there is a weak or no inflammatory reaction.

These observations might explain, at least in part, how an invader is able to ingraft in a tissue despite the effectors of natural or specific resistance. It is even reasonable to consider that one of the oldest mechanisms of pathogenicity is the ability to impede the local concentration of the effectors or resistance since one of the oldest phylogenic mechanisms of resistance in primitive metazoa is the mobilization of amoebocytes at the site of aggression. Such as immunorepulsion is mediated by immunorepellents synthesized by invaders. Among these products, some, like malignant cell factors, are not immunogenic. Furthermore, one can wonder, as is the case for some bacteria and malignant cells, if these immunorepellents are not produced mostly *in vivo* when the invaders are facing the resistance effectors of the host. These stratagems of some pathogens may also explain why so few vaccines are really effective against many bacteria and parasites. The same mechanisms may contribute also to explain why, despite the many weapons available in *in vitro* systems against malignant cells, they proliferate and metastasize *in vivo*.

In order to decrease or even to inhibit the proliferation and the metastasis of malignant cells in laboratory animals, it has been shown by many workers that endotoxin, BCG, polynucleotides, glucan and other substances can be used. Very often, following the treatment of laboratory animals with these "immunostimulants", an increased resistance against nonantigenically related pathogens is observed. Since following the injection of the more active immunostimulants granulomas occur, one can wonder if inflammation *per se* is not able to act on the host resistance against pathogens. As shown by Fauve and Hevin (1975), it was found that a local nonspecific inflammatory reaction may have great importance in the remote control of host resistance against *Listeria monocytogenes*.

Inflammation and the remote control of host resistance against invaders

As reviewed by Metchnikoff (1901), it has been known for nearly a century that animals are much more resistant to infections if bacteria are injected at the site of an acute inflammation. It is also well known that in the preantibiotic era, abcesses were induced in patients in order to stimulate their resistance against infectious diseases. However, these inflammatory reactions were produced following the injection of irritating substances (turpentine oil), bacteria or products now known to be able to diffuse from the injection site. For instance, as shown by Keller and Weiss (1972), the intraperitoneal injection of peptone, glycogen, starch, or polynucleotides, 5 days before the subcutaneous injection of malignant cells, is followed by a decreased growth of the Walker carcinoma in rats. Under these conditions, it is therefore difficult to dissociate the direct effect of these substances on the immune system from the effects of the inflammatory reaction *per se*. In order to investigate such effects, it was decided to induce inflammatory reactions with nonbiodegradable, nondiffusible and nonantigenic substances at a site distant from the site of aggression. For this purpose, mice were injected subcutaneously in the dorsal area with talc particles embedded in a gel of calcium phosphate (TCP). Care was taken during the preparation of this irritant and during its injection into mice to avoid the presence of pathogens and pyrogens. Later all the pathogens were injected intravenously or at sites distant from the site of inflammation.

As reviewed by Fauve (1978), it was found that such animals are more resistant against *Schistosoma mansoni*, *Plasmodium berghei*, *Candida albicans*, *Listeria monocytogenes*, *Salmonella typhimurium*, and the Lewis carcinoma.

When 8-week-old mice with a 3-day-old dorsal subcutaneous granuloma were infested transcutaneously following the immersion of the tail in water containing furcocercariae of *S. mansoni*, in nearly 100% no worms were found in the portal veins 45 days later. The same increased resistance was observed by Michel (1980) following the intravenous injection of merozoites from *P. berghei*. As shown by Hurtrel *et al.* (1980), such an inflammatory reaction was found to increase the resistance of mice against *Candida albicans*. The increased resistance following the inflammatory reaction was compared to the resistance of mice pretreated with different immunostimulants given at their respective optimal times and doses. It was found that whereas BCG, EBP and *Corynebacterium parvum* protected infected mice slightly, *Bordetella pertussis* vaccine, lipopolysaccharide and particularly TCP increased the resistance of mice very significantly. It was found that a correlation exists between the granulocytosis induced by these immunostimulants and the increased resistance against *C. albicans*.

Concerning the increased resistance against *Listeria monocytogenes*, it was found that in contrast with normal mice, all TCP treated mice survived a 5 LD_{50} intravenous inoculum of *Listeria* when they were infected between 4 and 11 days following the induction of the inflammatory reaction. The serum of such treated animals was not bactericidal and had no opsonizing effect. Following the fate of i.v. injected *Listeria* in the spleen and the liver of normal and treated mice, 1000 and 10 000 times fewer bacteria were found respectively in the spleens and the livers of mice injected 7 days before the infectious challenge. Studying the influence of the age of the granuloma on the fate of *Listeria* in the spleens, a significant increased bactericidal activity was found between days 3 and 11. The same increased resistance was found in germ-free and nude mice. More recently, Fontan and Fauve (1980) have shown that in a cell-free extract of a 5-day-old granuloma, it is possible to extract a fraction with a mol. wt around 50 000 with a pI of $5 \pm 0{\cdot}1$. Following the intravenous injection of this fraction in μg amounts, it is possible to increase significantly the resistance against *Listeria*.

The same increased resistance in TCP treated mice was recently reported by Zerial *et al.* (1980), but these authors observed that this inflammatory reaction exerted no influence upon the mortality of mice following their infection with herpes type 1, murine hepatitis, or encephalomyocarditis viruses.

In order to test the possible influence of an inflammatory reaction on experimental tumours, we used the Lewis carcinoma (3LL) which is one of the most malignant murine solid tumours. After *in vitro* culture and *in vivo* passages in pathogen-free C57Bl/6 mice, 3LL cells were checked for the absence of virus particle and mycoplasmas. Following the injection of 500 cells in the footpad, mice die some weeks later from lung metastases. If the inflammation is induced even 1 or 2 days following the inoculation of 3LL cells, the tumour growth is delayed and the number of lung metastases is strikingly decreased. As soon as 24 h after the induction of the inflammatory reaction, and during 7 days, as seen in tissue sections, the mitotic index is strikingly decreased. In contrast, following a pulse of ^{125}IUdR, the mitotic index is normal in testicles but from days 3 to 12, significantly increased in bone marrow, spleen, thymus, and popliteal lymph nodes. The serum of treated animals was found to stimulate the culture of bone marrow cells *in vitro*, to agglutinate malignant cells and to activate peritoneal cells against Lewis tumour cells. In this later case, it was indeed found, in several experiments, that the preincubation of mouse peritoneal cells with 10% of serum from treated mice is able, following contact with 3LL cells, to decrease the ^{125}IUdR incorporation in these cells between 93 and 99% of the control values. The same increased resistance against the Lewis carcinoma was observed in nude mice with a TCP induced inflammation.

Since this serum mediated activation of macrophages is found with serum samples obtained very early following the induction of the inflammatory reaction, one can wonder if such an activity is not the consequence of the release of acute mediators of inflammation. Among these mediators, kinins, following their injection into mouse 1 day after 3LL cells inoculation, were found to delay the growth of the tumour and to decrease the number of lung metastases. Furthermore, as shown by Fauve and Hevin (1979), mice pretreated with micrograms of bradykinin, lysylbradykinin or methionyllysylbradykinin are more resistant against *Listeria monocytogenes*. Since these products are rapidly destroyed, it was thought that the so-called inactive split products of kinins are possibly involved in the increased resistance. Preliminary experiments have shown that some of the split products of kinins, which are apparently devoid of the classic kinin's activity, are able to increase the resistance *Listeria* and the Lewis lung carcinoma.

It is evident from the results of these experiments that a local inflammatory reaction induced with nonbiodegradable, nondiffusible and nonantigenic substances is of great importance in the remote control of host resistance against invaders. It is also evident, as shown by Fauve and Hevin (1975), that the increased resistance is dependent upon the nature of the irritant. These differences are not surprising since it is very well known among aduvants, and even among different preparations of Freund's complete adjuvant, that their activity on the immune response is in some way related to their "physical state". As discussed by Fauve (1978), it is too early to present today a clear picture of the effects of a local inflammation on the host–invader interplay. Without doubt, as mentioned above, the possible activity of all factors released either from the granuloma or synthesized at distance from the host have to be taken into consideration. It was even found recently by Giroud *et al.* (1979) that an acute inflammatory reaction induced by intrapleural injection of calcium pyrophosphate not only protects mice against a *Klebsiella pneumoniae* infection, but that the transfer of protection against this pathogen is possible following the injection of serum from rats in which the same kind of inflammation was induced. Although it was not mentioned whether calcium pyrophosphate particles are not acting also in the reticuloendothelial system, this finding is of great interest since it is further confirmation that some serum factors might act as stimulants of host resistance. All these results indicate that following a local inflammatory reaction, mediators, in the broadest sense of the term, are able to act on the effectors of the host resistance. As mentioned before, the colony stimulating factor is one possible candidate. Other serum constituents whose purification is now in progress are other possible mediators. It is also possible, in some cases, that some activities found in the sera are not only related to well-defined substances but are the consequences of a modified ratio of some serum constituents.

Conclusions

As shown in this brief review, inflammation can be induced by different means, either following a mechanical trauma or when nonantigenic substances are introduced into the tissues. Once induced, inflammation is triggered following the release of products by the coagulation and complement systems and the interaction between clotting, fibrinolytic, complement and kinin systems. The different facets of the inflammatory process are the results of the interactions of endogenous mediators, not only *locally* with blood vessels, cells of the connective tissue and phagocytic cells, but also *at a distance* with the central nervous system, the haematopoietic tissue, the endocrine system and the cells involved in the synthesis of acute phase reactants.

In the inflammatory focus, an increased amount of phagocytic cells, of serum and tissue constituents can account for the local increased resistance against many invaders. Of these invaders, some are able to repel the effectors of natural resistance and such a property is often correlated with the virulence of pathogens. A local inflammation induced by nondiffusible, nonbiodegradable and nonantigenic substances is able to increase the host resistance against invaders at a site distant from the site of inflammation. This remote control of host resistance is mediated by substances which are able not only to stimulate the natural resistance of the host, but which are also able to pave the way for, and later to modulate, the specific response of the host against the antigenic determinants of the invaders.

References

Bata, J., Cordier, G., Revillard, J. P., Bonneau, M. and Latour, M. (1979). *In* "Transplantation and Clinical Immunology", Vol. 11, p. 59. Excerpta Medica, Amsterdam.

Cheung, H. T., Cantarow, W. D. and Sundharadas, G. (1979). *Int. J. Cancer* **23**, 344.

Chiu, K. M., Mortensen, R. F., Osmand, A. P. and Gewurz, H. (1977). *Immunology* **32**, 997.

Claus, D. R., Siegel, J., Petras, K., Skor, D., Osmand, A. P. and Gewurz, H. (1977). *J. Immunol.* **118**, 83.

Curie, G. A. (1978). *Nature* **273**, 758.

Donaldson, D. M. and Tew, J. G. (1977). *Bacteriol. Rev.* **41**, 501.

Fauve, R. M., Hevin, B., Jakob, H., Gaillard, J. A. and Jacob, F. (1974). *Proc. Natn. Acad. Sci., U.S.A.* **71**, 4052.

Fauve, R. M. (1976). *C. R. Acad. Sci., Paris* **282**, 1207.

Fauve, R. M. (1978). *In* "The Pharmacology of Immunoregulation" (G. H. Werner and F. Floc'h, eds), pp. 319–334. Academic Press, New York.

Fauve, R. M. and Hevin, B. (1975). *C. R. Acad. Sci., Paris* **281**, 2037.

Fauve, R. M. and Hevin, B. (1977). *Ann. Immunol.* (*Inst. Pasteur*) **128C**, 1079.

Fauve, R. M. and Hevin, B. (1979). *Ann. Immunol.* (*Inst. Pasteur*) **130C**, 743.

Fontan, E. and Fauve, R. M. (1980). *Ann. Immunol.* (*Inst. Pasteur*) **131C** (in prep.).

Giroud, J. P., Parant, M., Parant, F., Pelletier, M. and Chedid, L. (1979). *C. R. Acad. Sci., Paris* **289**, 1045.

Goldstein, I. M., Kaplan, H. B., Edelson, H. S. and Weissmann, G. (1979). *J. Biol. Chem.* **254**, 4040.

Gotschlich, E. C. and Edelman, G. M. (1967). *Proc. Natn. Acad. Sci., U.S.A.* **57**, 706.

Handman, E. and Burgess, A. W. (1979). *J. Immunol.* **122**, 1134.

Hovi, T., Mosher, D. and Vaheri, A. (1977). *J. Exp. Med.* **145**, 1580.

Hügli, T. E. and Müller-Eberhard, H. J. (1978). *Adv. Immunol.* **26**, 1.

Humbert, J. R., Miescher, P. A. and Jaffe, E. R. (1975). *In* "Neutrophil Physiology and Pathology". Grune and Stratton, New York and London.

Hurtrel, B., Lagrange, P. H. and Michel, J.-C. (1980). *Ann. Immunol.* (*Inst. Pasteur*) **131C**, 93, 105.

James, K. (1977). *In* "The Macrophage and Cancer", pp. 225–246. Econoprint, Edinburgh.

Johnson, J. A., Lau, B. H. S., Nutter, R. L., Slater, J. M. and Winter, C. E. (1978). *Infect. Immun.* **19**, 146.

Jong, E. C., Mahmoud, A. A. F. and Klebanoff, S. J. (1979). *Clin. Res.* **27**, 479.

Keller, R. and Hess, M. W. (1972). *Br. J. Exp. Path.* **53**, 570.

Klebanoff, S. J. and Clark, R. A. (1978). *In* "The Neutrophil: Function and Clinical disorders". North-Holland, Amsterdam.

Kof, A. (1974). *In* "Structure and Function of Plasma Proteins" (A. C. Allison, ed.), p. 73. Plenum Press, London.

Lepow, I. H. and Ward, P. A. (1972). *In* "Inflammation, Mechanisms and Control". Academic Press, New York.

Maillard, J. L. and Favreau, C. (1977). *Ann. Immunol.* (*Inst. Pasteur*) **128C**, 985, 999.

Mantovani, A., Jerrels, T. R., Dean, J. H. and Herberman, R. B. (1979). *Int. J. Cancer* **23**, 18.

Metchnikoff, E. (1892). *In* "Leçons sur la pathologie comparée de l'inflammation". Masson, Paris.

Metchnikoff, E. (1901). *In* "L'immunité dans les maladies infectieuses". Masson, Paris.

Michel, J. C. (1980). Submitted.

Mortensen, R. F. (1979). *Cell. Immunol.* **44**, 270.

Movat, H. Z. (ed.) (1979). *In* "Current Topics in Pathology". Springer-Verlag, Berlin and Heidelberg.

Müller-Eberhard, H. J. (1975). *Ann. Rev. Biochem.* **44**, 697.

Murphy, P. A., Simon, P. L. and Willoughby, F. (1980). *J. Immunol.* **124**, 2498.

Murray, H. W. and Cohn, Z. A. (1979). *J. Exp. Med.* **150**, 938.

Ogston, D. and Bennet, B. (eds) (1977). *In* "Haemostasis: Biochemistry, Physiology and Pathology". John Wiley & Sons, London.

Olds, G. R., Ellner, J. J., Kearse, L. A., Kazura, J. W. and Mahmoud, A. A. F. (1980). *J. Exp. Med.* **151**, 1557.

Osmand, A. P., Mortensen, R. F., Siegel, J. and Gewurz, H. (1975). *J. Exp. Med.* **142**, 1065.

Petrone, W. F., English, D. K., Wong, K. and McCord, J. M. (1980). *Proc. Natn. Acad. Sci., U.S.A.* **77**, 1159.

Rabatic, S., Jurin, M. and Dekaris, D. (1977). *Folia Biologica* (*Praha*) **23**, 317.

Razvorotnew, V. A., Lavrosky, V. A. and Vikslev, V. K. (1977). *Zh. Microbiol. Epidimiol. Microbiol.* **6**, 48.

Rifkin, M. R. (1978). *Proc. Natn. Acad. Sci. U.S.A.* **75**, 3450.

Rocha e Silva, M. and Garcia-Leme, J. (1972). *In* "Chemical Mediators of the Acute Inflammatory Reaction". Pergamon, Oxford.

Ryan, G. B. and Majno, G. (1977). *Am. J. Pathol.* **86**, 185.

Schutte, M., Dicamelli, R., Murhy, P., Sadoue, M. and Gewurz, H. (1974). *Clin. exp. Immunol.* **18**, 251.

Siegel, J., Osmand, A. P., Wilson, M. and Gewurz, H. (1975). *J. Exp. Med.* **142**, 709.

Stahl, K. W., Lambert, D., Rosenfeld, C., Muller, O. and Mathé, G. (1978). *Eur. J. Rheumatol. Inflamm.* **1**, 330.

Twumasi, D. Y., Liener, I. E., Galdston, M. and Levytska, V. (1977). *Nature* **267**, 61.

Tzehoval, E., Segal, S., Stabinsky, Y., Fridkin, M., Spirer, Z. and Feldman, M. (1978). *Proc. Natn. Acad. Sci. U.S.A.* **75**, 3400.

Vane, J. R. and Fereira, S. H. (eds) (1978). "Inflammation". Springer-Verlag, Berlin and Heidelberg.

Vogt, W. (1974). *Pharmacol. Rev.* **26**, 125.

Volanakis, J. E. and Kaplan, M. H. (1971). *Proc. Soc. Exp. Biol. Med.* **136**, 612.

Volanakis, J. E. and Kaplan, M. H. (1974). *J. Immunol.* **113**, 9.

Weiss, S. J., Lobuglio, A. F. and Kessler, H. B. (1980). *Proc. Natn. Acad. Sci. U.S.A.* **77**, 584.

Wilkinson, P. C. (1974). *In* "Chemotaxis and Inflammation". Churchill Livingstone, Edinburgh.

Zerial, A., Floc'h, F. and Werner, G. H. (1980). *Ann. Immunol.* (*Inst. Pasteur*) **131C** (in prep.).

Zweifach, B. W., Grant, L., and McCluskey, R. F. (eds) (1974). *In* "The Inflammatory Process", Vols 2 and 3, 2nd ed. Academic Press, New York.

Theme 11: Summary

Natural Immunity and Macrophages (including Immunity against Bacteria)

D. S. NELSON

Kolling Institute of Medical Research, Royal North Shore Hospital of Sydney, New South Wales, Australia

It was fitting that this Congress, held in the city in which Metchnikoff flourished, should include as one theme Natural Immunity and Macrophages. The title of the theme included immunity to bacteria. Immunity to viruses, protozoa, metazoa, allografts and cancer was discussed elsewhere, but it was inevitable that reference should be made to them in this theme.

By "natural immunity" we mean the resistance offered by an organisms—a host—to a parasite, tumour or organ graft, in the apparent absence of a specific immune response. Definitions are difficult in immunology and there is a grey area here. One is not sure how much the development of natural resistance mechanisms is influenced by exposure to micro-organisms and other environmental stimuli. Immune responses, overt or subliminal, may lead to change in, for example, the state of the mononuclear phagocyte system and the levels of activity of natural antibodies and natural killer cells.

Many different families of cells, molecules and biochemical systems contribute to natural immunity. Fauve (Chapter 42) illustrated the complexity of the interactions among the kinin, clotting and fibrinolytic and complement systems. Such humoral factors and natural antibodies received less attention in the workshops. As immunologists we are carried on the tides of fashion, though it is a moot point whether the tides roll onward or, like those of the sea, mainly up and down or to and fro. In this meeting attention was directed mostly to phagocytes, especially mononuclear phagocytes, natural killer (NK) cells, interferon and other regulatory factors.

Mononuclear and other phagocytes

The cells of the mononuclear phagocytic system are diverse in structure and function. Precursor cells, mainly in the bone marrow, give rise to monocytes, macrophages (which can vary widely in the degree to which they are activated or stimulated), to microglia and osteoclasts and to cells which are at present somewhat neglected: giant cells and epitheloid cells. Langerhans cells in the skin, veiled cells in afferent lymph, interdigitating cells in lymph nodes and the dendritic cells characterized *in vitro* by Steinman (11.2.12)* may be of similar lineage.

There was considerable discussion of the role of these cells, and of the Ia antigens which they may carry, in the induction of immune responses. The effective presentation of antigen requires Ia at the surface of the cell, but carriage of Ia is probably not the sole precondition for effective presentation. Macrophages which are Ia negative readily

* Reference numbers indicate Abstract numbers in: Abstracts 4th International Congress of Immunology, Paris, 1980.

become Ia positive under the influence of lymphokines, or after phagocytosis, or even simply after culture *in vitro*. The capacity to develop Ia, however, seems to be a thymus dependent process. Dendritic cells, which are nonphagocytic, appear to be phenotypically stable in their carriage of Ia. Excellent evidence was presented and discussed that both macrophages and dendritic cells could serve as antigen presenting cells and as nonspecific accessory cells. Their relative importance remains to be established, or at least agreed upon; this may well depend on the degree of purity of the separated populations of cells. Another interesting problem which remains to be solved is that while anti-Ia antibodies block the stimulation of specifically reactive T cells by antigen-presenting cells *in vitro*, antibodies to the antigen itself do not.

Of the newer tools for the study of macrophages, monoclonal antibodies and continuous macrophage cell lines received the most attention. Monoclonal antibodies have been used to define and separate populations of cells carrying particular determinants but their full potential has probably not yet been realized. Macrophage cell lines are convenient to use and interesting to study. Bloom (11.1.21) presented an intriguing example of the use of mutant cell lines in defining biochemical pathways essential for phagocytosis. I have reservations, however, about the extent of their value, for 2 reasons: firstly, because they are, like malignant haemopoietic cells, subject to differentiation anarchy; secondly, because whatever is found with cell lines must be related back to the behaviour of normal cells.

Effector mechanisms of phagocytic cells were reviewed by Klebanoff (Chapter 41). Most is known about oxygen dependent antimicrobial effector mechanisms in neutrophils. These pathways yield several highly reactive chemical species. Knowledge of similar mechanisms in eosinophils, mast cells and macrophages is expanding. Macrophages, however, are called on to function both as phagocytes and as anti-tumour effectors in areas of low oxygen tension. Some target tumour cells are, indeed, resistant to oxygen metabolites. The study of oxygen-independent mechanisms, a much more tedious affair, therefore requires more attention in the future. So, too, do other subjects raised in workshops: the effect of extracellular factors (both antibodies and other molecules) or intracellular killing; the relationship between biochemical activation and antimicrobial and antitumour activation; and the possibility of establishing simple biochemical criteria for activation. The full solution of these problems may well require the development of satisfactory clonal and single cell techniques for studying macrophage function.

NK cells

We are now in a position to consider that there exist natural resistance mechanisms not only to micro-organisms but to cancer cells and, as Cudkowicz pointed out (11.2.07), also to grafts of normal haemopoietic cells. The 2 best studied mechanisms are those involving macrophages (mostly discussed in Theme 10) and those involving NK cells. The latter were reviewed by Herberman (Chapter 39) and discussed in workshops.

NK cells are naturally occurring lymphoid cells which are cytotoxic to a broad though far from universal range of target cells, mostly malignant. They develop, apparently spontaneously, in most young individuals of most species and persist for varying periods of their lifespan. Though not T cells and not thymus-dependent they are related, in a way that is not clear, to T cells. Herberman presented evidence (Chapter 39) that they are, morphologically, large granular lymphocytes. Elsewhere, Lohmann-Matthes has shown that cells which are functionally macrophage precursors are NK cells. Once again the question of diversity has arisen. Evidence was presented that different NK cells have some broad specificity in their reactions with different targets; that NK cells killing sarcoma targets differ from those killing lymphoma targets; and that two physically different types of cell may interact to produce natural cytotoxicity. Clonal studies of the sort reported during the meeting should help to solve problems of specificity and recognition mechanisms.

Is NK cell activity a determinant of health or disease? There are parallels between NK activity and the progression of cancer in human patients, especially with melanoma. NK cells contribute to resistance to haemopoietic grafts. There may be NK cell defects in multiple sclerosis. There is a correlation between the susceptibility of mice to urethane carcinogenesis and the ability of urethane to depress NK cell activity in different strains of mice.

Among the most important problems posed by Herberman for further study are the susceptibility of primary (autochthonous) tumours to NK cells and, conversely, the effects of changes in NK cell activity on susceptibility to primary carcinogenesis. If normal animals offer some resistance to cancer it is likely that NK cells contribute to it. There are, however, tumours which resist NK cell attack; if there is natural resistance to their growth one must look elsewhere, probably to macrophages, for effectors. The second large set of problems for future study, for macrophages as well as for NK cells, concerns the regulation of their activity, both physiologically and, in terms of therapeutic intervention, pharmacologically.

Interferon

Is interferon the great regulator? Type I interferon (virus-induced, subclasses α and β) has been purified (to use the cynical phrase of a lymphokine chemist) to heterogeneity. This should allow rapid resolution of some problems concerning its biological role. Type II interferon (immune interferon, subclass γ) is now also well on the way to purification and may be more relevant to the internal regulation of the immune system.

In his review of interferon (Chapter 40), Gresser pointed out that it is among the most potent of biologically active molecules. Its role in natural immunity stems partly from its antiviral effect and partly from its effect on components of the immune system. In particular it can increase the activity of NK cells and macrophages as well as that of T cells and K cells. Its mode of action on NK cells was considered in workshop discussions. It seems to induce an increase in the frequency of actively cytotoxic cells (among otherwise differentiated precursors) as well as an increase in lytic efficiency of individual cells. For these effects a brief interaction with the cell membrane is required, as well as subsequent RNA and protein synthesis. It was suggested that interferon might act as a thiol oxidizing agent, by altering the intracellular ratio of oxidized to reduced glutathione. There was speculation that 2-mercaptoethanol might exert its beneficial effect on stimulated lymphocyte cultures by reversing an anti-proliferative effect of endogenous interferon.

Macrophages can be both targets for interferon, which increases their phagocytic and antitumour activity, and sources of interferon which in turn affects NK and other lymphoid cells. According to circumstances interferon may increase or decrease primary antibody formation and delayed type hypersensitivity. It can increase the surface expression of MHC antigens, including DR antigens on T cells. There exist in the mouse thymus cells which are susceptible to NK attack. It is difficult, however, to draw these disparate findings together to make a coherent case for interferon as a key immunoregulatory molecule. It may well have such a function, but workshop discussions made it clear that other substances often have similar effects. The properties of interferon eminently qualify it for candidature as a therapeutic agent. It seems likely to contribute, in nature, to resistance to virus infections. Its place in the treatment of virus infections, malignant diseases and perhaps immunodeficiency is, however, far from established. Gresser sounded a very necessary note of caution in view of certain experimental findings, notably the occurrence of runting and glomerulonephritis in nude mice and the exacerbation of autoimmune disease in NZB mice after interferon treatment. It may well be that its place in the therapeutic armamentarium against cancer in man will be determined by the definition of critical defects in individual patients, rather than by the desirability of global immunostimulation in all patients with a particular cancer.

Other factors modulating natural and acquired immunity

There is a rather daunting number of factors which are products, directly or indirectly, of inflammation and which have, again directly or indirectly, antimicrobial effects. Fauve (Chapter 42) pointed to changes in pH and temperature, complement components, high density lipoproteins, C-reactive protein and cationic proteins (such as β-lysin) as well as familiar molecules such as lysozyme and interferon. The number and degree of activation of macrophages are clearly subject to regulation by colony stimulating factor and lymphokines. Prostaglandins may provide a negative feedback and a factor increasing monocytopoiesis (FIM) a positive feedback effect on monocyte production. Fauve described a recently characterized factor produced by sterile talc granulomas in mice. It activated macrophages powerfully; it could account for the dramatic increase in the resistance of mice bearing granulomas to bacteria (*Salmonella typhimurium*, *Listeria monocytogenes*), fungi (*Candida albicans*, though here polymorphs may be more important), protozoa (*Plasmodium berghei*), metazoa (*Schistosoma mansoni*) and tumours. It remains to be seen whether this substance has an immunotherapeutic effect on established infections or tumours.

NK cells are also subject to other regulatory influences. Notably, prostaglandin (PGE_2) can reduce NK activity and antagonize the stimulating effect of interferon. Both are produced by macrophages which can thus exert a truly regulatory effect on NK cells.

Age and genetic factors have long been known to influence resistance to infection. Some progress was reported in delineating the immunological, quasi-immunological and frankly nonimmunological components involved.

One of the pressing problems for immunologists with a practical turn of mind is the need for further developments of adjuvants or immunomodulators for human use. There was some discussion of the mode of action of known agents such as BCG and muramyl dipeptide. There was a lively discussion of the effect of prior exposure to ubiquitous mycobacteria on reactivity to BCG vaccine, a highly practical problem in the control of tuberculosis and leprosy.

Reflections

Several developments are both desirable and likely in the near future. We may expect a clearer definition of the oxygen-independent ways in which macrophages exert antimicrobial and antitumour effects. It would be very helpful to be able to measure the intracellular microbicidal activity of macrophages quickly, easily and cheaply. We may also expect a clear delineation of the pathways of regulation of macrophage and NK cell activity. The new immunology, as least as far as postinduction events are concerned, will, I think, be a science of regulation and interaction, both specific (involving networks) and nonspecific (involving lymphokines, monokines and cytokines). We will probably not be able to offer effective immunological intervention in disease until we have a better molecular and biological understanding of regulation. I suspect that we have to face, as bravely as we can, the probability of discovering a good deal more complexity in the organization of the immune system before a new Pasteur or Metchnikoff sheds the light of inspiration on it.

Theme 12

Effector and Escape Mechanisms in Host–Parasite Relationships

Presidents:
B. H. WAKSMAN
A. CAPRON

Symposium Chairman:
K. S. WARREN

43

Humoral Responses to Protozoal Infections

SYDNEY COHEN

Department of Chemical Pathology, Guy's Hospital Medical School, London

Introduction

The protozoa comprise a phylum of unicellular organisms many of which are limited in their degree of independence and are found as parasites in a wide range of vertebrate and invertebrate hosts. Among several thousand parasitic species known only about 20 are significant pathogens of man, but these include the causative organisms of several major human diseases (Table I). The importance of these is illustrated by the estimates that 300 M people have amoebiasis, 12 M have South American trypanosomiasis and about 150 M suffer from malaria which carries a mortality, mainly among children, of over 1 M per year.

The potential importance of immunoprophylactic measures for protozoal diseases is obvious. There is much evidence that resistance to these infections can be acquired through mechanisms involving the effector pathways of specific

TABLE I
The major protozoal diseases of man

Causative organisms	*Disease*	*Pathogen location*	*Clinical immunity*
Rhizopodea			
Entamoeba histolytica	Amoebic dysentery	Lumen g.i.t.	None
Zoomastigophorea			
Trypanosoma gambiense	West and Central African sleeping sickness	Bloodstream	None
T. rhodesiense	East African sleeping sickness	Bloodstream	None
T. cruzi	South American trypanosomiasis (Chagas' disease)	Macrophages	Incomplete
Leishmania tropica	Cutaneous leishmaniasis (oriental sore)	Macrophages	Sterilizing
L. braziliense	Mucocutaneous leishmaniasis	Macrophages	Incomplete
L. donovani	Visceral leishmaniasis (kala-azar)	Macrophages	None
Sporozoa			
Plasmodium falciparum	Malaria (malignant tertian)	Bloodstream	Incomplete
P. malariae	Malaria (quartan)	Bloodstream	Incomplete
P. vivax	Malaria (benign tertian)	Bloodstream	Incomplete
P. ovale	Malaria (ovale tertian)	Bloodstream	Incomplete
Toxoplasma gondii	Toxoplasmosis	Macrophages	Incomplete

immunity. On the other hand, the characteristic chronicity of many of these infections and the progressive nature of some indicate an ability of protozoa to survive a potentially lethal immune attack. The complex and subtle balance between protozoan and host, characteristic of naturally occurring forms of obligate parasitism, is considered in this paper from the standpoint of humoral immunity. Discussion of so broad a topic is obviously limited in scope and very incomplete.

Clinical immunity in protozoal infections

Resistance to micro-organisms including protozoa is most frequently attributable to innate (natural) immunity; this is independent of previous discernible exposure to the pathogen and is usually characteristic of the species and sometimes of individual strains. The basis of host–parasite incompatibility is, for the most part, poorly understood, but where it has been elucidated it has generally proved independent of mechanisms mediating specific immunity. For example, a primary requirement for malaria infectivity is the presence of a specific red cell receptor for parasite attachment (Miller *et al.*, 1973; Butcher *et al.*, 1973). In the case of *Plasmodium knowlesi* and *P. vivax* this receptor is related to the Duffy blood group determinant (Mason *et al.*, 1977). This discovery explains the long-recognized resistance to *P. vivax* infection of West African Blacks and their descendents in the USA, since these populations have a high frequency of the Duffy negative genotype (Miller *et al.*, 1976).

Nonspecific acquired immunity

The progress of several protozoal diseases is inhibited by intercurrent bacterial infections as recognized, for example, in trypanosomiasis by Laveran and Mesnil in 1912. Mouse malaria is partially suppressed by pretreatment with endotoxin, Freund's complete adjuvant and Newcastle disease virus (see references in Cohen, 1979). The intravenous inoculation of BCG, *Corynebacterium parvum* or *Brucella abortus* protects mice against some babesia and plasmodial infections (Clark *et al.*, 1977; Herod *et al.*, 1978). It may be difficult to exclude cross-immunization in some such instances. However, mouse strains vary considerably with regard to the ease with which nonspecific immunity can be induced, and mechanisms including the activation of macrophages and induction of interferon synthesis and NK cell activity may be operative against protozoa.

Specific acquired immunity

Three categories of clinical response can be distinguished in protozoal diseases:

(a) Absence of an effective immune response. Human species do not usually develop effective immunity against *Trypanosoma rhodesiense* or *T. gambiense* infections, although healthy carriers are described (Ross, 1956; Blair *et al.*, 1968), nor is there discernible immunity in intestinal amoebiasis or amoebic meningoencephalitis (Carter, 1972). Individuals with Chagas' disease may harbour the parasites for life, often with progressive signs of debilitating disease. The same is true of human visceral leishmaniasis in which records of spontaneous cure are rare and acquired immunity usually becomes manifest only after drug therapy.

(b) Nonsterilizing (incomplete) immunity. Many parasitic infections include an immune response which results in clinical recovery and resistance to specific challenge, but is associated with persistence of the parasite at relatively low density. This has been referred to as "premunition" and its features were described in detail by Sergent (1963). Nonsterilizing immunity is characteristic of many human, simian and avian malarias. In some, such as *Plasmodium falciparum* in man, clinical resistance is associated with periodically detectable parasitaemia, while in others, like *P. inui* in the rhesus monkey, parasitaemia may persist with only minor fluctuations over a period of many years. Other examples of premunition are seen in the chronic relapsing form in human cutaneous leishmaniasis, *Trypanosoma cruzi* infections, many species of *Babesia* and *Theileria* in cattle and toxoplasmosis. Wild African ungulates may harbour potentially pathogenic trypanosomes, such as *T. rhodesiense*, without showing detectable symptoms, but the role of acquired immunity in controlling such infections has not been established.

(c) Sterilizing immunity. Immunity to some protozoal infections is associated with clinical care, complete elimination of the parasite and life-long specific resistance to challenge. Among the human protozoal diseases sterilizing immunity occurs only in cutaneous leishmaniasis. In the rat, *T. lewisi* and *P. berghei* infections induce sterilizing immunity.

The pattern of acquired immunity is not constant for a given protozoan, but may show wide variation in different hosts and among inbred strains of a species. In general, sterilizing responses are common in unnatural hosts subjected to laboratory infections, while incomplete immunity is characteristic of protozoal infections in naturally occurring hosts. It follows that immunological findings in experimental protozoal diseases may not have immediate relevance to the corresponding human disease.

Acquired immunity to protozoa, whether associated with premunition or a sterilizing response is, in general, species and strain specific. This has, for example, been established in some detail in human (Jefferey, 1966) and experimental malaria (Cohen and Mitchell, 1978). Acquired immunity in malaria is also stage specific since resistance to erythrocytic forms does not modify the exoerythrocytic development of parasites, but suppresses the subsequent phase of erythrocytic development. Conversely, sporozoite-immunized birds or rodents are fully susceptible to blood forms of the same parasite.

Humoral response to protozoal infections

The fact that clinical evidence for acquired immunity is often indecisive in protozoal infections led at one time to the belief that protozoa are poorly immunogenic. There is no basis whatever for this view since specific antibody has been demonstrated in every infection adequately studied. It is clear, however, that much of the antibody formed has no protective function.

Nonspecific immunoglobulin production

Immunoglobulins are considerably elevated in many protozoal infections. Only a small proportion may have demonstrable affinity for the pathogen and the increase may be attributable, at least in malaria, trypanosomiasis and Chagas' disease, to the occurrence of polyclonal lymphocyte activation.

West African adults living in hyperendemic malarial areas show elevated levels of IgG and IgM especially (Rowe *et al.*, 1968). In these clinically immune subjects the rate of albumin synthesis is similar to that of normal Europeans, but IgG production is almost 7 times greater. IgG synthesis was reduced by about 33% after malarial prophylactic therapy yet only 5% of immune adult IgG combines specifically with *Plasmodium falciparum* antigens (Cohen and Butcher, 1969). Some remaining IgG might be antibody against other serological variants of *P. falciparum* or against soluble malarial antigens present in serum. Nevertheless, it seems that chronic malarial infection stimulates nonspecific Ig and that this accounts for the unusually high incidence of heterophile and autoantibodies (Houba *et al.*, 1974; Greenwood *et al.*, 1971), cold agglutinins and immunoconglutinins (Coombs and Coombs, 1953) in hyper-γ-globulinaemic sera from subjects exposed to chronic malaria.

An even greater increase in γ-globulin involving mainly IgG is seen in visceral leishmaniasis. Concentrations above 5 g/100 ml are not unusual in human patients. The characterization of this IgG is incomplete, but a major part appears not to be specific antibody, and the stimulus for its production remains an intriguing and unanswered question. Equally remarkable is the elevation of IgM in African trypanosomiasis which is of diagnostic value since normal levels almost certainly rule out trypanosomal infection. The IgM contains trypanosome agglutinating antibody (Seed *et al.*, 1969), as well as antiglobulin and heterophil antibodies (Houba *et al.*, 1969; Klein *et al.*, 1970), increased levels of naturally occurring IgM antibodies (MacKenzie *et al.*, 1972) and autoantibodies (Kobayakawa *et al.*, 1979). IgM concentration may remain high long after exposure to infection has ceased and when tests for trypanocidal antibody are negative; it seems, therefore, that much of the IgM produced in trypanosomiasis is nonspecific. Increased levels of IgE characteristic of metazoan infections are not observed in protozoal diseases. Indeed *T. cruzi* infections have been shown to depress homocytotrophic antibody formation in mice (Mendes *et al.*, 1979).

Specific antibody

In all protozoan disease specific antibody can be demonstrated by a variety of serological techniques and by immediate or delayed hypersensitivity reactions. Many of these tests have been useful in diagnosis and in epidemiological surveys (Fife, 1971; Cohen and Sadun, 1976) but in general give poor correlation with clinical immune status. This indicates that, in addition to nonspecific Ig discussed above, protozoal infections stimulate the production of specific antibody having no protective function. Such antibody may be directed against serotypes of the organism present earlier in the infection, soluble serum antigens or various metabolites, degradation products and cell constituents not present on the surface of the intact living parasite, and therefore irrelevant to its specific destruction.

Protective antibody

The role of protective antibody in protozoal diseases has been demonstrated by passive immunization occurring either naturally (maternal–foetal transfer) or artificially and also by the use of bursectomized birds, μ-suppressed mice and Biozzi high and low responder mice. In addition, specific *in vitro* inhibition of protozoa by immune sera has been investigated by using a variety of tests (Table II). These various techniques have established a major role for antibody mediated immunity in malaria, African and South American trypanosomiasis and toxoplasmosis. Although resistance to leishmaniasis is predominantly dependent on mechanisms of cell-mediated immunity (Preston and Dumonde, 1976), recent experiments have shown that humoral antibody can transfer immunity to normal guinea-pigs when obtained from recently challenged animals (Poulter, 1980).

Immunity to malaria is strictly stage specific, no cross-protection occurring between exoerythrocytic and erythrocytic parasites. Immune sera from mice vaccinated with irradiated sporozoites of *Plasmodium berghei* contain antibodies reacting with a stage specific sporozoite surface antigen having a mol. wt of 44 000 (Nardin and Nussenzweig, 1978). The role of humoral antibody in sporozoite immunity is clearly demonstrated by the use of a monoclonal IgG_1 produced by a mouse hybrid cell line; this reacts with the stage specific surface sporozoite antigen and inoculation of 50–300 μg of antibody passively protects mice against sporozoite challenge (Yoshida *et al.*, 1980). The Fab fragment of this antibody is also active (Potocnjak *et al.*, 1980) suggesting that it acts by blocking the attachment of sporozoites to host receptor cells, presumably hepatocytes. The role of humoral antibody in immunity to the erythrocytic stage of malaria is evident from natural and artificial passive transfer and from the increased susceptibility to infection of bursectomized birds, μ-suppressed mice and Biozzi low responder mice (Table II). In human and rodent malarias antibody appears to act *in vivo* against extracellular merozoites (Cohen *et al.*, 1961; Diggs and Osler, 1975; Quinn and Wyler, 1979). This is supported by *in vitro* experiments which showed that antibody blocks the attachment of merozoites to red cells and prevents their subsequent invasion by either *P. knowlesi* (Cohen *et al.*, 1969; Miller *et al.*, 1975) or *P. falciparum* (Phillips *et al.*, 1972; Mitchell *et al.*, 1976). Merozoite inhibition is species specific, not complement dependent and is mediated by IgG and its $(Fab^1)_2$ fragment or IgM (Cohen and Butcher, 1970). Further confirmation of the role of antimerozoite antibodies in immunity to blood stage malaria comes from a study of five monoclonal immunoglobulins raised against *P. yoelii*. Two of these selectively reacted with merozoites and were protective when tested by passive transfer; the remaining three reacted with immature parasites or infected red cell membranes and provided no protection (Freeman *et al.*, 1980).

Pathogenic African trypanosomes present in the bloodstream have an outer glycoprotein coat which envelopes the surface membrane of the body and flagellum. Circulating organisms induce the synthesis of antibody which is

TABLE II

Demonstration of antibody-mediated immune protection in protozoal infections

	Passive transfer						
	Polyclonal antibody						
	Natural	*Artificial*	*Monoclonal antibody*	*Avian bursectomy*	*μ-chain suppression*	*Biozzi mice*	In vitro *inhibition*
Malaria—exoerythrocytic		− (8)	+ (29)				
erythrocytic	+ (1, 2, 3)	+ (9, 10, 11)	+ (30)	+ (18, 19)	+ (20)	+ (21)	+ (27)
Trypanosomiasis							
African	± (4)	± (12, 13, 14)					+ (12, 28, 40, 41)
S. American	± (5)	+ (15, 16, 22)				+ (22)	+ (25, 31, 32, 39)
Leishmaniasis	− (6)	− (17)				− (21, 23, 24)	− (36)
		+ (38)					
Toxoplasmosis	+ (7)	+ (37)					+ (26, 33, 34, 35)

+ = protection ± = variable protection − = no protection

1. Edozien *et al.* (1962)
2. Terry (1956)
3. Bruce-Chwatt and Gibson (1955)
4. Soltys (1967)
5. Ryckman (1965)
6. Rodjakin (1957)
7. Lewis and Markell (1958)
8. Spitalny *et al.* (1976)
9. Cohen *et al.* (1961)
10. Diggs and Osler (1969)
11. Phillips (1970)
12. Soltys (1957)
13. Watkins (1964)
14. Seed and Gamm (1966)
15. Culbertson and Kolodny (1938)
16. Kagan and Norman (1961)
17. Von Kretschmar (1965)
18. Longnecker *et al.* (1969)
19. Rank and Weidanz (1976)
20. Weinbaum *et al.* (1976)
21. Biozzi *et al.* (1979)
22. Kierszenbaum and Howard (1976)
23. Blum and Lioli (1978)
24. Hale and Howard (1980)
25. Krettli and Brener (1976)
26. Wilson *et al.* (1980)
27. Cohen and Butcher (1970)
28. Maseyeff and Gambert (1963)
29. Yoshida *et al.* (1980)
30. Freeman *et al.* (1980)
31. Krettli *et al.* (1979)
32. Budzko *et al.* (1975)
33. Anderson and Remington (1974)
34. Sabin and Feldman (1948)
35. Feldman (1956)
36. Mauel *et al.* (1975)
37. Hafizi and Modabber (1978)
38. Poulter (1980)
39. Kierszenbaum (1979)
40. Flemmings and Diggs (1978)
41. Stevens and Moulton (1978)

variant specific (see Section: Evasion of antibody-mediated immunity) and can mediate trypanosome lysis by complement (Flemmings and Diggs, 1978) and endocytosis by macrophages. Antibody-mediated immunity in trypanosomiasis is therefore variant specific and the prevention of relapse and death by passive immunization requires large amounts of immune serum and a small parasite challenge (Watkins, 1964). Variant specific antibody forms the basis of various *in vitro* tests of inhibition and neutralization of trypanosomes (Table II).

Trypanosoma cruzi, the cause of South American trypanosomiasis, gives rise to characteristically chronic infections and the protective role of humoral antibody has been controversial. However, passive protection by immune serum has been clearly demonstrated (Culbertson and Kolodny, 1938; Kagan and Norman, 1961; Kierszenbaum and Howard, 1976; McHardy, 1980). A protective role for humoral antibody is supported by the finding that Biozzi low-responder mice are more susceptible to infection with 2 distinct strains of *T. cruzi* than are high responders, while nonselected mice show an intermediate level of susceptibility (Kierszenbaum and Howard, 1976). The bloodstream forms of the parasite (trypomastigotes) are susceptible to complement-mediated immune lysis (Budzko *et al.*, 1975) which in some strains involves a combined action of the alternative and classical complement pathways (Krettli *et al.*, 1979). The role of C_3 in resistance is indicated by the increased parasitaemia and mortality of mice treated with cobra venom factor (Kierszenbaum and Howard, 1976). In addition, trypomastigotes isolated from the blood of infected mice are destroyed by human lymphoid cells, neutrophils or eosinophils in the presence of specific mouse immune serum (Kierszenbaum, 1979).

The extracellular trophozoites of *Toxoplasma gondii* are rapidly damaged and rendered nonviable by specific antibody in the presence of complement (Sabin and Feldman, 1948). The clinical significance of this reaction is uncertain since the major locus of infection is within macrophages of the host. Normal human monocyte-derived macrophages are readily infected *in vitro* by *T. gondii* and support intracellular replication of the parasite. However, if such normal cells ingest *T. gondii* trophozoites, which have previously been incubated with heat-inactivated homologous immune serum, then the intracellular parasites are killed (Anderson and Remington, 1974). Specific antibody is required to mediate this effect, which is manifest within one hour of cell entry (Wilson *et al.*, 1980) and involves fusion of lysosomes with phagosomes containing the parasite (Jones and Hirsch, 1972; Jones *et al.*, 1975) and the generation of reactive oxygen metabolites (Wilson *et al.*, 1980) An *in vivo* role for antibody-mediated immunity in toxoplasmosis is suggested by the enhanced virulence of infection observed in cytophosphamide treated mice (Gryzywinski, 1978) and its reversal by passive transfer of immune serum (Hafizi and Modabber, 1978).

Evasion of antibody-mediated immunity

It is apparent that several pathogenic human protozoa induce the synthesis of specific protective antibody, yet all those discussed above cause chronic infections with at best incomplete immunity. The analysis of mechanisms which enable these organisms to survive in the presence of potentially lethal humoral responses remains a central problem in the understanding of protozoal immunity (Table III).

TABLE III

Evasion of antibody-mediated protection in protozoal diseases

Immune evasion mechanisms	*Malaria*	*Trypanosomiasis* *African*	*S. American*	*Toxo-plasmosis*
Intracellular location	+ (1)		+ (44)	+ (42–46)
Antigenic variation	+ (2–8)	+ (28, 29)	+ (39)	
Antigenic complexity	+ (9, 10)			
Altered immune responsiveness				
Polyclonal lymphocyte activation	+ (11–16)	+ (17, 30–33)	+ (40)	
Immune suppression	+ (17–23)	+ (34–37)	+ (41)	
Lymphocytotoxic antibody	+ (24)			
Soluble antigen and immune complexes	+ (25–27)	+ (38)		

1. Krotoski *et al.* (1980)
2. Cox (1959)
3. Briggs and Wellde (1969)
4. Brown and Brown (1965)
5. Voller and Rossan (1969)
6. Butcher and Cohen (1972)
7. Butcher *et al.* (1978)
8. Wilson and Phillips (1976)
9. Deans and Cohen (1979)
10. Schmidt-Ulrich *et al.* (1979)
11. Cohen *et al.* (1961)
12. Greenwood (1974a)
13. Wyler and Oppenheim (1974)
14. Greenwood and Vick (1975)
15. Freeman and Parrish (1978)
16. Wyler (1979)
17. Greenwood (1974b)
18. Jayawardena *et al.* (1975)
19. Liew *et al.* (1979)
20. Loose *et al.* (1972)
21. Warren and Weidanz (1976)
22. Weinbaum *et al.* (1978)
23. Orjih and Nussenzweig (1979)
24. Wells *et al.* (1980)
25. Poels *et al.* (1977)
26. June *et al.* (1979)
27. Houba *et al.* (1976)
28. Cross (1978)
29. Vickerman (1978)
30. Hudson *et al.* (1976)
31. Corsini *et al.* (1977)
32. Mayor-Withey *et al.* (1978)
33. Clayton *et al.* (1979a)
34. Corsini *et al.* (1977)
35. Jayawardena *et al.* (1978)
36. Pearson *et al.* (1979)
37. Wellhausen and Mansfield (1979)
38. Allison and Houba (1976)
39. Krettli *et al.* (1979)
40. Ortiz-Ortiz *et al.* (1980)
41. Ramos *et al.* (1979)
42. Anderson and Remington (1974)
43. Jones and Hirsch (1972)
44. Nogueira (1974)
45. Nogueira and Cohn (1976)
46. Kress *et al.* (1975)

Immune evasion mechanisms have been most fully investigated in the case of African trypanosomiasis. These parasites, even when cloned from a single cell, can sequentially replace their surface coat glycoprotein (variant specific surface antigen—VSSA) with a larger number (probably hundreds) of alternative forms having distinct antigenic specificities and *N*-terminal amino acid sequences (Bridgen *et al.*, 1976). The variant specific host antibody response is therefore clinically ineffective and successive waves of parasitaemia represent the development of antigenically distinct trypanosomes. Host antibody was thought to induce variation, but new antigenic types are spontaneously generated during *in vitro* culture (Doyle *et al.*, 1980) and specific antibody now appears to have only a selective role. Individual clones of trypanosomes produce a characteristic series of VSSAs suggesting that the controlling genes are not generated by mutation, but are represented in the genome (Vickerman, 1978). Recent DNA hybridization experiments indicate that the sequential expression of alternative forms of the trypanosome surface antigen involves a rearrangement of genes (Williams *et al.*, 1979; Hoeijmakers *et al.*, 1980).

African trypanosomes exert a profound effect upon the host immune system. During the early stages of infection there occurs a polyclonal activation of B cells (Greenwood, 1974a; Hudson *et al.*; 1976, Corsini *et al.*, 1977) and of null cells (Mayor-Withey *et al.*, 1978) apparently triggered by the action of trypanosome products containing membrane components (Esuruosco, 1976; Mansfield *et al.*, 1976; Assoku and Tizard, 1978; Clayton *et al.*, 1979b; Sacks *et al.*, 1980). This leads to increased production of nonspecific Ig and of autoantibodies (Houba *et al.*, 1969; Kobayakawa *et al.*, 1979) and eventual exhaustion of antibody forming potential with loss of B and T cell memory (Askonas *et al.*, 1979). Functional T lymphocytes are not essential for mediating trypanosome mitogenicity which can be readily demonstrated in nude (athymic) mice (Clayton *et al.*, 1979). A direct action of trypanosomes or their products upon lymphocytes *in vitro* was reported (Esuruosco, 1976; Assoku and Tizard, 1978) but is not readily reproduced (Corsini *et al.*, 1977; Mansfield *et al.*, 1976). Normal spleen cell responses are actively suppressed by nonantigen specific T cells or by macrophages in trypanosome infected mice (Jayawardena *et al.*, 1978; Corsini *et al.*, 1977; Pearson *et al.*, 1979; Wellhausen and Mansfield, 1979). These diverse effects upon the immune system appear important in the pathogenesis of African trypanosomiasis since the virulence of distinct strains can be directly related to their inherently different immunosuppressive activities (Sacks *et al.*, 1980).

Plasmodial infections, especially in naturally occurring hosts, may be extremely long-lasting; for example, the human tertian malarias have a natural duration of 2–3 years while quartan *P. malariae* may persist for as long as 50 years. Several factors appear to promote long survival of *Plasmodia* (Table III). The initial phase of extraerythrocytic development within hepatic parenchymal cells excites no cellular reaction so that the surface of the infected liver cell probably does not express plasmodial antigens and the parasite is protected from immune attack by its intracellular location. While some mammalian malarias may produce secondary exoerythrocytic generations, such cyclical hepatic development appears to be exceptional (Garnham, 1977). On the other hand, hepatic forms which remain latent for many weeks (hypnozoites) occur in *P. cynomolgi* infections (Krotoski *et al.*, 1980) and probably also in human *P. vivax* infections especially those acquired in temperate zones. The interaction of sporozoites with specific antibody leads to capping of surface antigen—a reaction which could favour parasite survival. Although there is no evidence for antigenic variation in sporozoites the subsequent exoerythrocytic state has distinct serological specificity and this favours the survival of any parasites which escape antisporozoite immunity (Foley and Vanderberg, 1977). Malaria infected red cells carry surface plasmodial antigens (Deans and Cohen, 1979; Schmidt-Ulrich *et al.*, 1979) accessible to surface labelling and interaction with specific antibody. Although the red cell stages of several species of *Plasmodia* show serological variation between strains and in some species undergo antigenic variation, the effects of this in promoting parasite survival appear to be largely offset by the common antigenicity of variants (reviewed by Cohen, 1980).

Malaria is associated with notable alterations in the distribution of lymphocyte subpopulations and with marked changes in immune responsiveness. The percentage and absolute number of circulating T cells are depleted during infection while the percentage of both B cells and null cells is increased. Humoral responses to a variety of antigens are diminished during parasitaemia. Attempts to analyse the basis of immunosuppression have implicated adherent cells presumed to be macrophages apparently defective in their capacity to process antigens (Loose *et al.*, 1972; Brown *et al.*, 1977; Warren and Weidanz, 1976). In mice an interaction between macrophages and T cells is required to produce immunosuppressive mediators (Weinbaum *et al.*, 1978). Malaria infection also provides a potent stimulus for the synthesis of nonspecific Ig suggesting the association of a B cell mitogen with Plasmodia (Greenwood, 1974a). Plasmodial extracts or supernatants of *P. falciparum* cultures stimulate transformation of human peripheral lymphocytes and mouse spleen cells (Wyler and Oppenheim, 1974; Greenwood and Vick, 1975; Freeman and Parish, 1978). The mitogen appears to be a glycoprotein which acts on mouse B cells and human T or B cells taken from either immune or normal subjects (Wyler, 1979; Greenwood *et al.*, 1979). The importance of processes which compromise host immunity for promoting parasite survival has been demonstrated in sporozoite vaccinated mice previously infected with blood-stage *P. berghei* (Orjih and Nussenzweig, 1979). In animals carrying an erythrocytic infection the primary response to stage specific sporozoite surface antigen was short-lived, the response to secondary challenge was undetectable and vaccination did not induce protection. On the other hand, established antisporozoite immunity was unaffected by subsequent blood stage infection. These observations indicate that blood stage plasmodial infections impair humoral responses against sporozoites and so promote parasite survival.

Soluble malarial antigens have been detected in the serum of several host species infected with malaria. Some antigens could be of sporozoite origin since incubation with immune serum leads to accumulation on sporozoites of surface fibrillar material which caps posteriorly and is shed. Other serum plasmodial antigens are presumably derived from the merozoite coat which is stripped and shed during erythrocyte penetration (Bannister *et al.*, 1975). A wide diversity of circulating *P. falciparum* antigens has been identified (McGregor, 1972) and circulating immune complexes are detectable in rodent (Poels *et al.*, 1977; June *et al.*, 1979) and human (Houba *et al.*, 1976) malarias. Either free antigen or complexes in antigen excess or plasma inhibitory factors of unknown identity (Moore *et al.*, 1977) could block immune inductive or effector mechanisms in malaria, but their role in promoting parasite survival is not established.

Specific antibody in the presence of complement is lethal for blood stream forms (trypomastigotes) of *T. cruzi*, but has no apparent action against intracellular parasites. There is evidence for strain specific immunity against *T. cruzi* (Krettli *et al.*, 1979; McHardy, 1980) but the importance of antigenic diversity for survival of this protozoan in the mammalian host may be offset by the apparent invariance of a major cell surface glycoprotein (Snary, 1980). This protozoan is largely located within cells not normally phagocytic; its survival within mononuclear cells is associated with the passage of trypomastigotes from an initial location within phagosomes into the nonvacuolar cytoplasm where replication occurs (Nogueira, 1974; Kress *et al.*, 1975; Nogueira and Cohn, 1976). From the point of view of antibody-mediated immunity *T. cruzi* is undoubtedly protected by its intracellular location. Immune function is disordered in Chagas' disease, as evidenced by increased splenic suppressor cell activity associated with adherent cells (Rowland and Kuhn, 1978; Ramos *et al.*, 1979) and the occurrence of polyclonal B cell activation (Ortiz-Ortiz *et al.*, 1980) and this may favour survival of parasites.

The ability of *Toxoplasma* to survive within mononuclear cells has been related to the avoidance of phagosome-lysosome fusion and failure to stimulate production of reactive oxygen metabolites (Jones and Hirsch, 1972; Wilson *et al.*, 1980). These cytotoxic intracellular reactions are activated when ingested trypanosomes are antibody-coated, but a minority of the opsonized organisms do survive by somehow avoiding phagolysosome fusions and these presumably perpetuate infections.

Antibody-mediated immunopathology

Antibody-mediated immunopathology is a potentially important feature of several protozoal diseases including African and South American trypanosomiasis and malaria (Table IV).

It has frequently been pointed out that erythrocyte destruction in several malaria infections exceeds what could be accounted for by parasite rupture

TABLE IV

Some lesions possibly attributable to antibody-mediated immunopathology in protozoal diseases

Mechanism	*Malaria*	*S. American trypanosomiasis*	*African trypanosomiasis*
Direct cytotoxicity (Type 2)		*Cardiac lesions* *Gastro-intestinal lesions*	
Immune complex reactions (Type 3)	Anaemia Transient proteinuria Nephrotic syndrome		Myocarditis Encephalitis Proliferative glomerulonephritis
	Big spleen disease		

of infected cells. This has suggested the possibility that host red cells become sensitized by antired cell antibodies thus causing an autoimmune haemolytic anaemia. Although cold agglutinins have been found in rodent (Lustig *et al.*, 1977; Musoke *et al.*, 1977) and bird (Soni and Cox, 1975) malarias, similar antibodies of appropriate specificity present either in serum or erythrocyte eluates are rarely recorded in other species. Although antiglobulin tests are usually negative in human malaria (Greenwood *et al.*, 1978), the use of class-specific antisera did reveal IgG sensitization of red cells in West African children with *P. falciparum* infections (Facer *et al.*, 1979). This was attributed to the absorption of plasmodial antigen–antibody complexes onto erythrocyte surfaces (Facer, 1980)—a process which could promote red cell removal by the reticuloendothelial system and contribute to the anaemia associated with malaria. Transient nephropathy with glomerular immune deposits and proteinuria occur commonly in human and experimental malarias; however, only *P. malariae* is associated with progressive renal damage which presents as the nephrotic syndrome in human and monkey infections. The glomerular deposits associated with quartan malaria nephrosis contain Ig, most commonly IgG_2, IgM and IgG_3, complement components and *P. malariae* antigen (Allison and Houba, 1976).

The tropical splenomegaly syndrome (TSS) is characterized by massive enlargement of the spleen, having no obvious cause and associated with immunity to malaria, elevated levels of IgM, hepatic sinusoidal lymphocytosis and a favourable clinical response to malaria prophylaxis. Patients with TSS are thought to respond to malaria with excessive IgM production and this leads to the formation of high molecular weight immune complexes which become phagocytosed in the liver and spleen and cause eventual splenomegaly. A familial tendency to develop TSS suggests that the disease has a genetic basis possibly involving a disordered homeostasis of IgM synthesis (Greenwood and Fakunle, 1978).

In the chronic stage of Chagas' disease the characteristic gastrointestinal and cardiac lesions are associated with lymphocyte infiltration in the apparent absence of parasites and are generally thought to have an immunological basis. Some antigenic determinants of *T. cruzi* appear to have specificities common to various mammalian tissues and induce the formation of antibody which cross-reacts with membrane components of striated muscle and endothelial cells. Such antibodies are present in 95% of patients with Chagas' heart disease (Cossio *et al.*, 1974), but they fail to damage human foetal heart cells *in vitro* (Santos-Buch and Teixeira, 1974) and their pathogenic role is less certain than that of cytotoxic T cells (Teixeira *et al.*, 1978).

Human and experimental forms of African trypanosomiasis are associated with inflammatory and necrotic lesions including myocarditis and encephalitis and also with haemolytic anaemia. The participation of the host immune response in the genesis of these lesions is uncertain. The striated muscle damage observed in mice infected with *T. brucei* occurs concomitantly with the appearance of antitrypanosome antibodies and is associated with local Ig deposits while mice with immune deficiency have higher parasitaemias and few muscle lesions (Galvao-Castro *et al.*, 1978). Similarly, renal glomerular lesions in rats with *T. rhodesiense* infections are associated with Ig deposits (Lindsley *et al.*, 1978). These findings suggest that specific immune complexes play a role in the development of tissue pathology in African trypanosomiasis.

Conclusions

All the pathogenic protozoa of man induce a vigorous humoral response frequently associated with the production of nonspecific Ig which is sometimes confined largely to a single isotype. Specific antibodies are formed against a broad spectrum of protozoal determinants, but only a small proportion of these have a protective function. Nevertheless, humoral antibody has an experimentally established role in acquired immunity against several protozoa of major clinical importance. In malaria antibodies act against a stage specific sporozoite surface antigen to inhibit exoerythrocytic infection and also against free blood stage merozoites to prevent attachment to and invasion of erythrocytes. Protective antibody in African trypanosomiasis reacts with surface coat glycoprotein to produce agglutination, macrophage opsonization and complement mediated lysis of the circulating organisms. The bloodstream forms (trypomastigotes) of South American trypanosomiasis are susceptible to complement-mediated immune lysis and to antibody dependent cell-mediated cytotoxicity. The extracellular trophozoites of *Toxoplasma gondii* are also susceptible to complement-mediated immune lysis, while their prior coating with antibody triggers an intracellular killing reaction by monocyte derived macrophages involving phagosome-lysosome fusion. Despite these potentially lethal humoral responses demonstrable during the course of natural infection, each of the diseases mentioned has an extremely chronic course in the human host and immunity is either incomplete or not manifest clinically. The analysis of mechanisms which enable these organisms to survive in the presence of potentially lethal humoral responses is central for the understanding of immunity to protozoa.

The survival of African trypanosomes which circulate as free-living organisms in the bloodstream depends fundamentally upon their capacity to replace sequentially their surface antigen with probably hundreds of alternative forms having distinct amino acid sequences and antigenic specificities. Other free forms of protozoa apparently susceptible to antibody-mediated immunity include malaria sporozoites and merozoites, trypomastigotes of *T. cruzi* and trophozoites of *Toxoplasma*; some show a degree of antigenic diversity but in none of these organisms does this appear to constitute a fundamental means for evading humoral immunity. However, all are present only transiently in the bloodstream and each rapidly attains an intracellular environment which in most instances offers protection from the action of humoral antibody. In addition, the distinct specificities of successive stages of plasmodial development favours the survival of any parasites which escape the effects of antisporozoite immunity.

It is probably significant that those protozoa which present the most constant antigenic target for immune attack (free-living African trypanosomes and erythrocytic stages of plasmodia which express antigen on the host red cell membrane) have a particular capacity for interfering with host immune function. Products of these protozoa induce polyclonal lymphocyte activation severe enough in some experimental models to eventually exhaust immune responsiveness; in addition, suppressor cells are activated and there is direct experimental evidence that the immune disruption consequent to these processes promotes the survival of both African trypanosomes and plasmodia.

The structural and metabolic complexity of protozoa generate an enormous diversity of antigens and most specific antibody induced is irrelevant to protection. Such antibody by leading to the formation of immune complexes may, however, contribute to the pathogenesis of protozoal diseases. Thus several pathological manifestations of malaria, including anaemia, the nephrotic syndrome and tropical splenomegaly, appear to be attributable to Type III reactions mediated by complexes of malaria antigen with circulating antibody and the inflammatory lesions of African trypanosomiasis may have a similar origin.

The chronicity of protozoal infections reflects a complex and subtle balance between the immune reactivity of the host which generates potentially lethal humoral responses and the capacity of the parasite to evade these. Perhaps the most interesting question in protozoal immunology at present concerns the ability of purified antigen preparations of appropriate specificity to induce protective immune responses without activating mechanisms which permit parasite survival. The successful isolation of such antigens could ultimately lead to the development of effective methods for vaccination against several human protozoal infections.

References

Allison, A. C. and Houba, V. (1976). *In* "Immunology of Parasitic Infections" (S. Cohen and E. Sadun, eds) p. 436. Oxford Scientific Publications.

Anderson, S. E. and Remington, J. (1974). *J. Exp. Med.* **139**, 1154.

Askonas, B. A., Corsini, A. C., Clayton, C. E. and Ogilvie, B. M. (1979). *Immunology* **36**, 313.

Assoku, P. K. G. and Tizard, I. R. (1978). *Experientia* **34**, 127.

Bannister, L. H., Butcher, G. A., Dennis, E. D. and Mitchell, G. H. (1975). *Parasitology* **71**, 483.

Biozzi, G., Mouton, D., SantAnna, O. A., Passos, H. C., Gennari, M., Reis, M. H., Ferreira, V. C. A., Heumann, A. M., Bouthillier, Y., Ibanez, O. M., Stiffel, C. and Siqueira, M. (1979). *Curr. Topics Microbiol. Immunol.* **8**, 31.

Blair, D. M., Smith, E. B. and Gelfand, M. (1968). *Cent. Afric. J. Med.* **14**, 12.

Blum, K. and Cioli, D. (1978). *Eur. J. Immunol.* **8**, 52.

Bridgen, P. J., Cross, G. A. M. and Bridgen, J. (1976). *Nature* **263**, 613.

Briggs, N. T. and Wellde, B. T. (1969). *Milit. Med.* **134**, 1243.

Brown, I. N., Watson, S. R. and Sijivic, V. S. (1977). *Infec. Immun.* **16**, 456.

Brown, K. N. and Brown, I. N. (1965). *Nature* **208**, 1286.

Bruce-Chwatt, L. J. and Gibson, F. D. (1955). *Trans. R. Soc. Trop. Med. Hyg.* **50**, 47.

Budzko, D. B., Pizziment, M. C. and Kierszenbaum, F. (1975). *Infec. Immun.* **11**, 86.

Butcher, G. A. and Cohen, S. (1972). *Immunology* **23**, 503.

Butcher, G. A., Mitchell, G. H. and Cohen, S. (1973). *Nature* **244**, 40.

Butcher, G. A., Mitchell, G. H. and Cohen, S. (1978). *Immunology* **34**, 77.

Carter R. F. (1972). *Trans. R. Soc. Trop. Med. Hyg.* **66**, 193.

Clark, I. A., Cox, F. E. G. and Allison, A. C. (1977). *Parasitology* **74**, 9.

Clayton, C. E., Ogilvie, B. M. and Askonas, B. A. (1979a). *Parasite Immunol.* **1**, 39.

Clayton, C. E., Sacks, D. L., Ogilvie, B. M. and Askonas, B. A. (1979b). *Parasite Immunol.* **1**, 241.

Cohen, S. (1979). *Proc. R. Soc. Lond.* **203**, 323.

Cohen, S. (1980). *In* "Biochemistry of Parasites and Host Parasite Relationships" Janssen Research Federation (in press).

Cohen, S. and Butcher, G. A. (1969). *Milit. Med.* **134**, 1191.

Cohen, S. and Butcher, G. A. (1970). *Immunology* **19**, 369.

Cohen, S. and Mitchell, G. A. (1978). *Curr. Topics Microbiol. Immunol.* **80**, 97.

Cohen, S. and Sadun, E. (1976). *In* "Immunology of Parasitic Infections" (S. Cohen and E. Sadun, eds) pp. 498. Blackwell Scientific Publications, Oxford.

Cohen, S., Butcher, G. A. and Crandall, R. B. (1969). *Nature* **223**, 368.

Cohen, S., McGregor, I. A. and Carrington, S. C. (1961). *Nature* **192**, 733.

Coombs, A. M. and Coombs, R. R. A. (1953). *J. Hyg.* **51**, 509.

Corsini, A. C., Clayton, C. E., Askonas, B. A. and Ogilvie, B. M. (1977). *Clin. Exp. Immunol.* **29**, 122.

Cossio, P. M., Laguens, R. P., Diez, C., Szarfman, A., Segal, A. and Arana, R. M. (1974). *Circulation* **50**, 1252.

Cox, H. W. (1959). *J. Immunol.* **82**, 208.

Cross, G. A. M. (1978). *Proc. R. Soc. Lond.* **202**, 55.

Culbertson, J. T. and Kolodny, M. H. (1938). *J. Parasitol.* **24**, 83.

Deans, J. A. and Cohen, S. (1979). *Bull. WHO* **57**, Suppl. 1., 93.

Diggs, C. L. and Osler, A. G. (1969). *J. Immunol.* **102**, 298.

Diggs, C. L. and Osler, A. G. (1975). *J. Immunol.* **114**, 1243.
Doyle, J. J., Hirumi, H., Hirumi, K., Lupton, E. N. and Cross, G. A. M. (1980). *Parasitology* **80**, 359.
Edozien, J. C., Gilles, H. M. and Udeozo, I. O. K. (1962). *Lancet* **ii**, 951.
Esuruosco, G. O. (1976). *Clin. Exp. Immunol.* **23**, 314.
Facer, C. A. (1980). *Clin. Exp. Immunol.* **39**, 279.
Facer, C. A., Bray, R. S. and Brown, J. (1979). *Clin. Exp. Immunol.* **35**, 119.
Feldman, H. A. (1956). *Ann. N.Y. Acad. Sci.* **66**, 263.
Fife, E. H. (1971). *Exp. Parasitol.* **30**, 132.
Flemmings, B. and Diggs, C. (1978). *Infect. Imm.* **19**, 928.
Foley, D. A. and Vanderberg, J. P. (1977). *Exp. Parasitol.* **63**, 69.
Freeman, R. R. and Parish, C. R. (1978). *Clin. Exp. Immunol.* **32**, 41.
Freeman, R. R., Trejdosiewicz, A. J. and Cross, G. A. M. (1980). *Nature* **284**, 366.
Galvao-Castro, B., Hachmann, A. and Lambert, P. H. (1978). *Clin. Exp. Immunol.* **33**, 12.
Garnham, P. C. C. (1977). *Protozool. Abst.* **1**, 1.
Greenwood, B. M. (1974a). *Lancet* **i**, 435.
Greenwood, B. M. (1974b). *Ciba Foundation Symposium* **25**, 137.
Greenwood, B. M. and Fakunle, Y. M. (1978). *Trop. Dis. Res. Series* **1**, 229.
Greenwood, B. M. and Vick, R. M. (1975). *Nature* **257**, 592.
Greenwood, B. M., Playfair, J. H. L. and Torrigiani, G. (1971). *Clin. Exp. Immunol.* **8**, 467.
Greenwood, B. M., Stratton, D. and Williamson, W. A. (1978). *Transact. R. Soc. Trop. Med. Hyg.* **72**, 378.
Gryzywinski, L. (1978). *Acta Parasitol Poland* **25**, 275.
Hafizi, A. and Modabber, F. Z. (1978). *Clin. Exp. Immunol.* **33**, 389.
Hale, C. and Howard, J. G. (1980). *Parasite Immunol.* (in press).
Herod, E., Clark, I. A. and Allison, A. C. (1978). *Clin. Exp. Immunol.* **31**, 518.
Hoeijmakers, J. H. J., Frasch, A. C. C., Bernards, A., Borst, P. and Cross, G. A. M. (1980). *Nature* **284**, 78.
Houba, V., Brown, K. N. and Allison, A. C. (1969). *Clin. Exp. Immunol.* **4**, 113.
Houba, V., Page-Faulk, W. and Matola, Y. G. (1974). *Clin. Exp. Immunol.* **18**, 89.
Houba, V., Lambert, P. H., Voller, A. and Soyanwo, M. A. O. (1976). *Clin. Exp. Immunol.* **6**, 1.
Jayawardena, A. N., Targett, G. A. T., Leuchars, E., Carter, R. L., Doenhoff, M. J. and Davies, A. J. S. (1975). *Nature* **258**, 149.
Jayawardena, A. N., Waksman, B. H. and Eardley, D. D. (1978). *J. Immunol.* **121**, 622.
Jefferey, G. M. (1966). *Bull. WHO* **35**, 873.
Jones, T. C. and Hirsch, J. G. (1972). *J. Exp. Med.* **136**, 1173.
Jones, T. C., Len, L. and Hirsch, J. G. (1975). *J. Exp. Med.* **141**, 466.
June, C. H., Contreras, C. E., Perrin, L. H., Lambert, P. H. and Miescher, P. A. (1979). *J. Immunol.* **122**, 2154.
Kagan, I. G. and Norman, L. (1961). *J. Infect. Dis.* **108**, 213.
Kierszenbaum, F. (1979). *Am. J. Trop. Med. Hygiene* **28**, 965.
Kierszenbaum, F. and Howard, J. G. (1976). *J. Immunol.* **116**, 1208.
Klein, F., Mattern, P. and Bosch, H. J. K. (1970). *Clin. Exp. Immunol.* **7**, 851.
Kobayakawa, T., Louis, J., Izui, S. and Lambert, P. H. (1979). *J. Immunol.* **122**, 296.
Kress, Y., Bloom, B. R., Wittner, M., Rowen, A. and Tanowitz, H. (1975). *Nature* **257**, 394.
Krettli, A. U. and Brener, Z. (1976). *J. Immunol.* **116**, 755.
Krettli, A. U., Weiss-Carrington, P. and Nussenzweig, R. S. (1979). *Clin. Exp. Immunol.* **37**, 416.
Krotoski, W. A., Krotoski, D. M., Garnham, P. C. C., Bray, R. S., Killick-

Kendrick, R., Draper, C. C., Targett, G. A. T. and Guy, M. W. (1980). *Brit. Med. J.*. **280**, 153.
Laveran, A. and Mesnil, F. (1912). *In* "Trypanosomes et Trypanosomes" 2nd ed. Paris, Masson et Cie.
Lewis, W. P. and Markell, E. K. (1958). *Exp. Parasitol.* **7**, 463.
Lindsley, H. B., Nagle, R. B., Stechschulte, D. J. (1978). *Am. J. Trop. Med. Hyg.* **27**, 864.
Liew, F. Y., Dhaliwal, S. S. and Teh, K. L. (1979). *Immunology* **37**, 35.
Longnecker, B. M., Breitenbach, R. P., Congdon, L. L. and Farmer, J. N. (1969). *J. Parasitol.* **55**, 418.
Loose, L. D., Cook, J. A. and De Luzio, W. R. (1972). *Proc. Helminth. Soc. Wash.* **39**, 484.
Lustig, H. J., Nussenzweig, V. and Nussenzweig, R. (1977). *J. Immunol.* **119**, 210.
MacKenzie, A. R., Boreham, P. F. L. and Facer, C. A. (1972). *Trans. R. Soc. Trop. Med. Hyg.* **66**, 344.
McGregor, I. A. (1972). *Br. Med. Bull.* **28**, 22.
McHardy, N. (1980). *Parasitology* **80**, 471.
Mansfield, J. M., Craig, S. A. and Stelzer, G. T. (1976). *Infec. Immun.* **14**, 976.
Maseyeff, R. and Gambert, J. (1963). *Ann. Inst. Pasteur* **104**, 115.
Mason, S. J., Miller, L. H., Shiroishi, T., Dvorak, J. A. and McGinnis, M. H. (1977). *Br. J. Haem.* **36**, 327.
Mauel, J., Behin, R., Biroum-Noerjasin and Holle, B. (1975). *In* "Mononuclear Phagocytes in Immunity, Infection and Pathology" (R. von Furth, ed.) pp. 663. Blackwells Scientific Publications, Oxford.
Mayor-Withey, K. S., Clayton, C. E., Roelants, G. E. and Askonas, B. A. (1978). *Clin. Exp. Immunol.* **34**, 359.
Mendes, R. P., Takehara, H. A. and Mota, I. (1979). *Exp. Parasitol.* **48**, 345.
Miller, L. H., Dvorak, J. A., Shiroishi, T. and Durocher, J. R. (1973). *J. Exp. Med.* **138**, 1596.
Miller, L. H., Aikawa, M. and Dvorak, J. A. (1975). *J. Immunol.* **114**, 1237.
Miller, L. H., Mason, S. J., Clyde, D. F. and McGinnis, M. H. (1976). *New Engl. J. Med.* **295**, 302.
Mitchell, G. H., Butcher, G. A., Voller, A. and Cohen, S. (1976). *Parasitology* **72**, 149.
Moore, D. L., Heyworth, B. and Brown, J. (1977). *Immunology* **33**, 777.
Musoke, A. J., Cox, H. W. and Williams, J. F. (1977). *J. Parasitol.* **63**, 1081.
Nardin, E. and Nussenzweig, R. S. (1978). *Nature* **274**, 55.
Nogueira, N. (1974). *J. Cell Biol.* **63**, 246a.
Nogueira, N. and Cohn, Z. (1976). *J. Exp. Med.* **143**, 1402.
Orjih, A. U. and Nussenzweig, R. S. (1979). *Clin. Exp. Immunol.* **38**, 1.
Ortiz-Ortiz, L., Parks, D. E., Rodriguez, M. and Weigle, W. O. (1980). *J. Immunol.* **124**, 121.
Pearson, T. W., Roelants, G. E., Pinder, M., Lundin, L. B. and Mayor-Withey, K. S. (1979). *Eur. J. Immunol.* **9**, 200.
Phillips, R. S. (1970). *Exp. Parasitol.* **27**, 479.
Phillips, R. S., Trigg, P. I., Scott-Finnigan, T. J. and Bartholomew, R. K. (1972). *Parasitology* **65**, 525.
Poels, L. G., Van Niekerk, C., Pennings, L., Agterberg, J. and Van Elven, E. H. (1977). *Exp. Parasitol.* **43**, 255.
Potocnjak, P., Yoshida, N., Nussenzweig, R. and Nussenzweig, V. (1980). *J. Exp. Med.* **151**, 1504.
Poulter, L. W. (1980). *Clin. Exp. Immunol.* **39**, 14.
Preston, P. M. and Dumonde, D. C. (1976). *In* "Immunology of Parasitic Infections" (S. Cohen and E. Sadun, eds) pp. 167. Blackwells Scientific Publications, Oxford.
Quinn, T. C. and Wyler, D. J. (1979). *J. Immunol.* **123**, 2245.

Ramos, C., Schadtler-Siwon, I. and Ortiz-Ortiz, L. (1979). *J. Immunol.* **122**, 1243.
Rank, R. G. and Weidanz, W. P. (1976). *Proc. Soc. Exp. Biol. Med.* **151**, 257.
Rodjakin, N. F. (1957). *Inst. Sci. Res. Turkmenia S.S.R.* **242**.
Ross, R. (1956). *International Scientific Communications of Trypanosoma Research* **6**, 2.
Rowe, D. S., McGregor, I. A., Smith, S. J., Hall, P. and Williams, K. (1968). *Clin. Exp. Immunol.* **3**, 63.
Rowland, E. C. and Kuhn, R. E. (1978). *Infect. Immun.* **20**, 393.
Ryckman, R. E. (1965). *J. Med. Entomol.* **2**, 105.
Sabin, A. B. and Feldman, H. A. (1948). *Science* **108**, 660.
Sacks, D. L., Selkirk, M., Ogilvie, B. M. and Askonas, B. A. (1980). *Nature* **283**, 476.
Santos-Buch, C. A. and Teixeira, A. R. L. (1974). *J. Exp. Med.* **140**, 38.
Schmidt-Ullrich, R., Wallach, D. F. H. and Lightholder, J. (1979). *J. Exp. Med.* **150**, 86.
Seed, J. R. and Gamm, A. A. (1966). *J. Parasitol.* **52**, 1134.
Seed, J. R., Cornille, R. L., Risby, E. L. and Gamm, A. A. (1969). *Parasitology* **59**, 283.
Sergent, E. (1963). *In* "Symposium on Immunity to Protozoal Diseases" (P. C. C. Garnham, A. E. Pierce and I. Roitt, eds). Blackwell Scientific Publications, Oxford.
Snary, D. (1980). *Exp. Parasitol.* **49**, 68.
Soltys, M. A. (1957). *Parasitology* **47**, 375.
Soltys, M. A. (1967). *Can. J. Microbiol.* **13**, 743.
Soni, J. L. and Cox, H. W. (1975). *Am. J. Trop. Med. Hyg.* **24**, 206.
Spitalny, G. L., Rivera-Ortiz, C. and Nussenzweig, R. S. (1976). *Exp. Parasitol.* **40**, 179.
Teixeria, A. R. L., Teixeira, G., Macedo, V. and Prata, A. (1978). *Am. J. Trop. Med. Hyg.* **27**, 1097.
Terry, B. J. (1956). *Trans. R. Soc. Trop. Med. Hyg.* **50**, 41.
Vickerman, K. (1978). *Nature* **273**, 613.
Voller, A. and Rossan, R. N. (1969). *Trans. R. Soc. Trop. Med. Hyg.* **63**, 507.
Von Kretschmar, W. (1965). *Z. Tropenmed. Parasit.* **16**, 277.
Warren, H. S. and Weidanz, W. P. (1976). *Eur. J. Immunol.* **6**, 816.
Watkins, J. F. (1964). *J. Hyg.* **62**, 69.
Weinbaum, F. I., Evans, C. B. and Tigelaar, R. E. (1976). *J. Immunol.* **117**, 1199.
Weinbaum, F. I., Weintraub, J., Nkrumah, F. K., Evans, C. B., Tigelaar, P. E. and Rosenberg, Y. J. (1978). *J. Immunol.* **121**, 629.
Wellhausen, S. R. and Mansfield, J. M. (1979). *J. Immunol.* **122**, 818.
Wells, R. A., Pavanand, K., Zolyomi, S., Permpanich, B. and MacDermott, R. P. (1980). *Clin. Exp. Immunol.* **39**, 663.
Williams, R. O., Young, J. R. and Majiwa, P. A. O. (1979). *Nature* **282**, 847.
Wilson, C. B., Tsai, V. and Remington, J. S. (1980). *J. Exp. Med.* **151**, 328.
Wilson, R. J. M. and Phillips, R. S. (1976). *Nature* **263**, 132.
Wyler, D. J. (1979). *Bull. WHO* Suppl. 1, 239.
Wyler, D. J. and Oppenheim, J. J. (1974). *J. Immunol.* **113**, 449.
Yoshida, N., Nussenzweig, R. S., Potocnjak, P., Nussenzweig, V. and Aikawa, M. (1980). *Science* **207**, 71.

44

ADCC as Primary Mechanisms of Defence against Metazoan Parasites

ANDRÉ CAPRON, MONIQUE CAPRON and JEAN-PAUL DESSAINT

Centre d' Immunologie et de Biologie Parasitaire, Institut Pasteur, Lille, France

Introduction

Although there is now a great deal of circumstantial evidence for the acquisition in man of protective immunity against several helminth parasites, the most significant information concerning the effector mechanisms of immunity has come from the development of appropriate animal models together with considerable improvement of *in vitro* cultivation of metazoan parasites (Clegg and Smithers, 1972). The combined use of *in vitro* cytotoxicity assays and of cell or serum passive transfer experiments has allowed in many cases the identification of some of the immune mechanisms responsible for the acquisition of immunity to reinfection. It must, however, be emphasized that the major source of our knowledge is so far derived from *in vitro* observations for which the *in vivo* relevance has not always been precisely established. The main

Abbreviations
ADCC: antibody-dependent cell-mediated cytotoxicity; MBP: major basic protein; ECP: eosinophil cationic protein; ECF-A: eosinophil chemotactic factor of anaphylaxis.

purpose of this review will therefore be to consider the most recent advances in *in vitro* cytotoxicity mechanisms, without any prejudice of their real biological significance in the infected host. Although numerous studies have been made in several models of helminth infection, there is no doubt that schistosomiasis has provided so far the most precise information on effector mechanisms against a metazoan parasite. We shall therefore consider this particular model in this paper.

Schistosome infection is characterized by the presence of adult worms in the portal and mesenteric veins as the result of a complex migratory cycle initiated by cutaneous penetration of water-living infective larvae (cercariae), which transform into schistosomula under the skin of appropriate mammalian hosts. Schistosomiasis as a human disease affects 300 M people in the world and represents one of the major public health problems in developing countries. The use of rodent models such as the mouse or the rat and the possibility of maintaining schistosomula in *in vitro* culture have made possible a precise analysis of the immune mechanisms in this infection. As a whole, immune response to schistosomes is directed against the schistosomulum stage, whereas the adult population seems relatively unaffected by the immune effector mechanisms (concomitant immunity, Smithers and Terry, 1965). Although numerous evidences have been accumulated concerning the thymus-dependency of some essential features of the immune response, the demonstration has been made that cytotoxic T cells are not involved in killing mechanisms. Even though schistosomula do acquire MHC products (Sher *et al.*, 1978), which have been demonstrated on the surface of parasite, allo-reactive T cells of the Lyt-2 phenotype generated against MHC antigens adhere to schistosomula but do not induce any parasite killing (Butterworth *et al.*, 1979a). On the other hand, cell transfer experiments have generally led to rather equivocal results. Conversely, serum passive transfer experiments both in the mouse and the rat have indicated the important role played by the humoral response in the mechanisms of defence (Smithers and Terry, 1976). This is also supported by recent experiments in anti-μ treated neonate rats which entirely fail to develop immunity to a challenge infection (Bazin *et al.*, 1980). The most striking feature of the antibody response seems to be the massive production of anaphylactic antibodies, which is illustrated by a dramatic increase in IgE levels in both human and experimental schistosomiasis (Dessaint *et al.*, 1975; Rousseaux-Prevost *et al.*, 1978). Attempts to correlate this prominent humoral response with the biological activity of antibodies in *in vitro* cytotoxicity assays has led, firstly, to the demonstration that IgG antibodies from various immune host species were highly cytotoxic for schistosomula in the presence of complement (Clegg and Smithers, 1972). However, the passive transfer of these complement-fixing antibodies confers only partial resistance, whereas complement depletion by cobra venom factor only partially decreases immunity to reinfection (Capron and Capron, 1980). This indicates at least that other antibody-dependent mechanisms might be operative, justifying the numerous attempts which have been made to focus on antibody-dependent cell-mediated cytotoxicity (ADCC). Before going on to precise details concerning the most important ADCC mechanisms so far described (Table I), it seems necessary to point out that they do not involve conventional K cells but phagocytic cell populations, among which the participation of macrophages and eosinophils has particularly been stressed.

TABLE I
ADCC mechanisms to schistosomula

Effector cells	*Antibody*	*Models*	*First description*
Macrophages	IgE	Rat	A. Capron (1975)
		Man	Joseph (1978)
Monocytes	IgE	Baboon	
Eosinophils	IgG	Man	Butterworth (1974)
Eosinophils	IgG2a	Rat	M. Capron (1978)
Eosinophils	IgG	Mouse	Kassis (1979)
Eosinophils	IgE	Rat	M. Capron (1980)

ADCC involving macrophages

Killing mechanism

The hypothesis that macrophages participate in *in vitro* cytotoxicity mechanisms is supported by a series of experiments performed in our laboratory since 1974. It was initially shown that normal rat peritoneal cells with over 95% macrophages, preincubated for 3 h with immune rat serum were able to adhere strongly and to kill *Schistosoma mansoni* schistosomula. Important lesions were observed on the worm surface leading to a great many deaths in the parasite population (85·5 ± 3·1% killing at an effector to target ratio of 4000 : 1). Ultrastructural studies showed that only macrophages adhered to the target.

Investigation of the serum factor inducing macrophage cytotoxicity led to the conclusion that a heat labile, noncomplement-dependent specific antibody was involved. Various absorption tests allowed its characterization as IgE antibody to schistosomes (Capron *et al.*, 1975; 1977b). Experiments also indicated that the interaction between IgE and macrophages involves a cytophilic binding of the IgE molecule (Joseph *et al.*, 1977). This was further supported through the use of rosette formation or labelled IgE, by the identification of a saturable and specific binding site for aggregated IgE on the membrane of macrophages (Dessaint *et al.*, 1979). This observation was consistent with the characterization of IgE on the surface of macrophages from infected rats and with the finding that macrophage cytotoxicity was induced by IgE immune complexes which were shown to be present at preferen-

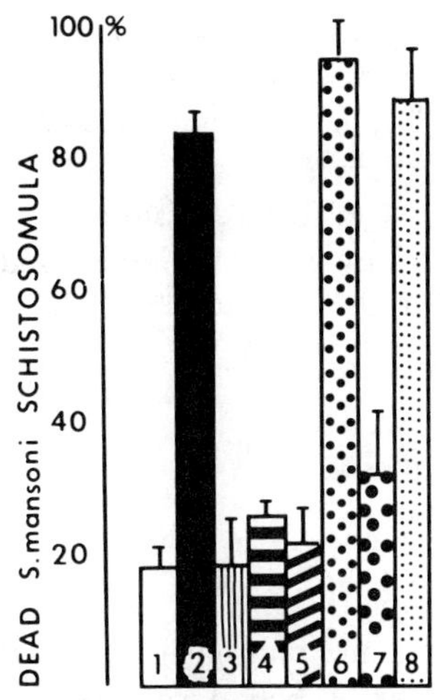

FIG. 1. *IgE-dependent macrophage cytotoxicity against* S. mansoni *schistosomula (1–5). Normal rat macrophages were for preincubated 3 h with normal or infected rat serum. Killing was assayed after 18 h contact between serum-incubated macrophages and schistosomula. Experiments 6–8 are inhibition experiments where the indicated monoclonal immunoglobulin was added to immune rat serum in the preincubation step.*

tial periods of infection (Capron *et al.*, 1977b). Macrophage cytotoxicity by IgE antibody can be competitively inhibited by chemically aggregated myeloma IgE protein but not by monomeric IgE. Aggregated or monomeric IgG did not inhibit either (Joseph *et al.*, 1977) (Fig. 1).

Macrophage activation by IgE

A particular study of macrophage activation by IgE showed that the binding of the aggregated molecules is followed within 30 min by a significant increase in the selective release and intracellular accumulation of lysosomal enzymes as well as superoxide production together with other classical parameters of macrophage activation (Dessaint *et al.*, 1980; Joseph *et al.*, 1980). It was moreover shown that IgE dimers represent the minimal molecular size required for macrophage activation, a process which was found to elicit a rapid cyclic GMP production and calcium uptake. The indirect participation of mast cells in this cytotoxicity mechanism could be ruled out by the very high degree of purification of macrophage monolayers, together with the persistance of macrophage activation by dimers of IgE when mast cell degranulation is prevented by an excess of monomeric IgE (Dessaint *et al.*, 1980).

Parallel observations have been made in human schistosomiasis. Human (normal) monocytes incubated with the serum from infected individuals are able to kill schistosomula. As in the rat model, IgE antibody was identified as the factor responsible for monocyte activation and cytoxicity (Joseph *et al.*, 1978). All these observations pointing to the role of IgE in an ADCC mechanism, and supporting evidence for a Fc_ϵ receptor on mononuclear phagocytes have recently been confirmed not only in other parasite models, namely in experimental filariasis (Haque *et al.*, 1980), but also in nonparasitic situations (Spiegelberg and Melewicz, 1980).

The *in vivo* relevance of this ADCC system is supported in rat schistosomiasis by the close correlation observed between the development of immunity and the evolution of specific IgE antibodies and IgE-dependent macrophage cytotoxicity (Capron *et al.*, 1977a).

ADCC involving eosinophils

Killing mechanism

Evidence that eosinophils can be implied in ADCC mechanisms came from the observation by Butterworth *et al.* (1974) that human polymorphonuclear leukocytes could kill schistosomula in the presence of *S. mansoni* infected human serum. A more precise study of the system allowed to identify eosinophils as the effector cells and IgG as the class of antibody involved (Butterworth *et al.*, 1977a, b). This killing mechanism is complement-independent and does not require the previous sensitization of the effector cell (Table II).

TABLE II
Eosinophil-dependent cytotoxicity mechanisms to S. mansoni *schistosomula*

Recognition factor	*Model*	*First description*
IgG	Man	Butterworth (1974)
IgG	Rat	MacKenzie (1977)
IgG2a	Rat	M. Capron (1978)
IgG	Mouse	Kassis (1979)
IgG1	Mouse	Ramalho-Pinto (1979)
IgE	Rat	M. Capron (1980)
Complement	Rat	Ramalho-Pinto (1978)
Complement	Man	Anwar (1979)

The mechanism of eosinophil-mediated damage has been elucidated by the elegant work of Butterworth and his colleagues and their various studies show that 3 successive steps can be considered.

Contact between eosinophils and targets
A strong adherence of eosinophils to the schistosomulum surface is required. This intimate contact can be obtained in the presence of antischistosomula serum, C3 or various ligands such as concanavalin A. The inhibitory role of cytochalasins on eosinophil-mediated damage suggests a role for the microfilaments. Vadas *et al.* (1980) have shown that antibody-dependent eosinophil adherence proceeds by at least two distinguishable phases. The first one, temperature-independent, is mediated by the Fc receptor and leads to

relatively weak adherence, whereas the second, a temperature-dependent step, leads to irreversible binding of eosinophils to schistosomula. The stable and irreversible adherence of human eosinophils to *S. mansoni* schistosomula, which is mainly induced by antibody, was shown to be attributable to the degranulation of eosinophils with the release of granule content, which serves as a ligand between the eosinophils and the parasite surface (Butterworth *et al.*, 1979c).

Degranulation step

This phase of degranulation, which only occurs for eosinophils in close contact to the target (Capron *et al.*, 1978a) is required both for binding stability and for target lysis, and contributes to the preferential killing capacity of eosinophils compared to neutrophils.

Presentation of the effector molecule.

The final step of lysis seems to be due to the release of molecules consequently to the degranulation of eosinophils. The first agent contained in the eosinophilic granule is a peroxidase which can be secreted onto the parasite surface, although no strong evidence suggests that this enzyme can damage this surface. The major basic protein (MBP) purified from eosinophil granules can be one of the granule components responsible for parasite lysis. Butterworth *et al.* (1979b) have shown that low concentrations of this molecule were able by themselves to kill schistosomula. They could also detect the local release of MBP at the parasite surface, while a small amount of MBP only was released into the supernatant of antibody-dependent eosinophil reaction. The release of MBP localized at the parasite surface can therefore be responsible for lytic activity of eosinophils to schistosomula. Similar effect of MBP has also been demonstrated against *Trichinella spiralis* newborn larvae (Wassom and Gleich, 1979). Other candidates for parasite lysis among the molecules contained in eosinophil granules can be the cationic proteins isolated from cytoplasmic granules, among which the eosinophil cationic protein (ECP) has been reported to be at least as active as MBP for schistosomula killing (Kay, 1979). The role of reductive products of oxygen such as superoxide or hydroxylradicals in eosinophil-dependent killing of helminthic parasites, is more speculative but the prolonged release of these molecules could explain the greater ability of eosinophils to damage nonphagocytable pathogens like helminths.

In conclusion, the eosinophil seems to be a highly specialized cell, able to damage tissue-stage helminths such as *Schistosoma* and *Trichinella*. This function may be due both to their particular property of degranulation when eosinophils come into contact with antibody-coated surfaces and to the unusual components of eosinophil granules which can directly be responsible for lysis.

Eosinophil activation

Investigations on the effector function of eosinophils have similarly been carried out in various experimental animals. In the rat, works in our laboratory have mainly been focused on the immune mechanisms leading to the activation and to the regulation of the eosinophil effector function.

Accessory role of mast cells

The study of eosinophil-mediated cytotoxicity in rat schistosomiasis led to the observation that besides eosinophils, mast cells were also present close to the surface of antibody-coated schistosomula. Their possible role in the cytotoxic reaction was therefore considered. Whereas mast cells by themselves could not kill the larvae, they participated as accessory cells in eosinophil-mediated cytotoxicity. Indeed, mast cell-depleted eosinophil populations showed a marked decrease in their killing activity which could be restored by the addition of a defined proportion of purified mast cells. The mechanism of mast cell-eosinophil co-operation was thus investigated. The presence of mast cells could be replaced by mast cell products obtained using various procedures of mast cell degranulation. Among the possible candidates in soluble preformed mast cell mediators, the role of the eosinophil chemotactic factor of anaphylaxis (ECF-A) was shown to be significant (Capron *et al.*, 1978b). The same level of cytotoxicity was obtained with intact mast cells, with unpurified mast cell mediators, or with purified ECF-A. In recent works, using EA rosette techniques, it was found that the preincubation of rat eosinophils with ECF-A tetrapeptides led to a significant enhancement of the expression of eosinophil surface Fc receptors, which was shown to be dose- and time-dependent. A significant correlation between EA-rosetting and the enhancement of eosinophil cytotoxicity strongly suggested that the effect of ECF-A on the expression of IgG Fc receptors and on the IgG-dependent eosinophil cytotoxicity may be fundamentally related. Similar observations could be made using human eosinophils (Capron and Capron, 1980).

Involvement of anaphylactic antibodies

Depending on the period of time following primary infection and the subsequent development of immunity, two different antibody isotypes were shown to be involved in the mechanism of eosinophil cytotoxocity. During the first 6 weeks of infection, solid-phase anti-immunoglobulin absorption procedures led to the demonstration that together with mast cell products, IgG2a (IgGa) antibody is responsible for eosinophil-mediated damage. IgG2a, the major subclass of IgG in the rat, is considered as the second class of anaphylactic antibody, able to induce histamine release from rat peritoneal mast cells. The role of IgG2a at this early period was very precisely confirmed by the production of monoclonal anti-schistosome IgG2a antibody, which was shown to elicit the same eosinophil-mediated cytotoxicity activity as 4-week-infected rat serum (Capron, M. *et al.*, 1978a; Verwaerde *et al.*, 1979). Interestingly, it was recently shown that mouse eosinophil-dependent antibody was of the IgG1 subclass (Ramalho-Pinto *et al.*, 1979), and IgG1 is able to mediate anaphylaxis in mice as well.

At the same time (first 6 weeks of infection), eosinophils collected from immune rats can kill schistosomula in the absence of opsonizing antibody. A *S. mansoni* antigen-rosette assay demonstrated the presence of cytophilic antibody on immune eosinophils (Capron *et al.*, 1979). A long term study of eosinophil effector function indicated that at certain later periods, immune eosinophils were no longer able to kill schistosomula, even in the presence of added antibody, and EA-rosette assay showed that eosinophil Fc receptors were blocked, whereas a blocking factor was identified in contemporary serum.

On the other hand, after 6 weeks of infection, a marked decrease in Ig2a antibody production was observed, raising therefore the question of the participation of another antibody isotype since unheated immune rat serum is still able to induce eosinophil cytotoxicity. It was indeed shown that a heat-labile, complement-independent antibody inducing eosinophil killing, was present in the immune serum 8 weeks after initial infection. As in the IgG2a-dependent system, the participation of mast cells or mast cell mediators was required. It could clearly be demonstrated that neither IgG2a-absorption of 8-week immune rat serum nor the preincubation of eosinophils with aggregated IgG led to a decrease in eosinophil cytotoxicity, when in the same conditions IgE-absorption or preincubation of eosinophils with aggregated myeloma IgE protein inhibit the cytotoxicity significantly (Capron and Capron, 1980). Thus, whereas an exclusive role can be attributed to IgG2a around 4 weeks of infection, later on IgE antibody appears exclusively involved in eosinophil ADCC (Table III).

TABLE III

Involvement of IgE in eosinophil-dependent cytotoxicity in the presence of unheated S. Mansoni *infected rat serum*

Treatment of	*% inhibition of cytotoxicity*[a]	P *value*
8 week-infected rat serum[b]		
IgE-absorbed (86% absorption)	65	<0·001
IgG2a-absorbed (75% absorption)	28	N.S.
Rat eosinophils		
preincubated with 0·2 mg/ml Aggr-IgE[c]	70	<0·02
preincubated with 1 mg/ml Aggr-IgG2a[d]	11	N.S.

[a] Compared to untreated infected rat serum or to eosinophils incubated with medium.
[b] Percentage of dead schistosomula after 24–48 h contact with effector cell (6000 : 1 target) and serum diluted 1/32 : 60·3 ± 6·6% (16·0 ± 5·7% with normal rat serum).
[c] Eosinophils preincubated 1 h with dimethylsuberimidate aggregated rat myeloma IgE protein (IR 162) before addition of infected rat serum and schistosomula.
[d] As in c except that heat-aggregated myeloma IgG2a protein was used for the preincubation step.

The presence of an IgE binding site at the eosinophil surface had therefore to be envisaged. Using a rosette assay with rat IgE-myeloma protein-coated erythrocytes, normal rat IgG-coated red cells as positive controls and rat serum albumin-coated erythrocytes as negative controls, around 45% of rat eosinophils formed IgE-rosettes. The specificity of the binding was confirmed as preincubation of eosinophils with aggregated IgE only led to a significant inhibition of IgE rosettes. No cross-inhibition was observed between IgE and IgG, suggesting no cross reactivity between the binding sites for IgE and IgG (Capron and Capron, 1980). Preliminary experiments using mixed rosettes indicate that the same eosinophil population or subpopulation expresses both receptors for IgG and IgE. It was again shown that preincubation of rat eosinophils with ECF-A significantly increased the number not only of IgG, but also of IgE-rosettes, supporting the hypothesis of an interaction between mast cells and eosinophils both for IgG and for IgE eosinophil receptors.

It appears from these studies that eosinophil cytotoxicity seems to result, in the rat at least, from two signals: one is provided by the binding of IgG or IgE anaphylactic antibodies to the corresponding Fc receptor of the eosinophil surface, the other by mast cell products of activation also resulting from the interaction of the cell with anaphylactic antibody of either isotypes.

The role of eosinophils *in vivo* is supported by the observation by Mahmoud *et al.* (1975) that antieosinophil serum decreases reinfection immunity in the mouse. In the recent years evidence has also been presented, that eosinophils could act as effector cells in other parasitic models. This is particularly the case for human and experimental filariasis, and for trichinosis where, in *in vitro* assays, eosinophils have been shown in close contact with the target, whereas in some instances killing was observed (Kazura and Grove, 1978; Mackenzie *et al.*, 1978; Haque *et al.*, 1980). However, in most instances the precise demonstration of an ADCC mechanism was not provided and the identification of the antibody class involved was not performed. Finally, it has been shown that eosinophils could kill schistosomula through the activation of the complement system at the parasite surface (Ramalho-Pinto *et al.*, 1978) and the adherence of eosinophils through their C3b receptors. This mechanism shown in rat and in human schistosomiasis was shown to involve complement either alone or acting in synergy with antibody (McLaren and Ramalho-Pinto, 1979; Anwar *et al.*, 1979).

Conclusion

Taken as a whole, the study of ADCC systems in helminth infections and more precisely in schistosomiasis points to several essential features of these in *in vitro* immune effector mechanisms.

(a) As already mentioned, phagocytic cell populations seem to play an essential function as the cellular component of the ADCC systems. In this regard, macrophages and eosinophils certainly represent the main effector cells in *in vitro* cytotoxicity assays. The possible role of neutrophils in the presence of IgG and/or complement has also been reported. However, though neutrophils can be shown in close contact with schistosomula, their direct killing activity is still debated (Vadas *et al.*, 1979). While the participation of phagocytic cells in *in vitro* assays appears certain, evidence for their *in vivo* function is still fragmentary.

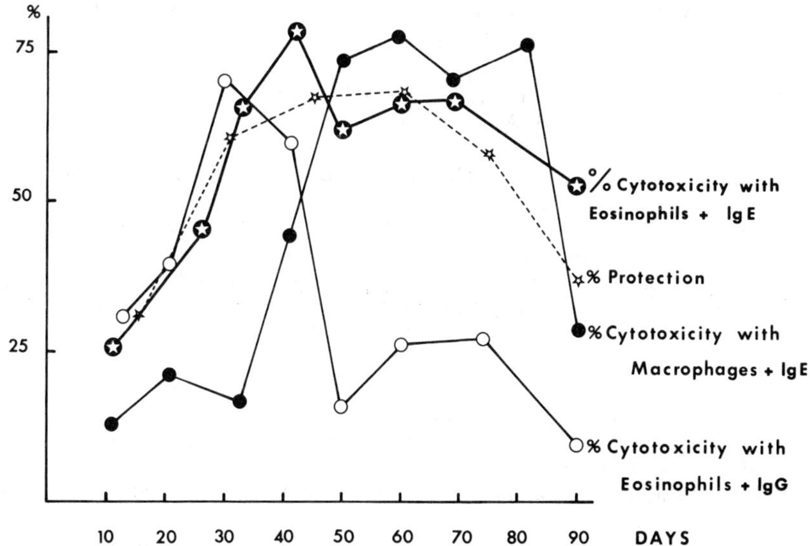

FIG. 2. *Comparative evolution of* in vitro *ADCC systems and of immunity to reinfection in rat* S. mansoni *schistosomiasis.*

(b) In contrast the role of antibodies and, more precisely, of the anaphylactic isotypes appears to be strongly supported both by their correlation with the development of immunity in experimental models (Fig. 2) and by passive transfer experiments performed after selective depletion of the immune serum of IgE or IgG2a antibodies in the rat (Capron *et al.*, 1980). These two kinds of data clearly stress the prominent role played by anaphylactic antibodies in ADCC mechanisms against various helminths and mainly schistosomes. In extending the area of ADCC systems from conventional K cells and IgG antibody to phagocytic cells and anaphylactic antibodies, parasite models have certainly contributed to improving our knowledge of these basic effector mechanisms. Moreover, the key role played by IgE antibody through the interaction of this molecule, not only with the conventional mast cell receptors, but also with specific receptors on macrophages and eosinophils, appears to give IgE a new and beneficial function in protective immunity.

References

Anwar, A. R. E., Smithers, S. R. and Kay, A. B. (1979). *J. Immunol.* **122**, 628.

Bazin, H., Capron, A., Capron, M., Joseph, M., Dessaint, J. P. and Pauwels, R. (1980). *J. Immunol.* **124**, 2373.

Butterworth, A. E., Sturrock, R. F., Houba, V. and Rees, P. M. (1974). *Nature* **252**, 503.

Butterworth, A. E., David, J. R., Franks, D., Mahmoud, A. A. F., David, P. H., Sturrock, R. F. and Houba, V. (1977a). *J. Exp. Med.* **145**, 136.

Butterworth, A. E., Remold, H. G., Houba, V., David, J. R., Franks, D., David, P. H. and Sturrock, R. F. (1977b). *J. Immunol.* **118**, 2230.

Butterworth, A. E., Vadas, M. A., Martz, E. and Sher, A. (1979a). *J. Immunol.* **122**, 1314.

Butterworth, A. E., Wassom, D. L., Gleich, G. J., Loegering, D. A. and David, J. R. (1979b). *J. Immunol.* **122**, 221.

Butterworth, A. E., Vadas, M. A., Wassom, D. L., Dessein, A., Hogan, M., Sherry, B., Gleich, G. J. and David, J. R. (1979c). *J. Exp. Med.* **150**, 1456.

Capron, A., Capron, M., Dupas, H., Bout, D. and Petitprez, A. (1974). *Int. J. Parasitol.* **4**. 613.

Capron, A., Dessaint, J. P., Capron, M. and Bazin, H. (1975). *Nature* **253**, 474.

Capron, A., Dessaint, J. P. and Capron, M. (1977a). *In* "Immunity in Parasitic Diseases" (Inserm, ed.) Vol. 72, pp. 217–230. Paris.

Capron, A., Dessaint, J. P., Joseph, M., Rousseaux, R., Capron, M. and Bazin, H. (1977b). *Eur. J. Immunol.* **7**, 315.

Capron, A., Dessaint, J. P., Capron, M., Joseph, M., and Pestel, J. (1980). *Am. J. Trop. Med. Hyg.* (in press).

Capron, M. and Capron, A. (1980). *Trans. R. Soc. Trop. Med. Hyg.* (in press).

Capron, M., Capron, A., Torpier, G., Bazin, H., Bout, D. and Joseph, M. (1978a). *Eur. J. Immunol.* **8**, 127.

Capron, M., Rousseaux, R., Mazingue, C., Bazin, H. and Capron, A. (1978b). *J. Immunol.* **121**, 2518.

Capron, M., Torpier, G. and Capron, A. (1979). *J. Immunol.* **123**, 2220.

Clegg, J. A. and Smithers, S. R. (1972). *Int. J. Parasitol.* **2**, 79.

Dessaint, J. P., Capron, M., Bout, D. and Capron, A. (1975). *Clin. Exp. Immunol.* **20**, 427.

Dessaint, J. P., Torpier, G., Capron, M., Bazin, H. and Capron, A. (1979). *Cell. Immunol.* **46**, 12.

Dessaint, J. P., Waksman, B. H., Metzger, H. and Capron, A. (1980). *Cell. Immunol.* **51**, 280.

Haque, A., Joseph, M., Ouaissi, M. A., Capron, M. and Capron, A. (1980). *Clin. Exp. Immunol.* **40**, 487.

Joseph, M., Dessaint, J. P. and Capron, A. (1977). *Cell. Immunol.* **34**, 247.

Joseph, M., Capron, A., Butterworth, A. E., Sturrock, R. F. and Houba, V. (1978). *Clin. Exp. Immunol.* **33**, 48.

Joseph, M., Tonnel, A., Capron, A. and Voisin, G. (1980). *Clin. Exp. Immunol.* **40**, 416.

Kassis, A. I., Aikawa, M. and Mahmoud, A. A. F. (1979). *J. Immunol.* **122**, 398.

Kazura, J. W. and Grove, D. I. (1978). *Nature* **274**, 588.

Kay, A. B. (1979). *J. All. Clin. Immunol.* **64**, 80.

MacKenzie, C. D., Ramalho-Pinto, F. J., McLaren, D. J. and Smithers, S. R. (1977). *Clin. Exp. Immunol.* **30**, 97.

MacKenzie, C. D., Preston, P. M. and Ogilvie, B. M. (1978). *Nature* **276**, 826.

Mahmoud, A. A. F., Warren, K. S. and Graham, R. C. (1975). *J. Exp. Med.* **142**, 805.

McLaren, D. J. and Ramalho-Pinto, F. J. (1979). *J. Immunol.* **123**, 1431.

Ramalho-Pinto, F. J., MacLaren, D. J. and Smithers, S. R. (1978). *J. Exp. Med.* **147**, 147.

Ramalho-Pinto, F. J., De Rossi, R. and Smithers, S. R. (1979). *Parasite Immunol.* **1**, 295.

Rousseaux-Prevost, R., Capron, M., Bazin, H. and Capron, A. (1978). *Immunology* **35**, 33.

Sher, A., Hall, B. F. and Vadas, M. A. (1978). *J. Exp. Med.* **148**, 46.

Smithers, S. R. and Terry, R. J. (1965). *Parasitology* **55**, 695.

Smithers, S. R. and Terry, R. J. (1976). *Adv. Parasitol.* **14**, 399.

Spiegelberg, H. L. and Melewicz, F. M. (1980). *Clin. Immunol. Immunopath.* **15**, 424.

Vadas, M. A., David, J. R., Butterworth, A. E., Pisani, N. T. and Sinogok, T. A. (1979). *J. Immunol.* **122**, 1228.

Vadas, M. A., Butterworth, A. E., Sherry, B., Dessein, A., Hogan, M., Bout, D. and David, J. R. (1980). *J. Immunol.* **124**, 1441.

Verwaerde, C., Grzych, J. M., Bazin, H., Capron, M. and Capron, A. (1979). *C. R. Acad. Sci.* **289**, 725.

Wassom, D. L. and Gleich, G. J. (1979). *Am. J. Trop. Med. Hyg.* **28**, 860.

45

T Cell Dependent Effects in Parasitic Infection and Disease

GRAHAM F. MITCHELL

Laboratory of Immunoparasitology, The Walter and Eliza Hall Institute of Medical Research, Melbourne, Victoria, Australia

Introduction

Immunoparasitology is the study of the immunological aspects of host–parasite relationships, the term "parasite" being restricted, arbitrarily, to metazoa (helminths), protozoa and arthropods, the latter usually occurring as ectoparasites. Most current research activities in the field fall into 5 categories (Fig. 1):

Abbreviations
B cell: bone marrow-derived precursor of antibody-secreting cells; BCG: Bacillus-Calmette-Guerin; DTH: delayed type hypersensitivity; HvP: host-versus-parasite; Ia and Ly: designations for alloantigenic markers on lymphocytes (Ly-1 and Ly-2 are locus designations); IEL: intraepithelial lymphocyte in intestinal mucosa; Igs: immunoglobulins; MMC: mucosal mast cells; RES: reticuloendothelial system; SEA: soluble egg antigens of *Schistosoma* spp.; T cell: thymus-influenced (derived) cell; T_{TDH}: T cells involved in DTH reactions; T_H: T cells involved in increasing antibody titres ("helpers'); T_S: T cells involved in suppression of immune responses.

(1) studies on the antigens of parasites, parasite products or parasitized cells;
(2) studies on effector cells, molecules and mechanisms of host-protective immunity;
(3) studies on mechanisms of evasion of host-protective immunities;
(4) studies on various accompaniments of parasitic infection (e.g. disease manifestations);
(5) development of immunodiagnostic reagents of high sensitivity and specificity.

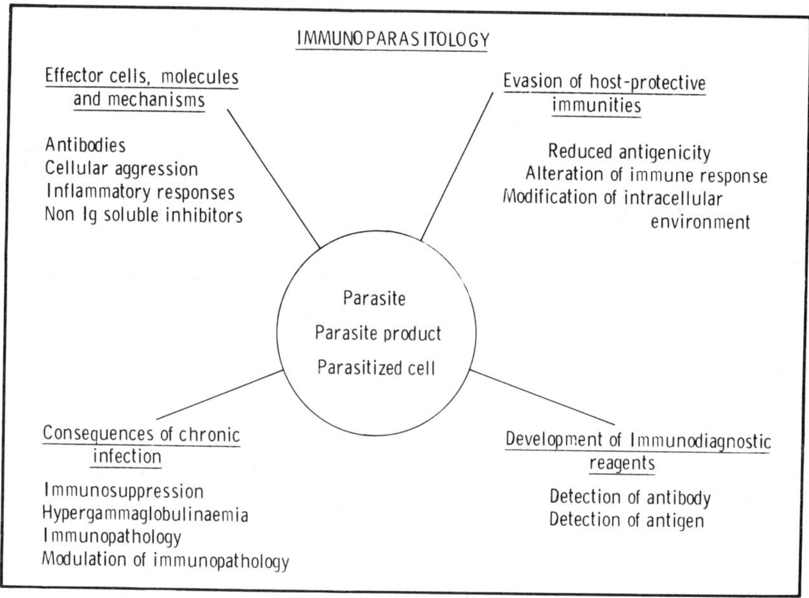

FIG. 1. *An indication of the scope of the topic area of immunoparasitology; most of the events listed on the left hand side of this figure are influenced by the presence of T cells.*

Studies embraced by categories 1 to 4, and the genetic aspects of variation within the components of these categories, are necessary in the development, by the rational approach, of vaccines against parasitic infection and disease. One small subsection of immunoparasitology which cuts across categories 2 to 4 is concerned with the activities of T cells in host-versus-parasite (HvP) reactions; these reactions include antiparasite immune responses. The information obtained in this type of investigation will be of broad immunological significance particularly with respect to antiparasite (effector) and disease consequences of T cell dependent inflammation plus lymphokine and antibody production.

Parasites induce a variety of HvP reactions in their biologically natural hosts as well as during the course of zoonotic infection in man and various unnatural infections in the laboratory. A large number of these reactions are influenced profoundly by the presence of activated T cells. In point of fact, the list of T cell dependent effects in parasitic infection and disease is so long that a demonstration of T cell dependence is often a useful, yet not particularly illuminating observation. Moreover, if, as is currently believed, the peripheral T cell population is a heterogeneous mixture of cell populations, each with very different biological functions, then the term "T cell dependence" loses much of its significance because it is imprecise. Studies on the broad immunoparasitological effects of T cells have been facilitated by the availability of hypothymic nude (nu/nu) mice and the capacity to fractionate reconstitutive T cell inocular into various subpopulations. It must be emphasized at the the outset, however, that interpretation difficulties may arise when the generalized epithelial defect of nude mice interferes with the induction or expression of HvP responses. Mucous membrane defects (in metazoan or protozoan parasitoses in the intestinal tract) and skin defects (in ectoparasitic arthropod or cutaneous leishmania infections) will influence the expression of local responses and the "accessibility" of parasites and their antigens (Mitchell and Anders, 1980).

A review on the use of nude mice in immunoparasitology is available (Mitchell, 1980). Most studies published to date have been confined to the assessment of the susceptibility of nude mice to infection: it is a simple task to count parasites, estimate parasitaemias, measure lesion sizes and compile mortality data in nude versus intact versus T cell injected (or thymus-grafted) nude mice. Nude mice will find particular use in immunoparasitology for:

(1) *Production of parasites.* Populations of parasites, parasitized cells and parasite products (such as eggs) in nude mice should be relatively unmodified by host immune responses. No studies have yet been reported on changes in the antigenic constitution of parasite populations after passage through nude versus immunologically intact mice. It can be anticipated that the lack of selection pressure imposed by T cell dependent immunities will lead to differences in the antigenic heterogeneity of parasite populations in nude mice. Such mice have already been used to rescue and maintain an irradiation-attenuated *Plasmodium berghei* parasite (Suzuki *et al.*, 1980). Differences in the larvae of the proliferating cestode parasite, *Mesocestoides corti* (Mitchell *et al.*, 1977a), and the trematode, *Fasciola hepatica* (Howard *et al.*, 1980), obtained from intact versus nude mice can be readily demonstrated. The larvae from intact mice contain, on their surface, much more immunoglobulin than parasites from nude mice. It has also been demonstrated that, for various antibody assays and hybridoma selection procedures, parasites derived from nude mice are a convenient source of antigen (Mitchell *et al.*, 1979). Parasitized nude mice may also prove useful for the determination of susceptibilities of parasites to chemotherapeutic agents *in vivo* without interference from the simultaneous action of an intact immune system.

(2) Analysis of *T cell dependent responses to parasitic infection*, i.e. cell

dependence of acquired or innate resistance, and T cell dependence of various parasitic disease manifestations such as chronic inflammation, immunosuppression and hyper-γ-globulinaemia.

(3) Studies on the broad *in vivo* immunoparasitological *activities of isolated T cell subpopulations*, isolated T cell dependent antibody isotypes, and isolated "accessory cells" such as eosinophils, mobile macrophages, mucosal mast cells and fibroblasts which seem to be responsive to T cell dependent stimuli (including antibodies) and/or T cell derived mediators.

There is one feature of experiments with reconstituted nude mice (or other T cell deficient animals) which is characteristic of many manifestations of chronic parasitic infection or the long lead-up time in the development of antiparasite effects. In the case of T cell deficient hosts injected with a particular T cell subpopulation especially, there is often ample time for a small and undetectable contaminant cell population in the inoculum to expand in the recipient. Obviously, assessment of the immunocompetence of the recipient at the time of assay is required. In several immunoparasitological studies, a negative effect with one or a few serum injections, and a positive with a mixed cellular inoculum, has been taken as evidence for cell-mediated effects (and against antibody-mediated effects) in HvP reactions or host protection against infection.

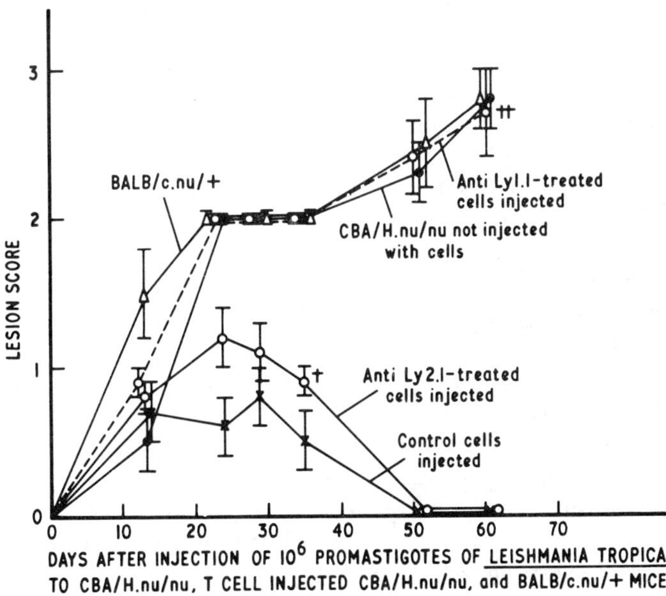

FIG. 2. *Reconstitution of the capacity to control cutaneous infection with an isolate of the intramacrophage protozoan parasite,* Leishmania tropica, *in CBA/H nude mice injected with no more than 2×10^6 syngeneic spleen cells treated with monoclonal anti-Ly-2, but not anti-Ly-1 hybridoma-derived antibodies plus complement. Lesion scores in control, as well as the genetically susceptible BALB/c mouse are indicated (4 or 5 mice per group). (Details in Mitchell* et al., *1980a).*

Reconstitution of resistance to infection back to the levels seen in intact mice may be difficult to achieve in nude mice injected with large numbers of T cells. This has proved to be the case in antilarval immunity, intestinal wall granuloma formation, and rejection of resident intestinal adults of the nematode, *Nematospiroides dubius* (Prowse *et al.*, 1978). On the other hand, in *Leishmania tropica* infections in mice, T cell injected BALB/c nude mice may be more resistant than either unreconstituted BALB/c nudes or intact BALB/c mice both of which invariably develop very obvious signs of cutaneous leishmaniasis (Mitchell *et al.*, 1980a). In the case of nude mice of relatively resistant genotype (e.g. CBA/H mice), very low numbers of Ly-1^+2^- cells are very effective in restoring resistance to infection (Fig. 2). Defects of the skin may render *L. tropica*-infected macrophages more vulnerable to T cell dependent antiparasite immune responses in T cell injected nude mice. Care should obviously be taken in the interpretation of observations in reconstituted nude mice in which generalized epithelial defects may influence the outcome of infection.

T cell dependence of susceptibility to parasitic infection in nude mice

In terms of the numbers of parasites in nude versus intact mice and rats, nudes may be:

(1) more susceptible to a primary infection and show a:
  (a) decreased innate resistance to infection
  (b) higher parasite numbers during infection
  (c) reduced ability to restrict the proliferative rate of parasites, or
  (d) failure to terminate a primary infection.

E.g. protozoans: *Pneumocystis carinii, Trypanosoma musculi, Trypanosoma congolense, Trypanosoma cruzi, Leishmania tropica, Giardia muris, Hexamita muris, Plasmodium yoelii* and *Babesia microti.*

Cestodes: *Taenia taeniaeformis, Mesocestoides corti, Hymenolepis nana* and *Hymenolepis diminuta.*

Nematodes: *Nippostrongylus brasiliensis, Nematospiroides dubius, Aspicularis tetraptera, Syphacia obvelata, Strongyloides ratti* and *Trichinella spiralis.*

(2) unable to develop high levels of resistance to reinfection (with or without drug cure of previous infection(s)).

E.g. Protozoans: *Eimeria* spp. and *Toxoplasma gondii.*

Nematodes: *Nematospiroides dubius, Nippostrongylus brasiliensis, Ascaris suum* and *Toxocara cans.*

(3) comparably susceptible or even marginally more resistant to a primary infection.

E.g Protozoans: *Plasmodium berghei, Babesia rodhaini, brucei vrucei* and *T. rhodesiense.*

Nematodes: *Ascaris suum* and *Toxocara canis.*

Trematodes: *Schistosoma mansoni* and *Fasciola hepatica.*

It can be seen that all parasites for which the mouse is a natural host (or which have not been modified by prolonged laboratory usage) are in categories (1) or (2). The findings using natural murine parasites in nude mice support the notion that T cell dependent HvP reactions have been a key ingredient in the evolution of balanced host–parasite relationships (discussed in Mitchell, 1979a, b). Full references for the above mentioned parasite systems (and those in the next section) are given in Mitchell (1980).

A listing of T cell dependent HvP reactions

When judged by defective responses in nude or other T cell deficient mice and rats relative to those in intact or T cell injected nude mice and rats, the T cell dependency of the following HvP reactions has been demonstrated or is suspected.

(1) Various antiparasite antibody responses as detected by binding assays.

(2) IgE antibody responses to antigens of metazoa.

(3) IgM antiphosphorylcholine responses to nematodes; other IgM responses (e.g. to *T. rhodesiense*) may be higher in parasitized nude versus intact mice.

(4) Host-protective IgG responses in *Taenia taeniaeformis* infection.

(5) IgG_1 antibodies on the surface of *Mesocestoides corti* larvae and circulating IgG_1 antibodies bearing a hybridoma idiotype in *M. corti* infection. Waki and Suzuki (1980) have reported a surprisingly high IgG_1 secondary antibody response in drug-cured *P. berghei*-infected mice).

(6) IgA antibodies to *Giardia muris* trophozoite extracts in serum and intestinal washings (Underdown, B. J., Anders, R. F., Mitchell, G. F. and Roberts-Thomson, I. C., unpub.).

(7) Ablastin production in *T. musculi* infections.

(8) IgM autoantibodies to enzyme-treated erythrocytes in *Plasmodium* and *Babesia* infections (see also Poels *et al.*, 1980); other autoimmune polyclonal antibody responses may be comparable in nude versus intact mice infected with *Trypanosoma* spp.

(9) Potentiated IgE production in metazoan infections.

(10) IgG_1 hyper-γ-globulinaemia in metazoan infections.

(11) Antihapten antibody responses to haptenated parasites.

(12) Mucosal mastocytosis in intestinal nematodiases.

(13) Circulating eosinophilia and tissue accumulations of eosinophils in metazoan infections. (In one study, Ly-1^+2^- T cells have been shown to be better than Ly-1^-2^+ T cells at promoting eosinophilia in parasitized nude mice (Johnson *et al.*, 1979)).

(14) Granuloma formation around *Schistosoma mansoni* eggs in liver and around *Nematospiroides dubius* larvae (or at sites of previous larval occupancy) in the intestinal wall.

(15) Faecal output of *Schistosoma mansoni* eggs.

(16) Inflammatory lung reactions to injected *Schistosoma mansoni* schistosomules.

(17) Granuloma modulation in chronic *Schistosoma mansoni* infections.

(18) Liver fibrotic reactions around *Mesocestoides corti* larvae.

(19) Impaired absorption of injected cells and molecules from the peritoneal cavity in *Mesocestoides corti* infection.

(20) Inflammatory muscle lesions in *Trypanosoma brucei* infections.

(21) Lymphodenopathy in intestinal nematodiases.

(22) Splenomegaly in haemoprotoxoal infections.

(23) Macrophage recruitment and "activation".

(24) Protection of hepatic parenchymal cells against morphological damage during *Schistosoma mansoni* infection.

(25) Intestinal goblet cell increases in *Nippostrongylus brasiliensis* infections.

(26) Architectural changes in the intestines during intestinal protozoan and metazoan infections.

(27) Nonspecific inhibitory influences on *in vitro* mitogenic responses of lymphocytes from parasitized mice.

(28) Induction of nonspecific resistance agains plasmodium infection using the immunotherapeutic biological BCG (in one study).

(29) DTH reactions to parasite antigens. (In leishmaniasis, DTH reactions may be host protective (e.g. Behin *et al.*, 1977), but theoretically they may also lead to accumulations of macrophages which are available for parasitization in the local site (Callow, L. L., pers. comm.; Sagher *et al.*, 1955).)

One major deficiency in our knowledge of the T cell dependence of tissue reactions to parasitic infection is the relative contribution of T cell dependent antiparasite antibodies versus T cell derived mediators (lymphokines) or T cell dependent mediators with no (or unknown) antigen specificity.

Considerable discussion on the T cell dependence of immunosuppression and the operation of suppressor T cells (T_S) has appeared in the recent literature. From a biological point of view, severe immunosuppression only "makes sense" if it reflects, or results in, partial inhibition of certain potentially host-protective antiparasite immune responses in *natural infection.* There would seem to be little for the parasite to gain by increasing the susceptibility of infected natural hosts to intercurrent infection and thereby threatening the life of the host. Thus the search for parasite antigen-specific T_S effects in immunosuppression is an active area of research in immunoparasitology. These investigations are plagued by interpretation problems. For example, there is a multitude of means by which the immune response to parasite antigens or nonparasite antigens may be reduced during parasite infection. Some proven or postulated mechanisms are: clonal anergy of T or B cells; cytotoxic or inhibitory parasite antigens; anti-idiotypic responses; lymphocyte receptor blockade; rapid antigen clearance and catabolism through RES hyperplasia, and macrophage activation; clonal exhaustive differentiation; accelerated catabolism of antibodies and mediators; architectural disruption of lymphoid tissues; and antimitotic effects during clonal expansion. With such a list it is obviously not very instructive simply to invoke "suppressor T cells", (or for that matter "antigenic competition" or other phenomena rather than mechanisms) as being responsible for immunosuppression in parasitic infections (discussed in Mitchell, 1979b).

Some investigations in immunoparasitology which are providing new information on T cell activities

There are numerous research endeavours in immunoparasitology in which the analysis of T cell dependent events and activities of various T cell subpopulations will be instrumental in the accumulation of knowledge on immunological phenomena. Examples are: granulomatous inflammation with fibrosis; other cellular aggregations in tissues (including skin and mucous membranes); autoimmunity; immunosuppression; hyper-γ-globulinaemia; activation of macrophages and expression of parasitocidal or parasitostatic effects; and differential antibody isotype induction (including IgE potentiation). Three are discussed below.

Granuloma formation and modulation

Nodular foci (granulomas) consisting of a mixed population of inflammatory cells are found around the eggs of *Schistosoma* spp. when such eggs are trapped in tissues (Boros, 1978; Phillips and Colley, 1978; Warren, 1972). The T cell dependence of the granulomatous reaction around *S. mansoni* eggs in liver and lungs of mice is well established (Byram and von Lichtenberg, 1977; Epstein *et al.*, 1979; Hsü *et al.*, 1976; Phillips *et al.*, 1977; Warren *et al.*, 1967) and some immunochemical data is available on the soluble egg antigens (SEA) involved in the elicitation of this tissue reaction (Pelley, 1977). The *S. mansoni*/egg granuloma/mouse system has the potential to provide a wealth of fundamental information on the activities, in chronic inflammation, of T cell subpopulations, T cell dependent antibodies, T cell derived (or dependent) mediators, and various accessory cells such as eosinophils, mobile macrophages and fibroblasts which are known to be affected by the presence of activated T cells. Similar T cell dependent inflammatory reactions are seen in the lungs of mice injected intravenously with schistosomules of *S. mansoni* (Sher, 1977) and in the intestinal wall of mice infected with the nematode, *Nematospiroides dubius*. In the latter case, granulomas are located at sites of previous larval encystment or, more persistently, at sites of presumed larval death in immune mice (Fig. 3). Macroscopically, these foci of cells are not obvious in *N. dubius*-infected nude mice (Prowse *et al.*, 1978) or other T cell deficient mice (Bartlett and Ball, 1974).

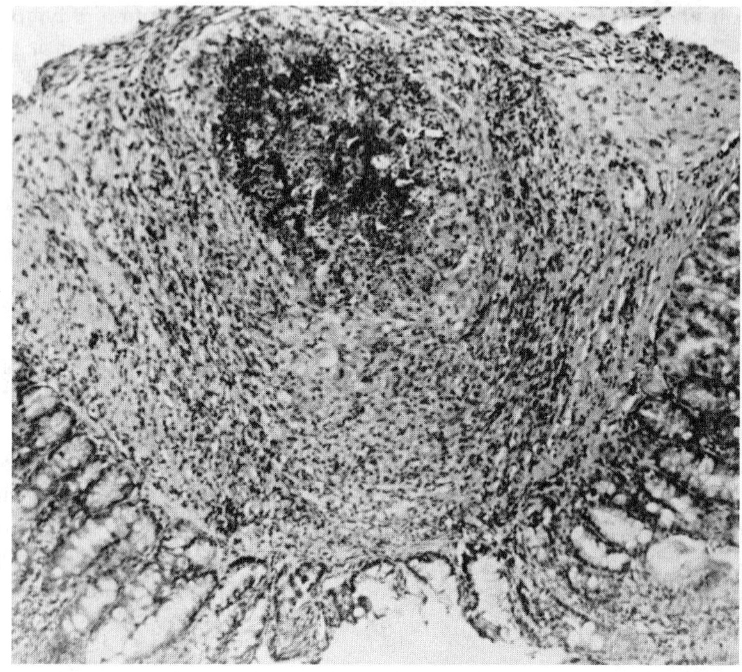

FIG. 3. *An intestinal wall granuloma at the site of previous larval occupancy in a sensitized BALB/c female mouse infected with the intestinal nematode,* Nematospiroides dubius. *This violent tissue reaction is not obvious in infected BALB/c nude mice.* (*Illustration from Hurley, J. C.* (*1980*). *B. Med. Sci.* (*thesis*), *University of Melbourne.*)

If the principal disease manifestations of schistosomiasis result from the immunopathologic response to eggs in organs such as the liver, then disease in infected nude mice should be less severe (Hsü *et al.*, 1976; Phillips *et al.*, 1977; cf. Buchanan *et al.*, 1973; Fine *et al.*, 1973). However, it has been proposed that products of eggs induce pathologic changes in parenchymal cells of the liver in nude mice and such mice are unable to sequester and neutralize (with antibody) such products in granulomas (Byram and von Lichtenberg, 1977; von Lichtenberg, 1977). Thus morbidity in infected T cell deficient mice (Doenhoff *et al.*, 1979; Byram *et al.*, 1979) may differ from that in infected intact mice in which the evidence that granulomatous inflammation and subsequent fibrosis result in disease is unequivocal. The type of T cell responsible for induction of granulomatous responses to eggs in the *S. mansoni*/mouse system is presumably an Ly-1^+2^- cell of the T_{DTH}/T_H type (Doughty and Phillips, 1980).

A diminution in the intensity of granulomatous inflammation occurs with increasing time of infection (Boros *et al.*, 1975; Pelley and Warren, 1978; Warren, 1974, 1977) and this *modulation of immunopathology* appears to be an active immunological event (e.g. Colley *et al.*, 1979; Colley, 1976). Much more work is needed before the relative contributions of antibody and T_S cells in this phenomenon are known. Antiparasite antibodies can have powerful inhibitory effects on T cell dependent antiparasite responses *in vivo* and *in vitro* (e.g. Ramalho-Pinto *et al.*, 1979a; Weiss, 1978; see also Colley *et al.*, 1977), and the lack of effect of passively administered serum antibodies versus an injection of a mixed population of cells with the capacity to proliferate in recipients, cannot be taken as strong evidence against a role for antibodies in mediating a particular event in transfer experiments. Considerable amounts of immunoglobulin (in particular, IgM) are present in granulomas in the baboon/*S. mansoni* system (Houba *et al.*, 1979) and increased numbers of B cells have been described in "modulated granulomas" in mice (Chensue and Boros, 1979b). There are two reports which implicate Ia^+ (Chensue and Boros, 1979a) and Ly-2^+ (Doughty and Phillips, 1980) T_S cells in the modulation of *S. mansoni*/egg granulomas *in vivo* and *in vitro* respectively. However, neither of these demonstrations can yet be taken as compelling evidence for the operation of T_S cells (distinct from T_H cells and antibody formation) in granuloma modulation *in vivo*.

T cell dependent intestinal mucosa reactions

Within this broad category of reactions are included mucosal mast cell (MMC) accumulations, goblet cell hyperplasia, and pathologic changes in villus: crypt ratios (reviewed in Mitchell, 1980), as well as intraepithelial lymphocyte (IEL) accumulations (Ferguson and MacDonald, 1977).

The relationship between T cells and MMC (cf. connective tissue mast cells) is unclear and hypotheses range from a direct lineage relationship to indirect effects (through T cell dependent antibodies or T cell derived mediators). Also unknown are the relationships between intraepithelial MMC (the globule leukocytes which in all probability are degranulated mast cells (MacDonald *et al.*, 1980)) and subepithelial MMC (controversies are discussed in Askenase, 1979), and the functions and cell lineage relationships of (T cell independent) granulated IEL and (T cell dependent) nongranulated IEL in MMC hyperplasia (Mayrhofer, 1980; cf. Guy-Grand *et al.*, 1978). The T cell dependence of MMC accumulations in the intestinal wall during intraluminal metazoan parasite infections has been demonstrated in mice, rats and guinea-pigs (see Askenase, 1979, for an excellent review of the work of Befus and Bienenstock, Mayrhofer, Miller *et al.*, Rothwell *et al.*, and Ruitenberg *et al.*). At least in rats, T cell dependent antibodies may be one of the critical factors involved in initiating MMC accumulations during *Nippostrongylus brasiliensis* infection (Befus and Bienenstock, 1979). As in the *S. mansoni*/egg granuloma system, dissection of T cell dependent inflammatory responses in the intestinal tract of parasitized hosts is likely to provide much new and detailed information on T cell activities and the consequences of such activities in the expression of disease and host resistance to infection (e.g. Manson-Smith *et al.*, 1979). It is anticipated that studies on tissue cellular accumulations in parasitic infections, and the activation status of accessory cells including macrophages, will lead to the identification of numerous T cell dependent soluble factors (e.g. James and Colley, 1978; Nogueira *et al.*, 1977; Shirata *et al.*, 1977).

T cell dependent induction of antiparasite antibodies of various isotypes

Although it has been known for many years that antibodies of various Ig isotypes (classes and subclasses) have different biological activities, there is a regrettable lack of detailed information on what particular antibody isotypes can and cannot do in the various mammalian species. Because various antibodies with differing antiparasite activities are induced during natural (or unnatural) parasitic infection, and because of the availability of methods for the isolation of Igs of various isotypes, it is anticipated that immunoparasitological studies will be an important source of information on the mechanisms of induction, immunpathologic activity, regulatory effects and effector potency of IgA, IgE, IgM and the various IgG antibodies. Hybridoma-derived monoclonal antiparasite antibodies of various isotypes will also be of enormous value in dissecting the biological and antiparasitic effects of antibody Igs (Freeman *et al.*, 1980; Mitchell *et al.*, 1979; Yoshida *et al.*, 1980).

Antibody responses in nude mice injected with unfractionated T cells may differ from those in intact mice possessing a full complement of such cells. This has been demonstrated quite clearly in the case of IgE (reaginic) antibody responses including those to parasite antigens. Circulating titres of IgE antibodies may be higher in T cell injected nude mice than in intact mice (Mitchell and Clarke, 1979), although indirect evidence that combining-site affinity may be low has been obtained (O'Donnell and Mitchell, 1978). IgE antibody production has long been considered a hallmark of many metazoan parasitic infections and the complex nature of T cell dependent IgE potentiation in such infections (but not systemic protozoan infections) remains a mystery (e.g. Jarrett and Ferguson, 1974; Jarrett *et al.*, 1980; Kojima *et al.*, 1980). Besides a role in immediate hypersensitivities, a function for IgE in macrophage-mediated schistosomule killing has been demonstrated in the rat/*S. mansoni* system (see Chapter 44).

A system well suited to the analysis of effector functions of antiparasite antibodies is provided by the *Taenia taeniaeformis*/mouse and *T. taeniaeformis*/rat systems. IgA antibodies adminstered orally (and perhaps directed against the secretory penetration enzymes of the invading oncosphere) will protect mice against infection (Lloyd and Soulsby, 1978). (One mode of action of IgA antibodies may be to delay penetration and thereby increase the susceptibility of the oncosphere to damage by intestinal contents as has been postulated for *Eimeria tenella* sporozoites (Davis and Porter, 1979).) Good evidence exists that T cell dependent complement-fixing IgG antibodies administered systemically will also protect rats (Musoke and Williams, (1975) and nude mice (Mitchell *et al.*, 1977b, 1980b). Certainly IgG rich fractions of "immune serum" will passively protect (provided they are injected early in infection) and decomplementation of recipients abolishes the protective effect of serum injection. In this system, the established cyst appears to protect itself from immune attack by elaboration of anticomplementary molecules (Hammerberg and Williams, 1978). Moreover, a combination of protein A-purified IgG_2 and IgG_1 fractions of "immune serum" are better than either alone at passively protecting nude mice (Mitchell *et al.*, 1980b). Does complement fixation by $IgG_2 + IgG_1$ (Ey *et al.*, 1979; James and Sher, 1980) lead to the death of the developing larvae whilst the non complement-fixing subfractions of IgG_1 neutralize the anticomplementary molecules of the larvae? In the *S. mansoni*/mouse system, Igs of various isotypes have different functions, protein A-purified IgG_1 being responsible for eosinophil plus antibody-mediated lethal effects on schistosomules, whereas IgG_{2a} is responsible for lethal effects mediated by complement fixation (Ramalho-Pinto *et al.*, 1979b). Other systems well suited to dissection of antibody isotype effects are the 7*s* antibody plus eosinophil mediated killing of newborn *Trichinella spiralis* larvae (e.g. Kazura and Aikawa, 1980) and those in which effects of antibodies (± cells) on infective helminth larvae and microfilariae have been demonstrated.

A role for helper T cells (T_H) reactive to common carrier determinants in the accelerated production of variant specific antibodies in *P. knowlesi* infection in rhesus monkeys has been postulated by Brown (1974, 1976). In this system, variant-specific schizont-agglutinating as well as opsonizing antibodies have been described. In addition to studies on T_H-dependent antibody production in malaria (plus babesiosis and African trypanosomiasis), those on the activities of T cells in the spleen in haemoprotozoal infections will certainly yield valuable new insights (WHO, 1979).

In experimental trypanosomiasis, selective suppression of certain Ig isotypes (Hudson and Terry, 1979; Sachs *et al.*, 1980) may have interesting consequences. Adequate IgM but defective IgG antitrypanosome antibody responses may enable blood parasites to be maintained at tolerable levels, yet enable antigenic variants to emerge in tissue locations where IgM is unable to penetrate (Campbell *et al.*, 1978; Seed, 1977; Terry, 1976).

Finally, hyper-γ-globulinaemias are a common feature of both metazoan and protozoan (systemic) parasitic infections, and the T cell dependence of IgG_1 hyper-γ-globulinaemias in high dose chronic metazoan parasitic infections in mice has been demonstrated (Chapman *et al.*, 1979). Again, dissection of T cell dependent events (including antigen versus mitogen effects) will provide new information on activation of B cells with the capacity to synthesize Igs of various isotypes *in vivo*, and the consequences of exaggerated responses on disease manifestations and phenomena such as immunosuppression. Like most studies on T cell dependent events in parasitic infection and disease, progress on T_H effects will be greatly accelerated by the availability of defined parasite antigens and specific methods and reagents for defining (and isolating) T cell subpopulations. It is obvious from the recent literature in immunology that immunoparasitologists may have to wait some some time for reliable methods to be developed for the identification and isolation of T cell subpopulations.

References

Askenase, P. W. (1979). *Springer Sem. Immunopath.* **2**, 1.
Bartlett, A. and Ball, P. A. J. (1974). *Int. J. Parasitol.* **4**, 463.
Befus, A. D. and Bienenstock, J. (1979). *Immunology* **38**, 95.
Behin, R., Mauel, J. and Rowe, D. S. (1977). *Clin. Exp. Immunol.* **29**, 320.
Boros, D. L. (1978). *Prog. Allergy* **24**, 183.
Boros, D. L., Pelley, R. P. and Warren, K. S. (1975). *J. Immunol.* **14**, 1437.
Brown, K. N. (1974). *In* "Parasites in the Immunized Host: Mechanisms of Survival" (R. Porter and J. Knight, eds), p. 35. Associated Scientific, Amsterdam.
Brown, K. N. (1976). *Nature* **259**, 525.
Buchanan, R. D., Fine, D. P. and Colley, D. G. (1973). *Am. J. Path.* **71**, 207.
Byram, J. E. and von Lichtenberg, F. (1977). *Am. J. Trop. Med. Hyg.* **26**, 944.
Byram, J. E., Doenhoff, M. J., Musallam, R., Brink, L. H. and von Lichtenberg, F. (1979). *Am. J. Trop. Med. Hyg.* **28**, 274.
Campbell, G. H., Esser, K. M. and Phillips, S. M. (1978). *Infect. Immunol.* **20**, 714.
Chapman, C. B., Knopf, P. M., Hicks, J. D. and Mitchell, G. F. (1979). *Aust. J. Exp. Biol. Med. Sci.* **57**, 369.
Chensue, S. W. and Boros, D. L, (1979a). *J. Immunol.* **123**, 1409.
Chensue, S. W. and Boros, D. L. (1979b). *Am. J. Trop. Med. Hyg.* **28**, 291.
Colley, D. G. (1976). *J. Exp. Med.* **143**, 696.
Colley, D. G., Hieny, S. E., Bartholomew, R. K. and Cook, J. A. (1977). *Am. J. Trop. Med. Hyg.* **26**, 917.
Colley, D. G., Lewis, F. A. and Todd, C. W. (1979). *Cell Immunol.* **46**, 192.
Davis, P. J. and Porter, P. (1979). *Immunology* **36**, 471.
Doenhoff, M., Musallam, R., Bain, J. and McGregor, A. (1979). *Am. J. Trop. Med. Hyg.* **28**, 260.
Doughty, B. L. and Phillips, S. M. (1980). Submitted for publication.
Epstein, W. L., Fukuyama, K., Danno, K. and Kwan-Wong, E. (1979). *J. Path.* **127**, 207.
Ey, P. L., Prowse, S. J. and Jenkin, C. R. (1979). *Nature* **281**, 492.
Ferguson, A. and MacDonald, T. T. (1977). *In* "Immunology of the Gut" (R. Porter and J. Knight, eds), p. 305. Elsevier, Amsterdam.
Fine, D. P., Buchanan, R. D. and Colley, D. G. (1973). *Am. J. Path.* **71**, 193.
Freeman, R. R., Trejdosiewicz, A. J. and Cross, G. A. M. (1980). *Nature* **284**, 366.
Guy-Grand, D., Griscelli, C. and Vassalli, P. (1978). *J. Exp. Med.* **148**, 1661.
Hammerberg, B. and Williams, J. F. (1978). *J. Immunol.* **120**, 1039.
Houba, V., Sturrock, R. F. and Butterworth, A. E. (1979). *In* "Function and Structure of the Immune System" (W. Müller-Ruckholtz and K. H. Müller-Hermelink, eds), p. 683. Plenum Press, New York
Howard, R. J., Chapman, C. B. and Mitchell, G. F. (1980). *Aust. J. Exp. Biol. Med. Sci.* **58**, 201.
Hsu, C-K., Hsu, S. H., Witney, R. A. Jr and Hansen, C. T. (1976). *Nature* **262**, 397.
Hudson, K. M. and Terry, R. J. (1979). *Parasite Immunol.* **1**, 317.
James, S. L. and Colley, D. G. (1978). *Cell. Immunol.* **38**, 48.
James, S. L. and Sher, A. (1980). *J. Immunol.* **124**, 1837.
Jarrett, E. and Ferguson, A. (1974). *Nature* **250**, 420.
Jarrett, E. E. E., Hall, E., Karlsson, T. and Bennich, H. (1980). *Clin. Exp. Immunol.* **39**, 183.

Johnson, G. R., Nicholas, W. L., McKenzie, I. F. C., Metcalf, D. and Mitchell, G. F. (1979). *Int. Archs Allergy Appl. Immunol.* **59**, 315.
Kojima, S., Kamijo, T. and Ovary, Z. (1980). *Cell. Immunol.* **50**, 327.
Kazura, J. W. and Aikawa, M. (1980). *J. Immunol.* **124**, 355.
von Lichtenberg, F. (1977). *Am. J. Trop. Med. Hyg.* **26**, 79.
Lloyd, S. and Soulsby, E. J. L. (1978). *Immunology* **34**, 939.
MacDonald, T. T., Murray, M. and Ferguson, A. (1980). *Exp. Parasitol.* **49**, 9.
Manson-Smith, D. F., Bruce, R. G. and Parrott, D. M. V. (1979). *Cell. Immunol.* **47**, 285.
Mayrohfer, G. (1980). *Blood* **55**, 532.
Mitchell, G. F. (1979a). *Immunology* **38**, 209.
Mitchell, G. F. (1979b). *Adv. Immunol.* **28**, 451.
Mitchell, G. F. (1980). *In* "The Nude Mouse in Experimental and Clinical Research" (2nd ed.) (Eds, J. Fogh and B. C. Giovanella) Academic Press, New York and London. (in press).
Mitchell, G. F. and Anders, R. F. (1980). *In* "The Antigens" Vol. 6 (Ed., M. Sela) Academic Press, New York and London. (in press).
Mitchell, G. F. and Clarke, A. E. (1979). *Int. Archs Allergy Appl. Immunol.* **58**, 391.
Mitchell, G. F., Marchalonis, J. J., Smith, P. M., Nicholas, W. L. and Warner, N. L. (1977a). *Aust. J. Exp. Biol. Med. Sci.* **55**, 187.
Mitchell, G. F., Goding, J. W. and Rickard, M. D. (1977b). *Aust. J. Exp. Biol. Med. Sci.* **55**, 165.
Mitchell, G. F., Cruise, K. M., Chapman, C. B., Anders, R. F. and Howard, M. C. (1979). *Aust. J. Exp. Biol. Med. Sci.* **57**, 287.
Mitchell, G. F., Curtis, J. M., Handman, E. and McKenzie, I. F. C. (1980a). *Aust. J. Exp. Biol. Med. Sci.* (in press).
Mitchell, G. F. Rajasekariah, G. R. and Rickard, M. D. (1980b). *Immunology* **39**, 481.
Musoke, A. J. and Williams, J. F. (1975). *Immunology* **29**, 855.
Nogueira, N., Gordon, S. and Cohn, Z. A. (1977). *J. Exp. Med.* **146**, 172.
O'Donnell, I. J. and Mitchell, G. F. (1978). *Aust. J. Biol. Sci.* **31**, 459.
Pelley, R. P. (1977). *Am. J. Trop. Med. Hyg.* **26**, 104.
Pelley, R. P. and Warren, K. S. (1978). *J. Invest. Derm.* **71**, 49.
Phillips, S. M. and Colley, D. G. (1978). *Prog. Allergy* **24**, 49.
Phillips, S. M. Deconza, J. J., Gold, J. A. and Reid, W. A. (1977). *J. Immunol.* **118**, 594.
Poels, L. C., van Niewkerk, C. C., van der Sterren-Reti, V. and Jerusalem, C. (1980). *Exp. Parasitol.* **49**, 97.
Prowse, S. J., Mitchell, G. F., Ey, P. L. and Jenkin, C. R. (1978). *Aust. J. Exp. Biol. Med. Sci.* **56**, 561.
Ramalho-Pinto, F. J., Smithers, S. R. and Playfair, J. H. L. (1979a). *J. Immunol.* **123**, 507.
Ramalho-Pinto, F. J., deRossi, R. and Smithers, S. R. (1979b). *Parasite Immunol.* **1**, 295.
Sachs, D. L., Selkirk, M., Ogilvie, B. M. and Askonas, B. A. (1980). *Nature* **283**, 476.
Sagher, F., Verbi, S. and Zuckerman, A. (1955). *J. Invest. Dermatol.* **24**, 417.
Seed, J. R. (1977). *Int. J. Parasitol.* **7**, 55.
Sher, A. (1977). *Am. J. Trop. Med. Hyg.* **26**, 30.
Shirata, T., Shimizu, K., Noda, S. and Suzuki, N. (1977). *Z. Parasitenkd.* **53**, 31.
Suzuki, M., Waki, S., Igarashi, I., Tamura, J., Imanaka, M. and Ishikawa, S. (1980). Submitted for publication.
Terry, R. J. (1976). *In* "Immunology of Parasitic Infections" (Eds, S. Cohen and E. H. Sadun) p. 203. Blackwell, Oxford.

Waki. S. and Suzuki, M. (1980). *In* "Proceedings of the Third International Workshop on Nude Mice". (in press).
Warren, K. S. (1972). *Trans. R. Soc. Trop. Med. Hyg.* **66**, 417.
Warren, K. S. (1974). *In* "Parasites in the Immunized Host: Mechanisms of Survival" (Eds, R. Porter and J. Knight) p. 243. Associated Scientific, Amsterdam.
Warren, K. S. (1977). *Am. J. Trop. Med. Hyg.* **26**, 113.
Warren, K. S., Domingo, E. O. and Cowan, R. B. T. (1967). *Am. J. Path.* **51**, 735.
Weiss, N. (1978). *Exp. Parasitol.* **46**, 283.
WHO Tropical Diseases Research Series 1 (1979). "Role of the Spleen in the Immunology of Parasitic Diseases". Schwabe, Basel.
Yoshida, N., Nussenzweig, R. S., Potocnjak, P., Nussenzweig, V. and Aikawa, M. (1980). *Science* **207**, 71.

Theme 12: Summary

Effector and Escape Mechanisms in Host-Parasite Relationships

ANTHONY C. ALLISON

Division of Cell Pathology, MRC Research Centre, Harrow, England

Paris is a city that has initiated fashions in dress, art and ideas for more than a century. Science is likewise influenced by fashion, and it is clear from the attendance at this meeting that immunology remains very much in vogue. Within immunology, research on parasites has become fashionable during the past decade, for excellent reasons. Parasitic diseases affect hundreds of millions of people and their domestic livestock, and the use of immunological methods for diagnosis and control of parasitic infections is obviously appealing. Moreover, the powerful immune responses to parasites can provide information of interest in other branches of immunology, for example the study of IgE.

As modern concepts and techniques are applied to analysis of parasite antigens and the immune responses which they elicit, the amount and quality of work in this field has increased greatly.

At this meeting the symposium and daily workshops on parasite immunology were well attended, and the subject was discussed in other workshops, for example on natural immunity and macrophages and genetic regulation of immune responsiveness.

There is space to summarize only the major trends in research on parasitic diseases that emerged during the meeting. One was the progress which has been made in purifying and characterizing parasite antigens. Surface labelling techniques have shown that only a limited number of major antigens predominate on the surface of parasites. The extreme example is the African trypanosomes, in which the surface consists almost entirely of a single glycoprotein molecule of about 65 000 daltons that is subject to antigenic variation. Several helminths were reported to have only a limited repertoire of antigens on their surface, sometimes stage-specific. The binding of these antigens by different subclasses of antibodies is genetically susceptible and resistant mice are providing interesting information about mechanisms of resistance. A major glycoprotein antigen of *Trypanosoma cruzi* has been used to increase the resistance of mice in acute infections.

A second major development is the use of monoclonal antibodies against parasite antigens. These are not only valuable diagnostic and analytical reagents. They can be used to define mechanisms of resistance against parasites and the antigens involved. For example, Yoshida and Nussenzweig (12.8.22)* have a monoclonal antibody reacting with antigen of 44 000 daltons in the membrane of *Plasmodium berghei* sporozoites. This antibody can passively protect mice against *P. berghei* infection by mosquitoes. Perrin

* Reference numbers indicate Abstract numbers in: Abstracts 4th International Congress of Immunology, Paris, 1980.

and colleagues (12.8.16) reported the finding that a monoclonal antibody against *P. falciparum* merozoites can block infection by this parasite in cultures of erythrocytes. A. Capron and coworkers (Chapter 44) have obtained a rat IgG_{2a} monoclonal antibody that can sensitize schistosomula to killing by eosinophils. The use of such antibodies will help to define antigens required for protection and effective mechanisms of immunity.

A major development has been the demonstration of ways in which antibodies and leukocytes can collaborate in immunity to parasites. For example, as shown by Butterworth and colleagues (12.4.02), schistosomula (schistosomes that have recently penetrated the skin) to which IgG antibodies are attached are killed by eosinophils. The eosinophils discharge the contents of their granules onto the surface of the schistosome, as shown by electron microscopy of peroxidase. The basic proteins of eosinophil granules can themselves lyse schistosomula by interacting with the single plasma membrane bilayer. Some evidence was produced that products of oxidative metabolism of eosinophils and neutrophils may be involved in killing of parasites to which these cells are attached, but the relevance of these mechanisms to protection is not yet established. Mast cell products may also contribute to resistance. The eosinophil chemotactic tetrapeptide ECF-A, can activate eosinophils, increasing their receptors for IgG, IgE and C_3. M. Capron (12.4.03) has found that an early response of rats to schistosomula is mediated by IgG and eosinophils whereas a later response is mediated by IgE eosinophils and macrophages. Attachment of IgE dimers or complexes to macrophages can activate these cells, as shown by several criteria. Thus cellular co-operation may confer protection against parasites.

Killing by IgG antibodies and eosinophils of the bovine lungworm *Dictyocaulus viviparus* and the liver fluke *Fasciola hepatica* was described. Irradiated L3 of *Dictyocaulus* are widely used to immunize cattle against this infection. *Fasciola* in the presence of antibodies shed antigen, and the continued presence of antibodies and eosinophils is required for effective killing.

The multiplicity of resistance mechanisms was again emphasized in studies of malaria. As already stated, antibodies are protective in some host–parasite combinations. However, μ-suppressed mice, which are unable to produce antibodies, recover spontaneously from *P. chabaudi* and *P. vinckei* infections and are fully immune to challenge (Weidanz: 12.8.21). If first infections with *P. yoelii* and *P. berghei* in μ-suppressed mice are terminated by chemotherapy, they become resistant to challenge with the same organisms. Mice and chickens deprived of T cells are unable to recover permanantly from or be immunized against malaria parasites. Thus thymus-dependent, antibody-independent mechanisms of protection against malaria parasites exist. The effectors may be the same as those activated by BCG, *C. parvum* and other agents that produce nonspecific resistance to haemoprotozoa. Since there is a correlation between natural killer activity and resistance to malaria and babesia infections in different strains of mice, these cells are thought by some investigators to participate in recovery from haemoprotozoan infections. It was also suggested that tumour necrosis factor and other mediators, probably liberated by activated macrophages, limit multiplication of malaria parasites in red cells.

T lymphocytes contribute to recovery from parasitic infections in several ways. They are helpers in antibody formation. Cytotoxic T lymphocytes can kill parasitized cells, the most striking example being the killing of lymphoblasts transformed by the parasite *Theileria parva* in immune bovines. This killing is confined to syngeneic parasitized cells, showing that the restriction established for virus infected cells in the mouse is applicable to parasitized cells in other species. Products of activated T lymphocytes can also increase the capacity of macrophages to prevent intracellular growth of parasites including *Leishmania tropica* and *Rickettsia tsutsugamushi* (Nacy: 12.2.09). Several mediators of different molecular weight may be involved. There may also be differences in the susceptibility of macrophage subpopulations to infection. For example, hamster resident peritoneal macrophages support multiplication of *Leishmania donovani* in cultures whereas bone-marrow-derived macrophages destroy ingested parasites (Schneider: 12.2.13).

An important tool for dissecting components of resistance is genetic analysis. A major gene for resistance to *L. donovani* is closely linked to another for resistance to *Salmonella typhimurium*, but the two appear to be distinct from one another and from genes for interferon production, sensitivity to interferon and sensitivity to endotoxin. A beginning has been made in the analysis of genes for resistance of mice to malaria (Borwell: 5.7.02). Some strains of mice which are relatively resistant to malaria can not be protected efficiently with *C. parvum* in spite of splenomegaly. Thus many genes conferring resistance to parasites, usually not associated with major histocompatibility loci, and some associated with production of, or sensitivity to mediators, are being identified.

For several years it has been known that *Entamoeba histolytica* activate complement by the alternative pathway, and the same is true of *Nagleria* and of early schistosomula of *S. mansoni*. At this meeting it was reported that trypomastigotes of *Trypanosoma cruzi* treated with proteasase or sialidase activate complement by the alternative pathway. The same is true of *T. brucei* or *T. congolense* cultured under conditions when the variant-specific glycoprotein coat does not develop and plasma can gain access to the parasite cell membrane. Thus coat components prevent complement activation in the absence of specific antibodies. Cuticle of the murine parasitic nematode *Nematospiroides dubius* can also activate complement by the alternative pathway (Prowse: 12.1.10). Recent studies of the binding to enzymatically modified red cell surfaces of activating and inhibiting components of complement provide models for what may happen on parasite surfaces. Complement activation may not only be involved in protection but also in pathology, e.g. formation of amoebic abscesses.

Immunopathological consequences of parasitic infections were also discussed. Participation of subpopulations of T lymphocytes reacting to schistosome egg antigens has been studied in an *in vitro* granuloma model (Doughty and Phillips: 12.6.09). Granulomas are modulated in chronically infected animals by a suppressor subpopulation of T lymphocytes, shown in the *in vitro* model to be Ly-1^+,2^- and to be sensitive to anti-I-J serum *in vivo* (Todd and Colley: 12.3.24).

Over the last 10 years there have been many reports of parasite-induced secondary immunodeficiencies, and the underlying mechanisms are now being analysed. Infection with African trypanosomes brings about polyclonal activation of host B cells and the ensuing clonal exhaustion may account for much of the associated immunodepression. Progress was reported in identifying a mitogenic agent which is associated with a membrane fraction of *T. brucei* (Sacks: 12.3.20). Immunodepression seems to affect the spleen most severely; other lymphoid organs are somewhat less affected. A specific T cell proliferative response is seen, but is rapidly inhibited as trypanosomes appear in the blood. Probably as a result of polyclonal activation, autoantibodies to splenocytes and thymocytes appears in the later stages of murine infections. Polyclonal activation and immunodepression was also reported for *T. cruzi*. Interestingly, immune responses are restored when the infection passes from the acute to the chronic stage. Evidence from *T. musculi* infections suggested that substances derived from the trypanosomes rendered B cells unresponsive. The position in schistosomiasis is complex. There is evidence for a low molecular heat stable factor, probably a peptidoglycan, which not only inhibits lymphocyte transformation but also mast cell degranulation and eosinophil-mediated cytotoxicity. Hatching fluid from eggs inhibits lymphocyte activation, as do immune complexes in men and baboons. Suppression of responses to schistosomal egg antigen may be brought about by macrophages. Suppressor cells were also reported in *Nippostrongylus* infections, and in *Pseudomonas* infections they appear to be B cells. During the intestinal phase of *Trichinella spiralis* infection, mice show strong suppression of the formation in the intestine of IgA antibodies against cholera toxin. Thus intestinal parasites could increase susceptibility to bacterial infections.

In summary, parasites appear to have evolved many ways of subverting the host's immune responses, and bringing about generalized as well as parasite-specific immunodepression. We must hope that an understanding of these mechanisms may lead to their reversal. For example, antibodies raised against chemically altered mitogens and suppressor factor, may prevent suppression and lead to an improved elimination of the parasites.

Theme 13

Immediate and Delayed-type Hypersensitivity

Presidents:
K. F. AUSTEN
A. DE WECK

Symposium chairman:
C. STEFFEN

46

Regulation of the IgE Response

KIMISHIGE ISHIZAKA

Johns Hopkins University, Baltimore, Maryland, USA

It is well established that IgE antibodies against allergens are a cause of hay fever and are probably involved in other allergic diseases. The crucial role of IgE antibody in reaginic hypersensitivity raised the possibility that regulation of IgE antibody formation is one of the fundamental treatments of allergic diseases. To achieve this goal, however, one has to study cellular events involved in the antibody response. In principle, mechanisms of the IgE antibody response are similar to those of IgM and IgG antibody responses to T dependent antigens. However, the IgE antibody response in experimental animals has certain characteristic features that are not easily demonstrated in the IgG antibody response. A series of experiments suggested that the IgE antibody response is more susceptible than IgG antibody response to regulatory mechanisms, and that immunocompetent cells involved in the IgE antibody response are different from those involved in the IgG antibody response. In this chapter I will discuss development of B lymphocytes committed for IgE antibody response, briefly summarize antigen-specific regulation and then discuss possible mechanisms of isotype-specific regulation.

This work was supported by research grants AI-11202 and AI-14784 from US Public Health Service. This paper is publication 396 from the O'Neill laboratories at the Good Samaritan Hospital.

Precursors of IgE-forming cells

Extensive studies, by many investigators, on the surface immunoglobulin on B cells in the mouse, showed that virgin B cells bear IgM, and that the lymphocytes bearing the other isotypes are derived from the virgin B cells. It is generally accepted that lymphocytes bearing IgG or IgA are already committed for the synthesis of respective isotype. This principle is applied to IgE system. The IgE-bearing lymphocytes were found in rat lymphoid tissues. In 2 different rat strains, the proportion of IgE-bearing lymphocytes in the mesenteric lymph nodes (MLN) was 2–5% of the total cells or 10–20% of B lymphocytes. It was also found that 1·5–3% of mouse spleen cells and about 2% of MLN cells bear IgE. The proportion of IgE-bearing lymphocytes markedly increase after infection of rats and mice with the nematode, *Nippostrongylus brasiliensis* (Nb) (Ishizaka *et al.*, 1976). We have also studied ontogenic development of IgE-bearing B cells in the rat (Ishizaka *et al.*, 1978). It was found that a significant number of IgE-bearing cells appeared in the spleen within 24–48 h after birth, and the proportion of these cells increased to adult level within 4 weeks after birth. More recent experiments in the mouse confirmed that IgE-bearing cells appear in the spleen within 48 h after birth. More than 95% of IgE-bearing cells in both neonatal and adult rats carry surface IgM. The results suggest that IgE–IgM double bearing cells are derived from IgM-bearing virgin B cells.

The development of IgE–IgM double bearing cells does not appear to require T cells. In the rat, neonatal thymectomy did not affect the appearance of IgE-bearing cells (Urban and Ishizaka, 1977). It was also found that athymic nude mice have IgE-bearing cells in their spleen. About 3% of total spleen cells or 5% of total B cells bore IgE on their surface.

A question to be asked is whether the IgE–IgM double bearing cells are actually precursors of IgE-forming cells. In order to answer this question, we set up an *in vitro* system in which Ig-forming cells can be developed from B lymphocytes (Suemura *et al.*, 1978). Thus, MLN cells from either normal or Nb-infected rats were cultured with pokeweed mitogen (PWM) and cytocentrifuge smears of the cells were examined by immunofluorescence. A substantial number of IgM, IgE and IgG2a forming cells developed when the cells from Nb-infected animals were stimulated with PWM. From normal lymph node cells, a significant number of IgM and IgE forming cells, but very few IgG2a forming cells developed. The development of Ig-forming cells was also obtained by stimulation of MLN cells from the infected rats with parasite antigens. As expected, the same antigen preparation failed to induce the development of Ig-forming cells from normal MLN cells.

In order to identify precursors of Ig-forming cells, we have depleted IgE-bearing cells in MLN cells and the rest of the cells were cultured with PWM or antigen. The results showed that depletion of IgE-bearing cells resulted in a marked decrease in IgE response but did not affect either IgM or IgG response. Since the majority of IgE-bearing lymphocytes carry IgM determinants, IgM-bearing cells in the same cell suspension were depleted, and the rest of the cells were cultured with PWM. As expected, depletion of IgM-bearing cells was accompanied by a marked decrease of IgE-bearing cells, and this procedure resulted in a significant decrease of both IgM-forming cells and IgE-forming cells. The results suggested that the majority of the precursors of IgE forming cells belong to IgE–IgM double bearing cells.

When these experiments were carried out, we did not know about rat IgD. Recently, however, Bazin *et al.* (1978a) obtained monoclonal IgD in Lou/c rats and demonstrated that the majority of rat B lymphocytes bear both μ and δ determinants. Therefore, we studied IgD-bearing lymphocytes in the MLN. The results confirmed that the majority of B cells bear both μ and δ determinants and showed that more than 90% of ϵ-bearing cells in both Nb-infected and normal rats bear δ determinants (Urban *et al.*, 1980). Since more than 95% of ϵ-bearing cells possess surface IgM, it appears that the majority of ϵ-bearing cells actually bear three isotypes, and that these cells are probably precursors of IgE-forming cells. Indeed, depletion of IgD-bearing cells resulted in a marked decrease in the *in vitro* IgE-forming cell response, without affecting the IgM response. Bazin *et al.* (1978b) have shown that anti-δ antibodies injected into neonatal rats suppressed subsequent IgE antibody response. All of these findings are in agreement with the idea that precursors of IgE-forming cells are triple bearing cells.

As expected, the Ig-forming cell response of rat MLN cells to PWM or Nb antigen is dependent on T cells. Purified B cells failed to respond to PWM for the development of IgE-forming cells. When a constant number of B cells from Nb-infected rats were mixed with various numbers of T cells from either Nb-infected rats or normal rats and the mixtures were cultured with Nb antigen, IgE-forming cells developed only with T cells from the infected animals.

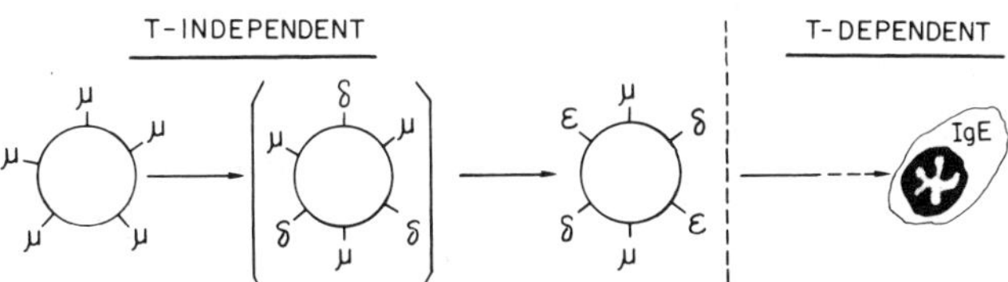

FIG. 1. *Schematic model of the development and differentiation of IgE-bearing B lymphocytes.*

Summarizing the findings described so far, it appears that a portion of virgin B cells, which bear μ determinants, differentiate to express μ, ϵ and δ determinants through T independent process, and these triple-bearing cells differentiate into IgE-forming cells through T dependent process (Fig. 1).

Antigen-specific regulation of IgE response

A question to be asked is how one can interrupt the differentiation. So far, there is no attempt to prevent the T independent process. All approaches to regulate the IgE response are either to tolerate IgE-B cells or to manipulate the population of T cells which regulate the differentiation of precursor B cells to IgE-forming cells. Major attempts by several investigators in the past 5 years are summarized in Table I. Katz *et al.* (1973) succeeded to induce B

TABLE I
Modified antigens for suppression of IgE response

Modified antigens	*Antigenic determinant*	*T cell priming*	*Suppression of Ig response*	*B cell inactivation*	*Suppressor T cells*
DNP-D-GL	DNP	−	All isotypes	+	−
DNP-polyvinyl alcohol	DNP	(+)	All isotypes	+	+
Anti-idiotype	Idiotype	−	(IgE)[a]	?	+
OA-D-GL	OA	+	IgE	−	−
Urea-denatured OA	−	+	IgE > IgG	-	+
OA-PEG[b]	−	+	IgE > IgG	−	+

[a] Suppression is more effective on the IgE than IgG antibody response.
[b] Ovalbumin-polyethylene glycol conjugates.

cell tolerance by injecting hapten coupled to nonimmunogenic carrier, such as *d*-glutamic acid *d*-lysine copolymer (dGL). Injections of such a dinitrophenyl derivative of dGL before immunization with DNP-ovalbumin (OA) completely suppressed the primary and secondary IgE anti-hapten antibody responses, and an injection of these materials into immunized animals terminated the ongoing antibody formation. The effect of the treatment was persistent and specific for haptenic group. Suppression of DNP-dGL is applied to all immunoglobulin isotypes including IgE and is due to inactivation of hapten-specific B cells. Suppressor cells were not detectable in the treated animals. More recently, Lee and Sehon (1979) employed DNP-conjugates of polyvinyl alcohol to terminate the anti-DNP IgE antibody response. Similar to DNP-dGL, polyvinyl alcohol conjugate inactivates hapten specific B cells. In addition, this material can induce DNP-specific suppressor T cells which regulate the antibody response of all isotypes.

Another approach to regulate the anti-hapten IgE antibody response is to induce anti-idiotypic antibodies. If the IgE anti-hapten antibody is restricted to a certain idiotype, one can expect that idiotype-specific regulation may be applied for the regulation of IgE antibody response. Indeed, Blaser *et al.* (1980)

reported that anti-idiotype antibody suppresses primary IgE antibody response and ongoing antibody formation to benzyl penicilloyl group. An interesting observation in their experiments is that the suppression obtained by the formation of anti-idiotype antibody is more effective on IgE system than the other isotypes.

From the practical viewpoint, the more important problem is to regulate the IgE response to allergens and protein antigens. In view of the tolerizing effect of DNP-dGL, Liu *et al.* (1979) prepared dGL conjugates with ovalbumin and ragweed antigen E, and studied the effect of the conjugates on the IgE response. As shown in Table I, treatment of mice with dGL-conjugates of ovalbumin suppressed both primary and secondary IgE antibody response to ovalbumin. However, mechanisms of suppression appears to be entirely different from those obtained by DNP-dGL. Ovalbumin-dGL conjugates failed to tolerize ovalbumin-specific B cells and to induce ovalbumin-specific suppressor T cells, and suppression is confined to IgE isotype.

The second approach to regulate the IgE production to protein antigen is to manipulate T cells. As the differentiation of IgE-B cells to IgE-forming cells is highly dependent on T cells, one can suppress the antibody formation by reducing helper T cell activity or by inducing suppressor T cells. This approach is based on the fact that antigenic determinants recognized by T cells are not necessarily the same as the major antigenic determinants in some antigens, such as ragweed antigen E and ovalbumin. For example, urea-denatured antigen E or ovalbumin do not react with antibodies against native antigen, or B cells specific for the major antigenic determinants, but can stimulate T cells specific for the antigen (Ishizaka *et al.*, 1974; Takatsu and Ishizaka, 1975). Indeed, immunization of mice with alum-absorbed urea-denatured antigen results in the priming of helper T cells. However, if one injects a relatively large dose of urea-denatured antigen without adjuvant, one can induce antigen specific suppressor T cells which regulate the IgE response (Takatsu and Ishizaka, 1976).

Ovalbumin polyethylene glycol conjugates prepared by Lee and Sehon (1978a, b) are an extension of this line. Their approach was to change an immunogen to nonimmunogen or tolerogen. Indeed, OA-polyethylene glycol conjugates do not react with antibodies against the native antigen. However, injections of the conjugate without adjuvant induce suppressor T cells specific for the native antigen molecules. In principle, this conjugate and urea-denatured antigen have common immunological properties, with respect to the loss of major antigenic determinants and the ability to induce suppressor T cells. Suppressor T cells induced by the urea-denatured antigen or OA-polyethylene glycol conjugates can suppress IgE antibody response better than IgG antibody response. Nevertheless, regulation of antibody response by these materials is not restricted to IgE class. Recently, modified allergens, such as dGL conjugates and polyethylene glycol conjugates of ragweed allergen are being applied to clinical trials. In principle, immunological effects of the modified antigens in atopic patients are similar to those obtained in inbred mice.

Although the treatment appears to be less effective in the patients than that obtained in animal experiments, it is hoped that further studies to prepare new tolerogenic conjugates will improve the effect of immunotherapy.

Isotype-specific regulation of IgE response

Attempts to regulate the IgE antibody response by modified antigen are based on the fact that the IgE antibody response is more susceptible than IgG response to antigen-specific regulation. A relatively high proportion of IgE-bearing cells or precursors of IgE forming cells in lymphoid tissues suggest that the differentiation of these precursors to IgE-forming cells is more strictly controlled than IgG antibody response. It is also known that the IgE antibody response is highly dependent on the nature and dose of antigen for immunization as well as adjuvant employed. These findings suggested the possibility that the IgE antibody response is controlled by isotype-specific regulatory mechanisms in addition to antigen-specific regulation. If this is actually the case, one can expect entirely new approaches to regulate the IgE response. Indeed, several investigators suggested possible mechanisms for the selective regulation of IgE response.

Discrepancies between the IgE and IgG response suggested the possibility that T helper cells for IgE-B cells may be distinct from T helper cells for IgG-B cells. Evidence for the hypothesis was obtained in the *in vitro* antibody response of rabbit mesenteric lymph node cells (Kishimoto and Ishizaka, 1973). In this system, helper function of carrier primed cells for the IgE response was highly dependent on the nature of adjuvant employed for carrier priming. Thus, T cells primed by immunization with alum-absorbed carrier had helper activities for both IgG and IgE antibody responses, whereas T cells primed by CFA immunization enhanced only IgG antibody response. More recently, Kishimoto *et al.* (1976) extended this hypothesis to antigen-specific suppressor T cells. In view of the fact that complete Freund's adjuvant is a poor adjuvant for the IgE antibody response, they primed Balb/c mice with DNP derivatives of tubercle bacilli (DNP-Tbc) and then immunized these mice with DNP-OA. The results clearly showed that the priming with DNP-Tbc suppressed anti-hapten IgE antibody response but enhanced IgG antibody response to DNP-OA. Furthermore, transfer of splenic T cells from the DNP-Tbc primed mice suppressed the primary IgE antibody response of the recipients to DNP-OA, without affecting the IgG antibody response. Suppressor T cells obtained from DNP-Tbc treated animals were specific for DNP group, and selectively regulated the IgE antibody response. Subsequently, these investigators incubated spleen cells from DNP-Tbc primed animals with DNP-heterologous carrier and obtained IgE-specific suppressive factor in the supernatant (Suemura *et al.*, 1977). This soluble factor was not DNP-specific, but treatment of B cells with the factor selectively regulated the IgE response (Kishimoto *et al.*, 1978). Subsequently, the same investigators established a

T hybrid cell line which spontaneously secrete suppressor factors specific for the IgE antibody response (Watanabe *et al.*, 1978). Their experiments do not necessarily mean that the factor is derived from DNP-specific suppressor cells, however, it is apparent that the IgE response is subjected to isotype-specific regulatory mechanisms.

It is generally accepted that regulatory T cells are antigen-specific. However, experiments on the IgE antibody response by several investigators suggest strongly that not only antigen-specific T cells but also nonspecific T cells are involved in the regulation of IgE antibody response. Levine and Vaz (1970) showed that some strains, such as SJL, produce a substantial amount of IgG antibody but gave no IgE antibody response to conventional protein antigens. Independent from their observations, it was found in several different systems that IgE antibody response was enhanced by exposure of animals to sublethal dose X-ray prior to immunization. Now we know that these two phenomena are interrelated. Watanabe *et al.* (1976) as well as Chiorazzi *et al.* (1976) demonstrated that enhancement of IgE response by irradiation is due to depletion of nonspecific suppressor T cells which selectively regulate the IgE response. Thus, an irradiation-enhanced IgE response in low IgE responders was suppressed by the transfer of normal thymocytes or splenic T cells into irradiated syngeneic animals. Subsequently, Katz and his associates have shown that the population of such suppressor cells expands by the treatment of the animals with CFA. They also demonstrated that the serum of the CFA-treated animals contained a soluble factor which selectively suppresses the IgE response (Tung *et al.*, 1978). Subsequently, the same investigators showed that the serum and ascites of CFA-treated animals contained not only suppressive factor but also a soluble factor which selectively enhances the IgE response (Katz *et al.*, 1979). Their more recent experiments showed that the suppressive factor could be obtained from both high and low IgE responder strains, and exerted selective effect on the IgE response across strain barriers (Katz *et al.*, 1980).

Another example of IgE specific regulation is the nematode infection which enhances IgE synthesis. It is well known that *Nippostrongylus* infection of antigen-primed rats selectively enhances the IgE antibody formation to the priming antigen without affecting the IgG antibody titre (Orr and Blair, 1969; Bloch *et al.*, 1973). Jarrett and Ferguson (1974) indicated requirement of T cells for IgE-potentiation. We anticipated that T lymphocytes from Nb-infected rats may have the ability to selectively enhance the differentiation of IgE-B cells, and tried to reproduce the IgE-potentiation phenomenon in an *in vitro* system (Suemura and Ishizaka, 1979). In the experimental system we employed, MLN cells of DNP-OA primed rats were cultured with the homologous antigen, and IgE-forming cells and IgG-forming cells were observed. As shown in Fig. 2, T cells from *Nippostrongylus* infected animals selectively enhanced IgE-forming cell response of DNP-OA primed cells, while T cells from normal animals failed to do so. The results show that the proportion of IgE response to IgG response is determined not only by antigen-specific

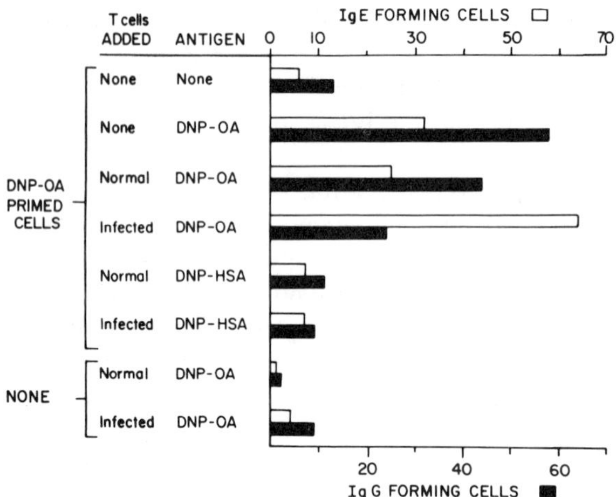

FIG. 2. *Selective enhancement of IgE-forming cell response of DNP-OA primed cells by T cells from Nb-infected rats. MLN cells from DNP-OA primed rats were mixed with an equal number of T cells from either normal or Nb-infected rats, and the mixtures were cultured for 5 days in the presence of 1 μg/ml DNP-OA or DNP-HSA. The number of IgE or IgG_2 forming cells represent those derived from 10^6 DNP-OA primed cells seeded.*

cell populations but also by bystander T cells. We wondered if T cells from Nb-infected animals may release a soluble factor which selectively potentiate the IgE response. Therefore, we cultured MLN cells (or T cells) from the infected animals, and added the culture supernatant to DNP-OA primed cells which were then stimulated by DNP-OA. It was found that cell free culture supernatant from the lymphocytes of the infected animals potentiated the IgE response of DNP-OA primed cells to homologous antigen, without affecting the IgG response. An effective substance for the enhancement of the IgE response is not a T cell replacing factor. The same culture supernatant failed to enhance the response of the DNP-OA primed cells to a DNP-heterologous carrier conjugate. Gel filtration of the culture supernatant indicated that the molecular size of the IgE-potentiating factor is between 10 000 and 20 000 and significantly smaller than the mol. wt of T cell replacing factor.

Evidence was obtained that the target of IgE-potentiating factor was IgE-bearing cells (Suemura *et al.*, 1980). The factor was absorbed by B cells but not by T cells. It was also found that the factor has affinity for IgE. In the experiment shown in Fig. 3, culture supernatant containing IgE potentiating factor was filtered through Amicon Diaflo membrane to remove all molecules having the molecular weight of 50 000 or higher. The filtrate was then absorbed with IgE-coated Sepharose and the supernatants were assessed for the ability to enhance the IgE response. The IgE-potentiating factor was specifically absorbed by IgE-Sepharose and was recovered by elution of the beads at acid pH. The affinity of IgE-potentiating factor for IgE may explain why this factor selectively enhances the IgE response. It is reasonable to speculate that the factor will bind to IgE-bearing B cells through surface IgE molecules, and

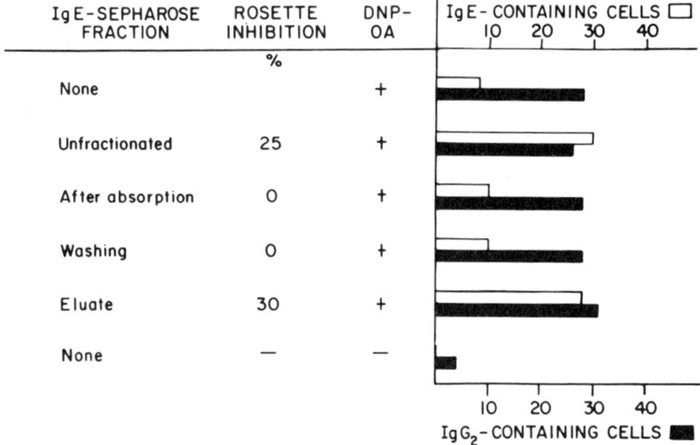

FIG.3. *Absorption of IgE-potentiating factor by IgE Sepharose. Culture supernatant containing IgE-potentiating factor was filtered through Diavlo CF 50A membrane. The filtrate was absorbed with IgE-coupled Sepharose which was then eluted with glycine HDl-buffer, pH 3·0. (IgE-binding factor in each fraction was detected by inhibition of rosette formation of* $Fc_\epsilon R(+)$ *cells. Numerals in the column represent the percentage of rosette inhibition). Each fraction was added to aliquots of DNP-OA primed cells which were then cultured with DNP-OA for 5 days. The IgE response was selectively enhanced by the addition of eluate fraction.*

enhances the differentiation of these cells to IgE-forming cells. As the factor does not bind to the other B cells, enhancing effect of the factor is IgE-specific.

At this stage, we could not figure out how T cells from the Nb-infected rats released a soluble factor which has affinity for IgE. However, separate experiments in our laboratory on Fc_ϵ receptor bearing ($Fc_\epsilon R(+)$) lymphocytes provided an explanation. Some years ago, it was reported that a subset of human and rat lymphocytes have receptors specific for IgE, which may be called Fc_ϵ receptors (Gonzalez-Molina and Spiegelberg, 1977; Fritsche and Spiegelberg, 1978). The majority of $Fc_\epsilon R(+)$ lymphocytes in normal animals are B cells. However, our studies have shown that the proportion of $Fc_\epsilon R(+)$ cells in the rat lymphoid tissues markedly increases after infection with Nb and that a subset of T cells in the infected rats bear $Fc_\epsilon R$ (Yodoi and Ishizaka, 1979). Furthermore, we found that T cells from infected animals release a soluble factor which inhibits rosette formation of $Fc_\epsilon R(+)$ cells with IgE-coated red cells (Yodoi and Ishizaka, 1980). In the experiment shown in Table II, MLN cells from either normal or infected rats were cultured for 24 h, and culture supernatants were assessed for the ability to inhibit rosette formation of $Fc_\epsilon R(+)$ cells. As can be seen, culture supernatants of lymph node cells from infected animals markedly inhibited IgE rosettes. Fractionation of the MLN cells into T cell and B cell fractions indicated that the factor is derived from T cells (Table II).

Demonstration of IgE-binding factors in the culture supernatants suggest strongly that IgE-potentiating factor is an IgE-binding factor. Both factors

TABLE II

Release of IgE-binding factor from lymphocytes of Nb-infected rats

Source	Fractions	S-Ig(+)	Rosette inhibition by CF[a] Dilution	IgE-RFC	Inhibition
		%		%	%
Normal	Lymphocyte	20	2	27·2	0
Nb-infected	Lymphocyte	20	2	8·1	70
			6	13·7	50
	T cell	4	2	6·4	77
			6	11·4	58
	B cell	74	2	19·0	31
			6	25·9	5
Medium control			—	27·4	—

[a] Culture supernatant was filtered through Diaflo CF 50A membrane. MLN lymphocytes from a Nb-infected rat was employed as a source of $Fc_{\epsilon}R(+)$ cells. Lymphocytes were mixed with IgE-coated erythrocytes (E′-IgE) in the presence of CF for rosette formation.

have affinity for IgE-Sepharose, and the molecular size of the two factors are comparable. Furthermore, the source of IgE potentiating factor was proved to be $Fc_{\epsilon}R(+)$ cells. In the experiment shown in Fig. 4, about 75% of $Fc_{\epsilon}R(+)$ cells were depleted and both unfractionated lymphocytes and $Fc_{\epsilon}R$-depleted fraction were incubated to recover culture filtrates. Culture supernatant of the $Fc_{\epsilon}R$-depleted fraction had much less IgE-binding activity and less potentiating activity than the culture supernatant of the unfractionated

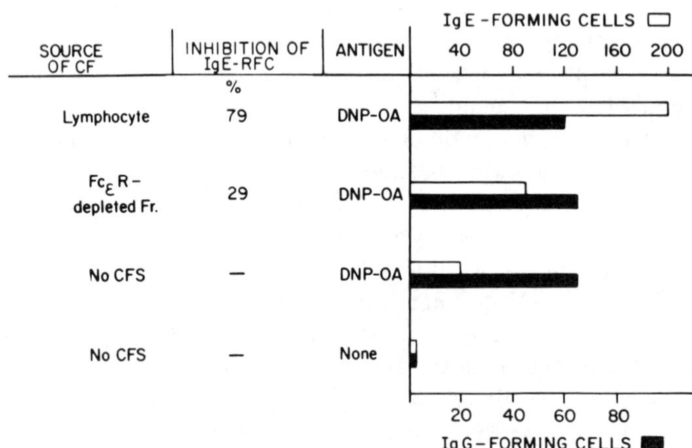

FIG. 4. *Effect of $Fc_{\epsilon}R(+)$ cell depletion on the formation of IgE-potentiating factor. $Fc_{\epsilon}R(+)$ cells in MLN cells were depleted by applying the cell suspension in IgE-coated dishes. Unfractionated lymphocytes and $Fc_{\epsilon}R(+)$-depleted fraction were incubated for 24 h to obtain culture supernatants. IgE-binding factor in the supernatants were assessed by inhibition of IgE rosettes.*

cells. More recent experiments suggested strongly that IgE potentiating factor is derived from $Fc_\epsilon R$ on T cells (Yodoi *et al.*, 1980).

In all of the experiments described above, we cultured lymph node cells obtained 14 days after infection when the proportion of $Fc_\epsilon R(+)$ cells reached maximum. However, further experiments on rat lymphocytes indicated that IgE-binding factors are heterogeneous with respect to their biologic activities and physicochemical properties. In the course of the experiments on the $Fc_\epsilon R(+)$ lymphocytes, we realized that the population of $Fc_\epsilon R(+)$ cells is regulated by the concentration of IgE in the environment. The proportion of $Fc_\epsilon R(+)$ cells was 2 to 3% in normal lymphocytes or those obtained 8 days after infection, and these cells did not release IgE binding factor. If one incubates these cells in 1 to 10 μg/ml of IgE, however, the proportion of the $Fc_\epsilon R(+)$ cells markedly increased and the supernatant obtained from the culture contained IgE-binding factor. In the experiment shown in Table III

TABLE III
Formation of rosette-inhibiting factor from normal lymphocytes

Source of MLN cells	*IgE in culture*	*$Fc_\epsilon R(+)$ cells*[a]	*Rosette inhibition*[b] *IgE-RFC*	*Inhibition*
		%	%	%
Normal	−	1·1	16·7	4
	+	8·1	9·5	46
8 days after infection	−	0·7	17·4	1
	+	16·1	4·6	74
Medium		—	17·6	

[a] The proportion of $Fc_\epsilon R(+)$ cells after 24 h culture with or without IgE.
[b] CFS were filtered through Diaflo 50A membrane and a 2-fold dilution of filtered CFS was added to E′-IgE to see inhibition of E′IgE-RFC.

culture filtrates were tested for the ability to inhibit rosette formation of $Fc_\epsilon R(+)$ cells. A filtrate from IgE-containing culture markedly inhibited the rosette formation, while culture filtrate from the IgE-free culture failed to do so. It was also found in a separate experiment that IgE-binding factor was formed by T cells. A reasonable question at this point is whether the IgE-binding factor in the culture supernatant may have IgE-potentiating activity. Thus, we cultured lymph node cells from the 8 day infected rats in the presence or absence of IgE, and culture filtrates were assessed for the ability to potentiate the IgE response of DNP-OA primed cells. As can be seen in Fig. 5, both culture filtrates failed to potentiate the IgE response, although the IgE-binding factor was detected in the filtrate from IgE containing culture. So, we added this culture filtrate to DNP-OA primed cells together with IgE-potentiating factor, and observed the Ig-forming cell response. It is apparent that the

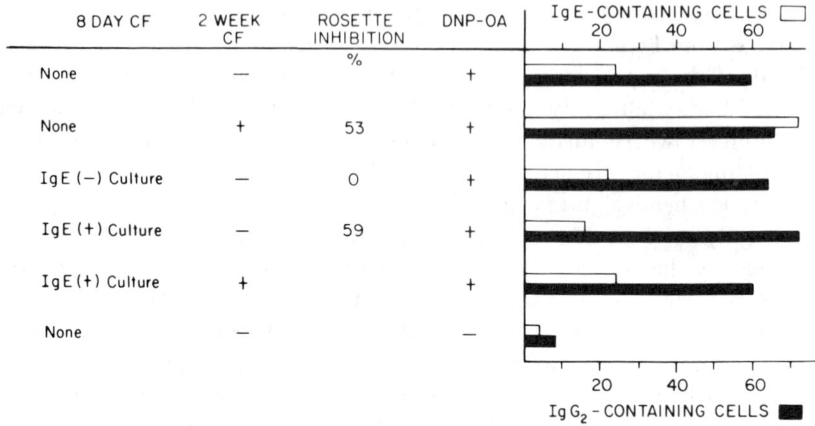

FIG. 5. *Demonstration of IgE-specific suppressive factor. MLN cells were obtained 8 days after Nb-infection and aliquots of the cell suspension were incubated for 24 h in the presence or absence of 10 μg/ml rat IgE. Culture supernatants were filtered through Diaflo CF 50A membranes and the filtrates were assessed for the ability to inhibit IgE rosettes. Each culture filtrate was added to DNP-OA primed cells together with DNP-OA and the cells were cultured for 5 days. Either culture filtrate preparation failed to affect the IgE and IgG_2 response of DNP-OA primed cells. However, addition of the filtrate from IgE(+) culture together with IgE-potentiating factor reversed the potentiating factor-enhanced IgE response back to control level.*

IgE-potentiating factor alone markedly enhanced the IgE response, but the addition of the culture filtrate of IgE containing culture reversed the potentiating factor-enhanced IgE response back to the control level. The results indicated that the filtrate of IgE-containing culture suppressed, rather than enhanced, the IgE response. Subsequent experiments actually showed that IgE-binding factor in the filtrate is responsible for the suppressive effect. The molecular size of IgE-specific suppressive factor is comparable to that of IgE-potentiating factor. Both factors have affinity for IgE and can be purified by using IgE-Sepharose. The main difference between the two factors is related to carbohydrate moiety. The IgE-potentiating factor was bound to lentil lectin Sepharose and was eluted from the lectin-coated beads with α-methyl mannoside (Yodoi *et al.*, 1980). In contrast, IgE-specific suppressive factor did not have affinity for lentil lectin (Hirashima *et al.*, 1980). The presence of the two IgE binding factors of opposite biologic functions will explain selective regulation of the IgE response.

Our recent experiments showed that the formation of IgE-binding factors is not confined to parasite infection. It was found that lymphocytes of rats treated with complete Freund's adjuvant (CFA) spontaneously released IgE-binding factors. The majority of IgE-binding factors was IgE-suppressive factor but culture filtrate contained a small amount of IgE-potentiating factor. It was also found that serum of CFA-treated animals contained both IgE-suppressive factor and IgE-potentiating factor and that the activity of the suppressive factor was much greater than potentiating factor. The presence of IgE-binding factors in the serum indicated that the factors are formed *in vivo*. We wondered that effect of adjuvant on the IgE antibody response may partly be explained by the formation of IgE-binding factors. As B. pertussis vaccine is the best adjuvant for the IgE antibody response in the rat, we injected 10^{10} pertussis vaccine into normal rats and examined the formation of IgE-binding factors by their lymphocytes. It was found that their peripheral lymphocytes form IgE-binding factor and their serum contained the same factor. Different from CFA-treated animals, however, essentially all IgE-binding factor in the serum of pertussis vaccine-treated animals was IgE-potentiating factor. The formation of the potentiating factor in the pertussis vaccine-treated animals, and the formation of IgE-suppressive factor in CFA-treated animals may partly be responsible for opposite effects of the two adjuvants on the IgE response. Table IV summarizes the nature and origin of

TABLE IV
Comparisons among IgE-specific suppressive factors

	IgE specific suppressor (Kishimoto)	*Suppressor factor of allergy (Katz)*	*IgE-suppressive factor*
Source	DNP-Tbc primed mouse T cells	CFA-treated mouse (T)	CFA-treated rat T cells
Target	B cells	?	IgE-B cells
Histo-compatibility	Restricted	Across barrier	Across barrier
Affinity for IgE	?	?	+
Mol. wt	45 000	150 000	10 000–20 000
Affinity for lectin	No affinity for lentil lectin	No affinity for conA	No affinity for lentil lectin

soluble factors which regulate the IgE response. As the molecular weight is entirely different from one factor to another, it is hard to believe that either Kishimoto's factor or Katz's factor is IgE-binding factor. It is possible, however, that IgE-binding factor may represent a portion of suppressive factor molecules as show by the other investigators. In any event, demonstration of IgE-specific regulator molecules indicates that IgE response is subjected to isotype-specific regulation, and this principle suggests a new approach to control the IgE response.

References

Bazin, H., Beckers, A., Urbain-Vansanten, G., Pauwels, R., Bruyns, C., Tilkin, A. F., Platteau, B. and Urbain, J. (1978a). *J. Immunol.* **121**, 2077.

Bazin, H., Platteau, B., Beckers, A. and Pauwels, R. (1978b). *J. Immunol.* **121**, 2083.

Blaser, K., Nakagawa, T. and deWeck, A. L. (1980). *J. Immunol.* **125**, 24.

Bloch, K. J., Ohman, J. L., Waltin, J. and Cygan, R. W. (1973). *J. Immunol.* **110**, 197.
Chiorazzi, N., Fox, D. A. and Katz, D. H. (1976). *J. Immunol.* **117**, 1629.
Fritsche, R. and Spiegelberg, H. L. (1978). *J. Immunol.* **121**, 471.
Gonzalez-Molina, A. and Spiegelberg, H. L. (1977). *J. Clin. Invest.* **59**, 616.
Hirashima, M., Yodoi, J. and Ishizaka, T. (1980). *J. Immunol.* (in press).
Ishizaka, K., Kishimoto, T., Delespesse, G. and King, T. P. (1974). *J. Immunol.* **113**, 70.
Ishizaka, T., Urban, J. F., Jr. and Isizaka, K. (1976). *Cell. Immunol.* **22**, 248.
Ishizaka, K., Ishizaka, T., Okudaira, H. and Bazin, H. (1978). *J. Immunol.* **120**, 655.
Jarrett, E. E. E. and Ferguson, A. (1974). *Nature* **250**, 420.
Katz, D. H. and Tung, A. S. (1979). *Immunology* **1**, 103.
Katz, D. H., Hamaoka, T. and Benacerraf, B. (1973). *Proc. Natn. Acad. Sci., U.S.A.* **73**, 2091.
Katz, D. H., Bargatze, R. F., Bogowitz, C. A. and Katz, L. R. (1979). *J. Immunol.* **122**, 2184.
Katz, D. H., Bargatze, R. F., Bogowitz, C. A. and Katz, L. R. (1980). *J. Immunol.* **124**, 819.
Kishimoto, T. and Ishizaka, T. (1973). *J. Immunol.* **111**, 720.
Kishimoto, T., Hirai, Y., Suemura, M. and Yamamura, Y. (1976). *J. Immunol.* **117**, 396.
Kishimoto, T., Hirai, Y., Suemura, M., Nakanishi, K. and Yamamura, Y. (1978). *J. Immunol.* **121**, 2106.
Lee, W. Y. and Sehon, A. H. (1978a). *Int. Arch. Allergy Appl. Immunol.* **56**, 159.
Lee, W. Y. and Sehon, A. H. (1978b). *Int. Arch. Allergy Appl. Immunol.* **56**, 193.
Lee, W. Y. and Sehon, A. H. (1979). *Immunology Letters* **1**, 31.
Levine, B. B. and Vaz, N. M. (1970). *Int. Arch. Allergy Appl. Immunol.* **39**, 156.
Liu, F. T., Bogowitz, C. A., Bargatze, R. F., Zinnecker, M., Katz, L. R. and Katz, D. H. (1979). *J. Immunol.* **123**, 2456.
Orr, T. S. C. and Blair, A. J. J. (1969). *Life Sci.* **8/II**, 1077.
Suemura, M. and Ishizaka, K. (1979). *J. Immunol.* **123**, 918.
Suemura, M., Kishimoto, T., Hirai, Y. and Yamamura, Y. (1977). *J. Immunol.* **119**, 149.
Suemura, M., Urban, J. F., Jr. and Ishizaka, K. (1978). *J. Immunol.* **121**, 2413.
Suemura, M., Yodoi, J., Hirashima, M. and Ishizaka, K. (1980). *J. Immunol.* **125**, 148.
Takatsu, K. and Ishizaka, K. (1975). *Cell Immunol.* **20**, 276.
Takatsu, K. and Ishizaka, K. (1976). *J. Immunol.* **116**, 1257.
Tung, A. S., Chiorazzi, N. and Katz, D. H. (1978). *J. Immunol.* **120**, 2050.
Urban, J. F., Jr. and Ishizaka, K. (1977). *J. Immunol.* **118**, 1982.
Urban, J. F., Jr., Ishizaka, K. and Bazin, H. (1980). *J. Immunol.* **124**, 527.
Watanabe, N., Kojima, S. and Ovary, Z. (1976). *J. Exp. Med.* **143**, 833.
Watanabe, T., Kimoto, M., Maruyama, S., Kishimoto, T. and Yamamura, Y. (1978). *J. Immunol.* **121**, 2113.
Yodoi, J. and Ishizaka, K. (1979). *J. Immunol.* **122**, 2577.
Yodoi, J. and Ishizaka, K. (1980). *J. Immunol.* **124**, 1322.
Yodoi, J., Hirashima, M. and Ishizaka, K. (1980). *J. Immunol.* (in press).

47

Effector Cells in Late and Delayed Hypersensitivity Reactions that are Dependent on Antibodies or T cells

PHILIP W. ASKENASE

Yale University School of Medicine, New Haven, Connecticut, USA

Abbreviations
DTH: delayed-type hypersensitivity; CFA: complete Freund's adjuvant; BCG: bacilli Calmette-Guérrin; PPD: purified protein derivative of tuberculin; CBH: cutaneous basophil hypersensitivity; JMR: Jones-Mote reaction(s); IFA: incomplete Freund's adjuvant; LPR: late phase reaction(s); MHC: major histocompatibility complex; CS: contact sensitivity; APC: antigen presenting cells; TNP: trinitrophenyl; LC: Langerhans cell; MΦ: macrophage: i.v.: intravenous; SRBC: sheep red blood cells; PEC: peritoneal exudate cells; TNBS: trinitrobenzene sulphonic acid; 5-HT: 5-hydroxy-tryptamine, serotonin.

Supported in part by grants from the American Cancer Society #IM-70F and the United States Public Health Service, National Institutes of Health #AI-12211, #AI-11707 and #AI-10497.

Introduction

Delayed-type hypersensitivity (DTH) reactions are the prototype of cell-mediated immunity. DTH was the first of the various functions of thymic derived or T lymphocytes to be identified and quantitated. We now know that T cells have other functions; such as helping B cells make antibodies, suppressing and regulating immune responses, and mediating cytotoxicity. However, DTH skin test responses still represent an easily measurable and quantifiable means of measuring T cell function *in vivo*. More importantly, DTH exemplifies the ability of T cells to recruit effector leukocytes to a tissue site, and this underlies many protective immune mechanisms, as well as some pathological conditions.

Recently it has been recognized that other immune reactions also have a delayed time course that can overlap with classical T cell dependent responses. This has led to a proliferation of confusing terms. In addition, newer data indicate that IgE-mediated immediate reactions can also have a delayed or late aspect. Conversely, basophils and mast cells, and their contained mediators such as histamine, which are ordinarily associated with immediate hypersensitivity, can also have prominent involvement in delayed reactions. This review will first attempt to sort out some of this new complexity and will then focus on the functions of various effector cells in late and delayed hypersensitivity reactions.

Terminology

Terms which encompass this entire area include: delayed onset hypersensitivity, delayed cutaneous reactions, and delayed-in-time reactions. These terms indicated a delayed time course immune hypersensitivity reaction, without prejudice as to whether they are T cell or antibody mediated, or as to whether basophils or mast cells participate.

The term delayed hypersensitivity (DH) or more precisely, tuberculin-type hypersensitivity is now reserved for the classical reaction, which is T cell dependent and associated with immunization augmented by water-in-oil emulsion adjuvant containing mycobacteria (complete Freund's adjuvant, CFA), or via infection with mycobacteria; such as bacilli Calmette-Guérrin (BCG). These reactions can either be elicited by purified protein derivative of tuberculin (PPD), which is the antigen in mycobacteria most relevant to elicitation of these responses, or by protein or cellular antigens that are administered with the mycobacteria. Subsequent reactions to antigens initially administered with mycobacteria share many characteristics of reactivity to PPD, and thus are called tuberculin-type hypersensitivity.

A histologic characteristic of most tuberculin-type reactions is that mononuclear cells predominate and there is a lack of significant basophil infiltration. Tuberculin-type reactions are related to the recruitment of macrophages as effector cells to resist infections and tumours. Delayed-type hypersensitivity (DTH) is a term that also refers to the T cell dependent delayed responses, but encompasses reactions induced with or without mycobacteria. Cutaneous basophil hypersensitivity (CBH) and Jones-Mote reactions (JMR) are delayed reactions that are induced without mycobacterial adjuvants. Strictly speaking, CBH refers to delayed cutaneous reactions that have a significant and often large accumulation of basophils. Many are T cell dependent, but, importantly, some are antibody mediated. JMR are a subcategory of CBH in that they are delayed onset reactions induced by injection of protein antigens in saline, or with incomplete Freund's adjuvant (IFA) (nonmycobacteria containing water-in-oil emulsions). They are rich in basophils, and can be dependent on T cells or antibodies.

Contact sensitivity (CS) reactions are a special case in that the immunogen is a simple haptenic reactive chemical that covalently links with host skin components to form a complete antigen that is necessary for induction of immune T cells and elicitation of responses. Contact reactions in humans and guinea-pigs are rich in basophils, and thus are a subset of CBH. In guinea-pigs, elicitation of CS can be dependent on T cells or antibodies.

It is now clear that some delayed cutaneous reactions can be mediated by antibodies. In humans, some of these antibody mediated reactions represent a newly recognized late phase of IgE mediated hypersensitivity and thus have been called late phase reactions (LPR) or late cutaneous reactions. The antibody aspect of CBH and JMR reactions in guinea-pigs is also mediated by anaphylactic homocytotrophic IgG_1 antibodies (and in more recent experiments in guinea-pig IgE antibodies), and thus are related to LPR.

In summary, it is proposed that the complex nomenclature of this field can be resolved if one first states that one is dealing with a delayed time course reaction that is dependent on T cells or homocytotropic antibodies. Then one can further subdivide reactions within these two broad categories according to whether the reaction does or does not contain significant infiltrates of basophils, and/or eosinophils, and/or deposits of fibrin, etc.

Effector cells in T cell aependent delayed onset reactions (DTH)

Effector cells in DTH can be divided into *recirculating cells*, *resident cells* and *recruited cells*.

Recirculating cells are sensitized T cells that are capable of specific recognition of antigen. Prior immunization provides clones of these effector T cells and of long-lived memory cells that can generate more effector T cells when antigen is encountered subsequently (Kojima *et al.*, 1979). The ability of these cells to interact specifically with antigen is dependent on surface molecules that are probably in part coded for by genes related to those coding for the variable region combining sites (idiotypes) of immunoglobulins.

Resident cells are already present in a given tissue. They become involved in DTH because of the interaction between sensitized recirculating T cells and specific antigen. They are of 3 types: (1) vascular endothelial cells, which must be traversed by the recirculating cells and by the recruited cells; (2) tissue macrophage-like cells, which take up and then present antigen to the T cells; and (3) mast cells which are activated by T cells to release vasoactive factors that alter the endothelial cells, allowing passage into the tissues of the recruited cells from their normal location in the circulation.

Recruited cells are bone marrow derived effector leukocytes (such as monocytes, basophils and neutrophils). The type of accessory leukocyte recruited into the tissues by T cells varies in at least 3 ways: (1) with the species: monocytes are the principal recruited cell in human reactions, while neutrophils are common in murine responses; (2) with the mode of immunization; basophils are preferentially recruited when immunization does not involve mycobacteria (Askenase, 1977; Galli and Dvorak, 1979) and ; (3) with the type of immunogen; eosinophils are recruited to DTH responses to helminthic parasites. Recruited cells comprise more than 95% of the infiltrate at a DTH reaction. They normally do not leave the intravascular space and enter the tissues. Recruitment of these cells into DTH reactions is probably mediated by chemoattractant and migration inhibitory lymphokine factors that are released by the T cells following activation by antigen. These factors act in synergy with mast cell dependent vasoactive factors that alter the vasculature to form gaps between endothelial cells through which the leukocytes emigrate into the tissues by diapedesis. Another new aspect of DTH is the presence of fibrin deposits. This probably accounts for much of the induration by which these reactions are characterized (Colvin and Dvorak, 1975).

Histocompatibility requirements and antigen presenting cells in DTH

In mice, DTH reactions are governed by recirculating T cells that bear the surface differentiation antigen Ly-1 (Huber *et al.*, 1976; Vadas *et al.*, 1976). Some Ly-1^+ T cells that mediate DTH are long-lived. These are recirculating cells that normally leave the circulation by passage directly through the cytoplasm of high endothelial cells of post capillary venules. This process is known as emperiopolesis. The molecular basis of this important phenomenon is not known, but could involve recognition based on interaction between endothelial and T cell surface moieties encoded by genes of the major histocompatibility complex (MHC). It is interesting to note that recognition of self-MHC is required for many T cell functions and becomes established in the foetal thymus (Zinkernagel, 1978) whereas developing thymic lymphocytes are similarly engulfed in emperiopolesis by huge thymic epithelial nurse cells (Wekerle and Ketelsen, 1980).

In addition to antigen specificity, recognition of self-MHC is a requirement in DTH. This is called dual specificity. As is true of other Ly-1^+ T cells, the MHC requirement of cells mediating DTH involves determinants encoded by the I region of the MHC (Ia antigens), rather than determinants encoded by the K or D regions, which are involved in the specificity of Ly-23^+ T cells, such as cytotoxic "killer" T cells (Cantor and Boyce, 1977). So far, this latter type of effector T cell has not been demonstrated to be involved in DTH. The requirement for interaction with homologous Ia antigens in DTH is exemplified by the work of Miller (1978) who showed that T cells could not transfer DTH across an MHC barrier. The locus of this histocompatibility requirement of T cells in DTH is probably associated with Ia antigens on the surface of macrophage-like cells now known as "antigen presenting cells" (APC). In fact, it is now clear that nearly all responses of T cells are critically dependent upon interaction with these adherent accessory cells. If cells used to study immune responses *in vitro* are thoroughly depleted of these cells, then responses fail to take place. Conversely, if antigen is first allowed to interact with these cells and then free antigen is removed, then these "antigen pulsed cells" substitute for antigen.

Much of the work pointing to the critical role of APC in T cell dependent immune responses is based upon *in vitro* systems (Unanue and Rosenthal, 1980). Recently, W. Ptak (1980) working in our laboratory, and others (Bach *et al.*, 1978; Green *et al.*, 1978) developed a simple system for studying the role of APC *in vivo* in a form of delayed hypersensitivity. These experiments involve contact sensitivity (CS) that is elicited by painting the ears of mice with a simple reactive chemical such as picryl chloride, and subsequently measuring ear swelling with a micrometer. CS is usually induced by prior painting of the abdominal and chest skin with the reactive hapten, but can also be induced by *in vitro* conjugation of autologous APC with a reactive hapten, such as trinitrobenzene sulphonate (TNBS), prior to injection of these cells. We found that intravenous injection of TNP-conjugated peritoneal exudate macrophages induced tolerance, but subcutaneous injection induced CS. However, these delayed reactions were weak and short-lived compared to the type of CS induced by skin painting with picryl chloride. We postulated that the latter form of CS might depend upon specialized APC in the skin. Thus, we prepared single cell suspensions from the epidermis of mouse skin and found that TNP-conjugated epidermal cells could induce potent contact sensitivity.

In subsequent experiments, epidermal cells were enriched for cells with surface receptors for the Fc portion of immunoglobulin by rosetting with antibody coated RBC. The Fc receptor enriched epidermal cells contained the APC, which we have tentatively concluded are related to Langerhans cells. These cells are known to be bone marrow derived, Ia$^+$ macrophage related cells, which are found in the epidermis and often pick up antigen on their surface and seem to deliver it to draining lymph nodes. Further studies demonstrated that Langerhans cells were especially potent in antigen presentation. Firstly, they induced a form of CS that was long-lived and, thus, analogous to that induced by contact painting. Secondly, they were active when given intravenously, which was not true of Ia bearing TNP-conjugated peritoneal exudate macrophages (TNP-MΦ) which induced tolerance when injected i.v. Lastly, when TNP-Langerhans cells (TNP-LC) and TNP-MΦ were coinjected i.v., the Langerhans cells were able to induce contact sensitivity even in the presence of suppression.

These studies demonstrated that the type of APC and the route of administration of these cells is critical to the induction of immunity. TNP-LC induce immunity via the i.v. route, TNP-MΦ induce tolerance if given i.v.—but induce CS if given subcutaneously, and TNP-LC induce immunity in the face of tolerance. Thus, TNP-LC seem to induce T cells that are resistant to suppression. Subsequent studies have shown that Ia antigens on the surface of the APC (in particular I-A and I-E/C) are important in these responses.

Antigen presenting cells and the mode of action of mycobacterial adjuvants in DTH

The ability of injected TNP-LC, or contact painting, to induce a form of long-lived CS, compared to the induction of a short-lived form of CS by subcutaneous injection of TNP-MΦ, seemed analogous to previous findings concerning DTH to SRBC in mice. In this latter system, a short-lived form of DTH is induced by i.v. or subcutaneous injection of optimal doses of SRBC in saline, while a more long-lived form of DTH is induced by coadministering SRBC with BCG or emulsifying with CFA (Askenase *et al.*, 1977; Mackaness *et al.*, 1974). Thus, we postulated that the immunoinducing quality of mycobacterial adjuvants could be based in part on their ability to alter APC. We found that peritoneal exudate MΦ induced by injections of IFA were similar to those induced by oil or thioglycollate in that they were able only to immunize for a weak and evanescent form of CS, after conjugation with TNP and injection subcutaneously. However, when peritoneal exudate MΦ were induced with CFA, or MΦ were harvested from mice treated with BCG, then these cells, when conjugated with TNP, were potent inducers of quantitatively greater CS, that was also long-lived (Britz *et al.*, 1980).

CS induced by TNP-CFA-PEC, like that induced by picryl chloride skin painting, was readily transferred to normal recipients with sensitized cells, while the weaker CS induced by TNP-IFA-PEC was not. Similar to LC, TNP-CFA-PEC were also resistant to suppression. Usually, i.v. injection of TNBS renders mice tolerant to picryl chloride CS, but injection of TNP-CFA-PEC in the face of coadministration of TNBS i.v., still induced CS. The potent antigen presenting capacity of CFA induced MΦ was not due to a cell dose or a hapten conjugation difference of these cells. These experiments demonstrate that potent APC, similar to Langerhans cells normally found in the skin, can be induced by treating mice with mycobacterial adjuvants.

The experiments summarized above indicate that APC are critical in determining whether DTH is induced, and whether the DTH that is induced is long-lived and resistant to suppression. Although these studies dealt with the role of APC in the induction of DTH, it seems likely that these cells also play an important role in the elicitation of DTH. Thus, in the extravascular tissues in the skin at the site of an evolving DTH reaction, it is likely that antigen associated with Ia determinants on Langerhans cells, triggers activation of rare, passing, sensitized, Ly-1^+ T cells that have entered the tissues by emperiopolesis as part of their normal recirculating migration.

Mast cells in DTH

The origin and development of tissue mast cells, and the details of their function in DTH have recently been elucidated in studies that have taken advantage of special attributes of mice. Kitamura and coworkers have employed three different kinds of unusual inbred lines of mice with defects in mast cell morphology, precursors, or differentiation. Through transfer and reconstitution studies, these workers have demonstrated that most connective tissue mast cells arise from bone marrow stem cells that circulate in the blood in a precursor state and then slowly differentiate into mast cells in the tissues. This differentiation is controlled by local microenvironmental influences, and is independent of a functional thymic influence. On the other hand, it is clear that tissue differentiation of a specialized subpopulation of mast cells is thymus dependent. These unusual mast cells are found in the intestinal mucosa of rats and mice that are expelling intestinal nematodes, such as *Nippstrongylus brasiliensis* and *Trichinella spiralis* (reviewed in Askenase, 1980). It is not clear whether these thymic dependent mucosal mast cells, which have several properties that distinguish them from thymus independent connective tissue mast cells, are also derived from bone marrow precursors, but need a thymic and a microenvironmental influence for differentiation; or whether they are actually derived from thymic cells. The thymic influence regulating differentiation of these unusual mast cells may in part be exerted via thymic dependent antibodies such as IgE.

The important functional role of mast cells in DTH has recently been elucidated. These studies were also performed in mice. In this species serotonin (5-HT) is stored in mast cells, and the local vasculature is quite sensitive to this vasoactive amine. In contrast, histamine, which is also stored in murine mast cells, has little effect on the vasculature (Schwartz *et al.*, 1977). These studies have taken advantage of the ability to alter the storage and effects of released 5-HT by pharmacological treatments, and the ability to follow (^{3}H)5-HT morphologically by radioautography. Initial experiments suggested that release of 5-HT by local tissue mast cells was required for the elicitation of

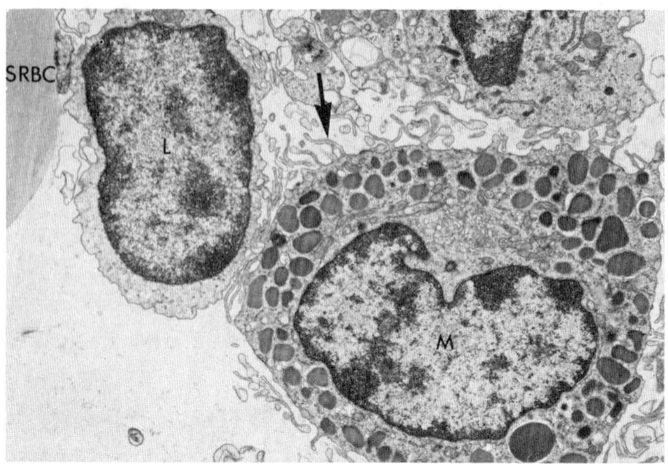

FIG. 1. *An electron micrograph of cells from the dermis of the footpad skin of an immunized mouse 6 h after challenge with SRBC. Note the surface contact between the antigen (SRBC), lymphocyte (L), mast cell (M) and monocyte. The surface filopodia of the mast cell are extended (arrow). The mast cell granules retain their homogeneous staining.* × *4788*

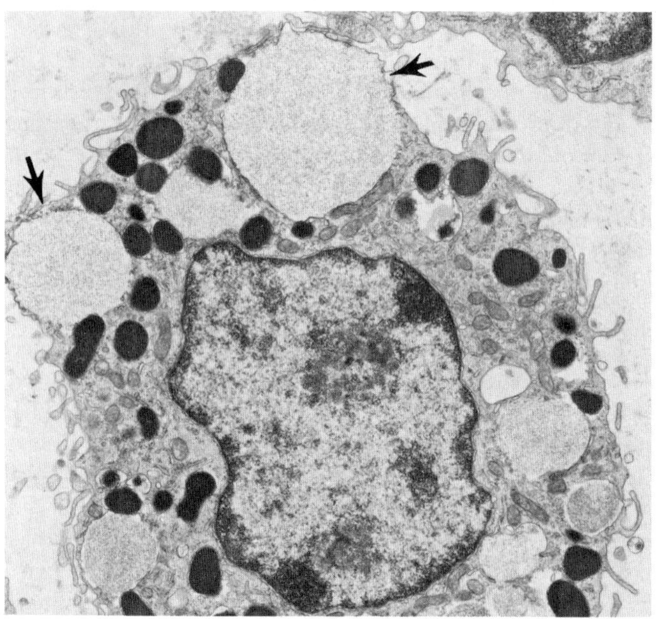

FIG. 2. *Electron micrograph of a mast cell from the dermis of the footpad skin of an immunized mouse obtained 18 h after challenge with SRBC. Fusion of granules has produced enlarged cavities. The matrix of these granules shows advanced dissolution. Only some of the granules are affected. However, there is no restriction of the process to any given region of the cell. The largest cavities (arrows) tend to occur near the plasma membrane. Extension of surface filopodia is again notable.* × *9072.*

DTH, since responses were preferentially elicited in those cutaneous sites of mice that were especially rich in 5-HT containing mast cells. Furthermore, administration of the 5-HT depleting agent, reserpine, abolished the ability to elicit DTH. Since the effect of reserpine could be prevented by administration of a monoamine oxidase inhibitor, the attribution of the action of reserpine to depletion of a monoamine (such as 5-HT) was confirmed (Gershon *et al.*, 1975). Subsequent studies, which have employed two additional and independent pharmacological manoeuvres (5-HT tachyphylaxis of the vasculature and the use of 5-HT antagonists), have been consistent with the hypothesis in murine DTH that specifically sensitized T cells interact with tissue mast cells leading to the release of 5-HT which acts on the local endothelium allowing the emigration of bone marrow derived leukocytes from the intravascular to the extravascular space.

More recent studies have directly demonstrated activation of mast cells to release 5-HT in murine DTH (Askenase *et al.*, 1980). Ultrastructural examination of mast cells revealed surface activation, indicated by extension of surface filopodia, and degranulation by fusion and exocytosis (Figs 1 and 2). Light microscopic radioautographs prepared from animals treated with (^{3}H)5-HT indicated that mast cells released 5-HT in DTH (Fig. 3a, b). Light and

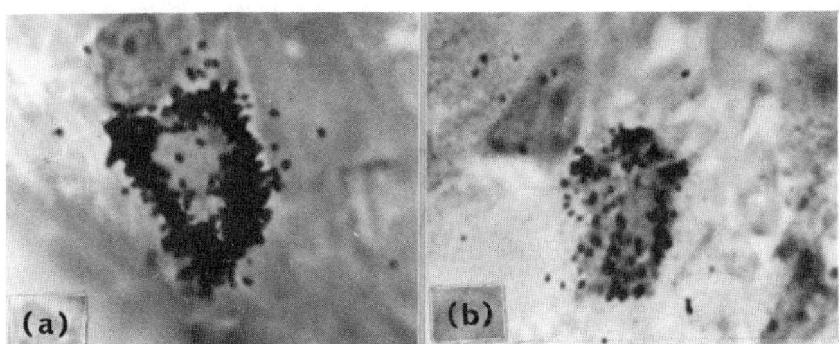

FIG. 3. *Light microscopic radioautographs of the dermis of the footpad skin removed 18 h following challenge with antigen (SRBC) to nonimmunized (a) or immunized (b) mice, that were previously injected with ^{3}H-5HT. Note the lower intensity of labelling of the mast cells fron the immunized animals. In the controls (a), the overlying silver grains are so numerous that th metachromasia of the mast cell granules is obscured. In immunized and challenged mice (b) the reduction in radiolabelling allows the granules to be seen.*

electron microscopic studies of the endothelium of postcapillary venules at sites of DTH revealed the development of gaps between adjacent cells that permitted extravasation of tracers and diapedesis of leukocytes (Figs 4 and 5). The gaps at endothelial junctions of post capillary venules were identical to those caused by infusion of 5-HT, and the extravasation of tracers was abolished by depletion or antagonism of 5-HT. Recipients of nonadherent, nonimmunoglobulin bearing sensitized lymphocytes (T cells) also demonstrated similar mast cell activation and degranulation, and the formation of endothelial gaps. This indicated that mast cell degranulation and 5-HT release in murine DTH were probably T cell dependent. Degranulation of mast cells

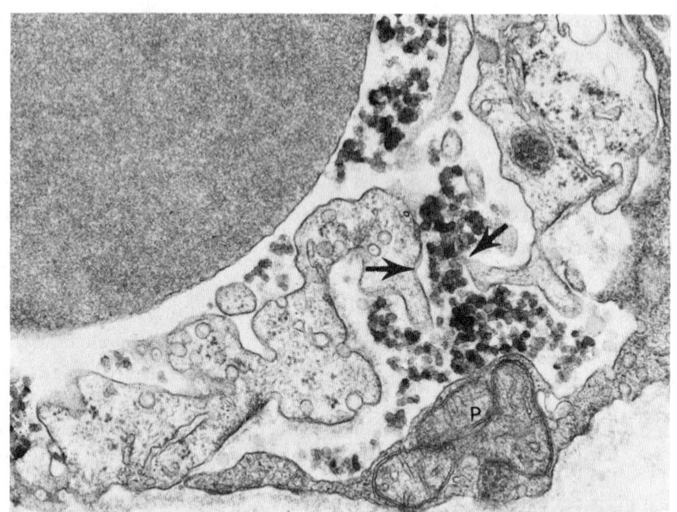

FIG. 4. *A postcapillary venule from the dermis of the footpad of an immunized mouse obtained 18 h after challenge with SRBC. The endothelial cells appear to have a corrugated surface, and contain cytoplasmic vesicles. A gap (arrows) has opened at the junction between endothelial cells allowing carbon particles, that were injected intravenously, to fill the resulting space and extravasate outside the lumen of the vessel. The carbon accumulates in contact with the process of a pericyte (P). × 27 000*

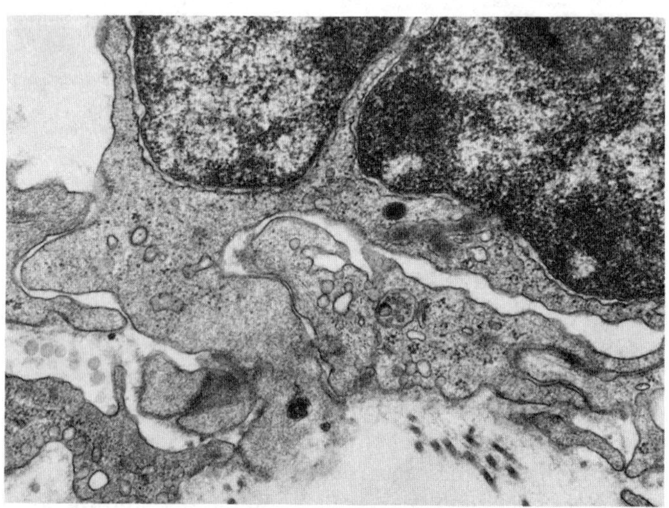

FIG. 5. *A mononuclear cell in the process of migrating through a gap between endothelial cells in the footpad skin 18 h after challenge of an immunized mouse with SRBC. × 10 800*

and formation of endothelial gaps in DTH of humans (Galli and Dvorak, 1979) suggest that an analogous process may be involved in reactions of this species.

Basophils in delayed reaction: cutaneous basophil hypersensitivity (CBH)

The widest definition of these reactions is that they are delayed time course immune reactions in which basophils are a major component of the recruited cells. CBH reactions can be mediated by T cells, by antibody, and via B cells (Askenase, 1979). They are classically elicited in animals or humans immunized with a protein antigen that was not coadministered with mycobacteria, but just injected in saline. In these Jones Mote Reactions, erythematous but mildly indurated delayed time course reactions are elicited about a week after immunization. Reactions are evanescent after elicitation and after immunization, and do not contain appreciable fibrin deposits. However, many other types of CBH reactions are long-lasting, particularly the biologically relevant ones such as contact sensitivity and reactions to viruses, parasites, and tumour cells. In fact, of all the various kinds of delayed reactions, only the tuberculin-type have a few basophils, and this is due to a regulatory phenomenon. Animals immunized with CFA have T cells that are capable of attracting basophils to the skin, but do not do so because of inhibitory factors. This can be demonstrated in transfer experiments in which basophil rich reactions are elicited in recipients of T cells from donors immunized with CFA, whose reactions were virtually devoid of basophils (Askenase, 1976). However, transfer of cells *plus* serum results in significant augmentation of the ability to elicit the macroscopic aspect of the delayed reaction in the recipient, and also results in a suppression of the basophil-rich histology. The macroscopic augmenter in the serum appears to be a specific IgG_2 antibody, and the alteration of the T cell dependent tissue basophilia appears to be due to a nonspecific basophil suppressing factor (Mitchell and Askenase, 1980). Examination of PPD reactions in patients with tuberculosis reveals that some have significant basophil accumulations while others have none. This could also be due to the action of similar regulatory factors.

Mechanistically, T cell dependent CBH reactions can be viewed as an extension of the remarks above for DTH. In this instance, specifically sensitized T cells interacting with antigen emit chemotactic factors and also factors that specifically augment chemotactic responsiveness of basophils. Such factors have been identified *in vitro* to account for the specific localization of basophils at CBH reactions (reviewed in Galli and Dvorak, 1979). The suppression of T cell CBH in animals immunized with mycobacteria could be due to interference with basophil chemotaxis.

Antibody-mediated CBH reactions in guinea-pigs are dependent on homocytotropic anaphylactic type 7S IgG_1 antibodies. Preliminary evidence indicates that antibody CBH represents an anaphylactic cascade reaction in which skin mast cells coated via surface Fc receptors with these antibodies (Graziano and Askenase, 1979) interact with injected antigen and release factors with late sequelae, some of which may be chemoattractant for basophils and eosinophils. Basophils in the circulation and, those arriving on the scene, are themselves coated with this type of antibody and may interact with residual antigen, releasing more factors, and thus, calling in more cells. These reactions may be related to human IgE mediated, late phase reactions (see below) in that homocytotropic antibodies are involved, the reactions are preceded by a wheal and flare response, and there are significant fibrin deposits (de Shazo *et al.*, 1979); in contrast to T cell mediated CBH in which fibrin is sparse (Colvin and Dvorak, 1975).

Having arrived at a CBH reaction, basophils are able to function and release mediators of immediate hypersensitivity amidst a DTH reaction. In CBH induced and elicited with soluble protein antigens, basophils that arrive 24 h after a single pulse of skin test antigen show minimal degranulation. However, if the immunizing protein antigen is reintroduced into a mature 24 or 48 h CBH reaction, basophils immediately degranulate and release mediators like histamine, and thus provide local augmented anaphylactic reactivity at a delayed cutaneous reaction site (Askenase *et al.*, 1978). In contrast to CBH reactions elicited by a single injection of a soluble protein antigen, at CBH reactions to tumours and parasites, basophils appear to be much more activated and to be releasing mediators. This is probably due to ongoing local release of antigens by the organisms or tumour cells. Antibody mediates the anaphylactic functional capacity of basophils in delayed reactions. Lymphocyte derived factors may also govern the secretory function of basophils at such sites, since basophil activating, histamine releasing factors have recently been described (Theuson *et al.*, 1979). The anaphylactic function of basophils at CBH is accompanied by classical degranulation by exocytosis. In addition, there is morphological evidence *in vivo* and kinetic evidence *in vitro* (Dvorak *et al.*, 1980) consistent with another slower mode of mediator release ("piecemeal degranulation") in which portions of basophil granules, and perhaps some accompanying mediators, are transported to the exterior of the cell via a system of cytoplasmic vesicles that bud off from the granules, and move towards and fuse with the cytoplasmic membrane.

The consequences of the release of mediators by basophils at CBH reactions may be protective, at sites where reactions are expelling tumours or parasites, or may have a regulatory role through the ability of mediators such as histamine to interact with histamine-2 receptors on various leukocytes (including regulatory T cells) leading to a net suppressive and/or anti-inflammatory effect, and contributing to the diminution of these reactions (reviewed in Askenase, 1977).

Effector function of basophils at CBH reactions

A crucial question is whether basophils at CBH reactions can serve as effector cells. The possibility that basophils might directly participate in immune resistance came initially from studies that demonstrated significant accumulations of basophils at skin sites of immune guinea-pigs inoculated with tumour cells (Dvorak *et al.*, 1973), or at skin sites penetrated by infective larvae of schistosomes, known as schistosomula (Askenase *et al.*, 1976). However, in either situation, it is unlikely that basophils act directly as effector cells. At skin responses to growing tumour cells, basophils comprise only 10–20% of the infiltrating cells. It is likely that activated MΦ, and cytotoxic killer T cells are more directly involved in resistance to tumour growth, although minor ultrastructural alterations in tumour cells have been noted following *in vitro* incubation with basophils. At the sites of skin penetration by schistosomula, basophils comprise up to 35% of the infiltrating cells. However, it is likely that recruited cells other than basophils, such as eosinophils, and MΦ, are the pertinent effector cells that contain and then destroy the invading parasites.

In these situations, basophils probably serve auxillary, rather than direct effector functions. Basophil release of chemotactic factors, to attract eosinophils, and of vasoactive amines, to also alter endothelium and aid in diapedesis of various recruited effector leukocytes would obviously be important. Additionally, basophils, like mast cells, could release factors able to activate the effector function of leukocytes recruited to the site, as was recently demonstrated *in vitro* for eosinophil-mediated antibody-dependent cell-mediated cytotoxicity of schistosomula (Capron *et al.*, 1978).

The study of immune cutaneous basophil resistance to ectoparasitic ticks has offered a unique opportunity to study the biological function of basophils that may be mediating an immune resistance mechanism. Guinea-pigs mount a potent immune resistance response to ticks that involve the ability of antibodies and/or sensitized lymphocytes to recruit unusual numbers of basophils to the skin site of tick feeding. Activation of these cells after arrival, with release of mediators, seems to lead to death of the ticks through a toxic effect on vital life processes of the arthropod, or interference with its feeding. In this system, basophils may play an important biological role, since up to 90% of the infiltrating cells are basophils. Nearly complete resistance (80–100% rejection of parasites) can be achieved, and resistance is transferable to normal animals with sensitized cells and/or immune serum (reviewed in Askenase, 1980).

The crucial question is whether the basophils are required to effect immune resistance to the ticks. This is being answered through the use of a potent and specific rabbit anti-guinea-pig basophil serum (ABS) (Galli *et al.*, 1978) in studies performed in collaboration with Stephen Brown in my laboratory and Stephen Galli from the laboratory of Harold Dvorak. Tick-sensitized guinea-pigs treated with ABS had complete loss of immune resistance to the parasites and a greater than 95% depletion of basophils from the bone marrow, the blood, and the sites of tick feeding. Controls that received normal rabbit serum or saline had unaltered resistance and normal numbers of basophil in the bone marrow, blood, and at the sites of tick feeding. In more recent experiments, immune resistance to ticks was abolished by treatment with either ABS or a specific rabbit anti-guinea-pig eosinophil serum (Gleich *et al.*, 1975). These results may indicate that immune resistance depends on a collaborative interaction between basophils and eosinophils. Release of mediators by basophils may be deleterious to the parasites, or basophils may be necessary to recruit and activate eosinophils to function as the principal effector cells. However, these results do establish that rejection of the ticks depends, at least in part, on the basophils.

Antibody dependent late phase reactions (LPR)

Recent evidence suggests that there is more to anaphylactic Type I hypersensitivity than can be observed immediately. Careful follow up of IgE mediated wheal and flare reactions in humans has revealed a late component with a delayed and prolonged time course. Many of these LPR follow strong wheal and flare reactions and are thus seen with higher allergen skin test doses, but LPR can be noted following ordinary responses (reviewed in Askenase, 1977).

Characteristically, as the immediate reaction begins to wane at 30–60 min, there is a slow emergence of another reaction. By 90 min after skin testing there is a large oedematous, erythematous and asymptomatic lesion which can then persist over the next few hours. Then at 4–5 h there is a new onset of pruritis and exacerbation of inflammation and burning which can peak at 6–12 h and consist of erythema, warmth, oedema, pruritis, burning, and tenderness. Initial 15–20 mm wheals are superseded at 6–12 h by 40–80 mm of oedema and erythema. The degree of erythema is less than in tuberculin reactions. By 24 h, lesions are fading, but some have not resolved until 48 h.

Such dual early and late phase reactions can be passively transferred with IgE antibody. Similar reactions can be elicited by injecting the nonspecific mast cell degranulator compound 48/80. But injection of histamine or bradykinin does not elicit such reactions. The histology of these LPR reveals a rather light, perivascular infiltrate consisting of mononuclear cells, eosinophils and some basophils. In addition, prominent fibrin deposits have been found (de Shazo *et al.*, 1979). Administration of corticosteroids suppresses the LPR but not the immediate wheal and flare aspect, and histamine-1 receptor antagonists inhibit the immediate—but not the LPR (Smith *et al.*, 1980), suggesting two separate mechanisms.

There are several similarities between IgE-mediated LPR in humans and antibody-mediated CBH in guinea-pigs. Both are mediated by antibodies that passively sensitize basophils and mast cells (homocytotrophic or anaphylactic antibodies), and both feature delayed time course erythema and skin swelling. Both are characterized by histologic infiltrates which include mononuclear cells, lymphocytes, eosinophils, and basophils, and both reactions contain fibrin deposits. In humans, they are mediated by IgE antibodies while in guinea-pigs these reactions are mediated by 7S IgG_1-type homocytotropic antibodies, and, in more recent studies, also by IgE (Graziano *et al.*, 1980). Fc competition experiments suggest that direct cytophilic binding of antibody to host cells, such as mast cells and basophils, is important in the human and guinea-pig reactions. If both of these reactions are mediated by anaphylactic antibodies that cause discharge of mediator-containing cells, then the late occurrence and delayed and prolonged duration of macroscopic and microscopic elements of inflammation implies that some of the following mechanisms may underlie these responses: (1) prolonged mediator release by local mast cells; (2) local persistence of active inflammatory mediators; (3) prolonged effects or consequences of earlier acting mediators; (4) a cascade in which antigen binding to mast cell bound antibody causes local mast cells to release factors leading to the tissue accumulation of inflammatory cells, and then subsequent triggering of newly arrived cells by residual antigen and/or nonspecific factors resulting in a prolonged and delayed reaction. Kaliner and coworkers (1980) have recently demonstrated that a peptide derived from mast cell granules may be responsible for some of the infiltrating cells at LPR.

Conclusions

It is now evident that the term delayed time course reactions describes a whole series of complex immune inflammatory responses that encompasses at one extreme, the classical T cell dependent tuberculin-type delayed hypersensitivity, and at the other extreme the newly recognized late and delayed components of classical IgE-mediated immediate hypersensitivity reactions. Thus, a new nomenclature is proposed to reflect primarily the T cell v. homocytotrophic antibody dependence of particular reactions. Secondary descriptive characteristics would then refer to the involvement of: mast cells, basophils, macrophages, fibrin deposits, etc.

This review has focused on the function of certain effector cells in delayed reactions. Although many of these responses are governed by a subpopulation of recirculating T cells, there is a requirement for resident cells which include: macrophage-type cells that present antigen; mast cells that release vasoactive factors; and responding endothelial cells that allow diapedesis of recruited effector cells. Basophils are one of these bone-marrow-derived cells that can be recruited via T cell or antibody dependent mechanisms. Importation of basophils brings to a particular tissue site the ability to release a variety of mediators that substantially broaden the biological potential of delayed reactions.

References

Askenase, P. W. (1976). *J. Immunol.* **117**, 741.
Askenase, P. W. (1977). *Prog. in Allergy* **23**, 199.
Askenase, P. W. (1979). *J. Allergy and Clin. Immunol.* **64**, 79.
Askenase, P. W. (1980). *Springer Seminars in Immunopathology* **2**, 417.
Askenase, P. W., Hayden, B. and Higashi, G. I. (1976). *Clin. Exp. Immunol.* **23**, 318.
Askenase, P. W., Hayden, B. J. and Gershon, R. K. (1977). *J. Immunol.* **119**, 1830.
Askenase, P. W., DeBernardo, R., Tauben, D. and Kashgarian, M. (1978). *Immunology* **35**, 741.
Askenase, P. W., Bursztajn, S., Gershon, M. D. and Gershon, R. K. (1980). *J. Exp. Med.* **152**.
Bach, B. A., Sherman, L., Benacerraf, B. and Greene, M. I. (1978). *J. Immun.* **121**, 1460.
Britz, J., Ptak, W., Askenase, P. W. and Gershon, R. K. (1980). *In* Abstracts of the IV Int. Congr. Immunology, Paris, 1980, No. 11. 202.
Cantor, H. and Boyce, E. A. (1977). *Cold Spring Harbor Symp. Quant. Biol.* **41**, 23.
Capron, M., Rousseaux, Mazique, C., Bazin, H. and Capron, A. (1978). *J. Immunol.* **121**, 2518.
Colvin, R. B. and Dvorak, H. F. (1975). *J. Immunol.* **114**, 377.
Dvorak, H. F., Dvorak, A. M. and Churchill, W. H. (1973). *J. Exp. Med.* **137**, 751.
Dvorak, A. M., Hammond, M. E., Morgan, E., Orenstein, N., Galli, S. J. and Dvorak, H. F. (1980). *Lab. Investig.* **42**, 263.
Galli, S. J. and Dvorak, H. F. (1979). *In* "Cellular, Molecular, and Clinical Aspects of Allergic Disorders" (S. Gupta and R. A. Good, eds) Vol. 6. Plenum Publishers, New York and London.
Galli, S. J., Colvin, R. B., Verderber, E., Galli, A. S., Monahan, R., Dvorak, A. M. and Dvorak, H. F. (1978). *J. Immunol.* **121**, 1157.
Gershon, R. K., Askenase, P. W. and Gershon, M. D. (1975). *J. Exp. Med.* **143**, 732.
Gleich, G., Loegering, D. A. and Olsen, G. M. (1975). *J. Immunol.* **115**, 950.
Graziano, F. and Askenase, P. W. (1979). *J. Immunol.* **123**, 1645.
Graziano, F. M., Gundersen, L. and Askenase, P. W. (1980). *Fed. Proc.* **39**, 2243.
Greene, M. I., Sugimoto, M. and Benacerraf, B. (1978). *J. Immunol.* **120**, 1604.
Huber, B., Devinsky, O., Gershon, R. K. and Cantor, H. (1976). *J. Exp. Med.* **143**, 1534.
Kitamura, Y., Go, S., Shimad, M., Matsuda, H., Hatanka, K. and Seki, M., (1979). *J. Exp. Med.* **150**, 482.
Kojima, A., Tamura, S. I. and Egashira, Y. (1979). *Cellular Immunol.* **45**, 61.
Mackaness, G., Lagrange, P. H. and Ishibashi, T. (1974). *J. Exp. Med.* **139**, 1540.
Mitchell, E. B. and Askenase, P. W. (1980). *Fed. Proc.* **39**, 1127.
Miller, J. A. F. P. (1978). *Immunol. Reviews* **42**, 76.
Ptak, W., Rozycka, D., Askenase, P. W. and Gershon, R. K. (1980). *J. Exp. Med.* **151**, 362.
Schwartz, A., Askenase, P. W. and Gershon, R. K. (1977). *J. Immunol.* **118**, 159.
de Shazo, R. D., Levinson, A. I., Dvorak, H. F. and Davis, R. W. (1979). *J. Immun.* **122**, 692.
Smith, J. A., Mansfield, L. E., de Shazo, R. D. and Nelson, H. S. (1980). *J. All. Clin. Immunol.* **65**, 118.

Tannenbaum, S., Oertel, H., Henderson, W. and Kaliner, M. (1980). *J. Immunol.* **125**, 325.

Theuson, D. O., Speck, L. S., Lett-Brown, M. and Grant, A. (1979). *J. Immunology* **123**, 626, 633.

Unanue, E. R. and Rosenthal, A. S. (eds) (1980). "Macrophage Regulation of Immunity". Academic Press, London and New York.

Vadas, M. A., Miller, J. A. F. P., McKenzie, I. F. C., Chism, S. E., Shen, F-W., Boyce, E. A., Gamble, J. R. and Whitelaw, A. M. (1976). *J. Exp. Med.* **144**, 10.

Wekerle, H. and Ketelsen, U-P. (1980). *Nature* **283**, 402.

Zinkernagel, R. (1978). *Immunol. Reviews* **42**, 224.

48

The Role of Cyclic Nucleotides in Mast Cell Activation and Secretion

STEPHEN T. HOLGATE,* ROBERT A. LEWIS and K. FRANK AUSTEN**

Department of Medicine, Harvard Medical School and the Robert B. Brigham Division of the Affiliated Hospitals Center, Inc., Boston, USA

Abbreviations

PG: prostaglandin; cyclic AMP: 3′,5′-cyclic adenosine monophosphate; cyclic GMP: 3′,5′-cyclic guanosine monophosphate; SRS-A: slow reacting substance of anaphylaxis; ATP: adenosine 5′-triphosphate; PIA: N^6-phenylisopropyladenosine; DDA: 2′,5′-dideoxyadenosine; 5′-AMP: 5′-adenosine monophosphate.

This work was supported in part by grants AI-07722, HL-17382, HL-19777 and RR-05669 from the National Institutes of Health, and in part by a grant from the Lillia Babbitt Hyde Foundation.

* Travelling Research Fellow of the British Medical Research Council and Wellcome Trust.

** Recipient of a Young Investigator Research grant HL-21089 from the National Heart, Lung and Blood Institute, National Institutes of Health.

Mast cells play an essential role in the initiation of host responses which are characteristic of the acute allergic reacion. The activation of rat mast cells by specific divalent antigen-induced dimerization of cell-bound IgE with secondary cross-bridging of IgE-Fc receptors stimulates a cascade of biochemical events which culminate in both the noncytotoxic release of preformed granule associated mediators and the generation of newly formed lipid mediators. A number of events which appear to follow bridging of IgE-Fc receptors, have been identified in rat peritoneal mast cells and are considered in this section because of their possible relationships to the activation of adenylate cyclase. As several of these events occur within 15 s of membrane receptor perturbation, kinetic studies do not distinguish parallel from sequential events. While pharmacologic intervention permits a recognition of parallel events and affords some circumstantial evidence for a sequence, this approach is not definitive unless the intervention is completely specific for the function of a single protein in the sequence.

After the perturbation of membrane IgE-Fc receptors, serine esterase activity is uncovered as inferred from the inhibition of mediator release by diisopropylfluorophosphonate (DFP) and by other irreversible inhibitors of serine esterases (Becker and Austen, 1966). As this intervention also prevents membrane phospholipid methylation (Ishizaka *et al.*, in press), it is compatible with the activation of serine esterase as part of the membrane signal. A rapid but transient increase of phospholipid methylation in the plasma membrane involving conversion of phosphatidylethanolamine to phosphatidylcholine occurs after immunologic challenge (Hirata *et al.*, 1979; Ishizaka *et al.*, 1980). That phospholipid methylation is obligatory for calcium influx and granule secretion is shown by the capacity of inhibitors of methyltransferase activity, namely, 3-deazaadenosine, its *S*-isobutyryl analogue (Ishizaka *et al.*, 1980) or 5′-deoxy-5′(isobutylthio)-3-deazaadenosine (Morita *et al.*, 1980) to inhibit in a parallel fashion methyl transferase activity, calcium ion influx and preformed mediator release. Newly generated phosphatidylcholine undergoes a reorientation in the membrane so that the polar head group is directed towards the outside (Hirata and Axelrod, 1978). The resultant change in membrane fluidity is believed to facilitate both the opening of calcium channels (Foreman *et al.*, 1977) and the increased availability of phospholipid substrate for the action of phospholipases (Kennerly *et al.*, 1979a; Lewis *et al.*, in press). While calcium influx or remobilization of intracellular calcium is essential for the progression of the secretory response to completion (Foreman *et al.*, 1977), the precise roles of calcium are, at present, speculative. Calcium, acting through its binding protein, calmodulin, is required for catalytic expression of a number of enzymes, including adenylate and guanylate cyclases, calcium-dependent protein kinases, phosphodiesterases, and Ca^{2+}/Mg^{2+}-activated ATPases, some or all of which may be necessary to the sequence of biochemical events leading to mast cell granule secretion. After uncovering of serine esterase activity or calcium ion influx, there is an energy requirement for glycolysis in that in the absence of glucose or in the presence of 2-deoxyglucose or other inhibitors of glycolytic enzymes, histamine release is suppressed. Inhibition of oxidative phosphorylation, either pharmacologically or by hypoxia, also suppresses histamine release, thereby implicating this pathway as an additional energy source.

Other intracellular events occurring during the release reaction in rat mast cells include phosphorylation of several mast cell proteins, organization of structural and contractile cytoskeletal elements and granule swelling before membrane fusion with partial solubilization before exocytosis. The crystalline structure of the human mast cell granule has allowed a definitive demonstration of its solubilization and of the association of the swollen granule with intermediate filaments after IgE-dependent activation and before granule movement, fusion of the perigranular with another perigranular and with plasma membranes, and exocytosis of the solubilized granule (Caulfield *et al.*, 1980).

Mast cell activation also results in profound elevations in the levels of intracellular cyclic 3′,5′-adenosine monophosphate (cyclic AMP) and cyclic 3′,5′-guanosine monophosphate (cyclic GMP). The relationship of changes in cyclic nucleotide levels to the process of mast cell coupled activation-secretion is the aspect to be considered.

Historical perspective of the relationship of changes in cyclic nucleotide levels to immunologic mast cell mediator release

Prior to the discovery of cyclic nucleotides, Schild (1936) demonstrated that high doses of adrenaline inhibited antigen-induced histamine release from actively sensitized guinea-pig lung. In 1968, Lichenstein and Margolis showed that classes of pharmacologic agents which elevate cellular levels of cyclic AMP, such as the β-adrenergic agonists isoprenaline and adrenaline, and inhibitors of phosphodiesterase, caffeine, theobromine and theophylline, were inhibitors of immunologic histamine release from sensitized human leukocytes. Subsequent studies on lung fragments from primates demonstrated that pharmacologic agents active in raising tissue levels of cyclic AMP inhibited both the IgE-dependent release of histamine and the generation and release of slow reacting substance of anaphylaxis (SRS-A) (Assem and Schild, 1969; Ishizaka *et al.*, 1970; Orange *et al.*, 1971; Lewis *et al.*, 1974). In addition, the relative inhibitory potencies of isoprenaline, noradrenaline, prostaglandin E_1 (PGE_1) and $PGF_{2\alpha}$, on mediator release from human lung fragments, closely correlated with their capacity to elevate tissue levels of cyclic AMP (Tauber *et al.*, 1973). Conversely, α-adrenergic agonists and muscarinic cholinergic agonists which lower tissue cyclic AMP levels and increase cyclic GMP levels, respectively, enhanced mediator release (Kaliner *et al.*, 1972; Kaliner, 1977). Thus, based on pharmacologic intervention, it seemed likely that mediator release from mast cells was dependent upon a fall in the cellular level of cyclic AMP, a rise in cyclic GMP, or both. To test this hypothesis, Hitchcock (1977) immunologically challenged sensitized guinea-pig lung fragments and showed a fall in whole tissue adenylate cyclase activity 2·5 min after challenge, when histamine release was approaching maximum. Other investigators, however, found that IgE-dependent mediator release from human (Platshon and Kaliner, 1978) and guinea-pig (Mathé *et al.*, 1977) lung fragments was associated with increases rather than decreases in cyclic nucleotide levels and suggested that these changes were secondary to the effects of released mediators such as histamine and prostaglandins.

As mast cells are a minor subpopulation in lung fragments, measurement of whole tissue levels of cyclic nucleotides cannot be employed to define the intracellular changes in cyclic nucleotides which accompany mast cell activation-secretion.

Changes in cyclic nucleotide levels associated with the immunologic activation of purified rat serosal mast cells

The intracellular concentrations of cyclic AMP in unstimulated rat mast cells measured by protein binding assay (Norn *et al.*, 1977; Fredholm *et al.*, 1976), protein kinase activation (Johnson *et al.*, 1974) and radioimmunoassay (Gripenberg *et al.*, 1974; Lewis *et al.*, 1979) fall in the range of 0·2–2 pmol/10^6 mast cells. However, considerable variations occur from one preparation to another which, in part, can be attributed to the effects of different buffer media, temperature, pH and calcium ion concentrations (Sullivan *et al.*, 1975a). By subcellular fractionation, more than 90% of the total cellular content of cyclic AMP was found in relation to the mast cell granules; and in morphologically intact rat mast cells, this cyclic AMP was protein-bound (Sullivan and Parker, 1976). This subcellular distribution of cyclic AMP is unusual since in other eukaryotic cells only about half of the total cellular content of cyclic AMP is bound to protein and that which is unbound is in the cytosol (Terasaki and Brooker, 1977). Unstimulated rat mast cells contain 0·1–0·5 pmol cyclic GMP/10^6 mast cells (Lewis *et al.*, 1979; Ishizaka *et al.*, in press) but at present its subcellular localization is unknown.

Early studies on the activation of rat serosal mast cells to release histamine by either the calcium inophore A23187 (Marquardt *et al.*, 1978), compound 48/80 (Gillespie, 1973; Sullivan *et al.*, 1957b) and antirat F(ab) (Kaliner and Austen, 1974) demonstrated a fall in the intracellular level of cyclic AMP in relation to histamine release. The possibility that these findings were the result of elevated resting levels of cyclic AMP, activation of phosphodiesterase or interaction of the agonist with cyclic AMP itself, were considered subsequently when detailed kinetic studies revealed that immunologic mast cell activation was associated with a rise rather than a fall in cellular levels of cyclic AMP. Activation of rat mast cells with either antirat IgE or concanavalin A, both of which also secondarily bridge IgE-Fc receptors, results in a monophasic increase in cyclic AMP within 15 s and a late monophasic increase at 2–5 min (Sullivan *et al.*, 1976; Lewis *et al.*, 1979; Ishizaka *et al.*, in press).

Preincubation and immunologic challenge of mast cells in the presence of 10 μM indomethacin, a reversible inhibitor of cyclo-oxygenase, completely ablated both mast cell prostaglandin production and the second monophasic increase in cyclic AMP, but had no effect on histamine release (Lewis *et al.*, 1979). After immunologic mast cell activation, newly formed phospholipids are cleaved by phospholipase A_2 (Ho and Orange, 1978) and phospholipase C (Kennerly *et al.*, 1979a, b) to generate arachidonic acid which is rapidly metabolized to PGD_2, the major product, and PGI_2 (Lewis *et al.*, in press). Since PGD_2 generation is largely complete within 30 s of mast cell activation (Lewis *et al.*, in press) and both PGD_2 and PGI_2 are able to transiently elevate mast cell levels of cyclic AMP (Holgate *et al.*, 1980a), the second monophasic increase in cyclic AMP observed with immunologic mast cell activation is attributed to these products. Thus, only the early indomethacin-resistant rise in cyclic AMP could represent a primary step in the mast cell degranulation process.

IgE-dependent mast cell activation also stimulated a 2- to 3-fold early monophasic increase in cyclic GMP which follows that of cyclic AMP in peaking 30 s after challenge (Lewis *et al.*, 1979; Ishizaka *et al.*, in press) and is itself followed by a smaller second monophasic increase in cyclic GMP after 3–5 min. Since indomethacin ablates both monophasic increases in cyclic GMP without influencing mediator release, alterations in mast cell cyclic GMP levels are unrelated to the primary events of mast cell secretion; rather, they are likely to be secondary to the generation of the prostaglandin endoperoxides PGG_2 and PGH_2 which, in the platelet, are activators of guanylate cyclase (Glass *et al.*, 1976).

That the immunologic stimulus activates membrane adenylate cyclase is indicated by the synergistic rise in cyclic AMP which accompanies IgE-dependent mast cell activation in the presence of the phosphodiesterase inhibitor, theophylline (Holgate *et al.*, 1980a). Both the initial monophasic increase in rat mast cell cyclic AMP and the stimulation of membrane phosphilipid methylation occur within 15 s (Lewis *et al.*, 1979; Ishizaka *et al.*, 1980), but nonetheless appear to be independent of one another. Inhibition of phospholipid methylation prevents mediator release but does not affect the early rise in cyclic AMP (Ishizaka *et al.*, in press); similarly, inhibition of mast cell adenylate cyclase activity with 2′,5′-dideoxyadenosine inhibits mediator release, but has no effect on membrane lipid methylation (Holgate, Lewis and Austen—unpublished observation). The recent report by Ishizaka *et al.* (in press), that DFP prevents the early increases in both cyclic AMP and phospholipid methylation after immunologic mast cell activation, suggests that both events are initiated by a membrane serine esterase which becomes activated by IgE-Fc receptor dimerization (Becker and Austen, 1966).

Biochemical and functional compartmentalization of the effects of cyclic AMP in the mast cell

The finding that the IgE-Fc receptor bridging on purified rat serosal mast cells to initiate mediator release is associated with a rise in the intracellular level of cyclic AMP appears to contradict the earlier studies showing that pharmacologically induced elevations in cyclic AMP levels suppressed release. More recent studies have demonstrated the limitations of measuring cellular cyclic AMP levels alone in that an increase may augment, suppress or have no effect on mediator release. Theophylline and aminophylline, inhibitors of phosphodiesterase, produce dose-dependent inhibition of rat mast cell mediator release which closely correlates with intracellular levels of cyclic AMP (Kaliner and Austen, 1974; Sullivan *et al.*, 1975a, b; Fredholm *et al.*, 1976; Norn *et al.*, 1977; Holgate *et al.*, 1980a). Further, when mast cell immunologic activation-secretion is inhibited by either dibutyryl cyclic AMP or theophylline, calcium ion influx is also inhibited (Foreman *et al.*, 1977). In contrast, these agents are without effect on mast cell secretion induced by the calcium ionophore A23187, suggesting that a site for the inhibitory effect of cyclic AMP on the immunologic release reaction is before calcium influx. Since both membrane lipid phosphorylation (Kennerly *et al.*, 1979b) and phospholipid methylation (Ishizaka *et al.*, in press) may be inhibited by intracellular elevations in cyclic AMP, one effect of cyclic AMP may be to prevent the opening of calcium channels in the cell membrane. Studies in other homogeneous cell systems demonstrate additional sites at which cyclic AMP may exert a regulatory action such as the inhibition of microtubule disassembly (Sloboda *et al.*, 1975) or the inhibition of myosin light-chain kinase, an enzyme which facilitates the energy-dependent interaction of myosin with actin in contractile filaments (Adelstein *et al.*, 1978).

Not all pharmacologic agents which elevate rate mast cell levels of cyclic AMP are inhibitory to the release reaction. The β-adrenergic agonists adrenaline, isoprenaline and salbutamol (Johnson *et al.*, 1974; Sullivan *et al.*, 1975b; Butchers *et al.*, 1979) and the phosphodiesterase inhibitor isobutylmethylxanthine (Norn *et al.*, 1977; 1979) not only fail to inhibit mast cell mediator release, but in some cases lead to enhancement. Both PGD_2 and PGI_2 produce transient (15–20 s) 2- to 3-fold increases in mast cell levels of cyclic AMP without inhibiting the release of mediators (Holgate *et al.*, 1980a). When theophylline was combined with PGD_2 to achieve a synergistic rise in cyclic AMP, the inhibition of mediator release was no greater than that obtained with theophylline alone. Therefore, if the inhibitory action of theophylline on mediator release from rat mast cells is due to increased levels of cyclic AMP, the inability of PGD_2, β-adrenergic agonists and isobutylmethylxanthine also to produce inhibition by increasing cyclic AMP suggests separate pools of cyclic AMP, only one of which decreases coupled activation-secretion.

Recent studies in this laboratory indicate that the early rise in cyclic AMP is essential to mediator release and thus cannot solely be a negative feedback step. The role of adenylate cyclase in IgE-dependent mast cell activation was probed utilizing analogues of adenosine which either directly inhibit the action of adenylate cyclase on adenosine 5′-triphosphate (ATP) or stimulate adenylate cyclase at a site independent of the immunologic stimulus. A receptor which stimulates adenylate cyclase in most cell types, the "R" site, is located on the external surface of the cell membrane, is activated by low concentrations of adenosine or adenosine analogues which have been modified in the purine ring and is inhibited by low concentrations of theophylline (Londos and Wolff, 1977; Haslam *et al.*, 1978; Fain and Malbon, 1979). The inhibitory effects of high concentrations of adenosine via its conversion of 5′-AMP or by ribose modified analogues on adenylate cyclase activity, are mediated via a site located on the intracellular face of the cell membrane. The latter receptor exhibits structural specificity for an intact purine and has thus been designated the "P" site.

Histamine release from rat mast cells activated by the calcium ionophore A23187, compound 48/80, concanavalin A, or anti-IgE was enhanced by 10^{-11}–10^{-5} M adenosine (Marquardt *et al.*, 1978; Welton and Simko, 1980). This effect of adenosine was characteristic of "R" site stimulation, since it was inhibited by low concentrations of theophylline (1–100 μM) which were insufficient to inhibit phosphodiesterase activity, was reproduced by purine analogues of adenosine which could not penetrate the cell membrane, and was unaffected by dipyridamole, an inhibitor of adenosine uptake. In studies where cellular levels of cyclic AMP were also measured, both adenosine and its purine analogue N^6-phenylisopropyladenosine (PIA) (10^{-8}–10^{-4} M) produced dose-related enhancement of immunologic mediator release which was paralleled by a stimulant effect on mast cell levels of cyclic AMP. While both adenosine and PIA elevated mast cell cyclic AMP, this elevation alone failed to induce mediator release over the range of drug concentrations studied. Differences in the ED_{50} values for the increase in mediator release and cyclic AMP levels (Table I), suggest that only 7–10% of adenylate cyclase activity stimulated by the adenosine analogues was at "R" sites linked to occupied IgE-Fc receptors.

Preincubation of purified rat mast cells with either the ribose modified adenosine analogue 2′,5′-dideoxyadenosine (DDA), or 9-(tetrahydo-2-furyl)

TABLE I

Effects of adenosine and N^6*-phenylisopropyladenosine on mast cell immunologic β-hexosaminidase release and cyclic AMP levels*

Pharmacologic agent	Maximum response, % of Control[a]		ED_{50} (M)	
	β-Hexosaminidase release	*Cyclic AMP*	*β-Hexosaminidase release*	*Cyclic AMP*
Adenosine	157 ± 4	323 ± 25	$2{\cdot}5 \times 10^{-7}$	$4{\cdot}0 \times 10^{-6}$
N^6-Phenyliso-propyladenosine	138 ± 3	315 ± 33	10^{-7}	$3{\cdot}3 \times 10^{-6}$

[a] Control refers to cells stimulated with anti-rat IgE alone; the data represent the mean of 5 experiments ± 1 s.e.

adenine (SQ22536), produced a dose-related inhibition of IgE-dependent mediator release from purified rat mast cells (Fig. 1). Assessment of cyclic

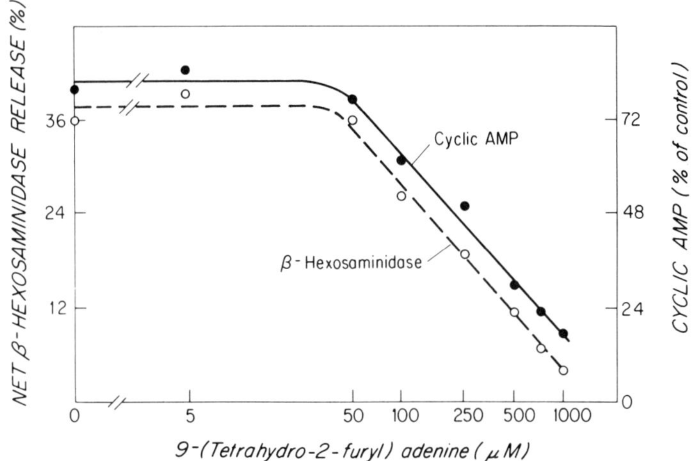

FIG. 1. *Dose-related effects of 9-(tetrahydro-2-furyl) adenine (SQ22536) on rat mast cell net percent β-hexosaminidase release (○- - -○) and on the increase in cyclic AMP associated with immunologic challenge with rabbit Ig antirat IgE (●——●). The results represent the mean of 2 experiments. The mean baseline level of cyclic AMP (260 fmol/10^6 mast cells) was not significantly altered by SQ22536.*

AMP levels measured 15 s after challenge showed that both analogues also caused a parallel dose-dependent suppression of the specific increase in cyclic AMP produced by immunologic activation (Fig. 1). The findings that independent stimulation of mast cell adenylate cyclase by adenosine and PIA acting at the "R" site enhance the release of mediators dependent upon the simultaneous bridging of IgE-Fc receptors and that inhibition of adenylate cyclase by DDA and SQ22536 acting at the "P" site suppress immunologic mediator release, indicate that stimulation of mast cell adenylate cyclase is an integral and obligatory event facilitating granule exocytosis.

Bridging of IgE-Fc receptors on the mast cell surface stimulates adenylate cyclase through a coupling protein which may equate to the DFP-inhibitable membrane serine esterase (Becker and Austen, 1966; Anderson *et al.*, 1978; Ishizaka *et al.*, in press). The activation sequence (Fig. 2), by analogy to adenylate cyclase in other cells, is completed by functional association by a guanosine 5′-triphosphate (GTP)-dependent mechanism of a regulatory protein with the catalytic protein of the cyclase converting the latter from a low to a high catalytic state. Termination of high catalytic activity occurs when all the bound GTP is converted to guanosine 5′-diphosphate (GDP) by the simultaneous uncovering of GTPase activity. The adenosine "R" site is precoupled to the regulatory protein of adenylate cyclase (Tolkovsky and Levitzki, 1978), and stimulation of this site also activates the catalytic subunit by a GTP-dependent mechanism. Occupation of the "P" site by ribose modi-

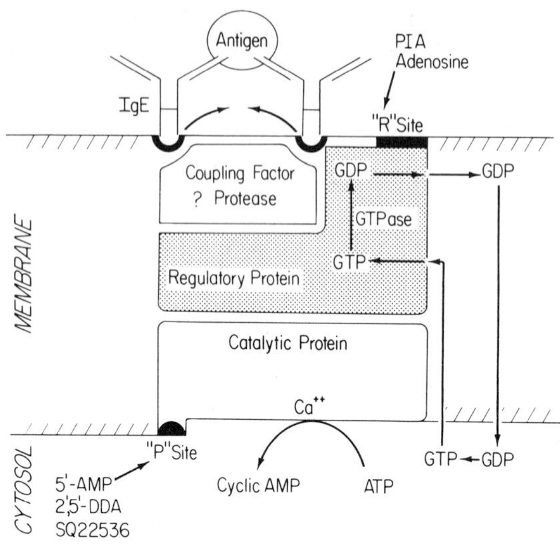

FIG. 2. *Schematic representation of the IgE-Fc receptor-linked adenylate cyclase complex in the plasma membrane of the rat serosal mast cell. Abbreviations used: PIA, N^6-phenylisopropyladenosine; 5′-AMP,-5′-adrenosine monophosphate; 2′,5′-DDA,-2′,5′-dideoxyadenosine; SQ22536, 9-(tetrahydro-2-furyl) adenine; "R" site, ribose requiring adenosine receptor; "P" site, purine requiring adenosine receptor.*

fied adenosine analogues inhibits the catalytic protein directly (Fain and Malbon, 1979). Thus, the net result of the transmembrane signal initiated by bridging of IgE-Fc receptors is the activation of a well-regulated membrane adenylate cyclase so as to yield a transient increase in cytoplasmic levels of cyclic AMP.

Cyclic AMP-dependent protein kinases of the rat mast cell and their differential activation

In eukaryotic cells the effects of cyclic AMP are mediated through the activation of cyclic AMP-dependent protein kinases. Cyclic AMP reversibly binds to a regulatory protein (R) and dissociates an active catalytic subunit (C) from inactive tetrameric holoenzyme (R_2C_2), as depicted by the following scheme:

$$\underset{\text{inactive}}{R_2C_2} + 2\text{ cyclic AMP} \rightleftharpoons (\text{R-cyclic AMP})_2 + \underset{\text{active}}{2C}$$

In the presence of Mg^{++}, the free catalytic subunit cleaves adenosine 5′-triphosphate (ATP) to phosphorylate serine and threonine residues of selective protein substrates (for review, see: Nimmo and Cohen, 1977). Protein kinase activity measured in highly purified rat serosal mast cell preparations by the incorporation of ^{32}P from γ-^{32}P-ATP into protamine sulphate amounted to

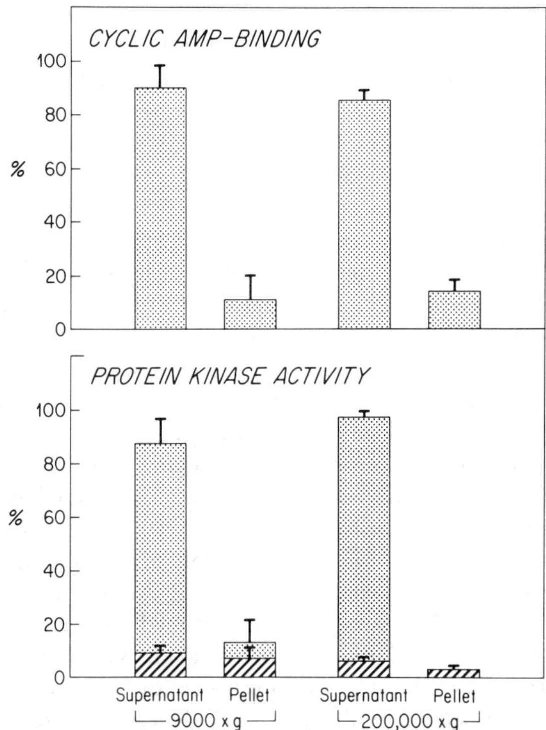

FIG. 3. *Subcellular distribution of rat mast cell cyclic AMP binding (upper panel) and of protein kinase activity assayed in the absence (hatched area) and presence (stippled area) of cyclic AMP (lower panel). The bars represent the mean of 4 experiments ± 1 s.d. in which cyclic AMP binding and protein kinase in the subcellular fractions are expressed as a percentage of the mean values obtained in the whole cell lysates.*

18·2 ± 3·9 (mean ± 1 s.d., n = 6) units of cyclic AMP-dependent activity, and 2·34 ± 0·46 units of cyclic AMP-independent activity/10^6 mast cells (Holgate *et al.*, 1980b). Subcellular fractionation of protein kinase activity from distilled water lysates of 30 × 10^6 rat mast cells of >95% purity revealed that more than 85% of the original activity remained in 9000 × *g* and 200 000 × *g* supernatants and was almost all cyclic AMP-dependent (Fig. 3). The remaining protein kinase activity identified in the 9000 × *g* and 200 000 × *g* cell pellets, and therefore membrane-bound, was predominantly independent of cyclic AMP for activity. When the cyclic AMP-binding capacity of the same subcellular fractions was assessed by the method of Gilman *et al.* (1970), it closely correlated with the cyclic AMP-dependent protein kinase activity (Fig. 3). Discrepancy in the apparent subcellular localization of cyclic AMP-binding proteins from the earlier findings using immunofluorescent detection of cyclic AMP (Sullivan and Parker, 1976) might arise if the cyclic AMP-dependent protein kinase is only loosely associated with the perigranular membrane and is leached off during distilled water lysis. Alternatively, if most of the protein kinase in the cytoplasm of the resting cell is present as holoenzyme, it would not be detectable with antibody to cyclic AMP.

The effect of immunologic activation of rat mast cells on the activity state of cyclic AMP-dependent protein kinase was investigated by Sephadex G-100 gel filtration which separates free catalytic subunit (C) from holoenzymes (R_2C_2) (Holgate *et al.*, 1980b). Rat mast cells activated with an IgG fraction of rabbit antirat $F(ab')_2$ at 37°C for 60 s, disrupted and filtered on Sephadex G-100 at 4°C, have a decrement in the cyclic AMP-dependent protein kinase activity filtering as holoenzymes and an increment in protein kinase activity filtering as free catalytic subunit (Holgate *et al.*, 1980b). In four experiments, immunologic mast cell activation caused a 3-fold increase in the ratio of free catalytic subunit to total enzyme activity ($R_2C_2 + C$) when compared to unstimulated cells. Furthermore, histamine release from mast cells challenged with increasing concentrations of rabbit antirat $F(ab')_2$ was related inversely to the residual cellular concentrations of holoenzymes.

The apparent discrepant findings that immunologic mediator release from mast cells requires the activation of adenylate cyclase to generate cyclic AMP, that elevations in cyclic AMP by inhibition of phosphodiesterase inhibit mediator release, and that elevations in cyclic AMP through activation of adenylate cyclase by PGD_2 have no effect on mediator release, may relate to the spatial and temporal relationships between adenylate cyclase, cyclic AMP-dependent protein kinases and the substrates for protein kinase. The mast cell contains two isoenzymes of cyclic AMP-dependent protein kinase which can be resolved by DEAE-cellulose chromatography (Holgate *et al.*, 1980b). Thus, the differential or failure of protein kinase activation by a stimulus acting via cyclic AMP could, in part, determine the physiologic effect of that stimulus. As shown in Fig. 4, unstimulated rat mast cells containing 400 fmol of cyclic AMP/10^6 mast cells, contain protein kinase activity representing the Type I and Type II isoenzymes. Pretreatment of cells with 7mM theophylline, which increased cellular levels of cyclic AMP to 900 fmol/10^6 mast cells, markedly reduced the quantity of both Type I and Type II holoenzymes identified by DEAE-cellulose chromatography. Comparison of the eluting activities revealed a 73% activation of Type I isoenzyme and a 36% activation of Type II as a consequence of theophylline treatment. The combination of theophylline with PGD_2, although raising total cyclic AMP levels to 1400 fmol/10^6 mast cells, failed to activate additional isoenzymes in that the activities of the isoenzymes eluted were identical to those obtained with cells treated with theophylline alone. Thus, the inability of PGD_2-mediated increases in cellular cyclic AMP to have a measurable biologic effect on mast cell coupled activation-secretion is explicable by a failure to activate a cyclic AMP-dependent protein kinase. In contrast, theophylline increases cyclic AMP, activates cyclic AMP-dependent protein kinase, and inhibits mediator release over the same dose range. Preliminary experiments in which mast cells were challenged with an IgG fraction of rabbit antirat IgE in the presence of 4mM theophylline, which alone had minimal effects on levels of cyclic AMP or

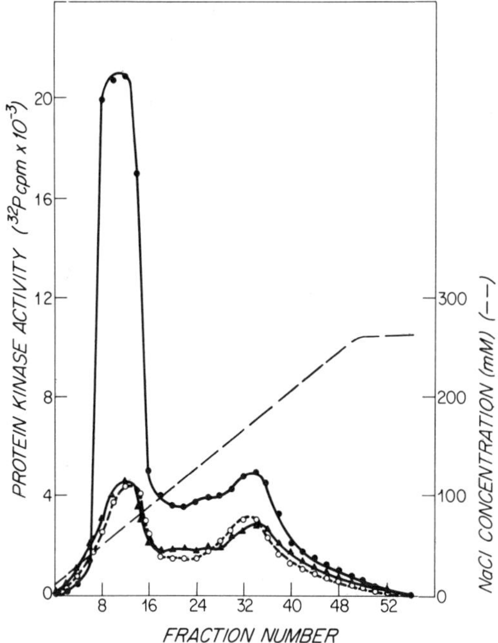

FIG. 4. *DEAE-cellulose chromatography of rat mast cell cyclic AMP-dependent protein kinase obtained from each of 3 preparations of 22·5 × 10^6 mast cells preincubated for 15 min at 37°C in either Tyrode's buffer (●——●), 7 mM theophylline (▲——▲), or 7 mM theophylline + 2 μM PGD_2 (○·····○). Each column was equilibrated in 10 mM KPh, pH 6·8, washed with equilibration buffer, and eluted with a 15 ml linear gradient of NaCl to 300 mM; 200 μl fractions were collected.*

protein kinase activation, revealed a preferential activation of the Type I isoenzyme by the immunologic stimulus. Thus, although the inhibitory action of theophylline on the release reaction could be due to cyclic AMP-dependent phosphorylation and inactivation of a critical protein in the reaction sequence, an alternative possibility is that depletion of the Type I cyclic AMP-dependent holoenzyme *per se* prevents progression of the mast cell activation-secretion process. The responses of mast cells to cyclic AMP are, thus, directed by more complex factors than can be appreciated by either the measurement of the total pool of cellular cyclic AMP or the activation state of the combined cyclic AMP-dependent protein kinase holoenzymes. The model that best fits the experimental data requires the presence of specific receptor-adenylate cyclase complexes, which, on stimulation, are capable of generating cyclic AMP at specific intracellular loci. This leads to the activation of specific protein kinase isoenzyme(s) and subsequent phosphorylation of proteins occurring either with or without translocation of the catalytic subunit.

Hypothetically, cyclic AMP could exert an agonist influence on the release reaction by enhancing calcium uptake and redistribution within the cell, as has recently been reported, for regulation of the contractile state of cardiac muscle by the cyclic AMP-dependent phosphorylation of a specific protein in the sarcoplasmic reticulum (Walsh *et al.*, 1979). Alternatively, cyclic AMP may stimulate anion transport across the mast cell perigranular membrane with subsequent granule swelling and partial solubilization of the granular matrix (Caulfield *et al.*, 1980). Permeable anions are obligatory for the energy-dependent degranulation of adrenal medulla cells, parathyroid cells and human platelets (Pollard *et al.*, 1977; Brown *et al.*, 1978), and it is well established that cyclic AMP, through phosphorylation of membrane proteins, is able to control ion permeability of both extracellular and intracellular membranes (Strewler and Orloff, 1977). The swelling of the granule may, in turn, be the signal for movement towards the cell surface, while the parallel events following upon phospholipid methylation and cleavage may elaborate principles which facilitate membrane fusion and final exposure of the granule contents to the extracellular environment.

References

Adelstein, R. S., Conti, M. A. and Hathaway, D. R. (1978). *J. Biol. Chem.* **253**, 8347.

Anderson, W. B., Janorski, C. J. and Vlahakis, G. (1978). *J. Biol. Chem.* **253**, 2921.

Assem, E. S. K. and Schild, H. O. (1969). *Int. Arch. All. Appl. Immunol.* **40**, 576.

Becker, E. L. and Austen, K. F. (1966). *J. Exp. Med.* **124**, 379.

Brown, E. M., Pazoles, C. J., Creutz, C. E., Auerbach, G. D. and Pollard, H. B. (1978). *Proc. Natn. Acad. Sci. U.S.A.* **75**, 876.

Butchers, P. R., Fullarton, J. R., Skidmore, I. F., Thompson, L. E., Vardey, C. J. and Wheeldon, A. (1979). *Br. J. Pharmacol.* **67**, 23.

Caulfield, J. P., Lewis, R. A., Hein, A. and Austen, K. F. (1980). *J. Cell Biol.* **85**, 299.

Fain, J. N. and Malbon, C. C. (1979). *Molec. Cell. Biochem.* **25**, 143.

Foreman, J. C., Hallett, M. B. and Mongar, J. L. (1977). *J. Physiol. (Lond.)* **271**, 193.

Fredholm, B. B., Guschin, I., Elwin, K., Schwab, G. and Uvnas, B. (1976). *Biochem. Pharmacol.* **25**, 1583.

Gillespie, E. (1973). *Experientia* **29**, 447.

Gilman, A. G. (1970). *Proc. Natn. Acad. Sci. U.S.A.* **67**, 305.

Glass, D. B., Carr, D. W., Gerrard, J. M., Townsend, D., White, J. G. and Goldberg, N. D. (1976). *Proc. Fed. Am. Socs. Exp. Biol.* **35**, 456.

Gripenberg, J., Härkönen, M. and Hansson, S. E. (1974). *Acta Physiol. Scand.* **90**, 648.

Haslam, R. J., Davidson, M. M. L. and Desjardins, J. V. (1978). *Biochem. J.* **176**, 83.

Hirata, F. and Axelrod, J. (1978). *Nature* **279**, 219.

Hirata, F., Axelrod, J. and Crews, F. T. (1979). *Proc. Natn. Acad. Sci. U.S.A.* **76**, 4813.

Hitchock, M. (1977). *J. Immunol.* **118**, 578.

Ho, P. C. and Orange, R. P. (1978). *Proc. Fed. Am. Soc. Exp. Biol.* **37**, 1667.

Holgate, S. T., Lewis, R. A., Maquire, J. F., Roberts, L. J. II, Oates, J. A. and Austen, K. F. (1980a). *J. Immunol.* (in press).

Holgate, S. T., Lewis, R. A. and Austen, K. F. (1980b). *J. Immunol.* **124**, 2093.

Ishizaka, T., Ishizaka, K., Orange, R. P. and Austen, K. F. (1970). *J. Immunol.* **104**, 335.

Ishizaka, T., Hirata, F., Ishizaka, K. and Axelrod, J. (1980). *Proc. Natn. Acad. Sci. U.S.A.* **77**, 1903.

Ishizaka, T., Hirata, F., Ishizaka, K. and Axelrod, J. (in press). *In* "Biochemistry of the Acute Allergic Reaction, Fourth International Symposium" (E. L. Becker and K. F. Austen, eds). Alan R. Liss, Inc., New York.

Johnson, A. R., Moran, N. C. and Mayer, S. E. (1974). *J. Immunol.* **112**, 511.

Kaliner, M. (1977). *J. All. Clin. Immunol.* **60**, 204.

Kaliner, M. and Austen, K. F. (1974). *J. Immunol.* **112**, 664.

Kaliner, M., Orange, R. P. and Austen, K. F. (1972). *J. Exp. Med.* **136**, 556.

Kennerly, D. A., Sullivan, T. J. and Parker, C. W. (1979a). *J. Immunol.* **122**, 152.

Kennerly, D. A., Sullivan, T. J., Sylwester, P. and Parker, C. W. (1979b). *J. Exp. Med.* **150**, 1039.

Lewis, R. A., Wasserman, S. I., Goetzl, E. J. and Austen, K. F. (1974). *J. Exp. Med.* **140**, 1133.

Lewis, R. A., Holgate, S. T., Roberts, J. L. II, Maguire, J. F., Oates, J. A. and Austen, K. F. (1979). *J. Immunol.* **123**, 1663.

Lewis, R. A., Holgate, S. T., Roberts, J. L. II, Oates, J. A. and Austen, K. F. (in press). *In* "Biochemistry of the Acute Allergic Reaction, Fourth International Symposium" (E. L. Becker and K. F. Austen, eds) Alan R. Liss, Inc., New York.

Lichtenstein, L. M. and Margolis, S. (1968). *Science* **161**, 902.

Londos, C. and Wolff, J. (1977). *Proc. Nat. Acad. Sci. U.S.A.* **74**, 5482.

Marquardt, D. L., Parker, C. W. and Sullivan, T. J. (1978). *J. Immunol.* **120**, 871.

Mathé, A. A., Yen, S. S., Sohn, R. and Hedqvist, P. (1977). *Biochem. Pharmacol.* **26**, 181.

Morita, Y., Cantoni, G. L. and Siriganian, P. (1980). *Proc. Fed. Am. Soc. Exp. Biol.* **39**, 695.

Nimmo, H. G. and Cohen, P. (1977). *Adv. Cyc. Nucl. Res.* **8**, 145.

Norn, S., Geisler, A., Stahl Skov, P. and Klysner, R. (1977). *Acta Allerg.* **32**, 183.

Norn, S., Geisler, A., Stahl Skov, P. and Klysner, R. (1979). *Ag. Act.* **9**, 64.

Orange, R. P., Austen, W. G. and Austen, K. F. (1971). *J. Exp. Med.* **134**, 136s.

Platshon, L. F. and Kaliner, M. (1978). *J. Clin. Invest.* **62**, 1113.

Pollard, H. B., Tack-Goldman, K., Pazoles, C. J., Creutz, C. E. and Shulman, N. R. (1977). *Proc. Nat. Acad. Sci. U.S.A.* **74**, 5295.

Schild, H. (1936). *Q. J. Exp. Physiol.* **26**, 165.

Sloboda, R. D., Rudolph, S. A., Rosenbaum, J. L. and Greengard, P. (1975). *Proc. Nat. Acad. Sci. U.S.A.* **72**, 177.

Strewler, G. J. and Orloff, J. (1977). *Adv. Cyc. Nucl. Res.* **8**, 311.

Sullivan, T. J. and Parker, C. W. (1976). *Am. J. Pathol.* **85**, 437.

Sullivan, T. J., Parker, K. L., Stenson, W. and Parker, C. W. (1975a). *J. Immunol.* **114**, 1473.

Sullivan, T. J., Parker, K. L., Eisen, S. A. and Parker, C. W. (1975b). *J. Immunol.* **114**, 1480.

Sullivan, T. J., Parker, K. L., Kulczycki, A. Jr. and Parker, C. W. (1976). *J. Immunol.* **117**, 713.

Tauber, A. I., Kaliner, M., Stechschulte, D. J. and Austen, K. F. (1973). *J. Immunol.* **111**, 27.

Terasaki, W. L. and Brooker, G. (1977). *J. Biol. Chem.* **252**, 1041.

Tolkovsky, A. M. and Levitzki, A. (1978). *Biochemistry (Washington)* **17**, 3811.

Walsh, D. A., Clippinger, M. S., Sivaramakrishnan, S. and McCullough, T. E. (1979). *Biochemistry (Washington)* **18**, 871.

Welton, A. F. and Simko, B. A. (1980). *Biochem. Pharmacol.* **29**, 1085.

49

Lymphokines in Delayed Hypersensitivity

STANLEY COHEN

University of Connecticut Health Center, Farmington, Connecticut, USA

Introduction

It is now generally accepted that, with the exception of cell-mediated cytotoxicity, most of the manifestations of cellular immunity are due to the effects of lymphokines. These lymphocyte-derived, soluble factors that are involved in effector functions are, in turn, related to other lymphocyte-derived macromolecules that participate in the afferent arm of the immune response. The latter include the myriad antigen-specific and nonspecific helper and suppressor factors described to date. The stimuli for both these kinds of lymphokines are antigens or mitogens. Originally it was thought that lympho-

Some of the work detailed here was supported by NIH grants AI-12358 and AI-12477.

kines were exclusively T cell products. In 1973, we demonstrated that B as well as T cells could make MIF provided that the appropriate stimulating agent was used (Yoshida *et al.*, 1973), and this capacity of B cells to make various lymphokines has been confirmed extensively in many laboratories (reviewed in Rosenstreich and Wahl, 1979). It has also been found that mediators with similar biologic activities (monokines) can be generated by macrophages stimulated by either phagocytosis or activation by lymphokines, and by a variety of nonlymphoid, noninflammatory cells activated by virus infection. These various factors, which we have collectively defined as "cytokines" (Cohen, 1977), have physicochemical properties that distinguish them from other biologic mediators such as complement components or products of anaphylactic reactions. In the case of lymphokines and virus-induced factors such properties include monosaccharide inhibition profiles (Amsden *et al.*, 1978) and cross-reactivity to certain antisera (Yoshida *et al.*, 1975a).

There is an almost overwhelming spectrum of biologic activities that are mediated by lymphokines as well as the other cytokines. Of these, the philogistic effects of lymphokines represent some of their more important manifestations, and these are seen in perhaps purest form in the traditional cutaneous delayed hypersensitivity reaction.

Delayed hypersensitivity

In general, the delayed hypersensitivity reaction is a slowly evolving inflammatory lesion at the site of antigen injection in suitable sensitized individuals. Usually the reaction takes 24–48 h to reach maximal intensity and size. It has the appearance of a raised, erythematous, indurated lump; a positive tuberculin reaction in man is a familiar example. Microscopically, at least in man and the guinea-pig, the reaction is characterized by a mononuclear cell infiltrate. However, there may be great variability in the histologic appearance. Of the mononuclear cells, most are macrophages. In addition, lymphocytes form a variable proportion of the infiltrating mononuclear cells in delayed reactions, ranging from less than 20% in tuberculin reactions in rats (Weiner *et al.*, 1965) to over 70% in guinea-pig delayed reactions to human γ-globulin (Turk *et al.*, 1966). Until about 15 years ago, it was assumed that the majority of the cells in these reactions were specifically sensitized to the antigen and that they were either attracted to the site or arrested there by the antigen. However, it is now known that only a very small percentage, usually less than 1–4%, of the infiltrating cells are specifically sensitized. Moreover, the bulk of the available evidence suggests that there is little, if any, preferential accumulation of sensitized cells at specific test sites. Most of this evidence is based on transfer studies with radiolabelled sensitized donor lymphocytes, or on experiments utilizing animals immunized with two unrelated antigens and injected with ^{3}H-thymidine in such a manner as to label only proliferating cells of one specificity. In these studies, preferential accumulation was assessed at skin test sites by autoradiography. These studies have been extensively reviewed (McCluskey and Cohen, 1972; McCluskey and Leber, 1974).

In addition to mononuclear cells, basophils, eosinophils and neutrophils accumulate to varying degrees in delayed hypersensitivity responses. In the guinea-pig and man it is possible to induce cell-mediated lesions in which the predominant cell is the basophil. This reaction, known as Jones-Mote or cutaneous basophil hypersensitivity (CBH), is commonly seen after immunization with low doses of antigen either in saline or IFA. CBH is also associated with contact sensitivity, tumour and allograft rejection and vaccinia infection (Dvorak, 1971; Dvorak and Hirsch, 1971; Dvorak and Dvorak, 1972).

Under special circumstances, delayed reactions can be characterized histologically by a striking accumulation of eosinophils. This is commonly seen when parasites serve as the antigenic stimulus or in "retest" reactions. The latter is a rapidly evolving reaction, usually appearing 2 h after antigen has been injected into a healed delayed reaction site that was elicited with the same antigen. This type of lesion reaches maximal size at 6–8 h, unlike the "classical" delayed reactions which usually require 24 h (Arnason and Waksman, 1963).

Neutrophils are observed early in most delayed hypersensitivity reactions and persist if necrosis occurs (Turk *et al.*, 1966; Turk, 1975). Interestingly, in the mouse, the neutrophil is a predominant cell type in all delayed reactions (Crowle, 1975; Cohen, 1977).

The previous examples demonstrate that the typical macrophage-rich reaction represents only one manifestation of delayed hypersensitivity. However, common to all these reactions is a small population of specifically sensitized lymphocytes that have been activated following local antigenic stimulation. As a consequence of this activation, lymphokines are liberated locally and a cellular infiltrate ensues.

The lymphokines

In vitro studies on delayed hypersensitivity were initiated by Rich and Lewis (1932). They demonstrated that antigen inhibited the migration of cells from tissue explants taken from sensitized animals. Thirty years later, George and Vaughan (1962) introduced a modification of the explant technique that utilized peritoneal exudate cells migrating out of capillary tubes. Using this method, Bloom and Bennett (1966) and David (1966) demonstrated that the inhibition of migration of the cells from such tubes was due to a soluble material released from sensitized lymphocytes following antigen stimulation. This soluble factor was called migration inhibition factor (MIF).

Since the description of the MIF assay, numerous other *in vitro* correlates of cellular immunity have been described and all of them, except lymphocyte-dependent cytotoxicity, are dependent on lymphokine activities for effector function.

At present, lymphokines affecting almost all cell types involved in inflammation have been reported. Most studies of mediators utilize supernatants from antigen- or mitogen-stimulated lymphocyte cultures as the lymphokine source and the mediators are defined by their effects on target cells *in vitro*. This methodology presents some difficulties in interpreting the available studies since lymphokines are not biochemically pure entities, but rather elusive molecules in a fluid that contains a *pot-pourri* of biologic activities. At present, at least 50 efferent lymphokines have been described, most of which influence inflammatory cells. The possibility exists that mediators identified by their behaviour in different *in vitro* assays are actually the same molecular species, but, depending on the nature of the assay, they express different activities. Thus, several of the named lymphokines may, in fact, represent artifacts of the assay system (artifactors). One alternative suggestion that has been reviewed in Adelman (1979) is that there is a (small) set of basic building block factors, the "mother factors" from which all of the observed lymphokines are derived. A third possibility is that the lymphokines possess a distinct subunit structure, and that the various possible permutations of a small number of discrete subunits give rise to the observed diversity. The experimental evidence related to this latter concept is largely circumstantial and beyond the scope of the present discussion. However, the recent finding that both monosaccharide inhibition profiles (Amsden *et al.*, 1978) and antilymphokine antibody activity (Kuratsuji *et al.*, 1976) are directed against regions of the lymphokine molecule that code for the target cell specificity, rather than biologic activity, support the possibility that these two lymphokine properties reside on distinct molecular sites.

With these various caveats in mind, it is possible to group lymphokines into well defined categories. Mediators have been described that affect cell surfaces, alter metabolic states, activate cells for enhanced phagocytosis and killing, and change cellular migration patterns. Additionally, there are lymphokines that are directly cytotoxic for various target cells. These kinds of activities suggest the following classification scheme, which encompass afferent as well as the efferent mediators discussed above:

(a) factors affecting cell motility;
(b) factors affecting cell proliferation;
(c) factors affecting cell activation;
(d) factors affecting cell viability.

Of the various efferent mediators known, those best studied are those that affect the behaviour of macrophages.

Lymphokines affecting macrophages

The mediators that affect macrophages represent the best studied group of lymphokines and are the only group that will be described in detail in this brief review.

The incubation of normal macrophages with MIF-containing supernatants or partially purified MIF has profound effects on cellular morphology on the light microscope level. During the first hour of incubation, inhibition of macrophage spreading on surfaces is commonly reported and by 24 h, the macrophages have rounded up, lost pseudopodia and are not very motile (David, 1966). Following 48 h of incubation, the cells exhibit increased spreading with formation of long pseudopods, and cellular aggregates are commonly seen (Lolekha *et al.*, 1970; Dvorak *et al.*, 1972). By 72 h, the macrophages are enlarged, show enhanced adherence to surfaces and demonstrate increased membrane ruffling and amoeboid movements (Nathan *et al.*, 1971). Additionally, there is an enrichment in vacuoles and lysosomal granules in activated cells.

Ultrastructurally, macrophages activated by incubation with MIF-rich fluids, or cocultured with sensitized lymphocytes and antigens, show some alterations, particularly in the plasma membrane. These cells tend to form complex cell aggregates characterized by intensive intercellular contact and loss of normal extramembraneous electron-dense material (Dvorak *et al.*, 1972). Also, these aggregated cells demonstrate an increase in microvilli (Smyth and Weiss, 1970). The observed aggregation may not be due to MIF, but rather to macrophage aggregation factor (MAF/MAgF), a high molecular weight factor which is separable from MIF and causes normal peritoneal macrophages to clump (Lolekha *et al.*, 1970; Postlethwaite and Kang, 1976).

The metabolic activities of macrophages following incubation with lymphokine-containing preparations are also considerably altered. Cellular metabolism studies demonstrate that activation of macrophages by MIF-containing media results in significant increases in glucose oxidation through the hexose monophosphate shunt (HMS) (Nathan *et al.*, 1971). This may be a major step in preparing macrophages for bactericidal activity since the HMS is indirectly involved in the generation of oxygen radicals which are bacteriocidal. Additionally, protein synthesis (Nathan *et al.*, 1971; Nath *et al.*, 1973) and uptake of glucosamine into membrane-associated materials are greatly enhanced (Hammond and Dvorak, 1972; Hammond *et al.*, 1975; Wilton *et al.*, 1975). The latter activity may reflect membrane repair of coat glycoproteins lost during activation or an increase in active membrane transport. Lysosomal enzyme levels are also affected by activation. However, there are conflicting reports on this aspect of macrophage activation. Pantalone and Page (1975, 1977) showed that 72-h incubation of normal mouse peritoneal macrophages with supernatants from mitogen-stimulated human peripheral blood leukocytes significantly enhanced the selective production and secretion of hydrolytic enzymes by these cells. Poulter and Turk (1975) also observed an increase in lysosomal activity following a 72-h incubation of guinea-pig macrophage and lymphokine preparations. This is in sharp contrast to the reports of Remold and Mednis (1972, 1975), which indicate that guinea-pig peritoneal exudate cells incubated in MIF-containing fractions show a consistent decrease in lysosomal enzymes measured after a 48-h incubation. Furthermore, the reduction in hydrolases in their experiments was not the result of enzyme secretion. The discrepancies among these reports are possibly due to the use of macrophages initially in different activation states. Other investigations have seen variation in the potential to activate macrophages *in vitro*, depending upon the level or prior activation achieved *in vivo* (Poulter, 1976; Unanue *et al.*, 1976).

MIF-rich fractions can also induce an increase in the levels of membrane-bound adenylate cyclase in the macrophage over the first 48 h of incubation, followed by a decrease at 72 h. The role of this enzyme in activated macrophages is unclear since MIF-inhibited macrophages do not show any increase in whole cell cAMP levels at any time during a 72-h incubation (Higgins *et al.*, 1973; Remold-O'Donnell and Remold, 1974).

Additional metabolic studies have shown that lymphokine-activated macrophages can secrete biologically active molecules that could be of considerable importance at an inflamed site. Wahl and coworkers (1975) reported that activated macrophages secrete collagenase into the milieu and Vassalli and Reich (1977) demonstrated that lymphokines could induce the synthesis of plasminogen activator by unstimulated peritoneal macrophages. Release of plasminogen activator could provide an important link between cell-mediated immune reactions and the powerful kinin system. Additionally, human monocytes incubated with lymphokines showed enhanced synthesis of the second component of complement relative to macrophages incubated in control medium. Interestingly, this synthesis could be partially blocked specifically by L-fucose, a sugar known to inhibit the response of macrophage to MIF (Littman and Ruddy, 1977). A recent report by Chao *et al.* (1977) provides supportive evidence that a lymphokine may be responsible for the release of endogenous pyrogen from guinea-pig exudate cells *in vitro*. An earlier report by Atkins *et al.* (1972) indicated the existence of this factor, but the cellular source of endogenous pyrogen was unclear. This lymphokine activity could explain the association between delayed hypersensitivity reactions and fever (von Pirquet, 1911).

Lymphokine treatment of macrophages *in vitro* can alter many functional parameters of these cells. Pinocytosis of colloidal gold (Meade *et al.*, 1974) and neutral red dye (Hammond, unpub. observation) is enhanced, while phagocytosis can either be stimulated or depressed. Nathan *et al.* (1971) reported that killed mycobacteria are readily engulfed by MIF-activated guinea-pig macrophages. Similarly, human monocytes demonstrate a rapid increase in phagocytosis of latex beads following activation (Schmidt *et al.*, 1973). In sharp contrast, Remold and Mednis (1972) found a depression in the uptake of aggregated, denatured haemoglobin, even though the protein adhered to the macrophage surface. Neta and Salvin (1971) also reported a reduction in the ability of mediator-activated macrophage to ingest *Candida albicans*. These results suggest that surface properties of both the particle and the activated cell play an important role in determining the kinetics of phagocytosis (David, 1975). Interestingly, a factor that is thought to alter the macrophage membrane has been reported. This activity, migration slowing factor (MSF), is defined by its ability to decrease macrophage motility in an electrical field (Caspary, 1971, 1972; Carnegie *et al.*, 1973) and requires protein synthesis on the part of the indicator macrophages for expression (Caspary, 1971). MSF is thought to act by changing the net electrical charge on the plasma membrane. The requirement for macrophage protein synthesis may reflect the addition of glycoproteins to the membrane or activities of activatable enzymes that either directly or indirectly remodel the membrane. In addition to changes in membrane electrical characteristics, Thrasher and coworkers (1973) demonstrated that MIF-rich fluids alter the "surface tension" of macrophage membranes. This physical property does not directly reflect the macrophage's surface charge, but rather the molecular composition and configuration of the membrane and any surface coats associated with it. These alterations could be seen following as little as 1 h of incubation of macrophage monolayers with lymphokine-containing culture fluids. This suggests that membrane remodelling is an early event in macrophage activation *in vitro*.

Lymphokines can also augment another important aspect of macrophage function; namely, the ability of these cells to deal with micro-organisms. *In* vitro incubation of macrophages with MIF-rich sources can enhance the bacteriostatic and bacteriocidal properties of these cells (Patterson and Youmans, 1970; Goda *et al.*, 1971; Krahenbuhl and Remington, 1971; Fowles *et al.*, 1973; Anderson and Remington, 1974). For example, Fowles *et al.* (1973) found that lymphokine-activated macrophages exhibit a 2- to 10-fold increase in bacteriostatic activity against *Listeria* and attributed this effect to MIF. Interestingly, in a few cases, the activated macrophages show enhanced capacities to deal with a specific organism; namely, the one used to stimulate the sensitized lymphocytes (Borgis and Johnson, 1974). However, in most cases the antigenicity of the micro-organism is irrelevant indicating the non-specific nature of the activation (Patterson and Youmans, 1970).

Recently, the function of activated macrophages in antitumour activities has received considerable attention (Alexander *et al.*, 1972; Hibbs, 1972; Gottlieb and Waldman, 1972). This activation is known to require an immune response since activated macrophages induced by the injection of nonspecific irritants into the peritoneal cavity are not cytotoxic (Hibbs *et al.*, 1972a, b). Several investigations reveal that lymphokine-rich supernatants can substitute for an immune response and render the macrophage tumouricidal *in vitro* (Nathan *et al.*, 1971; Krahenbuhl *et al.*, 1973; Churchill *et al.*, 1975; Fidler *et al.*, 1977). The specificity of the tumour killing by the activated macrophage is the subject of some controversy. In some *in vitro* systems, the killing is very specific, i.e. only tumour cells that are identical to the neoplastic cells used to activate the sensitized lymphocytes are destroyed (Evans and Alexander, 1970). In other systems, however, the activation seems to be nonspecific and all tumour cells, but not normal cells, are attacked (Piessens *et al.*, 1975). This controversy is probably the result of the independent activities of 2 lymphokines, the specific macrophage arming factor (SMAF) (Evans and Alexander,

1970) and MAF (Churchill *et al.*, 1975; Piessens *et al.*, 1975). SMAF is a product of stimulated T lymphocytes that have interacted with specific tumour antigen and the SMAF produced by the immune reaction activates macrophages to kill solely that tumour (Evans *et al.*, 1972; Lohmann-Matthes *et al.*, 1973). This arming is cytophilic and can be absorbed by macrophages. It can also be absorbed by the specific tumour used to induce it. SMAF may be a cytotoxic receptor shed into the culture medium by the activated lymphocytes (Lohmann-Matthes *et al.*, 1973) or a unique cytophilic antibody (Pels and Den-Otter, 1974). Although there is no direct evidence, it is tempting to speculate that SMAF is another version of the antigen-specific MIF described by Amos and Lachmann (1970). MAF is also a product of antigen-activated lymphocytes, but unlike SMAF, its tumouricidal activity is nonspecific (Piessens *et al.*, 1975; Churchill *et al.*, 1975). This factor is not cytophilic since activated macrophages can be trypsinized without affecting the tumouricidal activity. However, trypsinization of macrophage prior to incubation with MAF prevents acquisition of cytotoxicity (Hibbs *et al.*, 1977) suggesting that there may be a trypsin-sensitive receptor for MAF on the macrophage membrane.

Several additional aspects of macrophage behaviour *in vitro* can be modulated by lymphokines. The haphazard migration patterns of macrophages can be altered by monocyte–macrophage chemotactic factor (MCF). This factor, first described by Ward *et al.* (1969) and found in stimulated guinea-pig lymphocyte culture supernatants, can convert cell movement to enhanced migration in the direction of an increasing concentration gradient of MCF. Conventionally, chemotaxis is measured in Boyden chambers by quantitating the migration of target cells towards chemotactic substances across micropore filters of defined pore size (Boyden, 1962). Similar MCF activities have been defined in human, murine, rat and chicken systems and are reviewed by Altman (1978). As we shall see, this factor is the putative mediator responsible for attracting mononuclear cells to the site of local immune responses *in vivo*. Related to alterations in cell movement, stimulation of enhanced macrophage migration in conventional MIF assays is occasionally seen (David, 1966; Fox *et al.*, 1974; Svejcar and Johanovsky, 1961). This enhancement is attributed to lymphokines that are separable from MIF and MCF by physicochemical means. Several investigators have described this activity and dubbed it macrophage enhancement factor (MEF) (Weisbart *et al.*, 1974) or migration stimulation factor (MStF) (Aaskov and Anthony, 1976). It is quite possible that they are chemically identical. The occurrence of both MIF and MEF in the same supernatant re-emphasizes the difficulty of dealing with crude lymphokine preparations and bioassays.

Finally, two other alterations in the *in vitro* behaviour of macrophages are linked to macrophage activation by lymphokines. The first phenomenon is the occurrence of the proliferation of mature macrophages after incubation with antigen-stimulated lymphocyte culture fluids for 2–8 days (Godal *et al.*, 1971; Hadden *et al.*, 1975). The responsible lymphokine (macrophage mitogen factor or macrophage growth factor) appears to be distinct from MIF and may be implicated in the macrophage proliferation that occurs in delayed hypersensitivity reactions. The second phenomenon is the induction of macrophage fusion with the comcomitant formation of giant cells following incubation of normal macrophage cell-free fluids from BCG-stimulated lymphocyte cultures (Galindo, 1972; Galindo *et al.*, 1974). The relevance of MFF in the formation of giant cells and epithelioid sheets seen in granuloma formation *in vivo* is most intriguing and requires further investigation.

Lymphokines *in vivo*

The definition of the various lymphokine activities has been based solely on semi-quantative *in vitro* assays which utilize well defined target cell populations. It is generally assumed that the extrapolation from these *in vitro* results to *in vivo* conditions presents no problems. However, obtaining evidence to support this inference has been difficult and it has only been in the past few years that sufficient data have been amassed to substantiate a role for lymphokines *in vivo*.

Detection of lymphokine activity *in vivo*

One of the most convincing arguments for an *in vivo* role for the soluble mediators is the demonstration of lymphokine activity in appropriate settings; namely, at the sites of immune responses. Several investigators have found mediator activities in the blood, lymph, synovial fluid, exudates and tissue reaction sites in human and experimental animals. MIF or MIF-like activity was first described by Krejci *et al.* (1968) in the sera of sensitized guinea-pigs following i.v. challenge with high doses of antigen. This report was followed by several others documenting serum MIF in various experimental settings (Yamamoto and Takahashi, 1971; Salvin *et al.*, 1973; Yoshida and Cohen, 1974).

Several reports document the occurrence of MIF identical to conventional antigen-stimulated activity in the sera of humans with lymphoproliferative disorders. Cohen and coworkers (1974a) found serum MIF activity in the majority of patients studied with Hodgkin's disease, non-Hodgkin's lymphoma, chronic lymphocytic leukaemia and myelomas. The presence of this activity did not correlate with any clinical or laboratory measurements available, except possibly disease duration. In addition, these investigators examined patients with Sezary syndrome, a T cell leukaemia characterized by erythroderma, and found significant MIF in the sera of all individuals (Yoshida *et al.*, 1975b). In both studies, the lymphocytes from these patients also produced significant MIF *in vitro*. Normal individuals or patients with nonlymphoid proliferative disease used as controls rarely demonstrated serum lymphokine activity. It is unclear what triggers the release of MIF; possibilities include immunologic activation, a viral infection, the presence of nonspecific mitogenic factors or the proliferative response to the neoplastic cells itself. However, this production may be analogous to the synthesis of lymphokine activities by continuous lymphoblastoid cell lines in the absence of exogenous antigen stimulation (Yoshida *et al.*, 1976).

Recently, serum MIF has been found in patients under conditions that strongly suggest lymphokine liberation as the result of an immune reaction. Torisu *et al.* (1975) found MIF in the serum of all patients studied with posttransplantation hepatic dysfunction resulting from viral hepatitis infection. The release of the mediator preceded elevation of serum glutamic oxalacetic transaminase (SGOT) by approximately 5–10 days. These observations are suggestive of a destructive cellular immune event in the liver of these patients probably directed at virally infected cells. The MIF found in this study resembled conventional MIF produced in stimulated lymphocyte cultures both in biologic effect and physicochemical parameters.

Another lymphokine-like activity has been demonstrated in the sera of humans. Krüger *et al.* (1973) reported the occurrence of MAF-like activity (macrophage aggregation factor) in patients with erythrodema, erythema multiforme and erythema nodosum, but not in normal individuals or patients with other dermatologic diseases. In addition, all erythodermic patients manifested a substance in their sera that produced erythema in guinea-pig skin. No attempts were made to characterize these activities, hence their relationship to conventionally produced lymphokines cannot be assessed.

Stastny and Ziff in a series of reports (1971; Stastny *et al.*, 1973a, b) documented the presence of a MIF-like activity in the joint fluid of patients with rheumatoid arthritis and in rabbits with antigen-induced experimental arthritis. Additionally, they showed that the affected synovial tissues which contained intense mononuclear cell inflammatory infiltrates were capable of producing a similar substance when cultured without exogenous stimulation. The MIF-like activities from both sources resembled conventional rabbit MIF both in physical properties and elution patterns from Sephadex G-200 chromatography columns. Both the joint effusions and the supernatants from the cultured synovial tissues also stimulated ^{3}H-thymidine incorporation by mouse spleen cells indicating the presence of a mitogenic factor. Normal synovial fluid or joint effusion from rabbits with arthritis induced with urate crystals or from humans with osteoarthritis rarely contained any lymphokine-like activity. The presence of these activities in synovial fluid from diseased joints suggests that soluble mediators may be involved in the pathogenesis of certain disease states.

Several other investigators demonstrated lymphokine-like activity in exudates from experimental animals. MIF was detected in the peritoneal exudate fluids of animals undergoing the macrophage disappearance reaction (MDR), a documented manifestation of cell-mediated immunity (Sonozaki *et al.*, 1975). Postlethwaite and Synderman (1975) found monocyte chemotactic factor in the peritoneal fluids of sensitized guinea-pigs exhibiting delayed hypersensitivity following intraperitoneal antigen challenge. By repeated samplings from a permanent catheter placed in the abdominal cavity of these animals, the investigators were able to follow the kinetics of leukocyte accumulation and the production of chemotactic activity. They found that over the first 24 h the number of macrophages and chemotactic stimulus for macrophages in the peritoneal fluid increased significantly over control levels and that between 48 and 72 h the chemotactic activity returned to pre-challenge levels and the macrophages found in the cavity appeared to be actively phagocytic. No other lymphokine activities were evaluated. On the basis of chromatography results and physical properties, the chemotactic factor for macrophages produced *in vivo* is identical to the chemotactic lymphokine found in stimulated lymphocyte cultures.

Many other reports attest to the detectability of various lymphokines at sites of experimental cell-mediated immune responses (reviewed in Adelman *et al.*, 1979).

Injection of exogenous lymphokines

The converse of the experimental design described in the preceding selection, namely, the effect of *administering* lymphokines to animals instead of extracting them, has been tried and it too has yielded data supportive of an *in vivo* role for these mediators. This experimental approach takes advantage of the observation that cell-mediated immune responses can be triggered *in vitro* and the effector molecules synthesized by the activated lymphocytes are released into the surrounding *milieu*. The lymphokines can then be recovered from the culture fluids and administered to experimental animals to determine their effects. Numerous studies have demonstrated that injection of lymphokine-rich culture supernatants into normal animals results in inflammatory responses. Investigations of this type have already been described in the section on lymphokines that affect vascular permeability.

Bennett and Bloom (1968) were the first to report that MIF-rich culture fluids induced an inflammatory response upon intradermal injection into normal guinea-pigs. This activity, which they called SRF (skin reactive factor), was not dissociable from that of the other known lymphokines. This work provided a clue that soluble lymphocyte-derived mediators could be responsible for the evolution of inflammation following a cell-mediated immune response. This report was confirmed by several investigators using slightly modified systems (Dumonde *et al.*, 1969; Schwartz *et al.*, 1970; Pick *et al.*, 1970a, b; Maillard *et al.*, 1972; Yoshida *et al.*, 1973; Yoshida and Cohen, 1974). At present, the molecular make-up of SRF is unknown, but, as mentioned previously, it is probably a "blend" of chemotactic factors and an activity that can alter vascular permeability. Skin reactions induced by this activity start to evolve within 2 h following injection and reach maximal size within 12 h. The reactions fade slowly, but are still apparent at 24 h. The rapidity of SRF-induced reactions, as compared to delayed hypersensitivity reactions elicited by antigen in sensitized animals, probably reflects the fact that preformed mediators are being presented to the animals in high concentrations in the former situation, while in the latter situation *de novo* synthesis of inflammatory mediators must first be initiated.

The macrophage disappearance reaction (MDR) is an *in vivo* model of cell-mediated immunity characterized by the prompt disappearance of macrophages found in nonspecific peritoneal exudates following intraperitoneal antigen challenge in appropriately sensitized animals. Sonozaki and Cohen (1971a, b) demonstrated that passive transfer of an MDR could be effected by intraperitoneal injection of sensitized lymphocytes and specific antigen. Moreover, the MDR transfer was even successful when the lymphocytes were enclosed in micropore chambers that only permitted diffusion of soluble factors during the experiment. Finally, these investigators demonstrated that cell-free MIF-rich supernatants from antigen-stimulated lymphocyte cultures also passively transferred this reaction following intraperitoneal injection into normal guinea-pigs. The supernatants from unstimulated lymphocyte cultures reconstituted with antigen had no effect on the exudate macrophages, thus ruling out an effect of the antigen. Additionally, the supernatants used in these experiments were subjected to Sephadex chromatography to exclude the presence of immunoglobulin. Interestingly, the intraperitoneal injection of MCF extracted from dermal reaction sites did not affect the MDR, rather this activity induced a mononuclear exudate in the peritoneal cavity. This observation, coupled with the inability to isolate MIF from skin test sites, suggests that MIF is responsible for the MDR while MCF induces the infiltrate in cutaneous reactions. These investigators have confirmed this hypothesis in a recent study dealing with desensitization (Sonozaki *et al.*, 1975).

Additional studies involved with administering lymphokine-containing fluids to normal animals have strengthened the inference that these mediators play a role *in vivo*. Cohen and Ward (1971) demonstrated that the injection of activated ECF into normal guinea-pig skin resulted in the prompt formation of an inflammatory focus composed predominantly of eosinophils. The activity of this particular lymphokine may explain the pattern of association of these cells with experimental autoimmune thyroiditis.. Studies of this autoimmune disease model revealed that only animals with lymphocytic infiltration of the thyroid and circulating antibody develop eosinophil infiltrates in the thyroid. Animals with thyroiditis but no antibody did not demonstrate eosinophils within the gland. Neither did animals given antibody passively in amounts equal to those found in the positive experimental animals develop eosinophil infiltrates (Cohen *et al.*, 1974b). Interestingly, the eosinophils were not found within the areas of greatest lymphocytic infiltration but rather they were found between those areas and the connective tissue surrounding blood vessels. This pattern suggests that the eosinophils were appearing in an interface area where antibody was entering from the circulation and ECF was diffusing following local production by the lymphotic infiltrate. A similar picture is also seen in "retest" skin reactions (Leber *et al.*, 1973).

Another study by Ngan *et al.* (1976) demonstrated that the lymphokine interferon, although not an "inflammatory mediator" *per se*, suppressed heterologous adoptive cutaneous anaphylaxis in rat's skin when it was cotransferred with the murine lymphocytes actively synthesizing IgE. Controls demonstrated that the effect was not at the mast cell level. Most likely interferon actively suppressed antibody synthesis and/or its release *in vivo*.

One other report dealing with the administration of exogenous lymphokines to experimental animals implicated mediators in the development of a pathologic state. Andreis and coworkers (1974) reported that chronic synovitis could be induced in rabbits following 3 intra-articular injections of concentrated MIF-containing supernatants. The resulting synovitis was characterized by synovial effusion, hyperplasia of the lining layer, infiltration of the sublining layers with mononuclear cells and some fibroblasts. Injection of the concentrated control supernatant into the contralateral joint did not result in inflammation. This observation, coupled with the ones previously described, i.e. the presence of MIF activity in joint fluids of rheumatoid arthritis and the capacity of the synovial tissues from these individuals to produce MIF *in vitro*, strongly suggests that mediators are intimately involved in this disease state.

Regulation of lymphokine activity

A great deal is known about suppressor mechanisms operative in the induction of antibody responses. Such mechanisms, involving both cells and soluble factors, have also been shown to play a role in the induction of certain T cell mediated reactions as well. There is only very limited information, however, regarding the regulation and control of the various lymphokine-dependent reactions described above.

Since lymphokine-dependent reactions, such as cutaneous delayed hypersensitivity, are at the efferent portion of the immune response, regulation and control could theoretically occur at several stages. These can be divided into mechanisms that are operative at the stage of lymphokine production and mechanisms that are operative at the stage of expression of lymphokine activity. Our own studies have provided evidence that both kinds of mechanism exist.

The expression of lymphokine activity

In a previous section, our finding of serum lymphokine activity in a variety of diseases was described. In these various diseases, one may find cutaneous anergy as a clinical parameter. In particular, we have reported that the majority of patients with sarcoidosis have serum MIF (Yoshida *et al.*, 1979b) and in this condition, there is a correlation between such activity and the presence of cutaneous anergy.

These findings are reminiscent of our observations in experimental animals. We found that desensitizing doses of antigen, which induced cutaneous anergy, induced the transient appearance of MIF in the serum (Yoshida and Cohen, 1974). These findings, taken together, suggested that lymphokine activity itself could affect or limit the expression of lymphokine-dependent reactions.

In order to test the above hypothesis, we studied the effect of administering exogenous lymphokines to guinea-pigs. We found that intravenous injection of MIF-containing, but not control supernatants into normal guinea-pigs resulted in a monocytopenia (Yoshida and Cohen, 1974). Of even greater interest was the observation that such animals, if preimmunized, were markedly suppressed in their ability to produce a delayed hypersensitivity skin reaction on challenge with antigen. It should be stressed that in these experiments, the lymphokine source was a lymphoid cell suspension obtained from animals immunized with antigen unrelated to that used to immunize the recipients. Appropriate controls demonstrated that the observed suppression was also not due to antibody or to immune complexes.

This ability of MIF-containing supernatants to suppress cutaneous reactivity does not imply that MIF itself is this responsible factor, since, as indicated above, multiple activities are present in lymphokine preparations.

The suppressive effect of exogenous lymphokines is a transient one, lasting no more than 24–36 or 48 h. In contrast, active desensitization of an animal by the injection of large doses of antigen leads to a state of anergy that lasts for approximately 6–7 days. This model, and its relation to the above findings, will be discussed in the following section.

Desensitization

As indicated above, one can induce cutaneous anergy by a process known as desensitization. The procedure involves systemic administration of large doses of the sensitizing antigen. The anergic state is with respect to a variety of delayed hypersensitivity reactions as well as the cutaneous response.

Anergy is usually transient, nonspecific and occurs in the presence of serum antibodies against the antigen to which the individual or animal is anergic. Unlike tolerance, sensitization is a prerequisite for anergy and the maintenance of the desensitized or anergic state appears to involve an environmental factor in the anergic animal (Kantor, 1975). This concept is supported by the observation that the transfer of delayed hypersensitivity to unrelated protein antigens by immunocompetent lymphocytes is readily accomplished into normal recipients but not into desensitized ones. The presence of a circulating humoral factor capable of interfering with cell-mediated immune responses has been invoked to explain these findings. In support of this hypothesis is the demonstration that lymphocytes from desensitized animals can transfer delayed hypersensitivity reactions to normal animals. This transfer can even be accomplished with respect to the antigen used initially to desensitize the donor. These observations suggest that once lymphocytes are removed from the desensitized environment, they rapidly recover their antigen responsiveness (Dwyer and Kantor, 1975).

The concept of an anergic environment suggested that it might be possible to "transfer" anergy passively with serum from desensitized animals. Although initial attempts to do so were unsuccessful (Kantor, 1975), our finding that systemic administration of exogenous lymphokines induced anergy suggested a possible experimental strategy. As described above, desensitizing doses of antigen lead to serum MIF over a relatively limited period of time. Serum obtained during this critical time period should be capable of transferring the desensitized state. Indeed, we found that we could achieve up to 85% reduction in the intensity of skin reactions by passively transferring serums obtained 12 h after desensitization (Papermaster *et al.*, 1978). In those studies, we were also able to demonstrate inhibition of the macrophage disappearance reaction (MDR). This reaction, which will be described later, is a manifestation of cellular immunity. Appropriate controls excluded the possibility that the transfer of desensitization was mediated by antigen, antibody or immune complexes.

Suppressive factors for lymphokine production

All of the events in desensitization discussed so far occur within the first 24–48 h. Nevertheless, as indicated above, anergy can persist for 6–7 days. Little is known about the mechanisms operative in the latter period. One clue comes from a study involving active, antigen-induced desensitization of the macrophage disappearance reaction (MDR). The MDR is performed as follows: a previously immunized animal is given an intraperitoneal injection of a non-specific irritant such as mineral oil in order to induce an inflammatory exudate in the peritoneal cavity. Four days later, at a time when the exudate is composed mainly of macrophages, a small (microgram) dose of the immunizing antigen is injected intraperitoneally. A positive MDR is one in which there is an antigen-induced reduction in the macrophage content of the peritoneal exudate. This reduction occurs maximally within 4–6 h after antigen injection, and is a manifestation of cell-mediated immunity. During the course of the MDR, there is an appearance of MIF and other lymphokines in the peritoneal fluid (Sonozaki *et al.*, 1975), which appears to be due to local production by peritoneal lymphocytes. The important point here is that if the animal has been desensitized, and if the MDR is performed at a time when the serum MIF due to the desensitizing challenge is no longer detectable, then no lymphokines can be found in the peritoneal fluid as well. As expected, there is no change in macrophage content. Thus, at this stage of desensitization, the peritoneal lymphocytes appear to be incapable of responding to the challenging dose of antigen with local lymphokine production and the attendant redistribution of macrophages that characterizes the MDR. The most likely explanation for this state of affairs is that a suppressor cell or cell product is present. Although such a factor has not yet been conclusively identified, there is an interesting biological precedent for it, since T cells can produce a factor that inhibits the production of MIF by B cells (Cohen and

Yoshida, 1977). It may well be that T cells and/or other cell types such as macrophages can produce similar suppressor factors that interfere with the production of lymphokines by T cells themselves.

Two-stage model of desensitization

On the basis of the above considerations, we propose that desensitization in the guinea-pig is at least a two-stage process. In the first stage, the desensitizing antigen induces excess lymphokine production, and these mediators may be found systemically. There are two ways by which this situation can lead to loss of reactivity at a test site, as, for example, in anergy with respect to cutaneous delayed hypersensitivity. First, the inflammatory cells that are the targets for lymphokine effect are pre-empted systemically and may not be available for local reaction at the test site. Second, the presence of lymphokines in the general circulation prevents the establishment of the gradients of chemotactic factors that are involved in the accumulation of inflammatory cells at the test site. As delayed hypersensitivity reactions are composed predominantly of inflammatory infiltrates, these proposed mechanisms seem adequate to explain the experimental observations.

This first stage is transient and lasts for 1 or 2 days. Following this, we propose that a suppressor factor that inhibits lymphokine production plays a crucial role. Possible stimuli for suppressor factor production are the large desensitizing dose of antigen itself, or the "overproduction" of lymphokines that follow.

We have recently attempted a simple experimental test of this proposed model. In order to understand the protocol, it is necessary to digress and discuss a lymphokine known as skin reactive factor (SRF). It is known that lymphokine-containing, but not control, supernatants, can induce inflammatory reactions when injected into the skin (Cohen, 1977). These reactions mimic those of delayed hypersensitivity. The initiating agent in the supernatants has been defined as SRF; this probably consists of a mixture of the various inflammatory lymphokines. A comparison of reactivity to antigen and SRF (preformed lymphokine) during desensitization provides useful information. If an actively immunized animal is desensitized with antigen, skin reactions to antigens are suppressed for 6–7 days. According to the model, the initial suppression (1–2 days) is due to excess lymphokines exerting a paradoxical effect, as described above. Subsequently, as the excess lymphokine is cleared, the animal remains suppressed because a suppressor factor is produced, and this factor prevents the production of lymphokines at the local test site. If the animal is challenged with SRF, it should be nonreactive to the SRF during the first stage. However, it should respond to SRF during the second stage since SRF represents preformed lymphokine and should bypass the effect of the suppressor factor (which acts by preventing lymphokine production). This is exactly what is observed (Yoshida *et al.*, 1979a). Although the animal remains unresponsive to antigen for approximately 1 week, it begins to be responsive to SRF at 24 h postdesensitization, and is fully reactive by 48 h, a timing that correspond precisely to the kinetics of serum MIF.

Conclusion

Delayed hypersensitivity, in common with other forms of so-called cellular immunity, is mediated by soluble lymphocyte-derived mediators called lymphokines. These factors may be conveniently categorized into groups that affect cell viability, cell proliferation, cell motility and cell activation. The interactions between lymphokines and macrophages represent good models for all these kinds of activities.

Two topics of current concern are the role of lymphokines *in vivo*, and their regulation and control under both physiologic and pathologic conditions. Recent findings have demonstrated multiple pathways for control, affecting not only lymphokine production, but also the expression of lymphokine activity. These are important areas for future research as they provide the possibility for the development of novel forms of therapeutic intervention in the treatment of human disease.

References

Aaskov, J. G. and Anthony, H. M. (1976). *Aust. J. Exp. Biol. Med. Sci.* **54**, 527.
Adelman, N. E., Hammond, M. E., Cohen, S. and Dvorak, H. (1979). *In* "The Biology of the Lymphokines" (S. Cohen, E. Pick and J. J. Oppenheim, eds) p. 13. Academic Press, New York and London.
Alexander, P., Evans, R. and Grant, C. K. (1972). *Ann. Inst. Pasteur* **122**, 645.
Altman, L. C. (1978). *In* "Leukocyte Chemotaxis" (J. I. Gallin and P. G. Quie, eds) p. 267. Raven Press, New York.
Amos, H. E. and Lachmann, P. J. (1970). *Immunology* **18**, 269.
Amsden, A., Ewan, V., Yoshida, T. and Cohen, S. (1978). *J. Immunol.* **120**, 542.
Anderson, S. E. and Remington, J. S. (1974). *J. Exp. Med.* **139**, 1154.
Andreis, M., Stastny, P. and Ziff, M. (1974). *Arthritis Rheum.* **17**, 537.
Arnason, B. G. and Waksman, B. H. (1963). *Lab. Invest.* **12**, 737.
Atkins, E., Feldman, J. D., Francis, L. and Hirsh, E. (1972). *J. Exp. Med.* **135**, 1113.
Bennett, B. and Bloom, B. R. (1968). *Proc. Natn. Acad. Sci. U.S.A.* **59**, 756.
Bloom, B. R. and Bennett, B. (1966). *Science* **153**, 180.
Borgis, J. S. and Johnson, W. D. (1974). *J. Exp. Med.* **141**, 483.
Boyden, S. (1962). *J. Exp. Med.* **115**, 453.
Carnegie, P. R., Caspary, E. A., Dickinson, J. P. and Field, E. J. (1973). *Clin. Exp. Immunol.* **14**, 37.
Caspary, E. A. (1971). *Nature New Biol.* **231**, 24.
Caspary, E. A. (1972). *Clin. Exp. Immunol.* **11**, 305.
Chao, P., Francis, L. and Atkins, E. (1977). *J. Exp. Med.* **145**, 1288.
Churchill, W. H., Piessens, W. F., Sulis, C. A. and David, J. R. (1975). *J. Immunol.* **115**, 781.
Cohen, S. (1977). *Am. J. Path.* **88**, 501.

Cohen, S. and Ward, P. A. (1971). *J. Exp. Med.* **133**, 133.
Cohen, S. and Yoshida, T. (1977). *J. Immunol.* **119**, 719.
Cohen, S., Fisher, B., Yoshida, T. and Bettigole, R. E. (1974a). *New Eng. J. Med.* **290**, 882.
Cohen, S., Rose, N. R. and Brown, R. C. (1974b). *Clin. Immunol. Immunopathol.* **2**, 256.
Crowle, A. J. (1975). *Adv. Immunol.* **20**, 197.
David, J. R. (1966). *Proc. Natn. Acad. Sci. U.S.A.* **56**, 72.
David, J. R. (1975). *Fed. Proc.* **34**, 1730.
Dumonde, D. C., Wolstencroft, R. A., Panayi, G. S., Matthew, M., Morley, J. and Howson, W. T. (1969). *Nature* **224**, 38.
Dvorak, H. F. (1971). *J. Immunol.* **106**, 279.
Dvorak, H. F. and Dvorak, A. M. (1972). *Human Pathol.* **3**, 454.
Dvorak, H. F. and Hirsch, M. D. (1971). *J. Immunol.* **107**, 1576.
Dvorak, A. M., Hammond, M. E., Dvorak, H. F. and Karnovsky, M. J. (1972). *Lab. Invest.* **27**, 561.
Dwyer, J. M. and Kantor, F. S. (1975). *J. Exp. Med.* **142**, 588.
Evans, R. and Alexander, P. (1970). *Nature (Lond.)* **228**, 620.
Evans, R., Grant, C. K., Cox, H., Steele, K. and Alexander, P. (1972). *J. Exp. Med.* **136**, 1318.
Fidler, I. J., Darnell, J. H. and Budmen, M. B. (1977). *J. Immunol.* **117**, 666.
Fowles, R. E., Fajardo, I. M., Leibowitch, J. L. and David, J. R. (1973). *J. Exp. Med.* **138**, 952.
Fox, R. A., Gregory, D. S. and Feldman, J. D. (1974). *J. Immunol.* **112**, 1861.
Galindo, B. (1972). *Infect. Immun.* **5**, 583.
Galindo, B., Lazdins, J. and Castillo, R. (1974). *Infect. Immun.* **9**, 212.
George, M. and Vaughan, J. H. (1962). *Proc. Soc. Exp. Biol. Med.* **111**, 514.
Godal, T., Rees, R. J. W. and Lamvik, J. O. (1971). *Clin. Exp. Immunol.* **8**, 625.
Gottlieb, A. A. and Waldman, S. R. (1972). *In* "Macrophages and Cellular Immunity" (A. I. Laskin and H. Lechevalier, eds) p. 13. CRC Press, Cleveland.
Hadden, J. W., Sadlick, J. R. and Hadden, E. M. (1975). *Nature (Lond.)* **257**, 483.
Hammond, M. E. and Dvorak, H. F. (1972). *J. Exp. Med.* **136**, 1518.
Hammond, M. E., Selvaggio, S. S. and Dvorak, H. F. (1975). *J. Immunol.* **115**, 914.
Hibbs, J. B. (1972). *Science* **180**, 868.
Hibbs, J. B., Lambert, L. H. and Remington, J. S. (1972a). *Nature New Biol.* **235**, 48.
Hibbs, J. B., Lambert, L. H. and Remington, J. S. (1972b). *Science* **177**, 998.
Hibbs, J. B., Taintor, R. R., Chapasan, H. A. and Weinberg, J. B. (1977). *Science* **197**, 279.
Higgins, T. J., Winston, C. T. and David, J. R. (1973). *Fed. Proc.* **32**, 878 (Abstract).
Kantor, F. S. (1975). *New Eng. J. Med.* **292**, 629.
Krahenbuhl, J. L. and Remington, J. S. (1971). *Infect. Imm.* **4**, 337.
Krahenbuhl, J. L., Rosenberg, L. T. and Remington, J. S. (1973). *J. Immunol.* **111**, 992.
Krejci, J., Svejcar, J., Pekarek, J. and Johanovsky, J. (1968). *Z. Immunitstat.* **136**, 259.
Krüger, G. G., Weston, W. L., Thorne, E. G., Mandel, M. J. and Jacobs, R. J. (1973). *J. Invest. Dermat.* **60**, 284.
Kuratsuji, T., Yoshida, T. and Cohen, S. (1976). *J. Immunol.* **117**, 1985.
Leber, P. D., Milgrom, M. and Cohen, S. (1973). *Immunol. Comm.* **2**, 615.
Littman, B. H. and Ruddy, S. (1977). *J. Exp. Med.* **145**, 1344.
Lohmann-Matthes, M. L., Ziegler, F. G. and Fischer, H. (1973). *Eur. J. Immunol.* **3**, 56.
Lolekha, S., Dray, S. and Gotoff, S. P. (1970). *J. Immunol.* **104**, 296.
Maillard, J. L., Pick, E. and Turk, J. L. (1972). *Int. Arch. Allergy* **42**, 50.

McCluskey, R. T. and Cohen, S. (1972). *Pathobiol. Ann.* **2**, 111.
McCluskey, R. T. and Leber, P. E. (1974). *In* "Mechanisms of Cell-Mediated Immunity" (R. T. McCluskey and S. Cohen, eds) p. 1–24. J. Wiley and Sons, New York.
Meade, C. J., Lachmann, P. J. and Brenner, S. (1974). *Immunology* **27**, 227.
Nath, I., Poulter, L. W. and Turk, J. L. (1973). *Clin. Exp. Immunol.* **13**, 455.
Nathan, C. F., Karnovsky, M. L. and David, J. R. (1971). *J. Exp. Med.* **133**, 1356.
Neta, R. and Salvin, S. B. (1971). *Infect. Immun.* **4**, 697.
Ngan, J., Lee, S. H. S. and Kind, L. S. (1976). *J. Immunol.* **117**, 1063.
Pantalone, R. M. and Page, R. C. (1975). *Proc. Natn. Acad. Sci. U.S.A.* **72**, 2091.
Pantalone, R. M. and Page, R. C. (1977). *J. Reticuloendo. Soc.* **21**, 343.
Papermaster, V., Yoshida, T. and Cohen, S. (1978). *Cell. Immunol.* **35**, 378.
Patterson, R. J. and Youmans, G. P. (1970). *Infect. Imm.* **1**, 600.
Pels, E. and Den-Otter, W. (1974). *Cancer Res.* **34**, 3089.
Pick, E., Brostoff, J., Krejci, J. and Turk, J. L. (1970a). *Cell Immunol.* **1**, 92.
Pick, E., Krejci, J. and Turk, J. L. (1970b). *Nature* **225**, 236.
Piessens, W. F., Churchill, W. H. and David, J. R. (1975). *J. Immunol.* **114**, 293.
von Pirquet, C. E. (1911). *Arch. Intern. Med.* **7**, 383.
Postlethwaite, A. E. and Kang, A. H. (1976). *J. Immunol.* **117**, 1651.
Postlethwaite, A. E. and Synderman, R. (1975). *J. Immunol.* **114**, 274.
Poulter, L. W. (1976). *Cell Immunol.* **27**, 17.
Poulter, L. W. and Turk, J. L. (1975). *Cell. Immunol.* **20**, 25.
Remold, H. G. and Mednis, A. (1972). *Fed. Proc.* **31**, 753 (Abstract).
Remold, H. G. and Mednis, A. (1975). *Inflammation* **1**, 175.
Remold-O'Donnell, E. and Remold, H. G. (1974). *J. Biol. Chem.* **249**, 3622.
Rich, A. R. and Lewis, M. R. (1932). *Bull. Johns Hopkins Hosp.* **50**, 115.
Rosenstreich, D. L. and Wahl, S. M. (1979). *In* "The Biology of the Lymphokines" (S. Cohen, E. Pick and J. J. Oppenheim, eds) p. 210. Academic Press, New York and London.
Salvin, S., Younger, J. S. and Lederer, W. H. (1973). *Infect. Immun.* **7**, 68.
Schmidt, M. E., Douglas, S. D. and Rubin, A. (1973). *Cell. Immunol.* **9**, 45.
Schwartz, H. J., Leon, M. A. and Pelley, R. P. (1970). *J. Immunol.* **104**, 265.
Sonozaki, H. and Cohen, S. (1971a). *J. Immunol.* **106**, 1404.
Sonozaki, H. and Cohen, S. (1971b). *Cell. Immunol.* **2**, 341.
Sonozaki, H., Papermaster, V., Yoshida, T. and Cohen, S. (1975). *J. Immunol.* **115**, 1657.
Stastny, P. and Ziff, M. (1971). *In* "Immunopathology of Inflammation" (B. K. Forscher and J. C. Houck, eds) p. 66. Excerpta Medica, Amsterdam.
Stastny, P., Cooke, T. D. and Ziff, M. (1973a). *Clin. Exp. Immunol.* **14**, 141.
Stastny, P., Rosenthal, M., Andreis, M. and Ziff, M. (1973b). *Arthritis Rheum.* **16**, 572 (Abstract).
Svejcar, J. and Johanovsky, J. (1961). *Z. Immunitaetsforsch.* **56**, 398.
Symth, A. C. and Weiss, L. (1970). *J. Immunol.* **105**, 1360.
Thrasher, S. G., Yoshida, T., van Oss, C. J. Cohen, S. and Rose, N. R. (1973). *J. Immunol.* **110**, 321.
Torisu, M., Yoshida, T. and Cohen, S. (1975). *Clin. Immunol. Immunopathol.* **3**, 369.
Turk, J. L. (1975). "Delayed Hypersensitivity". Elsevier, New York.
Turk, J. L., Heather, C. J. and Diengdon, S. V. (1966). *Int. Arch. Allergy* **29**, 278.
Unanue, E. R., Kiely, J. M. and Calderon, J. (1976). *J. Exp. Med.* **144**, 155.
Vassalli, J. D. and Reich, E. (1977). *J. Exp. Med.* **145**, 429.
Wahl, L. M., Wahl, S. M., Mergenhagen, S. E. and Martin, G. R. (1975). *Science* **187**, 261.
Ward, P. A., Remold, H. G. and David, J. R. (1969). *Science* **163**, 1079.

Weisbart, R. H., Bluestone, R., Goldberg, L. S. and Pearson, C. M. (1974). *Proc. Natn. Acad. Sci. U.S.A.* **71**, 875.

Wiener, J., Spiro, D. and Zunker, H. O. (1965). *Am. J. Pathol.* **47**, 723.

Wilton, J. M., Rosenstreich, D. L. and Oppenheim, J. J. (1975). *J. Immunol.* **114**, 388.

Yamamoto, K. and Takahashi, Y. (1971). *Nature New Biol.* **233**, 261.

Yoshida, T. and Cohen, S. (1974). *J. Immunol.* **112**, 1540.

Yoshida, T., Nagai, R. and Hashimoto, T. (1973a). *Lab. Invest.* **29**, 329.

Yoshida, T., Sonozaki, H. and Cohen, S. (1973b). *J. Exp. Med.* **138**, 784.

Yoshida, T., Bigazzi, P. E. and Cohen, S. (1975a). *Proc. Natn. Acad. Sci. U.S.A.* **72**, 1641.

Yoshida, T., Edelson, R., Cohen, S. and Green, I. (1975b). *J. Immunol.* **114**, 915.

Yoshida, T., Kuratsuji, T., Takada, A., Takada, Y., Minowada, J. and Cohen, S. (1976). *J. Immunol.* **117**, 548.

Yoshida, T., Baba, T. and Cohen, S. (1979a). *In* "Second International Lymphokine Workshop: Biochemical Characterization of Lymphokines" Ermatingen, Switzerland (Abstract).

Yoshida, T., Siltzbach, L. E., Masih, N. and Cohen, S. (1979b). *Clin. Immunol. Immunopathol.* **13**, 39.

Theme 13: Summary

Immediate and Delayed-type Hypersensitivity

A. L. de WECK

Institut für Klinische Immunologie, Bern, Switzerland

Theme 13 was originally conceived as dealing only with immediate-type hypersensitivity. Various considerations have led the organizers of this congress to include delayed hypersensitivity in the theme. Strangely enough, events sometimes take their originally intended course despite attempts to thwart them. In fact, most of the work reported during the workshops of Theme 13 has been concerned primarily with immediate-type hypersensitivity reactions, reflecting at least in part the fact that a large number of advances have been made in this field at the molecular level during the past 3 or 4 years.

Immunoglobulin classes involved in immediate hypersensitivity

Undoubtedly IgE remains, from a functional point of view, the main immunoglobulin involved in immediate hypersensitivity reactions. While research on human IgE structure and the relationship between structure and function has been very much hampered in the past by the low amounts available, except for a few human myelomas, we now dispose of a large number of IgE myelomas in the rat model and of an increasing number of monoclonal mice IgE produced by the hybridoma technique by several groups (Barsumian *et al.*, 13.1.03; Eshhar *et al.*, 13.1.06; Fu-Tong *et al.*, 13.1.14).* Aside from potentially enabling quantitative evaluation of specific IgE reactivity by radioimmunoassay instead of by the cumbersome passive cutaneous anaphylaxis technique, the availability of larger amounts of pure IgE will undoubtedly help in assessing further the relationship between IgE and its receptors on various types of cells.

Despite the importance of IgE, there is an increasing awareness that other homocytotropic antibodies also play a role in immediate-type allergic reactions. At least two types of IgG subclasses may, in experimental animal models, bind to mast cells and basophils and are able upon challenge with antigen to lead to the release of mediators (Mota and Perini, 13.1.19). The existence of heat-stable homocytotropic IgG antibodies in man capable of sensitizing human skin for a short time (IgG-STS) was described several years ago. However, the nature of this IgG, in terms of current immunoglobulin classification, is still controversial. While several groups (Halpern *et al.*, 13.1.09, Shakib and Stanworth, 12.1.23) claim that IgG_4 or at least some immunoglobulin subgroup possessing IgG_4 determinants represent the second class of homocytotropic antibodies in man, other immunochemical studies fail to confirm this point of view (Aalberse and van Leeuwen, 13.1.01; van Toorenengeren *et al.*, 13.1.25). It is likely that the matter will only be settled by the availability of monoclonal antibodies directed against various IgG subgroups and classes and the isolation of allergen-specific IgG subclass

* These cross-references are to Abstract numbers—see *Abstracts 4th International Congress to Immunology*, Paris, 1980.

antibodies. It may well turn out that short-term sensitizing IgG antibodies are sensitizing when present in small amounts but have blocking capacity, when present in excess, either as free antibodies or on the mast cell membrane itself.

Regulation of the IgE response

As already reflected by the literature, the field of regulation of the IgE response has developed very interestingly during the last 3–4 years. It is generally admitted that the regulation of IgE responses is to be considered separately from the regulation of other immunoglobulin classes and obeys different rules, both theoretically and within the frame of experimental and clinical situations. A first point revisited by several groups (Bergstrand *et al.*, 13.2.03; Essani and Strejan, 13.2.06; Taylor and Sheldon, 13.2.24; Van der Straeten *et al.*, 13.2.26) is the role of various adjuvants in the IgE response. While a number of substances or bacterial products (e.g. *B. pertussis*, mycobacterial adjuvants) appear to foster IgE production when injected separately from antigen, covalent chemical coupling of the antigen to the adjuvant molecules or particles appears to exhibit a suppressive effect on IgE production. Analysis at the cellular level indicates this to be due to the induction of nonantigen specific T suppressor cells. It has become evident from the work of several groups (Ishizaka *et al.*, 13.2.11; Katz *et al.*, 13.2.13; Nakonishi *et al.*, 13.2.16) that stimulation of the lymphoid system, especially by some adjuvants, leads to the formation of factors which act in a nonantigen specific manner and which may either enhance or inhibit the IgE response, with very little or no effect on the other Ig classes. In several instances, the source of these factors appears to be T cells or a subset of T cells (Ishizaka *et al.*, 13.2.11). Some T cell hybrids producing such a factor have been clones (Nakanishi *et al.*, 13.2.16).

Knowledge about the origin and the molecular structure of such factors influencing across the board, and in some cases also across species, production of IgE is bound to have great practical consequences. However, the molecular identification of these factors is not yet completed (Katz *et al.*, 13.2.13; Ishizaka *et al.*, 13.2.11). One factor appears to have affinity for IgE and to possess H_2 determinants, it may therefore correspond to the IgE receptor (Nakanishi *et al.*, 13.2.16).

Another mechanism by which IgE and other Ig responses may be regulated is the idiotype–anti-idiotype network. It has been now demonstrated in several systems, as well in mice as in guinea-pigs, that active immunization with a mixture of idiotypes, encompassing the library of most common idiotypes against a definite antigen, is capable in a given strain of severely impairing subsequent IgE production towards the same antigen (de Weck *et al.*, 13.2.05). This suppression is specific and long-lasting; it appears to affect IgE production more than other Ig classes. Repeated passive administration of isologous anti-idiotypic antibodies also show suppressive effects even in animals exhibiting a so-called ongoing, well-established IgE response.

We must increasingly distinguish the regulation mechanisms operating during the early phase of an IgE response, such as primary and early secondary responses, which appear to be extremely T cell dependent, from those influencing the established late tertiary or ongoing response, which appears to follow quite different patterns. Many experimental manipulations which have spectacular suppressive effects on early IgE responses appear to be powerless in influencing the ongoing IgE response, which is of course the one which immunologists with practical goals in mind would be the most interested in suppressing. Chemical modifications of antigens by various means, such as covalent binding of polyethylene glycol, polyvinyl alcohol (Lee and Sehon, 13.2.14) phosphorylcholine groups (Singh *et al.*, 13.2.23) etc., have brought interesting experimental results, in terms of preferential induction of T suppressor activity, capable of suppressing the IgE response. Whether such modifications will be equally efficient in suppressing late ongoing responses and will be effective in man remains to be seen.

While most of the advances made in this field in recent years have been achieved in rodents, the goal of many of us remains to suppress excess IgE formation in man. Several groups have succeeded in the past years in studying IgE synthesis from human peripheral blood lymphocytes *in vitro* (Yanagihara *et al.*, 13.2.28; del Prete *et al.*, 13.2.04; Iwamoto *et al.*, 13.2.12; Ureña *et al.*, 13.2.25). In particular, a very efficient system of primary induction of human IgE response *in vitro* has been presented (Katz *et al.*, 13.2.13).

These systems may to some extent at least give clues as to whether rules established in experimental systems also apply to human IgE regulation. A word of warning, however, is requested here, since before jumping to conclusions based only on circulating lymphoid cells, there is no doubt in my mind that the study of human cell populations in various other lymphoid organs will be required. There is no general agreement yet about the demonstration and nature of human T cells in peripheral blood suppressing IgE synthesis *in vitro*. In particular, it seems that in ongoing responses B lymphocytes spontaneously secrete IgE without any longer requiring T cells or being influenced by their presence.

Mast cells and basophils

The tissue mast cells and blood basophils play a key role in immediate-type reactions and certainly also in many other types of allergic inflammatory reactions. From various lines of experimental work, several conclusions have emerged:

(a) Blood basophils and tissue mast cells, although functionally and morphologically similar when superficially considered, represent in fact markedly different populations of cells, both from the point of view of origin of ontogenesis and of functional capabilities (Denburg *et al.*, 13.3.07). Their development and differentiation appears to be under T cell control. There are also data suggesting that tissue mast cells in different tissues and localizations may not all react in the same way. This compartmentalization in terms of cellular elements capable of reacting to some specific or nonspecific stimuli may go a long way to explain various clinical forms of allergic reactions, such as the apparent independence of the skin expressing generalized urticaria from lung tissue mast cells in part responsible for bronchial obstruction.

(b) We have become increasingly aware that there are several pathways and triggering mechanisms by which mast cells and basophils may be induced to release their mediators. One also starts to doubt whether all possible mast cell mediators are being released as a whole after a triggering event (Dvorak, 13.9.08).

Cellular triggering processes (mast cells and lymphocytes)

This brings us to discuss the cellular triggering processes which have attracted increased attention. The availability of IgE meylomas has permitted to make great advances in assessing their binding to mast cells and also to identify the Fc_ϵ receptors present on mast cells and basophils. In the rat, the IgE receptor appears to be a 50 000 daltons glycoprotein, which is associated with a 30 000–35 000 polypeptide (Holowka and Metzger, 13.4.06; Kanellopoulos *et al.*, 13.4.10).

Antibodies directed against such receptors have permitted to better assess their functional sites (Ishizaka and Sterk, 13.4.08). While in previous years, modulation of mediator release following triggering was essentially attributed to cyclic nucleotides, 2 groups have recently investigated transmethylation phenomena within the cell membrane (Ishizaka and Sterk, 13.4.08; Morita *et al.*, 13.4.14). It has been shown that activation of phospholipids will lead to the production of arachidonic acid metabolites also modulating the release of intracellular mediators (König *et al.*, 13.4.11).

However, it is important to recognize that there are several other mechanisms than

IgE bridging which are capable of triggering mast cells, in particular C_{5a} and a number of peptides and drugs. These various triggering agents appear to function independently from one another, to act on different receptors and they may not all obligatorily lead to mediator formation and/or release by the same intracellular metabolic steps.

Interestingly, it is now well established that Fc_{ϵ} receptors for IgE are present not only on mast cells and basophils but also on macrophages (Joseph *et al.*, 13.4.09) and on some subsets of T and B lymphocytes (Spiegelberg and O'Connor, 13.4.16). Interaction between antigen and IgE on macrophages may lead to their activation and corresponding release of lysosomal enzymes. Whether this represents a link permitting to understand why in some circumstances IgE appears to be responsible not only for immediate but also for more protracted or delayed reactions remains to be more thoroughly investigated.

Primary (preformed) mediators

It has become apparent that, in the belief that IgE response automatically leads to allergic reactions, the intrinsic capacity of the mast cell to release its mediators (releasability) as well as the intrinsic sensitivity of target tissues to mast cell mediators has not been given sufficient attention. It increasingly appears that it is not enough to be a high responder in terms of IgE response to become at the same time a highly symptomatic allergic individual. Correlation studies between levels of free IgE, amounts of IgE molecules present on mast cells and release of mediators show fairly well that the differences in terms of releasability may even supersede in importance the immune response itself. This is giving new weight to those claiming that the allergic state is not only the result of an immune phenomenon but also the consequence of some pharmacological abnormalities. Breeding studies in rodents also start to show that releasability and sensitivity towards mast cell mediators may be a genetic trait (Pauwels *et al.*, 13.1.20). A possibly important new mediator has been described to be released from IgE-sensitized lung tissue and acting as prekallikrein activator (Newball *et al.*, 13.5.10).

Secondary mediators

Great progress has been achieved since the last international Immunology congress in the structural identification of at least two mediators which may well play a major role in immediate-type hypersensitivity reactions. One of them is the platelet activating factor (PAF), the structure of which has been characterized by two groups and the importance of which is now generally recognized (Arnoux *et al.*, 13.6.01; Polonsky *et al.*, 13.6.07). The platelet activating factor is certainly also produced by monocytes. Whether it is also produced by basophils and mast cells is still somewhat disputed. In any case, the involvement of platelets in immediate-type allergic reactions, which had for some time been considered as a secondary phenomenon, may well have to be more thoroughly considered, especially in asthma. The identification of the long elusive slow reacting substance of anaphylaxis (SRS-A) as arachidonic acid metabolites (collectively known as leucotrienes) and products of the lipo-oxygenase pathway is certainly one of the major achievements during the past years. Various reports suggest that there is some heterogeneity among the SRS-A molecules produced by different triggering mechanisms and further studies on this topic are progressing swiftly (Bach *et al.*, 13.6.02). Finally, there appears that eosinophil chemotactic factors formed in mast cells and basophils may not only be the classical tetrapeptide described a few years ago but that some arachidonic acid derivatives also have chemotactic activity on eosinophils (König *et al.*, 13.6.05).

Immunopathological mechanisms of hypersensitivity reactions

Eighteen years ago, Gell and Coombs published a classification of immunopathological reactions in tissues which for many years dominated the field. At the time, the division of immunopathological reactions in four types, together with the identification of separate tyes of cells and mediators involved in each one, made a great contribution to clarify the issues. It has become clear by now that this clarification was only possible by lack of knowledge, and that the reality is infinitely more complex. In terms of immunopathological mechanisms, I feel that the main point emerging during the past years is that each type of immunopathological reaction, whatever its initial triggering event, soon becomes embroiled in a network of complex interactions between various types of inflammatory cells on the one hand and soluble mediators affecting other cells as well as the mediator-producing cells themselves. Just to give one example: histamine was for a long time considered to be a hallmark of anaphylactic reactions, but it is now obvious that the release of histamine by mast cells has secondary effects on various types of inflammatory cells and plays thereby a role in many other types of allergic reactions than merely the anaphylactic ones. SRS-A may be quite prominent also in Arthus reactions (Jancar, 13.7.19), lymphokines appear to modulate basophil and mast cells activities (Lett-Brown *et al.*, 13. 7.23) the platelet activating factor shows links between basophil, mast cells, monocytes, platelets (Arnoux *et al.*, 13.6.01).

Most of the tissue induration characteristic of delayed-type allergic reactions is not due to infiltrating cells but to fibrin deposits, following activation of the coagulation systems (Geczy and Hopper, 13.7.13). It has also been shown that the deposition of fibrin on the membrane of macrophages activated by the macrophage migration inhibiting factor (MIF) may be the reason for the macrophage's reduced motility (Hopper *et al.*, 13.7.16).

It appears therefore that any modern classification of immunopathological reactions should encompass, on the one hand, the initial triggering event which may still to some extent correspond to the ones identified by Gell and Coombs (although even there a number of new subdivisions have to be made) and, on the other hand, an array of secondary events which are strongly influencing the final picture and the dynamics of the reaction. Investigators dealing with factors and mediators produced by lymphoid cell cultures *in vitro* have since long realized that various types of lymphoid cells involved interact with each other and that the mediators they produce initiate a kind of "ping-pong" game, which ultimately may have enhancing or inhibiting effects on the system. Immunopathologists become increasingly aware that the "ping-pong" game which we can monitor *in vitro* also occurs *in vivo*.

Lymphokines and monokines

The field of lymphokines and monokines—this ill-defined group of substances produced by lymphocytes or macrophages and encompassing effector mediators producing inflammatory reactions and regulatory factors influencing the functions of the immune system—is now emerging in force as a major new endeavour for molecular immunology. Most of the early difficulties in molecular characterization by classical means were due essentially to the low amounts of lymphokines available under laboratory conditions. Improvements in logistics and new technologies such as continuing cell line cultures and the establishment of lymphokine producing hybrids is starting to promote the field from alchemistry to biochemistry. We are also definitely moving away from the period where anyone detecting some kind of new biological activity in a crude culture supernatant would feel entitled to claim the discovery of a new factor, justifying the imposition of a new name and acronym. In fact, a marked process of concentration is taking place. Several factors previously described under different names by different groups have been shown by various criteria to be probably identical. Agreement on this point by the major groups involved has led for example to the recent characterization as interleukin-1 of a factor previously known as MP, HP-1, TRF, BAF, BDF, and of interleukin-2 for T cell growth factor, TMF, Costimulator, KHF and many other synonyms. However, arguments between so-called "lumpers" and "splitters" will certainly continue for some time. I have little doubt that this healthy process will continue and will be in particular fostered by the increasing availability of monoclonal antibodies recognizing such mediator molecules. Besides the monoclonal antibody against osteoclast activating factor described last year, a monoclonal antibody directed against lymphocyte activating factor was reported here (Otz *et al.*, 13.8.27). The term chosen of interleukin emphasizes that many of these molecules may play a role not only restricted to the lymphoid and immune system but also in a more general biological sense. The fact that a number of similar or identical molecules appear to be produced by tumour cells, fibroblasts and other cells not directly involved in immune reactions seems to show that we deal here with a general biological principle.

This brief summary in all its crudeness and superficiality should, I hope, have made clear that even in such classical fields of immunopathology as hypersensitivity reactions of the immediate or delayed-type, great changes are occurring, which are not less glamorous intellectually than some other more highly regarded fields of immunology, such as the molecular genetics of antibody production, the relationship between histocompatibility antigens and the generation of immunological diversity or the network aspects of immune regulation.

Theme 14

Mechanisms of Autoimmune Phenomena and Immune Deficiencies

Presidents:
M. D. COOPER
N. TALAL
J. P. REVILLARD

Symposium chairman:
P. GRABAR

50

Progress in the Mechanisms of Autoimmune Disease

N. TALAL, J. R. ROUBINIAN, HANNAH SHEAR*
JOANNE T. HOM* and N. MIYASAKA**

University of California, San Francisco, USA,
*New York University Medical Center, New York, USA**
*and Veterans Administration Medical Center, San Francisco, USA***

Abbreviations
MHC, major histocompatibility complex; SMLR, syngeneic mixed lymphocyte response; AMLR, autologous mixed lymphocyte response; SLE, systemic lupus erythematosus; SS, Sjögren's syndrome; LPS, lipopolysaccharide; con A, concanavalin A; EB, Epstein–Barr.

This work was supported in part by the Veterans Administration, and by a grant from the State of California (GA 77–101).

The autoimmune disorders have been intensively examined both in patients and in animal models during the past several years. These diseases are multifactorial and each may involve more than one pathogenetic mechanism. On one hand, this has complicated our understanding of autoimmunity; on the other hand, the multiple factors involved offer exciting new possibilities for therapeutic intervention.

This chapter will first review several theories proposed to explain autoimmunity, some of them now only of historical interest. The multifactorial nature of autoimmune diseases will then be discussed, with particular emphasis on genetic and hormonal factors in systemic lupus erythematosus (SLE). SLE is a disease in which T cell regulation is disturbed and much of the immunopathology is due to immune complex deposition in vascular sites. Finally, SLE will be contrasted with Sjögren's Syndrome (SS) in which abnormalities of B cells progressing to B cells neoplasia may be the major immunopathogenic mechanism.

Theories of autoimmunity (Table I)

The forbidden clone theory

If the immune system were to protect the host from potential threats in its environment, it must be endowed with mechanisms to prevent immunologic attack on its own tissues. Paul Ehrlich introduced the term "horror autotoxicus" to state his belief that the organism would not react against its own tissues. In the clonal selection theory, Burnet spoke of potentially self-reactive "forbidden clones" that were eliminated during foetal development.

TABLE I
Theories of autoimmunity

1. Forbidden clone
   A. Autoantigen binding cells exist in normal individuals
   B. Polyclonal B cell activation induces autoantibodies
2. Sequestered antigen
   A. Little experimental evidence
3. Autoantibodies are physiologic
   A. "Transporteurs"—carriers of cell debris
4. Cross-reactive antigens
   A. T cell bypass
   B. Viral-induced antigenic modification
5. Disordered immunologic regulation
   A. Imbalance of helper and suppressor T cells
   B. Intrinsic polyclonal B cell activation
   C. Self-recognition of idiotypic determinants
   D. Self-recognition of MHC determinants

The forbidden clone theory no longer seems appropriate in view of the view of the abundant evidence that autoantigen binding cells and perhaps even autoantibodies in low concentrations exist in normal invididuals. Lymphocytes capable of binding many different self-antigens, including DNA, have been found in healthy people. Furthermore, polyclonal B cell activators such as lipopolysaccharide (LPS) induce normal B cells to produce autoantibodies both *in vitro* and *in vivo*. Normal mice produce antibodies to DNA and even, in some circumstances, develop immune complex glomerulonephritis after repeated injections of LPS (Izui *et al.*, 1977).

Sequestered antigen

Certain antigens, e.g. thyroglobulin, spermatozoa, or lens protein, were once thought to be excluded from contact with lymphocytes by virtue of their sequestration in nonvascular sites. Autoimmunity could develop if these antigens came in contact with immunocompetent cells. There is little evidence today for the antigen sequestration theory. For example, normal individuals have antigen-binding lymphocytes with specificity for thyroglobulin.

Autoantibodies are physiologic

Grabar (1975) proposed that autoantibodies were preserved throughout evolution because they have a physiologic role. He suggested that autoantibodies are "transporteurs" or carriers of metabolic and catabolic tissue degradation products, and function as cleansing agents that eliminate waste products from the organism. The concept of a physiologic role for antiself deserves fresh consideration, particularly since immunologic regulation depends upon the recognition of self-antigens on cell membranes.

Cross-reactive antigens

Modified cross-reactive antigens or related foreign antigens can terminate a state of specific immunologic unresponsiveness (Weigle, 1977). For example, mice made tolerant to bovine serum albumin can be induced to make antibody ("escape from tolerance") by the injection of chemically modified bovine serum albumin or human serum albumin. This is an example of T cell bypass in which potentially responsive B cells are induced to make antibody even though the T cells are tolerant. This could be a model for autoimmunity. For example, viruses might induce antigenic modifications of self-antigens that permit stimulation of B cells and bypass the need for antigen-specific T cells.

Disordered immunologic regulation

The potential for autoimmunity is present but not expressed in healthy individuals due to the normal functioning of immunologic regulatory mechan-

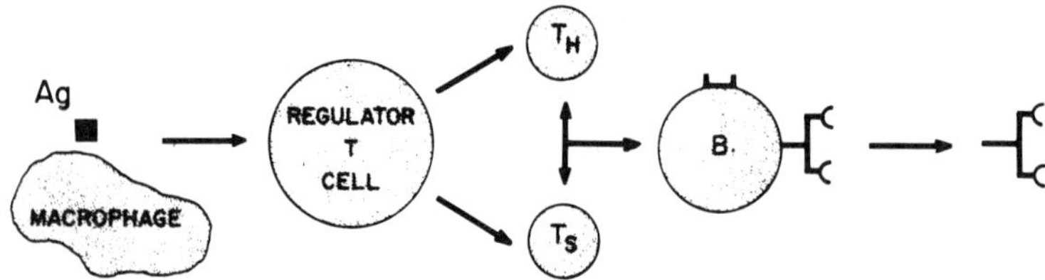

FIG. 1. *Schematic representation of the immune network as it normally functions to regulate the immune response. The combination of antigen and macrophage leads to T cell interactions which influence the activity of helper* (T_H) *and suppressor* (T_S) *T cells. Depending upon the regulatory balance established, B cells may be activated to synthesize antibody or suppressed and be made immunologically unresponsive.*

isms. The interactions between various T lymphocyte subpopulations are chiefly responsible for this regulation (Fig. 1). A disequilibrium resulting either in the generation of helper T cells or in a deficiency of suppressor T cells could trigger these potentially autoreactive B cell clones to produce autoantibody. Intrinsic polyclonal activation of B cells can also occur independent of T cell abnormalities (Fig. 2).

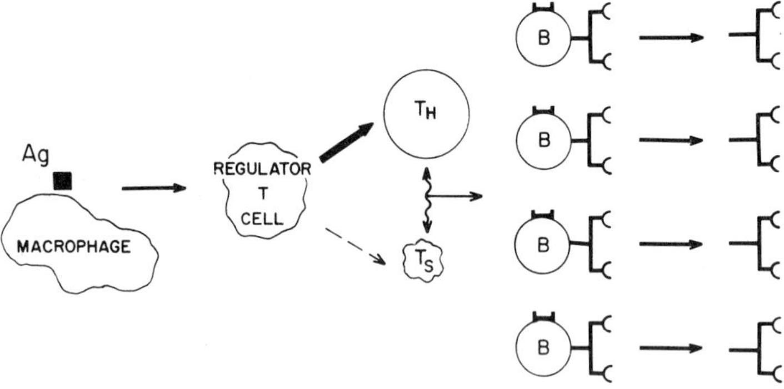

FIG. 2. *Schematic representation of the immune network as it functions abnormally in autoimmune disease. There may be overactivity of helper T cells, deficiency of suppressor T cells, and polyclonal activation of B cells.*

Recognition of self-antigens on cell membranes appears to be of profound importance in the immune response. Jerne (1974) proposed that immunologic control is mediated by a complementary network of membrane receptors that express idiotypic determinants of immunoglobulins. Idiotypes are present on both B and T cells, are closely related to the antigen-binding sites of immunoglobulin, and can function as cell surface receptors for antigen. Idiotypic determinants interact with complementary anti-idiotypic structures on immunoglobulins or lymphocytes. Anti-idiotypic antiserum can be either immunosuppressive or immunostimulatory, probably depending upon the nature of its interaction with the idiotypic cell receptor.

The immune system appears as a vast network of interacting cell surface receptors responding to signals that may be self, foreign, or often a combination of both. A hypothetical model that explains autoimmunity as an extension of normal self-recognition has recently been proposed (Talal, 1978). This model discriminates between a limited form of autoimmunity and autoimmune disease. The immunologic network of regulation is intact in autoimmunity, but fundamentally disturbed in autoimmune disease.

In clinical medicine, there are numerous examples of autoantibody production without autoimmune disease. Certain infectious disorders tending to chronicity, many drugs, and the process of ageing are associated with a limited form of autoimmunity. Upon successful eradication of the infection or discontinuation of the offending drug, the manifestations of autoimmunity disappear. The infectious agents or drugs may induce cell membrane changes that are recognized immunologically. For example, procainamide is a drug that can induce a lupus-like syndrome. The development of lupus is associated with the appearance of antilymphocyte antibodies, suggesting possible interaction of procainamide with the lymphocyte membrane (Bluestein *et al.*, 1979).

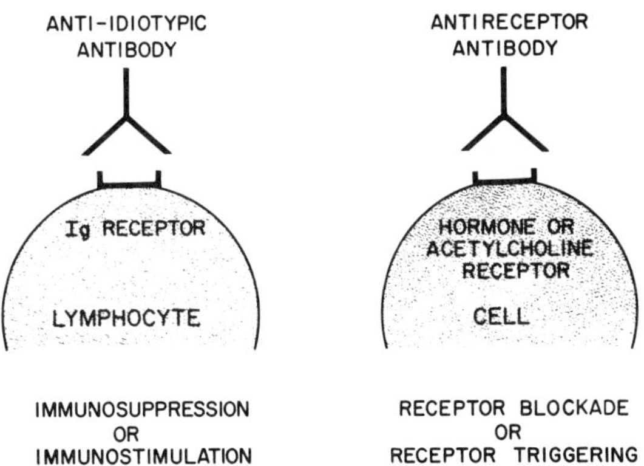

FIG. 3. *Modulation of cell surface receptors for hormones or neurotransmitters by antireceptor antibodies may be analogous to modulation of idiotypic receptors by anti-idiotypic antibodies.*

In the antireceptor autoimmune diseases (myasthenia gravis, Graves' disease, some forms of insulin-resistant diabetes mellitus), antibodies modulate cell surface receptors and influence receptor function. Either receptor blockade or receptor triggering may occur. An analogy can be made with anti-idiotypic antibodies which can result either in immune suppression or in priming (Fig. 3).

Systemic lupus erythematosus (SLE)

The multifactorial nature of autoimmune diseases is well demonstrated in SLE, where recent studies have demonstrated important genetic and endocrine factors (Table II).

TABLE II
Recent advances in understanding the pathogenesis of SLE

1. Genetic predisposition (HLA DRw2 and DRw3, Ia antigens).
2. Prolonged circulation of IgG-coated autologous RBC correlating with serum immune complexes.
3. Endocrine predisposition (altered metabolism of oestradiol).
4. Disordered immunoregulation with $\downarrow T_S$, $\uparrow T_H$ and polyclonal B cell activation.

Genetic factors

For many years, SLE was a disease in which an association with histocompatibility antigens was surprisingly absent. Reinertsen and colleagues (1978) provided the first substantial documentation of a histocompatibility antigen association in SLE. They found that the presence of HLA-DRw2 and DRw3 increased the relative risk for developing SLE by a factor of three. Even more, the presence of an antigen reactive with pregnancy serum Ia-715 increased the relative risk 18-fold. This antigen is present on B cells and macrophages. Serum Ia-715 reacted with cells from 70% of SLE patients, compared to 14% of normal subjects. This serum also reacts strongly with cells from patients with primary SS. Family studies in lupus suggest that two or more genes may be required for the full expression of disease.

Endocrine factors

An endocrine predisposition for the development of SLE was suggested by the demonstration from our laboratory (Roubinian *et al.*, 1977) and Dr Steinberg's laboratory (1979) that sex hormones modulate autoimmune disease in NZB/W F_1 mice. Androgens suppress and oestrogens accelerate immune complex glomerulonephritis and mortality. To understand the mechanism of sex hormone action, we recently studied the clearance of particulate immune complexes consisting of radiolabelled autologous erythrocytes sensitized with rabbit IgG antimouse erythrocytes.

There was a marked defect in the ability of old female and male mice to clear these IgG-coated red blood cells (Fig. 4). Female NZB/W mice at 3 months cleared the complexes completely in 1 h. At 7 months, clearance was impaired so that considerable radioactivity was still present at 2 h. Normal erythrocytes were not cleared by young or old mice.

Likewise, young male mice (3 months) cleared the particulate complexes rapidly while there was prolonged circulation in older male mice (Fig. 4). The defect appeared later in male than in female mice. Six-month-old males showed normal clearance patterns, which became abnormal by 13 months. The clearance of these sensitized eythrocytes was largely complement-dependent and mediated by the liver.

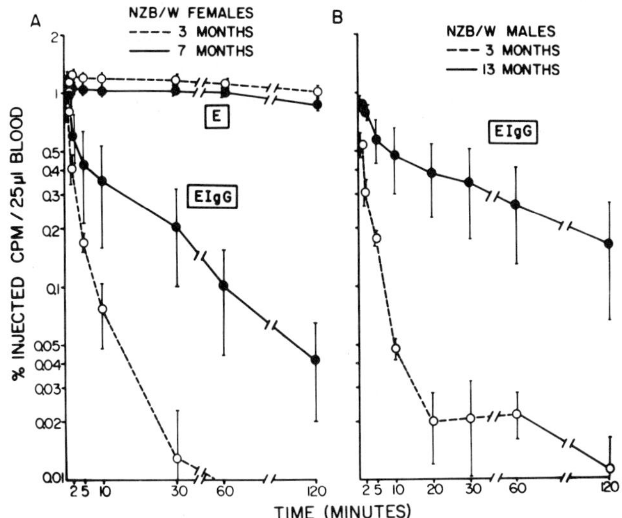

FIG. 4. *The clearance of* ^{51}*Cr-Ig coated autologous erythrocytes (EIgG) is shown over 120 min in NZB/W female (A) and male (B) mice. The circulation of noncoated erythrocytes (E) is also shown in the female mice. The data are presented as the percent of injected dose/25 µl of blood.*

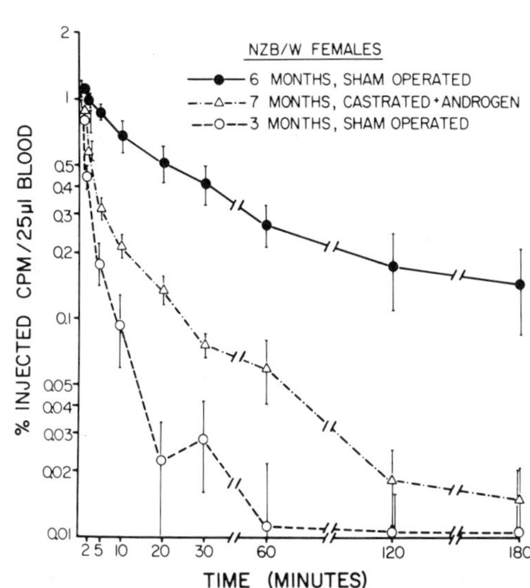

FIG. 5. *The clearance of* ^{51}*Cr-IgG coated autologous erythrocytes is significantly more rapid in castrated androgen-treated 7-month-old NZB/W female mice compared to 6-month-old sham-operated NZB/W mice. The clearance in 3-month-old NZB/W female mice is shown for comparison.*

Some NZB/W mice were castrated and treated with androgen or oestrogen to study the influence of sex hormones on this clearance function. Castration and androgen treatment of 7-month-old NZB/W female mice resulted in a greatly improved clearance of particulate immune complexes compared to sham-operated mice (Fig. 5).

Seven-month-old NZB/W male mice showed rapid clearance compared to 13-month-old NZB/W male mice (Fig. 6). Castration and oestrogen treatment of 7-month-old male NZB/W mice delayed the clearance (Fig. 6).

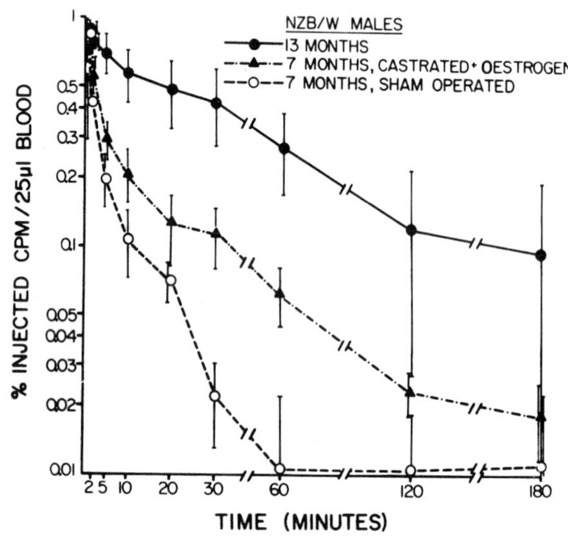

FIG. 6. *The clearance of* ^{51}*Cr-IgG coated autologous erythrocytes is prolonged in castrated-oestrogen treated 7-month-old NZB/W male mice compared to 7-month-old sham-operated NZB/W male mice. The clearance in 13-month-old NZB/W male mice is shown for comparison.*

Thus, androgen and oestrogen have opposite effects on the clearance of IgG-coated autologous erythrocytes by cells of the reticuloendothelial system. Androgen improved clearance; this may relate to the ability of androgen to retard immune complex glomerulonephritis. Oestrogen delayed clearance; this may relate to the enhanced immune complex glomerulonephritis seen in oestrogen-treated NZB/W mice.

Similar to these results in lupus mice, Frank and his colleagues at the NIH (1979) have shown that particulate immune complexes have a prolonged circulation time in SLE patients. They injected ^{15}Cr-labelled autologous red blood cells coated with anti-Rh antibody. In normal subjects, such particulate complexes were cleared within an hour as they were taken up by Fc receptors in the reticuloendothelial system (particularly in the spleen). In SLE, the complexes remained in the circulation for several hours. This defect correlated with disease activity and with the level of immune complexes as measured by C1q binding. The inefficient handling of immune complexes by the reticuloendothelial system in patients with SLE may lead to prolonged circulation of complexes and deposition in the kidneys and other tissues.

The marked female predominance of SLE, which can be as high as 15:1 (female:male) during the menstruating years, may be explained by an alteration of oestrogen metabolism that results in a hyperoestrogenic influence. Lahita *et al.* (1979) studied oestradiol metabolism in SLE patients and normal controls by measurements of urinary metabolites after injection of radiolabelled ^{3}H-oestradiol. They found a deviation in the metabolic pathway. Patients with SLE had increased hydroxylation of oestrone. Females had elevations of both 16α-hydroxyoestrone and oestriol, whereas male patients had an elevation only in 16α-hydroxyoestrone. These 16-hydroxylated metabolites bind to oestrogen receptors and retain oestrogenic activity. This diversion from normal 2-hydroxylated to 16-hydroxylated metabolities creates a hyperoestrogenic state in SLE that may augment immune reactivity. A similar defect in oestrogen metabolism has also been reported in Klinefelter's syndrome, an XXY state predisposed to SLE.

Miller *et al.* (1979) reported an abnormality of concanavalin A (con A), which induced suppression in SLE patients and in 13 first-degree relatives of these patients. Interestingly, 12 of these 13 healthy asymptomatic relatives were females. This abnormality was not present in normal females or in patients with discoid lupus, and was not related to the presence of antilymphocyte antibodies. The authors suggested that abnormalities of suppressor cell function may be a genetic marker for SLE.

T cell abnormalities

SLE patients have depressed T lymphocyte function and enhanced B lymphocyte activity. Several investigators (Abdou *et al.*, 1976; Breshnihan and Jasin, 1977; Horwitz *et al.*, 1977; Sakane *et al.*, 1978a; Morimoto, 1978; Fauci *et al.*, 1978) have found deficient suppressor T cell activity in SLE (Table III). Normal T cells activated by con A were able to suppress autologous T cell proliferation generated by mitogens or allogeneic cells (Sakane *et al.*, 1978b). However, con A-induced T cell suppression was defective in SLE. Further-

TABLE III

Evidence for decreased suppression in SLE

1. Impaired generation of suppressor T cells after exposure to con A
2. Sensitivity of suppressor T cells to thymocytotoxic antibody
3. Loss of a specific T cell subset revealed by FACS analysis
4. Decreased number of T_G cells
5. Decreased number of T cells reactive with T5 antiserum

Evidence for enhanced B cell activity in SLE

1. Increased spontaneous Ig synthesis
2. Decreased response to pokeweed mitogen
3. Increased plaque-forming cells to various haptens

more, con A activated T cells from normal individuals suppressed the response of SLE patients, whereas con A activated SLE T cells could not suppress normal responses. Thus, SLE patients could respond to normal suppressor signals. The defect in SLE was an inability to generate suppressor T cells and not in the response to suppressor cells.

T cell effector function is generally impaired in SLE. Thus, it is important to know whether the defect in suppression reflects a general T cell deficiency or whether it is more specific. SLE patients frequently produce, as part of their B cell hyperactivity, an autoantibody cytotoxic for T cells (Winfield *et al.*, 1975; Lies *et al.*, 1975). These antibodies are generally IgM, require complement for killing, and are associated with active disease and lymphopenia. The addition of active SLE plasma (containing antilymphocyte antibody) to normal T cells stimulated with con A inhibited the development of suppressor activity (Sakane *et al.*, 1979). Absorption of such inhibitory plasma with T cells eliminated the factor capable of blocking suppressor cell generation. The factor was an IgM and required complement for its inhibitory activity. This experiment appears to duplicate, using normal peripheral blood T cells and SLE serum, the findings generally present in patients with active SLE. Furthermore, if one dilutes SLE serum, it will selectively inhibit suppressor T cells with less effect on other T cell responses (Koike *et al.*, 1979). These results suggest that the *in vivo* loss of suppressor cell activity in SLE may be due, at least in part, to this anti-T cell antibody.

Further evidence for this mechanism was obtained using the fluorescence-activated cell sorter as an analytical tool (Steinberg *et al.*, 1979). When SLE serum was mixed with peripheral blood cells and then a fluorescent anti-IgM serum was added, SLE patients were found to have fewer brightly staining cells representing the suppressor T cell subset. These cells were presumably reduced in the patients due to the *in vivo* action of antilymphocyte antibodies.

SLE patients have a reduced number of T_G cells which contain a suppressor population (Fauci *et al.*, 1978; Hamilton and Winfield, 1979). Of antilymphocyte antibodies, 64% showed preferential reactivity with the T_G subpopulation (Okudaira, 1979). When T cells were depleted of the T_G subset by exposure to antilymphocyte antibody, and then cocultured with B cells, Ig synthesis by the B cells was enhanced. This result confirms the specificity of the antilymphocyte antibody for T_G cells, shows that T_G cells have suppressor activity, and suggests that B cells are more active in the absence of T_G cells.

SLE patients also have a decrease in T cells reactive with T5 antiserum which identifies the suppressor/cytotoxic T cell subset (Morimoto *et al.*, 1980).

Autologous mixed lymphocyte response (AMLR)

The generation of cytotoxic T cells is dependent upon recognition of both foreign and self-antigens on the target cells, but the exact mechanism of recognition is uncertain. Immune responses to modified self-antigens are controlled by genes contained within the major histocompatibility complex

(MHC). Recognition of these self-MHC antigens on cell membranes is often a necessary prerequisite for an immune response to foreign determinants such as viral or chemical antigens. Recognition of self occurs between lymphocytes themselves and also between lymphocytes and accessory cells such as macrophages. This response can be measured *in vitro* using a system called the autologous mixed lymphocyte response (AMLR), in which T cells respond to DR antigens expressed by non-T cells from the same individual (Weksler and Kozak, 1977; Hausman and Stobo, 1979). An analogous system in the mouse, in which splenic T cells respond to Ia antigens on non-T cells, is called the syngeneic mixed lymphocyte response (SMLR) (Smith and Pasternak, 1978).

The AMLR is decreased in SLE and is lowest in active disease (Sakane *et al.*, 1978b). The basis for this reduced response probably resides within the responding cells. In active SLE, both the T_G and T-non$_G$ responding cells gave a poor response. In inactive SLE, only the T_G cells were unresponsive. When a patient went from active to inactive disease, the responding T cells from that patient showed this transition in the AMLR (i.e. from poor response in both T cell populations to poor response only in the T_G suppressor population). Thus, the AMLR reveals a defect in the T_G suppressor population, even when disease is inactive (Sakane *et al.*, 1980).

One laboratory working with the AMLR produced evidence that the defect was in the stimulating and not the responding cell population (Kuntz *et al.*, 1979). This potential controversy has been partially resolved by studying identical twins where one twin had active SLE and the other inactive disease (Sakane *et al.*, 1979). Because the twins were identical, responding T cells and stimulating non-T cells could be mixed from one twin to the other without altering histocompatibility antigens. The twin with active disease had both defective responding T and stimulating non-T cells. The twin with inactive disease had a defect only in the responding T_G population. Thus, both responding and stimulating cells may contribute to a defective AMLR in SLE patients.

The SMLR, analogous to the human AMLR, is decreased in autoimmune-

TABLE IV

SMLR in various mouse strains

Strains	*Sex*	*Age (months)*	*Incorporation of H^3-dTr (cpm)* Unstimulated	*Stimulated*	*Net Incorporation*	*Stimulation index*
C57BL/6	F	2	2·525	11·741	9·216	4·6
C57BL/6	F	6	1·126	14·952	13·826	13·2
C57BL/6	M	2	2·171	8·765	6·594	4·0
CBA	F	2	1·781	13·567	11·786	7·6
B/W	F	7	5·446	2·955	−2·491	—
B/W	M	7	2·467	3·365	889	1·4
BXSB	M	6	17·195	16·968	−227	—
MRL/l	M	2	4·080	6·009	1·929	1·5

susceptible strains (NZB, NZB/W, BXSB and MRL/1) compared to normal mice (Table IV). The decreased SMLR correlates with disease activity. Murine lupus is more severe in NZB/W females and in BXSB males, by comparison with the opposite sex in each strain. The SMLR is abnormal earlier in NZB/W females compared to males, and in BXSB males compared to females. It is also lower in MRL/1 mice than in MRL/n mice, corresponding with the more severe disease in the former. The SMLR is decreased prior to the appearance of clinical disease. The decreased response is due to a selective abnormality in an Ly-1 positive responding T cell. It does not reflect a general T cell defect or a defect in the stimulating non-T cells (Hom and Talal, 1980). It may represent a common T cell abnormality predisposing to autoimmunity in mice and humans.

B cell abnormalities

The enhanced B cell activity in SLE (Jasin and Ziff, 1975; Morimoto *et al.*, 1977; Budman *et al.*, 1977; Nies and Louis, 1978; Bobrove and Miller, 1977) is demonstrated by increased spontaneous immunoglobulin synthesis, decreased response to pokeweed mitogen (because the B cells are already intrinsically activated), and increased numbers of plaque-forming cells to various haptens (Table III).

As a consequence of the disordered immunoregulatory system, SLE patients produce a large number of different autoantibodies. Many of these react with nuclear antigens. Antinuclear antibodies also occur in patients with other autoimmune diseases. The antigenic specificities of these various antinuclear antibodies are different and correlate in a general way with the clinical diagnosis (Table V).

Lerner and Steitz (1979) reported that Sm and RNP antibodies react with small nuclear RNAs complexed with nucleoproteins. They analysed immune precipitates formed by reacting these antibodies with radiolabelled nuclear

TABLE V
Antinuclear antibodies in autoimmune disease

Disease	*Antinuclear antibody*
SLE	Sm DNA SS-A (Ro) RNP (low titre)
Sjögren's syndrome	SS-A (Ro) SS-B (Ha, La)
Rheumatoid arthritis	RAP
Mixed connective tissue disease	RNP (high titre)

extracts from mouse Ehrlich ascites cells. Anti-Sm precipitated 6 small nuclear RNA molecules, and anti-RNP reacted with 2 of these. Each of the 6 small nuclear RNAs was complexed with and antigenic by virtue of association with nucleoproteins. These ribonucleoprotein complexes had a total mol. wt of approximately 175 000. These complexes may function as splicing enzymes to eliminate intervening sequences in DNA and allow the formation of intact and functional messenger RNA. Genes are separated by noncoding regions called introns or intervening sequences. An RNA copy of the entire gene is made, the introns are cleaved out, and RNA fragments rejoined with great specificity before the mature messenger RNA leaves the nucleus. The small nuclear RNP complexes may mediate these activities. An explanation as to why patients make antibodies to precisely these molecules is awaited with great interest.

Sjögren's syndrome (SS)

Primary and secondary SS

In SS, there is an autoimmune attack on lacrimal and salivary glands resulting in deficiency of tears and saliva. Approximately half of the patients have rheumatoid arthritis. The term "autoimmune exocrinopathy" has been applied to SS because there may be widespread involvement of the exocrine glands (Strand and Talal, 1980).

TABLE VI

Recent advances in understanding the pathogenesis of Sjögren's syndrome (SS)

1. Primary and secondary SS can be distinguished by clinical, genetic and serologic criteria.
2. Genetic predisposition (HLA B8 DRw3 in 1°, DRw4 in 2°, Ia antigens).
3. Antinuclear antibodies (Ha, SS-B, La in 1°, RAP in 2°).
4. Lymphocyte-aggressive disease can terminate in B cell neoplasia.
5. T cell and immune complex abnormalities may be less important than in SLE.

Recent studies suggest two forms of SS that can be distinguished by clinical, immunogenetic and serologic criteria (Moutsopoulos *et al.*, 1980). Primary SS is not associated with arthritis, is associated with HLA B8DRw3, and with the presence of a precipitating antinuclear antibody called SS-B (also called Ha or La). Secondary SS occurs in rheumatoid arthritis and is associated with HLA DRw4 and the autoantibody RAP (Table VI). The latter reacts with a nuclear antigen RANA which is related to infection with the Epstein–Barr (EB) virus. The exact relationship between rheumatoid arthritis and EB virus is not yet established. Certain Ia antigens occur in both primary and secondary SS. Reactivity with Ia-715 suggests a possible relationship between primary SS and SLE.

Benign and malignant lymphoproliferation

The salivary glands in SS show focal or diffuse infiltration by B lymphocytes and plasma cells which synthesize large amounts of immunoglobulin and rheumatoid factor. Germinal centres may develop in the infiltrated glands. T cells are present in severely involved glands. Similar immunopathologic events occur in the rheumatoid synovium.

Some patients develop a more severe lymphocyte-aggressive disease with infiltration of vital organs such as the lung or kidney. There may be generalized lymphadenopathy and splenomegaly. Biopsy of involved tissue shows atypical lymphoid infiltrates but it is usually difficult to make a diagnosis of lymphoid malignancy. The term "pseudolymphoma" has been used to describe such patients who may also have monoclonal macroglobulinaemia. Other patients develop a true lymphoma, at times accompanied by hypo-γ-globulinaemia.

Immunoperoxidase studies have shown that the benign salivary gland infiltrates and pseudolymphomas are polyclonal, containing B cells with cytoplasmic IgM, IgG, κ and λ chains (Zulman *et al.*, 1978). The malignant lymphomas, however, are monoclonal and consist of B cells with cytoplasmic IgM-κ. Thus, in SS, there can be a transition from a polyclonal autoimmune infiltrate to a monoclonal B cell neoplasm.

Although immune complexes occur in SS, they do not correlate with the extent of lymphoid infiltration or with other features of disease. For example, prolonged circulation of particulate immune complexes (Rh antibody coated autologous red blood cells) occurs in SS patients with extraglandular disease, indicative of Fc receptor abnormalities (Hamburger *et al.*, 1979). However, in contrast to SLE, this abnormality does not correlate with the presence of circulating immune complexes (Table VII).

Again, in contrast to SLE, there is no evidence of intrinsic B cell activation in SS, perhaps because the activated B cells are in the tissues and not in the peripheral blood (Moutsopoulos and Fauci, 1980b). In both diseases, there

TABLE VII
Comparison of abnormalities in SLE and SS

	SLE	*SS*
Increased immune complexes	+	+
Abnormal Fc receptor function	+	+[a]
Correlation of the above	Yes	No
Intrinsic B cell activation	+	−
Decreased PWM-induced anti-sRBC PFCs	+	+[a]
Decreased T_G cells	+	+
Decreased T_G cells is reversible due to serum blocking factors	No	Yes
Normal con A generated T_S of PWM-induced B cell proliferation	No	Yes
Decreased autologous MLR	+	+

[a] Extraglandular disease

is a decreased response to pokeweed mitogen. The decrease in the T_G population in SS is reversible and related to a serum blocking factor, again in contrast to SLE (Table VII). Con A generated suppressor cell function is normal in SS but abnormal in SLE. Antilymphocyte antibodies occur in only 20% of SS patients (Miyasaka *et al.*, submitted for publication). The AMLR is decreased in SS (Fig. 7) as it is in SLE. The mechanism of this defect could be different in each disease.

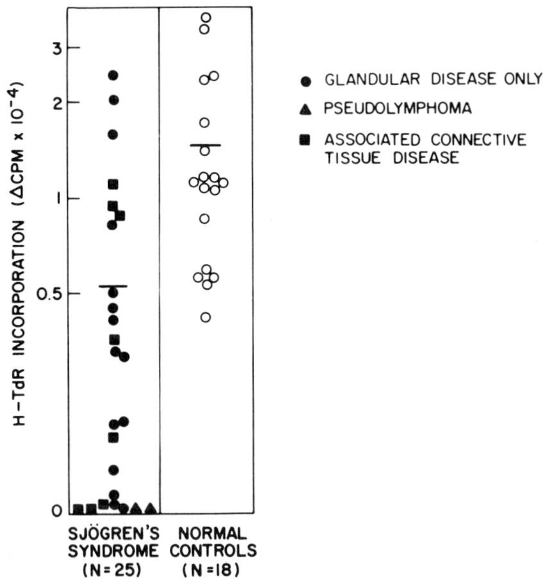

FIG. 7. *Decreased autologous mixed lymphocyte response was present in 60% of SS patients.*

Conclusion

Lewis Thomas (1980) in an essay entitled "Medical Lessons From History", writes that "for every disease there is a single key mechanism that dominates all others. If one can find it, and then think one's way around it, one can control the disorder."

Although his goal still seems far distant for the autoimmune diseases, it may now be possible to identify key immunopathogenic mechanisms responsible for the morbidity or mortality in any given disease. These key mechanisms should be distinguished from secondary immunologic mechanisms of lesser pathologic importance. Hopefully, specific forms of therapy will be devised to control the primary mechanisms and arrest or reverse the illness.

The decreased AMLR and SMLR in SLE, SS and in the several autoimmune strains of mice may speak for a common underlying mechanism.

Beyond that, however, SLE and SS seem to have different key immunopathogenic mechanisms. SLE is characterized by autoantibodies to T cells and loss of T cell regulation. The major consequence of the polyclonal B cell activation is related to immune complex disposition, particularly DNA containing complexes in the kidney. In SS, the B cell may be involved more directly resulting in excessive B cell proliferation, abnormal localization of B cells in parenchymal organs, and ultimately in B cell neoplasia.

References

Abdou, N. O., Sagawa, A., Pascual, E., Hebert, J. and Sadaghee, S. (1976). *Clin. Immunol. Immunopath.* **6**, 192.

Bluestein, H. G., Zvaifler, N. J., Weisman, H. M. and Shapiro, R. F. (1979). *Lancet* **ii**, 816.

Bobrove, A. M. and Miller, P. (1977). *Arth. Rheum.* **20**, 1326.

Breshnihan, B. and Jasin, H. E. (1977). *J. Clin. Invest.* **59**, 106.

Budman, D. R., Merchant, E. B., Steinberg, A. D., Doft, B., Gershwin, N. E., Lizzio, E. and Reeves, J. P. (1977). *Arth. Rheum.* **20**, 829.

Fauci, A. S., Steinberg, A. D., Haynes, B. F. and Whalen, G. (1978). *J. Immunology* **121**, 1978.

Frank, M. M., Hamburger, M. I., Lawley, T. J., Kimberly, R. P. and Plotz, P. H. (1979). *New Engl. J. Med.* **300**, 518.

Grabar, P. (1975). *Clin. Immunol. Immunopath.* **4**, 453.

Hamburger, M. I., Moutsopoulos, H. M., Lawley, T. J. and Frank, M. M. (1979). *Ann. Intern. Med.* **91**, 534.

Hamilton, M. E. and Winfield, J. B. (1979). *Arth. Rheum.* **22**, 1.

Hausman, P. B. and Stobo, J. D. (1979). *J. Exp. Med.* **147**, 1537.

Hom, J. T. and Talal, N. (1980). *In* "Proceedings of the Conference on Immunoregulation and Autoimmunity, Immunodynamics III" (R. S. Krakauer, ed.). Elsevier, N. Holland/New York (in press).

Horwitz, S., Borcherding, W., Moorthy, A. V., Chesney, R., Schulte-Wisserman, H., Hong, R. and Goldstein, A. (1977). *Science* **197**, 999.

Izui, S., Lambert, P. H., Fornie, G. J., Turler, H. and Miescher, P. A. (1977). *J. Exp. Med.* **145**, 1115.

Jasin, H. E. and Ziff, M. (1975). *Arth. Rheum.* **18**, 219.

Jerne, N. K. (1974). *Ann. Immunol.* (Paris) **125C**, 373.

Koike, T., Kobayashi, S., Hoshiki, T., Itoh, T. and Shirai, T. (1979). *Arth. Rheum.* **22**, 123.

Kuntz, M. M., Innes, J. G. and Weksler, M. E. (1979). *J. Clin. Invest.* **63**, 151.

Lahita, R. G., Bradlow, H. L., Kunkel, A. G. and Fishman, J. (1979). *Arth. Rheum.* **22**, 1195.

Lerner, M. R. and Steitz, J. A. (1979). *Proc. Natn. Acad. Sci. U.S.A.* (Washington) **76**, 5495.

Lies, R. B., Messner, R. P. and Williams, R. C. (1975). *Arth. Rheum.* **16**, 369.

Miller, P., Kenneth, B. and Schwartz, R. S. (1979). *New Engl. J. Med.* **301**, 803.

Miyasaka, N., Sauvezie, B., Pierce, D. A., Daniels, T. E. and Talal, N. (submitted for publication). *J. Clin. Invest.*

Morimoto, C. (1978). *Clin. Exp. Immunol.* **32**, 125.

Morimoto, C., Abe, T., Hara, M. and Homma, M. (1977). *J. Immunol.* **6**, 575.

Morimoto, C., Reinherz, E. L., Abe, T., Homma, M. and Schlossman, S. F. (1980). *Clin. Immunol. Immunopath.* (in press).

Moutsopoulos, H. M. and Fauci, A. S. (1980). *J. Clin. Invest.* **65**, 519.

Moutsopoulos, H. M., Chused, T. M., Mann, D. L., Klippel, J. H., Fauci, A. S., Frank, M. M., Lawley, T. J. and Hamburger, M. I. (1980). *Ann. Intern. Med.* **92**, 212.

Nies, K. M. and Louie, J. S. (1978). *Arth. Rheum.* **21**, 51.

Okudaira, K., Nakai, H., Hayakawa, T., Kashiwadao, T., Tanimoto, K., Horiuchi, Y. and Juji, T. (1979). *J. Clin. Invest.* **63**, 1213.

Reinersten, J. L., Klippel, J. H., Johnson, A. H., Steinberg, A. D., Decker, J. L. and Mann, D. L. (1978). *New Engl. J. Med.* **299**, 515.

Roubinian, J. R., Papoian, R. and Talal, N. (1977). *J. Clin. Invest.* **59**, 1066.

Sakane, T., Steinberg, A. D. and Green, I. (1978a). *Arth. Rheum.* **21**, 657.

Sakane, T., Steinberg, A. D. and Green, I. (1978b). *Proc. Natn. Acad. Sci. U.S.A.* (Washington) **75**, 3464.

Sakane, T., Steinberg, A. D., Arnett, F. C., Reinertsen, J. L. (1979). *Arth. Rheum.* **22**, 770.

Sakane, T., Steinberg, A. D. and Green, I. (1980). *Arth. Rheum.* **23**, 225.

Smith, B. and Pasternak, R. D. (1978). *J. Immunol.* **121**, 1889.

Steinberg, A. D., Melez, K. A., Raveche, E. S. and Reeves, J. P. (1969). *Arth. Rheum.* **22**, 1170.

Strand, V. and Talal, N. (1980). *Bull. Rheum. Dis.* (in press).

Talal, N. (1978). *Arth. Rheum.* **21**, 853.

Thomas, L. (1980). *In* "The Medussa and the Snail" p. 140, Bantom Books.

Weigle, W. O. (1977). *In* "Autoimmunity: Genetic, Immunologic, Virologic, and Clinical Aspects" (N. Talal, ed.), pp. 141–170. Academic Press, New York and London.

Weksler, M. E. and Kozak, R. (1977). *J. Exp. Med.* **146**, 1833.

Winfield, J. B., Winchester, R. J., Wernet, P., Fu, S. M. and Kunkel, H. G. (1975). *Arth. Rheum.* **18**, 1, 1975.

Zulman, J. I., Jaffe, R. and Talal, N. (1978). *New Engl. J. Med.* **229**, 1215.

51

Current Approaches to the Primary Immunodeficiencies

ROBERT A. GOOD, NEENA KAPOOR, RAJENDRA N. PAHWA, ANNE WEST and RICHARD J. O'REILLY

Sloan-Kettering Institute, Memorial Sloan-Kettering Cancer Center, New York, USA

Original studies described in this review were aided by grants CA-08748, CA-19267, CA-23766, CA-17404, AI-11843, and NS-11457 from the National Institutes of Health; the Sherman Fairchild Foundation New Frontiers Fund, the Zelda R. Weintraub Cancer Fund, the Judith Harris Selig Memorial Fund, the Fund for the Advanced Study of Cancer, and the National Foundation-March of Dimes.

Introduction

In recent years, the science of immunology has evolved at a prodigious rate. Primary disorders of the immunity system have stimulated perceptive interpretation by physicians and rigorous analysis in the laboratory, work which has revealed that the immunity network is made up of many interacting components. Abnormalities of cell-mediated or humoral immunity frequently reflect defects not simply of T and B cells, but of immunoregulation involving cell subpopulations and their molecular products, other biological amplification systems such as the components of the complement series, and fundamental effector mechanisms such as phagocytic cells. Recognizing these fundamental components enables us now to develop our therapeutic approaches to immunologically based disease in terms of cells and molecules.

This chapter will discuss the methods of treatment presently in use for the primary immunodeficiencies, a group which is likely to expand as we discover immunologic abnormalities linked with the pathogenesis of other diseases. We will consider disorders of the lymphoid system, aplastic anaemia, defects of the complement system and defects of the phagocytic system, along with our present capabilities for treating them. We will also consider several approaches which are being developed as therapeutic modalities for the future, not only for the treatment of immunologically based disease, but also for diseases like cancer which are not always associated with readily demonstrable immunodeficiency.

Transplantation of bone marrow for SCID

The bone marrow contains the pluripotent stem cell which differentiates into the haematopoietic, lymphoid, phagocytic, and megakaryocytic cell series. Thus, theoretically, bone marrow transplantation (BMT) could provide precursors for any of these cell systems. Successful achievements in allogeneic bone marrow transplantation were first made in patients with the class of primary immunodeficiency diseases called severe combined immunodeficiency (SCID). In these unfortunate children, both T and B lymphocyte systems are sometimes grossly deficient, leaving patients helpless against bacterial, viral and fungal infections, and likely to die if the situation is untreated.

Sibling donor, HLA-matched

The first successful bone marrow transplant was performed in 1968 on a child with SCID, using the marrow of a sister who was identical by histocompatibility typing, except at the HLA-A locus of the major histocompatibility complex. This transplant corrected the malfunctions of both the T and B immunity systems. Although the child developed aplastic anaemia following the procedure, probably due to the HLA-A mismatch, a second transplant from the same donor also cured the latter disease. This case, thus, also represented the first use of bone marrow transplantation from a matched sibling donor as successful treatment for aplastic anaemia (Gatti *et al.*, 1968; Good, 1969). The patient is in vigorous good health and immunologically normal 12 years later. The basic tenets of this achievement were quickly confirmed in both Holland and Boston for the autosomal recessive form of SCID (De Koning *et al.*, 1969; Levey *et al.*, 1971).

Shortly after this initial success, our Minnesota team performed a bone marrow transplantation for a child who, in addition to her combined immunodeficiency, entirely lacked the enzyme adenosine deaminase (ADA) (Biggar *et al.*, 1975). The donor, a sister, was matched at the major histocompatibility locus and had normal ADA. Mother and father had approximately one-half normal values of ADA, establishing the recessive nature of the inheritance of the immunodeficiency and enzyme defect in this case. Today, as a consequence of the marrow transplant from her matched sister, this girl remains well, immunologically normal, and in a fascinating chimaeric state: while her lymphoid cells now contain normal amounts of the enzyme, her peripheral red cells lack the ADA as before. Other patients with ADA deficiency have since been described who have benefited from this form of treatment, which has again produced this extraordinary chimaeric situation (Lewis *et al.*, 1977; Polmar, 1979).

TABLE I

Bone marrow transplantation for SCID using HLA-identical donors

Institution	*Patients Transplanted*	*Reconstitution T*	*Reconstitution B*	*Survival*
MSKCC, New York	5	4	4	4
U. Minnesota	8	6	5	5
U. Wisconsin	3	3	3	3
UCLA	3	3	3	3
Children's, Boston	8	4	4	3
Leiden	3	3	3	3
Lyon	5	3	3	3
Paris	6	5	5	4
Zurich	1	1	1	0
Beirut	2	2	1	1
Westminster, London	2	2	2	0
Ulm	1	0	0	0
U. Alabama	2	2	2	1
U. Washington	1	1	1	1
U. Albany	1	1	1	1
BMT Registry, other than above	5	1	0	0
Totals	57	41	38	32 (56%)

Since these original achievements, in which the availability of matched sibling donors permitted bone marrow transplantation without producing lethal graft-versus-host reaction (GVHR) or graft-versus-host disease (GVHD), at least 5 genetically distinct forms of SCID have been cured by bone marrow transplantation using a matched sibling donor. This method can now be said to represent the treatment of choice for SCID. Table I shows the results of BMT for SCID using a matched sibling donor, as reported by centres throughout Europe, England and the USA. Table II gives the results of the authors' own experience with this form of treatment at past and present institutions.

The next steps for medical immunologists were (a) to apply this therapy

TABLE II

Bone marrow transplantation for SCID, with matched sibling donor (combined Minnesota and New York experience)

Successful graft	12/13
Successful long-lived cure of disease	9/13 (69%)
GVHR present	5/13
GVHR severe	0/13
GVHR cause of death	0/13
Death from unrecognized pneumocystic pneumonia	1/13
Death from aspiration	1/13
Death from congenital GVHR and failure of graft	1/13
Not evaluable	1/13

TABLE III

Diseases now curable by bone marrow transplantation with HLA-matched donor

1. Severe combined immunodeficiency disease (SCID): X-linked recessive
2. SCID: autosomal recessive, both B and T cells absent
3. SCID: autosomal recessive, some B cells present
4. SCID: autosomal recessive, with ADA deficiency
5. SCID: autosomal recessive, with ADA inhibitor
6. SCID: autosomal recessive, with C1q deficiency
7. Wiskott-Aldrich syndrome
8. Diamond-Blackfan syndrome (primary red cell aplasia)
9. Cartilage hair hypoplasia with immunodeficiency
10. Fanconi's anaemia
11. Severe congenital neutrophil dysfunction
12. Severe congenital deficiency of neutrophills (Kostman's syndrome)
13. Chronic granulomatous disease of childhood
14. Osteopetrosis, infantile form
15. Osteopetrosis, tardive form
16. Aplastic anaemia, with defective stem cells
17. Leukaemia, acute myelogenous
18. Leukaemia, acute lymphoid
19. Leukaemia, chronic granulocytic
20. Burkitt's lymphoma

Reviewed by Good (1980)

TABLE IV

Lymphoid reconstruction of SCID following transplantation of marrow from donors other than genotypically identical sibling

Donor	*Degree of HLA compatibility*	*HLA incompatibility*	*Engraftment of donor cells*	*GVHD*	*T cell reconstruction*	*B cell reconstruction*	*Surviving*
Uncle	Genotypic	None	T cells	None	+ (Donor)	+ (Host)	Yes
Father	Genotypic	None	T cells	Mild	+ (Donor)	+ (Host)	Yes
Father	Phenotypic	None	Full	Severe	+	+ (Delayed)	Yes
Father	Phenotypic	None	Full	Mod	+	+	No
Uncle	Nonidentical	B7, B12	T cells	Mod	+	–	Yes
Sibling	Nonidentical	BW, 37	Full	Mod	+	+	Yes
Mother	Nonidentical	A2	Full	Severe	+	+	No
Father	Nonidentical	A2	Full	None	+	+	Yes
Father	Nonidentical	A, BC	T cells	Mod	+	–	Yes
Unrelated	Nonidentical	A2	Full	Severe	+	+	Yes
Father	Nonidentical	AW31, BW35	Full	Mod	+	+	Yes

Vossen *et. al.*, Geha *et al.*, Barrett *et al.*, Polmar and Sorensen, Koch *et al.*, Gatti *et al.*, Niethammer *et al.*, Ramsoe *et al.*, O'Reilly *et al.*, O'Reilly *et al.*, O'Reilly *et al.*

This table is updated from O'Reilly *et al.* (1978). The papers listed above appear in O'Reilly *et al.* (1980).

to other frequently fatal diseases, and (b) to extend their therapeutic resources beyond the availability of a histocompatible sibling. Both of these steps have been taken in several English and European facilities as well as in the USA, and have met with impressive success. Table III lists the otherwise fatal diseases which may now be cured by BMT. Table IV lists the cases in which BMT has been successful, i.e., produced immunologic reconstitution and long-term survival, when the donor was not a genotypically identical sibling.

Family donors, HLA-D matched

A triumphant recovery was made by a child with SCID, in Copenhagen, after treatment with bone marrow from an uncle who was discovered by tissue-typing to be matched with the boy at the HLA-D locus (Koch *et al.*, 1973). For a time after transplantation, the child showed a split chimaerism, i.e. while his T cell system developed fully, his B cell system was at first only partly reconstituted, and was comprised of recipient rather than donor cell type. However, he gradually recovered from moderate GVHD and developed progressively vigorous B cell function attributable to donor cells. When a younger brother was also born with SCID, he in turn was successfully transplanted with the father's marrow, a perfect HLA-D match, and has also developed a functionally normal immunity system (Copenhagen Study Group of Immunodeficiencies, 1976).

At least 9 infants with SCID have recovered after treatment with HLA-D matched marrow from related donors other than genotypically identical siblings (see Table IV). Mismatching at the HLA-A or B locus has generally resulted in more severe GVHD, associated with marrow suppression or aplasia, than when the HLA systems were completely matched and while lymphoid engraftment has been achieved, in some cases it has been limited to the T cell system (Pahwa *et al.*, 1978). It has also been possible to correct SCID in a child who was mismatched at both the A and B loci with the prospective sibling donor, whom we found to be haploidentical with the D-locus homozygous recipient. As we hoped and expected from experimental analysis in mice and dogs, the child tolerated marrow transplantation with only a moderate and readily controllable GVHR (Pahwa *et al.*, 1978).

Unrelated donors, HLA-D matched

This approach has been used when no related matched donor was available. Although there is evidence that it may not be the HLA-D locus itself, but rather a closely linked determinant between the B and D loci, perhaps DR, which is crucial to the success of bone marrow transplants (Dupont *et al.*, 1979), effective BMT has, until very recently, been limited to instances where donor and recipient were matched at the major histocompatibility complex. This match has nearly always required a family member. Thus, BMT using unrelated donors represents a true test of the limits of this type of treatment.

Horowitz and colleagues (1975) reported that after this procedure, in which they used an unrelated MLC-compatible donor who differed at one HLA locus, their patient did not develop the usual signs of GVHD. However, the child died of overwhelming interstitial pneumonia after only 30 days, too short a time for evaluation of immunologic competence. Our group has treated a child with SCID by transplantation of marrow from an HLA-D and HLA-B compatible unrelated donor (O'Reilly *et al.*, 1977). The child has achieved functional immunocompetent engraftment with haematopoietic and lymphoid elements entirely of donor origin. Although this boy has been afflicted with chronic and fairly severe GVHD of the skin and oral mucosa, no evidence of gastointestinal or hepatic GVHD has been present. Subsequently, both SCID and other immunodeficient diseases, including chronic gramulomatous disease (Westminster Hospital Bone Marrow Transplant Team, 1977) and aplastic anaemia (Barrett, pers. comm.) have undergone BMT using HLA-A, B- and D-compatible unrelated donors, and shown evidence of immunologic reconstitution along with impressive periods of survival.

HLA-incompatible marrow, treated to reduce their immunocompetence

Whole bone marrow from histocompatible donors has regularly produced fatal GVHD (van Bekkum *et al.*, 1972). Methods of treating histoincompatible marrow cells to reduce their immunocompetence, making them available for transplantation, are obviously crucial to the continuing expansion of cellular engineering as a therapeutic resource. To this end, several techniques are being explored in various laboratories. These methods have been reviewed elsewhere (Pahwa *et al.*, 1978) and have had, in some cases, dramatic success in animal models, although clinical applications to date have yielded inconclusive or disappointing results. They include:

(a) Physical separation of immunocompetent cells from stem cells either by discontinuous gradients of bovine serum albumin or by velocity sedimentation (Dicke *et al.*, 1970; Phillips and Miller, 1970).

(b) The depletion of proliferating alloantigen-responsive lymphocytes by treatment with 5-bromo-deoxyuridine and light (Rich *et al.*, 1972) or with ^{3}H-thymidine having high specific activity (Salmon *et al.*, 1970). This has not been consistently effective because the committed immunocompetent cells can differentiate to cells that initiate GVHR.

(c) Pretreatment with antilymphocyte or antithymocyte serum, absorbed so as to preserve stem cells undamaged while depleting lymphoid cells (Müller-Ruchholtz *et al.*, 1976; Joh and Good, unpub. data).

(d) *In vitro* treatment of marrow with anti-Thy-1, either with complement (Krown *et al.*, 1980) or with certain anti-Thy-1 preparations without complement (Onoé *et al.*, 1980).

(e) Removal of stem cells from other cells of thymus, marrow, or spleen by a process of differential agglutination, using peanut or soybean lectins (Reisner *et al.*, 1978).

(f) Maintenance of stem cells by culture *in vitro* for prolonged periods before use in transplantation (Dexter *et al.*, 1977).

In addition to these techniques of preparing haematopoietic material for transplantation, an ingenious new method of preparing the recipient has also been developed, based on total lymphoid irradiation (TLI), using 3400 rad given in fractionated doses over a 17-day period to all available lymph nodes and to the thymus, while shielding the bone marrow in the distal parts of the extremities. Slavin and associates have prepared chimaeric mice (1977), rats (1978), some dogs (1979), and even monkeys (Slavin, pers. comm.) in this way, and have tolerated the irradiation and transplantation of bone marrow (though *not* transplantation of spleen cells) without developing GVHD. Although the mechanism by which this method succeeds is not yet clear, there is evidence that animals subjected to TLI plus BMT preferentially develop a population of specific suppressor cells which inhibit the development of GVHD. This technique may prove to be especially useful in addressing the lymphomas, aplastic anaemias, and inborn errors of haematopoietic metabolism and function, as well as in inducing specific immunologic tolerance for organ transplantation. As all of these methods are refined and made applicable to human treatment, we will gain incalculable resources for recreating the immunity systems of children suffering from the primary immunodeficiency diseases (Lapointe and Meuwissen, 1970; Royal Marsden Hospital Bone Marrow Transplantation Team, 1972; Woodruff *et al.*, 1976; Thomas *et al.*, 1977).

At this time, however, GVHD remains the most imposing of the obstacles which still limit the application of BMT in treating the primary immunodeficiency diseases, as well as leukaemia and other haematopoietic diseases. Several teams have observed that transplant recipients are more subject to GVHD if they have been preconditioned with chemical immunosuppressants or total body irradiation, even when the donor is a haploidentical sibling. While several preparations have been tested in the laboratory for the control of GVHD—including antithymocyte globulin (van Bekkum *et al.*, 1972), cyclophosphamide and methotrexate (Owens and Santos, 1971), procarbazine (Glucksberg and Fefer, 1973), interferon (Pahwa, pers. comm.)—none of these has yet been sufficiently refined for clinical application. Other unresolved problems are the fact that B cell engraftment may fail even when a child gains T cell immune function after a transplant, and the continuing serious hazard of infection for posttransplant patients, whose immunologic functions may take a considerable time, of which we still cannot absolutely predict the length, to stabilize.

Transplantation of foetal liver, foetal thymus, and cultured thymic epithelium

Over 20 years have passed since Uphoff successfully achieved immunologic reconstitution in certain strains of mice by transplantation of allogeneic foetal liver following lethal irradiation (Uphoff, 1958). These experiments showed that foetal liver from foetuses which were young enough not to contain post-thymic T cells, but which did not possess precursors of haematopoietic cells, could be used as a source of allogeneic stem cells which did not induce GVHR (Tulunay *et al.*, 1975). The foetal liver of man contains a rich supply of haematopoietic and lymphoid precursors which can also be used as a source of allogeneic stem cells without producing GVHR or GVHD as long as the cells are taken from foetuses after less than 12 weeks' embryonation. However, unlike bone marrow, foetal liver does not induce differentiation of the recipient's thymus (Lewis *et al.*, 1977). For this reason, a thymus, preferably from the same foetus, must also be implanted in most cases for immunologic reconstitution.

TABLE V
Transplantation of bone marrow or foetal liver in treatment of SCID

Type	*Donor*	*Patients*	*Reconstitution* *T*	*B*	*Survival*
Marrow	Rel. HLA-Genotypic Identical	57	42	39	32 (55%)
	Rel. HLA-Phenotypic Identical	9	5	4	3 (33%)
	Rel. HLA-D Compatible	9	5	4	4 (44%)
	Unrel. HLA-D Compatible	4	2	1	1 (25%)
Foetal Liver	HLA-Mismatched	64 (44 evaluable)	2	1	11 (18%) (26% evaluable)

A small number of SCID babies have achieved viable immunity systems after being given fresh foetal liver (see Table V), especially when a foetal thymus transplant is also given (reviewed, Pahwa *et al.*, 1978). Transplantation of foetal thymus alone has not yet been adequate for full immunologic reconstitution of SCID except in rare cases; nor has foetal liver transplantation alone corrected immunodeficiency disease. In contrast, treatment by thymus transplantation of children born with DiGeorge's athymic syndrome has met with encouraging success. These children are born without a thymus, and have no T cells or any T cell mediated immune function. Of 8 such children who were given foetal thymic tissue, 7 have been reconstituted immunologically after varying lengths of time, and 6 remain alive and immunologically stable over a very long period (reviewed, Pahwa *et al.*, 1978) (see Table VI). Thymus transplantation or thymic hormone therapy may, in the future, provide effective supplementary therapy for SCID patients whose bone marrow responds to thymic hormones or thymic extracts by differentiating

TABLE VI

Thymus transplantation for the DiGeorge syndrome

	Age of patient		*Foetal thymus*			*Results*	
Authors	*Diagnosis*	*Transplant*	*Age*	*Route*[a]	*Reconstitution*	*How soon after treatment*	*Status when reviewed (1978)*
Cleveland	5 weeks	7 months	13 weeks	IM	Yes	3 weeks	Alive, 9 years neurol. deficit
August	9 months	21 months	16 weeks	IM	Yes	4 days	Alive, 9 years
Gatti	10 days	1·5 months	10–12 weeks	IM	Yes	4–7 months	Alive, 5 years
Steele	12 days	10 weeks	13 weeks	DC IM	Yes	6 hours	Died, 9 days post-transpl. penumocystis
Biggar	2 months	5 months	(1) 14 weeks (2) 15 weeks	IP IP	Yes	1 week	Alive, 4 years
Touraine	6 months	7 months	13 weeks	IM		10 days	Alive, 2 years
Pahwa	1 week	3 months	(1) 12 weeks (2) 14 weeks	IP IP	Yes (Partial)	7 months	Died, 2 years sudden death
Dooren	1 week	1 week	(1) 17 weeks (2) 12 weeks	IM IM	No	—	Alive?

[a] IM = intramuscular, usually into recturs abdominis muscle; IP = intraperitoneal; DC = diffusionchamber. Reviewed by Pahwa *et al.* (1978).

normally *in vitro*. Transplantation of cultured epithelial cells has been useful in correcting some of the immunologic defects in a few patients with SCID (see Table VII). Unfortunately, given the heterogeneity of this disorder, patients seen in a number of other centres have not responded satisfactorily to this form of therapy (see Table VIII).

TABLE VII

Transplantation of cultured thymic epithelium in treatment of SCID (Wisconsin group)

Total patients	*Engraftment (both B and T cell systems*	*Unsuccessful*
15	7	8[a]

[a] 3 = Moribund at time of transplant; 3 = Immunologically unresponsive to transplant; 2 = Some B cell response but no significant clinical benefit. Reviewed by Horowitz and Hong (1978, 1979).

TABLE VIII

Cultured thymic epithelium transplants in treatment of SCID

Reporting center	*Patients*	*Chimaerism*	*Reconstitution*		*Long-term survival*
			T	*B*	
Toronto	6	0	3	2	2
Zurich	2	0	1 (±)	0	0
Goteborg	2	0	1	1(±)	0
Ulm	1	1	1	1	1
Leiden	1	0	0	0	0
Memorial Sloan-Kettering	2	0	0	0	0
Univ. of Washington	1	0	0	1(±)	0
Univ. of Arizona	3	0	1(±)	1(±)	1
Totals	18	1	7(5)	6(3)	4

Thymic hormones as therapy for primary immunodeficiency

Recent experimental studies in many laboratories suggest that the potential use of thymic hormones and thymic extracts as a treatment for deficiency of thymus-derived immunity is rapidly becoming more feasible. Thymic molecules, including thymopoietin (G. Goldstein, 1975), ubiquitin (Schlesinger *et al.* 1975), Facteur Thymique Sérique (Bach *et al.*, 1975), thymosin α1 (A. Goldstein *et al.*, 1977), thymosin β3 and β4 (Pazmino *et al.*, 1978), and thymic humoral factor (Trainin *et al.*, 1975) all have a strong influence on cellular differentiation and function. Analysis of these hormones, including full amino acid sequencing with identification of comparatively short but potent amino acid sequences, has permitted synthesis of several active peptides, including thymopoietin pentapeptide (Schlesinger *et al.*, 1975b), FTS (Bach *et al.*, 1978) and thymosin $\alpha 4$ (Low and Goldstein, 1978).

The pentapeptide TP-5, produced by synthesis of the 32nd through 36th amino acid sequences of the thymopoietin molecule, has already been used to enhance T cell function in patients with partial DiGeorge syndrome (Aiuti *et al.*, 1979), while treatment with large doses of thymosin or the extract called TP-1 has also been successful in raising T cell numbers and improving T cell functions of patients with the DiGeorge syndrome (reviewed, Pahwa *et al.*, 1978). It has been reported that TP-5 alters the expression of antibody affinity by antibody-producing cells in ageing mice (Weksler *et al.*, 1978). Since the majority of patients with SCID have defective thymus-derived immunity, we anticipate that these cases will receive thymic hormone therapy as part of a therapeutic approach focused directly on the body's most fundamental components.

Aplastic anaemia

Aplastic anaemia (AA) remains, at the present time, a difficult and heterogeneous clinical problem which often defeats conventional forms of therapy, especially in the more severe cases (Thomas *et al.*, 1977). As we define more clearly the different pathogenic mechanisms which may be responsible for individual cases—inherently defective stem cells, defective developmental microenvironment for the cells, autoantibodies or suppressor cells which destroy or inhibit development of haematopoietic cells—cellular engineering may become increasingly useful as a therapeutic resource. Fortunately, agents that destroy this suppressor influence have been effective in treating such cases (reviewed, Pahwa *et al.*, 1978), including high doses of cyclophosphamide, antilymphocyte treatment and antithymocyte globulin, presumably because removal of the suppressors permits patients' cells to differentiate normally. In our clinic, a near-lethal dose of cyclophosphamide followed by a foetal liver transplant led to immunologic reconstitution in a patient with a most severe form of AA associated with potent suppressor cells (Pahwa *et al.*, 1977). This patient's own marrow elements reappeared without signs of suppressor activity or any other evidence of disease, and he has remained well with normal haematopoiesis.

So far, some 60% of patients whose disease is caused by defective stem cells, a group which represents the majority of cases of AA, have been saved by BMT using cells from a histocompatible sibling donor (reviewed, Good, 1979; Good *et al.*, 1980a, b). As long as patients are identified, the severity of the disease recognized, and treatment initiated before a series of supportive transfusions are given which sensitize the recipient and interfere with acceptance of a bone marrow transplant after immunosuppression, bone marrow transplantation points provides the treatment of choice for severe AA when a matched sibling donor is available. Suitably matched relative donors may also sometimes permit safe and effective bone marrow transplantation (Dupont *et al.*, 1979). In future years, cellular engineering may become refined to permit marrow stem cell transplantation even across major histocompatibility barriers without lethal GVHD, as a treatment for AA as well as for SCID. In 20–30% of cases of AA where the pathogenic mechanism appears to involve cells in the marrow which are capable of suppressing differentiation of stem cells (Ascensao *et al.*, 1976; Kagan *et al.*, 1976), marrow transplantation has failed even when the donor is an identical twin (Royal Marsden Hospital Bone Marrow Transplantation Team, 1972; Thomas *et al.*, 1977). Fortunately, agents that destroy this suppressor influence, including high doses of cyclophosphamide (Storb *et al.*, 1976), antilymphocyte treatment (Gluckman *et al.*, 1977) and antithymocyte globulin (Amare *et al.*, 1977) have all been effective in treating these cases (reviewed, Pahwa *et al.*, 1978), presumably because removal of the suppressors permits patients' cells to differentiate normally. In our clinic, a near-lethal dose of cyclophosphamide followed by a foetal liver transplant led to immunologic reconstitution in a patient with severe AA associated with a potent suppressor influence (Pahwa and Good, 1977). This patient's own marrow elements have reappeared without signs of suppressor activity or any other evidence of disease.

Defects of the complement system

Inherited or acquired deficiency of individual complement components has been associated with a number of diseases (reviewed, Day *et al.*, 1977), among which are mesenchymal, vascular, and autoimmune disorders as well as heightened susceptibility to infection, especially with bacteria or fungi. Hereditary angioneurotic oedema, or Osler's disease, was the first disorder in which deficiency of a complement component, in this case the inhibitor of C1 esterase, was recognized as playing a pathogenitic role (Donaldson and Evans, 1963). Several groups have found that infusions of normal plasma may provide an effective treatment or even prophylaxis for attacks of oedema in these patients, as well as therapy for patients with missing C3 inactivator, C5 dysfunction syndrome or Leiner's disease, and deficient C3 stabilizer (reviewed, Day *et al.*, 1977). However, Gelfand, Frank and colleagues have developed a treatment for hereditary angioneurotic oedema which goes beyond simply replacing the missing component, and which may, in fact, operate by activating a previously nonfunctional genetic mechanism; they give the anabolic steroid, danazol, which induces normal production by the liver of the missing molecule (Gelfand *et al.*, 1976). Several hundred patients have now been treated in this way by different groups, with the proper dose (up to 600 mg/day), individually titrated for each patient, and Frank's group has seen a success rate of greater than 95% (pers. comm.). In a case of C1r deficiency which had led to recurrent vascular attacks and ultimately endstage kidney disease, renal allotransplantation led to production of the missing component, presumably by providing the cells that synthesize this molecule (Day *et al.*, 1977).

Diseases of the phagocytic system

Impaired phagocytic function is being recognized as the basis for an increasing number of primary immunodeficiencies. The most extensively studied of these is fatal or chronic granulomatous disease of childhood (CGD), first defined as a distinct clinical entity in 1957 (Berendes *et al.*, 1957). An impairment in intracellular metabolism (reviewed, Pahwa *et al.*, 1978) makes the phagocytes incapable of killing catalase-positive bacteria which they have ingested, with the result that infections persist for a prolonged period of time, causing purulent granulocytic lesions. Different enzymatic abnormalities are associated with genetically different forms of this disease.

Since continuous or intermittent antibiotic therapy has, fortunately, made it possible to manage the diverse clinical manifestations of this disease, the pressure to assume the risks of attempting BMT has been less great than with other primary immunodeficiencies which were invariably fatal otherwise. However, BMT has been attempted in at least 7 instances at the present time, in 2 of which HLA-matched unrelated donors were used (Westminster Hospital Bone Marrow Transplant Team, 1977; Hobbs, pers. comm.). Three of the patients receiving grafts from matched sibling donors succumbed to intercurrent infection. Two of those receiving grafts from unrelated donors experienced some clinical improvement, but definitive evidence of engraftment was never obtained. Recently, Parkman and colleagues have succeeded in establishing complete haematopoietic chimaerism using a technique they developed for reconstituting the entire haematopoietic system, preparing the patient with procarbazine, antithymocyte globulin, and total body irradiation before transplanting marrow from a matched sibling donor (Parkman, pers. comm.).

The Chediak-Higashi anomaly (reviewed, Pahwa *et al.*, 1978) is characterized by ineffectual chemotactic responsiveness of the patient's phagocytes and consequent delayed killing of bacteria. Abnormal microtubule structure, associated with increased levels of intracellular cyclic AMP, has been linked with this abnormality of cellular "steering" (Boxer *et al.*, 1976). Ongoing controversy has surrounded the possibility that this defect may respond to treatment with vitamin C. While some studies have raised the hope that the cellular defects may be corrected both *in vitro* and *in vivo* by exposure to ascorbic acid (Boxer *et al.*, 1976) others have disputed these findings (Gallin *et al.*, 1979). In the most recent studies, improved chemotactic and bactericidal activity were observed after a Chediak-Higashi patient received treatment with ascorbate, although morphological abnormalities of the patient's cells were not affected (R. Weening and D. Roos, pers. comm.). Further investigations to explore this therapeutic possibility will be awaited with the greatest interest. It is possible that discrepant results may be explained by the existence of heterogeneous forms of this disease which were previously unrecognized and must be clarified by future studies. It would certainly be encouraging if vitamin therapy proved to be an effective measure against at least one form of this disease which, along with their highly increased susceptibility to infection, renders patients alarmingly vulnerable to lymphoid and lymphoreticular cancers.

The disorder of phagocytic function which has been treated with the most exciting and encouraging results has been the Wiskott-Aldrich syndrome. Based on an inherited defect in the monocyte-phagocyte system which has not yet been fully characterized, this disorder leaves patients with a broadly based immunodeficiency in which both antibody production and cell-mediated immunity are abnormal, and which, until recently, has led to high mortality among these children. Cellular engineering by BMT after immunosuppression with different preparations has now provided a complete cure for this lethal syndrome on several occasions (Bach *et al.*, 1968; Meuwissen *et al.*, 1978; Parkman *et al.*, 1978; Kapoor *et al.*, unpub.) (see Table IX). Splenectomy coupled with prophylactic antibiotics has also provided an impressive therapeutic resource in treatment of these patients, leading to improved immunologic status and a high rate of survival (Lum *et al.*, 1980), although splenectomy without antibiotic treatment may produce no improvement in immunologic parameters or prognosis.

Osteopetrosis, or Albers-Shönberg disease, is another disease involving cells related to the monocyte-macrophage system which is also usually fatal because defective function of the osteoclasts leads to abnormal bone development and gradual elimination of haematopoietic areas. Several recent efforts at BMT, using HLA-matched sibling donors, have apparently corrected the osteoclastic abnormality and saved these patients (reviewed, Good *et al.*, 1980a) (see Table IX). The successful treatment of osteopetrosis by marrow transplantation in man, as in experimental animals, demands that sustained haematopoietic chimaerism be obtained. When only osteoclasts and/or their immediate precursors are successfully transplanted, negative nitrogen balance is achieved, which is followed after a few months by loss of the graft. Immunodeficiency associated with cartilage hair hypoplasia or short-limbed dwarfism has also been treated successfully by cellular engineering, either with BMT alone or with BMT preceded by transplantation of foetal thymus (reviewed, Good *et al.*, 1980a).

Replacement therapy

One of the most encouraging areas of recent progress in treatment of the primary immunodeficiencies has been the development of safe and effective preparations of γ-globulin for intravenous administration. As recently as 2 years ago, no adequate preparations were commercially available, and

TABLE IX

Marrow transplantation for other immunodeficiencies[a]

Disease	*Deficiency*	*Patients*	*Preparative regimen*	*Engraftment*	*Surviving (with reconstitution)*
Wiskott-Aldrich syndrome	Lymphocytes, Platelets	4	Pcb, CTX + ATG, Ara-C	Lymphocytes	4 (4)
		5	ATG, TBI	Complete (4)[b] Partial (1)	4 (4)
		3	Busulphan, CTX	Complete	3 (3)
Congenital agranulocytosis	Neutrophil precursors	2	Cytoxan (1) ATG, TBI (1)	Lymphocytes (transient) (1) Complete (1)	2 (1)
Cartilage-hair hypoplasia	Neutrophils, Lymphocytes	2	Cytoxan, (Ara-C)	Complete with mixed chimaerism (2)	2
Chronic granulomatous disease	Neutrophils	3	Cytoxan	Not evaluable	0
		1	ATG, TBI	Complete	1
Neutrophil actin deficiency	Neutrophils	1		Not evauable	0
Severe neutrophil dysfunction	Neutrophils	1	ATG, TBI	Complete	1
Osteopetrosis	Osteoclasts, monocytes, natural killer cells	3	Cytoxan (1) ATG + TBI (1) Busulphan, CTX (1)	Transient complete with mixed chimaerism	3 (2)
		4	None	None (?)	3 (1?)

[a] Reviewed by O'Reilly *et al.* (1980).

[b] One of the completely reconstituted patients died of interstitial pneumonia and GVHD.

physicians had to rely instead upon intramuscular administration attended by the risk of infection, severe syncopal reaction, short periods of effectiveness and the necessity of painful intramuscular injection. Now, however, a substantial number of intravenous preparations are being refined in several countries (see Table X).

Infusions of fresh frozen plasma may serve as an alternative to γ-globulin, and in some cases may be the preferable choice. The advantages of plasma therapy over γ-globulin therapy are that: (a) higher serum immunoglobulin levels, including all classes of immunoglobulin, can be achieved more rapidly with more rapid equilibrium also between body fluid compartments; (b) catabolic losses due to local proteolysis by muscle enzymes are avoided; and (c) plasma donors can be immunized to provide high titres of specific antibodies. Disadvantages include the risk of serum hepatitis, transmission of cytomegalovirus, and transfusion reactions. Patients with complete IgA deficiency should not receive this form of treatment, since these patients frequently develop anti-IgA antibodies and serious reactions can follow when preparations containing IgA are subsequently given. Circumstances under which fresh frozen plasma administered intravenously has provided a useful alternative to γ-globulin treatment have been:

(a) In cases of immunodeficiency with severe life-threatening infection and refractory diarrhoea.

(b) With antibody-deficient patients who are either refractory to γ-globulin or for whom intramuscular γ-globulin therapy is contraindicated either by serious local or systemic reactions or because of thrombocytopaenia or extensive skin lesions.

(c) In instances when HLA-incompatible marrow transplantation is being carried out, when plasma therapy has been used as a possible source of enhancing antibodies.

(d) In certain cases of complement deficiency, such as Leiner's disease (associated with C5 dysfunction) and hereditary angioneurotic oedema (with deficiency or dysfunction of the C1 esterase inhibitor).

(e) In a few patients with the Wiskott-Aldrich syndrome and ataxia telangiectasia, when life-threatening infections have occurred (reviewed, Pahwa *et al.*, 1978).

Transfer factor, a dialysable substance extracted from lymphocytes, has also been brought forward as a possible resource for treating immunodeficiency diseases. Although we and others have found the influences of transfer factor to be for the most part nonspecific (Ballow *et al.*, 1975; Griscelli *et al.*, 1975), patients with chronic mucocutaneous candidiasis or with chronic fungal infections have sometimes responded startlingly well and apparently specifically to these extracts (reviewed, Kirkpatrick and Sohnle, 1980). Recently, more substantial evidence has been presented that both antigen specificity and degree of potency can be demonstrated *in vitro* for either dialysed leukocyte extract itself or for the antigen-specific moiety, using the leukocyte migration inhibition assay in agarose (Fudenberg *et al.*, 1980), while specificity of *in vivo*

TABLE X

Intravenous γ-globulin preparations[a]

Firm	*Treatment*	% *Monomer*	% *Aggregation*	% *Fragmentation*	*Antibody recovery*	*Other statements*
Biotest	β-Propiolactone	~85	dimer 13 polymer ~2	—	~90%	10 years clinical experience; good tolerance in immune deficients; intact Fc
Michigan	Plasmin	85–90	~3	7–12	~100%	5 years clinical trial—Cassidy; Univ. of Mich., Ann Arbor
Cutter	Reduced and alkylated	>80	<20	0	≥85% *in vivo* *in vitro*	Stable in 10% maltose solution for >6 months at 30°C; maintains opsonic activity; clinically safe and efficacious; anticomplement activity >2 mg per CH50
Green	1. Plasmin	50–60	<5	40–50	>90%	250 000 vials used in 1978
	2. ETOH-PEG	>95	<5	none	>95	3 years clinical experience
Continental	Cohn II + III + PEG 4000	~95	Dimer 5	0	~ 100%	Freeze-dried; safe clinically after 2 years of 5°C
Merieux	Plasmin	40–50	0	—	80–100%	Freeze-dried; 10 years experience; good tolerance
KABI	Cohn II-stabilized with HSA	> 80	Dimer 20 trace aggregates	—	~100%	
Swiss	pH 4	85	0	<5	5-fold	No anticomplementary activity; freeze-dried
Condie	SiO_2 QAE	98	<2	<2	3·5-fold	Stable at 5°C for 2 years
Austria	Nonmodified	98% 7S	≥40 mg 1 CH50	0	TAT 75%	Freeze-dried; opsonic characteristics unchanged
Scotland	None	>90	<10	0		
Behring	Pepsin	10–15 ≥7S	75–80 ~5S	5–10 ~3·5S	8-fold [5% solution]	No anticomplementary activity
Hyland	Plasmin	50–60	≤5	40–50	varies with specific antibody	Freeze-dried; low anticomplement titre
Winnipeg Rh Institute	None prepared by *DEAE-Sephadex column*	>96%	<2%	<2%	90%	Hyperimmune Rh, tetanus. Rh is Freeze-dried; low anticomplement titre 5 g% solution, 1 year dating
Japanese	Sulphonation nonmodified	?	Minimal	<2%	>90%	

[a] Based on information provided by the manufacturers.

activity has also been demonstrated by skin testing by Burger.

Deficiency of the enzyme adenosine deaminase (ADA) has been identified as one of the bases for an autosomal recessive form of SCID. Replacement of this enzyme by transfusions of frozen irradiated normal red blood cells has had remarkable success in several trials (reviewed, Polmar, 1979). Ten patients with SCID associated with ADA deficiency were reviewed by Polmar for their response to this form of treatment, and 5 of the 10 had evidence of restored immunologic responsiveness, which included lymphocytosis and some evidence of antibody formation. Three of these 5 individuals also received thymic factors or a graft of foetal thymus, and some of these patients would not respond to the replacement enzyme therapy until treatment with thymic factor was also given. It should be noted that each of the 5 who showed a significant response also had some evidence of immunologic activity, i.e. presence of some cells of both the T and B lineages, prior to transfusion.

Nutrients such as the trace metal zinc have also been identified as having pathogenetic significance for primary immunodeficiency (reviewed in Good *et al.*, 1979). Acrodermatitis enteropathica, defined as a clinical entity in 1942 (Danbolt and Closs, 1942) is usually fatal, presenting with a range of symptoms including severe skin lesions, devastating gastrointestinal malfunction, and central nervous system disturbances. All manifestations of the disease have been found to be attributable to an inborn error of metabolism which prevents normal absorption of zinc from gastrointestinal tract. Treatment with zinc in sufficient amounts, parenterally or in large doses orally, leads to complete correction of all symptoms and immunologic abnormalities, which include gross underdevelopment of the thymus, thymus-dependent areas of the lymphoid tissues, and T cell numbers and functions (Moynahan and Barnes, 1973). An experimental model for the same disease is represented by the A-46 mutant of black, pied, Danish cattle of the Holstein-Friesian line (Brummerstedt *et al.*, 1977). Calves born with this inherited defect are stunted, lethargic, and afflicted with skin lesions featured by hyperkeratosis and parakeratosis. Examination shows them to be profoundly immunodeficient, with severely underdeveloped thymus and thymus-derived immunity functions, as a result of which they frequently die of infection. A single metabolic defect underlies these animals' disease: just as in human acrodermatitis enteropathica, there is a failure to absorb zinc normally through the gastrointestinal tract, even though metabolism of this element is otherwise normal. Sufficiently large doses of zinc, either parenteral or oral, completely cures the immunodeficiency and all related symptoms.

Experimental studies of zinc restriction in mice (Fraker *et al.*, 1977; Fernandes *et al.*, 1979; Iwata *et al.*, 1979) have shown that thymic vigour, thymic hormone levels, and the immunologic functions of thymus-derived T lymphocytes are all highly dependent on the availability of zinc, as are many other biological processes (reviewed, Schloen *et al.*, 1979). Clinical investigations have revealed zinc deficiency in a number of patients with common variable immunodeficiency (Oleske *et al.*, 1979; Cunningham-Rundles *et al.*,

1979). Individuals with CVI who had deficient T cell immunity in addition to their antibody deficiency responded well to dietary zinc supplements, with improvement both of their symptoms and of their T cell abnormalities. Other work has shown that 20–30% of patients with epidermoid cancer of the head and neck, as well as with certain other cancers, are zinc deficient (Garofalo *et al.*, 1980). In the patients with epithelial cancers, inadequate diet was shown to be the basis of their zinc deficiency.

Future therapeutic approaches

In addition to the thymic hormone preparations mentioned briefly earlier, several new forms of immunotherapy for the primary immunodeficiencies, as well as other diseases, are being studied around the world. The growing science of immunopharmacology is exploring ways to harness fundamental biological substances such as thymic factors, lymphokines, and interferons, or to synthesize and to apply therapeutically molecules with similar biological effects. A number of thymic factors, including thymopoietin, thymosin $\alpha 1$, and FTS, have been well defined; these and several others are already in clinical trials, with encouraging early results (Good, 1980). Levamisole is one of the first chemically defined immunopotentiators to see extensive clinical testing, primarily in cancer patients (Renoux, 1978). It has been employed in several paediatric patients with congenital and acquired immunodeficiency, with encouraging results (Spitler *et al.*, 1977). A similar sulphur-containing compound, diethyldithiocarbamate (DTC) also discovered by Renoux (Renoux and Renoux, 1980) seems to have greater potency and safety in preliminary work. Isoprinosine, a synthetic nontoxic inducer of T cell differentiation and potentiator of mitogen-induced lymphoproliferative responses both *in vitro* and *in vivo*, may prove to be at least as effective in inducing immunologic responses as a natural substance (Hadden and Giner-Sorolla, 1980). NPT15392, a new immunopotentiator recently synthesized at the Memorial Sloan-Kettering Cancer Center, shows activity similar to isoprinosine, but with greater potency. It is only one of a number of powerful new immunomodulators which are currently being developed for clinical application (see Hadden *et al.*, 1980).

The several forms of interferon are receiving intense international attention, although the difficulty involved in obtaining sufficient quantities of these substances (as well as the lymphokines) have posed problems for investigators. In the case of both the interferons and the lymphokines, it remains to be determined which molecules are active and what the interactions are among the many active substances known to be present in the preparations currently in use. With increasing chemical characterization of these substances, the prospect of synthesizing effective analogues should steadily grow. All of these new preparations represent molecular engineering in a state of rapid progress, and are likely to provide powerful immunotherapeutic resources in the foreseeable future.

Comments and conclusions

Contemporary approaches to treatment of the primary immunodeficiencies have, to an increasingly great degree, been able to add forms of cellular and macromolecular engineering to the necessary traditional uses of careful antibiotic therapy and prophylactic measures. Our increasing knowledge, both clinical and experimental, of the fundamental components of the immunity networks, now frequently enables us to address these components directly when they are defective or absent. By reconstituting, replacing, or stimulating development or expression of ineffectual immunologic components, we can now treat diseases which have historically led to inevitable death. We look forward to continuing extension and refinement of the principles which we are successfully applying with these new forms of treatment, to prevent or cure with greater consistency an increasing number of these patients.

References

Aiuti, F., Ammirati, P., Fiorilli, M., D'Amelio, R., Franchi, F., Calvani, M. and Businco, L. (1979). *Pediatr. Res.* **131**, 797.

Amare, M., Abdou, N. L., Cook, J. D. and Abdou, N. I. (1977). *Clin. Res.* **25**, 333A (Abstract).

Ascensao, J., Pahwa, R., Kagan, W., Hansen, J., Moore, M. and Good, R. A. (1976). *Lancet* **i**, 669.

Bach, F. H., Albertini, R. J., Joo, P., Anderson, J. L. Y. and Bortin, M. M. (1968). *Lancet* **i**, 1364.

Bach, J. F., Bach, M. A., Charreire, J., Dardenne, M., Fournier, C., Papiernik, M. and Pleau, J. M. (1975). *In* "The Biological Activity of Thymic Hormones" (D. W. van Bekkum, ed.), p. 145. Kooyker Scientific Publications, Rotterdam.

Bach, J. F., Bach, M. A., Blanot, D., Bricas, E., Charreire, J., Dardenne, M., Fournier, C. and Pleau, J. M. (1978). *Bull. Inst. Pasteur* **76**, 325.

Ballow, M., Dupont, B., Hansen, J. and Good, R. A. (1975). *Birth Defects* **11(1)**, 457.

Berendes, H., Bridges, R. A. and Good, R. A. (1957). *Minn. Med.* **40**, 309.

Biggar, W. D., Park, B. H. and Good, R. A. (1975). *Birth Defects* **11(1)**, 385.

Boxer, L. A., Watanabe, A. M., Rister, M., Besch, H. R., Allen, J. and Baehner, R. L. (1976). *New Engl. J. Med.* **295**, 1041.

Brummerstedt, E., Basse, A., Flagstad, T. and Andresen, E. (1977). *Am. J. Pathol.* **87(3)**, 725.

Copenhagen Study Group of Immunodeficiencies (1976). *In* "International Cooperative Group for Bone Marrow Transplantation in Man, Third Workshop". Tarrytown, New York.

Cunningham-Rundles, C., Cunningham-Rundles, S., Garofalo, J. A., Iwata, T., Incefy, G., Twomey, J. and Good, R. A. (1979). *Fed. Proc. Fed. Am. Soc. Exp. Biol.* **38** (Abstract).

Danbolt, N. and Closs, K. (1942). *Acta Derm. Venereol.* (*Stockh.*) **23**, 127.

Day, N. K., Moncada, B. and Good, R. A. (1977). *In* "Biological Amplification Systems in Immunology" (N. K. Day and R. A. Good, eds) Vol. 2, p. 229. Comprehensive Immunology, Plenum Press, New York.

De Koning, J., Dooren, L. J., van Bekkum, D. W., van Rood, J. J., Dicke, K. A. and Radl, J. (1969). *Lancet* **i**, 1223.
Dexter, T. M., Moore, M. A. S. and Sheridan, A. P. C. (1977). *J. Exp. Med.* **145**, 1612.
Dicke, K. A., Lina, P. H. C. and van Bekkum, D. W. (1970). *Rev. Eur. Etud. Clin. Biol.* **15**, 205.
Donaldson, V. H. and Evans, R. R. (1963). *Am. J. Med.* **35**, 37.
Dupont, B., O'Reilly, R. J., Pollack, M. S. and Good, R. A. (1979). *Transplant. Proc.* **11**, 219.
Fernandes, G., Nair, M., Onoé, K., Tanaka, T., Floyd, R. and Good, R. A. (1979). *Proc. Natn. Acad. Sci. U.S.A.* **76**, 457.
Fraker, P. J., Haas, S. M. and Luecke, R. W. (1977). *J. Nutr.* **107**, 1889.
Fudenberg, H. H., Wilson, G. B., Gust, J. M., Nekam, K. and Smith, C. O. (1980). *In* "Proceedings of the Serono Symposium on Thymus, Thymic Hormones, and T Lymphocytes" (F. Aiuti, ed.). Academic Press, London and New York (in press).
Gallin, J. I., Elin, R. J., Hubert, R. T., Fauci, A. S., Kaliner, M. A. and Wolff, S. M. (1979). *Blood* **53**, 226.
Garofalo, J. A., Erlandson, E., Strong, E. W., Lesser, M., Gerold, F., Spiro, R., Schwartz, M. and Good, R. A. (1980). *J. Surg. Oncol.* (in press).
Gatti, R. A., Meuwissen, H. J., Allen, H. D., Hong, R. and Good, R. A. (1968). *Lancet* **ii**, 1366.
Gelfand, J. A., Sherins, R. J., David, W. A. and Frank, M. M. (1976). *New Engl. J. Med.* **296**, 1444.
Gluckman, E., Devergle, A. and Marty, M. (1977). *Exp. Hematol.* **5** (Suppl. 2), 104.
Glucksberg, H. and Fefer, A. (1973). *Cancer Res.* **33**, 859.
Goldstein, A. L., Low, T. L. K., McAdoo, M., McClure, J., Thomas, G. B., Rossio, J., Lai, C. Y., Chang, D., Wang, S. S., Harvery, C., Ramel, A. H. and Meienhofer, J. (1977). *Proc. Natn. Acad. Sci. U.S.A.* **74**, 725.
Goldstein, G. (1975). *Ann. N.Y. Acad. Sci.* **249**, 177.
Good, R. A. (1969). *Hosp. Pract.* **4**, 41.
Good, R. A. (1979). *New Engl. J. Med.*
Good, R. A. (1980). *In* "The Impact of Basic Research: Proceedings of the Sarasota Medical Awards Conference, 1979" (P. Bralow, ed.). McGraw Hill, New York (in press).
Good, R. A. and Day, N. K. (1980). *In* "New Trends in Human Immunology and Cancer Immunotherapy: Proceedings of the Montpellier International Symposium, 1980" (B. Serrou and C. Rosenfeld, eds). Editeur Dior (in press).
Good, R. A., Fernandes, G. and West, A. (1979). *Clin. Bull. Mem. Sloan-Kettering Cancer Center* **9(1)**, 3.
Good, R. A., O'Reilly, R. J. and West, A. (1980a). *In* "Proceedings of the Serono Symposium on Thymus, Thymic Hormones, and T Lymphocytes" (F. Aiuti, ed.). Academic Press, London and New York (in press).
Good, R. A., Pahwa, R. N. and West, A. (1980b). *In* "Immunodermatology" (B. Safai and R. A. Good, eds). Academic Press, New York and London (in press).
Good, R. A., West, A. and Fernandes, G. (1980c). *In* "Proceedings of the International Symposium on Infection in the Immunocompromised Host" (J. Verhoef, P. Peterson and P. G. Quie, eds). Elsevier-North Holland, New York (in press).
Griscelli, C. (1975). *Birth Defects* **11(1)**, 462.
Hadden, J. W. (1979). *Springer Sem. Immunopathol.* **2**, 35.
Hadden, J. W. and Giner-Sorolla, A. (1980). *In* "Augmenting Agents in Cancer Therapy: Current Status and Future Prospects" (M. Chirigos and E. Hirsch, eds). Raven Press, New York (in press).
Hadden, J., Chedid, L., Spreafico, F. and Mullen, P. (1980). "Advances in Immunopharmacology". Pergamon Press, Oxford (in press).
Horowitz, S. D. and Hong, R. (1978). *Lancet.*

Horowitz, S. D. and Hong, R. (1979. *Transplant. Rev.*

Horowitz, S. D., Groshong, T., Bach, F. H., Hong, R. and Yunis, E. J. (1975). *Lancet* **ii**, 431.

Iwata, T., Incefy, G. S., Tanaka, T., Fernandes, G., Menendez-Botet, C. J., Pih, K. and Good, R. A. (1979). *Cell. Immunol.* **47**, 100.

Kagan, W. A., Ascensao, J. A., Pahwa, R., Hansen, J. A., Goldstein, G., Valera, E. B., Incefy, G. S., Moore, M. S. and Good, R. A. (1976). *Proc. Natn. Acad. Sci. U.S.A.* **73**, 2890.

Kirkpatrick, C. H. and Sohnle, P. G. (1980). *In* "Immunodermatology" (B. Safai and R. A. Good, eds). Academic Press, New York and London (in press).

Koch, C., Henriksen, K., Juhl, F., Wiik, A., Faber, V., Anderson, V., Dupont, B., Hansen, G. S., Svejgaard, A., Thomsen, M., Ernst, P., Killmann, S. A., Good, R. A., Jensen, K. and Müller-Berat, N. (1973). *Lancet* **i**, 1146.

Lapointe, N. and Meuwissen, H. J. (1970). *Fed. Proc. Fed. Am. Soc. Exp. Biol.* **29**, 625 (Abstract).

Levey, R. H., Klemperer, M. R., Gelfand, E. W., Sanderson, A. R., Batchelor, J. R., Berkel, A. I. and Rosen, F. S. (1971). *Lancet* **ii**, 571.

Lewis, V., Twomey, J. J., Goldstein, G., O'Reilly, R., Smithwick, E., Pahwa, R., Pahwa, S., Good, R. A., Shulte-Wisserman, H., Horowitz, S., Hong, R., Jones, J., Sieber, O., Kirkpatrick, C., Polmer, S. and Bealmear, B. (1977). *Lancet* **ii**, 471.

Low, T. L. K. and Goldstein, A. L. (1978). *In* "The Year in Hematology" (R. Silber, J. LoBue and A. S. Gordon, eds) pp. 281–319. Plenum Publishing Corp., New York.

Lum, L. G., Tubergen, D. G., Corash, L. and Blaese, R. M. (1980). *New Engl. J. Med.* **302**, 892.

Meuwissen, H. J., Kiserman, M. A., Taft, E. G., Pollara, B. and Pickering, R. J. (1978). *Pediatr. Res.* **12**, 482 (Abstract).

Moynahan, E. J. and Barnes, P. M. (1973). *Lancet* **i**, 676.

Müller-Ruchholtz, W., Wottge, H. U. and Müller-Hermelink, H. K. (1976). *Transplant. Proc.* **8**, 537.

Oleske, J. M., Westphal, M. L., Shore, S., Gorden, D., Bogden, J. and Nahmias, A. (1979). *Am J. Dis. Child.* **133**, 915.

Onoé, K., Fernandes, G. and Good, R. A. (1980). *J. Exp. Med.* **151**, 115.

O'Reilly, R. J. and Good, R. A. (1980). *In* "Biology of Bone Marrow Transplantation: Proceedings of the ICN-UCLA Symposia on Molecular and Cellular Biology". Vol. 17 (R. P. Gale and C. F. Fox, eds). Academic Press, New York and London (in press).

O'Reilly, R. J., Dupont, B., Pahwa, S., Grimes, E., Smithwick, E. M., Pahwa, R., Schwartz, S., Hansen, J., Siegal, F., Sorell, M., Svejgaard, A., Jersilo, C., Thomsen, M., Platz, P., L'Esperance, P. and Good, R. A. (1977). *New Eng. J. Med.* **297**, 1311.

O'Reilly *et al.*, (1980). *In* "Immunodeficiency Diseases" (M. Seligmann and W. Hitzig eds). Elsevier/North Holland Publishing Co.

Owens, A. H. and Santos, G. W. (1971). *Transplantation* **11**, 378.

Pahwa, R. N., O'Reilly, R., Kagan, W. and Good, R. A. (1977). *Exp. Hematol.* **7** (Suppl. 6), 16 (Abstract).

Pahwa, R., Pahwa, S., O'Reilly, R. and Good, R. A. (1978). *Springer Sem. Immunopathol.* **1**, 355.

Park, B. H., Biggar, W. D. and Good, R. A. (1975). *Birth Defects* **11(1)**, 380.

Parkman, R., Rappeport, J., Geha, R., Belli, J., Cassady, R., Levey, R., Nathan, D. G. and Rosen, F. S. (1978). *New Engl. J. Med.* **298(17)**, 921.

Pazmino, N. H., Ihle, J. N. and Goldstein, A. L. (1978). *J. Exp. Med.* **147**, 708.

Phillips, R. A. and Miller, R. G. (1970). *J. Immunol.* **105**, 1168.

Polmar, S. H. (1979). *In* "Inborn Errors of Specific Immunity" (B. Pollara,

R. J. Pickering, H. J. Meuwissen and I. H. Porter, eds) pp. 343–352. Academic Press, New York and London.

Polmar, W. H., Wetzler, E. and Stern, R. C. (1975). *Lancet* **ii**, 743.

Reisner, Y., Itzicovitch, L., Meshorer, A. and Sharon, N. (1978). *Proc. Natn. Acad. Sci.* **75**, 2933.

Renoux, G. (1978). *Pharmacol. Ther.* **2**, 397.

Renoux, G. and Renoux, M. (1980). *In* "Augmenting Agents in Cancer Therapy: Current Status and Future Prospects" (M. Chirigos and E. Hirsch, eds). Raven Press, New York (in press).

Rich, R. R., Kilpatrick, C. H. and Smith, T. K. (1972). *Cell. Immunol.* **5**, 190.

Royal Marsden Hospital Bone Marrow Transplantation Team (1972). *Lancet* **ii**, 742.

Salmon, S. E., Smith, B. A., Lehrer, R. I., Mogerman, S. N., Shinefield, H. E. and Perkins, H. A. (1970). *Lancet* **ii**, 149.

Schlesinger, D. H., Goldstein, G., Scheid, M. P. and Boyse, E. A. (1975a). *Biochemistry* **14**, 2214.

Schlesinger, D. H., Goldstein, G., Scheid, M. P. and Boyse, E. A. (1975b). *Cell* **5**, 367.

Schloen, L. H., Fernandes, G., Garofalo, J. A. and Good, R. A. (1979). *Clin. Bull. MSKCC* **9(2)**, 63.

Slavin, S., Strober, S., Fuks, Z. and Kaplan, H. S. (1977). *J. Exp. Med.* **146**, 34.

Slavin, S., Fuks, Z., Kaplan, H. S. and Strober, S. (1978). *J. Exp. Med.* **147**, 963.

Slavin, S., Gottlieb, M., Strober, S., Bieber, C., Hoppe, R., Kaplan, H. S. and Grumet, F. C. (1979). *Transplantation* **27**, 139.

Sorell, M., Rosen, J. F., Kapoor, N., Kirkpatrick, D., Chaganti, R. S. K., Pollack, M. S., Dupont, B., Goossen, C., Good, R. A. and O'Reilly, R. J. (1979). *Pediatr. Res.* **13**, 481.

Spitler, L. E., Glogau, R. G., Nelms, D. C., Basch, C. M., Olson, J. A., Silverman, S. and Engelman, E. P. (1977). *In* "Control of Neoplasia by Modulation of the Immune System" (M. A. Chirigos, ed.) pp. 217–225. Raven Press, New York.

Storb, R., Thomas, E. D., Weiden, P. L., Buckner, C. D., Clift, R. A., Fefer, A., Fernando, L. P., Giblett, E. R., Goodell, B. W., Johnson, F. L., Lerner, K. G., Neiman, P. W. and Sanders, J. E. (1976). *Blood* **48**, 817.

Thomas, E. D., Fefer, A. F., Buckner, C. D. and Storb, R. (1977). *Blood* **49**, 671.

Trainin, N., Small, M., Zipori, D., Umiel, T., Kook, A. I. and Rotter, V. (1975). *In* "The Biological Activity of Thymic Hormones" (D. W. van Bekkum, ed.) p. 117. Kooyker Scientific Publications, Rotterdam.

Tulunay, O., Good, R. A. and Yunis, E. J. (1975). *Proc. Natn. Acad. Sci. U.S.A.* **72**, 4100.

Uphoff, D. (1958). *J. Natn. Cancer Inst.* **20**, 625.

van Bekkum, D. W. (1972). *Transplant. Rev.* **9**, 3.

van Bekkum, D. W., Balner, H., Dicke, K. A., van den Berg, F. G., Prinsen, G. H. and Hollander, C. F. (1972). *Transplantation* **13**, 400.

Weksler, M. E., Innes, J. B. and Goldstein, G. (1978). *J. Exp. Med.* **148**, 996.

Westminster Hospital Bone Marrow Transplant Team (1977). *Lancet* **i**, 210.

Woodruff, J. M., Hansen, J. A., Good, R. A., Santos, G. W. and Slavin, R. E. (1976). *Transplant. Proc.* **8**, 675.

52

Autoimmunity in Endocrine Disease

W. JAMES IRVINE

Endocrine Unit/Immunology Laboratories (Medicine), University Department of Medicine, Royal Infirmary, Edinburgh, Scotland

This work has been supported by grants from the British Medical Research Council, the British Diabetic Association and the Juvenile Diabetes Federation of the USA.

Introduction

Much of clinical endocrinology consists of a number of syndromes, each consisting of a number of different diseases. Some of these syndromes are shown in Fig. 1. Autoimmunity plays a significant, or sometimes the major, role in relation to certain of the constituent diseases. The objectives of the present chapter are to put the autoimmune endocrinopathies in perspective with the main clinical syndromes, and to compare and contrast the features of the principal autoimmune endocrinopathies.

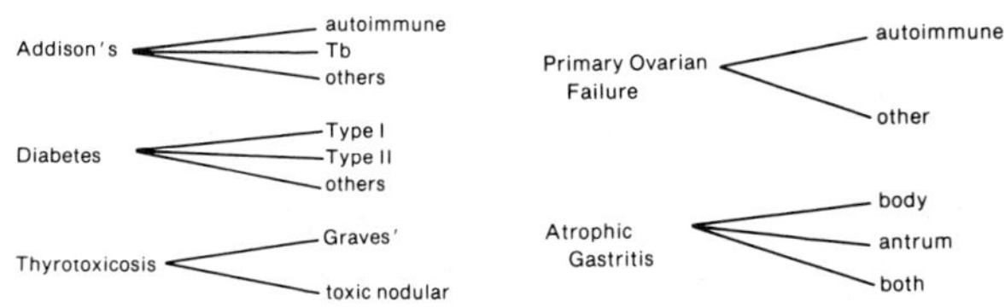

FIG. 1. *Heterogeneity within disease syndromes.*

Heterogeneity within disease syndromes

It is well known that primary adrenocortical failure (Addison's disease) may be caused by tuberculosis or rarely by haemorrhage, infarction, infection, carcinoma etc. (Irvine and Barnes, 1975). However, the commonest variety in developed countries has been referred to as "idiopathic", on account of the absence of any known cause. Autoimmunity to the adrenal cortex in the form of IgG antibodies in the serum reactive with adrenal cortex characterizes "idiopathic" Addison's disease, and in a study of an extensive series of cases these antibodies have not been described in unequivocal tuberculous Addison's disease or where other causes of adrenocortical destruction have been established (Irvine *et al.*, 1967). For this reason the idiopathic variety of Addison's disease is referred to as autoimmune Addison's disease. Cell-mediated immunity to adrenal extracts has been demonstrated using the peripheral blood lymphocytes and leukocytes from patients with "idiopathic" Addison's disease in the migration inhibition test (Nerup and Bendixen, 1969).

Only in the past few years has a reasonably definitive subdivision of the syndrome of primary diabetes been achieved (Irvine, 1977; NDDG, 1979; Irvine, 1980). This arose out of the recognition that diabetes occurred more commonly than expected in relation to the autoimmune endocrinopathies, and especially "idiopathic" Addison's disease. Not only that, but when diabetes did occur in clinical association with the autoimmune endocrinopathies it was predominantly of the insulin-dependent type (IDDM) (Irvine *et al.*, 1980a).

When the age at diagnosis of IDDM was correlated with the age at diagnosis of "idiopathic" (autoimmune) Addison's disease, a reasonably good correlation was achieved and the point securely made that the age at diagnosis of IDDM in this context at least was not restricted to juveniles (Fig. 2). It is recommended that the old classification of primary diabetes into "juvenile onset" and "maturity onset" be dropped; in preference to using the terms type I and type II diabetes. As will be emphasized later, type I diabetes is the end stage of the disease process that culminates in ketosis-prone insulin-dependent diabetes. Organ-specific autoimmunity is strongly implicated in type I diabetes, and not at all in type II diabetes. Type III primary diabetes

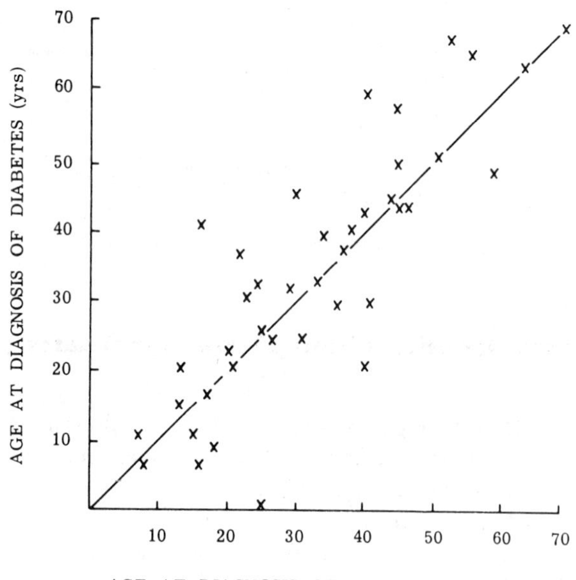

FIG. 2. *The age at diagnosis of insulin dependent diabetes correlated with the age at diagnosis of idiopathic Addison's disease in patients who developed both conditions. The information was extracted from a series of 350 cases of idiopathic Addison's disease.*

consists of a whole range of rare disorders, including the form of insulin-resistant diabetes associated with acanthosis nigricans and antibodies in the serum reactive with insulin receptors (Kahn *et al.*, 1980).

Within the syndrome of thyrotoxicosis there is Graves' disease (with diffuse involvement of the thyroid gland) and toxic nodular goitre, where the hyperthyroidism is due to the overactivity of one or more "hot" nodules. Thyroid stimulating antibodies are the probable cause of Graves' disease (Clague *et al.*, 1976; Davies *et al.*, 1977; Teng and Yeung, 1980), while they are absent in patients with toxic nodular goitre which has little or no association with autoimmunity (Bolk *et al.*, 1979).

Autoimmune primary ovarian failure is almost always associated with autoimmune Addison's disease. It probably accounts for the minority of cases of primary ovarian failure (failure of ovarian hormonal function associated with high gonadotrophin levels in the serum). The reason for the close association between autoimmune ovarian failure and autoimmune Addison's disease is the simple one that the antigens in the steroid-producing cells of the gonads are also present in the adrenal cortex, although not all antigens in the cortex are present in the steroid-producing cells of the gonads. Thus only a significant minority of patients with autoimmune Addison's disease get autoimmune gonadal failure (in terms of hormone production), but virtually all those with autoimmune gonadal failure have Addison's disease (Irvine *et al.*, 1978, 1979; Irvine, 1979). The reason why primary ovarian failure should be more conspicuous than primary testicular failure may be because the clinical features of the former are so readily apparent as amenorrhoea.

The syndrome of atrophic gastritis is included in this paper on autoimmune endocrinopathies, because it is closely associated with this group of diseases and because the gastric parietal cell in many ways behaves like an endocrine cell. The gastric parietal cells secrete intrinsic factor in response to local hormone stimulation (gastrin). Thus, although intrinsic factor is not a hormone, the way the parietal cell must function in order to secrete intrinsic factor must make it resemble the cells of an endocrine gland. Also, in the antrum of the stomach there are gastrin secreting cells. The subdivision of atrophic gastritis into its different constituent diseases is not as clear as initially thought. The classical autoimmune component of the syndrome is Addisonian pernicious anaemia (PA) with atrophy of the mucosa of the body of the stomach accompanied by achlorhydria and absent or virtually absent intrinsic factor secretion (in response to histamine or pentagastrin stimulation) leading to malabsorption of vitamin B12 and its consequences (Irvine, 1975; Wright, 1979). Again, classically the antrum of the stomach is spared so that the plasma gastrin levels are high. However, in some 25% of cases of otherwise classical PA the antrum is also atrophic and the plasma gastrin levels are low (Ganguli *et al.*, 1971). On the other hand, nonspecific atrophic gastritis may be caused by a multiplicity of factors unrelated to autoimmunity (e.g. alcohol, drugs, duodenal reflux, viruses, gastric ulcer, etc.). In this condition the antrum of the stomach is mainly affected with only variable involvement of the mucosa of the body of the stomach. Gastric parietal cell and intrinsic factor antibodies are absent. Nevertheless, Vandelli *et al.* (1979) have reported that some 5% of patients with nonspecific atrophic gastritis have antibodies to gastrin-producing cells in the antrum. These antibodies are not associated with autoimmune atrophic gastritis (with parietal cell antibody in the serum) or with other organ-specific autoimmune disorders. Strickland and MacKay (1973) have labelled these 2 main forms of atrophic gastritis as type A and type B respectively, but in my view it would be better to keep to more precisely descriptive terms: e.g. atrophy of the body or antrum or both associated or not associated with gastric autoimmunity in the form of parietal cell and/or intrinsic factor antibodies or antibodies to gastrin-producing cells. As collective terms "autoimmune atrophic gastritis" and "nonspecific atrophic gastritis" would be preferable to "A" and "B". It is not clear into which group the small number of patients with antritis and antibodies to gastrin-producing cells should fall as these patients do not have other stigmata of autoimmunity to suggest that they might belong to the family of organ-specific autoimmune disorders. Just how common the different forms of atrophic gastritis are depends on how hard one looks for them using endoscopy and gastric function tests. As described later there is a very substantial subclinical prevalence of autoimmune atrophic gastritis and probably of nonspecific atrophic gastritis. This must indicate that the rate of progression of atrophic gastritis to clinical disease with malabsorption of vitamin B12 is slow in many cases or stops before reserves of function have been seriously depleted (Irvine *et al.*, 1974).

Multiplicity of organ-specific antibodies in relation to each target organ

Each of the autoimmune endocrinopathies is characterized by a multiplicity of autoantibodies and usually supplemented with evidence of cell-mediated immunity using the migration inhibition test or transformation test. Cell-mediated immune reactions as evidenced by migration inhibition lack precision in terms of identifying positive reactions in individual patients as opposed to statistically significant results in groups of patients. Their interpretation is also somewhat confused by cross-reaction that appears to occur with extracts of liver mitochondria (Calder *et al.*, 1972; Wartenburg *et al.*, 1973).

The fact that autoantibodies are multiple in terms of their different specificities for antigens within the respective endocrine glands suggest that in terms of pathogenesis only one, or at most a few, of these antibodies may be of importance, while the others are of no particular relevance in terms of cytotoxicity or stimulation. What antibodies the immunologists describe depends on the characteristics and availability of the techniques being used. Thus it is easier to detect cytoplasmic antigens or antigens to secretions (e.g. thyroglobulin) than it is to detect surface antigens; it is easier to detect binding antibodies to extracts of cell membranes than it is to detect antibodies that stimulate intact cells or activate an enzyme system. Thus we should not be surprised that many of the autoantibodies detected in the autoimmune endocrinopathies appear not to correlate well with the onset or course of the disease in question. Even when we do identify the principle autoantibodies in relation to pathogenesis, then of course these antibodies may be operating in conjunction with other immunological mechanisms, such as K cells and immune complexes.

The number of different antibodies reacting at or near the TSH receptor on the thyroid cell membrane in Graves' disease is a good example of the multiplicity of antibodies (Table I) and how the initial description of one of these (LATS in the guinea-pig/mouse) created much initial interest (Adams

TABLE I
Multiple thyroid antibodies reacting on or near TSH receptors

Stimulating
Nonstimulating
Species specific
Species nonspecific

and Kennedy, 1967) only to be followed by some disappointment on account of its species specificity. LATS reacts poorly, if at all, with human thyroid. It was not until the use of both binding and function tests came into prominence that convincing data suggesting that thyroid-stimulating antibodies may indeed be the cause of Graves' disease was forthcoming.

Interrelationship between organ-specific autoimmune disorders

As shown diagrammatically in Fig. 3. the organ-specific autoimmune disorders are interrelated insofar that they overlap clinically and subclinically. The

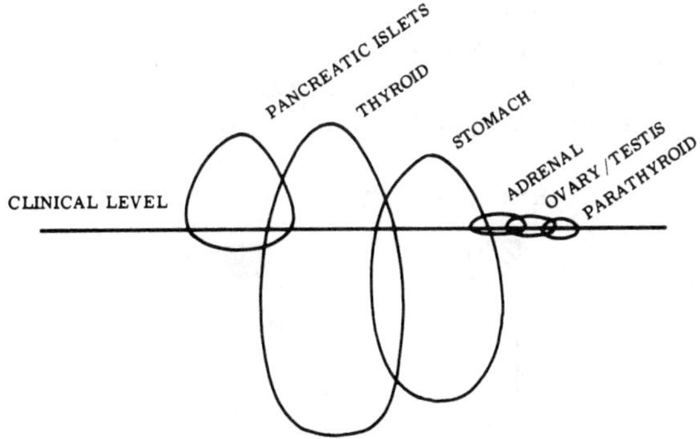

FIG. 3. *The organ-specific autoimmune diseases as icebergs. Only the tips of the icebergs represent clinical disease; the masses below the line represent subclinical disease. The volume of the icebergs represents the relative prevalence of autoimmune disease affecting each target organ clinically and subclinically.* (*From Irvine, 1979.*)

diagram should be 3-dimensional as the different diseases overlap with each other and not simply with its neighbour. The most striking overlap is seen in patients with autoimmune Addison's disease where approximately one third of the patients have at least one other clinical disorder associated with organ-specific autoimmunity (Table II). Figure 4 shows that the prevalence of both clinical and subclinical primary hypothyroidism (which correlates with the presence of antibodies to thyroid cytoplasm in the serum) is significantly higher in type I diabetics over the age of 50 years than in type II diabetics

TABLE II
Associated conditions in 383 patients with Addison's disease

	Idiopathic	*TB*	*Others*
Ovarian failure	40	1	
Thyroid disease			
Thyrotoxicosis	16	1	
Hashimoto	7	0	
Hypothyroidism	28	0	
Diabetes mellitus			
Type I	32	0	
Type II	6	2	
Hypoparathyroid	18	0	
Pernicious anaemia	12	0	
No. of patients affected	122	4	0
Total no. of patients	321	58	4

(From Irvine *et al.*, 1980a, b).

in the same age group (Gray *et al.*, 1979). Thyroid autoimmune disease includes the whole spectrum of Graves' disease, from Hashimoto goitre to primary atrophic hypothyroidism. There is a large subclinical component of autoimmune atrophic thyroiditis, as there is of autoimmune atrophic gastritis. This is associated with a substantial prevalence of thyroid and of gastric parietal cell antibodies in the serum of apparently normal individuals, rising with age and especially in females (Fig. 5). By contrast the prevalence of

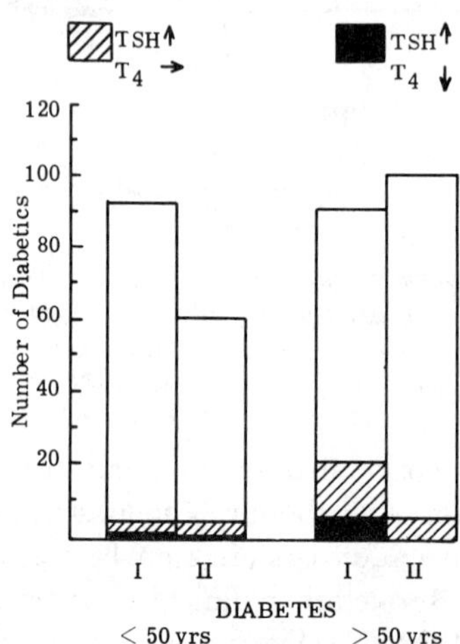

FIG. 4. *The prevalence of a raised serum TSH level (hatched) and of a low serum total T4 level (shaded) in type I (insulin-dependent) and in type II (noninsulin-dependent) diabetics according to their age at the time of the study. (From Gray* et al., *1979.)*

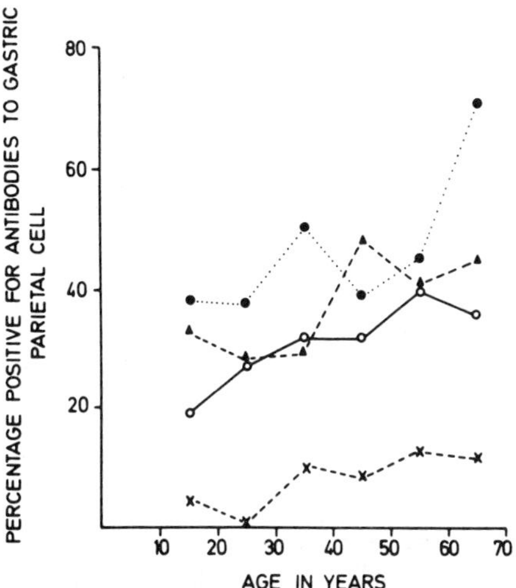

FIG. 5. *The incidence of parietal cell antibody in each decade in 753 female thyrotoxic patients* (○——○), *117 female euthyroid Hashimoto thyroiditis patients* (●.....●) *and 255 spontaneous hypothyroid patients* (▲-----▲) *compared to that in 443 control subjects* (X-----X). (*From Irvine, 1979.*)

subclinical autoimmune Addison's disease, hypoparathyroidism and ovarian failure is much less, in keeping with a very low prevalence of the corresponding antibodies in an apparently normal population. As will be described shortly with particular reference to islet cell antibodies, the presence of antibodies to these tissues in the serum of an apparently normal person tends to be associated with a high risk of that person subsequently developing the biochemical and clinical features of hypofunction of the corresponding endocrine gland. This striking contrast between the large amount of subclinical thyroid disease and of autoimmune atrophic gastritis and the small amount of subclinical adrenocortical or islet cell failure, may be related to the large amounts of thyroid tissues and gastric mucosa and the relatively small amounts of adrenocortical tissue, parathyroid tissue and β cells of the pancreatic islets. It would appear that once an autoimmune reaction starts in relation to the latter group it seems to have a reasonable chance of progressing, so that the relatively small reserves of function of these tissues are severely depleted before long.

While there is in general a fair degree of correlation between the age at diagnosis of autoimmune Addison's disease and the age at diagnosis of type I diabetes (Fig. 2), and of thyrotoxicosis, primary atrophic hypothyroidism, Addisonian PA and autoimmune ovarian failure (Nicol and Irvine, in prep.), it is very striking that within the same group of 350 autoimmune Addisonian patients idiopathic hypoparathyroidism occurred almost exclusively in young people, and more frequently than not was diagnosed before the adrenocortical

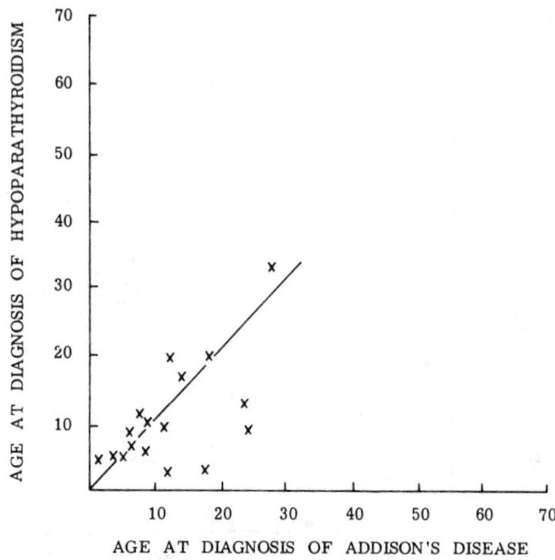

FIG. 6. *The age at diagnosis of idiopathic hypoparathyroidism correlated with the age at diagnosis of idiopathic Addison's disease when these 2 conditions occurred in the same patients. The information was extracted from the study of a series of 350 patients with idiopathic Addison's disease.*

failure (Fig. 6). This must indicate that the genetics of idiopathic hypoparathyroidism, and how that genetics interacts with the environment, must be different from that of the other autoimmune endocrinopathies, either quantitatively or qualitatively or both.

HLA and the autoimmune endocrinopathies

The difference in the genetics of the various diseases within the group of autoimmune endocrinopathies is also indicated by the findings of HLA studies (Table III). Autoimmune Addison's disease has the strongest association with

TABLE III
HLA and autoimmune endocrine disease

	B8	*DRW3*	*B15*	*DRW4*
Idio. Addison's	+ + +	+ + +	–	–
Graves' disease				
Persistent	+ +	+ +	–	–
Transient	–	–	–	–
Atrophic hypothyroid	+	?	–	–
Hashimoto goitre	–	?	–	–
Pernicious anaemia	–	–	–	–
Type I diabetes	+	+	+	+

HLA-B8 and DW3 (Thomsen *et al.*, 1975; Nerup *et al.*, 1980). With regard to Graves' disease the prevalence of HLA-B8 and of DW3 and DRW3 is related to the clinical course of the disease; it is those patients with the persistent or relapsing form of Graves' disease that have the highest prevalence of B8 and DW3, whereas the transient form of thyrotoxicosis has a much lower prevalence of these HLA antigens (Beck *et al.*, 1977; Irvine *et al.*, 1977a). McGregor *et al.* (1980) have observed that the accuracy of predicting whether or not a patient with Graves' disease is going to relapse or go into lasting remission after a 6 months course of antithyroid drugs is increased to 95% if the presence or absence of TSH-receptor antibodies is added to the presence or absence of DRW3. Thus if a patient is DRW3 or has TSH-receptor antibodies in the serum at this time, then he/she has a 95% chance of relapsing; whereas if the patient is not DRW3 and does not have TSH-receptor antibodies in the serum, there is a high probability that there will be a lasting remission when the antithyroid drugs are withdrawn. This must mean that DRW3 is not closely correlated with the production or the time course of production of TSH-receptor antibodies or that it is correlated with only one of the group of TSH-receptor antibodies (see Table I). Indeed, in relation to antibodies to thyroid cytoplasm or to thyroglobulin no correlation between the presence of these antibodies and HLA typing has yet been established. This is also true of gastric antibodies (Irvine *et al.*, 1978a).

It should be appreciated that, in the absence of ablative therapy, patients with Graves' disease may not only spontaneously remit, but after some years may progress to primary hypothyroidism (Irvine *et al.*, 1977b). This suggests that in the course of time thyroid-stimulating immune mechanisms may change to thyroid cytotoxic ones. Unusually, primary autoimmune hypothyroidism may be transient with the euthyroid state being restored spontaneously. A few cases have been described whereby unequivocal primary autoimmune hypothyroidism has turned into Graves' disease, presumably because of a change in the thyroid autoimmune mechanisms from cytotoxic to stimulating (Fig. 7) (reviewed by Irvine *et al.*, 1978a).

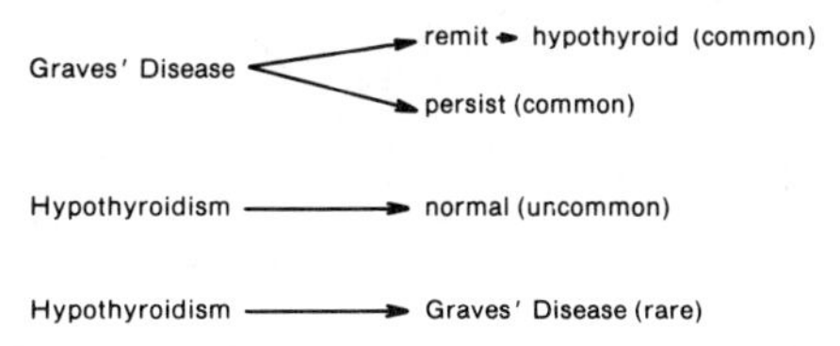

FIG. 7. *Natural history of thyroid autoimmune disease.*

Primary atrophic hypothyroidism is associated with an increased prevalence of B8, while Hashimoto goitre (whether hypothyroid or not) is not associated with B8 (Irvine *et al.*, 1978a) (Fig. 8). Addisonian PA in the absence of a clinical association with another autoimmune endocrinopathy is likewise not clearly associated with any known HLA group, although a slightly increased

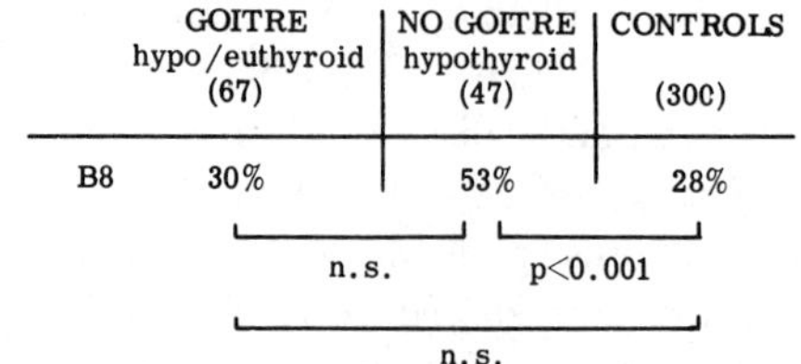

GOITRE
hypo/euthyroid
(67)
NO GOITRE
hypothyroid
(47)
CONTROLS
(300)
B8
30%
53%
28%
n.s.
p<0.001
n.s.

FIG. 8. *The increased prevalence of HLA-B8 in primary atrophic hypothyroidism, but not in Hashimoto goitre, compared to controls. NS = not significant.* (*Data from Irvine* et al., *1978a.*)

prevalence of A3 and B7 has been reported (Whittingham *et al.*, 1975; Goldstone *et al.*, 1976).

Type I diabetes mellitus is unique that it is associated in Caucasians with an increased prevalence of both B8, DW3 and of B15, DW4 (Nerup *et al.*, 1974, 1980; Cudworth *et al.*, 1980).

It is therefore apparent from HLA studies that although the autoimmune endocrinopathies may in some respects be closely interrelated, they are in other respects fundamentally different.

In the Japanese, HLA-B8 is much less common in the general population, compared to Caucasians (Wakisaka *et al.*, 1976). Figure 9 shows that in Japanese IDDM the prevalence of cytoplasmic ICAb is only 14% within 1 year after diagnosis as compared to some 50% in Caucasian IDDM, and that in Japanese IDDM no cytoplasmic ICAb was observed at more than 4 years after diagnosis. Thus there is little evidence so far of persistent ICAb in

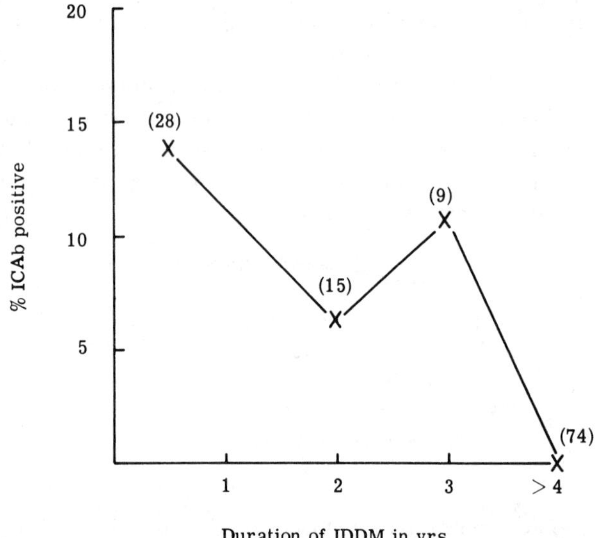

FIG. 9. *Prevalence of islet cell antibodies* (*ICAb*) *in insulin-dependent Japanese diabetics. Note the lower prevalence of ICAb at diagnosis and in the Caucasian population shown in Fig. 12 and the absence of any persistent ICAb at more than 4 years after diagnosis. IDDM = insulin-dependent diabetes mellitus.* (*Data from W. J. Irvine, K. Nagoaka and K. Nonaka.*)

Japanese type I diabetics. A weak autoimmune component in type I Japanese diabetes may contribute to the lower prevalence of IDDM in that ethnic group.

Type I diabetes mellitus

The study of primary diabetes with the unequivocal establishment that there are two main forms (type I and type II), and that in type I islet cell autoimmunity interacts with genetic and with environmental factors (such as viruses or chemicals), has proved to be one of the most exciting areas of research in recent years. The main characteristics of type I and of type II diabetes are shown in Fig. 10. Emphasis is placed on proneness to ketosis and

Type I

Insulin-dependent juvenile-onset diabetes
Insulin-dependent maturity-onset diabetes
ICAb positive diabetics initially controlled by OHA

Type II

Insulin-independent maturity-onset diabetes
Some insulin-independent juvenile-onset diabetes
(ICAb negative at diagnosis)

FIG. 10. *The classification of the 2 main types of primary diabetes.* (*From Irvine, 1977.*)

insulin dependency, and the presence or absence of islet cell antibodies (ICAb). It is stressed that age of onset should not be used as a reliable criterion for classification. No HLA type has a sufficiently high positive association with type I diabetes to help the classification of an individual diabetic as being type I or type II although statistically certain HLA antigens occur more commonly in type I diabetes.

The difficulty in this classification at the present time is the definition of the state of insulin dependency. This is clear when the patient is ketotic, but many physicians may consider insulin therapy to be indicated if the plasma glucose levels cannot be readily controlled by diet with or without oral hypoglycaemic agents. According to the physician's policy a patient may be "insulin-requiring" rather than truly "insulin-dependent". An objective assessment of islet cell function in terms of insulin secretion or C-peptide secretion (if the patient is already being given exogenous insulin) in response to glucagon stimulation should be helpful. However, proneness to ketosis within insulin dependency is the end-stage of type I diabetes, so that a low C-peptide or insulin secretion need not necessarily be present for a diabetic to be classified as type I. ICAb would appear to be the best *in vitro* marker for type I diabetes in the stage before insulin-dependency with proneness to ketosis becomes clinically manifest and before insulin or C-peptide secretion is severely impaired.

ICAb as a marker for secondary failure of OHA therapy

It has long been known that a significant proportion of diabetics treated with OHA satisfactorily for 3 months or more subsequently require insulin for good control, indeed some of them go on to develop classical ketosis-prone insulin-dependent diabetes. My colleagues and I have therefore studied what significance the presence of serum ICAb (reactive with the cytoplasm of all islet cells in the indirect immunofluorescence test using anti-IgG-FITC) may have in this context, while the patients were still controlled by OHA therapy (Irvine *et al.*, 1977a, b, 1979). Figure 11 illustrates the high risk that ICAb

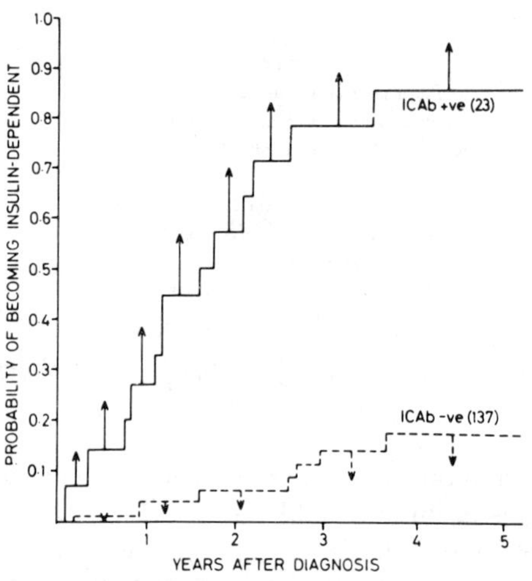

FIG. 11. *Probability of becoming insulin-dependent according to ICAb status in diabetics initially controlled on OHA. The continuous line represents ICAb positive patients. The interrupted line represents ICAb negative patients. The vertical arrows indicate standard errors. The numbers on OHA at 3 months and at yearly intervals thereafter are:*
ICAb positive: 14, 11, 6, 3, 2, 2 (total in group 23).
ICAb negative: 82, 64, 50, 34, 26, 22 (total in group 137).
(*From Irvine* et al., *1979b.*)

positivity confers on an OHA treated diabetic in terms of subsequent dependency on insulin using actuarial statistics. In view of the fact that ICAb is virtually absent from all classical diabetics treated with diet alone (type II) and has a very low prevalence in diabetics controlled by OHA who do not progress to insulin dependency within 5 years, it would appear that ICAb is characteristic only of type I diabetes (including the earlier stages of the disease). In other words, diabetics controlled by OHA should be subdivided into a majority that are type II (and who are ICAb negative) and a minority (who are ICAb positive) that are type I (see Fig. 10). This distinction is the best we can do at the present time, realizing that not all type I diabetics have

ICAb in the serum. Thus, although we have come a long way in terms of the classification of primary diabetes, the precision of that classification in terms of certain patients is not yet as clear as we would like it to be.

ICAb in the serum of subjects with impaired glucose tolerance of pregnancy

Although there is no general agreement as to what constitutes impaired glucose tolerance of pregnancy (IGT of pregnancy) (NDDG, 1979), Steel *et al.* (1980) took a 2 hour plasma glucose of >6·6 mmol/litre after 50 g oral glucose as indicative of it. As shown in Table IV a series of 50 such women were studied

TABLE IV
ICAb and impaired glucose tolerance in pregnancy

	2 h plasma glucose >6·6 mmol/litre		*ICAb*	*Develop*
	In pregnancy	*1 year postpartum*	*pos.*	*IDD*
No. of patients				
Nonobese	22	9	2	2
Obese	28	10	3	1
Totals	50	19	5	3

(From Steel *et al.*, 1980.)

prospectively to see what happened to their diabetes according to the presence or absence of ICAb in the serum during pregnancy. Nineteen of the women still had evidence of IGT 1 year postpartum and 3 of these developed IDDM. All three were included in the 5 of the total 50 who were ICAb positive during pregnancy. Of the 45 ICAb negative pregnant women, 14 required diet or OHA to control diabetes postpartum (type II diabetes). Again, ICAb appeared to be acting as a good *in vitro* marker for the subsequent development of IDDM (end-stage type I diabetes).

ICAb in the serum of subjects without clinical features of diabetes

Table V shows the results of a survey for serum ICAb in 1113 subjects without clinical diabetes. As mentioned above the prevalence of ICAb in control

TABLE V
ICAb in subjects without clinical diabetes

Organ-specific autoimmune diseases	29/522 (6%)
Nondiabetic first degree relatives of ICAb positive subjects	4/157 (3%)
Controls	2/434 (0·5%)

(From Irvine *et al.*, 1977d.)

subjects is very low at 0·5%. The prevalence in a large population of subjects with organ-specific autoimmune disease is significantly higher at 6% representing the area under "sea level" (i.e. subclinical disease) for the islet cell "iceberg" of Fig. 3. Serum ICAb was also found to be increased in the first degree relatives of prospositi who were positive for the antibody. This is in keeping with the observation that type I and type II diabetes appear to be inherited as separate diseases (Irvine *et al.*, 1977c).

In order to determine the value of ICAb as a predictor for the development of type I diabetes at sometime in the future, glucose tolerance tests were done in as many ICAb positive nondiabetic subjects as possible. The preliminary findings were reported by Irvine *et al.* (1976). The current findings are shown in Table VI. At the time of the initial glucose tolerance test 12 of the 42

TABLE VI

ICAb as a marker for type I diabetes

Initial GTT	*No.*	*Clinical follow-up at 1–5 yr*
Impaired	12	1 diabetic (diet) 1 diabetic (OHA) 1 diabetic (OHA → insulin) 1 diabetic (insulin)
Lag storage	4	1 prev. ab. GT → OHA 1 diabetic (insulin)
Normal	26	1 prev. ab. GT → diet 1 diabetic (diet) 1 diabetic (insulin)
Totals	42	9 clinically diabetic

Glucose tolerance tests (GTT) were done on 42 ICAb positive subjects without clinical diabetes, and then the subjects were followed up with further GTTs and clinically for 1–5 yr. The subjects in this study were mainly derived from a population of patients with one or more clinical organ-specific autoimmune diseases (but without clinical diabetes) and from the first degree relatives of subjects who were ICAb positive. (From Irvine, 1980.)

subjects in the study had evidence of impaired glucose tolerance. Four of the subjects had a lag storage form of GTT. The remaining 26 subjects had no evidence of any abnormality of their GTT. The clinical follow-up of these patients over the following 1–5 years is also shown in Table VI. Nine of the 42 subjects have become clinically diabetic. There is no other *in vitro* marker that can predict the onset of clinical diabetes with this degree of accuracy. It far exceeds that of any HLA type so far studied, including DR typing. It is interesting to observe the manner in which the diabetes develops clinically. IDDM may develop acutely or it may develop after a period of adequate control of glucose metabolism by diet or OHA. This further emphasizes that some diabetics controlled by diet and OHA belong to type I and not to type II diabetes. Two of the patients included in Table VI had previous episodes of glucose intolerance in relation to hyperthyroidism, which resolved when the thyrotoxicosis was treated. It will be of great interest to continue to follow-up these 42 patients to see how many of them eventually develop IDDM. However, like the other conditions depicted in Fig. 3, it is probable that subclinical impairment of β cell function of the islets may not always progress to the clinical stage or may even be transitory and resolve (forme fruste). In this context it is relevant to note that islet β cell function in nondiabetic ICAb positive subjects is significantly impaired in comparison with age and sex matched ICAb negative nondiabetics (Gray *et al.*, 1980a). Likewise, there is a greater impairment of islet β cell function in ICAb positive diabetics controlled by OHA in comparison with carefully matched diabetics controlled by OHA but whose serum was negative for ICAb (Gray *et al.*, 1980b). The function of the A cells producing glucagon was similar in the ICAb positive and in the ICAb negative groups and it was not significantly different from that in normal controls. This emphasizes the selectivity of the lesion in type I diabetes for the β cells of the islets, in keeping with histological observations (Gepts, 1980).

Heterogeneity within type I diabetes

Figure 12 shows the prevalence of ICAb in a large population of IDDM according to the duration from the start of insulin therapy (diagnosis of IDDM). It should be noted that at diagnosis the prevalence of the antibody is approximately 60% (Irvine *et al.*, 1977d). Some workers (Cudworth *et al.*, 1980) have claimed that the prevalence at diagnosis is almost 100% but the

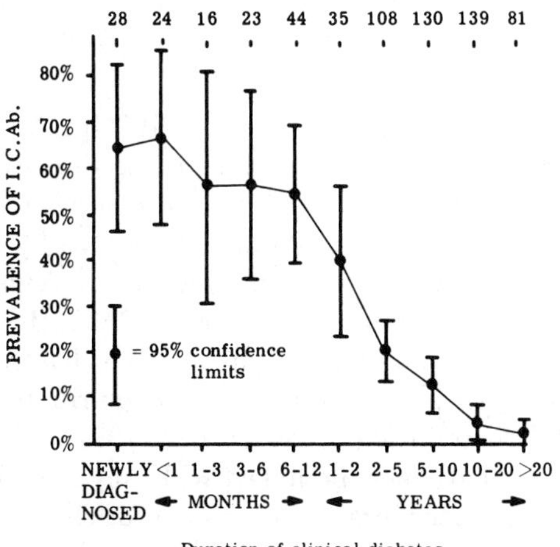

FIG. 12. *The prevalence of ICAb according to the duration of diabetes in 628 insulin-dependent diabetics. (From Irvine* et al., *1977a.)*

statistical evidence for saying this is very doubtful and they themselves have not been able to substantiate it (Bottazzo *et al.*, 1980). The graph shown in Fig. 12. is not characteristic of a "classical" organ-specific autoimmune disease. In idiopathic (autoimmune) Addison's disease, for example, the presence and even the titres of adrenocortical antibodies tend to be maintained over many years (Irvine, 1979); likewise, thyroid and gastric antibodies in primary atrophic hypothyroidism and Addisonian PA, respectively. The fall-off in prevalence of ICAb in IDDM with duration of the disease must therefore mean something. When one analyses the data included in Fig. 12 some IDDM are found to retain ICAb for many years, while others lose their ICAb in a matter of months if not weeks. In the majority the duration of ICAb in IDDM lies between these 2 extremes, and there is no clear segregation into "persisters" or "transients". The persistence of ICAb has been found to be related to the presence of HLA-B8 irrespective of whether or not other clinically associated

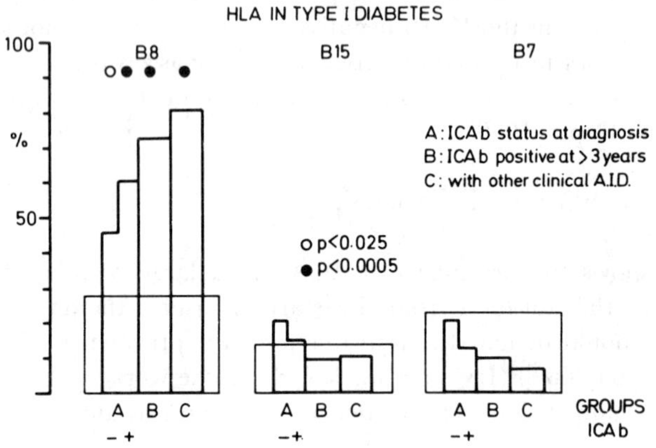

FIG. 13. *The positive association of the autoimmune aspect of type I diabetes with HLA-B8 and the lack of it with B15 and B7. Note especially the correlation between the persistence of ICAb in the serum and the prevalence of B8.* (*From Irvine, 1979.*)

autoimmune diseases are present (Irvine *et al.*, 1978b). As shown in fig. 13 HLA-B8 (but not BW15 or B7) is related to the persistence in the serum of ICAb. This means that the second HLA group of antigens (associated with each other through linkage disequilibrium) represented by B15 (Table III) is predisposing towards type I diabetes through some mechanism other than islet cell autoimmunity. As pointed out above, IDDM is the only member of the group of organ-specific autoimmune diseases that has a second group of HLA antigens associated with it, and apparently contributing in an additive way to the risk of developing IDDM (Nerup *et al.*, 1974). Obvious candidates for pathogenic factors that could be linked with this second group of HLA antigens are pancreatotrophic viral infections and/or chemicals. The work of Craighead (1975) and of Notkins (1977) indicate the involvement viruses in animal models of IDDM. Yoon *et al.* (1979) have isolated a diabetogenic variant of coxsackie B4 from the islet cells of a boy dying acutely of IDDM.

Streptozotocin is a chemical which can induce diabetes in animals in single dosage (if sufficiently large) or by repeated adminstration in small dosage (Rossini *et al.*, 1980). One could imagine therefore that there might be 2 forms of type I diabetes; one based on autoimmunity and the other based on viral or chemical damage to the islets. Indeed this has been proposed by Cudworth *et al.* (1980). However, in my view, this is not consistent with the facts so far recorded, except insofar that autoimmunity or viral-chemical damage may represent the extreme ends of the spectrum of interaction between these pathogenic factors (Fig. 14). Arguments in favour of the hypothesis shown in

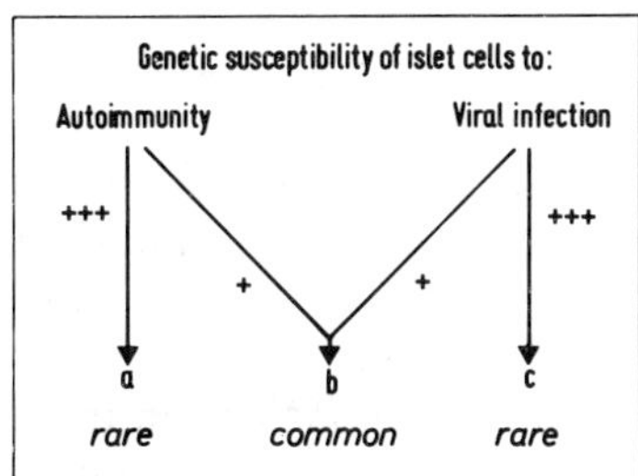

FIG. 14. *The concepts of an interaction between islet cell autoimmunity and viral infection in the pathogenesis of type I diabetes. Uncommonly one or the other may play the predominant role (i.e. types Ia and types Ic), but in most type I diabetes some genetic susceptibility to both probably exists (type Ib). (From Irvine, 1977.)*

Fig. 14 are that the persistence of ICAb in the serum is not grouped into short and long duration, but is continuously variable between these extremes; that the presence of B8/DRW3 and of B15/DRW4 has an additive effect on the risk of developing IDDM; and that there appears to be no clear clinical features (other than guesswork) that distinguish an autoimmune type of diabetes from a viral or chemical type except at the extremes of the spectrum shown in Fig. 14. As shown in Fig. 15 the genetic predisposition of islet cell autoimmunity and to islet cell damage by viruses or chemicals may vary quantitatively in different subjects. While the terminology of type Ia, b and c, is used, it is to be stressed again that there is believed to be a continuous

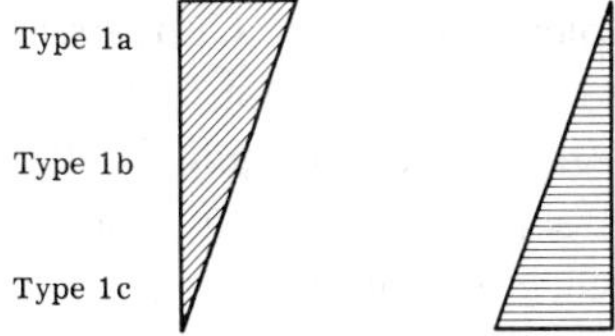

FIG. 15. *Illustration of the hypothesis that genetic susceptibility to islet cell autoimmunity (left) or to islet cell damage by virus or chemical (right) is not an all-or-none phenomenon, but may be present to different degrees in different individuals. The sum of the interaction between the 2 is a measure of an individual's susceptibility to type I diabetes. Thus, a mild viral infection or chemical damage of the islet cells may not lead by itself to clinical diabetes unless the islet cell damage is augmented by an autoimmune response to the islets in an individual with the appropriate immune response gene(s). (From Irvine, 1980.)*

spectrum representing different mixtures in terms of strength of genetic predisposition to islet cell autoimmunity or islet cell damage by exogenous factors. It is suggested that the terminology of Cudworth *et al.* (1980) of types a and b should be dropped to avoid further confusion, not least because they refer to the autoimmune component as type Ib. The hypothesis of Irvine (1977) has been adopted by the National Diabetes Data Group Report on the classification of diabetes (1979).

Cytotoxic mechanisms in autoimmune endocrine disease

Potential cytotoxic mechanisms include antibody, immune complexes (AgAb), K cells and T cells. Antibody may be shown to be avidly cytotoxic *in vitro* in the presence of complement. The clearest example of that is thyroid complement fixing antibodies (Irvine, 1962). Other examples are certain of the group of antibodies reactive with steroid-producing cells in the ovary when incubated with luteinized human granulosa cells *in vitro* in the presence of complement (McNatty *et al.*, 1975). This system has the advantage that no trypsinization or other enzymes are involved in getting granulosa cells into culture. In relation to type I diabetes it has been reported that serum from 11 out of 30 patients with "juvenile onset" diabetes had cytotoxic effects on isolated pancreatic cells from hamsters when guinea-pig complement was present, while this effect was not observed with the sera of 11 "maturity onset" diabetics or of 28 healthy adult controls (Rittenhouse *et al.*, 1980). One of the difficulties with islet cells in culture is being able to identify the different types of islet cells (A, B, D and polypeptide producing cells) and therefore to identify what type of cell may be involved in cytotoxicity. After all, it is necessary to explain why in type I diabetes it is only the islet B cells that are selectively damaged, whereas ICAb detected by indirect immunofluorescence using anti-IgG-FITC generally reacts with all cell types in the islets.

Using the fluorescent technique whereby an unfixed section of pancreas is incubated with test serum, followed by complement, followed by anti C_3-FITC (with appropriate washes in between), a proportion of ICAb positive sera can be shown to be complement fixing (Cudworth *et al.*, 1980; Bottazzo *et al.*, 1980). In contrast to the report by Cudworth *et al.* (1980) we have no incidence of any serum negative by anti-IgG-FITC that was positive by anti C_3-FITC (Irvine, 1980). In some cases the staining of the islets by anti C_3-FITC appears to be relatively selective for some cells in preference to others, but no one has demonstrated so far that this staining is selective for islet β cells. Bottazzo *et al.* (1980) have claimed that such antibodies tend to be present especially around the time of diagnosis of IDDM. This has been questioned by Rilay *et al.* (1980) and also by ourselves. Our own findings do not show any significant change in the proportion of ICAb positive serum that also have complement fixing ICAb over the first 12 months from the diagnosis of IDDM in a prospective study. Until it has been demonstrated that microsomal antigens present in the cytoplasm of islet B cells are also present in the plasma membrane of these cells, there is no *a priori* reason why complement fixing ICAb reactive with cytoplasm should necessarily be cytotoxic *in vivo*. Lernmark *et al.* (1978) have described antibodies in the sera of newly diagnosed IDDM that react with antigens in or on the plasma membrane of a proportion of cells isolated from rat pancreatic islets. These antibodies appear to be distinct from ICAb reactive with the cytoplasm of islet cells using anti-IgG-FITC (Irvine *et al.*, 1980) (Fig. 16). Nevertheless, it is to be remembered that the detection of ICAb (cytoplasm) and ICAb (surface) uses islet cells of different species. It is conceivable that if it were possible to use human islet cells for both tests that surface and cytoplasmic ICAb may be shown to be the same, as appears to be the case in thyroid autoimmune disease (Irvine and Butler, 1980) (Fig. 16).

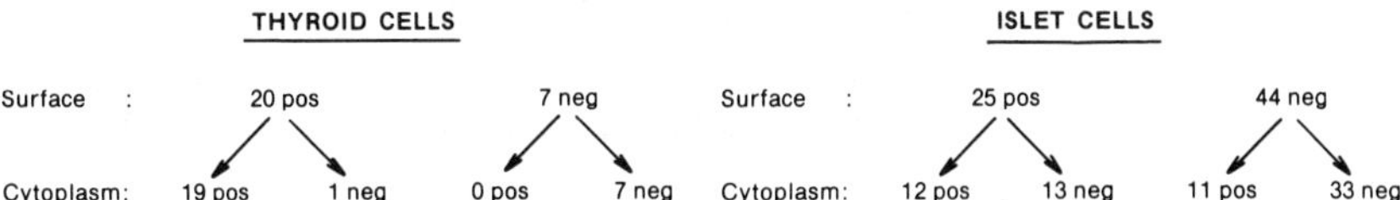

FIG. 16. *The correlation between thyroid cytoplasmic antibodies and antibodies reactive with antigens on the surface of thyroid cells; and the lack of a comparable correlation in relation to pancreatic islet cells.*

Claims have been made that T celis and K cells from "juvenile onset" diabetics are cytotoxic to insulinoma cells in tissue culture (Huang and MacLaren, 1976). However, in view of the fact that the "insulinoma" cells that were used had been in culture for many years and were no longer producing insulin (MacLaren and Huang, 1980), it is very difficult to place much credence in this report. Boitard *et al.* (1980) have observed that lymphocytes from patients with IDDM may suppress the release of insulin from isolated islet cells in response to glucose and theophylline *in vitro*.

K cell cytotoxicity has been studied *in vitro* using target cells coated with thyroid antigen (e.g. thyroglobulin) (Calder *et al.*, 1973; Wasserman *et al.*, 1974). In such circumstances the K cells in the presence of the corresponding antibody are highly cytotoxic. Immune complexes have been described in the sera of patients with thyroid autoimmune disease (Calder *et al.*, 1974; Al-Khateeb and Irvine, 1978; Brohee *et al.*, 1979).

K cell cytotoxic activity of peripheral blood lymphoid cells in patients with autoimmune thyroid disease is increased compared to age and sex matched controls when the duration of treatment for the thyroid condition was less than one year, when little or no goitre was present and when thyroid autoantibodies were in low titre (Calder *et al.*, 1976). Pozzilli *et al.* (1979) have reported that the number of K cells in newly diagnosed IDDM is increased. However, the measurement of K cell numbers by equating them with low affinity E rosetting cells has been questioned (Early and Ozer, 1979). In favour of a role of K cells is the observation that immune complexes are present in the sera of a significant number of newly diagnosed IDDM and that their presence correlates with that of ICAb (Fig. 17), suggesting that at least some of these complexes may consist of ICAg/ICAb in the presence of antibody excess (Irvine *et al.*, 1978c). That would be a situation in which K cells (whether or not they are increased in number) could be involved in islet cell cytotoxicity (Irvine *et al.*, 1978c).

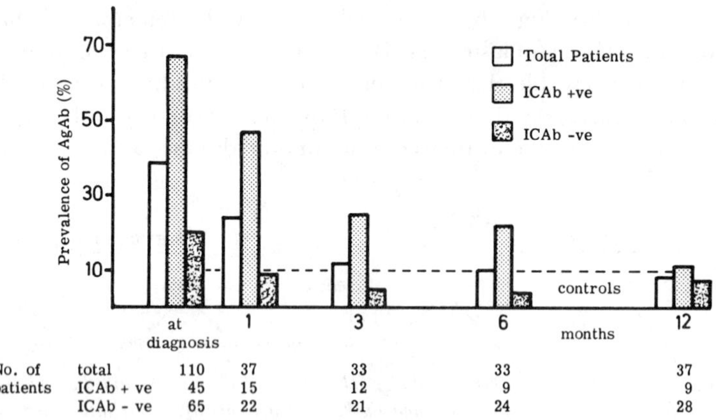

FIG. 17. *The prevalence of AgAb in newly diagnosed insulin-dependent (type I) diabetics and up to 12 months afterwards in some of the same patients as measured by sold phase Clq. The correlation between the prevalence of AgAb and ICAb in the serum at diagnosis and at one month afterwards is also illustrated.* (*From Irvine* et al., *1978c.*)

Muller *et al.* (1980) analysed T-lymphocyte subpopulations in well-established "juvenile-onset" diabetics, according to "low", "intermediate" and "high" affinity rosette forming cells by the use of 3 different lymphocyte: sheep red cell ratios. They concluded that only minor differences exist compared to controls. The depression of lymphocyte transformation to PHA is confined to diabetics in poor metabolic control, whereas the number of T cells in the peripheral blood of IDDM is not significantly different from that in control subjects irrespective of the metabolic state (MacCuish *et al.*, 1974).

With regard to the nature of the cells infiltrating the target organ, this has been studied in relation to the thyroid. Totterman *et al.* (1977) reported that the proportion of B cells is increased compared to the peripheral blood. No clear evidence concerning the number or function of K cells within Hashimoto goitre has been described to date.

Secondary effects on immunological function

In addition to the effect of poor metabolic control on PHA function already described, bacterial binding to peritoneal exudate cells in impaired in mice in which diabetes has been induced with alloxan (Weir *et al.*, 1980). Ptak *et al.* (1980), also in a study of alloxan-induced diabetes in mice, have shown that the expression of Fc receptors on macrophage surfaces is dependent on the *in vivo* insulin level. They consider that the generation and/or transmission of the Fc-dependent signal from the cell surface may be impaired in a hypoglycaemic environment.

Complications

The vascular complications in terms of microangiopathy constitute the most serious aspect of diabetes. Thus the commonest cause of blindness in young and middle-aged people is diabetes (Kohner and Dollery, 1975). Although Andersen (1975) has reported a positive association between severe proliferative retinopathy and insulin antibodies, my colleagues and I have argued that insulin–anti-insulin complexes are unlikely to have much biological activity (Irvine *et al.*, 1978d). Insulin is a bivalent antigen and is therefore

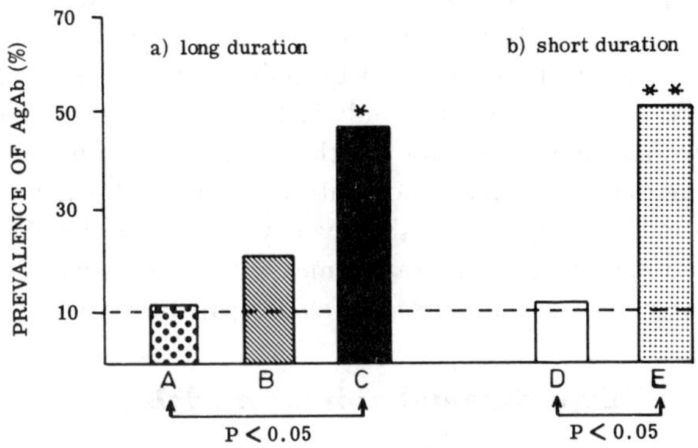

FIG. 18. (*a*) *The increased prevalence of immune complexes as detected by the solid phase Clq assay in diabetics of long standing with proliferative retinopathy* (*group C*) *compared to those with nonproliferative retinopathy* (*group B*) *and without retinopathy* (*group A*).
(*b*) *The increased prevalence of immune complexes in diabetics of short duration when retinopathy is present* (*E*) *compared to when it is absent* (*D*). (*Data from Irvine* et al., *1978c.*)

unlikely to form complexes that will effectively fix complement. On the other hand, we have shown that there is a positive association between the prevalence of soluble complement-fixing immune complexes and the severity of retinopathy, irrespective of whether the diabetic patient had received insulin or not. This association holds in relation to the development of diabetic proliferative retinopathy many years after the diagnosis of diabetes and also in relation to the early onset of diabetic retinopathy (Irvine *et al.*, 1978d) (Fig. 18).

Two papers have claimed that the microangiopathy of diabetes may be associated with B8 or that form of type I diabetes that has strong associations with autoimmunity (type Ia of Fig. 14), but in neither were there adequate controls. Barbosa *et al.* (1976) simply compared the prevalence of 22 HLA antigens in 110 IDDM with terminal glomerulosclerosis and retinopathy, who were being prepared for kidney transplantation. The "controls" were non-diabetic kidney transplant recipients and healthy subjects. Not surprisingly the authors found an increased frequency of antigens A1 and B8 which is characteristic of IDDM in Caucasians. The observation that the prevalence of B15 was not significantly different from controls yields little convincing information in relation to the microangiopathy. Bottazzo *et al.* (1978) felt that they could justify a similar claim from the observation that retinopathy or nephropathy, or both, was present in 10 diabetics, who were all members of "autoimmune families", in which one or more members had organ-specific autoantibodies. However, a direct comparison of the prevalence of retinopathy in IDDM of comparable age and duration of diabetes with and without thyroid autoimmune disease (thyrotoxicosis or thyroid failure) in a total of 329 subjects revealed no difference in the prevalence of retinopathy between the 2 groups (Gray and Clarke, 1979). It is therefore very unlikely that the association between immune complexes and retinopathy is related to autoimmunity or HLA-B8. Larkins *et al.* (1978) reported that the unusual pattern of B8-positive A1-negative was significantly increased in diabetics with proliferative retinopathy. This was not confirmed by Cudworth *et al.* (1980). Clearly detailed HLA studies are required, carefully matching diabetics with similar disease and with similar degree of metabolic control (as far as this is possible) and of similar duration, but differing in the severity of retinopathy. This must be done in conjunction with other laboratory measurements, such as the measurement of immune complexes in the serum as described above.

Experimental animal models

In experimental animals autoimmune thyroiditis has been produced in many species by immunization with thyroid antigen emulsified in Freund's adjuvant (Witebsky *et al.*, 1957). It is conceivable that thyroiditis produced in this way does not necessarily resemble human disease and may be T lymphocyte mediated in terms of the effector cell. Two other models are of particular interest: the spontaneous thyroiditis that occurs in Obese strain (OS) chickens (Wick *et al.*, 1974) and the thyroiditis that develops in PVG/c rats rendered partially T cell depleted by thymectomy followed by sublethal irradiation with the thyroid protected by a lead collar (Penhale *et al.*, 1975). Both these methods have the advantage that they are characterized by permanent (not transient) thyroiditis and that no initial injury to the thyroid or injection of thyroid antigen is involved. In the OS chickens the thyroiditis is bursa dependent, being made worse by thymectomy and prevented by bursectomy. In T cell depleted rats, the onset of thyroiditis can be prevented by reconstituting the animals with isologous (syngeneic) normal lymph node or spleen cells, whereas bone marrow cells, if anything, make the thyroiditis worse (Penhale *et al.*, 1976). The importance of genetic factors in this model is emphasized by the comparative ease with which thyroiditis may be induced in some strains of rats by this method, but not in others. It is possible that controlled auto-reactivity is a normal function of the immune system, possibly associated with the removal of tissue breakdown products. The fact that this autoreactivity is not generally expressed in terms of pathology is thought to be due to control mechanisms involving supressor T cells and helper T cells (Allison *et al.*, 1971; Irvine, 1974).

As already mentioned experimental diabetes can be induced in animals by chemical means (e.g. streptozotocin) or by viruses. Again the species and strain of animal are important. Rossini *et al.* (1980) have reported that when repeated small dosages of streptozotocin are used the development of diabetes may be prevented by the administration of antilymphocytic serum, indicating that an autoimmune element may be contributing to the islet cell damage initiated by the chemical. The claim by Buschard *et al.* (1978, 1980) that diabetes may be transferred from man to mouse by passive transfer of peripheral blood lymphocytes has not been substantiated (Lipsick *et al.*, 1979; Thurneyssen *et al.*, 1979; Rossini *et al.*, 1980).

Endocrine exophthalmos

There are probably 2 separate lesions in endocrine exophthalmos: myositis of the extraocular muscles and the increased bulk of the retro-orbital fat and/or connective tissues. Thyroglobulin is normally released from the thyroid, and patients with severe endocrine exophthalmos frequently have high titres of thyroglobulin antibody.

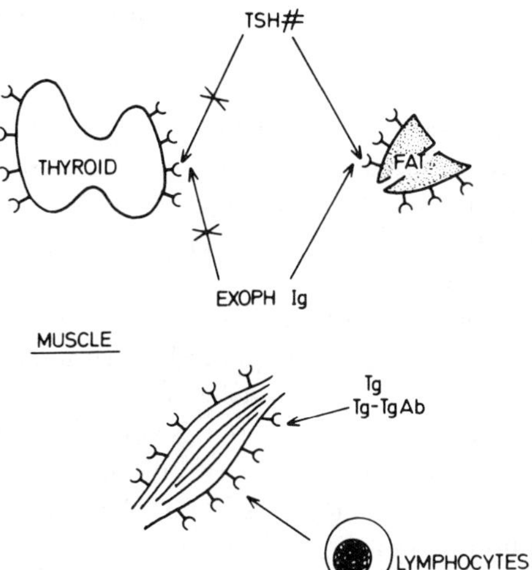

FIG. 19. *Summary of the present concept of relevant receptors on thyroid cells and retro-orbital fat and muscle cells in relation to the immunopathogenesis of endocrine exophthalmos. (From Irvine, 1981.)*

Isolated membranes from periocular tissues bind thyroglobulin–antithyroglobulin complexes about eight times more avidly than do membranes from heart muscle, liver or kidney cells (Konishi *et al.*, 1974) (Fig. 19). Furthermore, positive leukocyte migration inhibition tests have been obtained using retro-orbital tissue homogenates as antigen and the leukocytes of patients with endocrine exophthalmos (Munro *et al.*, 1973).

Receptors sensitive to TSH exist on adipocytes, harderian gland membranes, and human blood polymorphs and monocytes, so that it is possible that TSH-receptor antibodies react with and stimulate certain cells outside the thyroid gland (Hart and McKenzie, 1971; Bolonkin *et al.*, 1975) (Fig. 19). It is known that immunoglobulins from patients with severe endocrine exophthalmos can produce proptosis in animals by stimulating the harderian gland and other retro-orbital tissues (ophthalmic immunoglobulins, or O-Ig) (Dandona and El Kabir, 1970). Also, a fragment of the TSH molecule obtained by mild peptic digestion has been shown to have the properties of exophthalmos-producing substance (EPS) (Kohn and Winand, 1975), which was previously thought to be a separate pituitary factor. Apparently EPS can compete with TSH for receptor sites on these tissues, and it has been suggested that if O-Ig is added this enhances the attachment of EPS. Possible O-Ig's are antibodies that react both with EPS and part of the TSH receptor (Doniach and Florin-Christensen, 1975; Havard, 1979).

The use of immunosuppression

Prednisolone will rapidly reduce the size of many Hashimoto goitres so that a 10 day course may be used clinically in conjunction with thyroxine. Of theoretical interest only is the observation that some gastric acid secretion may be restored if patients with PA are treated with prednisolone (Jeffries *et al.*, 1962). However, the justification for using immunosuppressive therapy is very limited in autoimmune endocrine disease in view of the excellent replacement therapy and adequate means of controlling thyrotoxicosis that are available. The exception is rapidly progressive endocrine exophthalmos. Dandona *et al.*, (1979) reported the successful treatment of such a case with plasmaphoresis, prednisolone and azathioprine. In confirmation of this my colleagues and I have obtained good results with plasmaphoresis, prednisolone and cyclophosphamide in 3 severe cases of recent onset without subsequent relapse when maintained simply on a low dosage of prednisolone (Sawers *et al.*, in prep.). In the absence of a controlled trial (which would not be possible to do) one cannot differentiate between the benefits of plasmaphoresis, steroids or azathioprine/cyclophosphamide.

There has been much discussion about the possible use of immunosuppression so as to prevent the progression of type I diabetes and hopefully to revert it. However, until the pathogenesis of type I diabetes is better understood, especially in relation to the relative roles of autoimmunity and damage by exogenous agents (such as viruses) in individual cases, its use is probably inadvisable.

What is required is more precise ways of manipulating the immune response. In this regard the similarities and differences in the autoimmune aspects of the various endocrinopathies described in this review will need to be taken into account.

References

Adams, D. D. and Kennedy, T. J. (1967). *J. Clin. Endocrinol. Metab.* **27**, 173.

Al-Khateeb, S. F. and Irvine, W. J. (1978). *J. Clin. Lab. Immunol.* **1**, 55.

Allison, A. C., Denman, A. M. and Barnes, R. D. (1971). *Lancet* **ii**, 135.

Andersen, O. O. (1975). *Acta Endocrinol. (Copenhagen)* **78**, 723.

Barbosa, J., Noreen, H., Emme, L., Goetz, F., Simmons, R., De Levia, A., Najarian, J. and Yunes, E. J. (1976). *Tissue Antigens* **7**, 233.

Beck, K., Lumholtz, B., Nerup, J., Thomsen, M., Platz, P., Ryder, L. P., Svjgaard, A., Siersbaek-Nielsen, K., Hansen, J. M. and Larsen, J. H. (1977). *Acta Endocrinol. (Copenhagen)* **86**, 510.

Boitard, C., Debray-Sachs, M., Pouplard, A., Assan, R. and Hamburger, J. (1980). *Diabetologia* (in press).

Bolk, J. H., Elite, J. W. F., Bussenmaker, J. K., Haak, A. and Van Der Heide, D. (1979). *Lancet* **ii**, 61.

Bolonkin, D., Tate, R. L., Luber, J. H. and Kohn, L. D. (1975). *J. Biol. Chem.* **250**, 6516.

Bottazzo, G. F., Mann, J. I., Thorgood, M., Baum, J. D. and Doniach, D. (1978). *Brit. Med. J.* **2**, 165.

Bottazzo, G. F., Gorsuch, A. N., Dean, B. M., Cudworth, A. G. and Doniach, D. (1980). *Lancet* **i**, 668.

Brohee, D., Delespesse, G., Debisschop, M. J. and Bonnyns, M. (1979). *Clin. Exp. Immunol.* **36**, 379.

Buschard, K., Madsbad, S. and Rygaard, J. (1978). *Lancet* **i**, 908.

Buschard, K., Madsbad, S. and Rygaard, J. (1980). *In* "Immunology of Diabetes" (W. J. Irvine, ed) Ch. 9. Teviot Scientific Publications, Edinburgh.

Calder, E. A., McLennan, D., Barnes, E. W. and Irvine, W. J. (1972). *Clin. Exp. Immunol.* **12**, 429.

Calder, E. A., Penhale, W. J., McLennan, D., Barnes, E. W. and Irvine, W. J. (1973). *Clin. Exp. Immunol.* **14**, 153.

Calder, E. A., Penhale, W. J., Barnes, E. W. and Irvine, W. J. (1974). *Brit. Med. J.* **2**, 30.

Calder, E. A., Irvine, W. J., Davidson, McD. and Wu, F. (1976). *Clin. Exp. Immunol.* **25**, 17.

Clague, R., Muktar, E. D. and Pyle, G. A. (1976). *J. Clin. Endocrinol. Metab.* **43**, 508.

Craighead, J. E. (1975). *Prog. Med. Virol.* **19**, 161.

Cudworth, A. G., Bottazzo, G. F. and Doniach, D. (1980). *In* "Immunology of Diabetes" (W. J. Irvine, ed.). Teviot Scientific Publications, Edinburgh.

Dandona, P. and El Kabir, D. J. (1970). *Clin. Sci.* **38**, 2P.

Dandona, P., Marshall, N. J., Bidey, S. P., Nathan, A. and Havard, C. W. H. (1979). *Brit. Med. J.* **1**, 374.

Davies, T. F., Yeo, P. P. B., Evered, D. C., Clark, F., Rees-Smith, B. and Hall, R. (1977). *Lancet* **i**, 1181.

Doniach, D. and Florin-Christensen, A. (1975). *In* "Autoimmunity in Endocrine Disease" (W. J. Irvine, ed.) Vol. 4, p. 341. Saunders, Philadelphia, Pennsylvania.
Early, A. and Ozer, H. (1979). *Lancet* **ii**, 750.
Ganguli, P. C., Cullen, D. R. and Irvine, W. J. (1971). *Lancet* **i**, 155.
Gepts, W. (1980). *In* "Immunology of Diabetes" (W. J. Irvine, ed.) Ch. 15. Teviot Scientific Publications, Edinburgh.
Goldstone, A. H., Voak, D., Cawley, J. C. and Irvine, W. J. (1976). *Clin. Exp. Immunol.* **25**, 352.
Gray, R. S. and Clarke, B. F. (1979). *Brit. Med. J.* **2**.
Gray, R. S., Irvine, W. J., Toft, A. D., Seth, J., Cameron, E. H. D. and Clarke, B. F. (1979). *J. Clin. Lab. Immunol.* **2**, 221.
Gray, R. S., Irvine, W. J., Cameron, E. H. D. and Duncan, L. J. P. (1980a). *Diabetes* **29**, 312.
Gray, R. S., Irvine, W. J. and Buchanan, K. D. (1980b). (submitted).
Hart, I. T. and McKenzie, J. M. (1971). *Endocrinology* **88**, 26.
Havard, C. W. H. (1979). *Brit. Med. J.* **1**, 1001.
Huang, S. W. and MacLaren, N. K. (1976). *Science* **192**, 64.
Irvine, W. J. (1962). *Brit. Med. J.* **1**, 1444.
Irvine, W. J. (1974). *Proc. R. Soc. Med.* **67**, 548.
Irvine, W. J. (1975). "Clinics in Endocrinology and Metabolism", Vol. 4, p. 351. Saunders, Philadelphia, Pennsylvania.
Irvine, W. J. (1977). *Lancet* **i**, 638.
Irvine, W. J. (1979). *In* "Medical Immunology" (W. J. Irvine, ed.) Ch. 6. Teviot Scientific Publications, Edinburgh/McGraw-Hill, New York.
Irvine, W. J. (1980). *In* "Immunology of Diabetes" (W. J. Irvine, ed.) Ch. 1. Teviot Scientific Publications, Edinburgh.
Irvine, W. J. (1981). *J. Clin. Lab. Immunol.* **5** (in press).
Irvine, W. J. and Barnes, E. W. (1975). *Clinics Endocrinol. Metab.* **4**, 379.
Irvine, W. J. and Butler, S. (1980). *J. Clin. Lab. Immunol.* **4** (in press).
Irvine, W. J., Stewart, A. G. and Scarth, L. (1967). *Clin. Exp. Immunol.* **2**, 31.
Irvine, W. J., Chan, M. M. Y., Scarth, L., Kolb, F. O., Hartog, M., Bayliss, R. I. S. and Drury, M. I. (1968). *Lancet* **ii**, 883.
Irvine, W. J., Chan, M. M. W. and Scarth, L. (1969). *Clin. Exp. Immunol.* **4**, 489.
Irvine, W. J., Cullen, D. R. and Mawhinney, H. (1974). *Lancet* **ii**, 482.
Irvine, W. J., Gray, R. S. and McCallum, C. J. (1976). *Lancet* **ii**, 1097.
Irvine, W. J., Gray, R. S., Morris, P. J. and Ting, A. (1977a). *Lancet* **ii**, 898.
Irvine, W. J., Gray, R. S., Toft, A. D., Seth, J., Lidgard, G. P. and Cameron, E. H. D. (1977b). *Lancet* **ii**, 179.
Irvine, W. J., Toft, A. D., Holton, D. E., Prescott, R. J., Clarke, B. F. and Duncan, L. J. P. (1977c). *Lancet* **ii**, 325.
Irvine, W. J., McCallum, C. J., Gray, R. S., Cambell, C. J., Duncan, L. J. P., Farquhar, J., Vaughan, H. and Morris, P. J. (1977d). *Diabetes* **26**, 138.
Irvine, W. J., McCallum, C. J., Gray, R. S. and Duncan, L. J. P. (1977e). *Lancet* **i**, 1025.
Irvine, W. J., Gray, R. S., Morris, P. J. and Ting, A. (1978a). *J. Clin. Lab. Immunol.* **1**, 193.
Irvine, W. J., DiMario, U., Feek, C. M., Gray, R. S., Ting, A., Morris, P. J. and Duncan, L. J. P. (1978b). *J. Clin. Lab. Immunol.* **1**, 107.
Irvine, W. J., DiMario, U., Guy, K., Feek, C. M., Gray, R. S. and Duncan, L. J. P. (1978c). *J. Clin. Lab. Immunol.* **1**, 183.
Irvine, W. J., DiMario, U., Guy, K., Iavicolli, M., Pozziill, B., Lambruso, B. and Andreani, D. (1978d). *J. Clin. Lab. Immunol.* **1**, 187.
Irvine, W. J., Lambert, B. A., Cullen, D. R. and Gordin, R. (1979a). *J. Clin. Lab. Immunol.* **2**, 349.

Irvine, W. J., Sawers, J. S. A., Feek, C. M., Prescott, R. J. and Duncan, L. J. P. (1979b). *J. Clin. Lab. Immunol.* **2**, 23.

Irvine, W. J., Feek, C. M. and Nicol. F. (1980a). *J. Clin. Lab. Immunol.* **4** (in press).

Irvine, W. J., Feek, C. M., Freedman, Z. R., Lernmark, A., Rubenstein, A., Steiner, D. F. and Huen, A. (1980b). *J. Clin. Lab. Immunol.* **4** (in press).

Jeffries, G. H., Hoskins, D. W. and Sleisenger, M. H. (1962). *J. Clin. Invest.* **41**, 1106.

Kahn, C. R., Flier, J. S., Muggeo, M. and Harrison, L. C. (1980). *In* "Immunology of Diabetes" (W. J. Irvine, ed.) Ch. 12. Teviot Scientific Publications, Edinburgh.

Kohn, L. D. and Winand, R. J. (1975). *J. Biol. Chem.* **250**, 6503.

Kohner, E. M. and Dollery, C. T. (1975). *In* "Complications of Diabetes" H. Keen and J. Jarrett, eds) p. 71. Arnold, London.

Konishi, J., Herman, M. M. and Kriss, J. P. (1974). *Endocrinology* **95**, 434.

Larkins, R. G., Martin, F. I. R. and Tait, B. D. (1978). *Brit. Med. J.* **1**, 1111.

Lernmark, A., Freedman, Z. R., Hogman, C., Rubenstein, A. H., Steiner, D. F., Jackson, R. C., Winter, R. J. and Traisman, H. S. (1978). *New Engl. J. Med.* **299**, 375.

Lipsick, J., Beattie, G., Osler, A. G. and Kaplan, N. O. (1979). *Lancet* **i**, 1290.

MacCuish, A. C., Urbaniak, S. J., Campbell, C. J., Duncan, C. J. P. and Irvine, W. J. (1974). *Diabetes* **23**, 708.

McGregor, A. M., Smith, B. R., Hall, R., Petersen, M. M., Miller, M. and Dewar, P. J. (1980). *Lancet* **i**, 1101.

MacLaren, N. K. and Huang, S. W. (1980). *In* "Immunology of Diabetes" (W. J. Irvine, ed.) Ch. 10. Teviot Scientific Publications, Edinburgh.

McNatty, K. P., Short, R. V., Barnes, E. W. and Irvine, W. J. (1975). *Clin. Exp. Immunol.* **22**, 378.

Muller, R., Kolb, H., Kuschak, D., Jorgens, V. and Gries, F. A. (1980). *Clin. Exp. Immunol.* **39**, 130.

Munro, R. L., Lamki, L., Row, V. V. and Volpe, R. (1973). *J. Clin. Endrocrinol. Metab.* **37**, 286.

National Diabetes Data Group Report (1979). *Diabetes* **29**, 1039.

Nerup, J. and Bendixen, G. (1969). *Clin. Exp. Immunol.* **5**, 341.

Nerup, J., Platz, P., Andersen, O. O., Christy, M., Lyngsoe, J., Pulsen, J. E., Ryder, L. P., Staub Nielsen, L., Thomsen, M. and Svejgaard, A. (1974). *Lancet* **ii**, 864.

Nerup, J., Christy, M., Kroman, H., Andersen, O. O., Platz, P., Ryder, L. P., Thomsen, M. and Svejgaard, A. (1980). *In* "Immunological Aspects of Diabetes" (W. J. Irvine, ed.) Ch. 2. Teviot Scientific Publications, Edinburgh.

Notkins, A. L. (1977). *Arch. Virol.* **54**, 1.

Penhale, W. J., Farmer, A. and Irvine, W. J. (1975). *Clin. Exp. Immunol.* **21**, 362.

Penhale, W. J., Irvine, W. J., Inglis, J. R. and Farmer, A. (1976). *Clin. Exp. Immunol.* **25**, 6.

Pozzilli, P., Gorsuch, A., Sensi, M., Bottazzo, G. P. and Cudworth, A. G. (1979). *Lancet* **ii**, 173.

Ptak, W., Rewicka, M. and Hielecks, J. (1980). *J. Clin. Lab. Immunol.* **4** (in press).

Riley, W. J., Neufeld, M. and MacLaren, N. K. (1980). *Lancet* **i**, 1133.

Rittenhouse, H. G., Oxender, D. L., Pek, S. and Diane, A. R. (1980). *Diabetes* **29**, 317.

Rossini, A. A., Williams, R. M., Appel, M. C. and Like, A. A. (1980). *In* "Immunology of Diabetes" (W. J. Irvine, ed.) Ch. 18. Teviot Scientific Publications, Edinburgh.

Steel, J. M., Irvine, W. J., Feek, C. M. and Clarke, B. F. (1980). *J. Clin. Lab. Immunol.* **4** (in press).

Strickland, R. G. and MacKay, I. R. (1973). *Am. J. Dig. Diseases* **18**, 426.

Teng, C. S. and Yeung, R. T. T. (1980). *J. Clin. Endocrin. Metab.* **50**, 144.

Thomsen, M., Platz, P., Andersen, O. O., Christy, Y., Lyngsoe, J., Nerup, J.,

Rasmussen, K., Ryder, L. P., Staub-Nielsen, L. and Svejgaard, A. (1975). *Transpl. Rev.* **22**, 125.
Thurneyssen, O., Jansen, F. K., Vialettes, B., Vague, P. H., Selam, J. L. and Mirouze, J. (1979). *Lancet* **i**, 1291.
Totterman, T. H., Maenpaa, J., Gordin, A., Makinen, T. M., Taskinen, E., Andersen, L. C. and Hayry, P. (1977). *Clin. Exp. Immunol.* **30**, 193.
Vandelli, G., Bottazzo, G. F., Doniach, D. and Franceschi, F. (1979). *New Engl. J. Med.* **300**, 1406.
Wakisaka, A., Aizawa, M., Matsuura, N., Nagagawa, S., Nakayama, E., Itakura, K., Okuno, A. and Wagatsuma, Y. (1976). *Lancet* **ii**, 970.
Wartenburg, J., Doniach, D., Brostoff, J. and Roittz, I. M. (1973). *Clin. Exp. Immunol.* **14**, 203.
Wasserman, J., Stedinkg, L. V., Periman, P. *et al.* (1974). *Int. Arch. Allergy. Appl. Immunol.* **47**, 473.
Weir, D. M., Blackwell, C. C. and McLean, C. A. (1980). *J. Clin. Lab. Immunol.* **4** (in press).
Whittingham, S., Youngchaiyud, U., MacKay, I. R., Buckley, J. D. and Morris, P. J. (1975). *Clin. Exp. Immunol.* **19**, 289.
Wick, G., Sundick, R. S. and Albini, B. (1974). *Clin. Immunol. Immunopathol.* **3**, 272.
Witebsky, E., Rose, N. R., Terplan, K., Pain, J. R. and Egan, R. W. (1957). *J. Am. Med. Assoc.* **164**, 1439.
Wright, R. (1979). *In* "Medical Immunology" (W. J. Irvine, ed.) Ch. 7. Teviot Scientific Publications, Edinburgh/McGraw-Hill, New York.
Yoon, J. W., Austin, M., Onodera, T. and Notkins, A. L. (1979). *New Engl. J. Med.* **300**, 1173.

53

Murine SLE-Aetiology and Pathogenesis

FRANK J. DIXON, ARGYRIOS N. THEOFILOPOULOS SHOZO IZUI and PATRICIA J. McCONAHEY

Department of Immunopathology, Scripps Clinic and Research Foundation, La Jolla, California, USA

The authors wish to acknowledge the collaboration of Drs D. H. Katz, E. D. Murphy, J. B. Roths, R. A. Eisenberg, R. M. Zinkernagel, W. D. Creighton, B. S. Andrews, J. H. Elder, J. S. Crowell and S. Lee in certain parts of these studies. The expert technical assistance of D. L. Shawler, R. Balderas and L. Thor is also acknowledged. Ms Carolyn Honold expertly assisted in the typing of the manuscript.

The work in this chapter is supported by US Public Health Service grants AI-07007, NO1-CP-71078, CA-16600, CA-2322 and the Cecil H. and Ida M. Green Research Endowment.

This is publication No. 2206 from the Department of Immunopathology, Scripps Clinic and Research Foundation, 10666 North Torrey Pines Road, La Jolla, California 92037. USA.

Argyrios N. Theofilopoulos is supported by a Research Career Development Award, National Cancer Institute CA-00303.

Introduction

Autoimmunity observed in both clinical and experimental circumstances can best be defined as termination of the natural unresponsive state to self (Weigle, 1977). According to the original strict versions of the Clonal Selection Theory (Burnet, 1959) it has been postulated that self-tolerance is effected by elimination of self-reactive lymphocyte clones early in ontogeny. However, later investigators leave little doubt that such self-reactive clones are normally present in the intact immune system (Burnet, 1959; Clagett and Weigle, 1974; Cohen and Wekerle, 1973; Bankhurst *et al.*, 1973; Bankhurst and Williams, 1975; Sawada *et al.*, 1977; Wigzell, 1977; Katz, 1977).

In fact, in recent years it has been found that a common underlying element of immunity is self-recognition, which is based on the complementary properties of interacting structures on T cells, B cells and macrophages. Apparently, self-recognition is not a forbidden event, as thought, but the major principle upon which the immune and possibly other systems are founded. The prevailing current concept is that such self-recognition processes are normally controlled or damped by one or more mechanisms in order to avoid deleterious autoreactive consequences. A variety of events, either exogenous or endogenous, could tip the balance of such regulatory control thereby upsetting this normal damping mechanism with the consequence of harmful autoreactivity. In some instances, this imbalance may be only transient in nature after which time re-establishment of the normal damping mechanism brings the system back under control. In other instances, the defect may be permanent leading to a progressive increase in deleterious autoreactivity. This might explain the manifestations of chronic autoimmune phenomena seen in autoimmune strains of mice and in certain human diseases, most notably systemic lupus erythematosus (SLE), the prototype autoimmune disease.

Since the first comprehensive description of SLE by Osler (1895), there has been considerable progress in delineating the immunologic defects and pathogenic mechanisms of this disease. Nevertheless, its aetiology remains elusive. The availability of the New Zealand (NZ) mice, particularly the NZB and the (NZB × W) F_1 (NZB × W) (Howie and Helyer, 1968) which spontaneously develop a disease resembling human SLE, offered the unusual opportunity to study SLE at a preclinical stage that is only rarely possible in humans with this disorder. Considerable evidence has been generated in the past 20 years to indicate that a wide spectrum of immunologic abnormalities exist in such mice depending on the animals' age and sex and the assay system used to analyse such abnormalities (reviewed in Talal, 1976; Theofilopoulos *et al.*, 1980c). Glaringly absent among the voluminous data generated on such mice is a common thread that allows one to pinpoint with any certainty a clear-cut cause and effect relationship between most of the abnormalities observed and the aetiology/pathogenesis of the autoimmune component in these animals. Moreover, since these abnormalities derived from studying NZ mice only, it is extremely difficult to determine which are primary aetiologic factors in the murine SLE syndrome and which are epiphenomena or even incidental features of these unusual lines of mice. In view of this uncertainty, we have undertaken a detailed serologic, immunologic, virologic and genetic analysis of the NZ mice and of the two newly described autoimmune murine strains, BXSB and MRL (Murphy and Roths, 1979) in the hope of finding one or more common aspect of abnormality that might clarify the pathogenesis of murine and ultimately human SLE. A summary of our studies to date on the histopathologic, serologic, virologic, cellular and genetic characteristics of these mice is given below.

Derivation and mortality rate of SLE-prone murine strains

The derivation of the SLE-prone murine strains used in our studies are given in Table I. The development of the MRL and BXSB strains has been described

TABLE I
Derivation of SLE mice and genetic markers

Strain	*Derivation*	H-2	*Lymphocyte surface alloantigens*	*IgG allotype*
NZB	Inbred for colour from stock of undefined background	$H\text{-}2^d$	Thy-1·2, Ly-1·2, Ly-2·2, Ly-3·2, $Qa\text{-}1^a$, Mls^a	*e*
NZW		$H\text{-}2^z$	Thy-1·2	*e*
BXSB	Derived from (C57BL/6J × SB/Le) F_1	$H\text{-}2^b$	Thy-1·2, TL^-, Ly-1·2, Ly-2·2, Ly-3·2, $Qa\text{-}1^b$	*b*
MRL/l	Genome = 75% LG, 13% AKR, 12% C3H and 0·3% C57BL/6	$H\text{-}2^k$	Thy-1·2, TL^-, Ly-1·2, Ly-2·1, Ly-3·1, $Qa\text{-}1^b$	*a*

by Murphy and Roths (1979). These investigators have estimated from the breeding history that the composite genome of the MRL mice is derived 75·0% from LG, 12·6% AKR, 12·1% C3H, and 0·3% C57BL/6. In the 12th generation of the MRL inbreeding, due to a spontaneous autosomal recessive mutation, *lpr* (lymphoproliferation) gene, the MRL strain was subdivided into two substrains, one with the *lpr* gene and the other without, with the 2 substrains having at least 89% of their genomes in common. The *lpr* gene has been transferred to substrain MRL/n by 5 cycles of cross-intercross matings reducing the estimated residual heterozygosity from 11% to 0·4% and producing the congenic inbred strain MRL/Mp–lpr/lpr and +/+. The phenotype of MRL cell surface alloantigens include $H\text{-}2^k$, Ly-1·2, Ly-2·1, Ly-3·1, Thy-1·2, TL^- and $Qa\text{-}1^b$. The allotype of the IgG_{2A} subclass (*Ig-1* locus) for the MRL strains is *a*. The development of BXSB/Mp strain has been detailed elsewhere by Murphy and Roths (1979). This recombinant inbred strain was derived from a single cross between a C57BL/6 female and an SB/Le mouse homozygous for the linked mutant genes satin (*sa*) and beige (*bg*). The phenotype of BXSB cell surface alloantigens is $H\text{-}2^b$, Ly-1·2, Ly-2·2, Ly-3·2, Thy-1·2, TL^-, $Qa\text{-}1^b$ and the allotype of the IgG_{2A} subclass is *b*. The development of the NZB, NZW and NZB × W mice has been described elsewhere (Bielschowsky and Goodall, 1970). The NZB cell surface alloantigens include $H\text{-}2^d$, Thy-1·2, Ly-1·2, Ly-2·2, Ly-3·2, $Qa\text{-}1^a$, Mls^a and of the NZW are $H\text{-}2^z$, Thy-1·2. The allotype of the IgG_{2A} subclass for the NZB and NZW strain is *e*.

The survival rates of these autoimmune murine strains have been described elsewhere (Andrews *et al.*, 1978). NZB mice of both sexes have a 50% mortality by 16 to 17 months of age. In the NZB × W mice, the disease appears first in the female at about 6 months of age with 50% mortality at 8·5 months, while in the male 50% mortality is reached at 15 months. The MRL/Mp–*lpr*/*lpr* substrain (MRL/l) manifests early disease with 50% mortality in males and females at about 5 to 6 months, whereas the MRL/Mp–+/+ (MRL/n) which lacks the *lpr* gene has delayed disease with 50% mortality at 17 to 23 months for female and male, respectively. In contrast to NZB × W, the male BXSB/Mp (BXSB) is affected much earlier than the female with a 50% mortality for the male at around 6 months and for the female at 15 months.

Histoimmunopathologic and serologic features

Our immunopathologic studies on these mice have been presented in detail elsewhere (Andrews *et al.*, 1978; Accinni and Dixon, 1979) and are summarized in Table II. Immune complexes (IC) glomerulonephritis is a histopathologic feature in all of these autoimmune mice and is the major cause of death. Granular glomerular deposits of IgG and C3 and sometimes DNA and gp70 retroviral envelope antigens are present. Thymic atrophy, primarily of the cortex, is seen in all of these mice. However, the degree of lymph node hyperplasia varies considerably, ranging from normal to 2–3 times enlarged in

TABLE II

Histoimmunopathologic and serologic characteristics of SLE-mice

		Histopathologic features			
Strain	*IC-GN*	*Thymic atrophy*	*Lymphoid hyperplasia*	*Arteritis*	*Arthritis*
NZB	+	+	+	0	0
NZB × W	+ + +	+	+	0	0
MRL/l	+ + +	+	+ + +	+	+
BXSB	+ + +	+	+ +	0	0

Serologic features

Common	Hyper-γ-globulinaemia, ANA, anti-ds DNA, anti-ss DNA, antihapten antibodies, high levels of gp70, immune complexes, reduced complement levels (NZB is C-5 deficient).
Uncommon	Anti-Sm (MRL/n, MRL/l), IgG + IgM Rf (MRL/l), antierythrocyte (NZB, NZB × W), NTA (NZB, NZB × W, BXSB)

NZB × W females, 10–20 times above normal size in BXSB males, and up to 100 times enlarged in MRL/l mice. The proliferating cells in BXSB are of B type and those in MRL/l mice of T cell type (see below). Attempts to transplant enlarged lymph nodes to find evidence of malignancy in MRL/l mice have failed. Fifteen to 30% of mice in each SLE strain have acute and/or old myocardial infarction (Accinni and Dixon, 1979). Moreover, medium and small arteries and arterioles of hearts with and without infarcts have focal degenerative lesions consisting of PAS-positive or eosinophilic deposits in the intima and to a lesser extent in the media, without accompanying cellular inflammation. Granular deposits of mouse Ig, C3 and occasionally gp70 may be present in the walls of medium and small arteries, arterioles and venules of myocardium (Fig. 1). Apart from the degenerative vascular disease found in all strains, over half of MRL/l mice uniquely develop acute and/or necrotizing polyarteritis, most frequently involving renal and coronary arteries. About 25% of old, sick MRL/l mice also have swollen joints of the hind feet and lower legs (Fig. 2). There is destruction of articular cartilage, proliferation of synovium, pannus formation (Fig. 3) and at times joint effusions, which together present a picture not unlike that of rheumatoid arthritis.

Of the serologic abnormalities in SLE mice some are common to all strains and others are not (Andrews *et al.*, 1978; Izui *et al.*, 1978; Izui and Eisenburg, 1980; Eisenberg *et al.*, 1978; Eisenberg *et al.*, 1979a, b) (Table II). The common primary serologic abnormalities include: elevated concentrations of serum Ig frequently associated with monoclonal γ globulins, antinuclear antibodies, and anti-ds and ss-DNA antibodies. Additionally, all autoimmune mice at 2–4 weeks of age spontaneously produce 4–6 times more antihapten

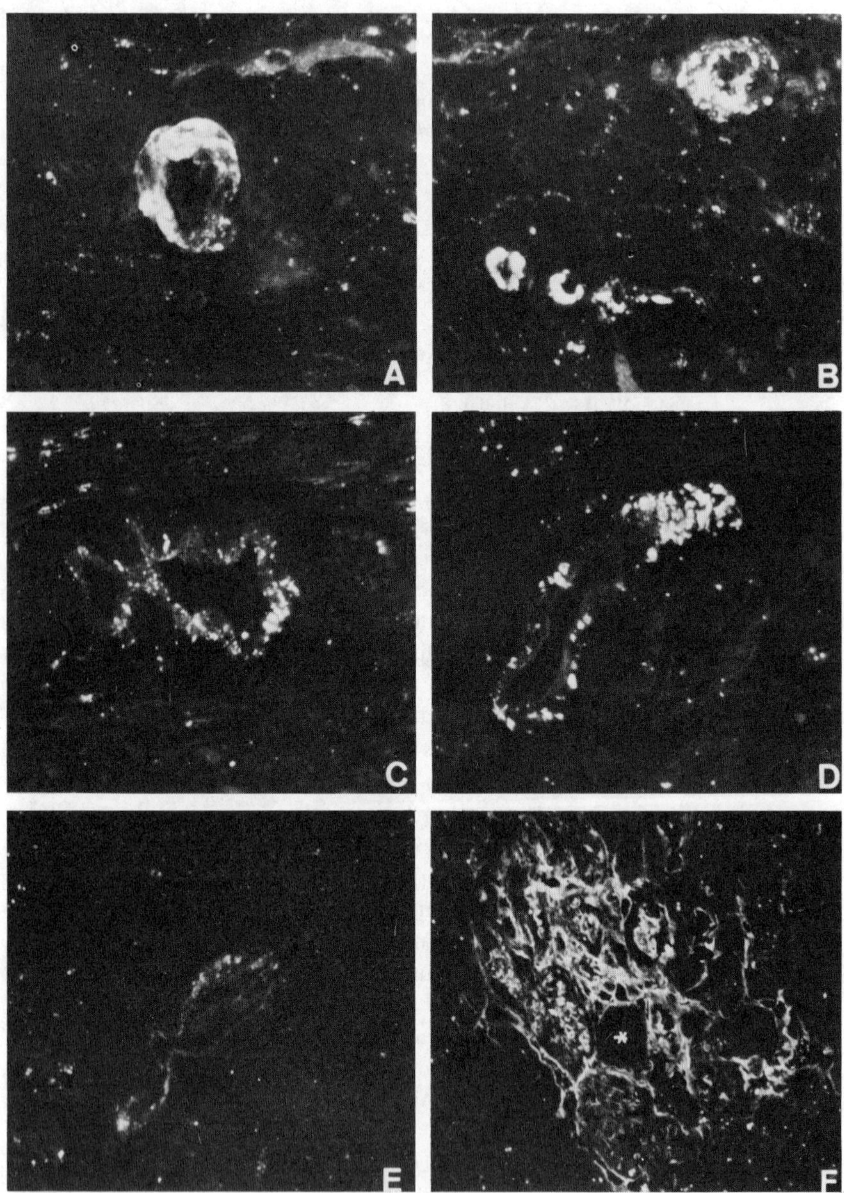

FIG. 1. *Frozen sections of NZB × W and BXSB myocardium, respectively, stained with FITC-conjugated antibody to murine IgG. Granular and patchy deposits are visible in the wall of small coronary arteries and arterioles (A and B). Section of NZB × W myocardium stained with FITC anti C3 (C and D). Section of MRL/l myocardium stained with anti-gp70 (F). Section of BXSB myocardium stained with FITC antifibrinogen (F). Fibrinogen is visible between necrotic myocardial fibres.*

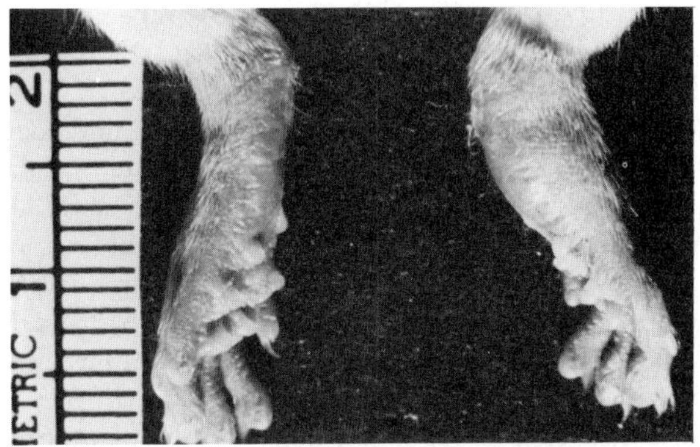

FIG. 2. *A 4-month-old MRL/l mouse with swollen joints of the hind feet and lower legs.*

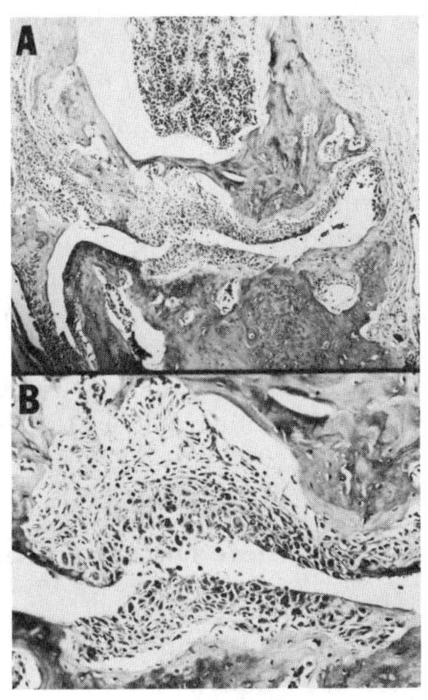

FIG. 3. *Destruction of articular cartilage, proliferation of synovium and pannus formation in sections of a swollen joint from MRL/l mouse.*

antibody-forming cells in spleens and have greater concentrations of antihapten antibodies in sera than age-matched immunologically normal strains of mice (Izui *et al.*, 1978). Significant levels of retroviral gp70 are also observed in all kinds of autoimmune mice, being highest in NZB and followed by NZB × W, MRL/l and BXSB mice (Andrews *et al.*, 1978). However, similar levels of retroviral gp70 are observed in sera of some immunologically normal mice (NZW, LG/J, 129/J, SM/J, DBA/2). Concentrations of serum gp70 do not increase with the autoimmune disease nor do they correlate with levels of anti-DNA and antihapten antibodies. Uncommon primary serologic abnormalities are: (a) antierythrocyte antibodies occurring frequently in the NZB and NZB × W (80%) but infrequently in MRL/l (11%) and BXSB (18%) mice; (b) antibodies against the nuclear glycoprotein Sm exclusively in older MRL/n (35% males, 45% females) and MRL/l mice (37% males, 10% females). The clinical signs of lupus are equally severe in anti-Sm positive and anti-Sm negative mice (20); (c) rheumatoid factors of both the IgM and IgG variety are present in sera of two-thirds of older MRL/l mice only (Andrews *et al.*, 1978; Izui and Eisenberg, 1980; Eisenberg *et al.*, 1979b). This finding is in accord with the arthritis occasionally observed in these mice and suggest that this strain may be a valuable animal model for the study of rheumatoid arthritis as well; (d) natural thymocytotoxic antibodies (NTA) are present in high levels and incidence in NZB and NZB × W mice, low in BXSB, very low or absent in MRL/l and MRL/n mice. A comprehensive survey (Eisenberg *et al.*, 1979a) showed similar incidences and serum titres of NTA in some immunologically normal strains (RF, SN, NC, 129-GIX$^+$, 129-GIX$^-$) as compared to NZ mice. Although the fine specificities of NTAs in the various murine strains remain to be determined, we may conclude that NTAs are neither necessary nor probably unique to SLE mice and that their mere presence does not indict the individual to become autoimmune. In fact, hereditarily asplenic (Dh/+) NZB mice develop autoimmune disease in the absence of NTA (Gershwin *et al.*, 1979) and NTAs could be expressed in recombinant NZB inbred strains in the absence of other types of autoantibodies or conversely anti-DNA and antierythrocyte antibodies could be expressed in the absence of NTAs (Rayeche *et al.*, 1980). Common secondary serologic features in all SLE strains are the appearance of circulating immune complexes (ICs) and a decrease in haemolytic complement as the disease progresses, especially in the older MRL/l mice. Interestingly, the NZB strain is genetically C5-deficient.

Nature of immune complexes in sera

Studies conducted to determine the nature of ICs detected by the Raji cell radioimmunoassay in sera of SLE-prone murine strains have demonstrated the presence of retroviral gp70-anti-gp70 complexes (Elder *et al.*, 1977). The sera of all older autoimmune murine strains, but not sera from several normal strains, are characterized by a rapidly sedimenting heavy form of gp70 (7-19S), in addition to 5S gp70 (Fig. 4). This heavy form of gp70, but not the 5S type, is specifically adsorbed with antimouse IgG antibody or *Staphylococcus aureus*, strongly suggesting that the heavy gp70 in serum is in the form of ICs. Immunoprecipitation analysis with antimouse IgG or adsorption to *Staphylococcus aureus* indicates that approximately one-fifth to one-half of the total serum gp70 in sera of older autoimmune mice is associated with IgG. Although the appearance of gp70-related ICs varies with age among the SLE susceptible strains, it parallels the onset of renal disease and the concentration of gp70 associated ICs increases with the progression of disease. IgG complexed gp70 is also found in renal eluates from the diseased kidneys of adult mice but not in those from 2-month-old mice.

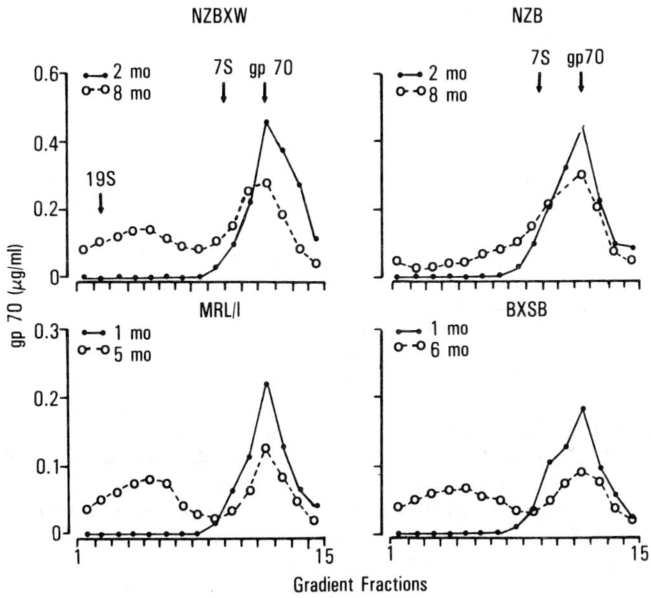

FIG. 4. *Sedimentation rate of serum gp70 from SLE-prone mice at various ages analysed by sucrose density gradient centrifugation. The concentration of gp70 was determined by a radioimmunoassay with anti-FeLV antiserum and* ^{125}*I-Rauscher MuLV gp70. The position of markers is indicated by the arrows.*

Since multiple immunologically related gp70s are produced in every mouse (Elder *et al.*, 1977), it is important to know what kind of retroviral gp70 is involved in the formation of ICs. Although the primary serum gp70 in all mice is similar to that found in the NZB xenotropic virus (Elder *et al.*, 1977) the lack of antibody formation against serum gp70 in normal mice raised the possibility that SLE mice might express a unique type of retroviral gp70 in their sera. However, immunochemical and tryptic peptide mapping analysis of the gp70 isolated from the circulating ICs revealed its xenotropic origin

(Izui *et al.*, 1980a). Moreover, studies of the immunologic specificity of isolated anti-gp70 antibodies from the ICs clearly showed that anti-gp70 antibodies have an affinity for NZB xenotropic viral gp70 approximately 10 times higher than that for AKR ecotropic viral gp70 (Fig. 5) indicating that the antibody involved is directed primarily to NZB xenotropic viral gp70. This is compatible with the fact that the presence of anti-AKR ecotropic gp70 antibodies in sera of mice does not correlate with formation of gp70 associated ICs (Izui *et al.*, 1979). Taken together, our studies indicate that mice which develop SLE do

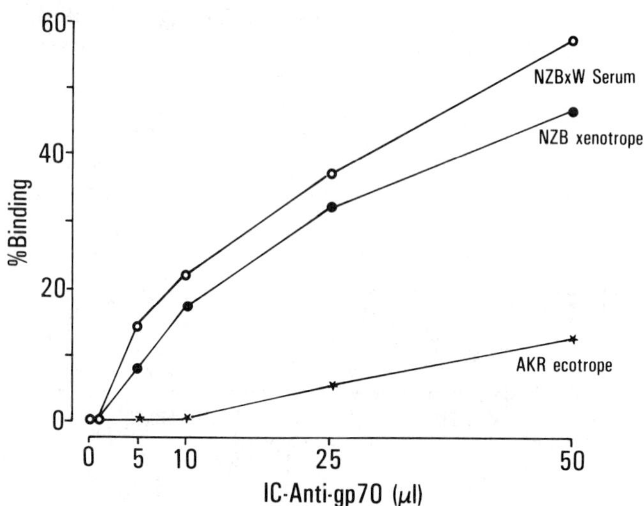

FIG. 5. *Binding of anti-gp70 isolated from serum immune complexes to free gp70 isolated from sera of 2-month-old NZB × W* (○——○), *NZB-XI gp70* (●——●) *and AKR ecotropic viral gp70* (*——*). *Constant amounts of gp70s were incubated with increasing amounts of immune complex-derived anti-gp70 at 4 °C overnight, and the per cent binding of these gp70s by the antibody was determined by using staphyloccocal protein A to precipitate the gp70-anti-gp70 complex.*

not have a unique kind of gp70, but instead have the unique ability to develop an antibody response to multiple available antigens, among them gp70, perhaps as a result of their immunologic dysfunction.

In addition to gp70–anti-gp70 complexes, sera of older MRL/l mice contained C-fixing IgG-IgG RF ICs of an intermediate sedimentation rate (Eisenberg *et al.*, 1979b). The role of these type of complexes in the pathogenesis of this strain's arthritis and polyarthritis is not yet known. Further studies (Izui and Eisenberg, 1980) indicate that part of the IgG RF-complexed IgG is anti-DNA antibody, apparently without associated DNA antigen.

Lymphocyte subsets in autoimmune mice and surface characteristics of their B cells

It has been reasoned that perturbations among the cellular components that participate and regulate immune responses, may be associated with the onset of autoimmune reactivity in experimental animals and man. Therefore, we have conducted a thorough analysis of the phenotypic expression of various surface markers on lymphocytes from lymphoid organs of the lupus mice with particular attention to the development of alterations in the T and B cell compositions of these mice around the time of onset of disease. Our results demonstrate that each strain of lupus mouse has some variations from the normal cellular distributions, but in no two of the strains are the abnormalities

TABLE III

B and T cells in SLE mice as determined by surface markers

B cells

(1) Low frequency and absolute numbers in NZB and NZB × W.

(2) Moderate proliferation in BXSB.

(3) Reduced frequency but normal numbers in MRL/l.

(4) Advanced maturity in all SLE mice (loss of surface Ig with age, high frequency of sIgG$^+$ cells, high frequency of complement receptor bearing cells, high ratio of sIgM/sIgD-bearing cells in NZ and BXSB but not MRL/l, high frequency of Ig secreting cells, high frequency of cells with intracytoplasmic Ig).

(5) Normal development isotype diversity in all SLE strains.

T cells

(1) Low frequency and number in NZB and NZB × W.

(2) Normal levels in BXSB.

(3) Massive proliferation in MRL/l.

(4) Normal content of I-J-bearing cells in BXSB and increased content in MRL/l.

the same (Theofilopoulos *et al.*, 1979a) (Table III). To summarize the following results were obtained:

(a) older NZ mice have low frequencies and absolute numbers of sIg$^+$ cells, male BXSB mice have a moderate proliferation of sIg$^+$ cells and MRL/l mice have reduced frequencies but not absolute numbers of sIg$^+$ cells;

(b) B cells of older NZB, NZB × W and BXSB mice are more mature than B cells of normal mice (high frequency of complement receptor-bearing cells, loss of sIg and high ratio of sIgM:sIgD-bearing cells with age);

(c) the developmental Ig-isotype diversity in autoimmune mice is normal with sIgM$^+$ cells present on spleen cells obtained immediately after birth, whereas sIgD$^+$ cells appeared for the first time 3 days after birth;

(d) there is a reduction of IgG FcR^+ cells in older autoimmune mice;
(e) there is a decline of T cells in NZB and NZB × W mice, normal levels of T cells in BXSB, and an overwhelming T cell proliferation in older MRL/l mice;
(f) the proliferating T cell in MRL/l mice is a Thy-1·2^+, Ly "null" or weakly Lyl^+ cell;
(g) MRL/l and BXSB mice have numerically a normal content of I-J alloantigen-bearing T cells (suppressor cells).

Experiments were performed in order to clarify further the surface characteristics of B cells from SLE-prone mice (Theofilopoulos *et al.*, in prep. b). The results can be summarized as follows:

(a) B cells from newborn SLE-prone mice, like B cells of normal strains, do not re-express sIg after modulation with $F(ab')_2$ anti-Ig;
(b) the rate of sIg-anti-Ig complex endocytosis and of sIg capping in autoimmune mice is similar to that of normal strains;
(c) at 2 months of age, B cells of autoimmune strains, like those of normal strains, can be stimulated mitogenically with IgG anti-μ as well as $F(ab')_2$ anti-μ.

Functional characteristics of B cells

The murine SLE syndrome is marked by B lymphocyte hyperactivity manifested by hyper-γ-globulaemia, spontaneous polyclonal antibody production, and secretion of various autoantibodies (Theofilopoulos *et al.*, 1980c). Because Ig secretion represents an indicator of the B cell maturational state and activity, we have investigated *in vitro* the magnitude and nature of the spontaneous and mitogen-induced secretion of Ig by splenic lymphocytes from these autoimmune mice (Theofilopoulos *et al.*, 1980a). Our results indicate that all of the above autoimmune murine strains do in fact have an increased frequency of mature, Ig-secreting (IgSC) or containing B cells in their spleens at one time or another as compared to age-matched, immunologically normal strains (Fig. 6). In the NZB and NZB × W mice, the high frequency of splenic IgSC was detectable as early as 1 month of age and increased somewhat thereafter. In contrast, in BXSB male and MRL/l female mice the high frequency of IgSC was first observed at or a little before the clinical onset of the disease. The secretion was due to the active synthesis of Ig. Spleen cells from young mice of all autoimmune strains secreted predominantly IgM, but with ageing and the appearance of disease, the cells switched to IgG secretion predominantly. Approximately 6–7% of the total spleen cells in the autoimmune mice versus 1% in normal mice stained for intracytoplasmic Ig. With advanced clinical disease, NZ mice had 5- to 10-fold and MRL/l mice had 30-fold higher number of Ig-containing cells than younger, syngeneic animals. Spleen cells from one-month-old NZB and NZB × W mice stimulated with low doses of LPS had 5- to 10-fold higher frequency of IgSC than spleen cells from the

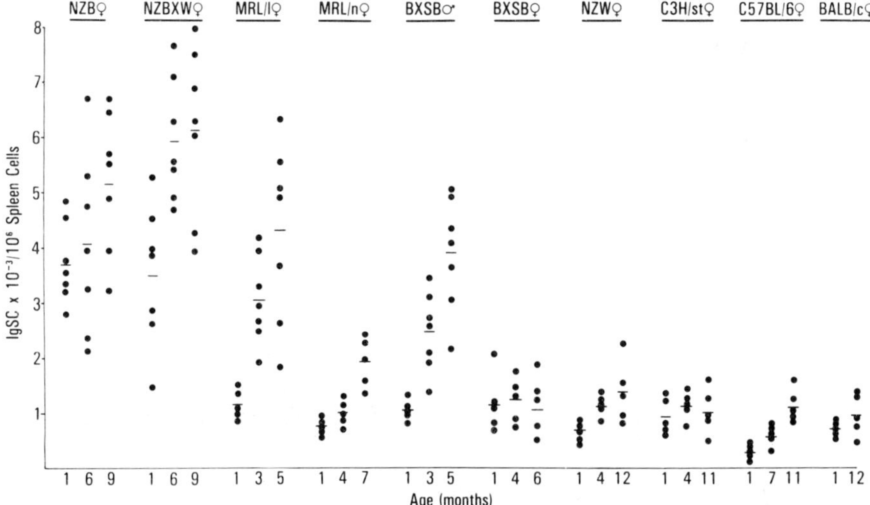

FIG. 6. *Spontaneous IgSC in spleens of autoimmune and normal murine strains at various ages. IgSC were identified by a reverse haemolytic plaque assay.*

two other autoimmune strains (MRL/l, BXSB) or several normal strains. It is not known whether this finding is due to an increased frequency of LPS responding B cells in the NZ mice or increased numbers of affinity of LPS receptors on their splenocytes. Certainly, this finding raises the possibility that the enhanced B cell maturity in NZ mice may result from the presence of low levels of endogenous polyclonal B cell activators. In accord with the studies of others (Cohen and Ziff, 1977), we found that the frequency of IgSC generated by LPS was greatly reduced in autoimmune mice of older age as compared to young autoimmune and young and old normal mice. This finding also indicates enhanced B cell maturity in older autoimmune mice since it suggests recruitment and differentiation of virtually all potentially LPS reactive B cells such that few B cells are available to generate antibody when challenged *in vitro* with this polyclonal B cell activator.

The early and advanced generalized maturity of the B cells in autoimmune mice was also shown by studying the frequency of antitrinitrophenyl (TNP) plaque forming cells in the spleens of these animals (Izui *et al.*, 1978). The results summarized in Fig. 7 indicate that all SLE strains, in contrast to normal strains, contained more PFC against TNP-SRBC than those of normal mice. Significant elevations occurred in the majority of NZB mice at 2 weeks of age whereas in the other three autoimmune strains (NZB × W, MRL/l, BXSB) the increase occurred at around 4 weeks of age. Further studies indicated that (a) increased polyclonal activation of B cells in spleens preceded the appearance of anti-DNP and anti-ssDNA antibodies in serum; (b) anti-ssDNA antibodies appeared in serum at the same time as anti-DNP antibodies increased with age, and (c) there was no correlation between serum levels of gp70 and of

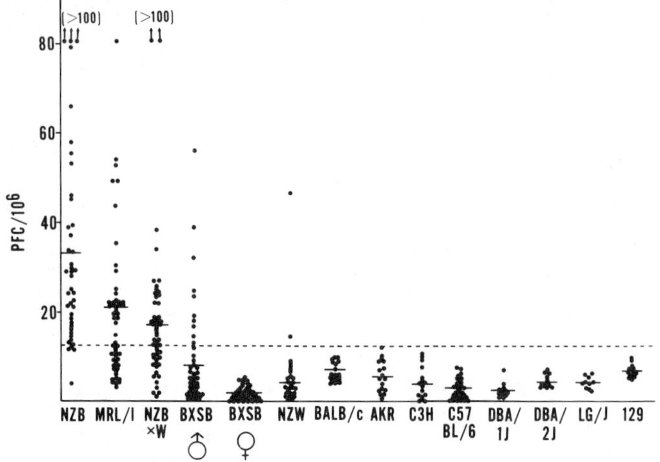

FIG. 7. *Spontaneous spleen PFC against TNP-SRBC in 1 to 2-month-old SLE and normal strains. The dotted line indicates the normal mean* ± 3 *s.d.*

anti-DNP antibodies. Additional studies have shown an increased frequency of B cell colony forming cells in spleens of all SLE strains as compared to normals (approximately 3000 colonies/10^6 cells in normal strains). All these results on Ig secretion, polyclonal antibody production and B cell colony formation strongly indicate that there is a generalized B cell activation in mice with autoimmune syndromes. Similar conclusions have been reached by others with NZ mice (Ohsugi and Gershwin, 1979; Kinkade *et al.*, 1979; Moutsopoulos *et al.*, 1977; Manny *et al.*, 1979; Tourog *et al.*, 1979).

Functional characteristics of T cells

Suppressor and helper T cells

The mechanisms responsible for the generalized B cell hyperactivity as well as the excessive production of autoantibodies in these mice remain unexplained. The cause may be one defect or combination of defects such as primary genetic or acquired B cell malfunction, the presence of endogenous or exogenous B cell activators, the lack of a negative influence by supressor T cells, an enhanced positive influence by helper T cells, defects in subsets of intra-T regulatory cells (i.e. Ly-123^+), and defects in other elements of the immune system such as macrophages. Evidence for functional or numerical inadequacies in antigen-nonspecific suppressor T cells (Krakauer *et al.*, 1976; Barthold *et al.*, 1974), lack of regulatory T cells (Cantor *et al.*, 1978; Cantor and Gershon, 1979) and lack of acceptor sites for suppressor messages on the surfaces of B cells (Primi *et al.*, 1978) has been reported in one or another of the susceptible strains. However, others have shown that thymocyte-mediated antigen-nonspecific suppression is not lost with age in autoimmune hereditarily asplenic (Dh/+) NZB mice (Gershwin *et al.*, 1979) or in conventional NZB mice (Manny *et al.*, 1979; Prini *et al.*, 1978). Moreover, suppressor cells, as defined with Ly-23 alloantigen expressing cells in NZB mice (Roubinian *et al.*, 1978) or I-J subregion controlled alloantigens in MRL/l mice (Theofilopoulos *et al.*, 1979a) are normal or higher in numbers. Therefore, we have performed studies to determine functionally the state of the antigen nonspecific and antigen-specific suppressor T cells and of the antigen-nonspecific helper T cells in the various autoimmune mice.

Antigen-specific suppression

We assessed antigen-specific suppressive mechanisms in young and old intact mice and in suppressor T cells from these mice after adoptive transfers into syngeneic recipients (Creighton *et al.*, 1979a). Suppressor cells were induced by intravenous injection of urea-denatured ovalbumin (UD-OVA) into ovalbumin (OVA) primed mice. All mice analysed, whether autoimmune or normal and irrespective of age, developed unmistakable OVA-specific supressive activities that diminished IgG and IgE antibody production. A representative experiment with BXSB mice is given in Fig. 8. To confirm the responsible cell type, T lymphocytes were isolated from the spleens of UD-OVA-treated donors by passage over nylon wool, cultured for 18 h with UD-OVA and then transferred into naive, syngeneic young recipients. Despite some strain variability in magnitude of suppressor T cell activity, clearly all of the autoimmune mice generated suppressor T lymphocytes that adoptively suppressed both IgG and IgE antibody responses (data not shown).

Antigen-nonspecific suppression

To determine the degree of antigen-nonspecific suppression, we examined the direct effect of concanavalin A (con A) on LPS-induced stimulation of Ig synthesis by cultured spleen cells (Theofilopoulos *et al.*, 1980a). Con A activated spleen cells from normal mice have been found to suppress polyclonal responses induced by several B cell mitogens, including LPS (Primi *et al.*, 1979). However, it has been reported that con A-treated spleen cells from old NZB and NZB × W mice, lack the ability to suppress polyclonal B cell mitogen-induced Ig secretion (Krakauer *et al.*, 1976). As shown in Fig. 9, high doses of con A effectively suppressed LPS-induced Ig synthesis by splenic cells not only from young and old normal mice but also from young and old autoimmune mice, including the NZB and NZB × W strain. These results were reassessed by incubating spleen cells from young and old mice with varying doses of con A, and then adding them to fresh syngeneic cells derived from both young and old animals to which a standard amount of LPS was added. After 3 days, the cocultures were examined for the frequency of IgSC. Spleen cells from both young and old autoimmune animals generated con A-induced suppressor cell activity, and LPS-responding B cells of young and old syngeneic animals were equally receptive to suppressor messages (data not shown).

The combined results on antigen-specific and antigen-nonspecific suppres-

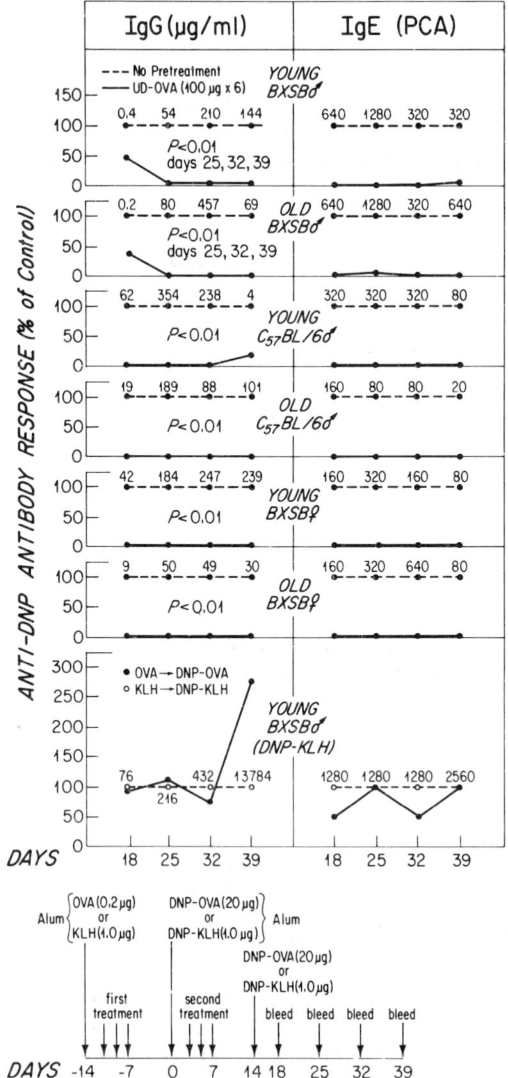

FIG. 8. *Induction of suppression in young and old BXSB and C57BL/6 mice with UD-OVA (for details see Creighton* et al., *1979). As summarized schematically at the bottom of the figure, groups of mice were immunized with 0·2 μg OVA* (*alum*) *or 1 μg DNP-KLH* (*alum*) *on day 14 and then given 100 μg UD-OVA i.v. on each of days −11, −9, −7, 3, 5, and 7. Primary and secondary immunization with 20 μg of DNP-OVA* (*alum*) *or 1 μg of DNP-KLH* (*alum*) *were given on days 0 and 14. Anti-DNP antibody responses were assayed on days 18, 25, 32, and 39. The IgE and IgG anti-DNP responses are presented as percentage of control responses with the control values given above the corresponding point.*

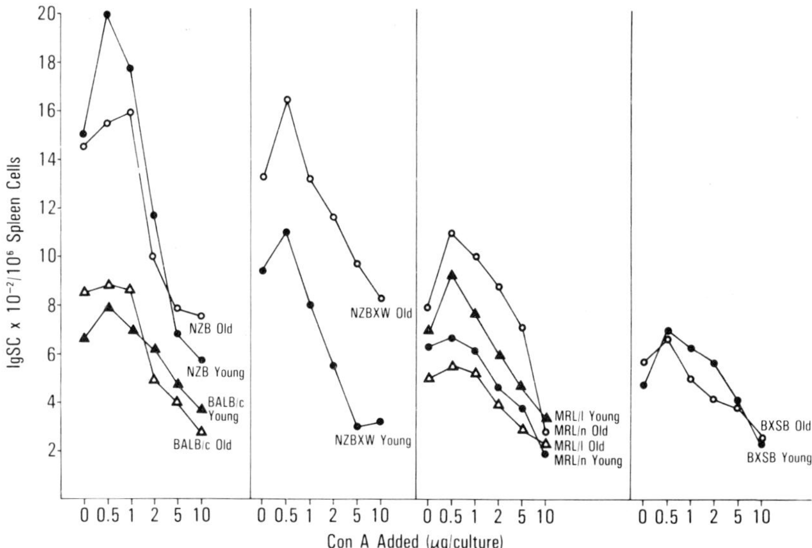

FIG. 9. *Direct suppression of LPS-induced IgSC by Con A. Cells from the indicated strains were cultured in the presence of a standard amount of LPS (20 μg/culture) and increasing concentrations of Con A. IgSC were assessed 3 days later.*

sion prompt us to question the assignment of a generalized defect of suppressor T cells as the cause of autoimmunity. However, our experiments do not exclude the presence of defects on subsets of immunoregulatory T cells that control responses to specific autoantigens nor do they exclude the possible presence of subtle abnormalities of suppressor T cells or the development of late, secondary suppressor T cell abnormality in these animals.

Antigen-nonspecific help

Because Ig hypersecretion is more prominent in old autoimmune mice than young, and because such hypersecretion may, at least in part, result from heightened T helper activity, we examined the degree of help provided by increasing numbers of isolated T cells from young and old animals to a standard number of LPS-stimulated syngeneic and allogeneic but *H-2* identical B cells isolated from spleens of young animals (Theofilopoulos *et al.*, 1980a). Increments of T cells from young and old NZB and BXSB autoimmune mice added to a standard number of B cells from syngeneic young mice provided—at all doses and at both ages—equal help in enhancing the frequency of IgSC after LPS stimulation (Fig. 10). Moreover, the help provided by T cells from these two autoimmune strains to their own B cells was not significantly different from that provided by T cells from young and old normal mice of the same *H-2* haplotype (BALB/c for NZB, C57BL/6 for BXSB). Similarly, in the reverse situation, when T cells from young and old NZB and BXSB mice were added to B cells from young, normal counterparts, the help was not significantly greater than that from T cells of the normal strains (data not shown). The

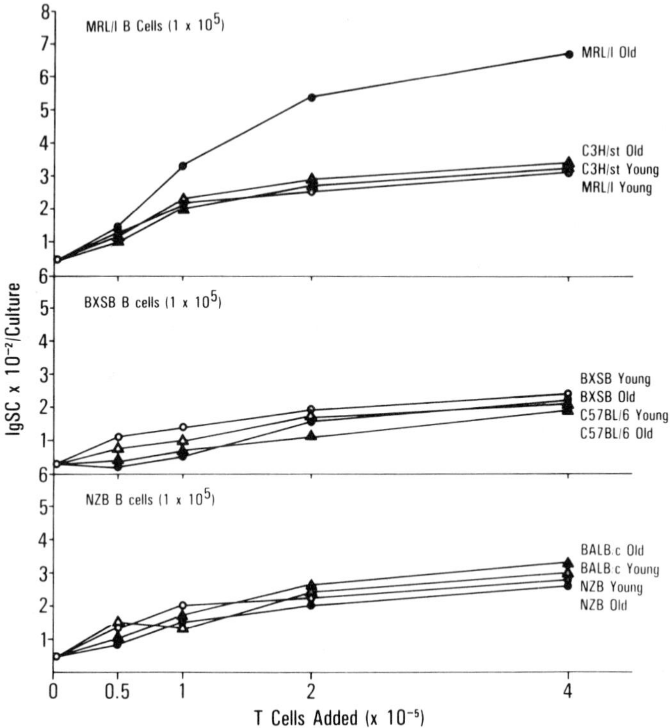

FIG. 10. *Antigen-nonspecific helper activity. Frequency of IgSC in B cell enriched spleen cell populations obtained from 1-month-old SLE mice to which increments of isolated T cells from syngeneic and allogeneic but* H-2 *identical young (1-month-old) and old (4–7-month-old) animals were added together with LPS.*

only notable exception was the MRL/l strain in which T cell enriched populations from old animals added at a 4:1 ratio to B cells from syngeneic young animals provided 2–3 times the help offered by equal numbers of T cells of young syngeneic animals or T cells from young and old normal mice of the same *H-2* haplotype (C3H/St) (Fig. 10). As we have demonstrated (Theofilopoulos *et al.*, 1979a), the ratio of T to B cells in MRL/l mice is significantly greater *in vivo* (10:1 in spleen 30:1 in lymph nodes) than the maximal ratio employed in these experiments *in vitro*. Therefore, one might well expect the helper activity observed *in vitro* to be greatly magnified in the intact animal. Thus, our experiments and those of others (Sawada and Talal, 1979) suggest that the advanced maturity of the MRL/l's B cells may be the result of a heightened helper T cell activity exerted by the proliferating Ly-1$^+$ T cells.

T cell mediated immune responsiveness

Several reports have described an age-dependent decline in certain T cell functions such as allograft rejection, graft versus host reaction, *in vitro* responses to phytohaemagglutinin or con A and killer cell activity against allogeneic tumour cells (reviewed in Zinkernagel and Dixon, 1977). Therefore, we assessed the age-dependent capacity of NZB, NZB × W and various normal strains to generate T cell mediated immune responses against alloantigens and virus infected target cells as well as cell-mediated immune protection against *Listeria* monocytogenes after systemic infection (Zinkernagel and Dixon, 1977). The results can be summarized as follows:

(a) no obvious hyper- or hyporesponsiveness was detectable when NZ and other mouse strains were tested for the generation of a cytotoxic T cell response against alloantigens in mixed lymphocyte cultures *in vitro*;

(b) the virus-specific cytolytic activity generated in NZ mice acutely infected with vaccinia virus was in no way different than that seen with similarly infected normal strains;

(c) the kinetics and the extent of the development of footpad swelling after lymphocytic choriomeningitis virus infection (a T dependent phenomenon) was comparable in NZ strains to that of normal strains; and

(d) recovery from *Listeria* infection, which is known to be dependent on generation of specific T cells that activate macrophages directly or via released lymphokines to increased bactericidal activity (Mackaness, 1969), was not different between NZ mice and other normal strains.

We then similarly studied young and old BXSB and MRL/l mice and found no difference in the kinetics of appearance or relative activity of cytotoxic T cells against alloantigens and viral antigens per spleen as compared to normal strains (Creighton *et al.*, 1979b). Thus overall cell-mediated immunity of SLE-prone mice as assessed in these functional models is within normal limits. Possible defects must therefore be selective and may not have been detected in these models.

Cytotolytic reactions against H-2 compatible and incompatible allogeneic cells

Recently, Botzenhardt *et al.* (1978) described the development of significant unidirectional primary T cell mediated lympholytic (CML) reactions by lymphoid cells of NZB mice against *H-2* identical allogeneic cells. These investigators speculated that such CML reactions represented an abnormality of NZB mice possibly associated with the pathogenesis of autoimmunity. Subsequently, studies performed by ourselves (Theofilopoulos *et al.*, 1979b) and Rich *et al.* (1979) confirmed the findings of Botzenhardt *et al.* in regard to the NZB mouse, but we failed to observe similar activity with lymphoid cells obtained from MRL/l and BXSB mice. Rich *et al.* studied the cross-reactivity patterns of NZB anti-$H\text{-}2^d$ effector cells and concluded that such cells exhibit specificity for antigenic determinants associated with the murine $Qa\text{-}1^b$ genetic locus. In subsequent studies (Theofilopoulos *et al.*, 1980b) we attempted to define the basis for the primary *in vitro* CML reactions exhibited uniquely by splenocytes from NZB mice against *H-2* identical allogeneic cells. These studies can be summarized as follows: (a) the NZB anti-*H-2*^{d} reactions appear not to be manifestations of autoimmunity nor manifestations of differences between the *H-2* complex of NZB mice and those of other *H-2*^{d} mouse strains; (b) following *in vitro* sensitization of NZB cells with irradiated BALB/c cells, NZB effector cells cross-react with target cells of varying *H-2* and *Mls* backgrounds (Table IV). Although such effector cells cause optimum lysis of targets bearing *Qa-1*^{b}

TABLE IV

Primary in vitro *CML reactions of SLE mice against* H-2 *identical allogeneic cells*

Effector	*Stimulator*	*Target* Strain	H-2	Qa-1	Mls	% *Specific release (mean ± s.d.)*
NZB	BALB/c	BALB/c	*d*	*b*	*b*	45·0 + 5·6
(*H-2*^{d}, *Qa-1*^{a}, *Mls*^{a})	(*H-2*^{d}, *Qa-1*β, *Mls*β)					
		DBA/2	*d*	*b*	*a*	49·2 ± 4·0
		B10.D2	*d*	*b*	*b*	46·8 ± 3·5
		DBA/1	*q*	*b*	*a*	55·5 ± 1·0
		AKR	*k*	*b*	*a*	46·9 ± 1·3
		ASW	*s*	*b*	*c*	55·6 ± 0·2
		C57BL/6	*b*	*b*	*b*	48·9 ± 5·9
NZB	BALB/c	B10.A	*k/d*	*a*	*c*	41·6 ± 3·2
		SJL	*s*	*a*	*c*	27·7 ± 4·1
		B10.A(5R)	*b/d*	*a*	*b*	25·7 ± 10·0
		NZB	*d*	*a*	*a*	15·3 ± 2·2
		SWR	*q*	*a*	*	14·4 ± 12·4
		A/J	*a*	*a*	*c*	13·7 ± 10·8
MRL/l (*H-2*^{k}, *Qa-1*^{b})	AKR	AKR	*k*	*b*	*a*	−1·0 ± 4·8
MRL/l (*H-2*^{k}, *Qa-1*^{b})	C57BR	C57BR	*k*	*a*	*	7·7 ± 1·7
BXSB (*H-2*^{b}, *Qa-1*^{b})	C57BL/6	C57BL/6	*b*	*b*	*b*	−2·4 ± 0·8
BXSB (*H-2*^{b}, *Qa-1*^{b})	B6.*Tl*^{a}	B6.*Tl*^{a}	*b*	*a*	*	3·0 ± 2·0

* Not known.

determinants, significant to modest degrees of specific lysis also occurs with certain targets bearing *Qa-l*^{a} antigenic determinants; (c) two other SLE-prone murine strains BXSB and MRL/l, do not display cytolytic activity against *H-2*-identical allogeneic cells irrespective of the *Qa-1* antigenic phenotype of the target cells (Table IV); (d) significant inhibition of NZB andti-*H-2*^{d} CML activity is observed when effector and stimulator cells are treated simultaneously, but not separately, with anti-Rauscher gp70 antibody, whereas independent treatment of the effector, stimulator or target cells is without effect. The inhibitory effect is specific since (a) $F(ab')_2$ anti-gp70 is as effective as whole IgG antibody; (b) anti-gp70 adsorbed with Sepharose-bound gp70 is ineffective; (c) nonimmune IgG, anti-p30, anti-Ig, anti-Thy-1·2 and a mixture of anti-Ig and anti-Thy-1·2 antibodies all are without effect (Fig. 11); (d) anti-gp70 inhibits only primary and secondary NZB anti-*H-2*^{d} responses, but not NZB responses against *H-2* incompatible cells or secondary responses among *H-2*^{d} compatible immunologically normal strains of mice. Anti-gp70 treatment of NZB effector and BALB/c stimulator cells inhibits the expression of NZB cytolytic cross-reactivity against both *Qa-1*^{b} and *Qa-1*^{a}-bearing target cells and cross-reactivities not only against *H-2* identical targets but also against *H-2* incompatible, *Qa-1*^{b} target cells (data not shown).

Thus, it appears that generation of NZB effector cells is solely dependent

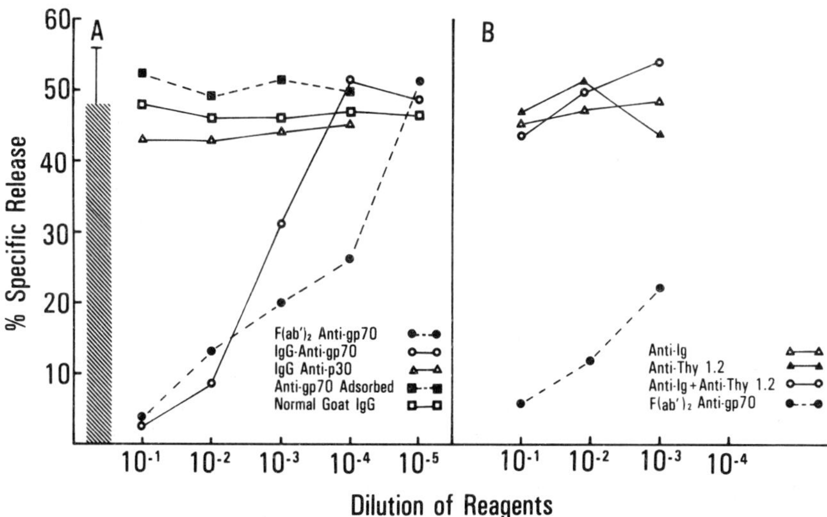

FIG. 11. *Specificity of anti-gp70 induced inhibition of NZB anti-*H-2^d *CML reactions. A mixture of NZB effector and BALB/c stimulator cells (6 × 10^6 each) were treated (30 min, 4°C) with 100 µl dilutions of the indicated reagents, washed once and then incubated for 5 days in triplicate cultures of 2 × 10^6 cells of each type. Untreated ^{51}Cr labelled target cells (1 × 10^5) were added at the final 4 hours of incubation. Dashed column indicates degree of lysis in untreated controls.*

in cognitive events occurring during incubation with BALB/c cells as well as the subsequent expression of gp70 in the culture, and not on the make-up of histocompatibility or other alloantigens on the target cells. It is postulated that due to minor histocompatibility differences between NZB and BALB/c cells, production of retroviruses or retroviral gp70 by the NZB cells is initiated. This, in turn, subsequently induces secondary memory-type responses by the NZB effectors against stimulator cells that cross-react with various target cells.

NZB mice are known to express a unique form of virion-associated gp70 (Elder *et al.*, 1980) and graft v. host reactions are known to induce expressions of retroviral antigens (Phillips *et al.*, 1975). That this interpretation concerning the basis for the anti-gp70 antibody-mediated inhbition of the NZB anti-$H\text{-}2^d$ responses is correct is supported by experiments currently in progress in our laboratory which have shown that Rauscher gp70 is capable of inducing NZB spleen cells to become cytotoxic for BALB/c targets (Theofilopoulos *et al.*, in prep. c). Moreover, other studies currently under way in our laboratory (Theofilopoulos and Altman, in prep.) and those of Botzenhardt *et al.* (1980) have shown that supernatants of NZB-BALB/c cultures contain soluble helper factor(s) capable of inducing BALB/c effector cells cultured together with DBA/2 stimulator cells to become cytotoxic for DBA/2 target cells. Perhaps such supernatants provide retroviral antigens which, together with interleukin II type molecules produced in the BALB/c anti-DBA/2 culture, effectively induce development of the cytotoxic cells as described recently in other systems (Wagner *et al.*, 1980). Although such reactions may play a role in the development of the NZB disease, our former conclusion that such CML reactions are not necessarily related to the development of murine SLE is still valid since as stated above BXSB and MRL/l SLE-prone strains do not exhibit such reactivities.

Tolerance susceptibility

It has been demonstrated that 6 to 8-week-old NZB and NZB × W mice are relatively resistant to induction of tolerance by bovine γ globulin (BGG) and human γ globulin (HGG) compared with many normal strains of mice (Staples and Talal, 1969; Golub and Weigle, 1979). One should be careful in interpreting these previous results since the induction and maintenance of tolerance to HGG is dependent on the preparation of deaggregated HGG (DHGG) and the sources of HGG (Cerottini *et al.*, 1969; Parks *et al.*, 1978). Nevertheless, this abnormality may be related to the pathogenesis of the disease of these mice since the spontaneous development of autoantibody might result from resistance, termination or breakdown of self-tolerance. Therefore, we conducted experiments to compare the previously reported findings in the NZ mice with the new SLE strains BXSB and MRL/l (Izui *et al.*, 1980b).

At 5 weeks of age, not only NZB and NZB × W mice but also MRL/l and male BXSB mice exhibited resistance to induction of tolerance to DHGG (Table V). Of interest, MRL/n and female BXSB, which are relatively immunologically normal compared with MRL/l and male BXSB, were sensitive to the induction of tolerance. Therefore, it appears that this abnormality of resistance to tolerance induction is a common feature of all autoimmune mice. In contrast, only SJL mice among several non-SLE stains similarly tested was found to be resistant to tolerance induction. However,

TABLE V

Effect of DHGG on induction of tolerance to HGG

Strain[a]	Anti-HGG ($\mu g/ml$)[b]		
	Control	DHGG	% of control
NZB	123 ± 20	79 ± 20	64
NZB × W	167 ± 45	123 ± 78	74
MRL/l	35 ± 16	34 ± 14	97
BXSB male	196 ± 138	263 ± 118	134
MRL/n	110 ± 19	20 ± 8	18
BXSB female	24 ± 13	2 ± 1	8
NZW	71 ± 16	5 ± 2	7
BALB/c	36 ± 13	1 ± 2	3
C57BL/6	27 ± 13	2 ± 1	7
C3H/St	33 ± 12	2 ± 0·3	6
SJL	>400	>400	100

[a] 5-week-old.

[b] 3 mg DHGG (160 000 × *g*, 150 min) were injected i.p. on day 0. 400 μg AHGG were injected i.v. on day 10 and anti HGG activity in sera was determined on day 17 or 24 by RIA.

one should note that SJL mice are known to exhibit certain immunologic abnormalities (Fujiwara and Cinader, 1974).

The hyperphagocytic activity of macrophages might account for the failure of ultracentrifuged DHGG to induce tolerance in SLE mice. BALB/c mice are relatively resistant to tolerance induction with BGG preparations except those preparations biofiltered through BALB/c mice, a process which renders the BGG effective in eliciting tolerance of subsequently challenged BALB/c mice (Staples *et al.*, 1970). Similar results are obtained in tolerance-resistant strain SJL mice (Fujiwara and Cinader, 1974). These experiments indicate that BALB/c and SJL mice are hyperphagocytic and are immunized by trace amounts of microaggregated IgG present in certain preparations of ultracentrifuged IgG. However, biofiltered DHGG still could not induce tolerance in SLE-prone mice, ruling out the possibility that the presence of microaggregates in ultracentrifuged DHGG preparations interfered with the induction of tolerance.

Role of thymus

It has been claimed that progressive imbalances in T cell function occur in NZ mice due to diminished production of thymic hormones. Administration of thymic hormones (i.e. extract of thymic tissue) (Dauphinee *et al.*, 1974) to

NZB mice or transplantation of thymuses from young NZB mice to old mice (Steinberg *et al.*, 1970) may temporarily prevent some of the immunologic defects and delay the onset of autoimmunity. In addition, it has been reported that adult NZB mice lack a serum activity thought to be a thymic hormone (Bach *et al.*, 1973). Previous studies of thymic histology in NZ mice have also disclosed premature thymic involution with prominent degeneration and vacuolization of epithelial cells (De Vries and Higmans, 1967). Moreover, significant age-dependent losses of both functional and morphologic characteristics of NZ thymic epithelial cells cultured *in vitro* have been observed (Gershwin *et al.*, 1978). Others have found that neonatal thymectomy inhibited the disease in NZB × W female mice but accelerated the disease in males (Roubinian *et al.*, 1977).

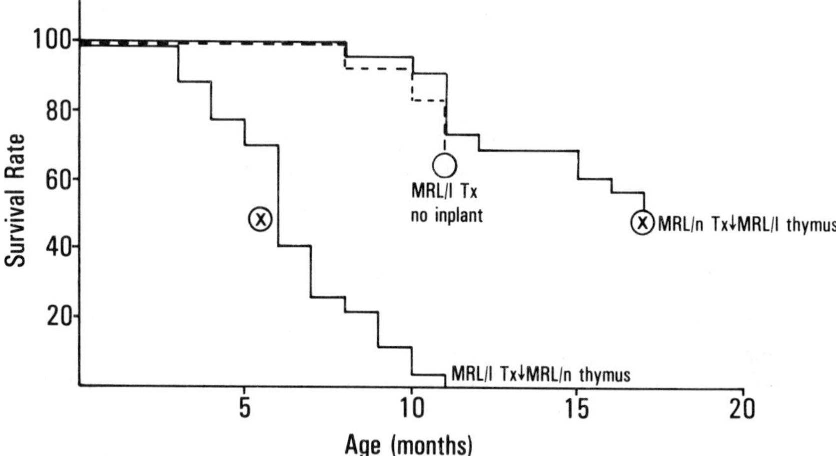

FIG. 12. *Survival rates of MRL/l mice thymectomized when newborn but not transplanted, MRL/l mice thymectomized and transplanted at 1 month of age with MRL/n thymus, and MRL/n mice thymectomized and transplanted at 1 month of age with MRL/l thymus. The asterisk depicts the time of 50% survival for control unmanipulated mice.*

Since there is a disparity in the time of disease onset between the congenic MRL/l and MRL/n mice and between male and female BXSB mice we have performed transplantation of thymuses among these strains in order to clarify whether there is an inherent thymic defect that contributes to the early appearance of murine SLE (Theofilopoulos *et al.*, in prep. a). As indicated in Fig. 12, MRL/l mice thymectomized when 1 day old and transplanted at 1 month of age with MRL/n thymus retained the disease phenotype of the unmanipulated MRL/l mice, including lymphoproliferation and a 60% mortality at 6 months of age. Similarly, thymectomized MRL/n mice transplanted with MRL/l thymus had a 50% mortality at 17 months of age like the unmanipulated controls. In contrast, MRL/l mice thymectomized when newborn but not transplanted with thymus did not develop lymphoid hyperplasia and autoimmune disease and 60% of them were alive by the 11th month of age (time of termination of the experiment), a point well beyond the 90% death rate of control unmanipulated mice (9 months of age). Serologically, the MRL/l recipients of MRL/n thymus behave like the unmanipulated MRL/l animals with hyper-γ-globulinaemia and high levels of autoantibodies. In contrast, MRL/l thymectomized but not transplanted had greatly reduced levels of serum IgG and background levels of anti-DNA antibodies.

These results indicate that: (a) T cell differentiation in the thymus is a necessary component in the MRL/l phenotype; (b) the genotype of the thymic microenvironment where differentiation occurs is irrelevant; (c) the differentiation of MRL/n T cells in a thymic microenvironment that possesses *lpr* genotype does not lead to abnormal T cell differentiation and early autoimmunity; and (d) the disease of the MRL/l mouse is possibly not due to an intrinsic B cell abnormality, although this cannot be concluded with certainty since T cells may be required for the expression of a putative B cell defect.

Similar experiments are in progress with the BXSB mouse strain. Preliminary results indicate again that the genotype of the thymus is irrelevant in the development of autoimmunity, since, newborn thymectomized male and female BXSB mice transplanted with male or female BXSB thymus displayed a disease pattern similar to the unmanipulated control animals.

Transfer of autoimmune disease

Transfer of autoimmune disease by specific tissue or tissue extracts derived from strains of mice having a genetic predisposition to autoimmunity into nonautoimmune recipients may be one of the most useful approaches in defining the humoral, cellular, microenvironmental and viral factors that influence and determine the development of autoimmunity. Others have reported the transfer of the NZB and NZB × W disease, as manifested by some autoantibody production, into lethally irradiated normal murine strains (Morton and Siegel, 1974; Akizuki *et al.*, 1978). However, the results have been inconclusive and sometimes difficult to interpret due to the use of normal recipients that are not congenic for NZ mice. The availability of the BXSB mice, the males and females of which differ substantially in mortality and expression of the disease, and of the MRL mice with like differences between the congenic MRL/l and MRL/n substrains makes possible the performance of histocompatible cell transfer experiments.

The failure to modify the male accelerated disease in BXSB mice by castration (Eisenberg *et al.*, 1980a) suggests that the male dominance of the BXSB autoimmune syndrome is not hormonally controlled. Further, genetic studies (see below) have indicated that this male dominant effect is linked to the Y chromosome, since the autoimmune phenotype is transmitted as a dominant trait to F_1 hybrids with an accelerated autoimmunity in male offsprings of BXSB fathers and mothers of other autoimmune strains. We have investigated the cellular basis of this male effect by transferring male and female bone marrow cells from 1-month-old mice into male and female lethally irradiated BXSB recipients of the same age (Eisenberg *et al.*, 1980b). As shown in Fig. 13, the disease transfer is dependent not on the sex of the recipient but on the sex of the donor cells with male bone marrow inducing early disease (glomerulonephritis and death) in both male and female recipients and female marrow inducing late disease in both male and female recipients. Similar results were obtained by transferring spleen cells from 4-month-old donors to 2-month-old lethally irradiated recipients. Again the type of the sex of the spleen cell donor determined the pace of disease development. The recipients

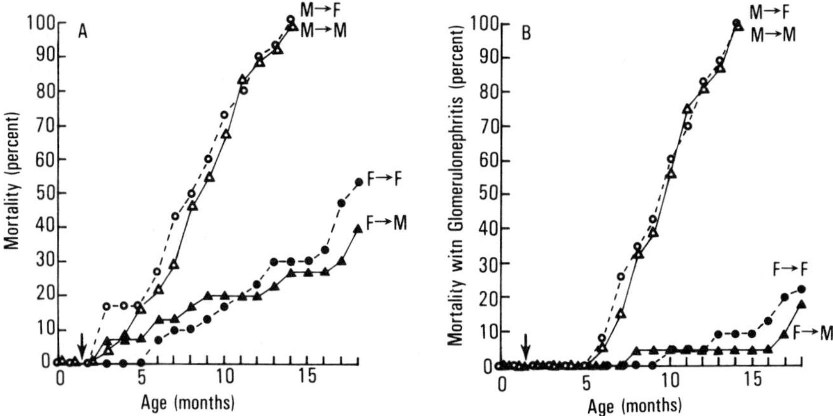

FIG. 13. (*A*) *Mortality from all causes in BXSB bone marrow chimaeras. Recipients were lethally iradiated (850R) and infused with donor bone marrow (5×10^7 cells) at 6 weeks of age, as shown by the arrow. Male recipients are depicted by triangles; females by circles. Male bone marrow is shown by open symbols; female by closed symbols. In summary* (△-----△) *M→M;* ((○-----○) *M→F;* (▲-----▲) *F→M; and* (●-----●) *F→F.* (*B*) *Mortality from documented glomerulonephritis in BXSB bone marrow sex chimaeras.*

expressed serologic markers similar to those seen in the donor strains. Thus, recipients of male bone marrow and spleen cells had higher IgG and anti-DNA antibodies than the recipients of female bone marrow or spleen cells and develop gp70-anti-gp70 complexes in their sera.

These results suggest that the male specific effect that accelerates autoimmune disease in the BXSB is not hormonally or environmentally mediated, but rather is expressed in the haematopoietic/lymphoid stem cell populations. Moreover, since transfer of spleen cells obtained from old male mice that already had manifest disease did not produce disease in the recipients any faster than transfer of bone marrow from premorbid mice, it can be suggested that (a) the active cell being transferred is the stem cell and not differentiated autoantibody secreting B cells, and (b) the development of BXSB disease does not appear to be the result of an accumulation of defects at the stem cell level, i.e., stem cells from male BXSB of any age are at the same stage of abnormality.

Genetic studies

The genetic analysis of SLE seen in NZB and NZB × W mice has revealed complex and as yet poorly understood genetic elements (Warner, 1977). It is clear that this disease is multigenic in nature and that a number of secondary factors influence the expression of its essential elements underlying autoimmunity. Recently, two new approaches have been shedding light on the genetics of this disease. The first compares the F_1 hybrids resulting from crosses between the several SLE-prone strains in search for common genetic denominators in this disease (Theofilopoulos *et al.*, 1980c). The second approach employs recombinant inbred strains to allow analysis of the interrelationships among individual immunopathologic traits related to SLE (Raveche *et al.*, 1980; Riblet, pers. comm.).

In view of the different origins, MHC, allotypes (see above) and other immunogenetic aspects of the various SLE mice, it is clear that several quite different genetic backgrounds are compatible with the disease. The disease seen in each of these strains consists of, or is associated with, numerous abnormal immunologic traits, some common to all strains and others found only in some (see above). Such multifactorial and variable pathogeneses make definite genetic analysis of all disease components extremely difficult, if not impossible. Since some members of each variety of SLE mouse, i.e., female BXSB, male NZB × W and MRL/n develop a late life disease (50% mortality from 14–20 months) and others, i.e., male BXSB, female NZB × W and MRL/l develop an early acute disease (50% mortality at 5–9 months) this natural division in the pace of disease can be used as a convenient phenotypic marker for genetic analysis and the gene or genes determining either late-life or early disease can be considered as two separate genetic units.

Late-life SLE

There appears to be multiple possible immunopathologic traits which can be important elements of late-life SLE. That the particular assortment or constellation of such traits varies from one strain of SLE mouse to another is clear from the immunopathologic features of the SLE in each (Andrews *et al.*, 1978; Theofilopoulos *et al.*, 1980c) and from the differences in the genetic interactions of SLE mice at the F_1 hybrid generation as seen in Table VI. In these crosses BXSB females are used since they carry only the late-life SLE traits and the MRL/l can be used since the *lpr* accelerator gene is known to be recessive (Murphy and Roths, 1979) and will not be expressed in F_1 hybrids leaving only the late-life traits to interact. BXSB and MRL/l hybrids of both sexes are relatively healthy having 50% mortalities at nearly 2 years and developing only a moderate glomerulonephritis suggesting little similarity between the genetic backgrounds of the late life SLE in these two strains. On the other

TABLE VI
F_1 hybrid crosses of late-life SLE

Crosses *Female Male*	*50% mortality (months)* *Female*	*Male*
BXSB × MRL/l	22	>24
BXSB × NZB	10	21
BXSB × NZW	9	16
NZB × NZW	9	14
BXSB × BALB/c	>24	>24
MRL/l × NZB	12	20
NZB × MRL/l	17	>24
MRL/l × NZW	16	>24
NZW × MRL/l	19	18
MRL/l × C57Bl/6	>24[a]	>24[a]

[a] Amyloid.

hand, BXSB × NZB and BXSB × NZW develop a severe SLE with early deaths from full-blown glomerulonephritis in the female. The character and timing of the SLE in BXSB × NZB or NZW hybrids are very similar to that seen in the classical NZB × W. Thus, it would appear that the BXSB late life SLE background can either complement or add to the NZB and NZW backgrounds in order to produce a typical SLE appearing early in the female. That being the case the BXSB should carry the equivalent of the genetic contributions of both NZB and NZW to the NZB × W SLE. Whether this BXSB contribution is qualitatively the same to the NZB and NZW or only quantitatively similar is not yet known. When the BXSB female is crossed with a normal strain such as the BALB/c, little or no disease is seen in the F_1 irrespective of the sex of the offspring. Taken together these data indicate X-linked recessive trait complementation between BXSB and NZB or NZW, similar to what may occur between NZB and NZW and possibly also NZB and MRL/l.

Crosses of the MRL/l with other SLE mice result, in general, in either late life or no SLE; the only possible exception is the MRL/1 × NZB cross where significant disease in the first year of life is seen. One possible explanation for the lack of disease in MRL/l F_1 hybrids could be that the SLE in the MRL/l is determined by homozygous recessive autoimmune traits the expression of which are lost in the F_1 hybrid of crosses with SLE strains lacking the same recessive genes.

Accelerating factors—early SLE

It seems clear that in each kind of SLE mouse there may be superimposed on the late-life SLE background a distinct, but in each case different, accelerating factor capable of changing the late-life disease to an early, acute form. While these accelerating factors are not completely understood, it appears that they are relatively straightforward, direct influences which can alter the course of a predetermined disease. In the BXSB mouse the accelerating factor is Y-linked and is both transmitted and expressed by the male (Murphy and Roths, 1979). In the MRL/l mouse the factor is determined by a recessive, autosomal gene *lpr* for lymphoproliferation (Murphy and Roths, 1979). In the NZB × W the accelerating effect is apparently mediated by female hormones (Roubinian *et al.*, 1978). In Table VII is shown the expression of

TABLE VII
BXSB Y-linked accelerating factor

Crosses *Female* *Male*	*50% mortality (months)* *Female* F_1	*Male* F_1
MRL/l × BXSB	16	6
MRL/n × BXSB	22	7
NZB × BXSB	8	6
NZW × BXSB	9	5
C3H × BXSB	>24	16[a]
BALB × BXSB	>24	>24
C57B1 × BXSB	>24	15[a]

[a] Amyloid.

the BXSB Y-linked accelerating factor in various F_1 hybrids. Most striking is the appearance of early, acute disease quite similar to that seen in the BXSB male in the F_1 males of all BXSB male crosses with SLE mice. Thus, the late-life SLE backgrounds of all SLE mice were accelerated by, or allowed the expression of, the BXSB Y-linked trait. This was true even with the MRL/l and MRL/n mice which did not complement the late-life SLE backgrounds of the BXSB female. As would be expected the F_1 females of these crosses with male BXSB had a disease similar to that seen in the F_1 offsprings of the crosses with female BXSB since the Y chromosome was not involved in these situations. In the crosses with normal strains (C3H, BALB/c, C57BL/6) since there was no late-life disease to accelerate there is little effect of the Y-linked factor. A potentially useful finding was the occurrence of early SLE in both males and females of the F_1 crosses of BXSB males with NZB or NZW. In terms of clinical characteristics and timing the disease observed in the females was quite similar to that in the NZB × W cross. In addition, an even earlier SLE occurred in the male offspring. Whether this disease is the same as that occurring in the BXSB male is being determined but these crosses offer the opportunity to study early SLE in both sexes which is not possible in the NZB × W.

Because *lpr* is a recessive gene it is not possible to observe its accelerating effect in hybrids. However, Murphy and Roths (pers. comm.) are establishing this gene in a homozygous state on a variety of murine strains where its effect can be observed. Their results indicate that *lpr/lpr* induces lymphoproliferation and accelerates onset and course of SLE in both MRL/n (50% mortality from 17 to 5 months) and NZB (50% mortality from 16 months to <5 months) in keeping with the expression of the BXSB accelerator trait in multiple SLE strains. But in spite of inducing lymphoproliferation, *lpr/lpr* causes no early SLE in C3H or AKR mice in which there is no SLE background to influence.

The acceleration of SLE in female NZB × W presumably by female hormones has been demonstrated by Talal and associates (Roubinian *et al.*, 1978). Early castration together with androgens given to females retarded the disease while early castration plus oestrogen administration accelerated the disease in males. That female hormones do not operate similarly in MRL/l and BXSB mice is evident although there is a slightly earlier disease in MRL/l females than males. Interestingly, the male first disease of the BXSB does not appear to be gonad or hormone dependent as shown by castration (Eisenberg *et al.*, 1980a) and cell transfer experiments (Eisenberg *et al.*, 1980b). Another kind of accelerating factor of murine SLE is chronic viral infection. LCM and polyoma (Tonietti *et al.*, 1970) and retrovirus (Croker *et al.*, 1974; Cannat and Varet, 1973) infections have all been observed to induce or elevate antinuclear antibodies and in the case of LCM and polyoma a SLE-like disease was associated. While these viruses probably act in part by causing virus-antivirus immune complexes, their stimulation of antinuclear and other autoantibody formation must be considered as potential enhancement of SLE. In the case of neonatal LCM infection the 50% mortality from SLE-like disease was changed from 15 to <5 months in NZB, from >24 to <6 months in NZW, from 9 months to 5 months in the female NZB × W, from 20 to 9 months in the female BXSB and from 18 to 12 months in the MRL/n. In normal mice, such as the C3H and SWR/J, with neonatal LCM infection no fatal SLE-like disease develops during the first 2 years of life.

SLE in F_2 hybrids and segregation of disease traits

Eight crosses between SLE and normal mice (BXSB × C3H, C3H × BXSB, BXSB × C57BL/6, C57BL/6 × BXSB, MRL/l × C3H, C3H × MRL/l, MRL/l × C57BL/6 and C57BL/6 × MRL/l) were carried to the F_2 generation to observe occurrence of SLE and segregation of various traits with each other and with disease. Only 26% of the F_2 males but no females of the C57BL/6 × BXSB and 12% of all offsprings from both MRL/l crosses with C57BL/6 had early life SLE whereas F_2 offspring derived from the other crosses listed above had no significant SLE. The overall low incidence or absence of SLE in most crosses suggests that the expression of disease must depend upon a critical number of genes which are reduced below the disease producing level in F_2 offspring. There was no convincing or consistent correlation of the amount of anyone of the immunologic or virologic parameters observed (IgM, anti-ssDNA, ANA, gp70 and lymphoproliferation) with the severity of disease as measured by the degree of glomerulonephritis at autopsy or by the age of death. Similarly there was relatively little correlation among the various immunologic or virologic abnormalities themselves. However, as might have been anticipated, the occurrences of the consequences of immune complex deposition, glomerulonephritis, vascular disease and myocardial infarction, were well correlated. The lack of any correlation among most of the immunologic features indicates an independent segregation of their responsible genetic factors. In addition, the failure of any of these traits to segregate convincingly with severity of disease suggests that disease is dependent upon the expression of multiple abnormal immunologic traits and that expression of various combinations of a critical number can cause disease while expression of only a few of these same traits does not produce disease.

These results are compatible with those of others that analysed a number of recombinant inbred strains derived from NZB crosses with DBA/2, ALN and C58J (Riblet, pers. comm.; Raveche *et al.*, 1980). These investigators found that the production of antierythrocyte, antithymocyte and anti-ssDNA antibodies as well as for syngeneic mixed leukocyte reactions and hyperdiploidy segregate separately and independently. Further, it appears that most if not all of these traits are determined by a single gene sometimes dominant as in the case of antierythrocyte and anti-DNA antibodies and sometimes recessive as in the case of the syngeneic mixed leukocyte reactions. These studies provide the clearest evidence to date for the independence of the various immunologic abnormalities in murine SLE at least as seen in the NZB. Further, they give no indication of any genetically determined across the board predisposition to autoimmune disease as it has been suggested (Miller and Schwartz, 1979).

Therapeutic manipulations

Effect of prostaglandin E

Prostaglandin E_1 (PGE_1) in pharmacologic quantities, has proven capable of altering many *in vivo* immune responses (Goodwin and Webb, 1980). Of considerable interest, recent studies indicate that PGE_1 prolongs survival in NZB × W mice (Zurier *et al.*, 1977). Our studies have confirmed the beneficial effects of PGE_1 in the disease of NZB × W mice (Kelly *et al.*, 1979) and have been extended to show similar beneficial effects on the MRL/l disease. In NZB × W mice therapy decreased the incidence of proteinuria, lessened renal pathology and prolonged survival. Maximum beneficial effects occurred when treatment began at 2 months of age. Of interest, in MRL/l mice PGE_1 treatment in addition to reducing glomerulonephritis also completely inhibited the massive T cell proliferation (Izui *et al.*, 1980c). However, despite the dramatic reduction of glomerulonephritis, in both NZB × W and MRL/l mice, PGE_1 treatment did not alter serum levels of antinuclear antibodies and anti-DNA antibodies in both animal models. Furthermore, no qualitative differences in the isotype or avidity of anti-DNA antibodies were observed between PGE-treated and untreated animals, suggestive that PGE achieves its therapeutic effect through mechanisms that do not directly involve the formation of anti-DNA antibodies. By contrast, the incidence and quantity of circulating gp70 immune complexes were greatly diminished in NZB × W and MRL/l mice treated with PGE compared with untreated mice. The mechanisms by which PGE suppress gp70 immune complex formation in serum have not been defined nor has it been determined whether the therapeutic effects of PGE_1 are due to diminishing levels of gp70-anti-gp70 complexes or other effects on the immune and phagocytic system.

Effect of whole body or total lymphoid irradiation

Recently, it was demonstrated that fractional total lymphoid irradiation (TLI) reduced proteinuria and increased the survival of NZB × W mice compared to untreated controls (Kotzin and Strober, 1979; Slavin, 1979). In these hybrids, the effects of TLI were apparent even when the disease was advanced. These results suggested that irradiation may be a new approach to treating SLE, and an aid in further defining the humoral and cellular abnormalities associated with this disease. We have now examined the effects of TLI as well as of subethal doses of whole body irradiation (WBI) on the progress of the MRL/l disease and the humoral and cellular parameters affected (Theofilopoulos, 1980d). As indicated above, MRL/l mice spontaneously develop massive nonmalignant T cell proliferation and autoimmune disease that kills 50% of them by 5 to 6 months of age. Of such mice, 100% given TLI (17 fractions of 200 rads each to achieve a total dose of 3400 rads during a 3 to 4 week period) at 3 months of age (time of clinical onset of disease) and 82% given WBI (a single dose of 300 rads) remained alive at 9 months old when the experiment was terminated (Fig. 14). At that age, 92% of unirradiated controls were dead with massive lymph node hyperplasia, splenomegaly and severe glomerulonephritis. In contrast, none of the TLI or WBI animals had enlarged nodes of splenomegaly and only 11 to 16% of them developed glomerulonephritis. Irradiated mice had less serum IgG and total immune complexes than controls, and no gp70-anti-gp70 complexes. However, levels of serum IgM and anti-double stranded DNA antibodies were minimally reduced in irradiated animals compared to controls and anti-single stranded DNA antibodies were the same in all groups. Owing to the lack of T cell proliferation, TLI and WBI mice had 100-fold fewer lymphocytes in their lymph nodes and 4 to 7-fold fewer mononuclear cells in their spleens. Moreover, TLI and WBI receiving mice had 14 to 33-fold, respectively, fewer spontaneous Ig secreting cells than age-matched unmanipulated diseased mice. At 6 months postirradiation, treated animals had normal suppressor T cell function (Con A-induced), but helper T cell activity on a cell to cell basis was much below that of the controls. To summarize, our results indicate that sublethal WBI as well as TLI inhibit the disease of the MRL/l mice much like the effect of TLI on NZB × W mice. It is of considerable interest that a single dose of

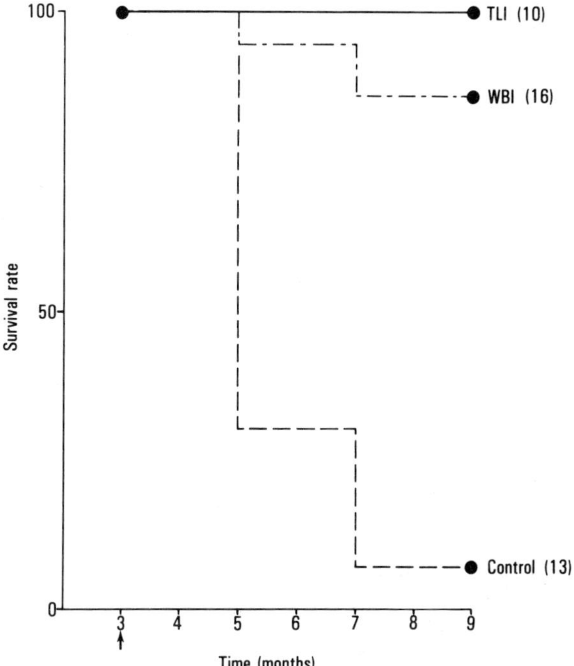

FIG. 14. *Survival rates of total lymphoid irradiation (TLI) or whole body irradiation (WBI) treated animals compared to controls. Numbers in parentheses indicate the numbers of mice included in each group. The arrow indicates the time of irradiation.*

WBI was nearly as effective as the TLI regimen. However, whether TLI and WBI have similar effects on long term survival of these mice was not determined since our study was terminated at 9 months. Nevertheless, our experiments suggest that alternative TLI regimens with only 2–3 fractions delivered, instead of 17, may be as effective in inhibiting murine SLE as the full sequence. Experiments are in progress to determine whether this is the case. If so, then current programmes to treat humans with SLE and other autoimmune diseases by using TLI may require considerably less than the total TLI regimen thereby becoming more practical and causing fewer side effects. Our present experiments with MRL/l mice and those of others in NZB × W mice (Slavin, 1979; Kotzin and Strober, 1979) clearly indicate that WBI and TLI have long lasting beneficial effects in murine SLE. Obviously, such an approach may be useful in treating humans with SLE who are currently receiving continuous treatment with high dose steroids and/or cytotoxic drugs. Apart from providing a potential means of treating SLE, irradiation should be useful in dissecting the humoral and cellular parameters associated with murine SLE.

Conclusions

The genetic autoimmune disease (lupus-like) in mice of several strains (NZB, NZB × W, MRL/l, BXSB) has been analysed in regard to histoimmunopathologic, serologic, virologic, lymphocytic and genetic characteristics. It is obvious from the discussion of these various parameters that the pathogenetic mechanisms underlying murine SLE are highly complex, apparently well programmed but still ill defined. Perhaps the most accurate statement that reflects where we stand in regard to delineating the pathogenesis of murine SLE is that we now have identified many of the fingerprints associated with this disorder and determine that different types of primary or secondary abnormalities can underlie SLE as a syndrome. If there is a common aetiology for the various defects associated with SLE it has not yet been defined. Future studies on the definition of the cellular basis of SLE via cell transfer studies and appropriate genetic manipulations may, hopefully, provide the answer.

References

Accinni, L. and Dixon, F. J. (1979). *Am. J. Path.* **96**, 477.
Akizuki, M., Reeves, J. P. and Steinberg, A. D. (1978). *Clin. Immunol. Immunopath.* **10**, 247.
Andrews, B. S., Eisenberg, R. A., Theofilopoulos, A. N., Izui, S., Wilson, C. B., McConahey, P. J., Murphy, E. D., Roths, J. B. and Dixon, F. J. (1978). *J. Exp. Med.* **148**, 1198.
Bach, J. F., Dardenne, M. and Salomon, J. C. (1973). *Clin. Exp. Immunol.* **14**, 247.
Bankhurst, A. D. and Williams, R. C. (1975). *J. Clin. Invest.* **56**, 1378.
Bankhurst, A. D., Torrigiani, G. and Allison, A. C. (1973). *Lancet* **i**, 226.
Barthold, D. R., Kysela, S. and Steinberg, A. D. (1974). *J. Immunol.* **112**, 9.
Bielschowsky, M. and Goodall, C. M. (1970). *Cancer Res.* **30**, 834.
Botzenhardt, V., Klein, J. and Ziff, M. (1978). *J. Exp. Med.* **147**, 1435.
Botzenhardt, V., Lemmel, E. M. and Stockinger, H. (1980). *Arthritis Rheum.* **23**, 656 (Abstract).
Burnet, F. M. (1959). *In* "The Clonal Selection Theory of Acquired Immunity", Vanderbilt University Press, Nashville, Tennessee.
Cannat, A. and Varet, B. (1973). *Immunol. Commun.* **2**, 527.
Cantor, H. and Gershon, R. K. (1979). *Fed. Proc.* **38**, 2058.
Cantor, H., McVay-Boudreau, L., Hugenberger, J., Naidorf, K., Shen, F. W. and Gershon, R. K. (1978). *J. Exp. Med.* **147**, 1116.
Cerottini, J. C., Lambert, P. H. and Dixon, F. J. (1969). *J. Exp. Med.* **130**, 1093.
Clagett, J. A. and Weigle, W. O. (1974). *J. Exp. Med.* **139**, 643.
Cohen, I. R. and Wekerle, H. (1973). *J. Exp. Med.* **137**, 224.
Cohen, P. L. and Ziff, M. (1977). *J. Immunol.* **119**, 1534.
Creighton, W. D., Katz, D. H. and Dixon, F. J. (1979a). *J. Immunol.* **123**, 2627.
Creighton, W. D., Zinkernagel, R. M. and Dixon, F. J. (1979b). *Clin. Exp. Immunol.* **37**, 181.

Croker, B. P., Del Villano, B. C., Jensen, F. C., Lerner, R. A. and Dixon, F. J. (1974). *J. Exp. Med.* **140**, 1028.

Dauphinee, M. J., Talal, N., Golstein, A. L. and White, A. (1974). *Proc. Natn. Acad. Sci. U.S.A.* **71**, 2637.

De Vries, M. J. and Higmans, W. (1967). *Immunology* **12**, 179.

Eisenberg, R. A., Tan, E. M. and Dixon, F. J. (1978). *J. Exp. Med.* **147**, 582.

Eisenberg, R. A., Theofilopoulos, A. N., Andrews, B. S., Peters, C. J., Thor, L. J. and Dixon, F. J. (1979a). *J. Immunol.* **122**, 2272.

Eisenberg, R. A., Thor, L. J. and Dixon, F. J. (1979b). *Arthritis Rheum.* **22**, 1074.

Eisenberg, R. A., Lee, S. and Dixon, F. J. (1980a). Effect of castration on male-determined acceleration of autoimmune disease in BXSB mice. *J. Immunol.* (Submitted).

Eisenberg, R. A., Izui, S., McConahey, P. J., Hang, L. M., Peters, C. J., Theofilopoulos, A. N. and Dixon, F. J. (1980b). Male determined accelerated autoimmune disease in BXSB mice: transfer by bone marrow and spleen cells. *J Immunol.* (in press).

Elder, J. H., Jensen, F. C., Bryant, M. L. and Lerner, R. A. (1977). *Nature* **267**, 23.

Elder, J. H., Gautsch, J. W., Jensen, F. C., Lerner, R. A., Chused, T. M., Morse, H. C., Hartley, J. W. and Rowe, W. P. (1980). *Clin. Immunol. Immunopath.* **15**, 258.

Fujiwara, M. and Cinader, N. (1974). *Cell Immunol.* **12**, 205.

Gershwin, M. E., Ikeda, R. M., Kruse, W. L., Wilson, F., Shifrine, M. and Spangler, W. (1978). *J. Immunol.* **120**, 971.

Gershwin, M. E., Castles, J. J., Ikeda, R. M., Erickson, K. and Montero, J. (1979). *J. Immunol.* **122**, 710.

Golub, E. S. and Weigle, W. O. (1979). *J. Immunol.* **102**, 389.

Goodwin, J. S. and Webb, D. R. (1980). *Clin. Immunol. Immunopath.* **15**, 106.

Howie, J. B. and Helyer, B. J. (1968). *Adv. Immunol.* **9**, 215.

Izui, S. and Eisenberg, R. A. (1980). *Clin. Immunol. Immunopath.* **15**, 536.

Izui, S., McConahey, P. J. and Dixon, F. J. (1978). *J. Immunol.* **121**, 2213.

Izui, S., McConahey, P. J., Theofilopoulos, A. N. and Dixon, F. J. (1979). *J. Exp. Med.* **149**, 1099.

Izui, S., Elder, J. H., McConahey, P. J. and Dixon, F. J. (1980a). Identification of retroviral gp70 and anti-gp70 antibodies involved in circulating immune complex in NZB × NZW mice (in prep.).

Izui, S., Hang, L. M., Thor, L. and Dixon, F. J. (1980b). Tolerance susceptibility in murine SLE strains (in prep.)

Izui, S., Kelley, V. E., McConahey, P. J. and Dixon, F. J. (1980c). Selective suppression of retroviral gp70-anti-gp70 immune complex formation by prostaglandin E_1 in murine systemic lupus erythematosus. *J. Exp. Med.* (Submitted).

Katz, D. H. (1977). *In* "Lymphocyte Differentiation, Recognition and Regulation" (F. J. Dixon and H. G. Kunkel, eds). Academic Press, New York and London.

Kelley, V. E., Winkelstein, A. and Izui, S. (1979). *Lab. Invest.* **41**, 531.

Kincade, P. W., Lee, G., Fernandes, G., Moore, M. A. S., Williams, N. and Good, R. A. (1979). *Proc. Natn. Acad. Sci. U.S.A.* **76**, 3464.

Kotzin, B. L. and Strober, S. (1979). *J. Exp. Med.* **150**, 371.

Krakauer, R. S., Waldmann, T. A. and Strober, W. (1976). *J. Exp. Med.* **144**, 662.

Mackaness, G. B. (1969). *J. Exp. Med.* **129**, 973.

Manny, N., Datta, S. K. and Schwartz, R. S. (1979). *J. Immunol.* **122**, 1220.

Miller, K. B. and Schwartz, R. S. (1979). *N. Engl. J. Med.* **301**, 803.

Morton, J. I. and Siegel, B. V. (1974). *Proc. Natn. Acad. Sci. U.S.A.* **71**, 2162.

Moutsopoulos, H. M., Boehm-Truitt, M., Kassan, S. S. and Chused, T. N. (1977). *J. Immunol.* **119**, 1639.

Murphy, E. D. and Roths, J. B. (1979). *In* "Genetic Control of Autoimmune Disease" (N. R. Rose, P. E. Bigazzi and N. L. Warner, eds), p. 207. Elsevier North Holland, Inc. New York.

Ohsugi, Y. and Gershwin, E. (1979). *J. Immunol.* **123**, 1260.
Osler, W. (1895). *J. Med. Sci.* **110**, 629.
Parks, D. E., Doyle, M. V. and Weigle, (1978). *J. Exp. Med.* **148**, 625.
Phillips, S. M., Hirsch, M. S., Andre-Schwartz, J., Solnik, C., Black, P., Schwartz, R. S., Merrill, J. P. and Carpenter, C. B. (1975). *Cell. Immunol.* **15**, 169.
Primi, D., Hammarström, L. and Smith, C. I. E. (1978). *J. Immunol.* **121**, 2241.
Primi, D., Hammarström, L. and Smith, C. I. E. (1979). *Cell. Immunol.* **42**, 40.
Raveche, S., Brown, L. J., Novotny, E. A., Tjio, J. H., Shreffler, D. C. and Steinberg, A. D. (1980). *Arth. Rheum.* **23**, 735 (Abstract).
Rich, R. R., Sedberry, D. A., Kastner, D. L. and Chu, L. (1979). *J. Exp. Med.* **150**, 1555.
Roubinian, J. R., Papoian, R. and Talal, N. (1977). *J. Immunol.* **118**, 1524.
Roubinian, J. R., Talal, N., Greenspam, J. S., Goodman, J. R. and Siiteri, P. K. (1978). *J. Exp. Med.* **147**, 1568.
Sawada, S. and Talal, N. (1979). *Arth. Rheum.* **22**, 655 (Abstract).
Sawada, S., Pillarisetty, R. J., Michalski, J. P., Palmer, D. W. and Talal, N. (1977). *J. Immunol.* **119**, 355.
Slavin, S. (1979). *Prof. Natn. Acad. Sci. U.S.A.* **76**, 5274.
Staples, P. J. and Talal, N. (1969). *J. Exp. Med.* **129**, 123.
Staples, P. J., Steinberg, A. D. and Talal, N. (1970). *J. Exp. Med.* **131**, 1223.
Steinberg, A. D., Law, L. D. and Talal, N. (1970). *Arth. Rheum.* **13**, 369.
Talal, N. (1976). *Transplant. Rev.* **31**, 240.
Theofilopoulos, A. N. and Altman, A. Production of helper factors in NZB anti-BALB/c cultures (in prep.).
Theofilopoulos, A. N., Eisenberg, R. A., Bourdon, M., Crowell, J. S., and Dixon, F. J. (1979a). *J. Exp. Med.* **149**, 516.
Theofilopoulos, A. N., Shawler, D. L., Katz, D. H. and Dixon, F. J. (1979b). *J. Immunol.* **122**, 2319.
Theofilopoulos, A. N., Shawler, D. L., Eisenberg, R. A. and Dixon, F. J. (1980a). *J. Exp. Med.* **151**, 446.
Theofilopoulos, A. N., Shawler, D. L., Balderas, R. S., Elder, J. H., Katz, D. H. and Dixon, F. J. (1980b). Specificities of NZB anti-H-2^d CML reactions: Role of Qa-1 and retroviral gp70 antigens. *J. Exp. Med.* (in press).
Theofilopoulos, A. N., McConahey, P. J., Izui, S., Eisenberg, R. A., Pereira, A. B. and Creighton, W. D. (1980c). *Clin. Immunol. Immunopath.* **15**, 258.
Theofilopoulos, A. N., Balderas, R., Shawler, D. L., Izui, S., Kotzin, B. L., Strober, S. and Dixon, F. J. (1980d). Inhibition of T cell proliferation and SLE-like syndrome of MRL/l mice by whole body or total lymphoid irradiation. *J. Immunol.* (in press).
Theofilopoulos, A. N., Shawler, D. L., Lee, S. and Dixon, F. J. Role of the thymus in murine lupus (in prep. a).
Theofilopoulos, A. N., Shawler, D. L. and Dixon, F. J. Studies on the surface characteristics of B cells derived from SLE-prone murine strains (in prep. b).
Theofilopoulos, A. N., Shawler, D. L., Elder, J. and Dixon, F. J. (NZB anti-H-2^d CML responses induced by retroviral gp70 (in prep. c).
Tonietti, G., Oldstone, M. B. A. and Dixon, F. J. (1970). *J. Exp. Med.* **132**, 89.
Tourog, J. D., Moutsopoulos, H. M., Rosenberg, Y. J., Chused, T. N. and Steinberg, A. D. (1979). *J. Exp. Med.* **150**, 31.
Wagner, H., Hardt, C., Heeg, K., Pfizenmaier, K., Solbach, W., Bartlett, R., Stockinger, H. and Röllinghoff, M. (1980). T-T cell interactions during cytotoxic T lymphocyte (CTL) response. *Immunol. Rev.* (in press).
Warner, N. L. (1977). *In* "Autoimmunity" (N. Talal, ed.), p. 33. Academic Press, New York and London.
Weigle, W. O. (1977). *In* "Autoimmunity" (N. Talal, ed.), p. 141. Academic Press, New York and London.

Wigzell, H. (1977). *In* "Autoimmunity" (N. Talal, ed.), p. 693. Academic Press, New York and London.

Zinkernagel, R. M. and Dixon, F. J. (1977). *Clin. Exp. Immunol.* **29**, 110.

Zurier, R. B., Damjanov, I., Sayadoff, D. M. and Rothfield, N. F. (1977). *Arth. Rheum.* **20**, 1449.

Theme 14: Summary

Mechanisms of Autoimmune Phenomena and Immune Deficiencies

MAX D. COOPER

The University of Alabama, Birmingham, USA

The frequency with which autoimmune disease (AID) occur and their diversity, complexity and unsolved nature have been reflected in the large number of papers devoted to this topic. Far fewer reports dealt with the related problem of primary immunodeficiencies. While many of the reports concerned autoimmune syndromes in humans, the emphasis on animal models in preference to human disease relates to the greater potential for genetic study, the ability to examine animals before and after AID development and the opportunity to sample any organ or tissue. In addition, most agree that the animal models are less complicated and lesson learned from them should in any case lead logically to understanding mechanisms of AID in humans.

The common denominator of AID is an immune response to self-antigens. In most AID, antibodies are formed to self-antigens and immune complexes lead to tissue damage. Interest has thus been focused on the question of what initiates and controls the autoantibody responses. Many studies have dealt with a dissection of the cellular basis for AID as one logical approach to the answers.

In recent years, attention has been centered on the role of the thymus and the various immunoregulatory T cells that begin their development in it and remain under its control via thymic hormones. Thymectomy may accelerate the onset of murine SLE, deficiencies of thymic hormones can exist in SLE prone mice; SLE manifestations may be favourably affected by treatment with thymic hormones, and thymic atrophy is consistently seen in SLE prone strains of mice. Moreover, thymic epithelial hyperkeratosis in the mutant rhino mouse is associated with T cell deficiency and autoantibodies.

Attention was directed early to an apparent deficiency of T cells with suppressor function in both mouse and human AID. This may occur as a primary deficit in Ts cells or possibly as the result of a reduction in Ly-1$^+$ inducers of Ts cells, as in the mutant hairless (hr/hr) strain of mice. On the other hand, other studies provide evidence for an excess of helper T cell activity as a genetically determined lesion. Thus, the idea has evolved that a variety of disturbances in the circuits of interacting immunoregulatory T cells could lead to abnormal triggering of self- and nonself-reactive clones of B cells leading to AID.

The significance of observations indicating that (i) a subpopulation of T cells with suppressor function may bear receptors for autologous erythrocytes and proliferate in response to autologous or syngeneic Ia$^+$ cells and (ii) this T cell subset may be deficient in human and murine SLE continues to be debated.

Several observations point away from the necessity for the thymus and deranged T cells in AID. The nude gene does not prevent NZB mice from producing autoantibodies, and abnormalities were not found in some extensive surveys of T cell numbers, function and cell membrane antigens in SLE-prone mice. Likewise, T cell abnormalities have not been consistently found in humans with AID, e.g. in rheumatoid arthritis or inactive SLE.

With regard to the latter point, the means for assessment of human T cells lag behind those available in mice, but this deficit is being corrected rapidly. In addition to the past use of sheep erythrocyte binding to detect human T cells and receptors for Fc and autologous erythrocytes for subpopulation identification, monoclonal antibodies have recently been made to a variety of surface antigens on human T cells of various types and stages of differentiation. These promise to be very valuable in assessment of human AID but, as in the mouse, early results from such studies indicate that simple answers to questions about pathogenesis of human AID may not be immediately forthcoming. In this regard it is noteworthy that most studies of human lymphocytes by necessity are performed on those obtained from circulating blood.

The B cell is viewed as the rising star in the case of cellular characters playing a role in AID. Polyclonal activation of B cell differentiation may be a consistent feature of AID in all species. This may antedate T cell alterations or even occur in the absence of thymic influence. For expression of the polyclonal B cell activation in murine SLE, it appears that the Ly-3^+ subpopulation of B cells must be present. While the polyclonal activation of B cells may be a central feature, which is genetically programmed at a stem cell level, extraneous polyclonal activators (viruses, various mitogens, etc.), immunoregulatory T cells, antigen presenting cells and hormonal regulators may still be important B cell modifiers in the pathogenesis of AID.

A relative newcomer to the cast of cellular characters involved in AID is the natural killer (NK) cell. A deficiency in functional NK cells and their physiologic inducer, interferon, may exist in certain AID. Finally, cells bearing receptors for the Fc portion of IgG antibodies, other than ones already mentioned, may be centrally involved in the pathophysiology of AID. For example, defective clearing of immune complexes by cells of the "RES" system may enhance the manifestations of AID. This may prove to be important in the treatment of AID by agents that enhance the cellular clearance of immune complexes.

Thus, it has become increasingly evident that a variety of cellular defects, which accumulate with age, may exist in experimental and human models of AID. Genetic analysis of inbred and recombinant strains of AID prone mice indicate that multiple gene defects may exist to account for the final array of abnormalities in AID. One theory put forward to explain this is the possibility of a common regulatory gene abnormality that results in the abnormal control of multiple defective structural genes. An alternative theory is that AID develops in individuals unlucky enough to inherit several defective structural genes, each of which may contribute one of the immune system defects associated with acquisition of AID. Included as an important feature of the latter theory is the existence of multiple acceleration factors. Candidates among the latter category for which evidence has been obtained include infection by xenotrophic and ecotrophic viruses, sex hormones, various drugs, and diet (i.e., increased caloric and fat intake). Some of the accelerating factors may have local effects on selective tissue targets for as yet poorly understood reasons.

Many investigators in the field believe that further genetic studies may soon lead to the ability to recognize specific features of the genetic makeup which predispose an individual to AID. This information might then be used to avoid factors accelerating the development of AID. For those individuals unfortunate enough to acquire AID, some therapeutic approaches beyond those involving conventional immunosuppressive therapy are now becoming evident. These include treatment with prostaglandin E, thymic hormones and either whole body or lymphoid tissue irradiation. Thus, while it is frustrating that no simple common mechanism for AID is yet in sight, and may not exist, there appears to be good progress towards new insight into the "genetic basis", accelerating factors and improved therapy of AID.

Immune deficiency syndromes (IDS) are also viewed traditionally as defects in development or in specific functions of cells comprising the immune system. This approach has led to the successful repair of congenital defects in development of stem cells along T and B cell lines by transplantation of histocompatible bone marrow cells. Bone marrow transplantation has also been used for successful treatment of other diseases of cells of haemopoietic stem cell origin. A great problem is the lack of HLA compatible donors for many patients who might benefit from stem cell transplantation. In a few such individuals, allogeneic foetal liver has been successfully used, often together with a thymus implant from the same donor. One major difficulty with the approach of transplanting healthy allogeneic stem cells is the paucity of information available on the MHC restrictions required for functional interactions between cells of the human immune system and for effective T cell recognition of virus-infected or otherwise altered cells not belonging to the immune system. Methods have now been developed for *in vitro* evaluation of HLA restrictions in T cell killing of virus-infected and haptenated cells. The system may also be applied to study cellular competence and MHC restrictions for antibody responses. These methods have already been used to study functional incompetence of T and B cells from individuals affected by certain immunodeficiencies.

A few human IDS have now been defined at a molecular level. An example is the autosomal recessive defect in adenosine deaminase activity. The effects of this enzyme abnormality may be caused by the resultant accumulation of deoxynucleotide triphosphates which inhibit ribonucleotide reductase leading to depletion of other triphosphates especially required for DNA synthesis in lymphoid cells.

There is accumulating evidence which suggests that defects in immunoregulatory T cells may lead to defective antibody production by B cells in certain human IDS. For example, an excess in suppressor T cell activity may be important in the pathogenesis of some panhypo-γ-globulinaemic states, while selective suppression of the differentiation of IgA producing cells may occur in other individuals. The precise mechanisms for such effects have not yet been elucidated, but future studies will surely be facilitated by the new reagents (e.g. monoclonal antibodies to lymphocyte and macrophage surface determinants) and methods for study of interactions between cells of the human immune system.

It is encouraging to note that γ-globulin preparations that are safe and effective for intravenous antibody replacement therapy have now been developed.

An interesting new IDS has been discovered in a child who was unable to produce immune interferon and had a secondary defect of NK activities. The repeated infections suffered by this individual surprisingly were both viral and bacterial in nature. Administration of human interferon was accompanied by a reversal of the impaired NK activity and the increased incidence of infections.

From the discussions during this congress and in a satellite meeting devoted to immune deficiencies (M. Seligmann and W. Hitzig, eds, in press), it is clear that much remains to be done before the pathogenesis of most IDS can be fully understood. The availability of useful new reagents, methods and concepts ensure rapid progress in this area.

Theme 15

Complement and Immune Complexes

Presidents:
C. G. COCHRANE
P. J. LACHMANN
A. P. PELTIER

Symposium chairman:
H. ISLIKER

54

Complement Reaction Pathways

HANS J. MÜLLER-EBERHARD*

Department of Molecular Immunology, Research Institute of Scripps Clinic, La Jolla, California, USA

This is publication number 2185 from the Research Institute of Scripps Clinic and was supported by United States Public Health Service Grants AI 07007, AI 13010 and HL 16411.

* Cecil H. and Ida M. Green Investigator in Medical Research, Research Institute of Scripps Clinic, La Jolla, Ca, USA.

Introduction

Complement has emerged as an integral part of the immune system. It reacts with immunoglobulins through C1q and is activated thereby. Cells of the immune system bear complement specific receptors which are important for their function. Complement is genetically linked to the major histocompatibility complex through its two C3 convertases, or the proteins C2, B and C4; certain cells of the immune system synthesize complement proteins.

Complement has also become a model of complex, molecular biological systems. Its reaction pathways involve protein–protein, protein–carbohydrate and protein–lipid interactions. They involve protein activation by highly restricted proteolysis or by conformational changes. And they utilize the novel strategy of the metastable binding site in order to attack targets.

Complement exercises its biological functions in three principal modes. (a) It forms ligand molecules such as C3b that can bind to biological particles through its metastable binding site and then link these particles to phagocytic cells by binding to their C3b receptors. (b) Complement elaborates hormone-like molecules. C3a, C4a, C5a and Bb elicit responses from a variety of cells that pertain to inflammation. For instance, C5a causes directed migration of monocytes, while Bb causes cessation of migration and cell spreading. And, (c) complement generates a unique membranolytic, multimolecular complex which is capable of weakening and disassembling lipid bilayers and of forming transmembrane channels.

All in all, the complement system comprises 20 plasma proteins. Six proteins constitute the classical pathway of activation: C1q, C1r, C1s, C2, C3 and C4, and 6 the alternative pathway: C3, B, D, β1H, C3b inactivator (C3bINA) and properdin. Whereas the latter 3 proteins are considered regulatory proteins, 2 of these, β1H and C3bINA, are essential for fruitful activation of the alternative pathway. Five proteins participate in the membrane attack pathway: C5, C6, C7, C8 and C9. This pathway is primarily regulated by the *S*-protein which is the inhibitor of the forming membrane attack complex. Classical pathway regulators are the C1 inhibitor (C1INH), the C4 binding protein (C4bp) and the C3bINA. The activation peptides of C3, C4, C5 and their anaphylatoxin activity are controlled by the serum carboxypeptidase B. Without question, C3 is the most versatile of these 20 proteins, as it fulfills many different functions in the system.

During the past several years major new insights have been gained, particularly into the molecular dynamics of the alternative pathway and the membrane attack pathway. This synopsis will therefore focus on these two subjects. Emphasis will be placed on the functional versatility of C3, on the nature of its metastable binding site, on a novel form of C3 which may explain the composition of the initial enzyme of the alternative pathway and on the recognition function of C3b bound to biological particles. The process of assembly of the membrane attack (MAC) will be illuminated with emphasis on subunit topology and the various modes of action of the MAC on target membranes will be analysed.

The versatility of C3

Properties of C3

C3 is historically the oldest complement protein. It was the first complement constituent to be recognized, isolated and described as a distinct protein (Müller-Eberhard and Nilsson, 1960; Müller-Eberhard *et al.*, 1960). Human C3 is a 9·5S β globulin containing 2·7% carbohydrate and having an $M_r = 180\,000$. It is composed of 2 non-identical polypeptide chains, α and β, the size of which is 110 000 and 70 000 daltons, respectively (Bokisch *et al.*, 1975; Nilsson *et al.*, 1975). Serine is the *N*-terminal amino acid residue of both chains, and the *C*-terminal residue of the α-chain. The *C*-terminal of the β-chain is occupied by alanine. Partial amino acid sequences of the α- and β-chain have been established (Hugli, 1975; Tack *et al.*, 1979). The protein is sensitive to treatment with amines such as hydrazine which inactivates it within minutes (Müller-Eberhard, 1961). Amines attack a putative thioester bond in C3 (Pangburn and Müller-Eberhard, 1980). C3 is synthesized as a single polypeptide chain, which, after translation, is processed in the cytoplasm to the 2-chain molecule that occurs in serum (Brade *et al.*, 1977).

Physiological fragments of C3 and their biological activities

C3 is the precursor of several biologically active fragments which arise during the process of activation and control of the molecule, and in its uncleaved form it is postulated to be a subunit of the initial C3 convertase of the alternative pathway (Table I). Activation of C3 occurs upon hydrolysis of peptide bond 77 (Arg–Ser) of the α-chain by C3 convertase (Hugli, 1975; Tack *et al.*, 1979). This cleavage leads to the formation of C3a (M_r† = 9000) which is one of the 3 anaphylatoxins (Dias Da Silva *et al.*, 1967; Cochrane and Müller-Eberhard, 1968; Gorski *et al.*, 1979b) and of the major fragment C3b ($M_r = 171\,000$). The primary structure of C3a is known (Hugli, 1975). Con-

† Molecular weight as determined by SDS gel.

TABLE I

Biological activities of C3 and its physiological fragments

Fragment	*Molecular weight*	*Polypeptide chains*	*Biological activity*
C3	180 000	2	Subunit initial C3 convertase (AP)
C3a	9000	1	Anaphylatoxin
			Histamine release
			Cellular enzyme release
			Smooth muscle contraction
C3b	170 000	2	Recognition (AP[a])
			Binding to biological particles
			Subunit C3/C5 convertase (AP)
			Subunit C5 convertase (CP[b])
			Receptor for activated properdin
			Ligand for cellular C3b receptor
iC3b	170 000	3	Ligand for cellular iC3b receptor
C3c	140 000	3 or more	Precursor of C3e
C3d	25 000	1	Ligand for cellular C3d receptor
C3e	12 000	1	Induction of leukocytosis

[a] Alternative pathway.
[b] Classical pathway.

comitant with the C3a–C3b cleavage, a metastable binding site is expressed on C3b through which C3b can firmly attach to a large variety of biological particles (Müller-Eberhard *et al.*, 1966). Particle-bound C3b has the following functions: (a) it is opsonic, i.e. it marks particles for ingestion by phagocytic cells and serves as a ligand to C3b specific cell surface receptors (Gigli and Nelson, 1968; Huber *et al.*, 1968); (b) it is the acceptor of activated factor B and thus a subunit of the target bound alternative pathway C3 convertase (Daha *et al.*, 1976; Medicus *et al.*, 1976; Vogt *et al.*, 1977); (c) it is the substrate modulator of the target-bound C5 convertase (Vogt *et al.*, 1978); (d) it serves as receptor for activated properdin (Schreiber *et al.*, 1975); (e) it binds β1H which results in blocking the factor B binding site or in dissociation of the b-fragment of factor B from the C3/C5 convertase (Weiler *et al.*, 1976; Whaley and Ruddy, 1976a; Conrad *et al.*, 1978; Nagaki *et al.*, 1978; Pangburn and Müller-Eberhard, 1978a, b) and in conformational adaptation of C3b to the action of C3bINA (Whaley and Ruddy, 1976a; Pangburn *et al.*, 1977); and (f) it appears to be capable of distinguishing between an activator and a non-activator of the alternative pathway (Pangburn and Müller-Eberhard, 1978a; Schreiber *et al.*, 1978; Pangburn *et al.*, 1980), which is reflected in a differential accessibility of bound C3b to the regulator β1H (Fearon and Austen, 1977a, b; Pangburn and Müller-Eberhard, 1978a, b; Kazatchkine *et al.*, 1979a). Control of the two primary fragments of C3 is exerted such that C3a is inactivated by the serum carboxypeptidase B which removes the essential *C*-terminal arginine residue (Bokisch and Müller-Eberhard, 1970; Budzko *et al.*,

1971) and C3b is inactivated by the C3bINA (Tamura and Nelson, 1967; Lachmann and Müller-Eberhard, 1968; Ruddy and Austen, 1971) which cleaves the α'-chain of C3b into a 67 000 and a 43 000 dalton fragment (Pangburn *et al.*, 1977). Since both α'-fragments are disulphide bonded to the β-chain, the cleaved molecule (iC3b) has the same molecular size as intact C3b. iC3b is highly susceptible to attack by tryptic enzymes which cleave the α'-chain in the *N*-terminal region and thereby produce the two fragments C3c (M_r = 140 000) and C3d (M_r = 30 000). The C3d portion contains the particle binding site of C3b and therefore remains bound when C3c is cleaved off (Ruddy and Austen, 1971; Bokisch *et al.*, 1975; Law *et al.*, 1979a). Further tryptic degradation of C3c produces the fragment C3e (M_r = 10 000) which is probably derived from the α'-chain and which has leukocytosis inducing activity (Ghebrehiwet and Müller-Eberhard, 1979).

Cell surface receptors for C3 fragments

Specific receptors for C3a are apparently present on smooth muscle cells, polymorphonuclear leukocytes and mast cells. Cells capable of phagocytosis such as polymorphonuclear leukocytes, monocytes, macrophages and mast cells have cell surface receptors for C3b. C3b molecules on the surface of target particles promote the adherence phase of phagocytosis. Receptors for iC3b have been described for polymorphonuclear leukocytes, monocytes (Ross and Rabellino, 1979) and mast cells (Vranian *et al.*, 1980). The iC3b receptor is distinct from the C3b and C3d receptors, the latter occurring apparently only on certain lymphocytes (Ross *et al.*, 1973). Engagement of particle-bound C3b with C3b receptors on phagocytes results in increased oxidative metabolic activity and production of superoxide anions, hydrogen peroxide, hydroxyl radicals and singlet oxygen (Curnette and Babior, 1974; Goldstein *et al.*, 1975). The same appears to be true for the interaction of iC3b with iC3b receptors on polymorphonuclear leukocytes (Schreiber and Müller-Eberhard, unpublished observations). All 3 of the C3 receptors are found among unfractionated human lymphocytes. About 11% of lymphocytes have receptors for C3b, 6% for iC3b and 2% for C3d. Most C3b receptor-bearing lymphocytes are distinct from those with iC3b- and C3d-receptors. Raji and Daudi lymphoblastoid cell lines are capable of reacting with iC3b and C3d, but not with C3b. Antibody dependent cellular cytotoxicity (ADCC) was markedly enhanced by C3 fragments on the target cells. Enhancement was strongest with iC3b, strong with C3d and moderate with C3b (Perlmann *et al.*, 1980). These observations indicate that all 3 fragments, and particularly iC3b, can participate in the ADCC reaction.

Evolutionary relationship between C3, C4 and C5

The 3 proteins are similar in several respects. Their molecular weights fall between 180 000 and 200 000 daltons. They exhibit similar electrophoretic mobilities. C3 and C5 have α- and β-chains of comparable size (Nilsson *et al.*, 1975) and although C4 is different in that it is a 3-chain protein (Schreiber and Müller-Eberhard, 1974), all 3 proteins are synthesized as single polypeptide chains (Ooi and Colten, 1980; Hall and Colten, 1977). Their activation peptides have anaphylatoxin activity, C3a and C4a addressing the same cell receptor, C5a a different one and, in addition, having chemotactic activity. The primary sequence of these α-chain fragments is very similar, C3a and C4a exhibiting 38% homology (Gorski *et al.*, 1980), and C3a and C5a 36% homology (Fernandez and Hugli, 1978). Approximately 45% α-helical content is present in C3a (Hugli *et al.*, 1975), C4a (Gorski *et al.*, 1980) and C5a (Morgan *et al.*, 1974). The b-fragments initially exhibit a metastable binding site through which C3b and C4b can bind to biological particles and C5b to C6. C4b (Cooper, 1969) and possibly C5b (Dierich and Landen, 1977) can react with the C3b-specific cell surface receptor. All 3 proteins are specialized in binding multiple proteins. C3 may be phylogenetically the older of the 3 proteins because it is most multifunctional, least specialized and confers upon the alternative pathway the capacity of target discrimination without enlisting antibody.

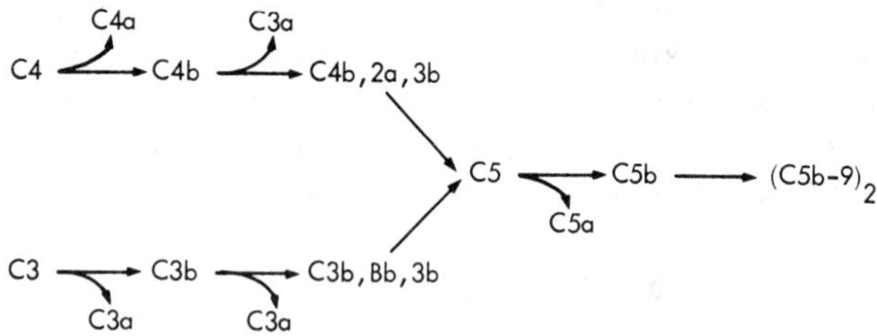

FIG. 1. *Comparison of the functions of the evolutionary relatives C3, C4 and C5. For explanation, see text.*

Viewing the respective positions of the 3 proteins in the 3 complement pathways reveals that each one fulfills key functions in one of the pathways (Fig. 1): C5 donates C5b which becomes the nucleus of the self-assembling MAC. C3 is part of the initial enzyme, donates C3b which establishes physical contact with the target, serves as a subunit of the alternative C3 convertase and as modulator of C5 in the classical and alternative C5 convertase. C4 donates C4b which establishes physical contact with the target and serves as subunit of the classical C3 convertase. Because C3b is an essential subunit of the activating enzyme of C3 in the alternative pathway, the pathway is endowed with a powerful positive feedback mechanism (Müller-Eberhard and Götze, 1972). Such feedback does not exist in the classical pathway.

A new form of C3 with functional properties of C3b

A putative thioester bond in native C3

That C3 loses its haemolytic activity upon treatment with amines such as hydrazine has been known (Müller-Eberhard, 1961). Nonenzymatic inactivation of C3 has also been accomplished using chaotropic reagents such as NaBr or KCNS (Dalmasso and Müller-Eberhard, 1966). In a recent study, native C3 was subjected to treatment with methylamine because this amine is readily available in radiolabelled form and has been used successfully for the inactivation of the plasma protease inhibitor α_2-macroglobulin (Swenson and Howard, 1979). The reaction with methylamine led to the stoichiometric, covalent incorporation of methylamine into the C3 protein, loss of haemolytic activity and the concomitant exposure of a sulphhydryl group which could be labelled with iodoacetamide (Pangburn and Müller-Eberhard, 1980). Both labelled sites were located in the C3d portion of the α-chain which is known to contain the metastable binding site of C3b. In α_2-macroglobulin methylamine was incorporated as methylamide of a glutamic acid residue and the sequence around the reactive glutamyl residue (denoted by asterisk) was determined to be –Gly–Cys–Gly–Glu–Glu*–Asn–Met– (Swenson and Howard, 1979). In the case of C3, methylamine is also incorporated as methylamide of a glutamic acid residue and the sequence around the reactive group was found to be identical to that described for α_2-macroglobulin (Tack, pers. comm.). The iodoacetamide–reactive cysteinyl residue was separated only by two amino acid residues from the methylamine–reactive glutamyl residue in C3. These findings suggest that native C3 contains an internal thioester bond and that this bond is essential for C3 haemolytic activity. While this bond is opened up by amines, it is likely that it can be hydrolysed by water under physiological conditions, although at a low rate. This possibility is suggested by the effect of chaotropic compounds which are known to perturb the tertiary structure of proteins and thus facilitate the reaction of water with relatively concealed groups. The $t_{1/2}$ of C3 haemolytic activity was 8 min at 37°C during treatment of C3 with 0·33 M KSCN and 12 min during treatment with 0·75 M guanidine (Pangburn and Müller-Eberhard, 1980).

Another observation supports the view that C3 contains a reactive carbonyl group, possibly preserved, in native C3, as a thioester. The α-chain of C3 is cleaved into two fragments, $M_r = 74\,000$ and $M_r = 46\,000$, by mere exposure of the protein to denaturants (Sim and Sim, 1980). This reaction occurs only with native C3, not with hydroxylamine treated C3 or with C3b. A similar reaction was observed with the α-chain of native C4. This autocatalytic denaturation-induced fragmentation suggests the presence of unusually reactive chemical groups in these proteins. It appears likely that these groups are the same as those involved in the reaction of the metastable binding site (see below).

The reactive carbonyl group may, upon denaturation of the protein, attack a nitrogen atom involved in a peptide bond resulting in eventual cleavage of the peptide bond (Howard *et al.*, 1980). In the case of C3, the affected bond could be identified as the Glu–Glu bond in the seven-residue sequence that contains the methylamine- and the iodoacetamide-reactive sites (Tack, pers. comm.).

Functionally C3b-like C3

Methylamine modified C3, designated C3(CH_3NH_2) has been found to be functionally C3b-like, although the C3a domain of the molecule remained covalently attached (Pangburn and Müller-Eberhard, 1980). C3(CH_3NH_2) exhibits affinity for factor B and β1H as evidenced by its ability to inhibit the binding of factor B to cell-bound C3b. It is cleaved by C3bINA in the presence of β1H. Addition of C3(CH_3NH_2) to human serum caused C3 consumption to a similar extent as the addition of C3b. C3(CH_3NH_2) formed a C3 convertase together with isolated factor B, D and Mg^{2+}, much like C3b. Anti-C3a removed the convertase forming material from C3(CH_3NH_2) and inhibited the C3 convertase formed with C3(CH_3NH_2). These studies showed that the C3(CH_3NH_2) induced C3 convertase contained a C3a bearing form of C3. Similar functional properties were exhibited by C3 exposed to KSCN or guanidine. It is suggested therefore that direct hydrolysis of the putative thioester bond in C3 may provide, under physiological conditions, a steady source of C3b-like C3, referred to as C3(H_2O), and that C3(H_2O) may give rise to the formation of the initial C3 convertase of the alternative pathway (Pangburn and Müller-Eberhard, 1980).

The metastable binding site and the putative thioester

The concept of the metastable binding site was originally developed to interpret the binding of C4 to unsensitized erythrocytes through the catalytic action of fluid phase C$\bar{1s}$ (Müller-Eberhard and Lepow, 1965) and was further elaborated on in order to explain the binding reaction of C3 (Müller-Eberhard *et al.*, 1966). The site effects the firm attachment of activated, metastable C3b to a wide variety of biological particles. It thereby enables C3b to fulfill its functions in the assembly of both activation pathways on the surface of target cells and in opsonization reactions. Present evidence indicates that C3b may be covalently linked to target particles through a hydroxylamine–labile bond and through hydrophobic interactions (Law and Levine, 1977). In these experiments, C3b was bound to zymosan by enzymatic activation of C3. While the bound C3b could not be eluted by treatment of the particles with detergent or acid, it was released by 1 M hydroxylamine (Law *et al.*, 1979b). That the hydroxylamine sensitive bond is an ester was suggested by the association of hydroxamate with the released protein. The bond formed between the metastable binding site and zymosan (Z) was thus proposed to be Z–O–CO–C3b (Law *et al.*, 1979b). By exposure of the bound C3b to β1H and C3bINA it was shown that binding of C3b occurs via the 67 000 dalton portion of the α′-chain and that this fragment is the precursor of the immunochemically defined C3d piece (Law *et al.*, 1979a). The covalent nature of the bond was further demonstrated by experiments in which serum containing radiolabelled C3b was incubated with ^{3}H-glucose-S-S-Sepharose. After removal of extraneous protein, the Sepharose beads were treated with a disulphide cleaving reagent which resulted in elution of C3b. Upon SDS gel electrophoresis of the reduced protein, ^{3}H was found to be associated with the α′-chain of C3b, strongly suggesting the formation of a covalent bond between the α′-chain and the carbohydrate (Mann *et al.*, 1980). Covalent binding of C3b to Sepharose could be inhibited by oxygen and nitrogen nucleophiles. Activation of C3 in the presence of radiolabelled phenylhydrazine, methylamine, glycerol or glucosamine resulted in apparent covalent incorporation of the nucleophile into the d-portion of C3b (Sim *et al.*, 1980). Like C3(CH_3NH_2), enzymatically derived C3b was shown to possess one reactive sulphhydryl group which is located in the d-domain (Tack *et al.*, 1980). Neither C3(CH_3NH_2) nor C3(H_2O) produced with chaotropic compounds are capable of entering the binding reaction, although with high concentrations of activating enzyme they may be cleaved (Pangburn and Müller-Eberhard, 1980). Thus, it is assumed that the putative thioester bond that is involved in the production of C3b-like C3 is also involved in the metastable binding site of C3b. The covalent binding

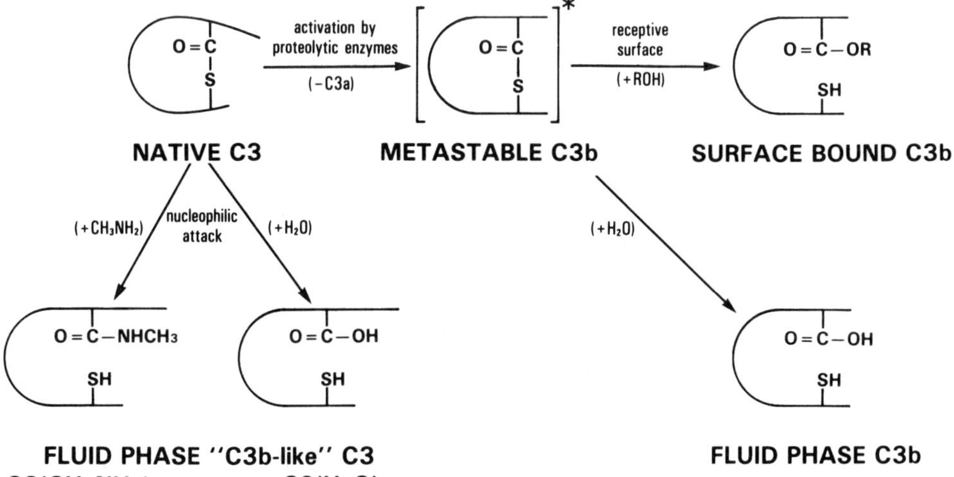

FIG. 2. *Proposed chemical reactions at the activated carbonyl site of C3. An internal thioester bond in the α-chain of C3 may undergo nucleophilic attack or water hydrolysis, thereby rendering the resultant altered C3 functionally C3b-like. Alternatively, the thioester becomes the active site of enzymatically formed metastable C3b and the carbonyl group of the thioester may form an ester bond with hydroxyl groups on the surface of complement targets (Pangburn and Müller-Eberhard, 1980).*

reaction of C3b is thought to occur by transfer of an electrophilic carbonyl group from the thioester bond in native C3 to an ester or amide bond with a receptive surface (Law *et al.*, 1979b; Sim *et al.*, 1980; Tack *et al.*, 1980).

Figure 2 summarizes the proposed chemical reactions at the reactive carbonyl site of C3 (Pangburn and Müller-Eberhard, 1980). The sensitivity of C3 to nucleophilic attack results from the scission of the reactive (thioester) bond and incorporation of the nucleophile. The methylamine product is shown. Water hydrolysis of the thioester would yield –OH in place of the methylamide. C3 altered by nucleophilic attack or water hydrolysis of the thioester becomes functionally C3b-like without proteolytic release of C3a. It can form an alternative pathway C3 convertase which proteolytically converts native C3 to metastable C3b by cleavage of peptide bond 77 of the α-chain. The active site of metastable C3b, according to the present hypothesis, is a highly reactive form of the thioester which is capable of undergoing transesterification with –OH groups. In establishing an ester bond with groups on the surface of biological particles, C3b becomes firmly bound. Failing to encounter an appropriate surface, metastable C3b reacts with water forming fluid phase C3b. These reactions explain the formation of the initial enzyme and the mechanism of C3b deposition which are essential ingredients of alternative pathway activation.

The alternative pathway

Biomedical significance

The biomedical significance of the alternative pathway is unquestioned today. Because the pathway may be activated by certain bacteria, viruses, virus-infected cells or parasites in total absence of specific antibody or immunoglobulins, it may constitute the molecular component of natural host defence mechanisms. Individuals with homozygous deficiencies of C3 or of the C3bINA have been described and found to suffer from life-threatening, recurrent infections. Homozygous deficiencies have not been described to date for factor B, D, β1H or properdin. On the other hand, the alternative pathway apparently participates in disease mechanisms. In hypercomplementemic, chronic glomerulonephritis and a number of skin diseases there exists immunohistochemical evidence for alternative pathway activation in the diseased tissues. Unclear to date is the biological meaning of the demonstrated genetic linkage of factor B to C2 (Alper *et al.*, 1972) and of both proteins to the major histocompatibility locus in man (Allen, 1974; Fu *et al.*, 1974). It is possible that factor B and C2 fulfill additional, as yet unknown functions.

The proteins

Table II lists the proteins of the alternative pathway and some of their

TABLE II
The proteins of the alternative pathway of complement activation

Protein	*Molecular weight*	*No. of chains*	*Electroph. mobility*	*Serum conc. (μg/ml)*
C3	180 000	2	β	1200
B	93 000	1	β	200
D	24 000	1	β-γ	1
C3bINA	88 000	2	β	34
β1H	150 000	1	β	500
P	224 000	4	γ	20

properties. B is the zymogen carrying the active site of the C3/C5 convertase. D is the activating enzyme of B and is always present in plasma in active form. Both enzymes are inhibitable by DFP and appear to be serine proteases. C3 participates in the formation of the initial enzyme and donates C3b. β1H and C3bINA are control proteins of the C3/C5 convertase generally suppressing its function. Properdin stabilizes the C3/C5 convertase, thereby enhancing its function. A detailed description of the six proteins has recently been published (Müller-Eberhard and Schreiber, 1980).

The initial enzyme and its function

Activation of the alternative pathway consists of initiation and amplification. Initiation itself is a two-step process, consisting of random deposition of C3b on the surface of biological particles and, secondly, of a discriminatory interaction of bound C3b with surface structures. Deposition requires enzymatic cleavage of C3 in the fluid phase and generation of metastable C3b that is capable of binding to biological particles. The obvious question, therefore, has been, what is the nature of the initial C3 convertase? It has been established that formation of the initial C3 convertase of the alternative pathway requires C3, B, D and Mg^{2+}, but not properdin or other factors (Medicus *et al.*, 1976; Schreiber *et al.*, 1978). Lachmann envisioned as the initiating event a spontaneous "tick-over" of C3, resulting in continuous low level C3b formation *in vitro* and *in vivo* without evoking the need for exogenous activation (Lachmann, 1979). Fearon and Austen (1975b) suggested that native C3 together with factors B, D and probably properdin can form a convertase capable of generating initial C3b. Because experimental evidence indicated that the initial enzyme is a fluid phase enzyme and that no extraneous proteases were involved in its formation (Schreiber *et al.*, 1978; Lesavre and Müller-Eberhard, 1978), it was concluded that uncleaved C3 served as critical subunit of the enzyme, perhaps in the form of a reversible conformer that expresses affinity for factor B (Müller-Eberhard and Schreiber, 1980).

The above described new observations strongly suggest that a hitherto unrecognized form of C3, that is distinct from native C3, constitutes the C3 derived subunit of the initial enzyme. Incubation of native C3 in water at pH 7·3 and 37°C effected a loss of C3 haemolytic activity of 0·5% per hour (Pangburn and Müller-Eberhard, 1980). Because of its concentration (55 M), the most effective nucleophile in plasma is probably water. Direct hydrolysis of the putative thioester bond in native C3 may provide, under physiological conditions, a steady source for functionally C3b-like C3. This form of uncleaved C3, C3(H_2O), which no longer contains a thioester bond, can bind and modulate factor B, thus allowing its activation by factor D (Fig. 3). The

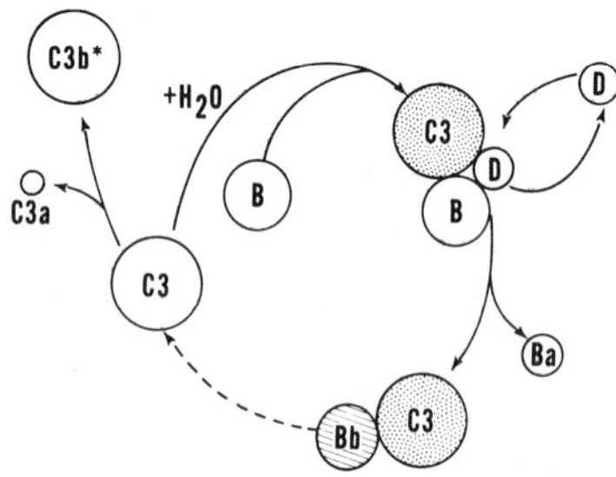

FIG. 3. *Initiation of the alternative pathway by formation of C3b-like C3. Spontaneous hydrolysis of the thioester bond in native C3 initiates a conformational change which exposes the binding site for factor B. Activation by factor D of the C3,B complex generates the first C3 convertase of the pathway, C3,Bb. The proteolytic action of this enzyme on native C3 subsequently generates the first molecule of metastable C3b (C3b*) (Pangburn and Müller-Eberhard, 1980).*

first molecule of C3b produced by the initial enzyme will then set in motion the C3b-dependent positive feedback reaction. The function of the initial enzyme is to transfer the alternative pathway from solution onto potential target particles by deposition of C3b via its metastable binding site.

Amplification, discrimination and control

Surface bound C3b is subject to two competing processes: amplification and control (i.e. inactivation). Amplification refers to deposition of additional C3b molecules around the original C3b molecule. This process commences with the binding of factor B to the first C3b molecule and its subsequent proteolytic cleavage into Ba and Bb by factor D. The resulting surface bound complex, $\overline{\text{C3b,Bb}}$, is a C3 convertase capable of generating C3b by cleavage of C3. Each subsequently bound C3b molecule can repeat this process of positive feedback (Müller-Eberhard and Götze, 1972). The alternative pathway feedback is relatively unique in that the product (C3b) of the substrate (C3) of the C3 activating enzyme ($\overline{\text{C3b,Bb}}$) becomes a subunit of that enzyme. Theoretically, the positive feedback must be of considerable biological importance. A very small event, insignificant by itself, such as deposition of one or a few molecules of C3b on a biological particle, may end up, given the appropriate microenvironment, in the formation of a molecule of C3 convertase, subsequent deposition of many more C3b molecules and thereby formation of many C3 convertase molecules. The feedback thus constitutes the driving force of the alternative pathway.

Without efficient control, this amplification system would deposit C3b indiscriminately on host cells and foreign particles alike. Control is primarily due to the binding of the plasma protein β1H (Whaley and Ruddy, 1976b) to a site on C3b distinct from, but competitive with the factor B binding site (Pangburn and Müller-Eberhard, 1978a). The resulting C3b, β1H complex is rapidly and irreversibly inactivated by C3bINA (Whaley and Ruddy, 1976b; Pangburn *et al.*, 1977). β1H also disassembles the convertase, dissociating Bb in inactive form (Conrad *et al.*, 1978).

The discriminatory event which allows this system to distinguish between host cells and activating particles lies in the dynamics of control versus amplification. Fearon and Austen (1977a, b) demonstrated that C3b bound to alternative pathway activators was more slowly inactivated than C3b bound to nonactivators. It was subsequently shown (Pangburn and Müller-Eberhard, 1978a, b; Schreiber *et al.*, 1978) that this effect was due to the ability of bound C3b rather than the control proteins to discriminate between activator and nonactivator. In the fluid phase or bound to nonactivators, C3b is inactivated before significant amplification occurs. Activators, however, restrict control without affecting amplification. Two hypotheses have been proposed to explain the mechanism of restricted control. It was suggested that negatively charged carbohydrates such as membrane bound sialic acid and heparin enhance control on nonactivators (Fearon, 1978; Kazatchkine *et al.*, 1979b). This mechanism does not explain the efficiency of control in the fluid phase. It was proposed therefore that a recognition site of C3b is capable of interacting with certain structures common to alternative pathway activators and that this interaction weakens or deactivates the β1H binding site of C3b (Pangburn *et al.*, 1980).

C3/C5 convertase and properdin

As the multiplicity of bound C3b molecules increases around each enzyme complex, the enzyme C5 convertase (C3b,Bb,3b) is formed from C3 convertase (Daha *et al.*, 1976; Medicus *et al.*, 1976). The additional C3b molecule is needed for modulation of C5 for enzymatic attack (Vogt *et al.*, 1978). The active site responsible for C3 and C5 cleavage resides in the Bb subunit of the enzyme. The C3/C5 convertase is innately labile and decays at 37°C with a half-life of 1·5 min (Fearon and Austen, 1975a; Medicus *et al.*, 1976). Decay is due to spontaneous dissociation of the Bb subunit in inactive form. Native properdin upon collision with the labile C3/C5 convertase becomes physically associated with it and "activated" in the process (Medicus *et al.*, 1976, 1980). Binding-activation of properdin results in stabilization of the enzyme such that its half-life at 37°C increases to 10 min.

The isolated cytolytic and bactericidal alternative pathway

Lysis of rabbit or neuraminidase-treated sheep erythrocytes

It has been possible to assemble the cytolytic alternative pathway entirely from 11 isolated proteins of human serum, the 6 proteins of the alternative pathway and the 5 proteins of the membrane attack pathway (Schreiber and Müller-Eberhard, 1978). The mixture containing physiological concentrations of the 11 proteins was stable during incubation at 37°C. When rabbit or neuraminidase-treated sheep erythrocytes were introduced into the mixture, the cells were rapidly lysed. Immunoglobulins were not present. Untreated sheep erythrocytes were neither lysed nor did they activate the purified system. It thus became clear that the 11 proteins constitute an intact cytolytic alternative pathway that is capable of coupling the initiation and amplification sequence with the cytolytic membrane attack sequence.

Killing of human lymphoblastoid cells

Lysis of Raji cells could be effected by the 11 proteins in complete absence of immunoglobulins (Schreiber *et al.*, 1980). The precise mechanism of Raji cell killing was investigated by correlating cellular binding of radiolabelled proteins with the release from the cytoplasm of radioactive markers and by measuring the effect of inhibition of protein synthesis on both events. A kinetic analysis of the measured events is shown in Fig. 4. Pathway activation was relatively rapid as evidenced by the fact that properdin uptake was maximal

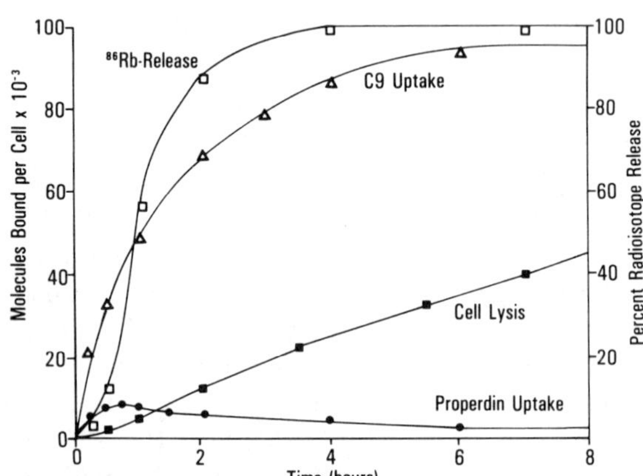

FIG. 4. *Injury and death of Raji cells caused by the purified cytolytic alternative pathway. Comparison of the kinetics of pathway activation (properdin uptake), membrane attack complex formation (C9 uptake), production of initial membrane lesion (^{86}Rb-release) and Raji cell lysis (^{51}Cr-release) (Schreiber* et al., *1980*).

at 1 h (8000 molecules per cell). Membrane attack complex formation was maximal at 4 h as indicated by C9 uptake (90 000 molecules per cell). Development of the initial membrane lesion (^{86}Rb-release) closely paralleled C9 uptake. However, cell death as measured by ^{51}Cr-release occurred slowly and reached completion only after 10–20 h. The rate of cell lysis was about 7 times lower than that of formation of the initial lesion. When cell metabolism was inhibited by puromycin, the kinetics of cell lysis paralleled that of C9 uptake and ^{86}Rb-release. The large lag between occurrence of the initial membrane lesion and cell lysis may be due to cellular defence against complement attack. This assumption is supported by disappearance of the lag following inhibition of cell metabolism. Nevertheless, it is remarkable that 90 000 C9 molecules per cell are not capable of effecting rapid cell death. Temporal resistance to lysis may not only be related to cellular defence, but also to the rate of accumulation of the membrane attack complex on the target cell. If this rate is high, the Raji cells lyse within minutes (Podack and Müller-Eberhard, unpublished observations).

Measles virus infected human cells also activate the alternative pathway and undergo subsequent lysis. This reaction was shown, however, to require antiviral antibody (Joseph *et al.*, 1975). Lately, it was found that while antibody is needed to effect lysis of measles virus infected cells, it is not required for the initiation of the alternative pathway as evidenced by C3b deposition on these cells (Sissons *et al.*, 1980).

Killing of Gram-negative bacteria

Utilizing the 11 isolated protein system it was shown that certain Gram-negative bacteria do activate the system in absence of immunoglobulin and are killed in the process. *E. coli* K12 W1485 introduced into the isolated system promptly lost viability (Schreiber *et al.*, 1979). Lysis of the bacteria required, in addition to the 11 proteins, lysozyme. Deletion of properdin reduced the killing or lytic activity of the system by 50%, indicating that properdin was not essential but enhanced the extent of the reaction. All other proteins including C9 were needed for bacterial killing and lysis. It appears therefore that maximal aggregation of the membrane attack complex is necessary to achieve the degree of reorganization of the outer lipid bilayer of the bacteria that effects killing.

Taken together, these applied studies indicate that the alternative pathway can be activated by a variety of cells in absence of antibody and that activation may proceed to lysis or killing erythrocytes, nucleated cells and bacteria.

The membrane attack pathway

Biomedical significance

The membrane attack complex (MAC) is exclusively responsible for the membranolytic activity of complement. For instance, the bactericidal activity of complement *in vitro* is entirely a function of the MAC. The ability of complement to abrogate the infectivity of viruses with a lipid membrane, including RNA tumour viruses, is due to the virolytic action of the MAC. Parasites in various stages of development are known to be susceptible *in vitro* to the killing action of the MAC. And cells of higher animals, including transformed or malignant cells, also succumb to MAC attack. Individuals with a homozygous deficiency of one of the MAC precursor proteins often suffer from repeated bacterial infections, particularly meningococcal meningitis and disseminated gonococcal infections.

The 5 MAC precursors are hydrophilic glycoproteins which are completely soluble in aqueous solutions. They have no affinity for lipids, detergents or biological and synthetic membranes. Upon activation of C5, they fuse in an orderly fashion into a unique tetradecamolecular complex. In the course of the fusion process, 2 novel events occur: a metastable membrane binding site is generated and a multiplicity of phospholipid binding sites are uncovered. It is through these sites that the MAC exerts its membranolytic effect. While the phospholipid binding function of the MAC has been firmly established, uncertainty prevails as to how the membrane permeability barrier is impaired by the MAC. There is no question as to whether the MAC forms a transmembrane channel. What is unanswered is whether the transmembrane ion flow caused by the MAC occurs through it or around it, that is to say, whether the hydrophilic channel is a protein or a lipid channel. In addition to forming channels, the MAC functions independent of channel formation. Some membranes such as viral envelopes that cannot be impaired by mere channel formers are practically disassembled or dissolved by MAC action.

The proteins

Some of the properties of the 5 MAC precursor proteins are listed in Table III. None of them has enzymatic activity. All have a carbohydrate moiety. C8 is somewhat unusual in that it has 3 nonidentical chains, 2 (α and γ) are linked by disulphide bridges, and the third (β) attached by noncovalent forces.

TABLE III
The proteins of the membrane attack pathway

Protein	*Molecular weight*	*No. of chains*	*Electroph. mobility*	*Serum conc. (µg/ml)*
C5	180 000	2	β_1	70
C6	128 000	1	β_2	60
C7	121 000	1	β_2	55
C8	154 000	3	γ_1	55
C9	72 000	1	α	60

As these 5 proteins function together, they display stereochemical affinity for each other. Reversible protein–protein interactions occur between C5 and C6, C7, C8 and between C8 and C9. This pattern of interactions reflects the eventual architecture of the MAC (Kolb *et al.*, 1973).

Assembly of the membrane attack complex

Assembly of the MAC is initiated by cleavage of peptide bond 74 of the α-chain of C5. Two complement enzymes are specialized to accomplish this task, the classical C5 convertase, C4b,2a,3b, and the alternative C5 convertase, C3b,Bb,3b. Both enzymes are exceedingly similar in subunit composition considering that C3 and C4 are homologous in primary structure and C2 and B are genetically linked. The reaction steps of MAC assembly are as follows:

$$\begin{aligned}
\text{C5} &\longrightarrow \text{C5a} + \text{C5b}^* \\
\text{C5b}^* + \text{C6} &\longrightarrow \text{C5b-6} \\
\text{C5b-6} + \text{C7} &\longrightarrow \text{C5b-7}^* \\
4\text{C5b-7}^* &\longrightarrow (\text{C5b-7})_4 \\
(\text{C5b-7})_4 + 4\text{C8} &\longrightarrow 4\text{C5b-8} \\
2\text{C5b-8} + 6\text{C9} &\longrightarrow 2\text{C5b-9} \\
2\text{C5b-9} &\longrightarrow (\text{C5b-9})_2
\end{aligned}$$

Nascent C5b forms a bimolecular complex with C6. The C5b-6 complex has a sedimentation rate of 11S, and by electron microscopic analysis, an elongated, slightly curved shape and dimensions of 16 nm × 6 nm × 6 nm. At protein concentrations > 1 mg/ml, and physiologic ionic strength and pH, the complex forms paracrystals that have the appearance of parallel strands. Equimolar quantities of C5b-6 and C7 mixed in the absence of lipids or detergents give rise to C5b-7 protein micelles which are soluble in aqueous media and have a sedimentation rate of 36S, suggesting a tetrameric composition. Ultrastructurally, C5b-7 protein micelles consist of 4 half-rings, each measuring 20 nm × 5 nm, which are connected to one another by short stalks extending from the convex side of the half-rings. C5b-7 bound to dioleoyl lecithin (DOL) vesicles has a similar ultrastructural appearance. After extraction with deoxycholate (DOC), C5b-7 has a sedimentation velocity of 36S which further suggests the occurrence of C5b-7 in the form of tetrameric protein micelles. Attachment of C8 to vesicle-bound C5b-7 results in dissociation of the protein micelles. An individual C5b-8 complex appears as a half-ring to the DOL-vesicle via a 10 nm long and 3 nm wide stalk. After extraction from the DOL-vesicles with DOC, C5b-8 has a sedimentation velocity of approximately 18S. Binding of C9 to DOL-vesicle bound C5b-8 induces the formation of the typical ultrastructural complement lesions. C5b-9 extracted from the vesicles with DOC has a sedimentation rate of 33S, which is characteristic of the C5b-9 dimer. It may be concluded that dimerization is a function of C9. C5b-9 monomers are visualized when a single C5b-9 complex or an odd number of complexes were bound per DOL-vesicle. The C5b-9 monomer has an ultrastructural appearance that is theoretically expected to be that of a half-dimer: a 20 nm × 5 nm half-ring which is attached to the DOL-vesicle by a 10 nm × 8 nm appendage. Extracted with DOC, the C5b-9 monomer has a sedimentation rate of 23S. At a higher multiplicity of MAC per DOL-vesicle, large structural defects in the lipid bilayer are seen which are attributed to direct physical destruction of membranes by the known lipid-binding capacity of the MAC. It is proposed that protein micelle formation at the C5b-7 stage of MAC assembly and dissociation of these micelles upon binding of C8 are events that facilitate dimerization of C5b-9 and thus MAC formation (Podack *et al.*, 1980). Similar studies utilizing erythrocytes rather than phospholipid vesicles were performed by Dourmashkin (1978). A schematic representation of dimeric MAC assembly is shown in Fig. 5.

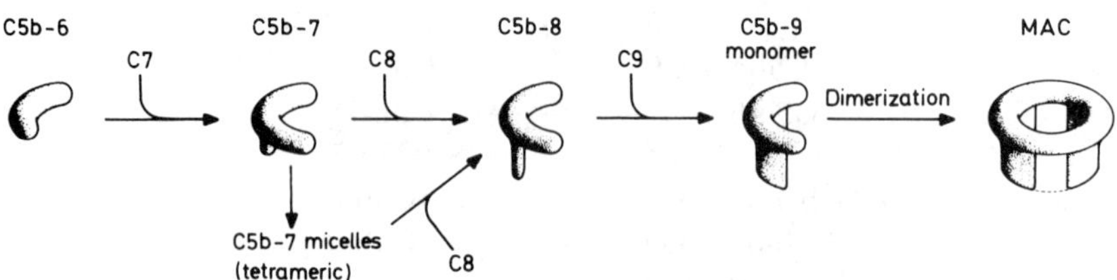

FIG. 5. *Schematic representation of structural aspects of MAC formation* (*Podack* et al., *1980*).

Thermodynamics and kinetics of formation of the membrane attack complex

The reaction of C5b-6 with C7, C8 and C9 was studied in cell free solution (Podack *et al.*, 1978a). Calculations indicated the binding of multiple C9 molecules per C5b-8 which contained equimolar amounts of C5b, C6, C7 and C8. The dissociation constants were calculated from Scatchard plots: K_D(C7) = 0·2 to 2·9 × 10^{-12}M, K_D(C8) = 0·9 to 8·6 × 10^{-12} M, and K_D (C9) = 0·1 to 0·5 × 10^{-12} M. The free energy for C5b-9 formation from C5b-6, C7, C8 and C9 was estimated to be −50kcal/mol. Inactivation of C5b-6 by C7 is a rapid, time and temperature dependent process following second-order kinetics. Complex formation at 37°C is diffusion controlled; at 4°C it is, in addition, controlled by activation energy requirement since the activation energy was 33·7 kcal/mol. Association of C5b-6 and C7 results in formation of a labile membrane binding site, C5b-7*, which decays rapidly to yield C5b-7_i. C5b-7 formation is the rate limiting step, decay of C5b-7* is rapid compared to the association reaction. The following thermodynamic parameters were obtained at 30°C for C5b-7_i formation from C5b-6 and C7: $\triangle G = -17$ kcal/mol, $\triangle H = +8{\cdot}6$ kcal/mol and $\triangle S = 77$ e.u. The data are compatible with the interpretation that the protein–protein interactions occurring upon complex formation are accompanied by release of protein-bound water or by conformational changes or both (Podack *et al.*, 1978a).

Control of membrane attack complex formation

MAC assembly is controlled by the *S*-protein of serum which binds to the forming complex and thus produces the hydrophilic, cytolytically inactive, decamolecular SC5b-9 complex. The *S*-protein, or MAC-inhibitor (Podack *et al.*, 1978b; Podack and Müller-Eberhard, 1978), is an acid α-glycoprotein having a molecular weight of 80 000 and a serum concentration of 0·5 mg/ml. Inhibition of MAC formation by the *S*-protein is expressed by the inhibition constant $K_i = 39\ \mu g/ml$ (Podack and Müller-Eberhard, 1979). A comparative electron microscopic analysis of the SC5b-9 complex and the MAC showed that while the MAC exhibited the above described structure, the hydrophilic SC5b-9 complex was strikingly similar to that of the amphiphilic C5b-9 monomer, showing a similar half-ring and perpendicular attachments. Proteolysis of SC5b-9 by trypsin and chymotrypsin in presence of 6 mM DOC led to dissociation of the *S*-protein and dimeric MAC formation. This observation suggests that *S*-protein binds to the forming C5b-9 complex at its membrane binding site and at sites involved in dimerization, thereby preventing membrane attack and MAC formation (Podack and Müller-Eberhard, 1980).

The dimer hypothesis

The conclusion that the MAC is the dimer of C5b-9 is based on two independent pieces of information. Compared to the hydrophilic SC5b-9 complex, the amphiphilic MAC extracted from complement lysed erythrocytes with 10% deoxycholate was approximately twice as large (Table IV) (Biesecker

TABLE IV

Physical evidence for MAC being the dimer of C5b-9

	s	*D*	*Mol. wt*
MAC	$33{\cdot}5 \times 10^{-13}$	$1{\cdot}79 \times 10^{-7}$	$1{\cdot}6 \times 10^{6}$
C5b-9	20×10^{-13}		$0{\cdot}76 \times 10^{6}$ [a]
SC5b-9	23×10^{-13}	$1{\cdot}98 \times 10^{-7}$	$1{\cdot}0 \times 10^{6}$

[a] SC5b-9 minus 3 × S.

et al., 1979). Second, in the electron microscope, the MAC had the appearance and dimensions that are characteristic for the complement produced ultrastructural membrane lesions (Biesecker *et al.*, 1979). By comparison, SC5b-9 and C5b-9 monomers attached to phospholipid vesicles (Podack *et al.*, 1980) appeared like half-dimers. Theoretically, the circular or cylindrical appearance (Tranum-Jensen *et al.*, 1978; Bhakdi and Tranum-Jensen, 1978) of the extracted MAC is readily explicable on the basis of a symmetrical structure. Since C5b-7 has the form of a half-ring which is lifted off the surface of target membranes by the attachment of C8 and C9, it may be concluded that the ring structure of the MAC is composed of two C5b-7 complexes and the vertical structure which is directly associated with the membrane is composed of two C8 molecules and 4 or 6 C9 molecules. A detailed delineation of the subunit topology of the MAC will require immunoelectron microscopic analysis which is in progress.

The mode of action

That the MAC can interact with lipid has been known for some time. Liposomes were shown to release internal markers (Haxby *et al.*, 1969) or to disintegrate (Lachmann *et al.*, 1970) under the influence of membrane attack by complement. MAC assembly on liposomes (Shin *et al.*, 1977) or gram-negative bacteria (Inoue *et al.*, 1977) was found to be accompanied by release of membrane lipid into the fluid phase. Mayer called this phenomenon "abortive insertion" of the MAC into the target membrane. Quantitation of the phospholipid binding capacity of the MAC documented its evolution as a function of progressing MAC assembly. Quantitative measurements of DOC binding showed increasing binding ability with the progression of complex assembly. C5b-6 and C5b-7 bound, respectively, 24 and 27 moles DOC/mole complex, C5b-8 and C5b-9 bound 63 and 86 moles DOC/mole complex, respectively, and the MAC bound 400 moles/mole. All complexes behaved as amphiphilic proteins upon charge shift electrophoresis (Podack and Müller-Eberhard, 1978). Using egg yolk lecithin for lipid binding studies, the molar phospholipid/protein ratios were found to be: C5b-7, 399 : 1; C5b-8, 841 : 1; C5b-9, 918 : 1; and C5b-9 dimer, 1460 : 1. Electron microscopy of the isolated phospholipid–protein complexes revealed no lipid bilayer structures. The magnitude of the phospholipid binding capacity of the MAC is consistent with the interpretation that the MAC forms phospholipid–protein complexes in lipid bilayers and biological membranes and thus causes formation of hydrophilic lipid channels (Podack *et al.*, 1979). Using spin-labelled derivatives of phospholipids and cholesterol and electron paramagnetic resonance spectroscopy, the penetration of the MAC into bilayers and its influence on the order of bilayers was measured. The MAC precursor components C5b-6, C7 and C9 did not exert any measurable influence on lipid membranes. Functional C5b-7 was shown to interact strongly with the bilayer surface without deep penetration into the bilayer. Formation of C5b-8 and especially C5b-9 caused a marked change in the anisotropy of spectra from probes located within the hydrocarbon phase. The spectral changes may be interpreted to be the result of reorientation of ordered bilayer lipids effected by strong binding of phospholipids to MAC proteins (Esser *et al.*, 1979a).

The effects of the MAC, nystatin and melittin were compared on the envelope of murine leukaemia viruses to determine if channel formation alone is sufficient to cause membranolysis. Nystatin is a channel former and melittin is not, although both are haemolytic. Whereas MAC and melittin disintegrated the viral membrane, nystatin had no effect on morphology, integrity and infectivity of the virus. These results are interpreted to indicate that virolysis by MAC is not caused by channel formation and, conversely, in the absence of colloid-osmotic effects, channel formation by itself is not sufficient to disassemble a viral membrane (Esser *et al.*, 1979b).

It may be concluded that the MAC exerts a direct physical effect on the target membrane which causes a weakening and eventual disassembly of the membrane through reorganization of bilayer lipids into more micellar domains. The simultaneous formation of hydrophilic lipid or protein channels facilitates target cell destruction provided an osmotic gradient is normally maintained across the target membrane.

Conclusion

C3 constitutes the pivotal protein of the complement system. An increasing understanding of its chemical structure has allowed the tentative definition of the initial events of the alternative pathway and the chemical mode of C3b binding to complement targets via its metastable binding site. C3b fulfills its biological functions by bringing into play 8 binding sites which specifically interact with certain proteins, carbohydrates or cell surface receptors. The distribution, specificity and function of these cellular C3 receptors have partially been elucidated. The C5 convertase formed as a consequence of classical or alternative pathway activation initiates the assembly of the tetradecamolecular MAC. The ability of the MAC to bind to and to disorganize biological membranes rests upon its phospholipid binding capacity. The ultrastructure and subunit topology of this unusual supramolecular organization as well as the question as to whether it causes the formation of transmembrane proteins or lipid channels have been presented.

Because of space limitations, the classical pathway of complement activation could not be treated. Attention should be directed, however, to the following topics: mechanism of antibody-independent C1 activation on murine leukaemia viruses (Bartholomew and Esser, 1980); antibody-dependent C1 activation by fluid and solid liposomes (Parce *et al.*, 1980); activation and control of the first complement component (Cooper and Ziccardi, 1977; Ziccardi and Cooper, 1979); modulation of the classical pathway C3 convertase by C4 binding protein and C3b inactivator (Gigli *et al.*, 1979) and C4a, a third anaphylatoxin (Gorski *et al.*, 1979a).

References

Allen, F. H., Jr. (1974). *Vox Sang.* **27**, 382.

Alper, C. A., Collen, H. R., Rosen, F. S., Rabson, A. R., Macnab, G. M. and Gear, J. S. S. (1972). *Lancet* **ii**, 1179.

Bartholomew, R. M. and Esser, A. F. (1980). *Biochemistry* (in press).

Bhakdi, S. and Tranum-Jensen, J. (1978). *Proc. Natn. Acad. Sci. U.S.A.* **75**, 5655.
Biesecker, G., Podack, E. R., Halverson, C. A. and Müller-Eberhard, H. J. (1979). *J. Exp. Med.* **149**, 448.
Bokisch, V. A. and Müller-Eberhard, H. J. (1970). *J. Clin. Invest.* **49**, 2427.
Bokisch, V. A., Dierich, M. P. and Müller-Eberhard, H. J. (1975). *Proc. Natn. Acad. Sci. U.S.A.* **72**, 1989.
Brade, V., Hall, R. E. and Colten, H. R. (1977). *J. Exp. Med.* **146**, 759.
Budzko, D. B., Bokisch, V. A. and Müller-Eberhard, H. J. (1971). *Biochemistry* **10**, 1166.
Cochrane, C. G. and Müller-Eberhard, H. J. (1968). *J. Exp. Med.* **127**, 371.
Conrad, D. H., Carlo, J. R. and Ruddy, S. (1978). *J. Exp. Med.* **147**, 1792.
Cooper, N. R. (1969). *Science* **165**, 396.
Cooper, N. R. and Ziccardi, R. J. (1977). *J. Immunol.* **119**, 1664.
Curnette, J. T. and Babior, B. M. (1974). *J. Clin. Invest.* **53**, 1662.
Daha, M. R., Fearon, D. T. and Austen, K. F. (1976). *J. Immunol.* **117**, 630.
Dalmasso, A. P. and Müller-Eberhard, H. J. (1966). *J. Immunol.* **97**, 680.
Dias Da Silva, W., Eisele, J. W. and Lepow, I. H. (1967). *J. Exp. Med.* **126**, 1027.
Dierich, M. P. and Landen, B. (1977). *J. Exp. Med.* **146**, 1484.
Dourmashkin, R. R. (1978). *Immunology* **35**, 205.
Esser, A. F., Kolb, W. P., Podack, E. R. and Müller-Eberhard, H. J. (1979a). *Proc. Natn. Acad. Sci. U.S.A.* **76**, 1410.
Esser, A. F., Bartholomew, R. M., Jensen, F. C. and Müller-Eberhard, H. J. (1979b). *Proc. Natn. Acad. Sci. U.S.A.* **76**, 5843.
Fearon, D. T. (1978). *Proc. Natn. Acad. Sci. U.S.A.* **75**, 1971.
Fearon, D. T. and Austen, K. F. (1975a). *J. Exp. Med.* **142**, 856.
Fearon, D. T. and Austen, K. F. (1975b). *J. Immunol.* **115**, 1357.
Fearon, D. T. and Austen, K. F. (1977a). *J. Exp. Med.* **146**, 22.
Fearon, D. T. and Austen, K. F. (1977b). *Proc. Natn. Acad. Sci. U.S.A.* **74**, 1683.
Fernandez, H. N. and Hugli, T. E. (1978). *J. Biol. Chem.* **253**, 6955.
Fu, S. M., Kunkel, H. G., Brusman, H. P., Allen, F. H., Jr. and Fotino, M. (1974). *J. Exp. Med.* **140**, 1108.
Ghebrehiwet, B. and Müller-Eberhard, H. J. (1979). *J. Immunol.* **123**, 616.
Gigli, I. and Nelson, R. A., Jr. (1968). *Exp. Cell Res.* **51**, 45.
Gigli, I., Fujita, T. and Nussenzweig, V. (1979). *Proc. Natn. Acad. Sci. U.S.A.* **76**, 6596.
Goldstein, I. M., Roos, D., Kaplan, H. B. and Weissmann, G. (1975). *J. Clin. Invest.* **56**, 1155.
Gorski, J. P., Hugli, T. E. and Müller-Eberhard, H. J. (1979a). *Proc. Natn. Acad. Sci. U.S.A.* **76**, 5299.
Gorski, J. P., Hugli, T. E. and Müller-Eberhard, H. J. (1979b). *Fed. Proc.* **38**, 1010.
Gorski, J. P., Hugli, T. E. and Müller-Eberhard, H. J. (1980). *Biochemistry* (submitted).
Hall, R. E. and Colten, H. R. (1977). *Proc. Natn. Acad. Sci. U.S.A.* **74**, 1707.
Haxby, J. A., Götze, O., Müller-Eberhard, H. J. and Kinsky, S. C. (1969). *Proc. Natn. Acad. Sci. U.S.A.* **64**, 290.
Howard, J. B., Vermeulen, M. and Swenson, R. P. (1980). *J. Biol. Chem.* **255**, 3820.
Huber, H., Polley, M. J., Linscott, W. D., Fudenberg, H. H. and Müller-Eberhard, H. J. (1968). *Science* **162**, 1281.
Hugli, T. E. (1975). *J. Biol. Chem.* **250**, 8293.
Hugli, T. E., Morgan, W. T. and Müller-Eberhard, H. J. (1975). *J. Biol. Chem.* **250**, 1479.
Inoue, K., Kinoshita, T., Okada, M. and Akiyama, Y. (1977). *J. Immunol.* **119**, 65.
Joseph, B. S., Cooper, N. R. and Oldstone, M. B. A. (1975). *J. Exp. Med.* **141**, 761.
Kazatchkine, M. D., Fearon, D. T. and Austen, K. F. (1979a). *J. Immunol.* **122**, 75.
Kazatchkine, M. D., Fearon, D. T., Silbert, J. E. and Austen, K. F. (1979b). *J. Exp. Med.* **150**, 1202.

Kolb, W. P., Haxby, J. A., Arroyave, C. M. and Müller-Eberhard, H. J. (1973). *J. Exp. Med.* **138**, 428.
Lachmann, P. J. (1979). *Behring Inst. Mitteilungen* **63**, 25.
Lachmann, P. J. and Müller-Eberhard, H. J. (1968). *J. Immunol.* **100**, 691.
Lachmann, P. J., Munn, E. A. and Weissmann, G. (1970). *Immunology* **19**, 983.
Law, S. K. and Levine, R. P. (1977). *Proc. Natn. Acad. Sci. U.S.A.* **74**, 2701.
Law, S. K., Fearon, D. T. and Levine, R. P. (1979a). *J. Immunol.* **122**, 759.
Law, S. K., Lichtenberg, N. A. and Levine, R. P. (1979b). *J. Immunol.* **123**, 1388.
Lesavre, P. and Müller-Eberhard, H. J. (1978). *J. Exp. Med.* **148**, 1498.
Mann, J., O'Brien, R., Alper, C. A., Rosen, F. S. and Babior, B. M. (1980). *J. Immunol.* **124**, 1531.
Medicus, R. G., Götze, O. and Müller-Eberhard, H. J. (1976). *J. Exp. Med.* **144**, 1076.
Medicus, R. G., Esser, A. F., Fernandez, H. N. and Müller-Eberhard, H. J. (1980). *J. Immunol.* **124**, 602.
Morgan, W. T., Vallota, E. H. and Müller-Eberhard, H. J. (1974). *Biochem. Biophys. Res. Comm.* **57**, 572.
Müller-Eberhard, H. J. (1961). *Acta Soc. Medi. Upsaliensis* **66**, 152.
Müller-Eberhard, H. J. and Götze, O. (1972). *J. Exp. Med.* **135**, 1003.
Müller-Eberhard, H. J. and Lepow, I. H. (1965). *J. Exp. Med.* **121**, 819.
Müller-Eberhard, H. J. and Nilsson, U. R. (1960). *J. Exp. Med.* **111**, 217.
Müller-Eberhard, H. J. and Schreiber, R. D. (1980). *Adv. Immunol.* **29**, 1.
Müller-Eberhard, H. J., Dalmasso, A. P. and Calcott, M. A. (1966). *J. Exp. Med.* **123**, 33.
Müller-Eberhard, H. J., Nilsson, U. R. and Aronsson, T. (1960). *J. Exp. Med.* **111**, 201.
Nagaki, K., Iida, K., Okubo, M. and Inai, S. (1978). *Int. Arch. Allergy Appl. Immunol.* **57**, 221.
Nilsson, U. R., Mandle, R. J., Jr. and McConnell-Mapes, J. A. (1975). *J. Immunol.* **114**, 815.
Ooi, Y. M. and Colten, H. R. (1980). *J. Immunol.* **124**, 1534.
Pangburn, M. K. and Müller-Eberhard, H. J. (1978a). *Proc. Natn. Acad. Sci. U.S.A.* **75**, 2416.
Pangburn, M. K. and Müller-Eberhard, H. J. (1978b). *J. Immunol.* **120**, 1791.
Pangburn, M. K. and Müller-Eberhard, H. J. (1980). *J. Exp. Med.* (in press).
Pangburn, M. K., Schreiber, R. D. and Müller-Eberhard, H. J. (1977). *J. Exp. Med.* **146**, 257.
Pangburn, M. K., Morrison, D. C., Schreiber, R. D. and Müller-Eberhard, H. J. (1980). *J. Immunol.* **124**, 977.
Parce, J. W., McConnell, H. M., Bartholomew, R. M. and Esser, A. F. (1980). *Biochem. Biophys. Res. Comm.* **93**, 235.
Perlmann, H., Perlmann, P., Schreiber, R. D. and Müller-Eberhard, H. J. (1980). *J. Exp. Med.* (submitted).
Podack, E. R. and Müller-Eberhard, H. J. (1978). *J. Immunol.* **121**, 1025.
Podack, E. R. and Müller-Eberhard, H. J. (1979). *J. Biol. Chem.* **254**, 9908.
Podack, E. R. and Müller-Eberhard, H. J. (1980). *J. Immunol.* **124**, 1779.
Podack, E. R., Biesecker, G., Kolb, W. P. and Müller-Eberhard, H. J. (1978a). *J. Immunol.* **121**, 484.
Podack, E. R., Kolb, W. P. and Müller-Eberhard, H. J. (1978b). *J. Immunol.* **120**, 1841.
Podack, E. R., Biesecker, G. and Müller-Eberhard, H. J. (1979). *Proc. Natn. Acad. Sci. U.S.A.* **76**, 897.
Podack, E. R., Esser, A. F., Biesecker, G. and Müller-Eberhard, H. J. (1980). *J. Exp. Med.* **151**, 301.

Ross, G. D. and Rabellino, E. M. (1979). *Fed. Proc.* **38**, 1467.
Ross, G. D., Polley, M. J., Rabellino, E. M. and Grey, H. M. (1973). *J. Exp. Med.* **138**, 798.
Ruddy, S. and Austen, K. F. (1971). *J. Immunol.* **107**, 742.
Schreiber, R. D. and Müller-Eberhard, H. J. (1974). *J. Exp. Med.* **140**, 1324.
Schreiber, R. D. and Müller-Eberhard, H. J. (1978). *J. Exp. Med.* **148**, 1722.
Schreiber, R. D., Medicus, R. G., Götze, O. and Müller-Eberhard, H. J. (1975). *J. Exp. Med.* **143**, 760.
Schreiber, R. D., Morrison, D. C., Podack, E. R. and Müller-Eberhard, H. J. (1979). *J. Exp. Med.* **149**, 870.
Schreiber, R. D., Pangburn, M. K., Lesavre, P. H. and Müller-Eberhard, H. J. (1978). *Proc. Natn. Acad. Sci. U.S.A.* **75**, 3948.
Schreiber, R. D., Pangburn, M. K., Medicus, R. G. and Müller-Eberhard, H. J. (1980). *Clin. Immunol. Immunopathol.* **15**, 384.
Shin, M. L., Paznekas, W. A., Abramovitz, A. S. and Mayer, M. M. (1977). *J. Immunol.* **119**, 1358.
Sim, R. B. and Sim, E. (1980). *Biochem. J.* (*Mol. Asp.*) (in press).
Sim, R. B., Twose, T. M., Patterson, D. S. and Sim, E. (1980). *Biochem. J.* (*Mol. Asp.*) (in press).
Sissons, J. G. P., Oldstone, M. B. A. and Schreiber, R. D. (1980). *Proc. Natn. Acad. Sci. U.S.A.* **77**, 559.
Swenson, R. P. and Howard, J. B. (1979). *Proc. Natn. Acad. Sci. U.S.A.* **76**, 4313.
Tack, B. F., Morris, S. C. and Prahl, J. W. (1979). *Biochemistry* **18**, 1497.
Tack, B. F., Janatova, J., Lorenz, P. E., Schechter, A. N. and Prahl, J. W. (1980). *J. Immunol.* **124**, 1542.
Tamura, N. and Nelson, R. A., Jr. (1967). *J. Immunol.* **99**, 582.
Tranum-Jensen, J., Bhakdi, S., Bhakdi-Lehnen, B., Bjerrum, O. J. and Speth, V. (1978). *Scand. J. Immunol.* **7**, 45.
Vogt, W., Dames, W., Schmidt, G. and Dieminger, L. (1977). *Immunochemistry* **14**, 201.
Vogt, W., Schmidt, G., vonButlar, B. and Dieminger, L. (1978). *Immunology* **34**, 29.
Vranian, G., Conrad, D. and Ruddy, S. (1980). *J. Immunol.* **124**, 1544.
Weiler, J. M., Daha, M. R., Austen, K. F. and Fearon, D. T. (1976). *Proc. Natn. Acad. Sci. U.S.A.* **73**, 3268.
Whaley, K. and Ruddy, S. (1976a). *J. Exp. Med.* **144**, 1147.
Whaley, K. and Ruddy, S. (1976b). *Science* **193**, 1011.
Ziccardi, R. J. and Cooper, N. R. (1979). *J. Immunol.* **123**, 788.

55

Involvement of Immune Complexes in Disease

URS E. NYDEGGER, M. D. KAZATCHKINE and P. H. LAMBERT

WHO Immunology Research and Training Center, Department of Medicine, University of Geneva and Central Laboratory of the Swiss Red Cross, Blood Transfusion Service, Berne, Switzerland

Introduction

Antigen-antibody complexes are involved in the pathogenesis of a large variety of human and animal diseases. Humoral and cellular immune responses co-operate in the formation of antibody efficiently complexing with antigen; therefore, the finding of circulating, or tissue-deposited immune complexes always reflects ongoing or past immune defence. There is no information, however, on the efficiency of the immune response which can be drawn from the detection of immune complexes; in one situation, or when present for a short time, such complexes reflect the successful removal of antigen; in another situation, their chronic presence could express inefficient antigen removal. The introduction into clinical medicine of new and more sensitive methods for the detection of immune complexes has led to the description of a large catalogue of diseases associated with circulating immune complexes, including systemic lupus erythematosus (SLE), rheumatoid arthritis (RA), necrotizing vasculitis, various bacterial, viral and parasitic diseases, a number of renal, haematologic, neoplastic, dermatological and some other rather rare conditions (Table I).

The role originally assigned to the presence of immune complexes in confirming or ruling out a working diagnosis has therefore lost some of its importance. Nevertheless, detection of immune complexes remains an important tool in clinical medicine for the following reasons:

(a) In the study of immune complexes it is hoped that, by identification of the antigen, it will be possible to define the cause of the disease. Tissue constituents, drugs and infectious (viral, bacterial and parasitic) antigens have been found in immune complexes.

(b) Study of the molecular composition of immune complexes may give an insight into their pathogenic potential. Thus, pathogenicity of immune complexes depends upon the physicochemical and biological properties of the antigen, antibody and their product, i.e. the mol. wt and antigenic valency of the antigen, the class, subclass and affinity of the specific antibody; the relative ratio of antigen to antibody within the complex; the ability of the complex to activate complement by the classical or alternative pathway, through the antigen or through the antibody, and its ability to react with rheumatoid factors or with various cellular receptor systems.

(c) The demonstration in a clinical sample of the presence of soluble immune complexes, together with that of a disequilibrium in the normal homeostasis of the complement system, strongly suggests their pathogenic role.

(d) Monitoring of serum immune complexes has become an important criterion during attempts to treat diseases associated with such complexes by means of plasma exchange or by means of *ex vivo* absorption of the complexes.

The purpose of this review is to define the conditions under which immune

TABLE I

Human diseases in which immune complexes have been observed

1. Idiopathic inflammatory diseases

SLE
RA, juvenile RA
Ankylosing spondylitis (seropositive form)
Essential cryoglobulinaemia
Scleroderma
Wegener's granulomatosis

2. Infectious diseases

Bacterial — streptococcal, staphylococcal, subacute endocarditis, pneumococcal, *Klebsiella*, *Mycoplasma pneumoniae*, *M. leprae*
Viral — hepatitis B, acute and chronic hepatitis, Dengue fever, infectious mononucleosis, cytomegalovirus disease of the newborn
Parasitic — malaria, trypanosomiasis, toxoplasmosis, leishmaniasis, filariasis, schistosomiasis

3. Renal diseases

Acute glomerulonephritis (GN)
Primitive GN with granular deposits
IgA nephropathy
Renal transplants

4. Haematological and neoplastic diseases

Acute lymphoblastic and myeloblastic leukaemia; chronic lymphocytic leukaemia
Hodgkin's disease
Solid tumours: lung, breast, colon, melanoma
Severe haemophilia
Immune haemolytic anaemia

2. Dermatological diseases

Dermatitis herpetiformis, pemphigus and bullous pemphigoig, urticaria
Pityriasis lichenoides

6. Diseases of the gastrointestinal tract

Coeliac disease, Chrohn's disease, ulterative colitis
Chronic active hepatitis. Primary biliary cirrhosis

7. Neurological diseases

Subacute sclerosing panencephalitis, amyotrophic lateral sclerosis
Guillain-Barré syndrome

8. Endocrinological diseases

Autoimmune thyroiditis (Hashimoto)
Juvenile diabetes

9. Iatrogenic diseases

Acute serum sickness
D-penicilline nephropathy
Gold nephropathy
Drug-induced thrombocytopaenia

10. Miscellaneous

Retinal vasculitis
Hereditary angioedema
Myocardial infarction
Milk allergy
Behçet's disease

complexes are formed, to discuss the biological implications of locally formed, as well as circulating, immune complexes, and to consider the various methods used for the detection of circulating immune complexes. Finally, some immunopathological aspects of immune complexes in human disease and some therapeutic possibilities will be discussed.

Antigen requirements for immune complex formation

Antigens are substances which can induce an immunologic response when introduced in a host. The term antigenicity encompasses two different capacities: (1) immunogenicity, i.e. ability to provoke an immune response regardless of specificity; and (2) antigenic specificity, i.e. the competence of a molecule to react specifically with an antibody. Antigens possess one or, mostly, several antigenic determinants, the number and density of which depend on both, chemical formula and molecular structure. Following contact with an antigen, the host organism may produce circulating antibody, may be primed without producing antibody, may develop delayed hypersensitivity, or become immunologically unresponsive. Persistent antigenaemia is more likely to induce an immune response than transient antigenaemia. Self-replicating *viruses*, which may be of low cytopathogenicity, e.g. hepatitis B virus, constitute a chronic source of antigen. This may easily lead, when coinciding with persistent antibody production, to formation of immune complexes. *Bacteria*, when chronically circulating or especially when growing in encapsulated inflammatory foci, may produce antigenic products that are immunogenic on their own. By changing antigenic subspecificities during a disease course, bacteria may also lead to simultaneous occurrence of immune complexes involving different specificities and thus behave pathogenetically different. Finally, in *parasitic* diseases, long-term formation of immune complexes involving antigens released from living or dying parasites would seem likely. The site of formation of such complexes depends on the distribution of parasites and their antigens in the host at the time of the immune response. It is probable that most of the immune complexes in parasitic diseases are formed in antibody excess at the site of parasitic localization.

Autologous antigens often participate in immune complex formation. In rheumatoid arthritis, the major antigen in immune complexes is the immunoglobulin molecule. Evidence was obtained, that some immune complexes found in patients with this disease may be a result of self-association of IgG molecules which have rheumatoid factor (RF) activity (Pope *et al.*, 1974). It has also been shown that anti-IgG molecules represent a high proportion of the antibodies produced in the rheumatoid synovium. Since it is known that synovium from a single joint can produce up to 90 mg of IgG per day, there is a high probability that such self-association may occur extensively. In SLE, antibody formation is directed at a large variety of native or altered autologous antigens. These antibodies are presumably involved in the pathogenesis of SLE through combination with soluble tissue antigens released in circulating blood or in extravascular spaces. Of several antigen–antibody systems, the deoxyribonucleic acid (DNA)–anti-DNA complexes have been observed to form a major part of immune complexes to be localized in renal and skin lesions (Koffler *et al.*, 1967). However, in view of recent findings in our laboratory, the presence of large amounts of DNA–anti-DNA complexes in circulating blood of SLE patients is unlikely and most of the complexes detected in SLE sera probably involve other antigen–antibody systems (Izui *et al.*, 1977b). Thus, some isologous plasma proteins are capable of eliciting the synthesis of anti-idiotypic antibodies; such antibodies may even occur naturally during the course of a humoral immune response. It has been observed in our laboratories that anti-idiotypic antibodies reacting with the corresponding idiotypic determinants on other antibody molecules may represent a source of circulating immune complexes (Rose and Lambert, 1980), and circulating idiotype–anti-idiotype antigen–antibody complexes have indeed been detected in normal human sera (Morgan *et al.*, 1979).

Physiological and pathogenetic role of immune complex formation

Although the term immune complex disease has become a routinely used designation in clinical nomenclature, we must consider the possibility that immune complex formation may often be a desirable phenomenon serving fast removal of the antigen. Theoretically, this eventuality is obvious; thus, formation of high affinity antibody of the IgG type during the secondary immune response should accelerate removal of antigen when compared to formation of low affinity IgM type antibody during the primary immune response.

Antibodies of low affinity may fail to form immune complexes with a stable lattice resulting in failure of immune elimination of antigen and giving rise to formation of relatively small, antigen excess immune complexes. It has been observed in murine experiments by Steward (1979) that immune complexes between human serum albumin (HSA) and anti-HSA were slightly larger and less heterogeneous in mice producing high affinity antibodies as compared to those observed in mice producing low affinity antibody. In low affinity mice, there was also a greater intensity of pathological immune deposits in the renal glomeruli as compared to high affinity antibody producing mice. These findings were consistent with earlier observations by Germuth and Rodriguez (1973), who found that small soluble immune complexes localize on the glomerular basement membrane as subepithelial deposits whereas larger slightly less soluble complexes were found mainly in the subendothelial mesangial region. Finally, it is well known that complex formation between antigen and antibody may lead to prolonged contact of the immune system with antigen, since it has been shown that such complexes deposit in the lymphoid organs, thus facilitating extensive immune recognition of the antigen.

Removal of immune complexes from the organism proceeds through at least two different mechanisms. The first is through interaction of complexes with the reticuloendothelial system, now also termed mononuclear phagocyte system, particularly through those of its cellular constituents which exhibit receptors for the Fc fragment of complexed immunoglobulins. Such receptors have been found on lymphocytes, macrophages and Kupffer cells, but also on the surface of "nonimmune" cells such as platelets, hepatocytes, cells of the human glomerulus, synoviocytes, chorioid plexus and some malignant cells. The integral function of these receptors for clearance of immune complexes has been stressed again recently, when it was proposed that their insufficiency may favour prolonged circulation of circulating immune complexes in SLE (Frank *et al.*, 1979). Binding of immune complexes to Fc receptors depends on various physicochemical properties of the complexes. Binding to lymphocytes is highest with complexes formed at equivalence or in slight antigenic excess. In addition, immunoglobulin aggregates, monomeric immunoglobulins and even their Fc fragments are able to bind to Fc receptors. Binding of monomeric immunoglobulins is more specific with respect to the different immunoglobulin classes but becomes unspecific with aggregation or immune complex formation. It is assumed that complexed or aggregated immunoglobulins bind with higher affinity to Fc receptors than their monomeric elements.

Accordingly, cells which are equipped with complement receptors, such as erythrocytes, lymphocytes, neutrophils, eosinophils and macrophages, could also assist in clearance of immune complexes which carry complement components on their lattic structure. Recent studies have shown phagocytosis of soluble immune complexes via C3 receptors without the necessity of Fc receptor participation (van Snick and Masson, 1978). The second removal mechanism for immune complexes is their clearance through filtering membranes, provided they are small enough to leave the circulation, which is the case when the antigen is small and when complexes are formed in large antigenic excess. This removal mechanism is likely to lead to tissue injury secondary to trapping of the complexes favouring local pathogenic effects such as complement activation.

Reaction of immune complexes with humoral receptors

The immune system features several mechanisms which can influence the pathogenetic effect of immune complexes. Rheumatoid factors (RF), complement and immunoconglutinin are the most efficient humoral receptors for modulating properties such as size, solubility and tissue affinity of complexes.

Rheumatoid factors are anti-IgG antibodies and react with the Fc portion of altered IgG (Johnson and Faulk, 1976), including IgG antibody which has reacted with its specific antigen. A number of *in vivo* studies have suggested that RF may play a role in the modification of immune complexes and immune aggregates. In one series of experiments, IgM-RF was regularly able to prevent the expected fall in serum complement levels in rats given intraperitoneal injections of aggregated IgG (Gough and Davis, 1966). RF appeared to block absorption of intact aggregates either through formation of larger aggregates or by facilitating the catabolism of aggregates. After intraperitoneal injection of labelled IgG, either alone or with IgM-RF, it was apparent that the level of radioactivity in sera and organs of rats also given RF was decreased compared to the controls: this suggested a protective function of IgM-RF. RF may alter the binding of immune complexes or aggregated IgG via the C3b receptor described in renal glomeruli (Schrock *et al.*, 1977). Also, IgM-RF was found to inhibit complement binding by red cell-bound aggregates.

Immunoconglutinin (IK) is another factor which might alter the immunopathogenetic characteristics of immune complexes. This is an antibody, primarily of the IgM class, which is directed at activated complement components, particularly C3b and activated C4. It reacts *in vitro* with antigen–antibody-complement complexes, markedly enhancing their clumping. In man it is produced in response to immunization, during certain infections, and in many patients with rheumatic diseases. This antibody may have an important bearing on immune complex metabolism, distribution and target organ effects. For example, on one hand it might enhance complement fixation; on the other hand, it might inhibit C3b binding to membrane receptors. Its role in augmenting aggregation of complement-containing complexes may be a balance to the recently described solubilization of complexes by C3b. Whether the net effect of IK is detrimental or beneficial to the host may depend on a delicate balance of certain specific factors.

Another autoantibody, of the IgG class, which has been identified for its specificity against bound complement, is nephritic factor (NeF). The specificity of NeF is directed towards the alternative pathway convertase C3b,Bb, and more precisely against antigenic determinants on Bb which are exposed after interaction of Bb with C3b (Daha and van Es, 1980). NeF considerably prolongs the half-life time of the C3 convertase protecting it from decay-dissociation by β1H (Daha *et al.*, 1977). NeF is found in some forms of membranoproliferative glomerulonephritis and in partial lipodystrophia (Sissons *et al.*, 1976).

The complement system is probably the most important humoral receptor for immune complexes to influence their pathogenicity inasmuch as the immune complex–complement interaction can be detrimental or beneficial for the host. Of course, complement activation by immune complexes is the hallmark and initial event in complex-induced damage giving rise to generation of the anaphylatoxins C3a and C5a. The highly active breakdown products of C3 and C5 lead to increased vascular permeability by causing mast cell degranulation and histamine release. This immune complex induced complement activation in inflammatory phenomenon has been extensively studied and reviewed (Cochrane and Dixon, 1976; Hugli and Müller-Eberhard, 1978).

Apart from its role in immune recognition, the complement system also has a regulatory function in immune phenomena. This is possible because the 20 plasma complement proteins features inbuilt control mechanisms, one of which is the "amplification loop" or alternative pathway. The dual role of this pathway in the initiation of complement activation and in the intrinsic regulation of the complement sequence is now well recognized. Because of the normal presence of $\overline{D}$, the interactions of the activating components of the alternative pathway must be equilibrated with regulatory proteins. Continuous low grade generation of C3b by the fluid phase interaction of purified native C3, B, P and $\overline{D}$ is normally prevented from advancing to C3b-dependent amplified C3 cleavage by the control proteins, C3bINA and β1H (reviewed in Fearon *et al.*, 1976). However, once amplification convertase C3b,Bb if formed, its spontaneous decay may be considerably retarded by properdin interacting with C3b to form the complex P,C3b,Bb, which is the stable and active form of the convertase. The combined actions of component proteins, which tend to assemble the amplification convertase, and of the control proteins, which tend to dissociate it, can be understood as a balance, where even very modest modifications in the concentration of proteins on either side can disturb its equilibrium (Nydegger *et al.*, 1978). One obvious implication of these findings which has practical importance became apparent when it was discovered by Miller and Nussenzweig (1975) that complement may lead to solubilization of immune complexes. Immune precipitates formed by bovine serum albumin (BSA) and antibodies to BSA dissolve rapidly when incubated in fresh serum. The key role of complement in immune complex solubilization capacity (ICSC) was postulated because treatments, such as heat inactivation, that destroyed complement in serum, also removed ICSC. Moreover, ICSC is mediated through the binding of C3b to the immune complexes and follows cleavage of native C3 mainly through activation of the alternative complement pathway, but activation of the classical $\overline{C42}$ C3 convertase could at least favour initial deposition of C3b on the complex.

It is possible that after spontaneous dissociation of antigen from antibody, the presence of C3 peptides on the antibody may prevent reassociation and cross-linking with antigen. Furthermore, C3b fragments may interfere with lattice formation by inhibiting the interactions between Fc fragments which occur during complex formation. That the ICSC phenomenon is pertinent also to human pathology has recently been confirmed in our laboratories, when formation of immune precipitates between tetanus toxoid and hepatitis B surface antigen and their corresponding antibodies was prevented by fresh serum, but not by complement depleted human serum (Casali and Lambert, 1979).

Methods for the detection of soluble immune complexes

Most of the methods for detection of soluble immune complexes are "antigen-nonspecific" as they deal with complexes of unknown specificity. "Antigen-specific" methods, on the other hand, only apply to those rare clinical circumstances where the complexed antigen has been identified. The reader is referred to several reviews which have appeared on this topic (Maini, 1977; Zubler and Lambert, 1977; Theophilopoulos and Dixon, 1979).

Physicochemical methods

The main advantage of this group of methods is that it is preparative, allowing, in addition to detection, further characterization of the complexes. Thus, search for cryoglobulins has often been used as a screening method for the presence of immune complexes. However, it lacks specificity and should be completed by demonstration of the presence of complement components, rheumatoid factor activity, or immunoglobulin of different classes (mixed cryoglobulinaemia) within the cryoprecipitate. Detection of soluble complexes can also be achieved by procedures which take advantage of their molecular weight, such as chromatography and ultracentrifugation in sucrose density gradients. Indeed, the demonstration of immunoglobulin or C3 in high mol. wt fractions from chromatographed or centrifuged sera, is very suggestive of their complexed nature (Amlot *et al.*, 1976). Polyethylene glycol (PEG) is known to enhance precipitation of antigen/antibody complexes and to fractionate plasma proteins according to the size of the molecules and their electric charge. For example, at 2% final concentration and at pH 7·4, PEG 6000 precipitates no more than 1–2% of plasma monomeric IgG. Thus, the presence of a higher amount of IgG in a PEG precipitate in the same conditions indicates that they are complexed. Therefore, specificity of the PEG assay for the presence of complexes is increased when the content of the PEG precipitate in immunoglobulins and/or complement components is assessed. The PEG method is also preparative and has been used for studying the specificity of complexed antibodies (Carella *et al.*, 1977).

Biological methods

Biological methods are based on the ability of antigen/antibody complexes to interact with humoral or cell receptor systems. C1q, rheumatoid factors, Fc receptors or macrophages and platelets, all recognize the Fc part of complexed (or aggregated) IgG. Other receptors such as conglutinin or C3 receptors on B lymphocytes recognize C3 bound to complexes.

Humoral receptors

The presence of antigen/antibody complexes which activate complement can be inferred from the inhibition of total haemolytic activity in a reference serum following its interaction with the test sample. However, various inhibitors such as bacterial products, acting at different stages of the complement system, cannot be easily distinguished from circulating immune complexes when using the haemolytic evaluation of anticomplementary activity.

In contrast, most of these inhibitors do not influence the tests which are based on the interaction of C1q with immune complexes. The C1q precipitation test (Agnello *et al.*, 1970) is based on the insolubility of the reaction product between C1q and immune complexes, visible as a precipitation line in agarose on a glass slide. The Clq binding test, developed by Nydegger *et al.* (1974) and modified by Zubler *et al.* (1976), is semi-quantitative and more sensitive. In this test, serum containing immune complexes is incubated with ^{125}I-C1q and PEG; separation of the immune complex-bound ^{125}I-C1q from free ^{125}I-C1q is achieved by selective precipitation with PEG (2·5% final concentration) and centrifugation, leaving free C1q in the supernate. A solid phase assay, analogous to the C1q binding test, has been developed by Hay *et al.* (1976) where the test serum is incubated in polystyrene tubes precoated with C1q; the tubes are then washed and the complexes bound to the insolubilized C1q are revealed using a radiolabelled rabbit antihuman IgG antiserum.

Complexed IgG is also recognized by rheumatoid factors (RF). Since the RF receptor site and the C1q receptor site located on the Fc part of complexed IgG differ, RF probably reveal complexes with different characteristics to those detected with C1q. The tests using RF include competitive inhibition by immune complexes from the test sample of the binding of radiolabelled aggregated IgG to insolubilized monoclonal RF (Luthra *et al.*, 1975), and inhibition by immune complexes of the agglutination of IgG-coated latex particles by purified RF (Lurhuma *et al.*, 1976).

Conglutinin is a bovine protein which specifically recognized C3bi, i.e. C3 bound to complexes. It can be insolubilized by coupling to Sepharose beads, or by coating polystyrene tubes (Casali *et al.*, 1977), so that it can bind complexes which, in turn, can be revealed using radiolabelled anti-IgG antibodies. Thus, conglutinin binding tests will detect a different group of soluble immune complexes compared to that detected by C1q or Rf binding tests.

Cellular receptors

Mononuclear cells also exhibit Fc receptors which have been used in 2 different tests: inhibition by immune complexes of K cell induced cytotoxicity (Jewell and McLennan, 1973); and inhibition of ingestion of radiolabelled aggregated IgG by guinea-pig peritoneal macrophages (Onyewutu *et al.*, 1974). Interpretation of the latter test is difficult when one considers its variability in such diseases as systemic lupus erythematosus (decreased ingestion) or rheumatoid arthritis (increased ingestion) (Mohammed *et al.*, 1977). The Raji cell assay uses an *in vitro* transformed lymphoblastoid (Raji) cell line (Theophilopoulos *et al.*, 1976). Raji cells exhibit receptors for C3d, and possibly C3bi and C3b. Complexes which are bound to the C3 receptors of the cells are revealed with radiolabelled anti-IgG. This test is presently the most widely used cellular assay for detection of soluble immune complexes.

Critical aspects of immune complex detection

Sensitivity and standardization

Most tests for detecting soluble immune complexes are semi-quantitative.

Sensitivity is usually expressed as an equivalent of μg/ml of *in vitro* heat-aggregated human IgG. However, aggregated IgG are difficult to standardize; they show more similarities with complexes in antibody excess than with complexes in antigen excess and their affinity for a humoral or cellular Fc receptor may differ from that of circulating complexes (Hughes-Jones, 1977). Moreover, optimal sensitivity of a test should allow optimal differentiation between normal and pathological values rather than the highest possible sensitivity.

Reproducibility

As a general rule, good reproducibility in cellular systems is more difficult to achieve than in humoral systems, except when a constant source of cellular receptor is available.

Specificity

Two main problems have to be considered about the specificity of methods for detecting immune complexes: (1) substances which interfere nonspecifically in a test can be responsible for false positive results; indeed, IgG, when aggregated by storage, by repeated freezing and thawing, or during a serum heat inactivation procedure, may interact in most of the test systems we have mentioned; endotoxin (Loos *et al.*, 1974), DNA and low mol. wt polyanions can react with C1q, and may require specific controls such as a limulus lysate test or DNase digestion. Similarly, warm reactive noncomplexed antilymphocyte auto- or alloantibodies may bind to Raji cells and should be adsorbed from the serum prior to the assay. Removal of cryoglobulins from immune complex containing serum diminishes its reactivity in both the Raji cell assay and the C1q binding test (Robinson *et al.*, 1979). Therefore, in order to avoid false negative results, care must be taken in the handling of serum, to ensure that cryoprecipitable complexes are not lost. (2) Only a restricted population of complexes is detected by a given test, so that a negative result in one assay system does not necessarily exclude the presence of soluble immune complexes. Most of the tests only detect complexes containing IgG and will select for the particular subtype of IgG complexes with which their receptor system can interact. In assays using C1q or receptors for C3, only complement-fixing immune complexes are detected such as complexes containing IgG_1 or IgG_3, large IgG complexes in slight antibody or antigen excess, or complexes containing complement fixing IgM antibodies. Tests which detect immune complex-bound C3 (C3b, C3bi, C3d), will also reveal those complexes which can activate complement by the alternative pathway. Even considering that complement-fixing complexes are more likely to be responsible for disease, a negative result in an assay using C1q or receptors for C3 should not eliminate the possible pathogenic role of noncomplement-fixing complexes. Therefore, additional and different tests should be performed on such a sample. Thus, in a minimal change nephrotic syndrome, some tests are negative whereas complexes can only be detected with assays involving RF (Levinsky *et al.*, 1978). In lupus or non lupus membranous glomerulonephritis (often considered as prototypes of immune complex disease), few circulating complexes have been detected (Robinson *et al.*, 1979). This could be due to their small size with respect to the assays which have been used, to small amounts or the intermittent presence of circulating complexes, or to their selective accumulation in the kidney on subepithelial receptors for C3b (in membranous nephritis) (Gelfand *et al.*, 1975) or within the basement membrane because they are formed *in situ* (Izui *et al.*, 1977a) (*vide infra*).

Characterization of complexed antigen or antibody

Identification of the complexed antigen or of the specificity of the complexed antibody could provide a rational basis for the treatment of immune complex disease, either by specific elimination of the causative antigen or *in vivo* modification of physicochemical characteristics of the complexes so as to facilitate their phagocytosis and elimination. The size of antigen excess complexes, for example, could be increased by addition of exogenous specific high affinity antibody. Characterization of complexes could also help in the understanding and pathophysiological classification of immune complex disease, and provide information on the nature of enhancing complexes found in transplant recipients (Paluoso *et al.*, 1976), or of circulating complexes detected in cancer patients (Sjögren *et al.*, 1971). Preparative techniques and more sophisticated methods (Lambert *et al.*, 1978) provide a partially purified material as a basis for further immunochemical and biochemical characterization of the complexes. Several techniques are now available for studying the composition of immune complexes in clinical research laboratories: (1) direct electron microscopic examination of a PEG precipitate, or of cryoglobulins; (2) dissociation of complexes at acid pH by urea or heat; (3) *in vitro* "manipulation" of complexes: by addition of the exogenous and purified suspected antigen, antibody-excess complexes can be shifted to antigen-excess, or slight antigen-excess to large antigen-excess complexes, so that the loss of their complement-fixing ability can be tested; (4) pepsin digestion of complexes in which the antigen is a protein will release $F(ab')_2$ fragments of the complexed antibody which can further be tested for their specificity; (5) absorption of immune complexes on conglutinin-coated polystyrene beads or tubes (Casali and Lambert, 1979).

Experimental immune complex disease

The classical experimental model of complex-induced vascular lesions is the Arthus reaction. For induction of this localized acute necrotizing vasculitis, relatively large amounts of antigen-antibody precipitates have to be localized in the vessel wall and in perivascular areas. One of the reactants, either antigen or antibody, circulates in peripheral blood and is also distributed in extravascular spaces; the other reactant is injected locally. Within a few hours, the injected antigen (active Arthus reaction) or the injected antibody (passive Arthus reaction) diffuses from the site of the injection forming a decreasing concentration gradient. Within the area of diffusion, immune precipitates will be formed where the antigen/antibody ratio is optimal. These locally formed immune complexes will react with complement and induce release of anaphylatoxins, such as C3a or C5a, which enhance vascular permeability and liberate other chemotactic factors attracting polymorphonuclear leukocytes to the site of the lesions. Upon contact with the immune complexes, polymorphonuclear leukocytes will liberate lysosomal enzymes accounting for necrosis at the site of their accumulation.

Another model for immune complex disease, particularly for its systemic manifestations, is the serum sickness syndrome, the pathogenic events in which have been elucidated in detail by Dixon and coworkers (Cochrane and Dixon, 1976). By i.v. injection in a rabbit of a single large dose of purified tracer-labelled serum protein from another species, it is possible to follow easily the disappearance of radioactivity from peripheral blood. In the early phase, injected antigen will equilibrate with extravascular spaces, which accounts for a rather rapid fall in its blood levels. This is followed by a short phase of physiological antigenic catabolism of the injected protein. Meanwhile, the thorough contact of the immune system with the injected protein will have allowed for formation of antibody which now, in a third phase (immune elimination), will react with antigen molecules in circulating blood and in interstitial fluids, thus forming antigen–antibody complexes.

The main pathogenic pathway in serum sickness disease was found to reside in the action of circulating immune complexes on vascular structures. Regarding the kidneys, these immune complexes may induce disease in certain conditions (low antibody responder animals forming circulating immune complexes in mild antigenic excess but still fixing complement). In these conditions, immune complexes are slowly deposited in the subepithelial layer of the glomerular loops. This deposition mechanism is similar to that observed in certain forms of leukopenia and thrombocytopenia where soluble immune complexes adhere to polymorphonuclear leukocytes and thrombocytes, leading to their destruction, especially following complement fixation at the cell surface.

Recently, an additional mechanism of immune complex damage to tissues and cells has been defined under the term "passive haemagglutination mechanism". Such a mechanism was clearly demonstrated by Levine, who first observed this mechanism in patients with immune haemolytic anaemia due to penicillin allergy (Levine and Redmond, 1967). In the first stage, the antigenic determinant, benzoyl penicilloyl, becomes attached to the surface of red cells; in the second stage, IgG-anti-BPO antibodies react with their antigenic target, inflicting damage on red cells. A few years ago, Izui in our laboratory defined a similar mechanism in DNA-anti-DNA induced glomerular nephritis in C57BL mice. During these experiments, DNA first became fixed to glomerular basement membrane in order then to absorb anti-DNA antibodies specifically from the circulation (Izui *et al.*, 1977a). This mechanism appears to prevail in patients with SLE kidney disease, where the majority of patients show subendothelial deposits typical of "the passive agglutination" type of mechanism, whereas only approximately 10% of lupus nephritis patients exhibit the subepithelial arrangement of serum sickness glomerular nephritis.

Evaluation of the *in vivo* pathogenic potential of circulating immune complexes

Serial estimations of circulating immune complexes in follow-up studies allow for evaluation of disease activity and of both the specificity and the efficiency of the treatment. However, correlations between levels of circulating immune complexes and the clinical status of a patient will only be possible when the detected complexes in the assay system which has been used are directly involved in the pathogenic process, or follow exactly the course of the disease. Such correlations are particularly valuable in the presence of complement-activating complexes where the clinical activity of the disease can be associated with variations in the level of circulating immune complexes, total haemolytic complement activity, functional activity of complement components, or the presence of increased levels of complement breakdown products. Evaluation of complement activation by "static" measurements of complement component levels may result in normal values despite active complement consumption. Indeed, C3, B and C3bINA at least are known to behave as acute phase reactants; therefore, in some instances complement catabolism can only be appreciated by turnover studies using purified radiolabelled proteins such as C3, B, Clq, β1H, or by measurement of levels of circulating complement breakdown products. Routine measurements of the C3d terminal cleavage fragment of C3 and of the Ba fragment of factor B can be achieved by radial immunodiffusion with specific antisera in the supernate of a 10% of 11% PEG precipitate separating them from the higher mol. wt C3, C3b, B and Bb molecules (Perrin *et al.*, 1975). A further way to assess complement activation in diseases in parallel with immune complex detection is to investigate the component and control proteins of the amplification convertase that amplifies the cleavage of C3 initiated by the classical or by the alternative pathway; such measurements have now been reported in SLE and chronic hypocomplementemic glomerulonephritis.

Both RA and SLE are well documented for the presence of circulating immune complexes and complement activation, which illustrates the relevance of immune complex detection and assessment of complement activation in clinical practice. We have shown in a large series of patients with RA (Nydegger *et al.*, 1977) that the amount of circulating Clq binding material is directly correlated with the level of circulating C3d.

To investigate further how the host is able to cope with formation of immune complexes, sera from patients with SLE have been chosen for evaluation of the alternative pathway protein levels. This has been done recently in a study by Whaley *et al.*, (1979), assaying 62 sera from 13 patients with SLE. In accordance with previous studies in our laboratory (Perrin *et al.*, 1973), significant reductions in the mean serum concentrations of C4 (classical pathway), factor B (alternative pathway) and of C3 (representing both pathways) were found. In addition, the mean levels of the control protein β1H, but not C3bINA, were reduced. This finding agrees well with the observation by Charlesworth *et al.* (1979), that the metabolism of β1H in patients with SLE may be clearly accelerated. Significant correlation existed between C3bINA and factor B levels, and between β1H and C4, C3, factor B and properdin levels (Whaley *et al.*, 1979). We have ourselves observed such correlations during serial studies in individual patients which further indicate that reductions in the serum concentrations of the regulatory proteins of the alternative complement pathway are inversely correlated with the levels of circulating immune complexes (Grandjean *et al.*, in prep.). One explanation for these correlations could be that C3bINA and particularly β1H are excessively consumed during immune complex formation in a way similar to that of factor B and C3.

Spontaneous immune complex disease in animals

Since the definition of serum sickness was formulated, a great variety of acquired diseases have been found to resemble the immune complex model described in rabbits. Particular attention was given to the autoimmune haemolytic disease and chronic membranous glomerulonephritis in New Zealand black mice, originally described by Bielschowsky *et al.* (1959). Hybridization between black-coated and white-coated strains resulted in a far more severe and fatal form of the same disease (review in Howie and Helyer, 1968). Many features of this disease in New Zealand mice are also found in SLE man, in particular the occurrence of circulating antibodies to DNA. One of the major issues in studying these mice has been the elucidation of the aetiologic factors in the immune response towards DNA. Particular interest has been focused on a possible infection with onconaviruses, but present knowledge, acquired mainly in studies involving transfer of virus-containing extracts to various strains of mice, fails to provide direct evidence for virus-triggered lupus in mice.

Other immune-complex-type diseases in animals involving viral antigens are Aleutian disease in mink (Ecklund *et al.*, 1968), lymphocytic choriomeningitis in which immune-complex-induced lesions develop (Oldstone and Dixon, 1967), and lactic dehydrogenase virus infection in mice with production of often lifelong levels of circulating immune complexes (Notkins, 1965).

Treatment of diseases associated with immune complexes

In those conditions where it is possible to establish clearly the pathogenetical role of circulating immune complexes it will become important to accelerate their removal (Table II). Theoretically, this can be accomplished by removal of antigen, removal of antibody or inhibition of its synthesis, by removal of antigen-antibody complexes or by a combination of all of these possibilities (Glassman, 1979).

TABLE II
Therapeutic possibilities in immune complex disease

Removal of antigen
e.g. anti-infectious treatment in parasitic, bacterial or viral diseases
Removal of antibody
immunosuppressive
cytapheresis (lymphapheresis)
Removal of immune complexes
plasma exchange
ex vivo filtration

Antigen removal will be easiest to achieve in infectious diseases by using antibacterial or antiparasitic drugs. Antibody removal may be achieved during treatments aimed at modification or suppression of the immune response. Among the immunosuppressant preparations used are alkylating agents (prototype: cyclophosphamide), antimetabolites (purine analogues, folic acid antagonists), corticosteroids and antilymphocyte globulin. Direct removal of antibody by extensive plasma exchange has also been successfully applied, and seems now to be clearly indicated in Goodpasture's syndrome (Lockwood *et al.*, 1976, Rosenblatt *et al.*, 1979; the latter reference contains a review of the literature).

With the recent development of continuous or intermittent flow cell separators it has become possible selectively to remove those blood components which carry (or participate in the production of) the pathogenetic factor(s). Based on a series of clearcut clinical improvements in a variety of diseases which are otherwise resistant to therapy, procedures such as lymphapheresis, plasma exchange therapy or plasmafiltration are now applied in a large number of medical centres. As an example, lymphapheresis has been used in the treatment of patients with severe, active rheumatoid arthritis during a 6-week period by the use of a continuous flow cell centrifuge and clinical improvement with regression of the synovitis was observed (Karsh *et al.*, 1979).

Rather than removing lymphocytes or some antibody-producing cells, direct removal of immune complexes has become a more broadly applied form of treatment in diseases associated with circulating immune complexes. Plasma exchange therapy has reduced the level of some types of immune complexes and has resulted in clinical improvement in patients with SLE (Jones *et al.*, 1976) or RA (Goldman *et al.*, 1979). With the application of sensitive techniques for their detection, circulating immune complexes are also detected with increased frequency in cancer patients, where they appear to correlate, at least in some patients, with the severity of the disease and with its prognosis (Carpentier *et al.*, 1977, Carpentier *et al.*, 1979).

Even more selective removal of antibodies and their complexes is achieved by extracorporeal filtration of plasma through cellulose diacetate hollow-fibre modules (Sieberth *et al.*, 1980) or through perfusion over *Staphylococcus aureus* paste in an extracorporeal filtration apparatus. Such plasma perfusion efficiently reduced the levels of IgG and immune complexes in the perfused plasma and was followed by clinical improvement and decrease of tumour size in a patient suffering from coloncarcinoma (Bansal *et al.*, 1978). The same procedure was also efficient in inducing necrosis and improvement of canine mammary adenocarcinoma (Terman *et al.*, 1980). All dogs in this latter study showed elevated levels of circulating immune complexes in serum before *ex vivo* absorption over *Staphyloccus aureus* cowan I and, most interestingly, these values transiently increased after completion of extracorporeal circulation over the absorbent. This demonstrates that the therapeutic effect of immune complex removal may not be based simply on their disappearance from the organism, but that such treatment may also (a) induce rapid formation of new immune complexes during the extracorporeal circulation due to compartmental redistribution of IgG, or (b) change the ratio of antigen to antibody in existing complexes in sera, hence increasing their possible detection by, in this case, the C1q binding test (Terman *et al.*, 1980).

In conclusion, circulating and tissue-deposited complexes between antibodies and a variety of antigens can, on the one hand, reflect efficient removal of undesired antigen; one may speculate that, in the healthy subject, such complexes appear quite frequently and for short periods until all antigen is removed. On the other hand, a large variety of diseases are associated with pathogenetically relevant, mostly chronically circulating immune complexes; these cases can be relived if successful removal of the complexes can be achieved.

References

Agnello, V., Winchester, R. J. and Kunkel, H. G. (1970). *Immunology* **19**, 909.

Amlot, P. L., Slaney, J. M. and Williams, B. D. (1976). *Lancet* **i**, 449.

Bansal, S. C., Bansal, B. R., Thomas, H. L. Siegel, P. D., Rhoads, J. E., Cooper, D. R., Terman, D. S. and Mark, R. (1978). *Cancer* **42**, 1.

Bielschowsky, M., Helyer, B. J. and Howie J. B. (1959). *Proc. Univ. Otago. Med. School* **37**, 9.

Carella, G., Digeon, M., Feldmann, G., Jungers, P., Drouet, J. and Bach, J. F. (1977). *Scand. J. Immunol.* **6**, 1297.

Carpentier, N. A., Lange, G. T., Fiere, D., Fournié, G. J., Lambert, P. H. and Miescher, P. A. (1977). *J. Clin. Invest.* **60**, 874.

Carpentier, N. A., Lambert, P. H. and Miescher, P. A. (1979) *In* "Current Trends in Tumor Immunology" (S. Ferrone *et al.*, eds) p. 165. Garland Publ. Inc., New York and London.

Casali, P. and Lambert, P. H. (1979). *Clin. Exp. Immunol.* **37**, 295.

Casali, P., Bossus, A., Carpentier, N. A. and Lambert, P. H. (1977). *Clin. Exp. Immunol.* **29**, 342.

Charlesworth, J. A., Scott, D. M., Pussell, B. A. and Peters, D. K. (1979). *Clin. Exp. Immunol.* **38**, 397.

Cochrane, C. G. and Dixon, F. J. (1976). *In* "Textbook of Immunopathology", (P. A. Miescher and H. J. Müller-Eberhard, eds) pp. 137–156. Grune & Stratton, New York.

Daha, M. R. and van Es, L. A. (1980). Abstr. V p. 7. European Complement Workshop, Lund, Sweden.

Daha, M. R., Austen, K. F. and Fearon, D. T. (1977). *J. Immunol.* **119**, 812.

Ecklund, C. M., Hadlow, W. J., Kennedy, R. C., Boyle, C. C. and Jackson, T. A. (1968). *J. Inf. Dis.* **118**, 510.

Fearon, D. T., Daha, J. M. and Austen, K. F. (1976). *Transplan. Rev.* **32**, 12.

Frank, M. M., Hamburger, M. I., Lawley, T. J., Kimberly, R. P. and Plotz, P. H. (1979). *New Engl. J. Med.* **300**, 518.

Gelfand, M. C., Frank, M. M. and Green, I. (1975). *J. Exp. Med.* **142**, 1029.

Germuth, F. G. and Rodriguez, E. (1973). "Immunopathology of the Venal Glomerulus". Little, Brown & Co., Boston.

Glassman, A. B. (1979). *Plasmatherapy* **1**, 13.

Goldman, J. A., Casey, H. K., McIlwain, H., Kirby, J., Wilson, C. H., Miller, S. B. (1979). *Arthritis Rheum.* **22**, 1146.

Gough, W. W., Davis, J. S. (1966). *Arthritis Rheum.* **9**, 631.

Hay, F. C., Nineham, L. J. and Roitt, I. M. (1976). *Clin. Exp. Immunol.* **24**, 396.

Howie, J. B. and Helyer, E. (1968). *Adv. Immunol.* **9**, 215.

Hughes-Jones, N. C. (1977). *Immunology* **32**, 191.

Hugli, T. E. and Müller-Eberhard, H. J. (1978). *Adv. Immunol.* **26**, 1.

Israel, L., Edelstein, R., Mannoni, P., Radot, E. and Greenspan, E. M. (1977). *Cancer* **40**, 3146.

Izui, S., Lambert, P. H., Fournié, G. J., Tuerler, H. and Miescher, P. A. (1977a). *J. Exp. Med.* **145**, 1115.

Izui, S., Lambert, P. H. and Miescher, P. A. (1977b). *Clin. Exp. Immunol.* **30**, 384.

Jewell, D. P. and McLennan, I. C. M. (1973). *Clin. Exp. Immunol.* **14**, 219.

Johnson, P. M. and Faulk, W. R. (1976). *Clin. Immunol. Immunopathol.* **6**, 414.

Jones, J. V., Cumming, R. H., Bucknall, R. C. and Asplin, C. M. (1976). *Lancet* **i**, 709.

Karsh, J., Wright, D. G., Klippel, J. H., Decker, J. L., Deisseroth, A. B. and Flye, M. W. (1979). *Arthritis Rheum.* **22**, 1055.

Koffler, D., Schur, P. H. and Kunkel, H. G. (1967). *J. Exp. Med.* **126**, 607.

Lambert, P. H., Dixon, F. J., Zubler, R. H., Agnello, V., Cambiaso, C., Casali, P., Jeremy Clarke, Cowdery, J. S., McDuffie, F. C., Hay, F. C., MacLennan, I. C., Masson, P., Müller-Eberhard, H. J., Penttinen, K., Smith, M., Tappeiner, G., Theofilopoulos, A. N. and Verroust, P. (1978). *J. Clin. Lab. Immunol.* **1**, 1.

Levine, B. B. and Redmond, A. P. (1967). *Int. Arch. All.* **31**, 594.

Levinsky, R. J., Malleson, P. N., Barrat, T. M. and Soothill, J. F. (1978). *New Engl. J. Med.* **298**, 126.

Lockwood, C. M., Rees, A. J., Pearson, T. A., Evans D. J., Peters, D. K. and Wilson, C. B. (1976). *Lancet* **i**, 711.

Loos, M., Bitter-Suermann, D., Dierich, M. (1974). *J. Immunol.* **112**, 935.

Lurhuma, A. Z., Cambiaso, C. L., Masson, P. L. and Heremans, J. F. (1976). *Clin. Exp. Immunol.* **25**, 212.
Luthra, H. S., McDuffie, F. C., Hunder, G. G. and Samayoa, E. A. (1975). *J. Clin. Invest.* **56**, 458.
Maini, R. N. and Holborow, E. J. (1977). *Ann. Rheum. Dis.* **36**.
Miller, G. W. and Nussenzweig, V. (1975). *Proc. Natn. Acad. Sci. U.S.A.* **72**, 418.
Mohammed, I., Thompson, B. and Holborow, E. J. (1977). *Ann. Rheum. Dis.* **36**, 49.
Morgan, A. C., Rossen, R. D. and Twomey, J. J. (1979). *J. Immunol.* **122**, 1672.
Notkins, A. L. (1965). *Bacteriol. Rev.* **39**, 143.
Nydegger, U. E., Lambert, P. H., Gerber, H. and Miescher, P. A. (1974). *J. Clin. Invest.* **54**, 297.
Nydegger, U. E., Zubler, R. H., Gabay, R., Joliat, G., Karagevrekis, Ch., Lambert, P. H. and Miescher, P. A. (1977). *J. Clin. Invest.* **59**, 862.
Nydegger, U. E., Fearon, D. T. and Austen, K. F. (1978). *J. Immunol.* **120**, 1401.
Oldstone, M. B. A. and Dixon, F. J. (1967). *Science* **158**, 1193.
Onyewutu, I. I., Holborow, E. J. and Johnson, G. D. (1974). *Nature (Lond.)* **284**, 156.
Paluoso, T., Kano, K., Anthone, S., Gerbasi, J. R. and Milgrom, F. (1976). *Transplantation* **21**, 312.
Perrin, L. H., Lambert, P. H., Nydegger, U. E. and Miescher, P. A. (1973). *Clin. Immunol. Immunopathol.* **2**, 16.
Perrin, L. H., Lambert, P. H. and Miescher, P. A. (1975). *J. Clin. Invest.* **56**, 165.
Pope, R. M. Teller, D. C. and Mannik, M. (1974). *Proc. Natn. Acad. Sci. U.S.A.* **71**, 517.
Robinson, M. F., Roberts, J. L., Verrier Jones, J. and Lewis, E. (1979). *Clin. Immunol. Immunopathol.* **14**, 348.
Rose, L. M. and Lambert, P. H. (1980). *Clin. Immunol. Immunopathol.* **15**, 481.
Rosenblatt, S. G., Knight, W., Bannayan, G. A. Wilson, C. B. and Stein, J. H. (1979). *Am. J. Med.* **66**, 689.
Schrock, J. H., Bolton, W. K., Godfrey, J. M. and Davis, J. S. (1977). *Clin. Res.* **25**, 25A.
Sieberth, H. G., Glöckner, W., Hirsch, H. H., Borberg, H., Dotzauer, G. and Mahieu, P. (1980). *Klin. Wschr.* **58**, 551.
Sissons, J. P. G., West, R. J., Fallows, J. Williams, D. G., Boucher, B. J., Amos, N. and Peters, D. K. (1976). *New Engl. J. Med.* **294**, 461.
Sjogren, H. O., Hellstrom, I., Bansal, S. C. and Hellstrom, K. E. (1971). *Proc. Natn. Acad. Sci. U.S.A.* **68**, 1372.
van Snick, J. L. and Masson, P. L. (1978). *J. Exp. Med.* **148**, 903.
Steward, M. W. (1979). *Clin. Exp. Immunol.* **38**, 414.
Terman, D. S., Yamamoto, T., Mattioli, M., Cook, G., Tillquist, R., Henry, J., Poser, R. and Daskal Y. (1980). *J. Immunol.* **124**, 975.
Theophilopoulos, A. N. and Dixon, F. J. (1979). *Adv. Immunol.* **28**, 89.
Theophilopoulos, A. N., Wilson, C. B. and Dixon, F. J. (1976). *J. Clin. Invest.* **57**, 169.
Whaley, K., Schur, P. and Ruddy, S. (1979). *Clin. Exp. Immunol.* **36**, 408.
Zubler, R. H. and Lambert, P. H. (1977). *Recent Adv. Clin. Immunol.* **1**, 125.
Zubler, R. H., Lange, G., Lambert, P. H. and Miescher, P. A. (1976). *J. Immunol.* **116**, 232.

56

Interaction Between Complement and Immune Complexes: Role of Complement in Containing Immune Complex Damage

VICTOR NUSSENZWEIG

New York University Medical Center, New York, New York, USA

Introduction

This chapter presents the arguments which support the idea that deficiencies in the complement system can aggravate and may even contribe to the development of immune complex (IC) diseases. This hypothesis was put forward a few years ago when, jointly with Dr Gary Miller, I found that immunoprecipitates could be solubilized by complement, and that the soluble complexes contained large amounts of tightly bound C3 and C4 peptides (Takahashi *et al.*, 1976, 1980). We reasoned that since phagocytic cells have complement receptors which recognize precisely those complement peptides, the *in vivo* clear-

Abbreviations
IC: immune complex or immune complexes; E: mouse erythrocytes; EIgG 10^{-3}: mouse erythrocytes sensitized with a 1/1000 dilution of rabbit IgG antibodies; EIgG 10^{-3} C: EIgG 10^{-3} after incubation with mouse complement *in vitro*; these cells bear C3b on their membranes; CVF: cobra venom factor.

Supported in part by NIH Grants AI-08499 and CA-16247.

ance and processing of immune complexes would be abnormal if the complement system is defective.

To facilitate the exposition, I will start by summarizing the evidence that immune aggregates are themselves the target of the complement cascade, then present data indicating that complement plays a major role in clearance of certain types of IC. To conclude, I will discuss some clinical observations which indicate that defects in the complement system may be involved in the pathogenesis of IC diseases.

Immune aggregates are the target of the complement cascade

Based on the observation that complement has a detergent-like effect on immune precipitates (Miller and Nussenzweig, 1975) we developed an assay to study the interaction between complement and IC prepared with various soluble antigens (Czop and Nussenzweig, 1976). Using this assay we found that every complement enzyme, from both the classical and alternative pathways, was assembled *on* the immune aggregates. Solubilization took place only when the immune aggregates bearing the alternative pathway C3-convertase ($\overline{\text{C3b,Bb,P}}$) cleaved fluid phase C3 and one of the products of this reaction (C3b peptide) accumulated on the lattice. Although solubilization occurred in the absence of C2, C4 or Ca^{2+} ions, it was greatly accelerated if the immune aggregates contained the classical pathway C3-convertase ($\overline{\text{C4b,2a}}$). The most probable role of the latter enzyme is to cleave C3 and generate a few lattice-associated C3b molecules, which in turn serve as seeds to initiate the assembly of the more vigorous alternative pathway C3 convertase $\overline{\text{C3b,Bb,P}}$ (Takahashi *et al.*, 1978; Fujita, 1979).

The participation of both pathways in solubilization is illustrated in the following experiment of Takahashi *et al.* (1980). They incubated at 37°C immune precipitates prepared with radiolabelled tetanus toxoid and human IgG antibody to tetanus toxoid with normal human serum or with serum from a patient with a genetically determined C2 deficiency. Solubilization of the precipitates was measured kinetically. At different times they removed samples from the tube containing the incubation mixture, and then subjected them to centrifugation. The resulting pellets and supernatants were counted in a gamma counter. In the absence of C2, solubilization was sluggish, and purified C2 accelerated the process at physiological concentrations (Fig. 1).

One of the implications of this and other experiments is that the processing of IC by complement, as measured by the solubilization assay, is greatly influenced by both C3-convertases, $\overline{\text{C4b,2a}}$ and $\overline{\text{C3b,Bb,P}}$. Therefore, deficiencies in any complement components or control proteins which result in the diminished activities of these enzymes will inhibit the processing of IC. It is also to be expected that IC prepared with IgA or IgE, which do not activate the classical pathway, should be processed and incorporate C3b very

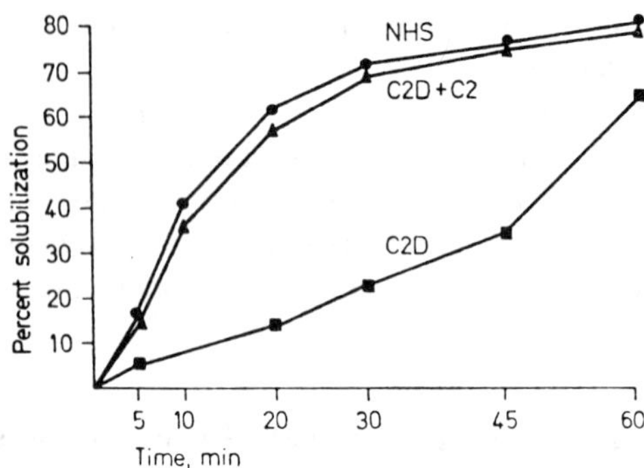

FIG. 1. *Solubilization of immune complexes is C2-dependent. 10 μl of an immune precipitate (tetanus-toxoid/*^{131} *I-labelled human antibody, IgG purified) containing 1 μg of complexed antibody was incubated at 37° C with 0·4 ml of 1/2 dilution of fresh human serum (NHS), C2-deficient human serum (C2D), and C2-deficient human serum plus purified human C2 (100 CH50 units) (C2D + C2). 50 μl samples were taken at various times at 37° C and diluted with cold buffer. Supernatants and pellets were separated by centrifugation at 1200* **g** *for 10 min and counted in a gamma counter. Solubilization was inefficient in C2D serum, and greatly enhanced by addition of C2 at physiological concentrations. (Reproduced with permission from Takahashi* et al., *1980.)*

inefficiently, and as a consequence will not be cleared from circulation as rapidly as IC prepared with IgG or IgM.

Solubilized complexes consist of antigen, antibody, C3- and C4-derived peptides, properdin, C4-binding protein and probably other complement components (Takahashi *et al.*, 1977, 1978; Scharfstein *et al.*, 1979). Although C5-convertase is assembled on the immune aggregates, the solubilized IC do not contain C5. Similar observations have been made by Nilsson and Müller-Eberhard (1965). Therefore, in contrast to nascent C3b and C4b, nascent C5b,6,7 appears to lack affinity for immunoaggregates. This is an important point because the implication would be that the presence of terminal complement components in the kidney of patients with nephritis results from local complement consumption and not from passive accumulation of IC containing C5–9.

On a quantitative basis, the most important complement peptides associated with complexes are derived from C3 and C4. The solubilizing effect of complement on IC results from the intercalation of the complement peptides in the lattice (Czop and Nussenzweig, 1976; Rajnavölgyi *et al.*, 1978; Kijlstra *et al.*, 1979a). The available evidence strongly suggests that they interfere, perhaps sterically, with the binding of antigen to antibody (Miller, 1977; Miller and Köhler, 1978). In fully solubilized complexes, the molar ratio of C3b to antibody is close to 1 (Takahashi *et al.*, 1977). Most of the C3 peptides derived from the α' chain are very tightly associated with the H chain of the immunoglobulins present in the IC. The α'-H chain bonds are broken after incubation in medium containing 8M urea and β2-mercaptoethanol. Furthermore, we found that the C3b molecules bound to the IC are very rapidly degraded by serum enzymes, most likely by C3b/C4b inactivator and cofactors. After less than 5 min of incubation of the solubilized complexes in serum at 37°C, the α' chain of the bound C3b was degraded, while the β chain appeared to be intact (J. Czop, B. Tack, V. Nussenzweig, unpublished observations). It is therefore likely that solubilized complexes are end-stage complexes in the sense that they are probably incapable of activating the terminal complement components, and therefore of generating new peptides with potential inflammatory activity.

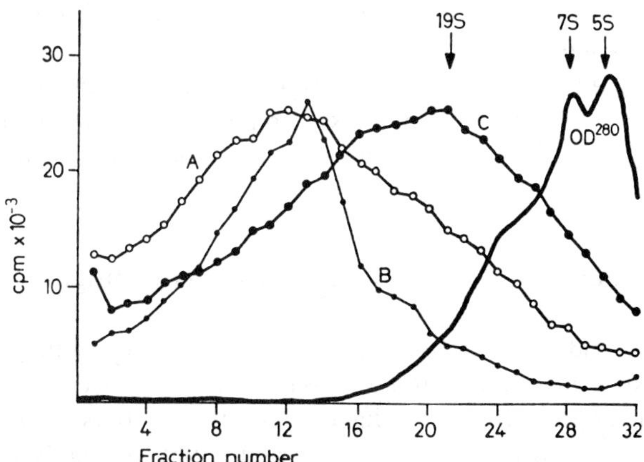

FIG. 2. *Sucrose gradient ultracentrifugation of solubilized IC. Immune precipitates were prepared with* ^{125}*I-labelled monomeric BSA, and rabbit anti-BSA at equivalence* (*A*), *2 × antibody excess* (*B*) *and 2 × antigen excess* (*C*). *10 μl of a suspension of precipitates containing 0·55–0·72 μg of complexed antibody were incubated with 0·4 ml of 1/2 dilution of fresh human serum at 37° C for 60 min. About 90% of the precipitates were solubilized at the end of the incubation. 20 μl of the supernatants were overlaid on 5 ml of 10–40% sucrose gradients and centrifuged in an SW 50·1 rotor at 50 000* **g** *for 14 h. After centrifugation, samples were collected and assayed for radioactivity. The arrows show the position of internal markers, IgM* (*19*s), *IgG* (*7*s) *and albumin* (*5*s), *monitored by double diffusion in agarose. The solubilized IC are heterogeneous in size. In the region of antibody excess or equivalence most solubilized IC have sedimentation coefficients greater than 19*s. (*Reproduced, with permission, from Takahashi* et al., *1980*).

That an end-stage in the solubilization process is reached as to the size distribution of IC is shown by the following experiments performed by Takahashi *et al.*, (1980). They incubated, in human serum for 1 h at 37°C, immunoprecipitates formed between ^{125}I-bovine albumin and rabbit antibodies. The mixture was subjected to ultracentrifugation in sucrose gradients (Fig. 2). The solubilized complexes were heterogeneous; their sedimentation coefficients varied from 11*s* to more than 19*s*. Interestingly, essentially the same patterns were obtained if the antigen–antibody–complement complexes were formed in conditions closer to those which are likely to occur *in vivo*; that is, if antigen was first mixed with fresh serum at 37°C and then the antibody was added. Nor did the ultracentrifugation patterns change when fractions containing solubilized complexes from previous runs were reincubated at 37°C for 1 h in fresh serum and recentrifuged.

Role of complement in the clearance and processing of immune complexes

Experiments dealing with the role of complement in clearance have led to opposite conclusions according to whether the IC used were prepared with particulate or soluble antigens. Investigators studying clearance of sensitized red cells or bacteria found that their removal from the circulation was complement-dependent. In contrast, it has been suggested that complement plays no role in the clearance of complexes prepared with soluble antigens. Some of the evidence on which these conclusions are based will be discussed in this section.

Clearance of complexes prepared with particulate antigens

The classic studies on the mechanisms of red cell destruction in haemolytic anaemias showed that the Kupffer cells in the liver remove from the circulation most of the erythrocytes which have bound both antibody and complement. It was found, however, that if the interaction with antibody did not lead to complement fixation, the red cells were cleared mainly in the spleen. When these studies were performed, the nature of the cell receptors in liver and spleen which recognize the targets was unknown (Mollison, 1970).

Further clarification of the mechanisms involved derived from two lines of investigation. On the one hand, studies on the mechanisms of phagocytosis showed that macrophages have membrane receptors for Fc and C3 and that the ingestion of sensitized erythrocytes depends on the interaction between these receptors and the red cell-associated ligands; that is, C3b and IgG (reviewed in Ehlenberger and Nussenzweig, 1977a). Furthermore, it was found that these receptors have synergistic roles in phagocytosis: C3 receptors mainly promote adherence of the sensitized particles to phagocytes and Fc receptors promote ingestion of the particles. When red cells are coated with C3b in the absence of IgG, they bind to the phagocyte membrane but are not readily internalized (Mantovani *et al.*, 1972; Ehlenberger and Nussenzweig, 1977b). An essential role for complement receptors in mediating the binding of sensitized particles to phagocytic cells *in vivo* was suggested by experiments showing that monomeric IgG at concentrations much below that found in normal serum can effectively inhibit the *in vitro* ingestion of red cells sensitized with IgG alone (Berken and Benacerraf, 1966; Lo Buglio *et al.*, 1967; Lay and Nussenzweig, 1968).

The elegant experiments in guinea-pigs and humans of Frank and his collaborators (1977) on the mechanism of clearance of autologous erythrocytes sensitized with IgG or IgM are the counterpart of these *in vitro* studies. Their observations and those of Brown *et al.* (1970) clearly demonstrated that both

C3 and Fc receptors are involved in the clearance of cells coated with immunologically active proteins.

Pappas *et al.* (1980) have recently adapted this experimental model of clearance to mice. They first studied the mechanisms of uptake from the circulation of ^{51}Cr-labelled autologous erythrocytes (E) sensitized with IgG antibodies produced in rabbits. Then they investigated the nature of a clearance defect found in malaria-infected mice, which, as previously shown by others, have clear manifestations of IC disease, including nephritis. Some of these findings are in full agreement with the main conclusions of Frank and his collaborators and can be summarized as follows.

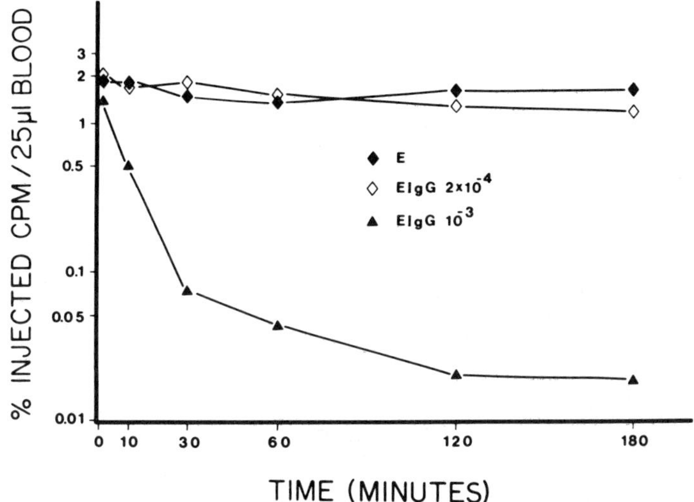

FIG. 3. *Clearance of ^{51}Cr-labelled mouse erythrocytes sensitized with different doses of rabbit antibody. Normal mice were injected with 4 × 10^7 nonsensitized cells (E) or erythrocytes sensitized with different dilutions of IgG. At indicated times, 25 µl of blood was obtained from each mouse and counted in a gamma counter.*

Clearance rates of IgG-sensitized autologous red cells were dependent on the antibody dose. As shown in Fig. 3, E sensitized with a 1:1000 dilution of IgG (EIgG 10^{-3}) were rapidly removed from circulation. These cells were sequestered mainly in the liver. Further dilutions of the antibody led to a very substantial decrease in blood clearance and a relative enhancement in spleen uptake.

The removal of the optimally sensitized cells from the circulation was complement-dependent. *In vivo* depletion of C3 with cobra venom factor (CVF) had two effects. It greatly retarded the clearance of EIgG 10^{-3}. In addition, those cells which were removed from the circulation were preferentially sequestered in the spleen. When EIgG 10^{-3} were preincubated in fresh mouse serum as a source of complement, washed by centrifugation and then injected into CVF-treated mice, the clearance defect and the abnormal sequestration patterns were not observed.

The preferential sequestration of complement-bearing red cells in the liver was confirmed in experiments in which mice were injected with autologous erythrocytes sensitized with complement in the absence of antibody. This was achieved by incubation of red cells in low ionic strength sucrose solution (Hartman and Jenkins, 1966) which leads to the deposition on their membranes of C3b and C4b. In normal mice or mice with malaria, these complement-sensitized red cells were taken up by the liver, but then gradually returned intact to the circulation. The release of red cells from the liver probably results from the cleavage of C3b or C4b by C3b/C4b inactivator (Frank *et al.*, 1977) and strongly suggests that the C3 receptor-C3b/C4b interaction by itself is not a potent stimulus for particle ingestion.

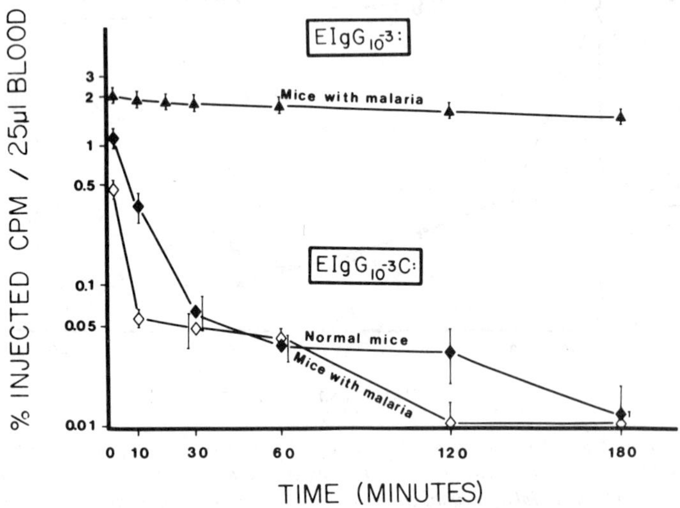

FIG. 4. *Clearance of 4 × 10⁷ ⁵¹Cr-labelled EIgG 10⁻³ and EIgG 10⁻³C in normal and* Plasmodium berghei-*infected mice, 14 d after infection. At indicated times, 25 µl of blood was obtained from each mouse and counted in a γ counter. Data points represent mean values ± 1 s.e. of 4 mice in 2 experiments. Note that, as compared to normal mice (Fig. 2), the clearance of EIgG 10⁻³ in malaria-infected mice is defective. However, the defect is corrected if the sensitized cells are coated* in vitro *with complement before injection (EIgG 10⁻³ C).*

When EIgG 10^{-3} were injected into malaria-infected mice the red cells were not cleared from circulation (Fig. 4). This profound defect was most likely the consequence of the hypocomplementemia observed in mice with malaria (Krettli *et al.*, 1976), since the sensitized erythrocytes were removed rapidly from their blood if coated with C3 *in vitro* before injection (EIgG 10^{-3} C). This is a direct demonstration that a major defect in clearance of complexes may occur in diseases in which an increased consumption of complement and/or defects in synthesis lead to hypocomplementemia. Complement-dependent alterations in the handling of particulate and soluble immune complexes have also been detected in old NZB/W mice, which have been used as a model for studying systemic lupus erythematosus (Miller *et al.*, 1975; Shear *et al.*, 1980).

Analogous conclusions supporting the important role of complement in the clearance of particulate complexes have been drawn in experiments involving the injection of sensitized bacteria into animals (Spiegelberg *et al.*, 1963; Brown *et al.*, 1980; Van Wick *et al.*, 1980). Again, the liver was the main site of complement-mediated sequestration, while the spleen accumulated poorly opsonized bacteria.

Clearance of complexes prepared with soluble antigens

The careful studies of Mannik and collaborators (reviewed in Mannik, 1980) in rabbits, mice and monkeys demonstrated that injected soluble complexes prepared with various antigens and IgG antibodies were sequestered mainly in the liver. Furthermore, they observed that in every case in which the complexes were rapidly cleared, they also activated the complement cascade. Complexes prepared in large antigen excess, consisting of $AgAb_2$, AgAb, Ag_2Ab or Ag_2Ab_2, or complexes prepared with reduced and alkylated antibodies, fixed complement very poorly and persisted for a long time in circulation.

With the exception, however, of instances in which the antigen within the complexes was IgM, decomplementation of the animals with CVF or aggregated immunoglobulin had no effect on clearance. On the basis of these results it would appear that, contrary to what has been demonstrated for red cells, bacteria, and soluble complexes containing IgM, the liver uptake of soluble complexes containing IgG is independent of the complement system, and is perhaps mediated solely by Fc receptors.

This unexpected conclusion rests on the premise that these IC could not have fixed C3b in the circulation of animals which had been decomplemented with CVF or with immune aggregates. However, since immune aggregates activate both complement pathways, it would be necessary to profoundly deplete an animal of both C3 and C4 to prevent the incorporation of a few C3b or C4b molecules in the injected complexes and their subsequent recognition by immune adherence receptors (Bianco and Nussenzweig, 1977). It should be pointed out that clearance is an extremely sensitive assay for the presence of C3b and C4b on particles. It takes very few C1-fixing units on red cells to promote their uptake by the liver (Frank *et al.*, 1977). Other complicating factors for the interpretation of the findings of Mannik and co-workers are the presence of receptors for C1q on lymphoid cells and monocytes (Gabay *et al.*, 1979; Tenner and Cooper, 1980) and the fact that the liver is one of the main sites of synthesis of complement. Therefore, in animals injected with CVF the concentration of complement proteins within the sinusoids of the liver may be higher than in serum at large. Whatever the explanation for these results, the conclusion that complement is not important for the clearance of soluble IC is not supported by recent observations that their processing *in vitro* by macrophages is markedly enhanced by complement. This effect appears to be mediated by increasing binding of the complement-treated complexes to the cell membranes, probably to C3 receptors, rather than by changes in the rate of intracellular degradation (Van Snick and Masson, 1978; Kijlstra *et al.*, 1979b).

Clinical observations

Acute and chronic IC diseases are characterized by the deposition of immunoglobulin and complement components in vessel walls, in the kidney, and in other sites. Deposits of IC in the walls of small veins or arteries, or in joints, cause local inflammation. This phlogistic effect of IC depends on the ability to activate complement and promote the local accumulation of neutrophils, as shown by Cochrane and others (reviewed by Cochrane and Janoff, 1974). For example, if rabbits manifesting serum sickness are treated with CVF to deplete C3, the arteritis associated with this disease is markedly inhibited, although the IC themselves are still found in the vessel walls.

The evidence that complement is one of the mediators of the inflammatory response which follows the local accumulation of immune complexes is very good. The issue which remains unresolved, however, is what causes the abnormal deposition of circulating IC; that is, the failure to be processed by complement while in the circulation, transformed into solubilized end-stage complexes, and taken up by the mononuclear phagocyte system.

Some clinical evidence indicates that complement deficiencies themselves may be part of the explanation. An ever-increasing number of observations document associations between IC diseases, including nephritis, and inborn deficiencies of C1r, C4, C2, C1-inhibitor (reviewed in Lachmann and Rosen, 1979), C1q (Thompson *et al.*, 1980) and C3 (Pussel *et al.*, 1980). It was initially thought that this association might be artefactual, and could be attributed to a sampling error resulting from the preferential evaluation of complement functions among the population of patients with IC diseases. However, from the accumulated experience of many clinical laboratories involved in the measurement of complement levels in large numbers of healthy individuals, or healthy relatives of patients with IC disease, this seems unlikely. Indeed, these studies suggest that complement deficiencies are more frequently found among patients with IC disease than in the general population. For example, in a controlled study, Glass *et al.*, (1976) found that C2 deficiencies were significantly higher in a group of unrelated lupus patients than among blood donors.

What abnormalities are expected to result from complement deficiencies? The absence of C1q, C1r, C2, C4 or C3 will lead directly to defects in the assembly of the C3-convertases of the classical and alternative pathways. A deficiency in C1-inhibitor has the same effect indirectly since it leads to an enhanced consumption of C4 and C2, and thus to low serum levels of these complement components. Defects in the assembly of C3-convertase, particularly of $\overline{\text{C3b,Bb}}$, as observed in individuals with C3 or C3b/C4b-inactivator deficiency, diminish the ability to deal with infectious agents, particularly pyogenic cocci, and perhaps certain viruses (Perrin *et al.*, 1976). In addition some RNA tumour viruses can directly trigger the classical complement cascade to be subsequently lysed (Cooper *et al.*, 1976). It could be argued, therefore, that patients with complement deficiencies will in general be more subject to infections, that they may consequently accumulate IC in the circulation, and that this will lead to IC diseases. The problem with this hypothesis is that, to my knowledge, there is no evidence that most individuals with defects in the assembly of the classical pathway C3-convertase have an unusual number of viral or bacterial infections.

It has also been suggested that the relationship between these genetically determined complement deficiencies and IC diseases is not direct, but that the diseases are caused by the presence of an abnormal allele in a closely linked genetic locus. For example, in the case of C4 and C2, whose structural genes map in the major histocompatibility complex, an *Ir* gene could be involved. This explanation, however, could not apply to other complement deficiencies which are not HLA-linked, such as C1r, or C1-inhibitor.

A simpler and more direct hypothesis is that these complement deficiencies lead to a defect in the processing of circulating IC found under pathological or even physiological conditions. Indeed, recent studies indicate that circulating IC occur in patients with a wide variety of clinical conditions and, at lower levels, in sera of many normal individuals. Several observations suggest that IC participate in the regulation of the immune system. In the context of the network hypothesis of Jerne (1974), reactions between idiotypes and anti-idiotypes occur continuously, and are the basic mechanism of the control of immune responses. Based on the experimental evidence presented in the previous sections and the observation that idiotype–anti-idiotype reactions can activate complement (Miller and Köhler, 1978) it is reasonable to postulate that the complement cascade and the mononuclear phagocyte system are fundamental mechanisms for their disposal. Whatever their origin, under normal circumstances, phagocytosis of complement-processed IC would prevent their pathological deposition in tissues. If they are incompletely processed or the phagocytes are incapable of ingesting them, tissue deposition will occur; once the complexes are deposited, local complement fixation may be harmful (Fig. 5).

Some additional clinical evidence, as well as results from experimental work in acute serum sickness in rabbits, lend support to the idea that primary or secondary complement deficiencies may lead to or aggravate IC glomerulonephritis. On the clinical side, Peters and his colleagues showed that in patients with partial lipodystrophy who develop mesangiocapillary glomerulonephritis, sometimes the serum complement levels diminish *before* any kidney involvement

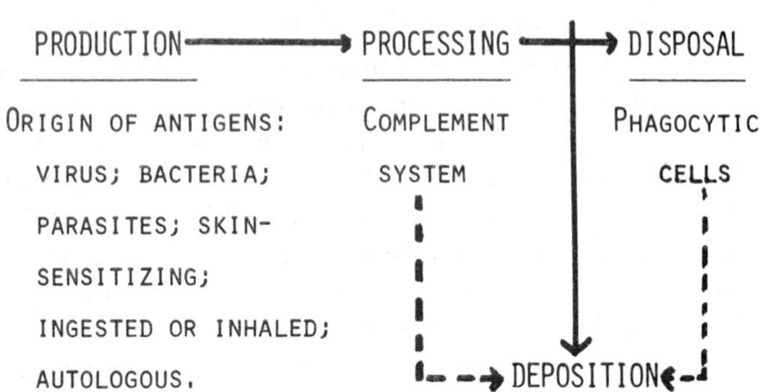

FIG. 5. *Schematic representation of the proposed mechanism for deposition of circulating complexes. IC are produced under physiological or pathological conditions. Physiological IC could originate from the interaction of antibodies with modified autologous constituents, with ingested or inhaled antigens, or from idiotype–anti-idiotype reactions. Under pathological conditions, IC could also contain viral, bacterial, or autologous antigens. These IC are normally processed through the complement system and ingested by phagocytic cells, in particular by the cells from the reticuloendothelial system. If either system is defective, IC are deposited. The incompletely processed, deposited IC still interact with the complement system, and this may cause local inflammation.*

(Peters and Williams, 1974). It is also well known that during flare-ups of systemic lupus erythematosus there are decreases in the levels of individual complement components, particularly of C4; however, it is not clear what the temporal relationship is between the appearance of clinically active disease and the diminution of complement in serum.

At the experimental level, Bartolotti and Peters (1978) made the intriguing observation that CVF-induced hypocomplementemia in rabbits with acute serum sickness results in delayed removal of IC from glomeruli. This finding, taken together with the observation that C3 appears to be deposited in large amounts in glomeruli during the healing phase of this disease (Wilson and Dixon, 1970) indicates that perhaps the deposited complexes are still accessible to the solubilizing or processing activity of the complement system.

In summary, we have reviewed the evidence that complement is involved in the solubilization and removal of IC from the circulation. The binding of circulating IC to the membrane receptors for Fc, C3b and C4b of the phagocytic cells depends primarily on whether the ligand is accessible in the immune aggregates. Complement fixation may affect this interaction in several ways. It changes the solubility, degree of aggregation and composition of the IC, and leads to the incorporation into the lattice of C4b and very large amounts of C3b. Moreover, after complement fixation, the interaction between IC and Fc receptors is inhibited, most likely because the complement peptides also bind to the Fc region of the immunoglobulin molecules (Eden *et al.*, 1973; Scharfstein *et al.*, 1979).

Antigen–antibody aggregates presumably have a limited number of sites which can trigger the complement cascade. Once they have interacted fully with the complement peptides and the lattice-associated enzymes are inhibited by the serum control proteins, the IC should be at an end-stage. In a situation of complement deficiency circulating complexes may not be fully processed, accumulate in tissues, and then the cascade could proceed locally. An inflammatory response and tissue damage may be consequences if the IC deposit in joints or vessel walls.

Also, during acute or chronic infections, when large amounts of soluble antigens may be released into the circulation, the capacity of the complement system and of the mononuclear phagocyte system may be overcome. Perhaps it is relevant that during acute infections the levels of various complement components in serum are elevated. This may be an adaptive reaction to cope with an increased load of potentially damaging IC. As pointed out by Peters and Lachmann (1974), in a situation of complement deficiency some infectious agents may not be eliminated. The persistence of antigen and of the antibody response to it will certainly aggravate the problem.

Finally, from the practical point of view, the present findings suggest that serious consideration should be given to the possibility that therapies which enhance complement levels could be used in some patients with circulating IC, in an effort to enhance their removal from the circulation and tissues and promote their ingestion by phagocytes. The measurement of the capacity of the serum of patients to solubilize complexes may be of diagnostic and prognostic value, if it is indeed an accurate reflection of a physiological defence function.

References

Bartolotti, S. R. and Peters, D. K. (1978). *Clin. Exp. Immunol* **32**, 199.

Berken, A. and Benacerraf, B. (1966). *J. Exp. Med.* **123**, 119.

Bianco, C. and Nussenzweig, V. (1977). *Contemporary Topics Mol. Immunol.* **6**, 145.

Brown, D. K., Lachmann, P. J. and Dacie, J. V. (1970). *Clin. Exp. Immunol.* **7**, 401.

Brown, E. J., Hosea, S. W. and Frank, M. M. (1980). *Clin. Res.* **28**, 362A.

Cochrane, C. G. and Janoff, A. (1974). *In* "The Inflammatory Process" (B. Zweifach *et al.*, eds) pp. 86–162. Academic Press, New York.

Cooper, N. R., Jensen, F. C., Welsh, R. M. and Oldstone, M. B. A. (1976). *J. Exp. Med.* **144**, 970.

Czop, J. and Nussenzweig, V. (1976). *J. Exp. Med.* **143**, 615.

Eden, A., Bianco, C. and Nussenzweig, V. (1973). *Cell. Immunol.* **7**, 459.

Ehlenberger, A. G. and Nussenzweig, V. (1977a). *In* "The Year in Hematology" (A. S. Gordon *et al.*, eds) pp. 221–240. Plenum Medical Book, New York and London.

Ehlenberger, A. G. and Nussenzweig, V. (1977b). *J. Exp. Med.* **145**, 357.

Frank, M. M., Schreiber, A. P., Atkinson, J. P. and Jaffe, C. J. (1977). *Ann. Int. Med.* **87**, 210.

Fujita, T. (1979). *Microbiol. Immunol.* **23**, 1023.

Gabay, Y., Pearlmann, H., Pearlmann, P. and Sobel, T. (1979). *Eur. J. Immunol.* **9**, 797.

Glass, D., Raum, D., Gibson, D., Stillman, J. S. and Schur, P. H. (1976). *J. Clin. Invest.* **58**, 853.

Hartman, R. C. and Jenkins, D. E. (1966). *N. Engl. J. Med.* **275**, 155.

Jerne, N. K. (1974). *Ann. Immunol., Paris* **125c**, 373.

Kijlstra, A., Leendert, A. van Es, and Daha, M. R. (1979a). *J. Immunol.* **123**, 640.

Kijlstra, A., Leendert, A. van Es and Daha, M. R. (1979b). *J. Immunol.* **123**, 2488.

Krettli, A. U., Nussenzweig, V. and Nussenzweig, R. S. (1976). *Am. J. Trop. Med. Hyg.* **25**, 34.

Lachmann, P. J. and Rosen, F. S. (1979). *In* "Immunodeficiency" (M. D. Cooper *et al.*, eds) pp. 105–120. Springer-Verlag, Berlin, Heidelberg and New York.

Lay, W. H. and Nussenzweig, V. (1968). *J. Exp. Med.* **128**, 991.

Lo Buglio, A. F., Cotran, R. S. and Jandl. J. H. (1967). *Science* **158**, 1582.

Mannik, M. (1980). *J. Investigative Dermatol.* **74**, 333.

Mantovani, B., Rabinovitch, M. and Nussenzweig, V. (1972). *J. Exp. Med.* **135**, 780.

Miller, G. W. (1977). *J. Immunol.* **119**, 488.

Miller, G. W. and Köhler, H. (1978). *Immunochemistry* **15**, 279.

Miller, G. W. and Nussenzweig, V. (1975). *Proc. Natn. Acad. Sci. U.S.A.* **72**, 418.

Miller, G. W., Steinberg, A. D., Green, I. and Nussenzweig, V. (1975). *J. Immunol.* **114**, 1166.

Mollison, P. L. (1970). *Brit. J. Haematol.* **18**, 249.

Nilsson, V. R. and Müller-Eberhard, H. J. (1965). *J. Exp. Med.* **122**, 277.

Pappas, M. G., Nussenzweig, R. S., Nussenzweig, V. and Shear, H. L. (1980). Submitted for publication.

Perrin, L. H., Joseph, B. S., Cooper, N. R. and Oldstone, M. B. A. (1976). *J. Exp. Med.* **143**, 1027.

Peters, D. K. and Lachmann, P. J. (1974). *Lancet* **i**, 58.

Peters, D. K. and Williams, D. G. (1974). *Adv. Nephrol.* **4**, 67.

Pussel, B. A., Bourke, E., Nayef, M., Morris, S. and Peters, D. K. (1980). *Lancet* **i**, 675.

Rajnovölgyi, E., Füst, G., Ember, J., Medgyesi, G. A. and Gergely, J. (1978). *Immunochemistry* **15**, 335.

Scharfstein, J., Correa, E. B., Gallo, G. R. and Nussenzweig, V. (1979). *J. Clin. Invest.* **63**, 437.

Shear, H. L., Roubinian, J., Gil, P. and Talal, N. (1980). Submitted for publication.

Spiegelberger, H. L., Miescher, P. A. and Benacerraf, B. (1963). *J. Immunol.* **90**, 751.

Takahashi, M., Czop, J., Ferreira, A. and Nussenzweig, V. (1976). *Transplant. Rev.* **32**, 121.

Takahashi, M., Tack, B. F. and Nussenzweig, V. (1977). *J. Exp. Med.* **145**, 86.

Takahashi, M., Takahashi, S., Brade, V. and Nussenzweig, V. (1978). *J. Clin. Invest.* **62**, 349.

Takahashi, M., Takahashi, S. and Hirose, S. (1980). *Prog. Allergy* **27**, 134.

Tenner, A. J. and Cooper, N. R. (1980). *Fed. Proc.* **39**, 361.

Thompson, R. A., Haeney, M., Reid, K. B. M., Davies, J. G., White, R. H. R. and Cameron, A. H. (1980). *New Engl. J. Med.* **303**, 22.

Van Snick, J. L. and Masson, P. L. (1978). *J. Exp. Med.* **148**, 903.

Van Wick, D. B., Witte, M. H., Witte, C. L. and Kintner, K. (1980). *Clin. Res.* **28**, 381A.

Wilson, C. B. and Dixon, F. J. (1970). *J. Immunol.* **105**, 279.

Theme 15: Summary
Complement and Immune Complexes

M. DIERICH

Institut für Med. Mikrobiologie, Mainz, West Germany

Under Theme 15 "Complement and Immune Complexes" we had 8 workshops with 197 contributions: it is therefore impossible to report on all of them. I will first summarize the complement-related contributions and then those related to immune complexes.

In contrast to past meetings, no new complement component was described. It appears that with about 20 factors known today, the serum system is complete.

Activation of the classical pathway of complement starts off by activation of C1 through binding of C1q to the CH_2 domain in the Fc portion of antibodies fixed to antigens. Binding may occur without activation (Hughes-Jones *et al.*, 15.1.11)*. Possibly C1q, in addition to binding by its globular heads, has to interact with a lysin residue in the Fc portion. Human C-reactive protein (CRP) can interfere with C1q binding (Drahovsky, 15.3.06). Bound C1q allows activation of C1r, which can also be studied with the purified proenzyme. Concomitant with activation, dimerization and cleavage of C1r is observed (Arland *et al.*, 15.1.01). Whether this cleavage is an autocatalytic process or depends on proteolysis (Bauer *et al.*, 15.1.03) from outside remains controversial.

The C1 inactivator (C1In) dissociates the C1r-dimer; it also forms complexes with C1s (Chesne *et al.*, 15.1.05). Binding of C1q or C1 occurs not only to antibody but also directly to surfaces of Gram-negative bacteria (Betz *et al.*, 15.2.01; Bub *et al.*, 15.3.03). Activated C1 generates the classical pathway C3 convertase C$\overline{42}$. This labile enzyme is further destabilized by the C4 binding protein which enhances the dissociation of C2. The decay is counteracted competitively by antibodies found in some patients with lupus erythematosus (Daha *et al.*, 15.1.07). This stabilization is responsible for a prolonged C3 consumption by a stabilized C$\overline{42}$ enzyme.

The C$\overline{42}$ enzyme not only acts on C3 but one a $\overline{\text{C4b,2a,3b}}$ complex is formed on the surfaces, it also cleaves C5. Similar conditions to the surfaces can be provided in the fluid phase by a high concentration of C3 allowing, probably transiently, for high enough concentrations of nascent metastable C3b in the fluid phase (Vogt *et al.* 15.1.24).

The activation of C3 by the classical pathway is achieved by the splitting off from the NH_2-terminus of the α chain of C3 a 9000 dalton fragment, C3a. The remaining 180 000 dalton fragment C3b can bind via a metastable site to cell surface sites, the C3 acceptors. On mononuclear blood cells C3 acceptor sites were found close to or on Fc receptors (Füst *et al.* 15.3.08). The potential of C3 to bind via a metastable site can be destroyed with increasing effectiveness by treatment with reagents of increasing nucleophilicity (Twose *et al.*, 15.1.22). From detailed analyses the understanding of the essential role of a thioester site in C3 for the activation of C3 and its binding to C3 acceptors has evolved (Tack *et al.* 15.1.19).

* Reference numbers indicate Abstract numbers in: Abstracts 4th International Congress of Immunology, Paris, 1980.

The thioester site in native C3 becomes "exposed" upon cleavage of C3. By reaction with OH groups of C3 acceptors, an SH group appears, which can be titrated with iodoacetamide. OH groups not only on cell surfaces but also from water may serve as acceptors. By the use of methylamine native C3 can be transformed into a C3b-like state; this can also occur spontaneously with H_2O. Such a "C3b-like" C3 is haemolytically inactive, but it interacts with factor B and also with β_1H. Therefore a "C3b-like" C3 may actually contribute the very first C3 convertase of the alternate pathway activation (Müller-Eberhard, see Chapter 54).

Studies of alternate pathway C3 convertases such as the one constituted from cobra venom factor and factor B are now performed with respect to their detailed enzymatic kinetics (Vogel *et al.*, 15.1.23) and their inhibition by small peptides like leupeptin (Ac LeuLeuArginal) (Caporale *et al.*, 15.1.04). Heparin can interfere with the build-up of such a convertase. It was found that *O*-sulphation and *N*-substitution of heparin are critical structural requirements for its ability to inhibit formation of the amplification convertase. *N*-substitution (SO_3- or acetyl) was discriminating between the pathway of coagulation and of complement (Kazatchkine, 15.1.13). The opsonization of particles with C3 seems to be influenced by a large molecular weight factor (Hawkins, 15.1.10). The relationship to another factor is not known (Kawakami *et al.*, 15.8.05).

The convertase once formed can be modulated: thus a high salt extract from Raji cells but not from Daudi cells could remove Bb from EAC4b,3b,Bb (Conrad *et al.*, 15.1.06), while nephritic factor, an antibody against the convertase, stabilizes this enzyme. It was shown that neuraminidase and periodate reduce the stabilizing potential of the antibody (Scott *et al.*, 15.1.18).

Activation of C3 either via the classical or via the alternate pathway allows then the activation of C5 and consecutively of C6, C7, C8 and C9 resulting in the formation of the C5b–C9 complex, the membrane attack complex (MAC). The activation of C5 can also be induced by mild acidification of serum (Hänsch *et al.*, 15.2.06). The effect on the structure of C5 remains to be clarified. This complex can be assembled in fluid phase or on the membrane. After binding to the membrane a second step, namely insertion, ensues accompanied by rearrangements of the components. The process from binding to lysis of cells shows distinct temperature dependency (Boyle *et al.*, 15.2.02). That the complex is actually inserted into the membrane, earlier shown with enzymatic stripping, is now more definite, supported by results from experiments with a particular photoaffinity label (Hu *et al.* 15.2.07). New information was also presented on modulation of target membranes with unsaturated phospholipides (Yoo *et al.*, 15.2.12) and with A_2C, an amphiphilic agent with a strong bend due to a cyclopropyl ring in the middle of the acyl chain (Shin *et al.*, 15.2.09). These membrane fluidizing modulations are believed to increase the efficiency of insertion of hydrophobic complement peptides.

The actual mechanism of lysis by complement has not been finally elucidated. It is a complexity of channel formation (Mayer, Johns Hopkins) and micellar deformation (Müller-Eberhard and coworkers, La Jolla) of the membrane. Depending on the particles, for instance erythrocytes versus viruses, and the dose of membrane attack complex, the channel formation or the detergent-like effects of the complex may prevail. There is now evidence that the complement lysis is a modified osmotic lysis since the cells lyse clearly below the critical volume (Valet *et al.*, 15.2.11). Circular lesions in target cells like in complement lysis are observed also in ADCC (Dourmashkin *et al.*, 15.2.03). But these circles are larger and measure 16–18 nm.

Several papers were presented indicating a synergistic cytotoxic effect involving complement and granulocytes, monocytes or lymphocytes (Grewal *et al.*, 15.2.04; Muchmore *et al.*, 15.2.08, Bridges *et al.*, 15.3.02; Joisel *et al.*, 15.3.10). During the activation of the complement system biologically active fragments arise. The spasmogenicity of C3a appears to be independent of histamine while spasmogenicity of $C5a_{desarg}$ is dependent on histamin (Damerau *et al.*, 15.3.05). Time course experiments in rabbit skin of PMN leukocyte sequestration and vascular permeability haemorrage established an *in vivo* role of the anaphylatoxin (Renker *et al.*, 15.3.20).

Several papers dealt with the possible involvement of complement components in the activation of lymphocytes. Evidence was presented suggesting a role for surface associated complement proteins in lymphocyte activation (Sundsmo *et al.*, 15.3.28). C3 was found to increase Con A induced blastogenesis, even in mouse spleen cells deprived of C3 receptor cells (Erdei *et al.*, 15.3.07). Complement was deposited on the lymphoblasts. Lymphoblasts induced by allogeneic stimulation were also shown to fix complement in normal serum (Martin *et al.*, 15.3.13), as did virus-infected cells (McConnell *et al.*, 15.3.14). In serum-free cultures purified C3 suppressed MLR dependent DNA synthesis (Needleman *et al.*, 15.3.17). Interaction of Raji cells with C3b-carrying cells was shown to be accompanied by, and dependent on, release of C5, B_1H and C3b from the Raji cells (Ross *et al.*, 15.3.22). It was hypothesized that C5 and the regulator proteins might be critical for lymphocyte activation.

In macrophage activation the macrophages' own C3 plays a central role (Schorlemmer *et al.*, 15.3.25). Triggering of macrophages was also shown to occur by primary aliphatic amines such as methylamine which at the same time induce complement activation (Riches *et al.*, 15.3.21). This might be due to generation of a "C3b-like" C3. Phagocytosis of complement coated particles was shown to be inhibitable by the carbohydrate portion of α_1-antitrypsin (Mod *et al.*, 15.3.16). Evidence for the role of carbohydrates was also derived from a different system (Hawkins *et al.*, 15.8.03).

A series of papers were devoted to genetic aspects of the complement system. Total defects of Clq (Leyva-Cobiani *et al.*, 15.4.05), C3 (Roord *et al.* 15.4.12) and C9 (Yukiyama *et al.*, 15.4.20) were detected in families without linkage to HLA. The C3 defect was associated with repeated pneumococcal infections associated with meningitis. Functional defects of C8 were described (Matthews *et al.*, 15.4.06; Spira *et al.*, 15.4.13). In spite of unimpaired opsonization by his serum one patient was particularly susceptible to attacks of meningococci. The defect in serum bactericidal activity seems to be critical in the handling of *Neisseria*. A functional defect of C4 due to cleavage (Day *et al.*, 14.4.01) and a functional defect of C4 accompanied by the absence of the Rodgers antigen (O'Neill *et al.*, 15.4.10) were not linked to HLA. This raises the possibility that there may be genes outside the MHC which to some degree regulate C4 expression. Studies on mouse C4 showed that there are variations in the γ and α chain of C4 and that the C4d fragment only of γ_1-C4 carries the H-2·7 determinant. This antigenic determinant on cell surfaces might be acquired secondarily by binding C4 to these cells (Ferreira *et al.*, 15.4.02). Based on various methods the conclusion was reached that the gene for human C4 is located between HLA-D/DR and HLA-B, probably closer to the latter. The genes for B and C2 then are in the same area (Teisberg *et al.*, 15.4.17). A progress report was given concerning the effort to establish cloning of cDNAs for mouse C3 and C4. An identification of 3 different C3 cDNA clones has been achieved (Fey *et al.*, 15.4.03).

The antibody response in a C4-deficient patient and in C4-deficient guinea-pigs was shown to be impaired. The secondary response lacked amplification and showed no switch from IgM to IgG (Wedgwood *et al.*, 15.4.18). C4 deficiency also appeared to have a negative impact on the stimulatory function of human lymphocytes in MLRs (Tappeiner *et al.*, 15.4.15). C8 deficient mice displayed increased susceptibility to crytococcus neoformans (Wicker *et al.*, 15.4.19). An increased frequency of the C3 Fast variant of C3 in patients with membranoproliferative glomerulonephritis and partial lipodystrophy was reported (McLean *et al.*, 15.4.07).

The second group of papers dealt with immune complex related aspects. The studies confirmed and extended previous observations on the role of complement for solubilizing immune complexes (Schifferli *et al.*, 15.3.24; Malasit *et al.*, 15.3.13). The β_1H globulin was shown to have an inhibitory effect (Nydegger *et al.*, 15.3.18). Degradation of immune complexes by macrophages was enhanced by complement (Kijlstra *et al.*,

15.3.11). No correlation was found between C3 conversion products, circulating IC (CIC) and the half-life of injected labelled C3 in a group of patients (Swaak *et al.* 15.3.29).

In the workshop concerned with spontaneous and experimental animal disease associated with immune complexes, 2 main questions were discussed. The first concerned the role of antigen in the initiation and perpetuation of the immune response (Alexander *et al.* 15.5.01). Experiments were presented showing that polyclonal B cell stimulation, produced *in vivo* by injecting into mice B cell activators such as LPS or dextransulphate, resulted in formation of CIC and the production of anti-antibodies (Niembro *et al.*, 15.5.14). Also, applying phosphorylcholine in another system, production of specific antibodies carrying a particular idiotype and anti-idiotypic antibodies were observed (Rose *et al.*, 15.5.15). This could explain the difficulties in identifying the antigen contained in the IC. It also reminds one of the situations in which CIC seems to persist long after the disappearance of the antigen. It has been proposed that, in such cases, IC could contain antibodies directed against other long-lasting antigens, such as autoantigens.

The second question referred to the pathogenic role of CIC and of inflammation mediators. The pathogenic effect has been questioned (Das *et al.*, 15.5.04); Sindrey *et al.*, 15.5.17) as CIC are absent in some diseases considered as "immune complex disease" and are present in apparently normal situations. The size of the complexes, the affinity of the antibodies, and their biological properties and the type of antigen (Finbloom *et al.*, 15.8.02) are critical factors (Hamashima *et al.*, 15.5.08). Attention should be paid not only to IgG but also to IgM and IgA (Digeon *et al.*, 15.7.11; Kauffmann *et al.*, 15.7.22). In spite of the general heterogeneity of the results obtained in different immunopathological systems (Capron *et al.*, 15.5.02) it has been suggested that various inflammatory mediators (Sanchez-Crespo *et al.*, 15.5.16) and cells (Seehra *et al.*, 15.8.07; Mathison *et al.*, 15.8.08; Morrison *et al.*, 15.8.09; Kavai *et al.*, 15.7.23) are involved and that complement aside from destructive effects might play a protective role (Day *et al.*, 15.5.05).

There are several assays used to detect soluble immune complexes. The C1q binding test, the solid phase C1q binding assay, the conglutinin binding test and the Raji cell assay have been the most popular for several years. Modifications of some assays were described (Nineham *et al.*, 15.6.18; Eisenberg *et al.*, 15.6.08) and pitfalls were pointed out such as interference of fibrinogen with C1q (Faaber *et al.*, 15.6.09) and direct binding of antibodies to Raji cells (Anderson *et al.*, 15.6.03; Horsefall *et al.*, 15.7.19). Some new assays were also presented (Witkin *et al.*, 15.6.29). As a result of a WHO collaborative study (Agnello *et al.*, 15.6.01) standard reference preparations for IC-testing will now be available from the Swiss Red Cross (Nydegger: Chapter 55): one containing aggregated IgG and the other tetanus toxoid–antitoxoid preparations.

A great deal was discussed concerning the relevance of IC detection. A long catalogue of diseases including malignancies accompanied by appearance of CIC has been compiled (most papers of workshop 15.7). It is obvious that detection of CIC has very little, if any, value for the discrimination of diseases. Nevertheless, it was generally agreed on in the discussion, that the search for CIC is of great value in carefully selected circumstances: (1) single patients, not large groups, might be followed since the amount of IC might reflect the severity of the underlying disease. In longitudinal studies of cancer patients with bad prognosis high IC concentrations have been observed (Manro *et al.*, 15.7.31). There is an indication that relapses are preceded by an increase of CIC-concentration (Kristensen *et al.*, 15.7.26). (2) Therapeutic regimens can be monitored. (3) Isolation of IC may allow the identification of the antigen. Particularly binding of IC to conglutinin is used as a tool (Maine *et al.*, 15.7.30).

Besides the detection of IC, the evaluation of a patient's serum capacity for IC-solubilization can be of value (Agnado *et al.*, 15.7.01). In SLE patients, solubilization correlated better with alternative pathway activation than with classical pathway activation. But as well as complement, other factors may well interfere with the solubilizing process.

Finally, I would like to extend my sincere gratitude, particularly to Professor Dr Peltier, the president of Theme 15, to Dr Lise Halbwachs, Dr Hauptman and to Dr Michael Kazatchkine, the French co-ordinators. They have been of great assistance. I also thank the chairmen for their kind help.

Theme 16

Immunology of Reproduction and Embryonic Development

President:
R. E. BILLINGHAM
G. A. VOISIN

Symposium chairman:
K. BRATANOV

57

Auto- and Isoimmune Reactions to Antigens of the Gonads and Genital Tract

P. RÜMKE

Division of Immunology, The Netherlands Cancer Institute, Plesmanlaan 121, Amsterdam, The Netherlands

I thank the following colleagues who helped me generously by sending me their preprints of recent work and reviews: Drs N. J. Alexander, M. D'Almeida, B. Boettcher, E. Goldberg, R. J. T. Hancock, W. F. Hendry, T. Hjort, S. Jager, W. R. Jones, Z. H. Marcus, A. C. Menge, C. B. Metz, D. B. Morton, M. G. O'Rand, G. F. B. Schumacher, C. A. Shivers, S. Shulman, K. S. K. Tung, F. Toullet and G. A. Voisin. I gratefully acknowledge Drs B. Boettcher, C. P. Engelfriet, A. Hekman and Marie Anne van Halem for help with the preparation of the manuscript.

Introduction

This chapter will deal with various aspects of auto- and isoimmune reactivity against gonadal antigens. (The prefix "iso" is, as proposed by Voisin *et al.* (1975) used to indicate reactivity of the female against male substances of the same species). Since most experimental and clinical work has been done on the testis and spermatozoa, the main part of this chapter is devoted to the male reproductive antigens. Immunology of other gonads and antigens of the genital tract will only be discussed briefly.

A long-existing gap between experimental and clinical research is reason to treat the 2 fields separately. In particular, this gap concerns on the one hand the virtual nonexistence of immunological research on ejaculates of experimental animals, in contrast to a longstanding and extensive knowledge of mechanisms playing a role in autoimmune syndromes of the testis, and on the other hand the lack of knowledge about testis immunopathology in man, while much is known of immune phenomena in ejaculates of some infertile men. Although these aspects are treated separately, it is hoped that this chapter will contribute to a better orientation of experimentalists on clinical problems, and vice versa to a better application by clinicians of experimental knowledge, in order to solve still existing questions in the diagnosis and treatment of infertility.

Autoantigens of testis and spermatozoa

Autoantigens of testis and spermatozoa in animal models

Sperm and testis autoantigens have been studied in experimental models by using antisera from animals immunized with allogeneic, syngeneic or autologous testis or sperm homogenates, or extracts thereof. Since orchitis leading to aspermatogenesis is often the result of autoimmunization, at least when the animals are immunized with a proper adjuvant, these autoantigens are also called aspermatogenic antigens. Immunohistological studies, mainly carried out in the guinea-pig and the rabbit, showed that the autoantigens occur only in postmeiotic stages of spermatogenesis. The same was found by studying antibody binding to fractionated germ cells from the testis (Johnson, 1970; O'Rand and Romrell, 1977). Earlier it had been demonstrated that no autoimmune syndrome could be induced in the adult male with neonatal testicular tissue containing only primitive spermatogenic and Sertoli cells (Katsh, 1960; Pokorná and Vojtísková, 1964), and newborn guinea-pigs immunized with adult testicular homogenate incorporated in complete Freund's adjuvant, did not show any sign of testicular abnormality until after spermatogenesis was fully developed (Bishop *et al.*, 1961). Some of the aspermatogenic autoantigens are membrane antigens, others are acrosomal enzymes and still others are differentiation products appearing at different stages of spermatogenesis (O'Rand, 1980). Several of these antigens have been semi-purified and partly characterized. A highly soluble acrosomal small protein (mol. wt 15 000) evokes a mild autoimmune orchitis in an amount as low as 0·2 μg (Jackson *et al.*, 1975). A protein, called P, two glycoproteins (S and Z) and a membrane-linked protein (called T antigen) have been studied extensively (Toullet *et al.*, 1973; Voisin *et al.*, 1975). All induce spermatogenesis, but seemingly by different immunopathological mechanisms due to different immunogenic properties of the antigens. For instance, only the water-insoluble T antigen induces complement dependent cytotoxic antibodies against spermatozoa, while the water-soluble glycoprotein S induces delayed hypersensitivity and anaphylactic antibodies, and the water-soluble protein P anaphylactic as well as complement fixing antibodies. The most purified preparation of T consists of 5 polypeptides, and the antigen itself is possibly a lipoprotein (Lefroit-Jolly *et al.*, 1979). Two other guinea-pig aspermatogenic glycoproteins have been purified by other workers (Hagopian *et al.*, 1976). Recent work on rabbit sperm membrane autoantigens by O'Rand and his coworkers (reviewed by O'Rand, 1980) has revealed at least 5 protein-staining bands by polyacrylamide gel electrophoresis. A single autoantigen (RSA-1) was shown to be a sialoglycoprotein of mol. wt 13 000. RSA-1 appears first on the surface of pachytene spermatocytes. On the mature spermatozoa it is concentrated in the postacrosomal and middle-piece regions but may occur in isolated patches over the acrosome and tail regions. Two subclasses of surface autoantigens could be identified, the one appears only on pachytene spermatocytes and the other does not appear until midspermatid stage. The subclass appearing early contains molecules of larger molecular weight which are not present on spermatozoa. Other autoantigens are intracellular at the pachytene stage and do not appear on the surface until later stages, while still others, like RSA-1, appear on the surface of pachytene spermatocytes and remain throughout spermatogenesis.

Autoantigenic acrosomal enzymes are hyaluronidase (Metz, 1979) and possibly acrosin (Morton, 1977). The testis specific cytoplasmatic enzyme lactate dehydrogenase (LDH-X or LDH-C_4) is also autoantigenic (Goldberg, 1974).

It is thus clear that various organ-specific sperm antigens exist. They are differentiation products as well as acrosomal substances and enzymes, and appear at different postmeiotic stages of spermatogenesis.

Sperm autoantigens in man

Sperm-specific autoantibodies, found in the serum of some naturally infertile and of vasectomized men, produce different patterns of agglutination which suggests that distinct surface antigens occur on the head, the tail and the tip of the tail. Recently Hjort *et al.* (1978) found that $F(ab)_2$ fragments of the IgG of certain sera, revealing both agglutination and complement dependent immobilization, would block the immobilization caused by the intact antibodies of the same serum, but not always that caused by those in other sera. By cross-experiments it was shown that there are at least two tail antigens. It was surprising that $F(ab)_2$ of pure head-to-head agglutinating sera could block immobilization by tail-to-tail agglutinating sera, whereas antitail $F(ab)_2$ could not block immobilization by head-to-head agglutinins. It was concluded that there are at least 4 different specific membrane antigens, 1 involved in head-to-head agglutination which is also present on the tail, 2 involved in tail agglutination, which are also located in the posterior part of the head, and 1 in tip of the tail agglutination. Jager *et al.* (1980b) made similar observations in another way: with the mixed antiglobulin test they found that, irrespective of the direct agglutination type, the adherence of the sensitized erythrocytes used in the test in most cases were found on all sites of the spermatozoa.

Recently Poulson and Hjort (1980) with the aid of human sera containing agglutinating and immobilizing antibodies, isolated 3 polypeptides from human sperm membranes, one with a molecular weight of about 45 000 and 2 with molecular weights of about 77 000. De Almeida (1980) found at least 3 distinct antigenic fractions that either inhibited head-to-head agglutination or tail-to-tail agglutination or spermotoxicity.

Earlier it was found that 2 strongly basic nuclear proteins—protamines—isolated from human spermatozoa could be identified as autoantigens (Kolk and Samuel, 1975). Antibodies to these protamines in sera of some infertile patients and some vasectomized men, cross-react with fish protamines, and vice versa, antibodies against salmon protamines, found in diabetic patients treated with protamine-Zn-insulin, cross-react with protamine from human spermatozoa (Samuel, 1977). Such sera do not react with the nuclei of somatic cells. Autoantibodies have also been found against a sperm-specific DNA polymerase (Witkin *et al.*, 1978).

LDH-X is probably isoantigenic since, according to results in a radioimmunoassay, the serum of a single infertile woman contained antibodies to LDH-X (Kolk *et al.*, 1978). So far no men have been found with antibodies against LDH-X.

Relevant nonorgan-specific sperm antigens

Histocompatibility and blood group antigens

Histocompatibility antigens have been demonstrated in low concentrations on spermatozoa of men and mice. Some evidence exists for a haploid expression of HLA antigens on spermatozoa in man (Festenstein *et al.*, 1978), but this finding needs confirmation in other laboratories. Blood group substances A and B which are present in the seminal plasma of secretors adhere to spermatozoa. Whether weak A and B also occur on the spermatozoa of nonsecretors is still controversial, but most investigators could not detect A and B as intrinsic antigens on human spermatozoa (for references see Hekman and Rümke, 1976).

Sperm-coating antigens

In any discussion on the antigens of spermatozoa it must be realized that ejaculated spermatozoa are coated by substances derived from the adnexal glands, which are hard to remove without damaging the spermatozoa. When in the analysis of semen heterologous antisera are used, these sperm-coating antigens (SCA) can be the cause of cross-reactions between antibodies to ejaculated spermatozoa or to seminal plasma. The major SCA in man is lactoferrin which originates from the seminal vesicles. Possibly other coating antigens are contributed by the prostate and epididymis (for references see Hekman and Rümke, 1976). It has been recently shown that a monoclonal antibody against one of the SCA, present in seminal plasma as well as in milk, but which was different from lactoferrin, could strongly immobilize but not agglutinate spermatozoa (Shigeta *et al.*, 1980).

The normal immunological unresponsiveness to sperm antigens

In men

Until recently it was believed that because of the sequestration of spermatozoa, no autoimmunity to sperm antigens could normally develop. Indeed, a strong barrier at the level of the seminiferous tubules is provided by the Sertoli cells and the tight junctions between them. During all steps of spermatogenesis the germ cells, excluding spermatogonia and preleptotene spermatocytes, are sequestered behind this barrier. However, at the rete testis and the tubuli efferentes the barrier is less tight, and "physiological" leakage of sperm antigens would here be possible. It has been postulated that in this way a physiological state of tolerance might be induced (Tung, 1980). Recently Hurtenbach *et al.* (1980) found that germ cells isolated from testis were able to suppress lymphocytic proliferation, whereas somatic cells from the same testis were not able to do so. This inhibition appeared to be the result of activation of non-specific T suppressor cells. The authors suggest that germ cells have immunoregulatory functions which may operate via embryonic antigens. Overt autoimmunity to sperm would then only occur if immunoregulatory mechanisms are circumvented, for instance after excessive resorption of sperm antigens or leakage of whole sperm such as it occurs after vasectomy, or when the immunoregulatory mechanisms themselves fail. The latter may occur in the A-line beagle dog in which genetically dependent testicular pathology resembling orchitis, occurs spontaneously, sometimes together with lymphocytic thyroiditis (Fritz *et al.*, 1976), and in the Lewis rat in which thymectomy can lead to autoimmune orchitis and sperm antibody formation (Lipscomb *et al.*, 1979). For proof of a physiological leakage of sperm antigens, sensitive assays of isolated sperm antigens have yet to be developed.

In women

The fate of spermatozoa in the female differs in various species. For a detailed discussion and references the reader is referred to a review by Austin, 1976). In man, most of the ejaculated spermatozoa flush from the vagina, and only a relatively small proportion of them enter the uterus. They are scavenged by macrophages and neutrophils in the uterus, and macrophages of the peritoneum, but may also enter other cells, such as metaplastic epithelium of the cervix. Whether phagocytosis is only confined to dead spermatozoa is not clear. Artificial insemination may result in pregnancy when performed 6 days before ovulation, indicating that viable spermatozoa can remain unaffected in the genital tract for an appreciable time.

The reason why phagocytosis of spermatozoa does not lead to an overt immune response is not known. One of the possibilities is that the amount of antigens is low and that rather than an overt humoral antibody response, low-dose immune tolerance is induced. Roberts *et al.* (1977) found in mice that cell-mediated immunity (CMI) against sperm, as measured in leukocyte adherence and migration inhibition tests, was not demonstrable in virgin females, while after mating these tests became positive. The same was found in women: 6/7 nonvirgin nulliparous and 6/7 multiparous, and 0/7 virgins revealed positive CMI tests. Other mechanisms that might operate in a maintenance of unresponsiveness of the female genital tract to spermatozoa involve the coating of sperm by substances like lactoferrin that may prevent antigenic recognition (Boettcher, 1968) and the immunosuppressive action of spermatozoa themselves. Intact spermatozoa as well as seminal plasma components inhibit PHA and Con A induced blast formation of human lymphocytes (Marcus *et al.*, 1978). Also, inhibition of E-rosette formation is demonstrable (Marcus *et al.*, 1979). Whether mature spermatozoa are able to activate T suppressor cells, as has been found with testicular germ cells (Hurtenbach *et al.*, 1980), has not been studied.

It has also been proposed that natural antibodies against spermatozoa may play a role in the maintenance of tolerance to spermatozoa in the female. Various aspects of unresponsiveness to sperm in the female have been discussed by Hancock (1978).

Experimentally induced autoimmune aspermatogenic orchi-epididymitis

After its discovery in 1951 by Voisin *et al.* (1951) experimentally induced autoimmune disease of the testis became one of the first models of the immunological mechanisms in autoimmune syndromes. An excellent detailed review, in which references can be found, has recently been published by Tung (1980). Only the main points derived from experimental work in several species, but mostly in guinea-pigs, will be discussed here.

Immunopathology and pathogenesis

Immunization with crude extracts of allogeneic sperm or testis, or with purified sperm-specific antigens, will lead to autoimmune aspermatogenic orchi-epididymitis (AIAO), but in general only when an appropriate adjuvant is used. Without an adjuvant multiple large does of antigen are needed to induce AIAO, and the disease will be milder. The histopathological findings are complex, and begin to appear after 6 to 9 days with degenerative changes of spermatids and exfoliation of germinal epithelium. Perivascular or peritubular infiltration of inflammatory cells is not consistent at this stage. The morphological abnormalities are not specific for immunologically induced lesions since they can also be found after various injuries. Focal clusters of lymphocytes and macrophages are early signs of AIAO. These cells enter the seminiferous tubules through holes in the tubular basement membrane and between the Sertoli cells. Adjacent to these infiltrations the germinal epithelium desquamates, which results in local aspermatogenesis. Neutrophil-rich lesions are seen in the efferent duct, the epididymis and the vas deferens. Later lesions include large abscesses, granulomata and periductal fibrosis. In the end-stage, complete aspermatogenesis with atrophy of the seminiferous tubules and interstitial fibrosis, together with signs of regeneration, can be found but without infiltration of mononuclear cells.

Distinct differences in the immunopathological patterns are found after immunization with different isolated sperm-specific autoantigens. Thus, the disease does not develop in a unified manner, nor do all the lesions always develop. Various immunological mechanisms may operate in different degrees. Differences are not only dependent on the antigens involved, but also on the genetic background of the animal. The lesions can be induced in normal animals after passive transfer of either antibodies alone, provided that they are from hyperimmunized animals, or by T cell enriched lymphocytes, but not B cell or macrophage enriched cells from immunized animals, indicating that both humoral and cellular immunity play a role in the pathogenesis of the disease. How AIAO is initiated is still a matter of debate. Central is the question of how the blood-testis barrier is passed by antibodies and immune cells. As already discussed the barrier has its weakest spots in the rete testis. It may be there that soluble sperm antigens leak outside the tubules where reactions with antibodies and cells may first occur, after which the inflamed barrier becomes weaker allowing immune reactants to enter the lumen of the efferent ducts. From there, in a retrograde way the seminiferous tubules are reached. A predominantly antibody response will lead to desquamative lesions without much orchitis, whereas a strong cell-mediated immune response will lead to severe orchitis. Immune reactants may also reach the epididymis where inflammatory lesions are elicited.

Another type of experimentally induced autoimmune orchitis, concerns orchitis in rats after passive transfer of rabbit antiserum against a collagen-free soluble fraction of the basement membrane of seminiferous tubules of rat testis (Denduchis and Lustig, 1981).

Autoimmune pathology of the testis has been found to occur after injury of the testis and after vasectomy. Unilateral burning by electrocoagulation of guinea-pig testis resulted in the formation of testis specific autoantibodies, and histological abnormalities were sometimes seen in the other testis (Rapaport *et al.*, 1969). An autoimmune response was recorded after mechanical pressure to such an extent that the normal consistency was lost, and histological abnormalities were found in the contralateral untreated testis (Mancini, 1974). In the rabbit, testis pathology 8 to 10 months after vasectomy resembles experimental AIAO, and peritoneal exudate cells from vasectomized guinea-pigs could adoptively transfer the testicular lesions. In mice and rhesus monkeys orchitis and/or aspermatogenesis was found significantly more frequently in vasectomized animals than in matched controls (Alexander and Anderson, 1979; Anderson and Alexander, 1980). For these reasons it might be expected that autoimmune orchitis can occur naturally in man, the more so since experiments in man suggest that autoimmune orchitis can be induced by injections of testicular homogenates or extracts in Freund's adjuvant (Mancini, 1976).

Auto- and isoimmunity to sperm in human infertility

Since 1954, when Wilson and Rümke independently reported on the occurrence of sperm autoantibodies in infertile males, and later, when Franklin and Dukes in 1964 reported on sperm isoantibodies in infertile women, an extensive literature has appeared on the immunology of infertility in men and women. For references and details the reader is referred to Shulman (1975), Hekman and Rümke (1976), Rümke and Hekman (1977), Rümke (1978), Shulman (1978), Boettcher (1979), Jones (1980) and Menge (1980).

Test systems currently in use for the detection of sperm antibodies in men

Technical aspects of the detection of sperm antibodies in men and women can be found in the following reviews: Rose *et al.* (1976), Boettcher *et al.* (1977), Shulman (1978) and Menge (1980).

The conventional test systems for the detection of antibodies against surface antigens of spermatozoa are the agglutination and the complement-dependent immobilization and cytotoxicity tests. The agglutination test in gelatin-containing medium in tubes (GAT), which is read macroscopically and the micro-test in trays (TAT), which is read microscopically, are the most widely used agglutination tests. The GAT and TAT, in general, give comparable results, although the chance of nonimmune agglutination, as for instance due to β macroglobulin in some sera, is greater in the TAT than in the GAT. The advantage of the TAT is the microscale application and the possibility of recording the type of agglutination, i.e. head-to-head, tail-to-tail, tailtip-to-tailtip and mixed forms. Fortunately, in spite of the presence of blood group A and B antigens as SCA, neither anti-A nor anti-B agglutinate spermatozoa from individuals, positive for the corresponding antigen(s). Therefore, every donor sample of semen of good quality can be used as substrate in these tests. The immobilization test is applied with various modifications. Whereas the agglutinins are most often semiquantitated by titration, the immobilization test as well as the cytotoxicity test often is performed with undiluted serum and the strength of the reaction is expressed in an index. The qualitative and quantitative differences between the immobilization and cytotoxicity test are minimal. The same antibodies are detected by both these techniques. A particular advantage of the latter tests is that, because of their complement dependency, positive results can be more reliably ascribed to the activity of antibodies. An advantage of the agglutination tests is their higher sensitivity. With few exceptions, immobilizins (including cytotoxic antibodies) are found only when agglutinins are present in the same serum. The higher the agglutinin titres, the more frequently immobilizins are also present. The relationship is irrespective of the agglutination type, with the exception of the rarely occurring tailtip type that has been found in high titres in the absence of immobilizins. Because of its anticomplementarity it is difficult to detect immobilizins or cytotoxic antibodies in seminal plasma.

Recently, a number of other tests for antispermatozoal antibodies have been developed. The mixed haemabsorption test is feasible for routine testing and has the advantage that the microglobulin class of the antibodies is automatically determined. In particular, the test has been used to detect and classify antibodies bound to spermatozoa in ejaculates of patients (Jager *et al.*, 1978, 1980b), but it can also be applied for the detection of serum antibodies (Mathur *et al.*, 1979).

Tests with direct biological relevance are the sperm–cervical mucus penetration test (S-CMPT) (Kremer, 1965) and the sperm–cervical mucus contact test (S-CMCT) (Kremer and Jager, 1980). They are both applied in cases of male as well as female infertility. The S-CMPT measures the degree to which spermatozoa, sensitized by autoantibodies from the seminal plasma or by isoantibodies in the cervical mucus, are inhibited in their migration through a capillary filled with cervical mucus. The S-CMCT measures the percentages of spermatozoa that display jerking movements without progressive motility. This type of flagellation-in-place was called the "shaking phenomenon" and is found to be associated with agglutinating antibodies in high titre. It is caused by adherence of the sensitized spermatozoa to the micelles of the cervical mucus. Since spermatozoa sensitized with $F(ab)_2$ derived from autoantibodies do not adhere, and also since $F(ab)_2$ of antibodies against the Fc part of IgG can inhibit the phenomenon, it is likely that the adherence is due to an interaction of the Fc part with the micelles (Jager *et al.*, 1980a). An interesting new approach is the technique based on the inhibition of the penetration of human spermatozoa into zona-free hamster ova (Menge and Black, 1979).

The indirect immunofluorescence test, usually applied on sperm smears has not found a wide application, not only because positive results were often obtained with control sera and the correlation with the result of agglutination and immobilization tests was poor, but also because of a lack of interlaboratory reproducibility (Boettcher *et al.*, 1977). An exception can be made for the detection of antiprotamine antibodies on swollen spermatozoa. This test is reproducible and does not give positive reactions in the controls.

New techniques

Most of the tests discussed so far are semiquantitative, subjective and liable to experimental error. There is therefore a need for objective assays such as those in which radiolabelled anti-antibody is quantitatively measured. A recently developed solid phase indirect microradioimmunoassay in which washed spermatozoa are fixed to the bottom of the wells of microtitre trays (Young, 1978) may be promising. Also a test involving nuclear binding of ^{3}H-actinomycin-D after membrane damage by complement-dependent cytotoxic antibodies is advantageous for testing many samples at the same time (Sung *et al.*, 1977; Boettcher and Boettcher, 1979). A test based on the difference in ATP content between damaged and undamaged spermatozoa gave satisfactory results in the assay for cytotoxic antibodies, and appeared simpler and faster than the conventional staining methods, allowing 200 samples to be tested within one day (Suominen *et al.*, 1980). Nanogram amounts of IgG bound to guinea-pig testicular cells could be detected using radiolabelled staphylococcal protein A (Han and Tung, 1979).

Autoimmunity against spermatozoa in infertile men

Depending on the selection of patients, the technique used and the subjective appreciation of the lowest serum dilution in which a positive result can still be recorded, the incidence of sperm antibodies in different reports varies considerably. Roughly estimated, 10% of the husbands of infertile couples in whom no organic cause can be found (so called "unexplained" infertile couples) have sperm agglutinating (mainly of the tail-to-tail type) and often also immobilizing antibodies. Sera containing such antibodies do not react in the immunofluorescence test with other organs, and absorption studies have shown that only testis or spermatozoa, and not seminal fluid, can absorb the antibodies. Therefore it may be concluded that, in general, agglutinating and immobilizing antibodies in men are directed against testis-specific sperm antigens and not against SCA. They are most often of the IgG class, although IgM antibodies can also occur. (If agglutinin titres are low, i.e. less than 20, and immobilizins are not present, there is often no proof of the antibody nature of the agglutinating factor).

The higher the titre in the serum, the higher the chance that the seminal plasma also contains agglutinating antibodies. With a serum titre of 64, 50% of the men and, with a titre of 512 nearly 95%, have seminal plasma agglutinins (Rümke, 1978). The agglutinins in seminal plasma can be of the IgG and IgA or sIgA type. Although 1 or 2% of circulating IgG transudates via the prostate into the seminal compartment, most of the antibodies are locally formed somewhere in the genital tract. It is proposed that sIgA is produced in the genital tract distal to the vasa deferentia (Boettcher, 1977). Agglutinins are practically never found in the seminal plasma if they are not present in the serum. The levels of immunoglobulins in the seminal plasma of patients with sperm antibodies in the seminal plasma are not increased (Friberg, 1980).

For the discussion of the mechanism by which autoantibodies can be related to infertility, the patients can be divided in 2 categories. In the first category are the majority of the men in whom spermatogenesis apparently is not impaired, because ejaculates contain a normal number of spermatozoa. A normal morphology and a normal initial motility moreover show that in these patients there is no obvious defect in the function of the genital organs. The only problem is the autoantibody present in the seminal plasma. The other category is comprised of patients in whom the infertility can be explained by oligo- or azoospermia, whatever the cause of these conditions may be. In relation to their case the question arises whether autoimmune orchi-epididymitis exists in man. The normospermic men will be discussed first.

Judged by postcoital and cervical mucus invasion tests *in vitro*, a parallel between the inability to invade cervical mucus and serum agglutination and immobilizing titres was found (Fjällbrant, 1968). The relationship of serum agglutinin titres with prolonged infertility was shown in a follow-up study (Rümke *et al.*, 1974) comprising 254 men in whom serum titres of 4 to over 1024 had been determined at an earlier date. In the subsequent years 36 men became fathers. Thirty of them belonged to a group of 137 normospermic men. An inverse relationship with the titre was evident, since 48% of the men with titres of 4–16 became fathers, whereas of those with a titre of 32–128,

16% and of those with a titre > 128 only 12%. Occasionally however men become fathers even in the presence of a serum agglutinin titre as high as 1024. Of better predictive value are the seminal plasma titres. I have never come across a man who became fertile when his seminal agglutinin titre was higher than 16. In a series of 26 patients Husted and Hjort (1975) did not see any paternity in 15 patients with titres of 64 or higher, whereas the wives of 4 of 11 patients with titres of 4 to 16 became pregnant. A direct relationship was found between autoagglutination in the ejaculates of the normospermic men and the seminal titre. Also, the chance of the remaining nonagglutinated spermatozoa becoming immobilized after penetration in the cervical mucus increases with the seminal plasma titres. Jager *et al.* (1979) found that with titres of 32 and higher, the nonagglutinated spermatozoa did not have a normal migration pattern as measured in the sperm penetration meter test and, also, in the sperm–cervical mucus contact test the vast majority of the spermatozoa showed the "shaking phenomenon", indicating adherence of sensitized spermatozoa to the glycoprotein micelles in the cervical mucus. Even if some spermatozoa loaded with sperm antibody would escape through the cervix, animal experimental work shows that they might not be able to adhere to the ovum, since spermatozoa incubated with Fab of sperm antibodies were not able to adhere to ova (Metz and Anika, 1970).

The second category of patients, i.e. those with an insufficient number of spermatozoa in the ejaculate, can be divided in two groups: one in whom there is complete azoospermia with an anatomical obstruction of the efferent pathways, and one to which the oligozoospermic patients mainly belong, in whom anatomical obstruction is not evident at all. In the first group testis biopsies most often show a normal spermatogenesis. These patients are comparable to vasectomized men. From longitudinal studies in vasectomized men it is known that 60–80% of them form sperm antibodies within one year after the operation and therefore it can be concluded that pathological resorption of spermatozoa or antigenic fragments as a result of obstruction in the efferent pathways, is a major cause of sperm autoantibody formation. The fact that high-titred sperm autoantibodies occur, on the one hand, in the group of normospermic men already discussed and, on the other hand, in azoospermic men with normal spermatogenesis, shows that sperm antibodies as such do not necessarily interfere with spermatogenesis. As discussed earlier, the same has been found in animals: after immunization with the use of incomplete Freund's adjuvant sperm antibodies are formed, but there is no indication of the development of AIAO.

The last group of infertile men with sperm autoantibodies to be discussed comprises patients with a low output of spermatozoa, or those azoospermic men in whom a testis biopsy shows abnormalities of the spermatogenesis. The incidence of such patients among the total of oligozoospermic patients is probably less than 10% or even 5%. Nevertheless, from the point of view of immunopathology, they form an intriguing group of patients. In spite of the fact that the testis was one of the first target organs in experimental animal work in which mechanisms of autoimmunopathology were studied, in the clinical situation autoimmune diseases of the testis and/or epididymis are ill-defined and their existence has not been unequivocally proven. Immunological studies in suspected patients are scanty and often do not deal with more than one possible criterion. A difficulty in recognizing autoimmune orchi-epididymitis by a testis biopsy is undoubtedly that, as was shown in experimental animals, no pathognomonic histological criteria exist other than early clustering of macrophages and lymphocytes. This stage might easily be missed the more so since, as was already shown in the experiment, Leydig cells are not affected, so that patients will have no hormonal deficiency that brings them to the doctor at a sufficiently early stage. A prerequisite for the existence of the syndrome seems to be demonstrable sperm immunity, but it has to be anticipated that in the case of complete azoospermia due to autoimmune aspermatogenesis in an end stage, antibodies may have disappeared, with the result that the syndrome in an end stage is difficult to recognize.

Because the importance of T lymphocytes and delayed hypersensitivity against sperm antigens in the animal model, several investigators attempted to demonstrate cellular immunity against sperm antigens. Various techniques have been used, and in several disorders of the testis indications of cellular immunity were found. However, a formal proof that the reactivity was against sperm antigens has not yet been given. Boettcher *et al.* (1979) showed that whole semen could stimulate allogeneic lymphocytes, whereas the same amount of isolated motile spermatozoa from the same semen sample did not stimulate. Also Lucas and Rose (1978) mention nonspecific stimulatory activity or sometimes spontaneous lymphocyte toxicity by whole semen or sperm extracts. Nevertheless, in several studies patients much more often had indications of cell-mediated immunity to sperm than controls (Dondero *et al.*, 1980), and also autologous sperm sometimes proved to be stimulatory in lymphocyte transformation tests (Thestrup-Pedersen *et al.*, 1976). Since indications of cell-mediated autoimmunity also occurred in some normospermic men, a positive reaction cannot be considered to be specific for autoimmune orchitis. A positive finding, as is the case with humoral sperm antibodies, only indicates that the patient at one time became immunized against his own sperm.

The proof for an effect of autoimmunity at the level of testis will probably have to come from immunohistological studies of testis biopsies. Indeed there are several reports on tissue bound immunoglobulin or C3 in the testis, but most often these concern immunoglobulins bound to the interstitium and the tubular walls and seldom to their contents. In the few cases in which germ cells sealed off from the walls showed immunohistological staining, no attempts were undertaken to relate the findings with the various types of sperm antibodies (Wall *et al.*, 1975; Donat and Morenz, 1979; Jadot-van de Casseye *et al.*, 1980). No comprehensive studies on such cases have ever been carried out.

Nevertheless, studies in which oligozoospermic patients were treated with corticosteroids, do give evidence for the existence of the syndrome in man.

Four of 13 oligo- or azoospermic patients, all having indication of cellular immunity against sperm, showed a considerable increase of the sperm output during treatment, whereas 11 such patients, who did not have a positive blastoid transformation test did not benefit from the therapy (Bassili and El-Alfi, 1970). Hendry *et al.* (1979) found a considerable improvement of the sperm output during or after treatment with corticosteroids in some oligozoospermic patients with sperm antibodies, while at the same time the sperm antibodies in the serum and seminal plasma decreased in titre. It was remarkable that in 3 oligozoospermic men with high titres of antisperm antibodies, testis biopsies showed an adequate spermatogenesis. The authors pointed out that testicular biopsies are always taken from the body of the testis, and thus they are unlikely to detect forms of autoimmune orchitis, which cause oligozoospermia by affecting transport in the efferent passages, such as can be induced experimentally. Since corticosteroids have no influence on hormonal factors related to spermatogenesis, it may tentatively be concluded that, when sperm counts rise and sperm antibody titres fall, it is likely that the patient had an autoimmune orchi-epididymitis. For further immunological studies related to oligozoospermia the reader is referred to a recent review (Rümke, 1981).

Therapy of infertile men with sperm autoantibodies

Corticosteroid therapy has been tried in normo- and oligozoospermic men with sperm antibodies. High doses of methylprednisolone (96 mg per day given in courses of one week, synchronized with the last week of the menstrual cycle of the wife) has resulted in a 35% pregnancy rate (Shulman *et al.*, 1978). With the same regime Hendry *et al.* (pers. comm.) achieved 12 paternities in 43 men who received 1 to 3 courses in alternate months. In the successful cases the immobilization test became negative, whereas the agglutinin titre sometimes decreased, but was not well-correlated with paternity. Katz and Newill (1980) had a success rate of 4 out of 7, and in all the 4 successful cases were the patients treated in the first week of the wife's menstrual cycle, and in 3 of them only one course was sufficient. These data suggest that with a high dose of corticosteroids a rapid fall of locally produced antibodies in the genital tract may occur. In some cases the decline may continue, in others antibody levels may soon rise again (Hendry, pers. comm.). De Almeida (pers. comm.) treated 14 patients with 2 to 3 mg dexamethasone for 2 to 3 months with a gradual decrease thereafter. She saw 4 pregnancies between 2 to 24 weeks of treatment when serum-spermatotoxic antibodies and seminal sperm agglutinins had become negative, while agglutinin titres in the serum remained high. From both studies it may be concluded that tests in which complement-dependent antibodies are measured, give a better predictive answer than the agglutination test.

Another approach of therapy is the administration of antibiotics in cases in which it is believed that antibody formation is related to prostatitis.

Fjällbrant and Nilsson (1977) noted a considerable decrease or even the complete disappearance of sperm antibodies in 8 men, of whom 5 became fathers.

Since sensitized but not agglutinated spermatozoa stick to the micelles of the cervical mucus, Kremer *et al.* (1978) inseminated the wives by the intrauterine method, and in 3 of the 15 cases a pregnancy was achieved.

Immunological implications of vasectomy

In vasectomized men 60–80% form sperm antibodies within a year after the operation. Since sperm antibodies do not cross-react with other somatic antigens, there is no direct risk of harm to other organs or cells. However, indirect side-effects are not excluded. Preliminary reports in rodents show that a patchy orchitis may develop and also that immune complexes may deposit in the ductuli efferentes as well as on the basement membrane of the renal glomerulus. In rhesus monkeys atherosclerosis may be enhanced, possibly because of the deposition of immune complexes in plaques and T cell reactivity might be reduced (see reviews: Alexander and Anderson, 1979; Lepow and Crozier, 1979). On the other hand, it was shown in a recent study (Anderson and Alexander, 1980) that in spite of the development of sperm antibodies in 100% of BDF_1 mice within one month after vasectomy, tests for immunecompetence performed up to 2·5 years postvasectomy, revealed no differences in the mitogenic responsiveness in the course of time in age-matched operated and sham-operated animals, nor in lymphocyte responses to mitogenic or allogenic stimulation *in vitro*, nor to an *in vivo* challenge with picrylchloride or humoral responses to foreign protein. Autoimmune reactivity at the level of the testis was however found: orchitic lesions characterized by immune complex deposition and lymphocyte infiltration were found in 3 out of 15 long-term vasectomized mice as compared to none in the sham-operated group. So far, no adverse effect in long-term vasectomized men have been recorded, and epidemiological studies have not revealed differences in disease incidence between vasectomized and nonvasectomized men (Goldacre and Vessey, 1979). Since in guinea-pigs, rabbits, mice, rats and rhesus monkeys patchy autoimmune orchitis may develop, and since also the autoimmune response is genetically determined, it may be anticipated that in certain vasectomized men not only sperm antibodies will develop but also a mild asymptomatic patchy orchitis. Such men may not become fertile after a reanastomosis operation, not only because ejaculated sperm are coated by sperm antibody, but also because of a decreased spermatogenesis. It has already been demonstrated that after vasovasostomy sperm antibodies can appear in the semen at levels high enough to be expected to be detrimental. Such an occurrence has been observed in 4 out of 29 reoperated men (Linnet and Fogh-Andersen, 1979). In 9 out of the 29 men the sperm counts after the vasovasostomy were between > 0 and 10×10^6/ml, in 7 of them sperm antibodies were present in the serum and in 5 in the semen. Further clinical research is needed to evaluate whether in such cases an autoimmune orchi-epididymitis induced by the vasectomy is the cause of the oligozoospermia and the continuing infertility after the vasovasotomy.

Isoimmunity to spermatozoa in experimental female animals

Intravaginal injections of foreign antigens elicit local antibody formation in the cervix of various species. In rabbits, for instance, systemic immunization with horseradish peroxidase resulted in antibodies in the circulation and in the reproductive tract of the IgG class, but none of the IgA class, whereas vaginal immunization produced IgA and IgG antibodies in the reproductive tract and also IgG antibodies in the serum. Cell-mediated immune responses occurred after systemic and not after local immunization. Intrauterine immunization was not effective at all (McAnulty and Morton, 1978). Oviductal fluid antibodies are related to serum titres and not to transvaginal immunization (Collins *et al.*, 1979). Many other references to the existence of a local immune system in the female genital tract can be found in a WHO workshop report (Cinader and de Weck, 1976).

The immune response after vaginal application of foreign antigens has recently also been studied in rhesus monkeys. Antibodies in the cervical mucus appeared after local booster applications. In 3 of the 4 cases the levels were higher in the mucus than in the serum. Systemic immunization resulted in high circulating and low cervical mucus titres. Alum as an adjuvant enhanced the local immune response. A characteristic decrease in cervical mucus antibodies after both local and systemic immunization was usually observed at midcycle. More than 90% of the antibodies to one antigen could be removed by anti-IgG antiserum. The lymphocyte response to the antigens was weak or absent after local immunization, whereas they were high after systemic immunization (Yang and Schumacher, 1979). In oviductal fluids antibody titres were about 10 times less than in serum and were apparently derived from the serum, since there was no relationship with the local immunization (Schumacher *et al.*, 1980b).

Whether the formation of antibodies to homologous spermatozoa can also be induced by vaginal application is controversial: both positive and negative results have been reported (see Hekman and Rümke, 1976). Guinea-pigs immunized parenterally with guinea-pig sperm form sperm antibodies that gradually decrease in titre. Even after the disappearance of these antibodies, mating caused a subsequent immediate rise of the titre (Isojima and Ashitaka, 1964; Behrman and Nakayama, 1965). This experiment shows that a pre-existing immunity may be boosted by mating, whereas mating itself is usually not sufficient to induce a primary response. Apparently the immunogenicity of sperm absorbed under normal conditions is low, or immunoregulatory functions maintain unresponsiveness as has been discussed above. However it could be possible that under pathological conditions a primary response may occur spontaneously. One reason for an increased immunological response may be the presence of lesions in the epithelium of the vagina, cervix and the uterus as shown in cows by Bratanov (1969) and indicated by the results of El-Maghoub (1972) who found a much higher incidence of sperm agglutinins in the sera of women with cervicovaginal schistosomiasis than of those with other forms of this infection. A significantly higher incidence of antispermatozoal antibodies was found in sera from females who were to undergo hysterectomy for various lesions of the reproductive tract than in sera from controls (Boettcher, 1974). Further, a significantly greater incidence of sperm agglutinins in serum was found with women with carcinoma of the cervix than in women with other forms of genital cancer, showing that perhaps the cervix is more important in the induction of immunity to spermatozoa (Jones *et al.*, 1973).

Immunization of females with homologous sperm or testis homogenate has resulted in a reduction of fertility in guinea-pigs, rats, mice, rabbits, cattle and hens (references in Hekman and Rümke, 1976). In general a prolonged immunization or the use of an adjuvant was necessary to obtain an effect on fecundity, although also intraperitoneally injected homologous epididymal sperm in female mice induced the formation of isoantibodies together with infertility (Tung *et al.*, 1979). Female rabbits immunized with subcellular sperm fractions became infertile. The sera of these animals contained sperm agglutinating and immobilizing antibodies as well as precipitating antibodies against the extracts (Munoz and Metz, 1978). Attempts to induce subfertility with purified sperm-specific antigens such as enzymes were less successful. Female sheep immunized with ram acrosin and hyaluronidase remained infertile (Morton and McAnulty, 1979). In the guinea-pig no impairment of fertility occurred after immunization with the earlier described aspermatogenic antigens P, S and T (De Almeida and Voisin, 1979). More successful were isoimmunization experiments with LDH-X, also called LDH-C_4. Rabbits immunized with LDH-X become infertile (Goldberg, 1973, 1974). Inhibition of sperm transport by antibodies in the oviductal fluids was probably a major factor in contributing to the infertility (Kille and Goldberg, 1980). Antibody levels against LDH-X which were of the IgG class in oviductal fluid rose after the application of whole sperm (Kille and Goldberg, 1979). Also in mice and baboons infertility has been achieved after immunization with LDH-X (Goldberg, 1979). Since LDH-X lacks species-specific antigenicity, it can be widely used in animal experiments and even may be a potential fertility control vaccine (Goldberg, 1979). So far, it has not been demonstrated that infertility induced by immunization with whole sperm is related to the development of antibodies against LDH-X.

It has been shown that semen treated with antispermatozoal antiserum prior to insemination loses the capacity to fertilize, even when incubation took place with nonagglutinating univalent antibody fragments (Menge, 1971). One of the feasible mechanisms involved is the inhibition of attachment of spermatozoa to the zona pellucida. Other mechanisms concern the interference of sperm penetration and migration in the cervical mucus, as found in man (Kremer and Jager, 1980). The interference of isoimmunity to sperm with infertility can also act after fertilization. Depending on the immunogenic function of rabbit spermatozoa used to immunize female rabbits, infertility was either the result of pre- or postfertilization effects, the latter mediated by IgA antibodies in the uterine fluids that react with blastocysts as well as with swollen sperm heads (Menge *et al.*, 1979; Menge and Peegel, 1980).

Immunoglobulins have been shown to be present in various fluids of the genital tract of different species. IgG, IgA and sometimes IgM and secretory IgA were found in the cervical mucus of women at mid-cycle, in concentrations of the order of 1% of the serum levels. The capacity of human cervical tissue to produce immunoglobulins has been demonstrated both *in vitro* and *in situ* (Insler and Bettendorf, 1977). Although human mid-cycle cervical mucus has virtually no lytic complement activity (Cinader and De Weck, 1976), limited amounts of complement factors were shown to be present and to be partly able to immobilize sensitized spermatozoa (Price and Boettcher, 1979). With the blotting method human endometrial fluid was found to contain IgG, IgA and IgM in 20–50% of the serum concentrations. Surprisingly IgD sometimes occurred in a concentration twice that in the serum. Lytic complement activity was virtually absent (Schumacher *et al.*, 1980a). Also follicular fluid contains IgG, even though only slightly less than in serum (Menge, 1980).

It can be concluded that interference with fertility by sperm isoantibodies if they are present in the female, can occur at different levels by various mechanisms. Sensitized spermatozoa can adhere to the micelles in cervical mucus; they can be killed if the antibodies are of the most common, i.e. complement binding, IgG type and if complement is present, which is probably the case in uterine, oviductal and follicular fluids; and adherence and penetration in the ovum can be inhibited. Lastly, cross-reactivity of spermatozoa with blastocysts might make it possible that even fertilized egg development is inhibited. Little is known, however, about the circumstances under which local or systemic immunization against sperm could occur under natural conditions.

Isoimmunity to spermatozoa in infertile women

Again, as in men, the incidence at which sperm antibodies are found in the serum of infertile women varies considerably. In unexplained infertility, the incidence of relevant antibodies is estimated between 5 and 20% by most authors. Details can be found in recent published reviews (Jones, 1980; Menge, 1980). In studies on large series of patients (Lehmann *et al.*, 1977; Ingerslev and Hjort, 1979; Ingerslev and Ingerslev, 1980; Jones, 1980) the reproductive performance subsequent to testing for antisperm antibodies indicated that, irrespective of the titre, patients with agglutinins had nearly a 50% chance of being fertile, which is about the same percentage as that for women without sperm antibodies. However in one study, in those women who have antibodies the infertile period was longer (Ingerslev and Ingerslev, 1980). The immobilization test might have a better predictive value since in the study of Jones (1980) 53% of 309 negative women became pregnant, compared with

35% in 23 positive women whose infertility was unexplained. This difference was even more pronounced if only patients were compared who were infertile for at least 3 years. Using serum dilutions of 1 : 4 and higher to detect the antibodies, Lehmann *et al.* (1977) found that 12% of 32 positive women became pregnant and 40% of 344 negative women. With the agglutination test only Menge (1980) found an influence of the titre: a decrease in the chance to become fertile was seen with titres of 16 and higher. Also based on the comparisons of fertile and infertile women, the immobilization test is generally accepted as a more predictive test in women than the agglutination test. For instance, Isojima *et al.* (1972) found 19% of 74 women with unexplained infertility to possess immobilizins whereas only 1 of 100 women with known causes of infertility and none of 131 other controls were positive. Such a difference has never been found with agglutinins in undiluted serum. However, using dilutions of 1 : 32 or higher the agglutination test also discriminates clearly. Using this threshold none of 266 controls had agglutinins in the serum, but 11 out of 326 infertile women did (Ingerslev and Hjort, 1979). The reason why the agglutination technique applied on undiluted serum discriminates less well between fertile and infertile women is that head-to-head agglutination can be caused by factors other than immunoglobulins, such as a $\beta 2$ macroglobulin that is often present in the serum of pregnant women (Boettcher, 1974). Ingerslev and Hjort (1979) found in 10 out of 29 infertile women that agglutination was due to this factor.

Probably more relevant to an immunological cause of infertility is the presence of antibody activity in the cervical mucus. In most of the studies the incidence of complement dependent immobilizins in the cervical mucus among unexplained infertile women is 25–30% which is much higher than the incidence in serum. The appearance of immobilizing and agglutinating antibodies in cervical mucus is unrelated to the serum titres of these antibodies (Moghissi *et al.*, 1980). Kremer and Jager (1980) found a high correlation between a strongly positive shaking phenomenon in the sperm–cervical mucus contact test, a disturbed penetration in cervical mucus, and sperm agglutinin titres in the cervical mucus. This was confirmed by Menge (1980). Immobilizins and agglutinins can occur independently of each other in the cervical mucus. Their possibly different roles in the mechanism of inhibition of penetration or migration is not yet clear. Although the immunofluorescence technique has been applied on cervical mucus (Eyquem and De Almeida, 1973; Coelingh Bennink and Menge, 1974) this technique is considered less reliable than the immobilization technique for the detection of antibodies in cervical mucus.

So far, a causal relationship between isoimmunity to sperm and infertility in women is indicated by the inhibition of sperm migration through the cervical mucus. Whether sperm antibodies could act elsewhere, for instance in the uterine and oviductal fluids in patients with serum antibodies in whom mucus penetration tests are normal, has still to be investigated.

Therapy of infertile women with sperm isoantibodies

On the assumption that regular sperm resorption sustains the production of sperm antibodies, several investigators have prescribed the use of condoms for a period of at least 6 months. In some of these studies, decreased serum antibody titres were observed, and a number of pregnancies occurred after unprotected intercourse was resumed. However agglutinins may also disappear without therapy (Lehmann *et al.*, 1977). Others have been unsuccessful with "condom" therapy (Jones, 1975). It may well be that in some women the antibodies do disappear, but this may perhaps take as long as 12 months (Shulman *et al.*, 1978).

Immunosuppressive therapy with high doses of corticosteroids has been claimed to result in a 16% success rate (Shulman *et al.*, 1978). Kremer *et al.* (1978) inseminated 5 women by the intrauterine route and one became pregnant. Jones (1980) reported 4 pregnancies out of 7 attempts, but raised the point that it is impossible to distinguish between therapeutic success and pregnancies occurring during one of the many nadirs of the sperm antibody titre which have been recorded in long-term studies by S. Isojima.

Isoimmunity to seminal plasma components

In infertile women

Experimental work shows that seminal plasma components can be autoantigenic, for instance the rabbit produces autoantibodies after immunization with rabbit seminal plasma (Chen, 1979). Relatively little is known about antibodies in human serum against seminal plasma components. Using a technique involving passive haemolysis, Carretti (1974) found serum antibodies to human seminal plasma antigens in 33% of women with unexplained infertility, whereas negative results were obtained with sera of pregnant and other women. With the use of the counter immunoelectrophoresis technique Chen (1979) showed that infertile women as well as prostitutes could have antibodies to seminal plasma. A fraction of seminal plasma modified by bacteria appeared to be the antigen to which some infertile, but not fertile, women had antibodies (Chen and Simons, 1977).

According to Isojima (1969) agglutinating and immobilizing antibodies found in the serum of some infertile women could be absorbed by seminal plasma, indicating that the antibodies are directed against seminal plasma antigens that coat spermatozoa. Two semipurified glycoproteins of human seminal plasma from azoospermic and vasectomized men could absorb immobilizing activity of sera of infertile women with immobilizins (Koyama *et al.*, 1979).

Postcoital allergy

Separate from its bearing on infertility stands the rare condition of allergy to seminal plasma. A few cases of urticaria, pharyngeal and vaginal oedema, cardiovascular symptoms and loss of consciousness immediately after intercourse have been described. Seminal plasma and prostate extracts, but not spermatozoa and testis extracts, revealed immediate types of hypersensitivity by skin testing. IgE antibodies appeared to be involved (for references: Hekman and Rümke, 1976; Chen, 1979).

Autoantibodies to antigens of the female gonads in women

Autoimmune ovarian failure

Clinical studies have shown that organ-specific autoantibodies reacting against ovarian granulosa and theca interna cells as well as against steroid-producing cells in other organs, such as adrenals and testis, were related to primary or secondary amenorrhea in some women. This syndrome occurs especially as secondary to autoimmune adrenal failure, but has also been found together with autoimmune disorders of the thyroid, parathyroid and the stomach, and less frequently with other autoimmune syndromes (Friedman *et al.*, 1972; Irvine and Barnes, 1975; Jones, 1976; Donat and Morenz, 1979).

Autoantibodies to the zona pellucida

The zonae pellucidae around mammalian eggs have one or more antigens that appear important in fertilization. Experimentally induced antizona autoantibodies have been shown to be potent inhibitors of fertilization, provided the antibody has access to the zona *in vivo*. Zona antigen appears to be organ specific and cross-reactivity has been shown to occur between human, pig and other mammalian zona. In the sera of some infertile and a large number of postmenopausal women antibodies were found reacting with pig zona antigen. Sperm attachment to eggs is blocked to a certain extent after exposure of the eggs to antizona antibodies and, moreover, the eggs could not be fertilized (Shivers, 1979). Also, autoantibodies from postmenopausal women could drastically reduce the number of human spermatozoa attaching to human zonae (Trounson *et al.*, 1980). The incidence of specific antizona antibodies in sera of women as detected in the indirect immunofluorescence test on pig zona, may have been overestimated since it was recently found that in most cases the antibodies could be removed with pig erythrocytes (Mori *et al.*, 1979). Nevertheless, it may yet be possible that infertility in some women can be due to autoantibodies against zona antigens. More research has still to be done to show that this is definitely the case.

Some suggestions for further research

Sperm auto- and isoantigens

Various surface and subsurface autoantigens of spermatozoa and their postmeiotic precursors have been shown to exist. Some are easily released, others are not. Their isolation and characterization in different species may serve various purposes. Some of the antigens might leak into the circulation, even under normal conditions, and if so they might induce a low-dose tolerance to sperm. Sensitive techniques should be developed to detect these antigens in the circulation. If they are released from germ cells in different stages of spermatogenesis, these antigens might be used as markers in seminal plasma in order to classify different forms of functional azoospermia. Attempts should be made to use antisera to pure sperm antigens for the recognition of precursor germ cells in ejaculates. Also their different roles in the induction of autoimmune orchi-epididymitis and in the induction of isoimmune infertility in the female should be studied further. The sperm-specific antigens are potential candidates for contraceptive vaccines. On the other hand, since it has been shown that seminal substances and germ cells can display immunosuppressive activity, some of the pure antigens could probably activate nonspecific suppressor T cells and therefore be used as immunosuppressive agents.

Experimental autoimmune orchi-epididymitis

Different immunological mechanisms play a role in the induction of autoimmune orchi-epididymitis. The dependence of these differences on different immunogenicity of the various autoantigens should be studied further. The weakest sites of the blood–testis barrier are localized at the rete testis and tubuli efferentes; these are the places where the syndrome is initiated. More studies are needed to investigate the exact mechanism of the initiation. The epididymis may be involved in the syndrome and the circumstances under which this occurs should be studied further. Chronic forms of the syndrome are not yet well investigated and virtually no studies have yet been directed to the question as to whether the ejaculates of the affected animals can be used for diagnostic purposes. It should be investigated whether blood plasma components and markers for autoimmune reactions appear in the ejaculates. Cells desquamated from the tubuli might be recognized in the ejaculates. Such investigations should help clinicians to make a better use of patients' ejaculates in order to diagnose testicular pathology. Cells other than the postmeiotic germ cells should be studied in regard to weak autoantigenic properties. Little is known about the immunological properties of Sertoli cells and even spermatogonia. The basement membrane of the seminiferous tubuli might even have some specific antigenic determinants.

Natural autoimmune orchi-epididymitis in animals and man

Further studies of this syndrome in certain A-line beagle dog families and in thymectomized Lewis rats should be carried out, in relation to genetically determined immunoregulatory defects as well as to concurrent abnormalities of the blood–testis barrier.

In man, certain cases of oligozoospermia may be due to autoimmune orchi-epididymitis. Comprehensive immunological studies involving: (a) the specificity and class of the sperm antibodies; (b) the specificity and character of a possible cell-mediated component; (c) the binding of immunoglobulins and complement factors to cells in the tubules or their walls (of testis biopsies); (d) abnormalities of the semen with respect to sensitized spermatozoa, precursor germ cells, immunoglobulins, antibodies, macrophages and leukocytes and blood plasma markers; and (e) the response on immunosuppressive therapy, are urgently needed in such cases.

Normospermic men with sperm autoantibodies

It is well established that in these men autoantibodies in the seminal plasma sensitize spermatozoa in such a way that they agglutinate, or, if not agglutinated, are rendered incapable of migrating through cervical mucus. The mechanism of the latter phenomenon has still to be clarified. It should also be studied why some spermatozoa agglutinate and others not. More than half of the men with autoimmunity to sperm are idiopathic cases. Do they have an abnormal leakage of sperm antigens outside the sperm compartment? Virtually nothing is known about the sites in the genital tract where sIgA antibodies are produced; the prostate may be involved, but it can also be elsewhere. Corticosteroid therapy helps some of these men; further studies are needed to improve results and diminish side-effects.

Immunological implications of vasectomy

In monkeys and rodents patchy autoimmune orchitis was shown to be a result of vasectomy. Many vasectomized men form sperm antibodies within a few months after the operation. These antibodies and probably also patchy autoimmune orchitis, might be the cause of functionally unsuccessful reanastomosis operations; further studies are needed to prove this. In monkeys atherosclerosis is enhanced and the formation of immune complexes seems to play a role in this phenomenon. Although in men circulating immune complexes have never consistently been found after vasectomy, further research is needed to investigate whether this could occur in some rare cases. Further epidemiological studies are needed to evaluate long-term risks, such as enhancement of atherosclerosis.

Isoimmunity to sperm in infertile women

There is ample evidence that sperm isoantibodies in cervical mucus can block the migration of spermatozoa and therefore cause infertility. How often this occurs among women with unexplained infertility is still a matter of debate. We need routine techniques that *prove* the presence of antibodies, since agglutination and immobilization as such do not sufficiently prove the antibody nature of the factors involved. Also uterine fluids should be investigated for the presence of sperm antibodies in order to explain infertility in case of normal cervical mucus penetration. The pathogenesis of sperm isoantibody formation should be further investigated, especially in relation to infections and IUDs. The role of seminal plasma components either as sperm-coating antigens or as soluble substances should be explored further.

Autoimmune infertility in women

Autoimmune ovarian failure has been shown to be related to other autoimmune diseases. Further clinical research is needed to evaluate whether autoimmunity to organ-specific ovarian components can occur.

The significance of antibodies to zona pellucida antigens is not yet clear. Further research is needed to explore the possibility that such antibodies are involved in infertility.

References

Alexander, N. J. and Anderson, D. J. (1979). *Fert. Steril.* **32**, 253.

De Almeida, M. (1980). *In* "Abstracts 4th International Congress of Immunology", Paris.

De Almeida, M. and Voisin, G. A. (1979). *J. Reprod. Immunol.* **1**, 237.

Anderson, D. J. and Alexander, N. J. (1980). *Clin. Exp. Immunol.* (in press).

Austin, C. R. (1976). *In* "Development of Vaccines for Fertility Regulation", WHO Symposium Varna, Bulgaria, 1975, pp. 63–80. Scriptor, Copenhagen.

Bassili, F. and El-Alfi, O. S. (1970). *J. Reprod. Fert.* **21**, 29.

Behrman, S. J. and Nakayama, M. (1965). *Fert. Steril.* **16**, 37.

Bishop, D. W., Narbaitz, R. and Lessof, M. (1961). *Develop. Biol.* **3**, 444.

Boettcher, B. (1968). *In* "Immunology and Reproduction" (R. G. Edwards, ed.) pp. 148–154. Int. Planned Parenthood Federation, London.

Boettcher, B. (1974). *J. Reprod. Fert. Suppl.* **21**, 151.

Boettcher, B. (1977). *In* "Immunological Influence on Human Fertility" (B. Boettcher, ed.) pp. 105–110. Academic Press, Sydney.

Boettcher, B. (1979). *Clin. Obstet. Gynaecol.* **6**, 385.

Boettcher, B. and Boettcher, M. J. (1979). *In* "Immunology of Reproduction" (K. Bratanov *et al.*, eds) pp. 331–335. Bulgarian Academy of Sciences, Sofia.

Boettcher, B., Hjort, T., Rümke, Ph., Shulman, S. and Vyazov, O. E. (eds) (1977). *Acta Pathol. Microbiol. Scand.* Section C, Suppl. **258**, 1.

Boettcher, B., Misko, I. S., Roberts, T. K., Kay, D. J., Hicks, L. and Gruszyński,

R. (1979). *In* "Immunology of Reproduction" (K. Bratanov *et al.*, eds) pp. 201–204. Bulgarian Academy of Sciences, Sofia.

Bratanov, K. (1969). *In* "Immunology and Reproduction" (R. G. Edwards, ed) pp. 175–189. Int. Planned Parenthood Federation London.

Carretti, N. (1974). *In* "Immunology in Obstetrics and Gynecology" (A. Centaro and N. Carretti, eds) pp. 71–77. Excerpta Medica, Amsterdam.

Chen, C. (1979). *Clin. Obstet. Gyn.* **6**, 403.

Chen, C. and Simons, M. J. (1977). *In* "Immunological Influence on Human Fertility" (B. Boettcher, ed.) pp. 255–261. Academic Press, Sydney.

Cinader, B. and De Weck, A. (eds) (1976). Proceedings of a WHO Workshop, Geneva, January 9–11, 1975. Scriptor, Copenhagen.

Coelingh Bennink, H. J. T. and Menge, A. C. (1974). *Eur. J. Obstet. Gyn. Reprod. Biol.* **4**, 147.

Collins, S., Menge, A. C., Archie, J. T. and Behrman, S. J. (1979). *Int. J. Fert.* **24**, 149.

Denduchis, B. and Lustig, L. (1981). *In* "Recent Progress in Andrology", Proceedings International Symposium on Oligozoospermia, L'Aquila, Italy, June 30–July 2, 1980. (G. Frajese, ed.). Raven Press, New York (in press).

Donat, H. and Morenz, J. (1979). *In* "Immunology of Reproduction" (K. Bratanov *et al.*, eds) pp. 921–929. Bulgarian Academy of Sciences, Sofia.

Dondero, F., Lenzi, A., Picardo, M., Pastore, R. and Valesini, G. (1980). *Andrologia* **12**, 25.

El-Mahgoub, S. (1972). *Am. J. Obstet. Gyn.* **112**, 781.

Eyquem, A. and De Almeida, M. (1973). *In* "Immunology of Reproduction" (K. Bratanov, ed.) pp. 344–350. Bulgarian Academy of Sciences, Sofia.

Festenstein, H., Halim, K. and Arnaiz-Villena, A. (1978). *In* "Spermatozoa, Antibodies and Infertility" (J. Cohen and W. F. Hendry, eds) pp. 11–16. Blackwell Scientific Publications, Oxford.

Fjällbrant, B. (1968). *Acta Obstet. Gyn. Scand.* **47**, 102.

Fjällbrant, B. and Nilsson, S. (1977). *Int. J. Fert.* **22**, 255.

Friberg, J. (1980). *Obstet. Gyn.* **136**, 671.

Friedman, S., McCormick, J. N., Fudenberg, H. H. and Golfien, A. (1972). *Clin. Immunol. Immunopathol.* **1**, 94.

Fritz, T. E., Lombard, L., Tyler, S. A. and Norris, W. P. (1976). *Exp. Mol. Pathol.* **24**, 142.

Goldacre, M. and Vessey, M. (1979). *In* "Vasectomy: Immunologic and Pathophysiologic Effects in Animals and Men" (I. H. Lepow and R. Crozier, eds) pp. 567–579. Academic Press, New York.

Goldberg, E. (1973). *Science* **181**, 458.

Goldberg, E. (1974). *Acta Endocrinol.* **78**, Suppl. 194, 202.

Goldberg, E. (1979). *In* "Recent Advances in Reproduction and Regulation of Fertility" (G. P. Talwar, Ed.) pp. 281–290. Elsevier/North-Holland Biomedical Press, Amsterdam.

Han, B. L.-P. and Tung, K. S. K. (1979). *Biol. Reprod.* **21**, 99.

Hancock, R. J. T. (1978). *In* "Spermatozoa, Antibodies and Infertility" (J. Cohen and W. F. Hendry, eds) pp. 1–9. Blackwell Scientific Publications, Oxford.

Hagopian, A., Limjuco, G., Jackson, J. J., Carlo, D. and Eylar, E. H. (1976). *Biochim. Biophys. Acta* **434**, 354.

Hekman, A. and Rümke, Ph. (1976). *In* "Textbook of Immunopathology" (P. A. Miescher and H. J. Müller-Eberhard, eds) pp. 947–962. Grune & Stratton, New York.

Hendry, W. F., Stedronska, J., Hughes, L., Cameron, K. M. and Pugh, R. C. B. (1979). *Lancet* **ii**, 498.

Hjort, T., Hansen, K. B. and Poulson, F. (1978). *In* "Spermatozoa, Antibodies and

Infertility" (J. Cohen and W. F. Hendry, eds) pp. 101–115. Blackwell Scientific Publications, Oxford.
Hurtenbach, U., Morgenstern, F. and Bennett, D. (1980). *J. Exp. Med.* **151**, 827.
Husted, S. and Hjort, T. (1975). *Int. J. Fert.* **20**, 97.
Ingerslev, H. J. and Hjort, T. (1979). *Fert. Steril.* **31**, 496.
Ingerslev, H. J. and Ingerslev, M. (1980). *Fert. Steril.* **33** (in press).
Insler, V. and Bettendorf, G. (eds) (1977). "The Uterine Cervix in Reproduction". George Thieme Publishers, Stuttgart.
Irvine, W. J. and Barnes, E. W. (1975). *Clin. Endocrinol. Metabol.* **4**, 379.
Isojima, S. (1969). *In* "Immunology and Reproduction" (R. G. Edwards, ed.) pp. 267–279. International Planned Parenthood Federation, London.
Isojima, S. and Ashitaka, Y. (1964). *Am. J. Obstet. Gyn.* **88**, 433.
Isojima, S., Tsuchiya, K., Koyama, K., Tanaka, C., Naka, O. and Adachi, H. (1972). *Am. J. Obstet. Gyn.* **112**, 199.
Jackson, J. J., Hagopian, A., Carlo, D. J. and Limjuco, G. A. (1975). *Biol. Chem.* **250**, 6141.
Jadot-van de Casseye, M., de Bled, G., Gepts, W. and Schoysman, R. (1980). *Andrologia* **12**, 122.
Jager, S., Kremer, J. and Van Slochteren-Draaisma, T. (1978). *Int. J. Fert.* **23**, 12.
Jager, S., Kremer, J. and Van Slochteren-Draaisma, T. (1979). *Int. J. Andrology* **2**, 117.
Jager, S., Kremer, J. and Kuiken, J. (1980a). *In* "Proceedings IVth International Congress of Immunology, Paris" (Abstr.).
Jager, S., Kremer, J., Kuiken, J. and Van Slochteren-Draaisma, T. (1980b). *Int. J. Andrology* **3**, 1.
Johnson, M. H. (1970). *J. Pathol.* **102**, 131.
Jones, W. R. (1975). *Acta Endocrinol.* **78**, Suppl. 194, 376.
Jones, W. R. (1976). *In* "Immunology of Human Reproduction" (J. S. Scott and W. R. Jones, eds) pp. 375–413. Academic Press, London/Grune & Stratton, New York.
Jones, W. R. (1980). *Fert. Steril.* **33**, 577.
Jones, W. R., Kaye, M. D. and Ing, R. M. Y. (1973). *Am. J. Obstet. Gyn.* **116**, 883.
Katsh, S. (1960). *Int. Arch. Allergy* **16**, 241.
Katz, M. and Newill, R. (1980). *Lancet* **i**, 1306.
Kille, J. W. and Goldberg, E. (1979). *Biol. Reprod.* **20**, 863.
Kille, J. W. and Goldberg, E. (1980). *J. Reprod. Immunol.* **2**, 15.
Kolk, A. H. J. and Samuel, T. (1975). *Biochim. Biophys. Acta* **393**, 307.
Kolk, A. H. J., Van Kuyk, L. and Boettcher, B. (1978). *Biochim. J.* **173**, 767.
Koyama, K., Kubota, K., Ikuma, K. and Isojima, S. (1979). *In* "Immunology of Reproduction" (K. Bratanov *et al.*, eds) pp. 889–894. Bulgarian Academy of Sciences, Sofia.
Kremer, J. (1965). *Int. J. Fert.* **10**, 209.
Kremer, J. and Jager, S. (1980). *Int. J. Andrology* **3**, 143.
Kremer, J., Jager, S., Kuiken, J. and Van Slochteren-Draaisma, T. (1978). *In* "Spermatozoa, Antibodies and Infertility" (J. Cohen and W. F. Hendry, eds) pp. 117–127. Blackwell Scientific Publications, Oxford.
Lefroit-Jolly, M., Lebar, R. and Voisin, G. A. (1979). *Mol. Immunol* **16**, 327.
Lehmann, F., Stripling, K., Büdel, B., Krebs, D. and Masson, D. (1977). *In* "The Uterine Cervix in Reproduction" pp. 204–211. George Thieme, Stuttgart.
Lepow, I. H. and Crozier, R. (eds) (1979). "Vasectomy: Immunologic and Pathophysiologic Effects in Animals and Man". Academic Press, New York.
Linnet, L. and Fogh-Andersen, P. (1979). *J. Clin. Lab. Immunol.* **2**, 245.
Lipscomb, H. L., Gardner, P. J. and Sharp, J. G. (1979). *J. Reprod. Immunol.* **1**, 209.
Lucas, P. L. and Rose, N. R. (1978). *Ann. Immunol. (Paris)* **129**, 301.

Mancini, R. E. (1974). *In* "Immunology in Obstetrics and Gynecology" (A. Centaro and N. Carretti, eds) pp. 16–25. Excerpta Medica, Amsterdam.
Mancini, R. E. (1976). *In* "Human Semen and Fertility Regulation in Men" (E. S. E. Hafez, ed.) pp. 287–307. C. V. Mosby, St. Louis.
Marcus, Z. H., Freisheim, J. H., Houk, J. L., Herman, J. H. and Hess, E. V. (1978). *Clin. Immunol. Immunopathol.* **9**, 318.
Marcus, Z. H., Hess, E. V., Herman, J. H., Troiano, P. and Freisheim, J. (1979). *J. Reprod. Immunol.* **1**, 97.
Mathur, S., Williamson, H. O., Landgrebe, S. C., Smith, C. L. and Fudenberg, H. H. (1979). *J. Immunol. Meth.* **30**, 381.
McAnulty, P. A. and Morton, D. B. (1978). *J. Clin. Lab. Immunol.* **1**, 255.
Menge, A. C. (1971). *Proc. Soc. Exp. Biol. Med.* **138**, 98.
Menge, A. C. (1980). *In* "Immunological Aspects of Infertility and Fertility Regulation" (D. S. Dhindsa and G. F. B. Schumacher, eds) Elsevier/North-Holland, New York (in press).
Menge, A. C. and Black, C. S. (1979). *Fert. Steril.* **32**, 214.
Menge, A. C. and Peegel, H. (1980). *Arch. Andrology* **4**, 171.
Menge, A. C., Peegel, H. and Riolo, M. L. (1979). *Biol. Reprod.* **20**, 931.
Metz, C. B. (1979). *In* "Contraception: Science, Technology and Application" (E. V. Jensen, ed.) pp. 180–220. National Academy of Sciences, Washington, D.C.
Metz, C. B. and Anika, J. (1970). *Biol. Reprod.* **2**, 284.
Moghissi, K. S., Sacco, A. and Borin, K. (1980). *Am. J. Obstet. Gyn.* **136**, 941.
Mori, T., Nishimoto, T., Kohda, H., Takai, I., Nishimura, T. and Oikawa, T. (1979). *Fert. Steril.* **32**, 67.
Morton, D. B. (1977). *In* "Immunobiology of Gametes" (M. Edidin and M. H. Johnson, eds) pp. 115–155. Cambridge University Press, Cambridge.
Morton, D. B. and McAnulty, P. A. (1979). *J. Reprod. Immunol.* **1**, 61.
Munoz, M. G. and Metz, C. B. (1978). *Biol. Reprod.* **18**, 669–678.
O'Rand, M. G. (1980). *In* "Immunological Aspects of Infertility and Fertility Regulation" (D. S. Dhindsa and G. F. B. Schumacher, eds). Elsevier/North-Holland, New York (in press).
O'Rand, M. G. and Romrell, L. J. (1977). *Develop. Biol.* **55**, 347.
Pokorná, Z. and Vojtísková, M. (1964). *Folia Biol. Praha* **10**, 392.
Poulson, F. and Hjort, T.(1980). *In* "Abstracts 4th International Congress of Immunology, Paris".
Price, R. J. and Boettcher, B. (1979). *Fert. Steril.* **32**, 61.
Rapaport, F. T., Sampath, A., Kano, D., McCluskey, R. T. and Milgrom, F. (1969). *J. Exp. Med.* **130**, 1411.
Roberts, T. K., Tumboh-Oeri, A. G., Dorsman, B. G., Hall, R. and Lewins, E. (1977). *In* "Immunological Influence on Human Fertility" (B. Boettcher, ed.) pp. 271–273. Academic Press, Sydney.
Rose, N. R., Hjort, T., Rümke, Ph., Harper, M. J. K. and Vyazov, O. (eds) (1976). *Clin. Exp. Immunol.* **23**, 175.
Rümke, Ph. (1978). *In* "Spermatozoa, Antibodies and Infertility" (J. Cohen and W. F. Hendry, eds) pp. 67–79. Blackwell Scientific Publications, Oxford.
Rümke, Ph. (1981). *In* "Recent Progress in Andrology. Proceedings Internation Symposium on Oligozoospermia, L'Aquila, Italy 1980" (G. Frajese, ed.). Raven Press, New York (in press).
Rümke, Ph. and Hekman, A. (1977). *Clin. Obstet. Gyn.* **20**, 691.
Rümke, Ph., Van Amstel, N., Messer, E. N. and Bezemer, P. D. (1974). *Fert. Steril.* **25**, 393.
Samuel, T. (1977). *Clin. Exp. Immunol.* **30**, 181.
Schumacher, G. F. B., Holt, J. A. and Reale, F. (1980a). *In* "Biology of the Fluids

of the Female Genital Tract" (F. K. Beller and G. F. B. Schumacher, eds). Elsevier/North-Holland, New York (in press).

Schumacher, G. F. B., Yang, S. L. and Broder, K. H. (1980b). *In* "Biology of the Fluids of the Female Genital Tract" (F. K. Beller and G. F. B. Schumacher, eds) Elsevier/North-Holland, New York (in press).

Shigeta, M., Watanabe, T., Maruyama, S., Koyama, K. and Isojima, S. (1980). *Clin. Exp. Immunol.* (in press).

Shivers, C. A. (1979). *In* "Animal Models for Research on Contraception and Fertility". (N. Alexander, ed.) pp. 314–325. Harper and Row, Hagerstown.

Shulman, S. (1975). "Reproduction and Antibody Response". CRC Press, Cleveland.

Shulman, S. (1978). *In* "Spermatozoa, Antibodies and Infertility" (J. Cohen and W. F. Hendry, eds) pp. 81–99. Blackwell Scientific Publications, Oxford.

Shulman, S., Harlin, B., Davis, Ph. and Reyniak, J. V. (1978). *Fert. Steril.* **29**, 309.

Sung, J. S., Shizuya, H., Block, D. D. and Mumford, D. M. (1977). *Clin. Exp. Immunol.* **27**, 469.

Suominen, J. J. O., Multamäki, S. and Djupsund, B. M. (1980). *Arch. Andrology* **4**, 257.

Thestrup-Pedersen, K., Husted, S. and Hjort, T. (1976). *Int. J. Fert.* **21**, 218.

Toullet, F., Voisin, G. A. and Nemirovsky, M. (1973). *Immunology* **24**, 635.

Trounson, A. O., Shivers, C. A., McMaster, R. and Lopata, A. (1980). *Arch. Andrology* **4**, 29.

Tung, K. S. K. (1980). *In* "Immunological Aspects of Infertility and Fertility Regulation" (D. S. Dhindsa and G. F. B. Schumacher, eds) Elsevier/North-Holland, New York (in press).

Tung, K. S. K., Goldberg, E. H. and Goldberg, E. (1979). *J. Reprod. Immunol.* **1**, 145.

Voisin, G. A., Delaunay, A. and Barber, M. (1951). *Ann. Inst. Pasteur* **81**, 48.

Voisin, G. A., Toullet, F. and D'Almeida, M. (1975). *Acta Endocrinol.* **78**, Suppl. 194, 173.

Wall, J. R., Stedronska, J., David, R. D., Harrison, G. F., Goriup, D. and Lessof, M. (1975). *Fert. Steril.* **26**, 1035.

Witkin, S. S., Higgins, P. J. and Bendich, A. (1978). *Clin. Exp. Immunol.* **33**, 244.

Yang, S. L. and Schumacher, G. F. B. (1979). *Fert. Steril.* **32**, 588.

Young, L. G. (1978). *J. Cell Biol.* **79**, 257.

58

Immunology of the Maternofoetal Relationship

W. PAGE FAULK

Blond McIndoe Centre for Transplantation Biology, East Grinstead, England

Introduction

Three points must be made at the outset of this chapter. Firstly, it is quite impossible to cover every immunological aspect of the maternofoetal relationship in the space allowed, so the information presented has been selected and distilled to represent an overview, inasmuch as that is possible. Secondly, this report contains a heavy bias on the role of placentae in normal and abnormal pregnancies, because this organ stands at the interface between mother and foetus, creating much of the phenomenology which collectively comprises maternofoetal immunology. Thirdly, the contents of this document relate almost exclusively to immunological aspects of the maternofoetal relationship in human pregnancy, and the following reasons are put forward to exonerate this somewhat idiosyncratic approach. It can be defended without reserve that mammals arise from one-celled eggs, pass through a blastocyst stage and thereafter develop their embryonic body from a disc on the floor of an amniotic cavity within an outer trophoblastic shell, but these events are subject to an almost infinite number of variations. The programme of development is not the same in any 2 species as, for instance, represented by differences in blastocyst shape or the mechanisms of amnion formation. The yolk sac may be large or small, open or closed, functional or atrophic, and the allantois can be absent, small, large or enormous. Although Corner (1944) proposed a conventionalized diagram of a mammalian embryo and its membranes for teaching purposes, such a creature does not exist. Even the method and depth of implantation varies markedly among the primates (Ramsey *et al.*, 1976). Not only are there gross and microscopical dissimilarities, but functional differences such as IgG transport are well known (Brambell, 1970) and the architecture of maternofoetal vascularity bears scant similarity between species. It is a usual reflex to ascribe these differences to Darwinian evolution, relating more specialized structure and function to evolutionary progress, but Wislocki put this prejudice to rest in 1929 by showing a lack of correlation in placental types and evolutionary relationships as derived from the comparative anatomy of living and fossil mammals. Thus in placentology and development, unlike contemporary investigations of livers, kidneys and brains, it does not necessarily follow that the results of studies obtained from one species can be extrapolated to another, and for these reasons this review is primarily limited to the human.

Maternal considerations

Humoral considerations

Nonimmunoproteins

Immunological considerations of the maternofoetal relationship can best be brought into focus by first concentrating on those substances identified in maternal blood which are thought to be placenta-specific. A large number of proteins are associated with either pregnancy or the foetus without being immunoregulatory or placenta-specific (Horne and Nisbet, 1979). Several foetal proteins, such as carcinoembryonic antigen and alpha-1-foeto protein are not found in human placentae (Faulk and Johnson, 1977), and a large number of other proteins such as the steroid-binding β_1-globulin (SP2), pregnancy-associated α2-glycoprotein (α2-PAG, SP3) and the placental proteins PP-1, PP-2, PP-3, PP-4, PP-6 and PP-7 (Sedlacek *et al.*, 1976) are pregnancy-associated proteins which do not seem to be limited to the placenta (Horne and Rosen, 1978). In contrast, human chorionic gonadotropin (hCG), placental lactogen (hPL), placental alkaline phosphatase, perhaps PAPP-A and PAPP-B, pregnancy-specific β_1-glycoprotein (PSBG), SP1 and the placental protein PP-5 are placenta-specific, and much is already known about their physiology and biochemistry (Klopper, 1980). There is not, however, a clear body of evidence to indicate that any of these are clearly involved in maternofoetal immunity, and there are some indications that foetal antigens are on balance poor (Chism *et al.*, 1979).

Several placental or trophoblast-specific proteins can be measured in maternal plasma, some of which have proven to be accurate and useful indices of pregnancy. Concentrations of hCG increase follow implantation so rapidly that detection in maternal blood or urine form the basis of widely used methods for pregnancy diagnosis. Values for hCG tend to decline as pregnancy progresses, while both hPL and SP1 increase (Letchworth, 1976). Maternal concentrations of SP1 provide useful indices of foetal and placental weight (Tatra *et al.*, 1975), and maternal SP1 concentrations are closely correlated with foetal growth retardation (Gordon *et al.*, 1977). Morton *et al.* (1977) have described an early pregnancy factor in maternal serum that is measured by a rosette inhibition assay, but the site of synthesis for this factor is not known. Some trophoblastic as well as nontrophoblastic tumours have been shown to produce pregnancy-specific proteins, and this is particularly true for hCG. The concentration of hCG is related to the total mass of tumour (Bagshawe, 1976), thus providing a predictive index for the growth or regression of tumour cells. Other placental proteins such as hPL and SP1 are also produced by some nontrophoblastic tumours.

Immunoglobulins and complement

There are not a large number of reports detailing results of quantitative studies of immunoglobulins (Ig) in pregnancy, but such information as is currently available indicates no major shifts in IgG, IgA and IgM throughout gestation (Gusdon, 1969), but there is some evidence that IgG values tend to decrease during the latter half of normal pregnancy (Maroulis *et al.*, 1971). Although difficult to interpret due to ambivalance about its function, Gusdon and Prichard (1972) found IgD values to be elevated at term. Measurements of IgE would be of interest because human pregnancy has been likened to a successful host-parasite relationship, and it is common knowledge that IgE values are raised as a consequence of certain parasitic infestations. Other non-specific indices of possible immune responses to foetal growth and development are progressive elevations of total complement as well as the third component of the blood complement system (Kitzmiller, 1976).

Antibody responses

A mass of clinical and experimental evidence (reviewed by Rocklin *et al.*, 1979 and Gill and Repetti, 1979) indicate that the capacity to mount an antibody response during pregnancy is not significantly impaired. On the contrary, a substantial amount of foetal and neonatal disease is caused by maternal antibody to incompatible paternal antigens on foetal cells which enter the mother's circulation and against which she produces IgG antibody that crosses the placenta to attack and kill the foetal cells in question. Common clinical examples of this are erythroblastosis foetalis due usually to maternofoetal Rh incompatibility and neonatal thrombocytopenia due to maternofoetal incompatibility of platelet antigens. Although of probably no clinical importance other than the provision of typing reagents, mothers commonly produce antibodies to histocompatibility antigens on incompatible foetal cells that enter their circulation. This phenomenon is so predictable that several diseases, including spontaneous abortion and pre-eclampsia have been thought to supervene in conditions where antibodies to transplantation antigens do not occur.

Most maternal antibodies to antigens of the HLA system are IgG and as such they are capable of being actively transported across the placenta by an elegant system of Fc-receptors originally envisioned and proposed by Brambell (1970). These maternal antibodies are known to increase with parity but they are not always found in cord blood. When the antibody is directed towards an HLA specificity which is not manifest by the present pregnancy, cord blood will contain maternal antibody, but, cord bloods do not contain maternal anti-HLA when the specificity of the antibody is the same as that represented by the present pregnancy (Jeannet *et al.*, 1977). The reason for this discrepancy lies in the fact that most cells other than the trophoblast have HLA antigens, so the HLA antigens of incompatible foetal cells within placentae such as fibroblasts and endothelia will tend to bind anti-HLA and as such serve as an immunoadsorbent removing maternal antibody and thus denying their entrance into the foetus. In contrast, maternal anti-HLA directed towards HLA antigens not represented by the present pregnancy will pass unimpeded to enter the foetal circulation, but they can have no effect in this circulation by virtue of the fact that they find no cell surface antigens with which to react. Faulk and Johnson (1980) have referred to this as the placental "sink", vindication of which stems from the observation that maternal anti-HLA can be eluted from placenta of HLA incompatible but not from HLA compatible pregnancies (Jeannet *et al.*, 1977).

At least 4 other types of anticellular antibodies have been identified during pregnancy, the most studied of which is the maternal antifoetal (paternal) B cell alloantigen. This reagent has allowed for the development of anti-B-cell sera to map and eventually describe the polymorphism of B cell and B cell related antigens. The effect of these antibodies on the normal course of human pregnancy is not presently known. A second group of antibodies which have been described during pregnancy has specificity for so-called non-HLA antigens. Ferrone *et al.* (1976) reported that 46% of their patients who lacked anti-HLA had cytotoxic antibodies to human cultured lymphoblastoid cells, and they speculated that these had specificity for antigens which were associated with immune-response genes. A third group of antibodies described by Tal (1965) are found in pregnancy sera and react with certain nonlymphoid transformed cells maintained in culture. Although these results stand largely unconfirmed, the basis for their reactivity may be due to the appearance of embryonic antigens on the transformed cells, because experimental studies reported by Salinas *et al.* (1978) described antibodies in pregnant mice that reacted with normal foetal mouse liver cells *in vitro*. Fourthly, many authors have reported supposedly antibody-mediated *in vitro* phenomenology whereby maternal blood causes a generalized suppression of lymphocyte function (Buckley *et al.*, 1972), and these observations have been extended to similar reactions caused by IgG eluted from human placentae as well as by $F(ab')_2$ fragments of eluates prepared from human (Faulk *et al.*, 1974) or mouse (Voisin and Chaouat, 1974; Chaouat *et al.*, 1979) placentae. Inasmuch as the basic test system used by many of these investigators involved blockade of the mixed lymphocyte culture (MLC) reaction, a jargon developed among reproductive immunobiologists in which the materials that were responsible for MLC blockage became known as "blocking factors". Substances released during MLC reactions were also used as assay systems to monitor blocking activity, and using modifications of this assay both Rocklin *et al.* (1976) and Stimson *et al.* (1979) have significantly extended contemporary knowledge about the role of blocking factors in normal and abnormal pregnancies.

In addition to maternal anticellular immunity, pregnant mothers also produce antibodies to certain viruses (Hirsch *et al.*, 1978) and incompatible serum protein allotypes. This phenomenon is perhaps best studied in the so-called Gm (genetic marker) system of IgG heavy chain antigens (Nathenson *et al.*, 1971). Such maternal immunization during pregnancy has reportedly caused a condition associated with a curious type of haemolytic disease of the newborn (Fudenberg and Fudenberg, 1964). Maternal immunization to incompatible foetal light chain alloantigens inherited from the foetus have also been reported (Faulk and Johnson, 1980) and in this case the first-born child was diagnosed as having congenital nephrosis. The circumstances of maternal immunity to allotypically determined immunoglobulin antigens could be relevant to the phenomenon of allotype suppression reported in rabbits and mice, because many maternal antifoetal allotypes will be IgG and as such they should theoretically be transported across the placentae to immunosuppress the production of certain foetal immunoglobulin classes. This type of transport is, however, subject to involvement in the placental sink, because maternal antifoetal immunoglobulin allotypes will, in all probability, meet their antigens in the mesenchymal stromata of chorionic villi where they will either bind to form immune complexes as shown by Johnson *et al.* (1977) or be coprecipitated by complement fixation as reported by Faulk *et al.* (1980). If the allotype-antiallotype complexes escape precipitation or complement-mediated coprecipitation and enter placental vessels, the immune complexes will be trapped and prevented from entering the foetal circulation by a dense array of Fc-receptors found on the plasma membranes of foetal stem vessel endothelium (Johnson and Faulk, 1977), thus placing into some doubt the possibility that maternal anti-immunoglobulin allotypic immunity is responsible for the suppression of foetal immunoglobulin production in human pregnancy.

Cellular considerations

A large number of investigators have studied the possible manifestations of altered cellular immunity in human pregnancy, but no clear pattern of lymphocyte responses have emerged from these reports. For example, Blecher and Thompson (1976) maintain that maternal lymphocyte responses to phytohaemagglutinin (PHA) during pregnancy are depressed while Birkeland and Kristoffersen (1977) find no effect caused by pregnancy on the ability of lymphocytes to respond to this lectin. Similarly, mixed lymphocyte culture (MLC) responses of pregnant mother's lymphocytes to stimulation from allogeneic lymphocytes have been found to be either decreased (Petrucco *et al.*, 1976) or normal (Carr *et al.*, 1974), although experimental studies by Chaouat and Voisin (1979) have shown MLC suppressing cells in the spleens of mice after several allogeneic pregnancies. Skin grafts seem to remain intact somewhat longer during human pregnancy (Anderson and Monroe, 1962) although this is more obvious for first than for second set grafts (Peer, 1958). Consistent with the grafting data is the observation that delayed hypersensitivity reactions as measured by skin testing with PPD is depressed in pregnancy (Smith *et al.*, 1972) but this is more apparent in the latter half of gestation (Birkeland and Kristoffersen, 1977). A final note of confusion concerns the populations of T and B lymphocytes in human pregnancy, because Campion and Currey (1972) report normal numbers of T cell rosettes whereas Finn *et al.* (1972) and Strelkauskas *et al.* (1975) find fewer circulating T cells up to 20 weeks gestation followed by a compensatory increase in B cells and eventual normal T:B ratio. Regarding leukocytes in normal human pregnancy, Mitchel *et al.* (1970) have found that they demonstrate significantly increased rates of phagocytosis and bactericidal activity, possibly accounting for the clinical impression that most infections are not more common in pregnant patients.

Placental considerations

The trophoblast

Research to clarify whether human trophoblast expressed major histocompatibility complex (MHC) antigens was first done by using monospecific antisera to human β2-microglobulin, a protein noncovalently associated with HLA-A, B and C determinants on cell membranes. Nontrophoblastic placental cells such as fibroblasts and endothelia were found to be positive but β2-microglobulin could not be demonstrated on the trophoblast (Faulk and Temple, 1976), nor could it be exposed by culture of placental tissues or by treatment of placental sections with various chemicals and enzymes. HLA and B cell alloantigens were also found to be absent from human trophoblast (Faulk *et al.*, 1977). This is supported by biochemical studies of placental (Goodfellow *et al.*, 1976) and syncytiotrophoblastic plasma membranes (Ogbimi *et al.*, 1979) as well as by the absence of anti-β2-microglobulin antibody in antisera raised to human trophoblast membranes (Faulk *et al.*, 1978). These observations may contribute to a broader understanding of how trophoblast break away from the placenta to enter the mother's circulation and lodge in her lung without causing histopathological signs of inflammation (Park, 1959). Such reports should not however lead to a conclusion that the trophoblast is immunologically inert, because Taylor and Hancock (1975) have shown that maternal lymphocytes are cytotoxic for trophoblast *in vitro*. This cytotoxicity is inhibited by maternal serum suggesting an involvement of the blocking phenomenon. Two important immunological events must thus take place to insure the successful completion of pregnancy: firstly, a specific mechanism to impede maternal recognition or rejection of the allogeneic trophoblast, and secondly blocking factors must be mounted. A need for blocking factors in normal pregnancy has been shown by their absence in the blood of chronic aborters (Stimson *et al.*, 1979).

Immune responses to placental antigens

Although mothers often mount immune responses to foetal HLA antigens inherited from the father, the lack of trophoblastic HLA antigens may serve to protect the placenta from recognition by maternal lymphocytes. This finds an analogy in cytotoxic reactions to virus-infected cells, because Zinkernagel and Doherty (1977) have shown that these depend upon the presence of MHC antigens on target cells, indicating that the absence of MHC antigens on human trophoblast might frustrate maternal immune recognition by denying maternal cells the HLA target needed for cell-mediated immune reactions. Other antigens such as the ABO and Rh blood groups cannot be shown on trophoblast (Szulman, 1973). The PP_1 p^k complex is a blood group which could be important in maternofoetal interactions, especially in view of the increased incidence of abortions in women of genotype pp, but it is presently not known whether P antigen is represented on trophoblast. A relatively weak histocompatibility antigen is the male marker H-Y; evidence from laboratory animals has indicated that zygotes which are antigenically dissimilar from the mother are favoured at implantation, prompting the suggestion that H-Y antigens of the zygotes may play a role in sex determination through its obvious difference with maternal cells. It has been additionally proposed that H-Y should be present on the blastocyst, but there are no studies of human fertilized eggs to evaluate this point.

Is there then any evidence that trophoblast themselves manifest antigens, and have maternal antibodies been identified to placental membranes? A small proportion of mothers with pre-eclamptic toxaemia reportedly produce haemagglutinating antibodies to a placental polysaccharide (Levanon and Rossetini, 1968), and immunohistological methods have reportedly been used to identify antitrophoblast antibodies in postpartum sera (Hulka and Brinton, 1963) but these reports have yet to be confirmed. Other trophoblastic glycoproteins have been isolated and maternal antibodies to some of these have been reported (Gaugas and Curzen, 1974). The interrelationship between these antigens and antibodies has not yet been studied and no attempt has been made to introduce a uniform nomenclature for trophoblast antigens.

Specialized processes must have arisen during evolution and natural selection which allowed for the coexistence of genetically dissimilar tissues during pregnancy. A possible explanation for this is that the trophoblast developed an ability to produce a substance that impaired maternal rejection reactions. Several suggestions have been advanced to explain maternal acceptance of the placental homograft, but none of these account for specificity of maternal tolerance of the placenta. The mother's immune system is not clinically compromised during pregnancy, making it difficult to assign any meaning to reports of generalized suppression of lymphocyte function caused by factors identified in maternal and cord blood or in immunoglobulins eluted from human placentae (Faulk *et al.*, 1974). It should, however, be pointed out that reports of immunobiological activity in placental eluates support the general hypothesis that mothers do respond immunologically to trophoblast antigens.

Research into the antigens of trophoblast membranes has been assisted by the development of techniques for isolating syncytiotrophoblast microvillous plasma membranes (Smith and Brush, 1978), making it possible to resolve solubilized trophoblast membranes into chromatographically defined peaks. Studies with antisera to trophoblastic fractions have allowed Faulk *et al.* (1978) to propose the presence of at least 2 serologically defined antigen groups which have been tentatively designated as TA_1 (trophoblast antigens, peak 1) and TA_2 (trophoblast antigens, peak 2). Interestingly, antisera to peak 1 block the MLC reaction without affecting nonspecific responses of lymphocytes to phytohaemagglutinin (PHA) or pokeweed mitogen (PWM) and these same antitrophoblast sera inhibit human:human MLC without affecting either human:baboon or baboon:baboon MLC reactions (McIntyre and Faulk, 1979a). Anti-peak 1 serum is organ and species specific and only recognizes the trophoblast (Faulk *et al.*, 1979).

Antigens contained in peak 1 preparations inhibit intraspecies MLC without affecting lymphocyte responses to mitogens (McIntyre and Faulk, 1979b). Allogeneically-stimulated human lymphocytes, but not mitogen-stimulated cells, manifest trophoblast cross-reactive antigens on their plasma membranes, and these antigens seem to be involved in early recognition responses in MLC reactions (McIntyre and Faulk, 1979c). Not only do peak 1 antigens affect responding T cells in the MLC reaction, but this inhibitory property seems to be associated with the clotting system inasmuch as coagulation removes inhibition. Indeed, specific allogeneic inhibition is mediated by autologous pregnancy plasma and not serum (McIntyre and Faulk, 1979d). This finding is compatible with the observation that plasma is the only biological medium relevant in *in vivo* reactions. That the MLC inhibiting material arises from trophoblastic microvilli is also consistent with the fact that trophoblast forms the interface of the maternofoetal relationship, and any biological mechanism would be expected to have its maximum effectiveness at this juncture. Finally, inhibition of MLC is most pertinent to studies of the maternofoetal relationship because pregnancy represents the only biological circumstance in which lymphocytes from allogeneic individuals are mixed and cocultured *in vivo*.

Maternofoetal interface antigens

The embryonic F9 antigen in experimental animals is expressed by teratocarcinoma cells and Jacob (1977) has shown that F9 promotes antibody responses in syngeneic adult recipients as well as expressing some reciprocal relationship with the expression of MHC antigens on developing embryonic cells, raising the possibility that analogous antigens may be expressed on the human trophoblast. Some human breast tumour cells do manifest cross-reactive cell membrane antigens with trophoblast (Faulk *et al.*, 1979), opening the speculation that pregnancy could sensitize young women to these antigens and abrogate the subsequent development of breast tumours, thereby lending support to the observation that early pregnancy tends to protect against this disease. In contrast, pregnancy later in life might provoke blocking immunity which could enhance the establishment of trophoblast cross-reactive antigen-bearing cells, and account for the increased incidence of breast cancer in women who become pregnant later in life (Doll, 1975).

Other placental proteins have known biological functions, examples being hCG and hPL and the enzyme alkaline phosphatase, but many other so-called trophoblast proteins such as SP1, PP5, PAPP-A and PAPP-B, are currently of unknown function. Placentae obviously take a part in the maternofoetal relationship, but the role of these proteins in pregnancy is very poorly defined. Nevertheless, because the operational interface between maternal and foetal tissues is the trophoblast, one must look to this membrane for factors which may modulate the immunological balance between mother and foetus, especially with the knowledge that throughout gestation pieces of syncytiotrophoblast break away and enter the maternal circulation (Ikle and Gallen, 1964). It was several years ago proposed that hCG served an immunomodulating function, but this was found to be due to impurities in the hCG preparations. Similar considerations of systemic effects and possible contaminants may also apply to some of the other placental proteins and steroids, though oestrogens do seem to play a special role in maternal resistance during pregnancy by increasing the number and activity of neutrophils (Harkness, 1980).

Receptors at the maternofoetal interface

IgG is selectively transported across the human placenta, and this transport process is responsible for the transmission of immunity from mother to foetus. Brambell (1970) proposed that selectively transported plasma proteins may be protected from enzymatic degradation by binding to plasma membrane receptors during pinocytotic vesicle formation and intracellular transport, an idea which has been further developed by Wild (1975) to include a selective role for cell surface vesicular formation. Micropinocytotic vesicles normally fuse with lysosomes and degrade their protein content, but "coated" micropinocytotic vesicles evade fusion with lysosomes and thus are able to transport their protein content intact. Coated vesicles are an important component of the micropinocytotic system and have been demonstrated within human syncytiotrophoblast (Ockleford and Whyte, 1977). Virtually nothing, however, is known about the release of IgG on the foetal side of trophoblast or of its transfer through trophoblast basement membrane to enter the foetal circulation.

Another feature of the maternofoetal interface is that the apical aspect of syncytiotrophoblast contains a uniform distribution of transferrin (Faulk and Johnson, 1977). This has been confirmed by immunoelectron microscopy and immunofluorescence, and extended to studies of immature placentae (Johnson and Faulk, 1978) as well as to certain monkeys and baboons with haemochorial placentae (Faulk and Galbraith, 1979). This has been shown to be due to trophoblast transferrin receptors which may participate in several biological functions in addition to their more traditional role of iron transport. Maternal transferrin bound by foetal receptors restrict the amount of iron available within the placental intervillous spaces, thus serving as a nonspecific factor of resistance against several infectious organisms in which iron has been implicated in proliferation and toxin production. Trophoblastic transferrin may also exert a local effect on maternal lymphocytes because transferrin is required for lymphocyte proliferation, indicating that placental control of maternal transferrin concentrations could influence the responses of maternal lymphocytes within placentae. Finally, trophoblast transferrin receptors could function in an analogous way to the surface receptors of schistosomes that bind and cover the parasites with host proteins, presumably disguising the invertebrate's own antigens (Goldring *et al.*, 1977). The transferrin receptors of trophoblast (the "parasite") may exert a similar effect by binding transferrin from the mother (the "host"), thus "masking" trophoblast antigens from maternal immune recognition.

Within the context of pregnancy as an example of well-balanced host-parasite relationship, IgE becomes quite important. Under normal circumstances of host-parasite interaction there is an increase in IgE synthesis by the host. This is specially true for those hosts who are infected with parasites that use mucosal surfaces as their portal of entry. Since human blastocysts implant in the uterine mucosa, it would not be surprising to find that during normal pregnancy IgE levels increase above those of nonpregnant controls, but what role IgE plays is not yet known. A role for IgE may be relevant to pregnancy insofar as this immunoglobin has only been described in mammals, and mammals are the only animals which have placentae, raising an intriguing speculation that the development of IgE might have been an evolutionary step that in part allowed the coexistence of genetically dissimilar tissues during mammalian gestation.

A result of maternal IgG transfer across human trophoblast is the formation of soluble immune complexes within chorionic villi which consist of maternal IgG antibody and foetal alloantigens. Fc receptors in placenta are located on placental endothelia and villous macrophages, suggesting that they may help protect the foetus from immune complex mediated tissue damage (Johnson and Faulk, 1977). As stated above, the concept of maternal antibody binding within placentae also includes maternal antibody bound to paternally-derived histocompatibility antigens on HLA-positive cells such as fibroblasts within chorionic villi. Maternal anti-HLA antibody with specificity for the present pregnancy can be detected in placental eluates and not in neonatal sera (Jeannet *et al.*, 1977), and the opposite of this situation is true for maternal anti-HLA antibody which results either from a previous pregnancy or from an incompatible blood transfusion. This concept can also be extended to rhesus antigens, because erythrocyte lysis by maternal antibody results in the release of complexes which are bound by Fc receptors on placental endothelium, and placental endothelial cell damage has been reported in placentae from cases of maternofoetal rhesus incompatibility (Fox, 1978). It would thus appear that placental antigen-bearing cells and Fc receptors tend to bind certain maternal antibodies and immune complexes and deny their entrance into the foetal circulation. The effects of such complexes on the growth and development of placental tissues have not been studied, but it is thought that they in part account for the immunopathology found in normal placentae (Faulk *et al.*, 1980).

Maternofoetal immunopathology

Trophoblast is separated from the villous stroma of the placenta by the trophoblastic basement membrane (TBM) and this structure presents a formidable barrier across which maternal components are transported into placental connective tissues to eventually reach the foetal circulation. These membranes show a progressive thickening in the later stages of pregnancy to $1000–3000 \times 10^{-1}$ nm and are further thickened in pathological disorders such as maternal malaria (Galbraith *et al.*, 1980b), pre-eclamptic toxaemia, maternal diabetes, rhesus incompatibility and prolonged pregnancies (Fox, 1978). These changes could be ascribed to placental ischaemia, but immunological reactions may be involved. Immunologically mediated basement membrane damage and cell lysis results from complement activation, and the identification of activated complement components within lesions has come to be associated with the presence of immunopathological damage. Complement components have been identified in normal preterm and term placental tissues (Faulk *et al.*, 1980), but there is no evidence for significant complement activation in normal pregnancy serum, suggesting that complement activation in pregnancy may be limited to immunopathology within the placental bed. Most complement components have characteristic locations in normal human placentae, indicating that they are either synthesized or deposited in response to specific events during pregnancy.

IgG eluted from well-washed human placental tissue and labelled with FITC will react with a TBM antigen (McCormick *et al.*, 1971), suggesting that TBM antigens may be important in the maternofoetal relationship. Analogies can be drawn between TBM and glomerular basement membranes (GBM) in terms of protein transport, but the observation of immunoproteins on TBM in normal pregnancy contrasts sharply with the results of similar studies on GBM, because IgG and C3 are not usually deposited on GBM unless there are immunopathological disturbances in the kidney. Although an activation of maternal complement would not seem to be to the advantage of the foetus, this apparently occurs in all normal pregnancies because C1q can be regularly observed in vessel walls, endothelia, and on certain stromal cells. That this represents the presence of immune complexes is supported by studies with antisera to human IgG allotypes which show both maternal and foetal IgG in and around placental vessels and within stromal cells (Johnson *et al.*, 1977). The likely composition of some of these complexes is maternal antibody to foetal immunoglobulin heavy and light chain alloantigens, since both anti-Gm and anti-Km antibodies with specificity for foetal (paternal) alloantigens have been identified in maternal blood (Faulk and Johnson, 1980).

Immunohistological studies using antisera to many complement components have confirmed and extended earlier reports of complement fixation on TBM of normal placentae. C3 activation on TBM may involve the alternative pathway because C1q and C4 are absent. The nature of complement-activating material associated with TBM remains unknown but this could involve tissue glycoproteins or trophoblastic enzymes. The only other complement component that has been consistently identified on TBM is C9, and this can sometimes be identified in foetal stem vessel walls, often in association with C1q. Although the presence of C1q and C9 might suggest classical pathway activation, it should be emphasized that C4 is rarely found in these vessel walls. The same distribution for C3 and C9 is found on TBM of baboon chorionic villi, suggesting similarities in the immunobiology of the maternofoetal relationship in humans and baboons. A certain amount of complement activation in specific areas of human placentae thus seems to be an immunobiological necessity of normal pregnancy, representing activation by tissue-bound immune complexes as well as activation through the alternative pathway.

Placental transport

The human placenta is classed as being haemochorial, meaning that the syncytiotrophoblastic mantel is in direct contact with maternal blood in the intervillous spaces (Amoroso, 1961). Some substances in maternal blood are concentrated for transport onto the syncytiotrophoblast by specific receptor binding, and Brambell (1970) has proposed that trophoblast receptors for IgG are somewhat unusual from other Fc-receptors inasmuch as they bind monomeric, uncomplexed IgG for transport whereas macrophage, endothelial and B cell Fc-receptors tend to bind only immune complexes (Papamichail *et al.*, 1979). It is also interesting that the human placenta transports very few allotypically determined maternal proteins other than IgG while many of these allotypes are allowed passage through amnion into amniotic fluid, and this fluid is circulated through the foetal gastrointestinal tract by swallowing, thus passing maternal antigens over mucosal surfaces which are also capable of selective absorption into the foetal circulation. It is not clear why the placenta is so rigorous and amnion so wanton in their criteria for passage, while transport by either route could theoretically carry a maternal antigen into the foetal blood.

The passage of maternal antibody to the foetus can have several biological consequences, the first and most obvious of which is the passive transfer of temporary immunity from mother to child (Brambell, 1970). This property has been utilized by public health workers in certain countries where tetanus neonatorum is a problem with the effect of virtual control of the disease. This is done by immunizing the mother with tetanus toxoid to produce antitoxin in her which will be transported into the developing baby and available for protection against tetanus at the time of birth. Maternal antibody can also increase the immune response (Levi *et al.*, 1969), presumably through an additive or adjuvant effect (McBride and Schierman, 1971). The presence of maternal antibody in the neonate can, however, have other not wholly beneficial effects, such as either interfering with early immunization or, in the case of respiratory syncytial virus, cause a particularly unpleasant or dangerous form of immune complex disease. For the sake of completion, a word will also be said about the possibilities of allotype suppression and immune-regulation by anti-idiotype antibodies transferred from mother to foetus; although both conditions have been shown to occur in experimental animals (Jacobson and Herzenberg, 1972; Weiler *et al.*, 1977), neither have been convincingly demonstrated in humans. Similarly, not much is known about antigen transport across the human placenta (for review see Gill and Repetti, 1979), a potentially important aspect of maternofoetal immunology.

Foetal considerations

Human foetal lymphocytes not only have a much greater rate of spontaneous turnover *in vitro* than adult cells (Faulk *et al.*, 1973) but their capacity to initiate DNA synthesis subsequent to lectin stimulation is also more rapid than that found in the adult (Yoffey *et al.*, 1978). Conflicting results have, however, been reported concerning their ability to respond to PHA compared to adult lymphocytes, the reports ranging from decreased (Ayoub and Kasakura, 1971), equivalent (Schechter *et al.*, 1977) or increased (Harina *et al.*, 1980) values. Carr *et al.* (1972) maintain that the variation in these results is due to an inconstant approach to dose-response requirements of foetal lymphocytes for PHA. Carr and his colleagues (1974) have also shown that perinatal lymphocytes respond and stimulate in mixed lymphocyte culture reactions, and several reports have subsequently pointed out that stimulated foetal mononuclear cells release a soluble substance which inhibits the proliferative response of adult lymphocytes (Olding *et al.*, 1977). In addition, they can manifest cell-mediated lympholysis (Granberg *et al.*, 1976) and are capable of responding to sheep erythrocytes at 17–26 weeks in plaque forming cell assays (Koros *et al.*, 1978) and can respond to an array of soluble antigens, though less well than adults (Harina *et al.*, 1980).

The ontogeny of immunoglobulin, antibody and complement synthesis and the maturation of cellular populations involved in host defences have been reviewed by Cooper and Dayton (1977), Gill and Repetti (1979) and Rocklin *et al.* (1979), but a contemporary interest has centred on the possible function of suppressor cell activity in the immunobiology of the maternofoetal relationship in human pregnancy. As mentioned above, male cord blood lymphocytes are able to inhibit maternal lectin and MLC responses (Olding *et al.*, 1977) and this inhibition seems to be much less manifest by older children than by neonates (Finn *et al.*, 1977). It appears that the cells in cord blood which are responsible for suppressor activity are IgG Fc-receptor bearing T lymphocytes (Olding and Oldstone, 1976; Oldstone *et al.*, 1977) which release a membrane-permeable soluble suppressor factor (Olding *et al.*, 1977). A dialysable suppressor factor which is not cytotoxic for target cells can also be obtained from the culture supernates of cord but not adult monocytes, and this soluble mediator inhibits lymphocyte responses to PHA as well as MLC reactions and leukocyte inhibitory factor production (Wolf *et al.*, 1977). It is not possible to speculate on the importance, or lack thereof of these factors in human pregnancy until more information is available.

Disordered maternofoetal relationships

Pre-eclampsia

Efforts to conduct critical studies in pre-eclampsia (PE) are plagued by inaccuracies in the clinical diagnosis, particularly because PE is often associated with so many other diseases. PE is more common during the first pregnancy, it tends to occur in certain families, and the disease can develop subsequent to changes in mating partners (Need, 1979). Anatomically, the uterine spiral arteries normally undergo changes throughout pregnancy causing an increase in the arterial lumen as a result of the erosive interaction of trophoblast with maternal endothelial cells, but this process extends less far into the uterus in PE resulting in diminished luminal size and decreased perfusion of the intervillous space (Brosens *et al.*, 1972). Reports of fibrinoid necrosis, lipid-laden foam cells and infiltration of lymphocytes and plasma cells in and around these vessels are reminiscent of vascular lesions which are often found in certain connective tissue diseases and rejected kidney grafts. Evidence in support of immune reactions within spiral arteries comes from reports of IgM and C3 in the vessel walls (Kitzmiller, 1976), but similar findings can also be obtained from some women with chronic hypertension or diabetic nephropathy. In other words, the chorionic villous in PE is neither normal nor characteristic. An unusually large amount of villous cytotrophoblastic proliferation is found, although this is also seen in essential hypertension, in pregnancy above the age of 30, as well as in grand multiparae. Chorionic villi contain increased numbers of fibrinoid necrotic areas, but these can also be found in placentae from cases of diabetes mellitus and rhesus incompatibility and occasionally even in normal placentae (Fox, 1978), suggesting that the increased numbers of fibrinoid areas in PE may represent an amplification of an as yet undefined normal process in maternofoetal immunology.

Ultrastructural studies of PE trophoblastic basement membranes have also revealed them to be thickened and scarred, but no evidence for immune complexes has been found by using traditional transmission electron microscopy (Jones and Fox, 1980). In contrast, IgG and fragments of the first component of complement activation have been identified within chorionic macrophages of PE placentae with the use of fluorochrome labelled antisera (Keane *et al.*, 1980), but neither the specificity of the IgG nor the nature of the antigens responsible for their synthesis have been determined. The concept of immune processes being important in PE placentae is strengthened by immunohistological studies of trophoblastic basement membranes in normal and PE placentae; both contain C3d and C9, but the number of positive villi is greater in PE tissues than in normal placentae (Faulk and Johnson, 1980). Total blood complement levels have been reported to be both depressed and increased, but individual complement components could increase in the face of a falling haemolytic titre. Measurements of maternal IgG in PE have usually detected depressed values but maternal IgM has been reported as being both lower and higher than nontoxaemic controls and one report has even recorded the provocative finding that cord blood IgM is increased in infants from PE mothers (Yang *et al.*, 1975), suggesting some as yet undefined stimulation to the foetal immune system. Maternal IgA seems to not significantly vary and IgD values are thought to fall as proteinuria increases. Data on IgE are almost nonexistent.

The percentage of T and B lymphocytes in peripheral blood do not show predictable changes in nonpregnant, pregnant and PE women (Gusdon *et al.*, 1977). Other studies have been unable to show differences in the spontaneous uptake of tritiated thymidine by lymphocytes from PE and normally pregnant patients (Petrucco *et al.*, 1976). Similarly, the response of PE lymphocytes to nonspecific stimulation by lectins such as PHA is only marginally depressed and these cells seem to respond normally to both cord blood and paternal lymphocytes in MLC reactions. Birkeland and Kristofferson (1979) have however, associated PE with low T and B lymphocyte counts and impaired T lymphocyte function in mothers and increased B cell counts in their children. Although both maternal and cord blood normally contain large numbers of suppressor cells (Oldstone *et al.*, 1977), there are currently no data available on the role of this important subpopulation of lymphocytes in PE.

Immune complexes can be identified in the maternal circulation during normal pregnancy (Masson *et al.*, 1977), and some investigators have reported that the amount of immune complexes in PE blood is greater than in normal pregnancy (McLaughlin *et al.*, 1979), although these findings have been challenged (Knox *et al.*, 1978). Whether this discrepancy is due to the physical-chemistry of the complexes or to a peculiar characteristic of the antigen or antigens is presently not clear. Immune complex formation in human pregnancy may be a normal manifestation of maternal responses to allotypically incompatible plasma proteins, but the physiological deportation of trophoblast membranes into the maternal circulation may also be important, particularly the idea that deportation is increased in PE. This is important because any increase in the flux of trophoblast membranes would also increase the amount of trophoblast antigens to the mother, thus running a risk of upsetting the immunological balance of the maternofoetal relationship. Early investigations of maternal glomeruli showed deposits of fibrinogen in the absence of immunoglobulins and complement, but more recent studies have reported the presence of fibrinogen plus immunoglobulins and complement (Kincaid-Smith and Fairley, 1976). Alterations in the clotting system may also be relevant to immune complexes in normal and abnormal pregnancies, as certain complexes can interact with complement and clotting factors. Several clotting abnormalities are known to be associated with PE, especially factor VIII cleavage (Thornton and Bonnar, 1977) and the production of fibrinogen-degradation products. The trigger mechanism for the activation of clotting is not clear. Chorionic villi from PE placentae contain more plasminogen and fibrinogen than do normal placentae, and human placental tissues maintained in culture for several days begin to manifest plasminogen reactive cells (Matter and Faulk, 1980) raising the possibility that hypoxia or ischaemia may initiate fibrinolysin synthesis with the subsequent appearance of fibrinogen-degradation and factor VIII cleavage products. Finally, one group has reported a greater than expected incidence of HLA homozygosity in mothers who developed severe pre-eclampsia (Redman *et al.*, 1978), but immunogenetical studies do not indicate that PE is associated with a particular HLA type (Editorial, 1980). Whatever the genetical explanation might be, development of the syndrome seems to be impeded by prior blood transfusion (Feeney *et al.*, 1977).

Abortion

An impression that immunology may participate in the pathophysiology of spontaneous abortion has been drawn from clinical observations. For example, some women who habitually abort for no detectable gynaecological reason have conceived normally by another mate and successfully carried to term a live child. There are also many instances where a clearer role for immunology in abortion has come from patients with antisperm antibodies and immunological infertility, systemic lupus erythematosus, and classical immunological disorders such as blood group incompatibilities that sometimes result in abortion as originally pointed out by Levine and Stetson (1939). There is in fact a relative deficiency of blood group A children produced by group O mothers and group A fathers, and a higher than expected incidence of ABO incompatibility has been reported between husbands and aborting mothers. There is also good evidence for a high incidence of abortions in women of genotype pp who have anti-P antibodies as a result of a previous pregnancy (Levine, 1978).

Differences in the histocompatibility antigens on lymphocytes have been studied by several groups, but there is no evidence that HLA incompatibility between man and wife is associated with an increased incidence of abortion. A different approach to the role of HLA in spontaneous abortions is the idea of a higher frequency of shared antigens at A and B loci by both partners (Komlos *et al.*, 1977), suggesting an increased incidence of homozygosity in the aborted foetuses. Why homozygosity for HLA within the foetus should result in abortion is not presently clear. A working hypothesis has been advanced that matings between partners who have similar trophoblast antigens may produce fertilized eggs which, after implantation, will not be able to stimulate immunological enhancement, thus enabling the mother to recognize and reject foreign trophoblast antigens on the blastocyst (Faulk *et al.*, 1978). Such an hypothesis of course suffers from the present rudimentary knowledge about the chemistry and genetics of trophoblast antigens, but contemporary information on blocking factors in human pregnancy does tend to support this idea.

The natural history of pregnancy in humans seems associated with the production of blocking factors in maternal blood, the absence of which has been described in women who repeatedly abort. Maternal lymphocytes do not produce a particular lymphokine when cocultured with paternal lymphocytes in the presence of maternal autologous serum, but lymphokine production proceeds normally from coculture of lymphocytes from a mating couple when the wife has sustained an abortion (Rocklin *et al.*, 1976). Although this has generally been confirmed (Stimson *et al.*, 1979), it has also been reported that MLC reactions done in the presence of normal maternal serum do not proceed as vigorously as the same reactions performed in the presence of sera from women who have experienced an abortion (Halbrecht and Komlos, 1976).

Blocking factors that inhibit maternal lymphocyte responses to paternal cells in autologous plasma but not serum have also been reported (McIntyre and Faulk, 1979d). A picture thus seems to be emerging that indicates maternal blocking factors are of particular importance in maintaining normal pregnancy, but, as with blocking factors in cancer research and organ transplantation, very little is currently known about the biology or chemistry of these factors.

Maternal diabetes mellitus

Burstein *et al.* (1963) observed that γ globulins and insulin were localized to characteristic structures in diabetic placentae, and Galbraith and Faulk (1979) have found trophoblastic basement membrane immunopathology in chorionic villi of insulin dependent as well as insulin-independent diabetic placentae, both having increased numbers of plasminogen reactive areas as identified by indirect immunofluorescence with antiplasminogen sera. Studies with the electron microscope of insulin-dependent and gestational diabetic placentae by Jones and Fox (1976a, b) revealed several morphological abnormalities such as necrotic foci in syncytiotrophoblast, cytotrophoblast proliferation and basement membrane thickening, yet these findings are neither unique to diabetes nor are they more characteristic of insulin-dependent than gestational diabetics. The placenta is of foetal origin, so there is no reason that it should manifest the lesions of a metabolic disease in the mother, but Harrison and colleagues (1977) have reported that the insulin receptors of syncytiotrophoblastic membranes of placentae from diabetic mothers bind less insulin than controls causing them to query whether maternal responses could affect certain foetal metabolic processes. Some diabetic patients do have immunological aberrations, and Flier *et al.* (1977) have identified the presence of autoantibodies to insulin receptors in a small proportion of insulin resistant patients. In view of this report of immune responses to isogeneic receptors, one is prompted to ask whether allogeneic (i.e. foetal) insulin receptors could stimulate immunological recognition and responses in the mother, but no information on this point is available.

Intra-uterine growth retardation

Inaccuracies in the diagnosis all too often pose an impediment to researchers who are interested in studying this condition of unestablished aetiology. Not only have no immunological studies been done, but it is not even generally accepted that the placenta in cases of this syndrome have characteristic morphological detail (Fox, 1978). Intrauterine growth retardation (IUGR) offspring do not however thrive as well as age-matched controls, and Chandra (1976) has reported that they have certain immunological deficiencies which persist for varying periods of time, but these are neither characteristic nor constant. Immunological methodology has assisted somewhat in the diagnosis of IUGR by providing quantitative measurements of a pregnancy-specific β-1-glycoprotein (Gordon *et al.*, 1977). This is one of the several glycoproteins of unknown function which are thought to be made by trophoblast (Horne and Nisbet, 1979) and which might eventually be found to be important in maternofoetal immunology (Klopper, 1980).

Immunological diseases in pregnancy

In cases of women with underlying immunological diseases who become pregnant, it is of interest to learn the effect of pregnancy on the disease as well as the effect of the underlying disease upon the pregnancy. These interactions have been reviewed by Scott (1976). The placenta in patients with systemic lupus erythematosis (SLE) is pathologically and immunopathologically abnormal (Grennan *et al.*, 1978), and pregnant women with this disease tend to abort much more frequently than expected. Some SLE patients produce a cold-reactive lymphocytotoxin which cross-reacts with trophoblast membranes, putting forward yet another example of maternal immune recognition of trophoblast antigens (Bresnihan *et al.*, 1977). The causal relationship between these antibodies and abortion in SLE needs further investigation. Sera from these patients may provide a valuable source of antitrophoblast sera which can hopefully be used as typing reagents in the continuing search for trophoblast antigens.

Maternal malaria

Malaria is an extremely common disease in certain parts of the world, and its impact on the maternofoetal relationship is probably of greater social and economic importance than realized hitherto. Although infection of the foetus is rare, parasites are commonly found in the placental bed (Wislocki, 1930; Blacklock and Gordon, 1925; Garnham, 1938). Placentae have no specific immune mechanism to protect themselves from infestation, but mothers with malaria have reasonably high titred IgG anti-malarial antibody (McGregor *et al.*, 1966), the placental transport of which probably offers protection to the foetus and placenta. These maternal antiplasmodial antibodies encounter plasmodial antigen within the placental bed and result in the formation of malarial pigment (Galbraith *et al.*, 1980a), immune complexes, and an activation of the clotting system (Galbraith *et al.*, 1980b). These events, coupled with the inevitable maternal anaemia, could account for the high incidence of foetal growth failure and unsatisfactory morbidity and mortality statistics from areas of heavy malaria infection (Jeliffe, 1967). Ultrastructural studies of chorionic villous damage in maternal malaria have revealed the striking findings of large numbers of monocytes in the intervillous spaces and badly damaged syncytiotrophoblastic membranes (Galbraith *et al.*, 1980b). The actual extent of damage seems to vary with the burden of infection. Contemporary information from *in vitro* studies of placental cultures indicate that damaged syncytiotrophoblastic membranes tend to repair themselves (Clint *et al.*, 1978). Maternal malaria thus provides a model for the study of trophoblast damage and repair, the resulting immunopathology could be in part responsible for the large number of perinatal accidents in areas where malaria is still a public health problem.

Choriocarcinoma

Choriocarcinoma is a unique tumour insofar as it is a neoplastic allograft of the reproductive system, and the processes which allow it to grow are probably pertinent to an understanding of the maternofoetal relationship in normal pregnancy. It has been suggested that there is a particular tendency for choriocarcinoma to develop where there is a close antigenic compatibility between the mating partners (Iliya *et al.*, 1967), but it has not been subsequently shown that there is any excess of ABO compatibility in couples in which the female has developed a choriocarcinoma (Mittal *et al.*, 1975; Tomoda *et al.*, 1976). A determining risk factor in choriocarcinoma does however appear to be the paternal blood group (Bagshawe, 1976), although the immunological implications of this finding are presently unclear. Choriocarcinoma was also thought to be likely to develop when the conceptus was compatible with maternal tissues at one or more HLA loci (Lewis and Terasaki, 1971) but studies by Lawler (1976) have shown no evidence that choriocarcinoma is preferentially associated with a conceptus that is HLA compatible with the mother.

Elston (1976) found cellular infiltrates consisting predominantly of plasma cells and lymphocytes in the uteri of 57 women with choriocarcinoma, 33 of whom were classed as having a mild inflammatory cellular response and 24 of the responses were considered to be severe. A good correlation existed between the intensity of the inflammatory reaction and the response to treatment, 70% of those with mild reactions succumbed to the disease while only 12% of those with severe reaction died. Elston and Bagshawe (1973) suggested that the cellular infiltrate into tumour-bearing uteri represents an attempt at tissue rejection on an immunological basis, and this has some support from the experimental work of Lewis *et al.* (1969) who found that the administration of heterologous antilymphocyte serum resulted in an increased growth rate and a diminished response to chemotherapy of choriocarcinoma transplanted to the cheek pouch of the Syrian hamsters. Whether the maternal immune response is directed against tissue-specific trophoblastic antigens, to antigens related to malignant transformation or to paternal transplantation antigens is currently unknown.

Some patients with trophoblastic disease in their first pregnancy, who have never received a blood transfusion, have anti-HLA antibodies with specificity for the HLA type of their mate (Lawler *et al.*, 1976). This is particularly challenging because contemporary understanding of the human trophoblast suggests that it lacks MHC antigens, thus raising the question of how these women become immunized. It is important to appreciate that all researchers who have reported the absence of histocompatibility antigens from trophoblast have used only normal placentae to establish their findings. Relevant to this point is the report by Arce-Gomez *et al.* (1978) that Daudi cells, which also lack β-2-microglobulin and HLA, can be stressed to manifest these antigens by hybridizing them with either HeLa cell derivatives or mouse lymphocytes. The possibility thus remains that an early trophoblast could be metabolically stressed, as for instance by hypoxia or virus infection, and manifest paternal HLA to which the mother would normally respond by the production of paternal specific anti-HLA. It however still remains to be determined if choriocarcinomata cells manifest antigens of the major histocompatibility complex. Further observations on abnormal trophoblastic tissues indicate that tissues from hydatidiform moles are genetically unstable because they seem to be androgenetic in origin (Wake *et al.*, 1978).

Conclusions

Research in maternofoetal immunology will no doubt continue to segregate itself into the traditional compartments of studies on the mother, placenta and foetus, and the following conclusions are a personal statement of what efforts in which compartment are likely to produce useful information. First and perhaps foremost is of course the largely technical contributions which can be expected to accrue from progress in basic immunological research. This is best demonstrated in the area of maternal components by blocking factors, a point of as much importance for transplantation and cancer research as for reproduction; but progress in this field awaits more precise identification of the antigens which give rise to blocking factor synthesis, particularly whether they are related to trophoblast membranes. Indeed, the process of trophoblast deportation into maternal blood requires more complete characterization in normal and abnormal pregnancies. The biological and immunological effects of trophoblast membranes on maternal defences should receive more attention, and it might be expected that research on the chemistry and biology of trophoblast and amnion antigens will be one of the most active and productive avenues of future investigation. It is quite likely that the many reports of viruses in placentae will be extended to pathophysiological significance, and it would seem that pre-eclampsia would be one condition where this might be important. Finally, research on foetal aspects of immunity and how these responses are adapted to organogenesis and vivipara require more study.

References

Amoroso, E. C. (1961). *Br. Med. Bull.* **17**, 81.
Andersen, R. H. and Monroe, C. W. (1962). *Am. J. Obstet. Gyn.* **84**, 1096.
Arce-Gomez, B., Jones, E. A., Barnstable, C. J., Solomon, E. and Bodmer, W. F. (1978). *Tiss. Ant.* **11**, 96.
Ayoub, J. and Kasakura, S. (1971). *Clin. Exp. Immunol.* **8**, 427.
Bagshawe, K. D. (1976). *Cancer* **38**, 1373.
Birkeland, S. A. and Kristoffersen, K. (1977). *Clin. Exp. Immunol.* **30**, 408.
Birkeland, S. A. and Kristoffersen, K. (1979). *Lancet* **i**, 934.
Blacklock, B. and Gordon, R. M. (1925). *Ann. Trop. Med. Parasitol.* **19**, 37.
Blecher, T. E. and Thompson, M. J. (1976). *J. Clin. Path.* **29**, 727.
Brambell, F. W. R. (1970). *In* "Frontiers of Biology" Vol. 18. North-Holland Publishing Company, Amsterdam.
Bresnihan, B., Grigor, R. R., Oliver, M., Lewkonia, R. M., Hughes, G. R. V., Lovins, R. E. and Faulk, W. P. (1977). *Lancet* **ii**, 1205.
Brosens, I., Robertson, W. B. and Dixon, H. G. (1972). *In* "Obstetrics and Gynaecology Annual" (R. M. Wynn, ed.) p. 177. Appleton-Century-Crofts, New York.
Buckley, R. H., Schiff, R. I. and Amos, D. B. (1972). *J. Immunol.* **108**, 34.
Burstein, R., Berns, A. W., Hirata, Y., and Blumenthal, H. T. (1963). *Am. J. Obstet. Gyn.* **86**, 66.
Campion, P. D. and Currey, H. L. F. (1972). *Lancet* **ii**, 830.
Carr, M. C., Stites, D. P., and Fudenberg, H. H. (1972). *Cell. Immunol.* **5**, 21.
Carr, M. C., Stites, D. P., and Fudenberg, H. H. (1973). *Cell. Immunol.* **8**, 448.
Carr, M. C., Stites, D. P., and Fudenberg, H. H. (1974). *Cell. Immunol.* **11**, 332.
Chandra, R. K. (1976). *In* "Maternofoetal Transmission of Immunoglobulins" (W. A. Hemmings, ed.) p. 77. Cambridge.
Chaouat, G., Voisin, G. A., Escalier, D. and Robert P. (1979). *Clin. Exp. Immunol.* **35**, 13.
Chaouat, G. and Voisin, G. A. (1979). *J. Immunol.* **122**, 1383.
Chism, S. E., Burton, R. C. and Warner, N. L. (1979). *Clin. Immunol. Immunopath.* **11**, 346.
Clint, J. M., Wakely, J., and Ockleford, C. D. (1978). *Proc. R. Soc. Lond.* (*B*) **204**, 345.
Cooper, M. D. and Dayton, D. H. (eds) (1977). "Development of Host Defenses". Raven Press, New York.
Corner, G. W. (1944). "Ourselves Unborn". Yale University Press, New Haven.
Doll, R. (1975). *Scot. Med. J.* **20**, 305.
Editorial (1980). *Lancet* **i**, 634.
Elston, C. W. (1976). *J. Clin. Path.* **29**. (Royal College of Pathologists) **10**, 111.
Elston, C. W., and Bagshawe, K. D. (1973). *Br. J. Cancer* **28**, 245.
Faulk, W. Page, Goodman, J. R., Maloney, M. A., Fudenberg, H. H. and Yoffey, J. M. (1973). *Immunology* **8**, 166.
Faulk, W. Page, Jeannet, M., Creighton, W. D. and Carbonara, A. (1974). *J. Clin. Invest.* **54**, 1011.
Faulk, W. Page, Sanderson, A., and Temple, A. (1977). *Transplant. Proc.* **9**, 1379.
Faulk, W. Page, Temple, A., Lovins, R., and Smith, N. C. (1978). *Proc. Natn. Acad. Sc. U.S.A.* **75**, 1947.
Faulk, W. P., Yeager, C., McIntyre, J. A., and Ueda, M. (1979). *Proc. R. Soc. Lond.* (*B*) **206**, 163.
Faulk, W. P., Jarret, R., Keane, M., Johnson, P. M. and Boackle, R. (1980). *Clin. Exp. Immunol.* **40**, 299.
Faulk, W. P. and Galbraith, G. M. P. (1979). *Proc. R. Soc. Lond.* (*B*) **204**, 83.

Faulk, W. P. and Johnson, P. M. (1977). *Clin. Exp. Immunol.* **27**, 365.
Faulk, W. P. and Johnson, P. M. (1980). *Adv. Clin. Immunol.* **2**, (in press).
Faulk, W. P. and Temple, A. (1976). *Nature* **262**, 799.
Feeney, J. G., Tovey, L. A. C. and Scott, J. S. (1977). *Lancet* **1**, 874.
Ferrone, S., Mickey, M. F., Terasaki, P. I., Reisfeld, R. A. and Pellegrino, M. A. (1976). *Transplantation* **22(1)**, 61.
Finn, R., St. Hill, C. A., Govan, A. J., Ralfs, I. G., Gurney, F. J. and Denye, V. (1972). *Br. Med. J.* **3**, 150.
Finn, R., Davis, J. C., St. Hill, C. A., and Hipkin, L. J. (1977). *Lancet* **ii**, 1200.
Flier, J. S., Kahn, C. R., Jarrett, D. B. and Roth, J. (1977). *J. Clin. Invest.* **60**, 784.
Fox, H. (1978). "Pathology of the Placenta". W. B. Saunders Company Ltd., London.
Fudenberg, H. H. and Fudenberg, B. R. (1964). *Science* **145**, 170.
Galbraith, R. M., Faulk, W. P., Galbraith, G. M. P., Holbrook, T. W. and Bray, R. S. (1980a). *Trans. R. Soc. Trop. Med. Hyg.* **74**, 52.
Galbraith, R. M., Fox, H., Hsi, B., Galbraith, G. M. P., Bray, R. S., and Faulk, W. P. (1980b). *Trans. R. Soc. Trop. Med. Hyg.* **74**, 61.
Galbraith, R. M. and Faulk, W. P. (1979). *In* "The Diabetic Pregnancy: A Perinatal Perspective" (I. R. Merkatz and P. A. J. Adams, eds) pp. 111–121. Grune & Stratton, London and New York.
Garnham. P. C. (1938). *Trans. R. Soc. Trop. Med. Hyg.* **32**, 13.
Gaugas, J. M. and Curzen, P. (1974). *Br. J. Exp. Path.* **55**, 570.
Gill, T. J. and Repetti, C. F. (1979). *Am. J. Path.* **95**, 465.
Goldring, O. L., Kusel, J. R. and Smithers, S. R. (1977). *Exp. Parasitol.* **43**, 82.
Goodfellow, P. M., Barnstable, C. J., Bodmer, W. F., Snary, D. E. and Crumpton, M. J. (1976). *Transplantation* **22**, 595.
Gordon, Y. P., Jeffrey, D., Grudzinaskas, T., Chard, T. and Letchworth, A. T. (1977). *Lancet* **i**, 331.
Granberg, C., Manninen, K. and Toivanen, P. (1976). *Clin. Immunol Immunopath.* **6**, 256.
Grennan, D. M., McCormick, J. N., Wojtacha, D., Carty, M. and Behan, W. (1978). *Ann. Rheum. Dis.* **37**, 129.
Gusdon, J. P. Jr. (1969). *Am. J. Obstet. Gyn.* **103**, 895.
Gusdon, J. P., Heise, E. R. and Hervst, G. A. (1977). *Am. J. Obstet. Gyn.* **129**, 255.
Gusdon, J. P. Jr. and Prichard, D. (1972). *Am. J. Obstet. Gyn.* **112**, 867.
Halbrecht, I. and Komlos, L. (1976). *Acta Europ. Fertil.* **7**, 249.
Harina, B. M., Gill, T. J. III, Rabin, B. S., and Taylor, F. H. (1980). *J. Immunogen.* (in press).
Harkness, R. A. (1980). *J. R. Soc. Med.* **73**, 161.
Harrison, L. C., Billington, T., Clark, S., Nichols, R., East, I. and Martin, F. I. R. (1977). *J. Clin. Endocrinol. Metabol.* **44**, 206.
Hirsch, M. S., Kelly, A. D., Chapin, D. S., Fuller, T. C., Black, P. H. and Kurth, P. (1978). *Science* **199**, 1337.
Horne, C. H. W. and Nisbet, A. D. (1979). *Invest. Cell Path.* **2**.
Horne, C. H. W. and Rosen, S. W. (1978). *Scand. J. Immunol.* Supplement **8**, 55.
Hulka, J. F. and Brinton, V. (1963). *Am. J. Obstet. Gyn.* **86**, 130.
Ikle, F. A. and Gallen, S. T. (1964). *Bull. Schweiz. Akad. Med. Wiss.* **20**, 62.
Iliya, F. A., Williamson, S. and Azar, H. A. (1967). *Cancer* **20**, 144.
Jacob, F. (1977). *Immunol. Rev.* **33**, 3.
Jacobson, E. B. and Herzenberg, L. A. (1972). *J. Exp. Med.* **135**, 1151.
Jeannet, M., Werner, Ch., Ramirez, E., Vassalli, P. and Faulk, W. P. (1977). *Transplant. Proc.* **9**, 1417.
Jeliffe, E. F. P. (1967). *In* "Nutrition and Infection. CIBA Foundation Study Group No. 31". (G. E. W. Wolstenholme and M. O'Connor, eds) pp. 18–35. J. A. Churchill, London.

Johnson, P. M., Natvig, J., Ystehede, U. A. and Faulk, W. P. (1977). *Clin. Exp. Immunol.* **30**, 145.
Johnson, P. M. and Faulk, W. P. (1977). *In* "Immunological Influence on Human Fertility". (B. Boettcher, ed.), p. 161. Academic Press, London & New York.
Johnson, P. M. and Faulk, W. P. (1978). *Immunology* **34**, 1027.
Jones, C. J. P. and Fox, H. (1976a). *J. Path.* **119**, 91.
Jones, C. J. P. and Fox, H. (1976b). *Obstet. Gyn.* **48**, 274.
Jones, C. J. P. and Fox, J. (1980). *Placenta* **1**, 61.
Keane, M., Sinha, D., Hsi, B. and Faulk, W. P. (1980). *J. Immunol. Reprod.* (in press).
Kincaid-Smith, P. and Fairley, K. F. (1976). *Perspect. Nephrol. Hypertension* **5**, 157.
Kitzmiller, J. L. (1976). *Clin. Obstet. Gyn.* **20**, 717.
Klopper, A. (1980). *Placenta* **1**, 77.
Knox, G. E., Stagno, S., Valanakis, J. F. and Huddleston, J. F. (1978). *Am. J. Obstet. Gyn.* **132**, 87.
Komlos, L., Zamir, R., Joshua, H. and Halbrecht, I. (1977). *Clin. Immunol. Immunopath.* **7**, 330.
Koros, A. M. C., Szulman, A. E., Hamill, E. C. and Merchant, B. (1978). *Vox Sanguinis* **35**, 234.
Lawler, S. D. (1976). *J. Clin. Path.* **29**, Supplement (Royal College of Pathologists) **10**, 132.
Lawler, S. D., Klouda, P. T. and Bagshawe, K. D. (1976). *Brit. J. Obstet. Gyn.* **83**, 651.
Letchworth, A. T. (1976). *In* "Plasma Hormone Assays in Evaluation of Foetal Well-being" (A. Klopper, ed.) pp. 147–173. Churchill Livingstone, Edinburgh.
Levanon, Y. and Rossetini, S. M. O. (1968). *Archiv. Dumonoforschung* **136**, 178.
Levi, M. I., Krautzov, F. E., Levova, T. M. and Fomenko, G. A. (1969). *Immunology* **16**, 145.
Levine, P. and Stetson, R. E. (1939). *J. Am. Med. Assoc.* **113**, 126.
Levine, P. (1978). *Sem. Oncol.* **5**, 25.
Lewis, J. L., Davis, R. C. and Parker, J. T. (1969). *Cancer Res.* **29**, 1988.
Lewis, J. L. and Terasaki, P. I. (1971). *Am. J. Obstet. Gyn.* **111**, 547.
Maroulis, G. B., Buckley, R. H., and Younger, J. B. (1971). *Am. J. Obstet. Gyn.* **109**, 971.
Masson, P., Delire, M. and Cambiaso, C. C. (1977). *Nature* **266**, 542.
Matter, L. and Faulk, W. P. (1980). *In* "Fibrinogen degradation products and factor VIII consumption in pre-eclamptic toxemia: Role of the placenta in Pregnancy Hypertension" (J. Bonnar, ed.) M. T. P. Press, Ltd., Lancs.
McBride, R. A., and Schierman, L. W. (1971). *J. Exp. Med.* **134**, 833.
McCormick, J. N., Faulk, W. P., Fox, H. and Fudenberg, H. H. (1971). *J. Exp. Med.* **133**, 1.
McGregor, I. A., Hall, P. J., Williams, K. Hardy, C. L. S. and Turner, M. W. (1966). *Nature* **210**, 1384.
McIntyre, J. A. and Faulk, W. P. (1979a). *J. Exp. Med.* **149**, 824.
McIntyre, J. A. and Faulk, W. P. (1979b). *Proc. Natn. Acad. Sci. U.S.A.* **76**, 4029.
McIntyre, J. A. and Faulk, W. P. (1979c). *Transplant. Proc.* **11**, 1892.
McIntyre, J. A. and Faulk, W. P. (1979d). *Lancet* **ii**, 821.
McLaughlin, P. J., Stirrat, G. M., Redman, C. W. G. and Levinsky, R. H. (1979). *Lancet* **i**, 934.
Mitchell, G. W., Jacobs, A. A., Hadad, V., Paul, B. B., Straus, R. R., and Sbama, A. J. (1970). *Am. J. Obstet. Gyn.* **108**, 805.
Mittal, K. K., Kachru, R. B. and Brewer, J. I. (1975). *Tiss. Ant.* **6**, 57.
Morton, H., Rolfe, B. & Clunie, G. J. A. (1977). *Lancet* **i**, 394.
Nathenson, G., Schorr, J. B., and Litwin, S. D. (1971). *Ped. Res.* **5**, 2.
Need, J. A. (1979). *Clin. Obstet. Gyn.* **6**, 443.

Ockleford, C. D. and Whyte, A. (1977). *J. Cell. Sci.* **25**, 293.
Ogbimi, A. O., Johnson, P. M., Brown, P. J. and Fox, H. (1979). *J. Reprod. Immunol.* **2**, 127.
Olding, L. B. and Oldstone, M. G. A. (1976). *J. Immunol.* **116**, 682.
Olding, L. B., Benirschke, K. and Oldstone, M. G. A. (1974). *Clin. Immunol. Immunopath.* **3**, 79.
Olding, L. B., Murgita, R. A. and Wigzell, H. (1977). *J. Immunol.* **119**, 1109.
Oldstone, M. B. A., Tishon, A. and Moretta, L. (1977). *Nature* **269**, 333.
Park, W. W. (1959). *Ann. N. Y. Acad. Sci.* **80**, 152.
Papamichail, M., Faulk, W. P., Gutierrez, C., Temple, A. and Johnson, P. M. (1979). *Clin. Immunol. Immunopath.* **12**, 436.
Peer, L. A. (1958). *Ann. N. Y. Acad. Sci.* **73**, 854.
Petrucco, O. M., Seamark, R. F., Holmes, K., Forbes, I. S. and Symons, R. G. (1976). *Br. J. Obstet. Gyn.* **83**, 245.
Ramsey, E. M., Houston, M. L. and Harris, J. W. (1976). *Am. J. Obstet. Gyn.* **124**, 647.
Redman, C. E. G., Bodmer, J. G., Bodmer, W. F., Beilen, L. J. and Bonnar, J. (1978). *Lancet* **i**, 397.
Rocklin, R. E., Kitzmiller, J. C., Carpenter, C. B., Garovoy, M. R. and David, J. R. (1976). *New Engl. J. Med.* **295**, 1209.
Rocklin, R., Kitzmiller, J. and Kaye, M. (1979). *Ann. Rev. Med.* **30**, 375.
Salinas, F. A., Silver, H. K. B., Sheikh, K. M. and Chandor, S. B. (1978). *Cancer* **42** (Suppl.) 1653.
Schechter, B., Handzel, Z. T., Altman, Y., Nir, E., and Levin, S. (1977). *Clin. Exp. Immunol.* **27**, 478.
Scott, J. S. (1976). *In* "Immunology of Human Reproduction" (J. S. Scott and W. R. Jones, eds). p. 229. Academic Press, London and New York.
Sedlacek, H. H., Rehkopf, R. and Bohn, H. (1976). *Behring Institute Mitteilinger,* **59**, 81.
Smith, J. K., Caspary, E. A., and Field, E. J. (1972). *Am. J. Obstet. Gyn.* **113**, 602.
Smith, N. C. and Brush, M. G. (1978). *Med. Biol.* **56**, 272.
Stimson, W. H., Strachan, A. F. and Shepherd, A. (1979). *Br. J. Obstet. Gyn.* **86**, 41.
Sterlkauskas, A. J., Wilson, B. S., Dray, S., and Dodson, M. (1975). *Nature* **258**, 331.
Szulman, A. E. (1973). *New Engl. J. Med.* **286**, 1028.
Tal, C. (1965). *Proc. Natn. Acad. Sci. U.S.A.* **54**, 1318.
Tatra, G., Placheta, P. and Breitenecker, G. (1975). *Wien. Klin. Wschr.* **87**, 279.
Taylor, P. V. and Hancock, K. W. (1975). *Immunology* **28**, 973.
Thornton, C. A. and Bonnar, J. (1977). *Br. J. Obstet. Gyn.* **84**, 919.
Tomoda, Y., Fuma, M., Miwa T., Saiki N. and Ishizuka, N. (1976). *Gyn. Invest.* **7**, 280.
Voisin, G. A. and Chaouat, G. (1974). *J. Reprod. Fertil.* (Supp.) **21**, 89.
Wake, N., Takagi, N. and Sasaki, M. (1978). *J. Natn. Cancer Inst.* **60**, 51.
Weiler, I. J., Weiler, E., Sprenger, R. and Cosenza H. (1977). *Eur. J. Immunol.* **7**, 591.
Wild, A. E. (1975). *Phil. Trans. R. Soc.* (B) **271**, 395.
Wislocki, G. B. (1929). "Contributions to Embryology". Carnegie Institution of Washington, **20**, 51.
Wislocki, G. B. (1930). *Johns Hopkins Hosp. Bull.* **47**, 157.
Wolf, R. L., Lomnitzer, R. and Rabson, A. B. (1977). *Clin. Exp. Immunol.* **27**, 464.
Yang, S.-L., Kleinman, A. M. and Wei, P.-Y. (1975). *Am. J. Obstet. Gyn.* **122**, 727.
Yoffey, J. M., Ron, A., Prindull, G. and Yaffe, P. (1978). *Clin. Immunol. Immunopath.* **9**, 491.
Zinkernagel, R. M. and Doherty, P. C. (1977). *Cold Spring Harbor Symp. Quant. Biol.* **41**, 505.

59

Hormones and Antibodies in the Study and Control of Reproductive Processes

G. P. TALWAR*, S. K. MANHAR, A. TANDON, S. RAMAKRISHNAN and S. K. GUPTA

All-India Institute of Medical Sciences, Ansari Nagar, New Delhi, India

Hormones in reproduction

ormal fertile subjects

A characteristic feature of mammalian reproduction is its heavy dependence on hormones. Figure 1 is a schematic representation of the hormones involved in the function and maintenance of the reproductive system. The hypothalamic–pituitary–gonad axis is mediated by 3 sets of hormones. Hypothalamus secretes a decapeptide LHRH, which acts on the basophil cells of the anterior pituitary to release the gonadotropins, FSH and LH. These in turn act on the gonads. FSH stimulates the development and maturation of the follicle in the female. In the male, recent evidence points to its role in the development

The work was supported by grants from IDRC of Canada, Family Planning Foundation of India, Rockefeller Foundation and ICCR of Population Council.

*Jawahar Lal Nehru Fellow.

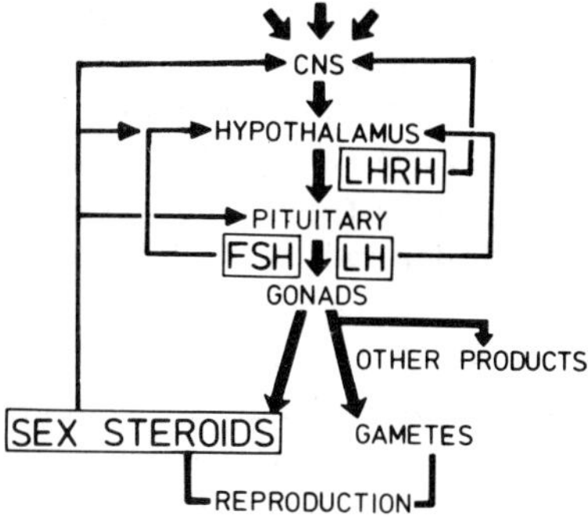

FIG. 1. *Hormones involved in regulation of the reproductive system in normal fertile subjects.*

of the germinal cells, at least in the primates. A surge of LH in the females brings about ovulation. LH has an important role in steroidogenesis in both male and female. The steroid hormones in turn act on the secondary reproductive organs, e.g. uterus, vagina, cervix, seminal vesicles, prostate and epididymis, the normal function of these organs being critically dependent on sex steroids. A sequential interdependence of the hormones can be discerned in the forward direction. There are also feedback controls. LHRH and gonadotropins have short loop negative feedbacks on the hypothalamus directly, and indirectly through certain brain centres. Steroids exercise both positive and negative feedbacks at the pituitary and at the hypothalamus. It is thus obvious that immunological neutralization *in vivo* of any one of *these* hormones will have *primary* as well as *secondary* effects by cutting off the hormonal support to the target organs of the putative hormone, followed and accompanied by secondary effects arising ouf of the disregulation of the circuit.

Hormones in pregnancy

The early embryo (blastocyst) requires an appropriate hormonal milieu for implantation. The uterus has to be primed with oestradiol followed by progesterone to be in a state of "receptivity" for implantation. Progesterone support to the endometrium needs to be sustained to prevent its shedding. Pregnancy provides a signal for rescue of the corpus luteum and continuation of the steroid synthesis. The message obviously emanates from either the early embryo, and or from the interaction of the embryo with the endometrium.

The trophoblast is the source of several hormones. Amongst these, human chorionic gonadotropin (hCG) is detectable in circulation at about the 8th day postfertilization (Saxena *et al.*, 1974, Catt *et al.*, 1975). Its levels rise steeply, attaining a peak at 8–10 weeks of pregnancy (Braunstein *et al.*, 1976), at which time approximately 4·6 mg of hCG is present per litre of serum with an equivalent amount excreted in the urine. The functions performed by hCG are partially understood. It has no doubt a gonadotropic action and is presumably responsible for progesterone production by the ovary in the first 5 to 7 weeks of pregnancy. Pregnancy may engender an additional factor, which sustains the corpus luteum function along with hCG (Talwar, 1979). hCG has also been implicated as a shield against immunological rejection by virtue of its presence on the trophoblast (Borland *et al.*, 1975). A fall in hCG titres during the first 5 to 7 weeks of pregnancy is usually accompanied by abortion (Crosignani *et al.*, 1974; Kunz, 1976). Antibodies neutralizing hCG also bring about the termination of pregnancy. These observations suggest an important role of hCG in the maintenance of early pregnancy, whether it be due to the above mentioned functions, or others to be discovered.

Another trophoblastic hormone hPL is perceptible in maternal serum from about 6 weeks of pregnancy, with a progressive rise in course of pregnancy (Fig. 2). The level of this hormone is an index of the normal growth and functioning of the foeto-placental unit. Its role in pregnancy is not clearly established. Antibodies against hPL interrupted pregnancy in rats and rabbits (El Tomi *et al.*, 1970, 1971). However, these were not abortifacient in baboons (Stevens, 1976).

Pregnancy is characterized by high levels of oestriol and progesterone in

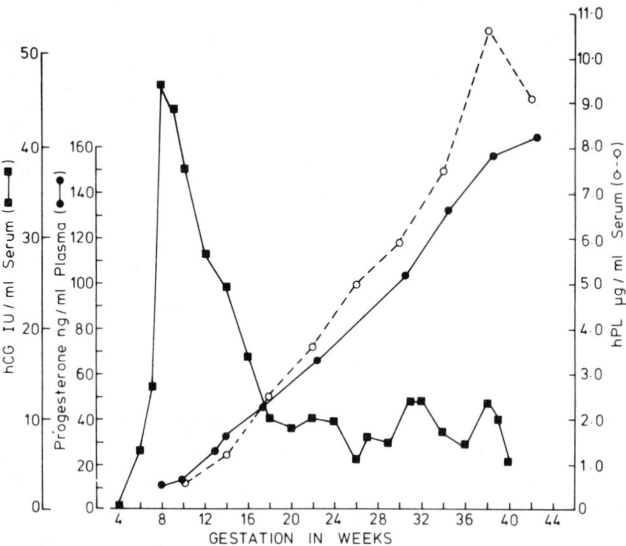

FIG. 2. *Major hormones produced in pregnancy. Their levels in blood at different stages of pregnancy are given. hCG appears early, rises steeply to attain peak values around week 8–10 of pregnancy after which it declines to a low level persisting throughout the period of gestation. hPL and progesterone increase progressively with pregnancy. Oestrogens, which are also produced by the foeto–placental unit, are not shown in the figure (data from Braunstein, G. D.* et al. *(1976)* Am. J. Obstet. Gyn., **12**, *679; Josimovich, J. B.* et al. *(1970)* Obstet. Gyn. **36**, *244; Johansson, E. D. and Jonasson, L. E. (1971)* Acta Obstet. Gyn. Scand. **50**, *339*).

contrast to luteal phase (Klopper and Fuchs, 1977). A fall in both progesterone and oestriol are indicative of abnormal pregnancy and could spell abortion. Besides the above mentioned principal hormones, the placenta is considered to make a number of others, such as thyrotropin, corticotropin, LHRH, somatostatin and endorphins.

Antibody response to reproductive hormones

The reproductive hormones fall in two categories—large molecular weight proteins and small molecular weight steroids and short polypeptides. The former are immunogenic in heterospecies but seldom in homo- or isospecies. Both categories can be rendered immunogenic by conjugating them with a carrier protein. Methods for conjugation of steroids to carriers have been worked out by insertion of an activating handle at a desired position in the steroid molecule (Bauminger *et al.*, 1974). All hormones can be made immunogenic in isospecies by either insertion of haptenic groups (Stevens and Crystle, 1973; Dubey *et al.*, 1976) or carriers such as the tetanus toxoid (Talwar *et al.*, 1975, 1976a, b).

Applications of antibodies against reproductive hormones

At least three important uses of antihormone antibodies can be listed:

(1) Development of assays with extreme sensitivity for hormones.
(2) Provision of clinching evidence for the role and site of action of the hormones.
(3) Control of fertility.

High sensitivity methods for determination of hormones

Radioimmunoassays (RIA) brought in a new dimension in quantitative determination of hormones in biological fluids. Measurements became possible with microvolumes and frequent samples could be analysed. The new body of data helped considerably in better understanding of the body endocrinology in health and disease. While RIA have become widespread, a still larger utilization of immunoassays can be expected from the recent introduction of the enzyme-linked immunoassays (EIA). An enzyme with a high turnover number giving easy colour reactions, substituting the radioisotopic marker, renders these estimations cheaper and widely applicable. It is not unlikely that EIA will replace many conventional clinical chemistry assays in hospital laboratories. A particular advantage of these highly sensitive assays may be the putting in evidence of early pathological changes, providing clues to clinically latent abnormalities.

Antibodies as a tool for recognition of a hormone have also given rise to a variety of immunodiagnostic kits. Not long ago, the diagnosis of pregnancy demanded a large number of frogs and rabbits. It required large volumes of urine and several days of experimentation before the apprehension of a woman having become pregnant could be confirmed. Today, the diagnosis of pregnancy can be made in minutes by a slide test utilizing immunological reagents.

Role of hormones in the biological processes, location and mode of action

It is not infrequent in biological research that controversies arise on the precise role of a hormone, specially in processes dependent on the interplay of more than one hormone. For example, many investigators felt that LH was the principal hormone stimulating steroidogenesis but others obtained steroidogenic effects with FSH. The presence of one or the other hormone as contaminant in preparations could not be excluded, as the source of the two hormones was the same tissue. Availability of monospecific antibodies reacting with one and not the other hormone made possible the decision (Moudgil, 1975). Antibodies have also been extremely valuable in demarcation of the sites at which the hormone binds in the target tissue. Immunofluorescence, immunoenzymatic and immunoradioisotopic methods have enabled the delineation of the cell types in a tissue binding the hormone and the subcellular location of receptors for different hormones.

Antihormonal antibodies in control of fertility

Theoretically, antibodies neutralizing the action of one or more of the reproductive hormones would produce a block of fertility. The practicability of this approach will, however, be determined by (a) the ease with which neutralizing antibodies of sufficient titres against a hormone can be produced and (b) their noninterference in body functions other than reproduction. Active immunization against most of the hormones represented in Fig. 1 will entail undesirable side-effects and is thus *a priori* excluded for human applications except in special circumstances (such as menopause and cancers). A reserve may, however, be expressed over the possible utility of immunization against the pituitary gonadotropins and in particular against FSH.

FSH

Anti-FSH antibodies lead to an arrest of spermatogenesis in monkey. The block was reversible and the animals regained fertility in course of time on withdrawal of the anti-FSH antibodies (Sairam and Madhwa Raj, 1980; Murty *et al.*, 1980). Active immunization may eventually be conceivable through the use of the β-subunit of FSH, on the analogy of utilizing the β-gCG for immunization against hCG. So far, studies against FSH have been carried out in one male subhuman primate. It should be of interest to extend these to apes and also to evaluate the effect in the female. A method inhibiting the development of the follicle without the loss of sex steroid production would be of considerable value.

LH

LH has a definite role in induction of ovulation and steroidogenesis by luteal cells. Antibodies against LH will counteract both these activities and would lead to infertility. However, the clinical use of this approach can only be made if the procedure is modulated so as to cause the insufficiency of the luteal phase without completely abolishing the production of progesterone. This is apparently attainable in two different ways: (i) partial inhibition of FSH action and follicular cell maturation; and (ii) partial but not complete neutralization of the pituitary LH. Hodgen and collaborators have observed that inhibin or porcine follicular fluid given over the first 3 days of the cycle diminish the follicular growth and maturation in the monkey in a manner so that the granulosa cells are less responsive to LH/hCG. Immunization of rhesus monkey with β-oLH rendered them infertile, although the animals were ovulating (Sundaram *et al.*, 1976). Infertility was considered to be due to cross-reaction of the antibodies with the monkey chorionic gonadotropin. Further studies have also revealed the insufficiency of the luteal function in these animals (Thau *et al.*, 1979). Immunization against a heterospecies LH can thus be visualized to be useful for control of fertility, if the present observations in rhesus monkeys can be confirmed in higher primates. Ovine LH is a remarkable gonadotropin possessing immunological cross-reaction with both the pituitary and the chorionic gonadotropin of a large number of animal species varying from mouse to human. The pregnant mare serum gonadotropin (PMSG) has also cross-reactions with the rodent, primate and human hormones and could also be explored as an antigen for fertility control. The main concern in these approaches will be the impact of long-term presence of antibodies in circulation cross-reacting with pituitary hormones. Immune complexes and their deleterious effects as well as the possible pituitary pathology would have to be excluded.

LHRH

Immunization against LHRH can cut off the gonadotropins, which are key hormones for both gametogenesis and steroid hormone production. Indeed, active immunization against LHRH leads to infertility in sheep (Fraser *et al.*, 1977) and marmosets (Hodges and Hearn, 1977). The block is reversible and fertility is regained on decline of antibody titre. Bulls immunized against LHRH have diminished spermatogenesis and androgen production (Robertson *et al.*, 1979). In our laboratory LHRH was conjugated to tetanus toxoid. The conjugates were immunogenic in a variety of test animals without recourse to the use of the Freunds Complete Adjuvant (FCA). Mice actively immunized with LHRH-TT had disturbed oestrus cycles. Preliminary studies also indicate the suppression of the periodic heat in bitches and cats by anti-LHRH immunization (Fig. 3). Animals with periodic oestrus cycles may be particularly suitable for immunization with vaccines provoking anti-LHRH response. Such animals may withstand, without undue side-effects, the impact of

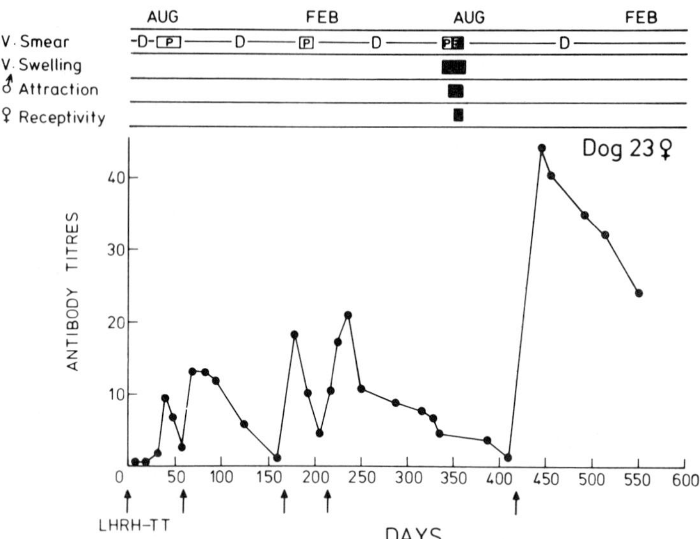

FIG. 3. *Immunization of female dogs against LHRH. A new conjugate LHRH-TT was effective in inducing anti-LHRH titres without the use of Complete Freund's Adjuvant. High titres suppressed oestrus cycle.*

deprivation of steroid hormones, a resultant of blocking the activity of this hormone. Hypothalamus may not be the only site of LHRH synthesis nor pituitary the sole target tissue. The peptide has recently been observed to exercise an effect beyond the pituitary; such as a direct action on the gonads (Labrie *et al.*, 1979) and on the reproductive tract organs. Receptors for LHRH are also located in the brain and LHRH administration has been claimed to increase libido in rodents (Moss and Dudley, 1980).

Steroid hormones

Antibodies have been raised against androgens, oestrogens and progestogens. The effects are, however, complex. The antibodies, by binding with the hormone, prolong significantly their metabolic clearance. A compensatory hypersecretion of gonadotropins is produced, which in turn induces an increased production of the steroids. Nieschlag *et al.* (1975) noted 30 to 100-fold increase in serum testosterone in animals immunized against testosterone. There was a marked rise in LH and FSH with increase in number of Leydig cells and weight of the testes but there was a loss of sexual activity. Ferin *et al.* (1975) reported high levels of oestrogens in monkeys immunized against oestradiol. Ovulation was blocked with loss of cyclicity. Sheep immunized against androstenedione had increased ovulation rate, and the number of follicles $\geqslant 3$ mm in diameter were higher (Scarmuzzi *et al.*, 1980). The latter approach may have veterinary applications.

Human chorionic gonadotropin

Although hCG has been reported recently to be synthesized in very small amounts by a variety of extraplacental tissues (Braunstein *et al.*, 1979; Chen *et al.*, 1976; Yoshimoto *et al.*, 1977), hCG is principally a hormone of pregnancy and its detection in urine has served for many years as a faithful criteria for the confirmation of pregnancy. In selecting this as a target antigen, the aim was to intercept an event beginning with pregnancy, thus avoiding undue interference in normal endocrinology of the non-pregnant female. It is not surprising that a major part of research on the antifertility vaccines has centred around hCG.

hCG is composed of two nonidentical subunits α and β. The α subunit is nearly identical to the alpha of FSH, LH and TSH (Pierce *et al.*, 1976). It is thus obvious that the entire molecule of hCG cannot be used as an antigen, even though the conformation of the intact hormone is optimal to provoke the formation of antibodies with maximal neutralization capacity. The next reductive possibilities are: (a) β-subunit of hCG, (b) derivatives of β-hCG; and (c) enzyme cleaved or synthetic subfragments of β-hCG.

Chemistry and molecular anatomy of β-hCG

The β subunit of hCG is a glycopeptide of 145 amino acids with 6 sugar moieties, 2 linked to asparagine and 4 to serine residues (Morgan *et al.*, 1975). The carbohydrate content of the subunit is comparatively higher than β-hLH, which is presumably responsible for the longer biological half life of hCG. β-hCG has 12 half-cystine residues but no free titrable SH group. There exist, therefore, 6 intrachain S–S linkages. The position of these linkages are not defined, except for the suggestive evidence for Cys 93 to Cys 100 S–S link (Pierce *et al.*, 1976). These linkages play a crucial part in the native conformation; reduction and alkylation of hCG results in the loss of biological activity. This modification alters also the immunological properties of the molecule drastically.

An extra strand of 30 amino acids is present at the C-terminal end of β-hCG, which is nonexistent in β-hLH. This β-hCG unique strand is particularly rich in serines (8 in number) and prolines (9 in number). There are

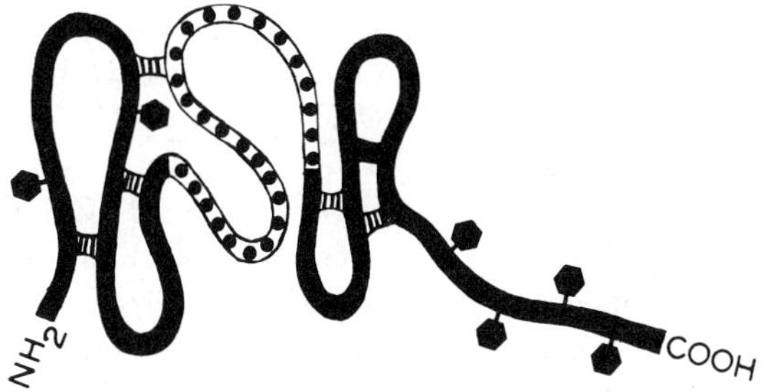

FIG. 4. *A conceptual diagram of β-hCG. The 145 amino acid long glycopeptide has 6–S–S–linkages which are largely unmapped and which confer important conformational characteristics to the molecule. Reduction and alkylation results in the loss of its ability to recombine with a subunit and biological activity. The C-terminal 35 amino acid β-hCG unique region is rich in serines and prolines, has no aromatic amino acids and carries 4 of the 6 carbohydrate residues.*

no aromatic amino acids, or cystine in this part of the molecule. Circular dichroism studies on the C-terminal synthetic peptides of β-hCG (31-CTP; 35-CTP and 45-CTP) indicate the absence of any ordered secondary structure, such as the α-helix and β-structures (unpublished data). These features are represented conceptually in Fig. 4.

Determinants involved in target tissue recognition

For optimal bioactivity, association of the α and β subunits is required. The possible sites at which the subunit association takes place are known to some extent for oLH but not for hCG; in oLH, an association between Lys at position 49 of the α-subunit with Asp at position 111 of β-subunit is indicated (Weare and Reichert Jr., 1979). The β-subunit in dissociated state, has some intrinsic bioactivity, though 400-fold less than the associated native hormone (Ramakrishnan *et al.*, 1978a). Within the subunit, the peptide 39–71 is capable of stimulating dose-dependent steroidogenesis in the mouse Leydig cells (Figs. 5a, b). The C-terminal peptides consisting of the last 31, 35 and 45 amino acids did not manifest any activity in this system, suggesting thereby that the C-terminal, β-hCG unique strand, may not be involved in recognition of the receptors in the target tissue.

Immunodeterminants

A question of prime concern for immunological application is the region(s) of the β-hCG which are (a) immunodominant, (b) capable of eliciting hCG-specific antibodies, non cross-reacting with hLH. It has been possible in the past year to obtain sera against β-hCG with fairly high specificity for hCG and low cross-reactivity with hLH (Vaitukaitis *et al.*, 1972; Salahuddin *et al.*, 1976). Such sera have been used in RIA for measuring hCG in presence of hLH. The affinity of antibodies raised against β-hCG-conjugated to TT were 5 to 10-fold higher for binding with hCG than for hLH (Shastri *et al.*, 1978). The antibodies neutralized preferentially the bioactivity of hCG, sparing hLH and oLH activity *in vivo* and *in vitro* (Das *et al.*, 1978; Ramakrishnan *et al.*, 1978b). These observations demonstrate the presence in the β-hCG of conformations peculiar to hCG, besides of course those common to hLH. What are these determinants? At first thought, it would appear that the C-terminal region should *a priori* constitute the immunospecific part of β-hCG. Sera against the C-terminal peptides are no doubt devoid of reactivity with hLH. However, when immunization is carried out with β-hCG, there are seldom antibodies formed with properties of binding with the C-terminal β-hCG unique peptide. Neither SB_6 serum, nor about 33 other sera raised in monkeys and baboons against β-hCG in our laboratory reacted with labelled C-terminal peptide. Swaminathan and Braunstein (1978) have suggested that a major antigenic site of β-hCG resides in the region 21–31 with a disulphide bond connecting cysteine 23 or 26 with cysteine at position 72 or 110.

Anti-hCG vaccines

The human female is immunologically nonresponsive to hCG. Tolerance against hCG was abrogated by two different approaches: (1) by modification

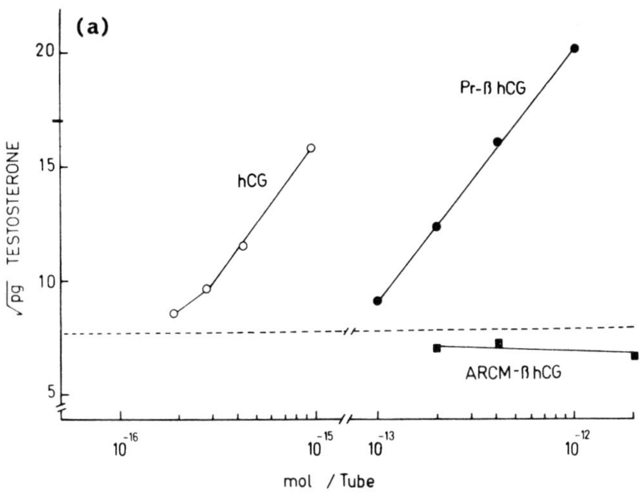

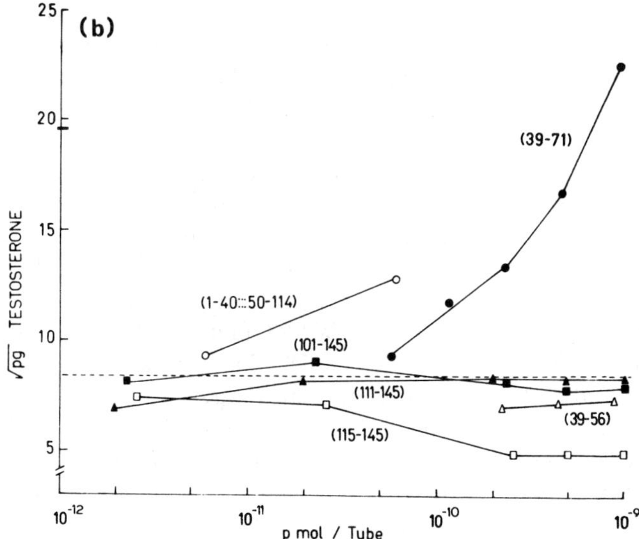

FIG. 5. *Recognition of determinants in β-hCG by tissue receptor: a dose dependent production of testosterone by the mouse Leydig cells was measured in presence of hCG, immunologically purified β-hCG (Pr-β-hCG) and various synthetic or enzymatically cleaved peptides. The subunit retained bioactivity though 400-fold lower than the native hormone in the system (a). The C-terminal 31, 35 and 45 amino acids long peptides as well as asialo reduced carboxymethyl β-hCG (ARCM-β-hCG) failed to stimulate steroidogenesis. One of the core peptides 39–71 gave a dose dependent steroidogenic response (b). (Data from Ramakrishnan* et al., *1978.)*

with haptenic groups, such as sulphanolic acid residues (Stevens and Crystle, 1973; Pala *et al.*, 1976) and DNP (Dubey *et al.*, 1976); (2) conjugation with an immunogenic carrier such as tetanus toxoid (TT) (Talwar *et al.*, 1975, 1976a, b). Conjugation with this carrier was accompanied by additional benefits of *adjuvanticity* and concurrent formation of *antibodies protective against tetanus*.

TABLE I

Properties of hCG vaccines based on CTP and β-hCG

	C-terminal peptide (CTP)	*β-hCG*
Immunogenicity	Low	High
Antibodies	Sequence reading	Conformations recognizing
Neutralization	Low	High
Valency	Monovalent	Polyvalent
Cross-reaction with hLH	None	Low

Vaccines based on C-terminal peptides (CTP) of β-hCG. Peptides conforming to the C-terminal sequence of β-hCG have been synthesized and investigated by 3 groups: at the NIH, the WHO Task Force and the AIIMS-ICCR-Population Council scientists. These were linked to either TT or other carriers. Immunization was carried out almost in every case with FCA, as without FCA the peptides were not immunogenic. The antibodies, as and when obtained, bound the homologous peptide, β-hCG and hCG. The binding to hCG was about 100-fold lower than to the C-terminal peptide. The slopes of competitive inhibition curve in RIA were either parallel (Stevens, 1976) or non-parallel (Ramakrishnan *et al.*, 1979). The binding site of the antibodies resided in the last 15 amino acids (131–145), and was primarily contributed by the dipeptide Pro-Gln (144–145) and the tetrapeptide Arg–Leu–Pro–Gly (133–136) (Matsuura *et al.*, 1978). The antibodies were devoid of cross-reaction with hLH. Antibodies against the last 23 amino acids did not neutralize the bioactivity of hCG (Louvet *et al.*, 1974). The neutralization potential tested *in vivo* was also absent in antibodies raised against the 30 amino acids CTP (Matsuura *et al.*, 1979). However, another group of investigators has reported that the antibodies against the 35 amino acid CTP raised in baboons, neutralized not only hCG but also the baboon chorionic gonadotropin (bCG) (Stevens, 1976). These conflicting observations need to be resolved, especially in view of the report by Chen and Hodgen (1976), on the absence of β-hCG analogous C-terminal regions in bCG.

We have studied four C-terminal synthetic peptides of β-hCG consisting of the last (a) 31, (b) 35, (c) 45 and (d) 53 amino acids. In each case these were conjugated to TT. The conjugates were by and large poor in their antigenicity as compared to β-hCG-TT. With the increase in size of the peptide, the immunogenicity improved and sera with reasonable titres were obtained with 45-CTP and 53-CTP. Both sera retained the characteristics of specificity with lack of cross-reactivity with hLH. They neutralized the bioactivity of hCG in mouse Leydig cell assay, but the neutralization capacity did not withstand dilution when compared to anti-β-hCG sera of similar titres (Ramakrishnan *et al.*, 1979). The possible reason for this trait is the monovalent character of the antibodies, in contrast to 2-3 antibody binding epitopes in sera against β-hCG (Fig. 6). The neutralization capacity was not very much improved

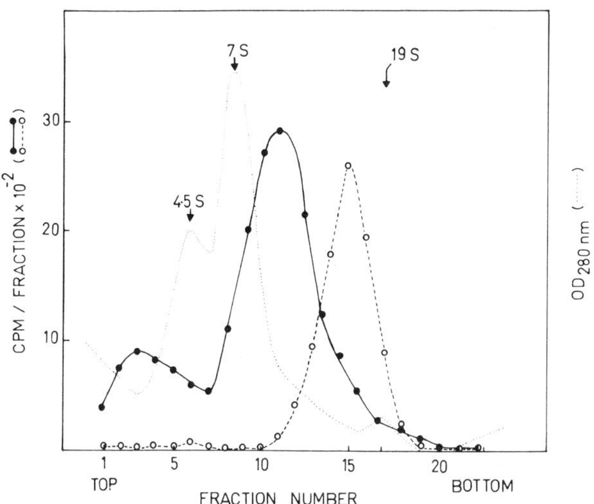

FIG. 6. *Antibodies against Pr-β-hCG-TT* (O ..... O) *and anti 45 CTP-TT* (●—●) *were incubated with* ^{125}*I-hCG and analysed on sucrose density gradients. The radioactivity profiles show the sedimentation behaviour of immune complexes formed by the two types of antisera with hCG (about 9S and 17S respectively). In case of anti-45 CTP, a portion of radioactivity was measured as free hCG, while the anti-β-hCG-TT antibodies bound all the added hCG (Ramakrishnan* et al., *1978).*

by lengthening of the peptide to 53-CTP. To sum up, the C-terminal peptides are primarily of interest for generation of highly specific antibodies utilizable for various types of assays. Their poor immunogenicity, coupled with low neutralization capacity, render them as unlikely candidates for anti-hCG vaccines destined for fertility control. Table I summarizes the merits and limitations of different types of anti-hCG vaccines.

Vaccines utilizing chemically modified β-hCG. Although a number of derivatives like nitro, ethylglycyl, O-acetyl, carboxymethyl have been prepared, the most interesting ones from an immunological point of view are the reduced alkylated derivatives of β-hCG. By controlled treatment, the disulphide bonds can be broken partially or fully (Giudice and Pierce, 1978). The reduced carboxymethyl derivatives of β-hCG (RCM-βhCG) as such do not bind substantially to anti-hCG antibodies. They do, however, generate sera with binding properties similar to 45-CTP (unpublished data) and are thus highly specific. Their utility for practical purposes may be similar to those of CTP.

Vaccines based on β-hCG. Active immunization with β-hCG renders marmosets infertile (Hearn, 1979). The block is exercised throughout the period of detectable antibody titres; thereafter a period follows when the animals conceive but abort, the prevailing antibody titres at this stage being very low. This phase is followed by normality of conception and regain of fertility. High titres are often, but not always, accompanied by prevention of fertility (Stevens, 1976; Talwar *et al.*, 1980a, b), perhaps because bCG has a variable low cross-reaction with anti-hCG antibodies. The most convincing evidence for the effectiveness of the anti-β-hCG-TTantibodies is provided by the termination of pregnancy consequent upon their administration to a pregnant baboon (Fig. 7). The effect was not due to nonspecific proteinic load, as instillation of an equivalent amount of immunoglobulins from nonimmunized animals did not bring about the termination of pregnancy.

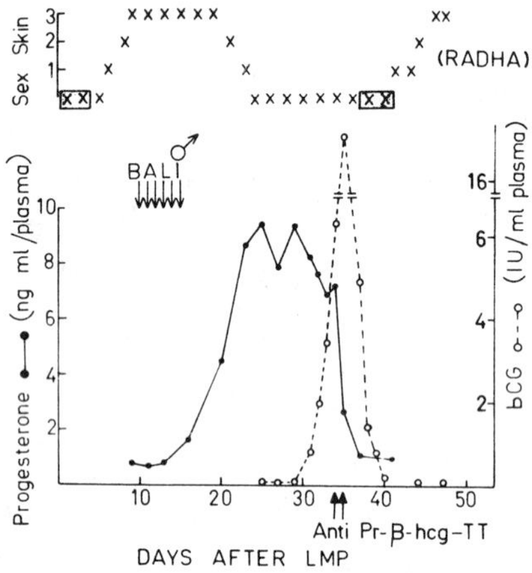

FIG. 7. *Termination of pregnancy in a baboon by anti-Pr-β-hCG-TT antibodies. Two injections were given when baboon chorionic gonadotropin was measurable in plasma. The administration of antibodies resulted in sharp decline of bCG, progesterone and loss of pregnancy* (*Talwar* et al., *1980a*).

Immunization of monkeys and baboons with the vaccine Pr-β-hCG-TT does not lead to any apparent side-effects. The animals keep ovulating. The hormonal profiles are normal, endocrine, metabolic and organ functions are not disturbed (Sharma *et al.*, 1976). The autopsy of immunized animals challenged repeatedly with hCG did not show any gross or morphological abnormality (Nath *et al.*, 1976a; Gupta *et al.*, 1978). There was no evidence for the deposition of immune complexes in kidney and chorioid plexus, nor was any pathology seen in pituitary, adrenal, thyroid and other organs.

Phase I clinical trials with this vaccine were initially carried out in New

Delhi in 4 women of reproductive age who had completed their families (Talwar *et al.*, 1976a, b; Hingorani and Kumar, 1979). These were extended and conducted subsequently in 5 more centres in Bombay, Helsinki, Uppsala, Santiago, Bahia under eminent clinical scientists. In all, 63 women were immunized. To most of them, a regimen consisting of 4 fortnightly injections of Pr-β-hCG-TT (80–100 μg β-hCG coupled to 10 LF of TT) in alum, was given (Fig. 8). In some women, a monthly schedule of 3 injections of 160 μg βhCG was applied.

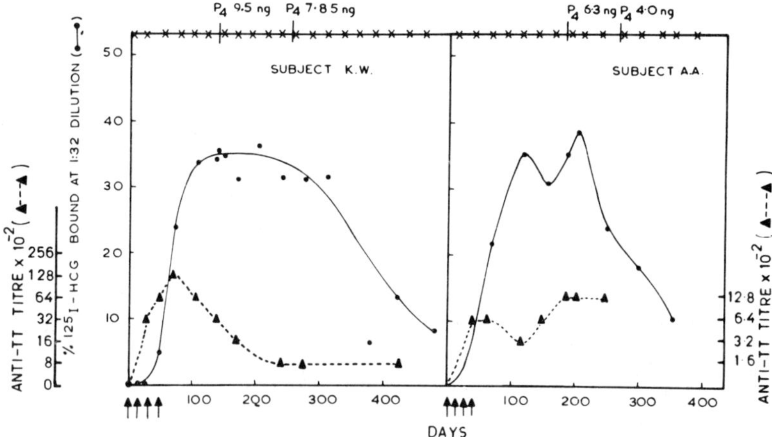

FIG. 8. *Antibody response to hCG (●——●) and tetanus toxoid (▲------▲) in two women given 4 fortnightly injections of Pr-β-hCG-TT. The subject KW was immunized in New Delhi and AA at Uppsalaa. The crosses on the upper abscissa denote the menstruation which remained undisturbed. Plasma progesterone* (P_4) *values in the leuteal phase were indicative of normal ovulation. The antibodies in both cases declined to near zero levels after 400 days.*

Sixty-one out of 63 women responded with the formation of anti-hCG and antitetanus antibodies. The antibody titres among the responders were variable, about 13% of women made antibodies above 20 ng/ml, some having as high as 70–100 ng/ml hCG binding capacity. Others (about 15%) were moderate responders (10–20 ng/ml). The rest produced antibody titres below 10 ng binding/ml serum. The duration of antibody response was variable. In women with adequate titres, the antibody response lasted between 300 and 500 days (Talwar *et al.*, 1976a, b). In all cases, the titres declined to subdetectable levels in course of time indicating the complete reversibility of the immune response. All women ovulated normally as gauged by the plasma progesterone level during luteal phase, as well as by information from endometrial biopsies in some cases. Libido was intact in all cases. The menstrual regularity and bleeding remained unchanged. Haematological and biochemical constituents in blood remained within the normal limits in all cases. Endocrine (thyroid, adrenal, ovarian, pancreatic, hypothalamic, hypophysial) and organ (kidney, liver) functions remained undisturbed. No DNA reacting, rheumatoid factor and other tissue reacting antibodies were detectable in circulation (Nath *et al.*, 1976b), nor were any undue hypersensitivity reactions reported. Phase I clinical pharmacology studies carried out with the same vaccine in different centres have given evidence of safety and lack of toxicity of Pr-β-hCG-TT (Hingorani and Kumar, 1979; Shahani *et al.*, 1979; Nash *et al.*, 1980).

Is the anti-hCG approach feasible for control of fertility?
Two modalities can be employed, e.g. active immunization with vaccines such as Pr-β-hCG-TT and passive intervention with preformed anti-hCG antibodies. The active immunization approach when successful in eliciting adequate antibody response produces a state of surveillence lasting over the duration of the antibody response, e.g. about a year, thus conferring protection for a reasonably long duration. Active immunization is practicable on a mass scale. The major limitation of this approach at the moment is the large variability of immune response and susceptibility to pregnancy of those with inadequate antibody titres. Although variability is not unique to this vaccine, but is also a feature of other vaccines used against communicable diseases, the saving factor in the latter is the statistical improbability of everyone in a community receiving high infection, whereas every woman opting for antifertility vaccine would be of proven fertility. It is thus imperative that ways and means are found for (a) enhancing the general threshold of the antibody response with such vaccines, and (b) counteracting variability of individual immune response, before these vaccines can be practically employed. For the former, nontoxic immunopotentiating agents will be required, and for the latter, development of novel strategies for immunization, exploiting the available knowledge on regulation of the immune apparatus. Active research is in progress to develop adjuvants. Amongst those holding promise are (a) MDP (Audibert *et al.*, 1976) and (b) derivatives of lipopolysaccharides. Liposomes, BCG and perhaps other agents may also find utility in this context. Problems related to toxicity of these adjuvants have not been fully resolved and a number of chemical derivatives of these compounds are being prepared to achieve the desired end.

Another question that may arise at this stage is the possible long-term impact of anti-hCG immunization on normal and cancerous tissues making hCG. The effect of anti-hCG antibodies on a choriocarcinoma making hCG has been studied *in vitro* and *in vivo*. Anti-hCG antibodies in the presence of complement are cytotoxic to normal and malignant trophoblast cells cultured *in vitro* (Currie, 1967; Morisada *et al.*, 1976; Talwar *et al.*, 1978). High titres of anti-hCG antibodies, however, fail to suppress the *in vivo* growth of the BeWo choriocarcinoma cells in hamster cheek pouch (Knecht, 1980).

While research must continue to develop satisfactory anti-hCG vaccines with enhanced immunogenicity and devoid of contraindications, passive use of anti-hCG antibodies may find useful application as self-administered mode of menstrual regulation. With the development of hybridoma technology, it seems possible to obtain monoclonal antibodies of high titres. Passive, in contrast to active immunization, does not confer long-lasting immunity but has the advantage over the latter of providing, in an insured way, the requisite amount of antibodies to interrupt pregnancy. Due to the limited period over which the passively administered antibodies circulate, the safety requirements will be less stringent.

Summary and conclusions

Reproductive system is dependent on the interplay of a number of hormones. Antibodies neutralizing one or more of these hormones can interfere in the reproductive processes. Immunointervention of the hypothalamic–hypophysial–gonadal hormones, though effective, will be accompanied in most cases by undesirable side effects, e.g. lack of sex steroid hormones. These, therefore, will not be the approaches of choice for control of human fertility except in special circumstances such as menopause and cancers. Immunological approaches against some of these hormones may, however, find useful applications in farm animals and domestic pets. Recent reports on the arrest of gametogenesis in the primates by β-FSH immunization demands further study on the possible potentiality of this intervention not only in the male, but also in the female. Active immunization against normal reproductive hormones made and secreted continuously by the endocrines may entail the problem of immune complexes and endocrinopathies, which would require careful safety studies. It is due to this reason that immunization against hormones made only in special situations such as pregnancy would be preferable.

hCG is predominantly a hormone of pregnancy and is produced by the implanting blastocyst. Neutralization of hCG by anti-hCG antibodies brings about the termination of pregnancy. The possibility of producing large quantities of high titre antibodies through hybridomas has opened out a potential application of anti-hCG antibodies for menstrual regulation, e.g. a self-administered method for termination of pregnancy.

A number of anti-hCG vaccines are under development. The merits and limitations of these vaccines have been discussed and summarized above. Some advances have been made in delineation of the immunodominant parts of β-hCG, the portion of the molecule recognized by the tissue receptors and the cardinal role of the disulphide bonds. Maximal progress has been achieved on the β-hCG based vaccines whose efficacy and reversibility has been tested in more than one subhuman primate species. Pr-β-hCG-TT has undergone early phase I clinical trials in 5 countries. The vaccine was competent to produce in almost all women anti-hCG and antitetanus antibodies, without disturbance of ovulation, hormonal profiles, libido and menstrual regularity. Extensive investigations have shown the safety and lack of side-effects of the procedure. The major shortcoming of this vaccine was the large variability in immune response from individual to individual. Those with low titres were prone to pregnancy. The large-scale practical application of this (and other antifertility vaccines) is thus dependent on the development of potent, non-toxic adjuvants, as well as new immunization strategies overriding the individual variability of immune response.

Besides fertility control, 3 other major applications of antibodies against hormones have been in (a) development of highly sensitive methods for assay of hormones (RIA, EIA); (b) immuno-diagnostic kits; and (c) the elucidation of the biological role and subcellular location of the hormone by use of the hormone specific antibodies.

References

Audibert, F., Chedid, L., Lefrancier, P. and Choay, J. (1976). *Cell. Immunol.* **21**, 243.

Bauminger, S., Kohen, F. and Lindner, H. R. (1974). *J. Steroid Biochem.* **5**, 739.

Borland, R., Loke, Y. W. and Wilson, D. (1975). *In* "Immunology of Trophoblast" (R. G. Edwards, C. W. S. Howe, M. H. Johnson, eds) pp. 157–164. Cambridge University Press, Cambridge.

Braunstein, G. D., Rasor, J., Adler, D., Danzer, H. and Wade, M. E. (1976). *Am. J. Obstet. Gyn.* **12**, 676.

Braunstein, G. D., Kamdar, V., Rasor, J., Swaminathan, N. and Wade, M. E. (1979). *J. Clinical Endocr. Meta.* **49**, 917.

Catt, K. J., Dufau, M. L. and Vaitukaitis, J. L. (1975). *J. Clin. Endocr. Metab.* **40**, 537.

Chen, H. C., Hodgen, G. D., Matsuura, L. J., Birken, S., Canfield, R. E. and Ross, G. T. (1976). *Proc. Natn. Acad. Sci. U.S.A.* **73**, 2285.

Chen, H. C. and Hodgen, G. D. (1976). *Proc. Natn. Acad. Sci. U.S.A.* **73**, 2885.

Crosignani, P. G., Trojsi, L., Attanasio, A. E. M. and Lambroso, F. (1974). *Obstet. Gyn.* **44**, 673.

Currie, G. A. (1967). *J. Obstet. Gyn.* **74**, 845.

Das, C., Talwar, G. P., Ramakrishnan, S., Salahuddin, M., Kumar, S., Hingorani, V., Coutinho, E., Croxatto, H., Hemmingson, E., Johansson, E., Luukkainen, T., Shahani, S., Sundaram, K., Nash, H. and Segal, S. J. (1978). *Contraception* **18**, 35.

Dubey, S. K., Salahuddin, M., Shastri, N. and Talwar, G. P. (1976). *Contraception* **13**, 141.

E. Tomi, A. E. F., Boots, L. and Stevens, V. C. (1970). *Endocrinology* **87**, 1181.

El Tõmi, A. E. F., Crystle, C. D. and Stevens, V. C. (1971). *Am. J. Obstet. Gyn.* **109**, 74.

Ferin, M., Dyrenfurth, I., Schwartz, U. and Vande Wiele, R. L. (1975). *In* "Immunization with Hormones in Reproduction Research" (E. Nieschlag, ed.) pp. 119–137. North-Holland, Amsterdam.

Fraser, H. M., Clarke, I. J. and McNeilly, A. S. (1977). *J. Endocrinol.* **75**, 45.

Giudice, L. C. and Pierce, J. G. (1978). *Biochim. Biophys. Acta* **533**, 140.

Gupta, P. D., Nath, I. and Talwar, G. P. (1978). *Contraception* **18**, 91.

Hearn J. P. (1979). *In* "Recent Advances in Reproduction and Regulation of Fertility" (G. P. Talwar, ed.) pp. 427–438. Elsevier/North-Holland Biomedical Press, Amsterdam.

Hingorani, V. and Kumar, S. (1979). *In* "Recent Advances in Reproduction and Regulation of Fertility" (G. P. Talwar, ed.) pp. 467–472. Elsevier/North-Holland Biomedical Press, Amsterdam and New York.

Hodges, J. K. and Hearn, J. P. (1977). *Nature* **265**, 746.

Klopper, A. and Fuchs, F. (1977). *In* "Endocrinology of Pregnancy" (F. Fuchs and A. Klopper, eds) pp. 99–122. Harper & Row, Hagerstown, Maryland, U.S.A.

Knecht, M. (1980). *Endocrinology* **106**, 150.

Kunz, J. (1976). *Brit. J. Obstet. Gyn.* **83**, 640.

Labrie, F., Auclair, C., Cusan, L., Lemay, A., Kelly, P. A., Belanger, A., Pelletier, G., Seguin, C., Ferland, F. and Raynaud, J. P. (1979). *In* "Recent Advances in Reproduction and Regulation of Fertility" (G. P. Talwar, ed.) pp. 57–72. Elsevier/North-Holland Biomedical Press, Amsterdam, New York.

Louvet, J. P., Ross, G. T., Birken, S. and Canfield, R. E. (1974). *J. Clin. Endocr. Metab.* **39**, 1155.

Matsuura, S., Chen, H. C. and Hodgen, G. D. (1978). *Biochemistry* **17**, 575.

Matsuura, S., Ohashi, M., Chen, H. C. and Hodgen, G. D. (1979). *Endocrinology* **104**, 396.

Morgan, F. J., Birken, S. and Canfield, R. E. (1975). *J. Biol. Chem.* **250**, 5247.

Morisada, M., Yamaguchi, H. and Iizuka, R. (1976). *Am. J. Obstet. Gyn.* **125**, 3.

Moss, R. L. and Dudley, C. A. (1980). *In* "Proceeding VI International Congress of Endocrinology", Australian Academy of Science (in press).

Moudgil, N. R. (1975). *In* "Immunization with Hormones in Reproduction Research" (E. Nieschlag, ed.) pp. 83–93. North-Holland, Amsterdam.

Murty, G. S. R. C., Sheela Rani, C. S. and Moudgil, N. R. (1980). *In* "Proceedings VI International Congress of Endocrinology" Australian Academy of Science (in press).

Nash, H., Talwar, G. P., Segal, S., Luukkainen, T., Johansson, E. D. B., Vasquez, J., Coutinho, E. and Sundaram, K. (1980). *Fertility and Sterility* (in press).

Nath, I., Gupta, P. D., Bhuyan, U. N. and Talwar, G. P. (1976a). *Contraception* **13**, 213.

Nath, I., Whittingham, S., Lambert, P. H. and Talwar, G. P. (1976b). *Contraception* **13**, 225.

Nieschlag, E., Usadel, K. H., Wickings, E. J., Kley, H. K. and Wuttke, W. (1975). *In* "Immunization with Hormones in Reproduction Research" (E. Nieschlag, ed.) pp. 155–170. North-Holland, Amsterdam.

Pala, A., Ermini, M., Caranza, L. and Benagiano, G. (1976). *Contraception* **14**, 579.

Pierce, J. G., Faith, M. R., Giudice, L. C. and Reeve, J. R. (1976). *In* "Polypeptide Hormones: Molecular and Cellular Aspects" pp. 225–242. Ciba Foundation Symposium **41**.

Ramakrishnan, S., Das, C. and Talwar, G. P. (1978a). *Biochem. J.* **176**, 599.

Ramakrishnan, S., Das, C. and Talwar, G. P. (1978b). *Contraception* **18**, 51.

Ramakrishnan, S., Das, C., Dubey, S. K., Salahuddin, M. and Talwar, G. P. (1979). *J. Reprod. Immunol.* **1**, 249.

Robertson, I. S., Wilson, J. C. and Fraser, H. M. (1979). *Vet. Rec.* **105**, 556.

Sairam, M. P. and Madhwa Raj, H. G. (1980). *In* "Non-Human Primate Models for Study of Human Reproduction" (T. C. Anand Kumar, ed.) S. Karger, Basel.

Salahuddin, M., Ramakrishnan, S., Dubey, S. K. and Talwar, G. P. (1976). *Contraception* **13**, 163.

Saxena, B. B., Hasan, S. H., Haour, F. and Gollwitzers, S. M. (1974). *Science* **184**, 793.

Scaramuzzi, R. J., Baird, D. T., Clarke, I. J., Martensz, N. D. and Van Look, P. F. A. (1980). *J. Reprod. Fert.* **58**, 27.

Shahani, S. M., Kulkarni, P. P. and Patel, K. L. (1979). *In* "Recent Advances in Reproduction and Regulation of Fertility" (G. P. Talwar, ed.) pp. 473–476. Elsevier/North-Holland Biomedical Press, Amsterdam.

Sharma, N. C., Goel, B. K., Bajaj, J. S. and Talwar, G. P. (1976). *Contraception* **13**, 201.

Shastri, N., Dubey, S. K., Vijaya Raghavan, S., Salahuddin, M. and Talwar, G. P. (1978). *Contraception* **18**, 23.

Stevens, V. C. (1976). *In* "Development of Vaccines for Fertility Regulation", WHO Symposium, Varna 1975, pp. 93–110. Scriptor, Copenhagen.

Stevens, V. C. and Crystle, C. D. (1973). *Obstet. Gyn.* **42**, 485.

Sundaram, K., Chang, C. C., Laurence, K. A., Brinson, A. O., Atkinson, L. E. and Segal, S. J. (1976). *Contraception* **14**, 639.

Swaminathan, N. and Braunstein, G. D. (1978). *Biochemistry* **17**, 5832.

Talwar, G. P. (1979). *J. Steroid Biochem.* **11**, 27.

Talwar, G. P., Sharma, N. C., Dubey, S. K., Das, C., Ramakrishnan, S., Kumar, S. and Hingorani, V. and Bloom, B. (1975). *In* "VIII World Congress of Fertility and Sterility", Buenos Aires, Excerpta Medica Series No. 394, pp. 224–232.

Talwar, G. P., Sharma, N. C., Dubey, S. K., Salahuddin, M., Das, C., Ramakrishnan, S., Kumar, S. and Hingorani, V. (1976a). *Proc. Natn. Acad. Sci. U.S.A.* **73**, 218.

Talwar, G. P., Dubey, S. K., Salahuddin, M. and Shastri, N. (1976b). *Contraception* **13**, 153.

Talwar, G. P., Ramakrishnan, S., Das, C., Gupta, S. K., Salahuddin, M., Viswanathan, M. K., Gupta, P. D., Pal, P., Buckshee, K. and Frick, J. (1978). *In* "Proceedings 6th Asia and Oceania Congress of Endocrinology", Singapore, Vol. 2, pp. 472–476.

Talwar, G. P., Das, C., Tandon, A., Sharma, M. G., Salahuddin, M. and Dubey, S. K. (1980a). *In* "Non-Human Primate Models for Study of Human Reproduction" (T. C. Anand Kumar, ed.) pp. 190–201. S. Karger, Basel.

Talwar, G. P., Ramakrishnan, S., Das, C., Tandon, A., Gupta, S. K., Shastri, N., Singh, O., Kumar, S., Hingorani, V., Shahani, S., Luukkainen, T., Johansson, E., Croxatto, H., Coutinho, E., Frick, J., Nash, H. and Segal, S. J. (1980b). *In* "Proceedings VI International Congress of Endocrinology", Australian Academy of Science (in press).

Thau, R. B., Sundaram, K., Thornton, Y. S. and Seidman, L. S. (1979). *Fert. Steril.* **31**, 200.

Vaitukaitis, J. L., Braunstein, G. D. and Ross, G. T. (1972). *Am. J. Obstet. Gyn.* **113**, 751.

Weare, J. A. and Reichert, L. F. (1979). *J. Biol. Chem.* **254**, 6972.

Yoshimoto, Y., Nolfsen, A. A. and Odell, N. D. (1977). *Science* **197**, 575.

Theme 16: Summary

Immunology of Reproduction and Embryonic Development

ALAN E. BEER

University of Michigan, Ann Arbor, USA

The immunology of reproduction and embryonic development is a very new field. Only 16 years have elapsed since the first critical, comprehensive review by Professor Billingham of the various explanations advanced to account for the remarkable immune system exemption of germ cells mammalian foetoplacental units from rejection by their mothers as allografts.

Until a few years ago, as eloquently stated by Professor Billingham, "the successful survival of the allogeneic foetus to term remains like a rock in a fomenting sea of immunological endeavour, still provocatively unbroken after 50 years' assault by waves of experimentation and armchair speculation". The question was put: "is it not absurd to ask whether the various immuno-regulatory processes demonstrable following mating and during pregnancy, most of them on the basis of *in vitro* models, are not just irrelevant consequences of or events associated with one simple central mechanism, the immunologically privileged status of the trophoblast—no more essential for the protection of the foetus than is natural prophylactic immunization for animals raised and maintained in gnotobiotic environments". Since this time we have learned a great deal more regarding the success of the foeto-placental allograft due to major progress in immunology, immunogenetics, embryology and endocrinology. During this meeting we have learned of many new techniques that have been developed and applied, especially *in vitro* assays for immunosuppressive agents, immunosuppressed, immunostimulated and immunosuppressive lymphocytes, the activities of maternal and foetal proteins, and hormones on immune responses and alloantigens on cell surfaces. In addition, our horizons have been broadened in that immunological interchange between the mother and her offspring does not stop with parturition in that the mammary gland, descriptively, the "puerperal placenta" initiates an immunological and nutritional bond of a nature quite different than that associated with the placenta.

The immune system is the most complex product of evolution. The major aim of immunologic research has been to dissect the complex cellular network involved in responses of the system and to elucidate the fine-grained structures of the cell surfaces involved as well as the molecular products of these cells. It is obvious that reproductive biology has intruded firmly into the science of immunology. Certainly a complete understanding of the immunology of reproduction and embryonic development remains one of our greatest challenges today. Based on new and exciting information exchanged during this meeting it is not absurd to ask the following questions.

(a) Is the complexity and manipulability of our immunological response machinery, orchestrated in part by genes associated with the major histocompatibility complex, necessary to allow the safe production, storage and passage of germ cells and preserve maternal-foetal immunological co-existence and the survival of the species?

(b) With the immunological information now in hand, can we look forward to a safe and efficient immunological method, not only of fertility regulation but also of fertility restoration?

Auto- and isoimmunizations against gamete and genital tract antigens

Our knowledge of immune responses is based upon studies utilizing experimental immunization with foreign antigens presented with complex adjuvants or coupled with haptens or carriers.

Recently we have become aware of immune responses on the part of both the female and the male to antigens of ova and its investments and to semen. During this congress many well planned and executed studies have been presented that shed light on both the immunologic hazards of viviparous reproduction as well as the physical and molecular components of semen as oocytes that in most circumstances avert purposeless immunological responses in a quest to preserve the continued viability of the species and assist in the immunoprotection of germ cells and embryo during all stages of the reproductive process. From the turn of the century with the inception of modern immunological thinking, investigators focused on the potential biological effects of immunological responses to spermatozoa. Although the testes, accessory organs and their products are uniquely designed to ensure isolation from the attentions of the immune system, nonetheless they can become immunologic targets. Modern medicine with the introduction of new procedures in quest of fertility control has aided in our understanding of the above. The defining of the immunopathologic effects of vasectomy is a recent example. During this Congress we have learned the following:

The "Sperm Wars" continue. There is still much "immunological noise' in our assays and not all investigators agree as to the nature of the antigens involved nor to the type or effects of the antibodies elicited. Nonetheless progress is being made. d'Almeida (16.1.05)* in fractionating extracts from human spermatozoa has shown the antigen eliciting antibodies for head-to-head agglutination is different from that responsible for tail-to-tail agglutination and different from those inciting cytotoxic antibody formation.

Shigeta (16.1.20) using hybridoma monoclonal antibody was able to isolate a single pure antigen relevant to sperm immobilizing antibody.

Hjort (16.1.08) in a series of sophisticated experiments with $F(ab')_2$ antibodies identified 2 discrete antigens of spermatozoa involved in immobilization. His studies confirmed the immunologic noise in our present systems in that the pattern of agglutination seen was in no way indicative of the antigen(s) involved.

Mathur (16.1.14) showed that antisperm antibodies cross-reacted with T lymphocytes and occasionally led to decreased numbers of circulating T cells. These findings alert us to the possibility of future autoimmune complications in patients and should prompt investigations to look for sperm cytotoxicity in individuals with antilymphocyte antibodies.

Hurtenbach and Shearer (16.1.09) showed that alloantigen or mitogen activated lymphocyte proliferation was strongly suppressed by autologous germ cells. Operationally the generation of suppressor cells were involved in that the suppression could be abrogated by Ly-2·2 serum and complement. The natural immunoprotective consequences of this process on germ cells is obvious and exciting. We now must ask what determinants, products or molecules of germ cell origin stimulate suppressor T cell production.

Jager *et al.* (16.1.10) utilizing antisperm $F(ab')_2$ and Fab fragments of the IgG

* Reference numbers indicate Abstract numbers in: Abstracts 4th International Congress of Immunology, Paris.

molecule showed that sperm immobilization was achieved only when the Fc portion of the immunoglobulin could interact with molecules of cervical mucous. The identification of Fc "receptors" associated with cervical mucus has not been done.

With the natural barriers and suppressive factors tuned to preventing immune reactivity to germ cells the question was raised as to why does it ever occur? d'Almeida has shown no association with a specific HLA phenotype. One must question however; are females inseminated by males who share HLA antigenic determinants or immune response genes more prone to react to tissue or organ specific antigens of spermatozoa? Does HLA incompatability protect against antisperm immunization much in the same manner that ABO erythrocyte incompatibility protects women from seeing the Rh (D) antigen on erythrocytes? Preliminary findings by Marcus (16.1.13) and Beer (work in progress) suggest that studies addressing this question may yield new and useful data. Areas most in need of future research efforts are:

(a) Purification and characterization of the obviously multiple aspermatogenic antigens.

(b) Careful scrutiny of the MHC and its role in allowing immunoreactivity to reproductive organs and their products. This should include studies addressing the possibility that immunoreactivity to semen may be more or less common when sexual partners share MHC antigens or immune response genes clustered there.

(c) We are in need of sensitive radioimmunoassays for assessing immune factors to antigens associated with the reproductive tract and its products.

(d) Critical experiments are needed to study molecules or products of the reproductive organs prone to elicit suppression responses.

(e) Unlike the gut and the bronchus the mucosal surfaces of the reproductive tract of the female have eluded critical immunological studies. An understanding of the immune responses native there is needed. Experiments designed to capture the cells in the uterine lamina propria or lumen to assess their *in vitro* reactivity will certainly advance our understanding of responses resident there.

(f) Cell hybridization experiments and the production of monoclonal antibodies to spermatozoal and ovum antigens will continue to rapidly assist us in clearing the "immunological noise" from our systems.

Placental antigens and hormones

The chorionic epithelium; the dialysis membrane between the mother and the foetus has truly become an "immunological treadmill". This Congress has presented us with an explosion of data allowing us to understand more fully the unique antigenic nature of this lipid bilayer that qualifies an immunological privileged tissue.

The papers presented fell into 2 categories:

(a) those describing or identifying antigens;

(b) those studying functional aspects of antigen expression.

The studies of Yane *et al.* (16.2.15) on retrovirus expression on trophoblast provided the exciting finding that antibodies eluted from placentas of pre-eclamptic patients were cytotoxic for virus infected cells, while those from normal pregnant patients were not and blocked the action and antibodies from patients with toxaemia.

Several trophoblastic molecules were described as placental-specific antigens including:

(a) A phase specific antigen found only on early human placenta (Botev, 16.2.01).

(b) An antigen isolated from human syncytiotrophoblast microvillus membrane preparations and absent or normal tissues assayed.

(c) An antigen unique to ectoplacental cone tissue of mice not found on other tissues and having species specificity (Searle, 16.2.10). A similar type antigen was described on human placentae that disappears with transformation.

Placental hormonal antigens HCG and HPL were localized to the syncytiotrophoblast while that placental lactogen appeared to be produced by the giant cells. Finally the pregnancy associated glycoprotein was found localized in both trophoblast and amnion cells.

There was general agreement on a number of markers on trophoblast including the presence of Fc receptors, transferrin, IgG,α_2 macroglobulin and alkaline phosphatase. β_2 microglobulin appears to be absent.

Difficulties in defining many of these antigens as trophoblast specific were summarized by Galbraith. A primary problem of weak immunogenicity renders antibody production difficult. In addition Thomson cautioned that although heterologous antisera can be raised in rabbits it does not mean females of the species will react during normal gestation.

MHC-coded antigens on trophoblast was reported by Lala (16.2.03) using a radio autographic technique to collagenase-derived cell suspensions. Ia antigens were not found. The question of cell purity, cell identity on trophoblast was raised. All agreed that the placenta is a complex mixture of regions and cell types and precise identity of trophoblast versus foetal mesenchyme versus decidual cells is difficult.

The presence or absence of MHC antigen on trophoblast remains a heated issue. Nature simply and reasonably could have made her immunologic work easy by omitting them, however it appears that she chose an alternative course, placed them there and engineered scholarly processes to modulate and mask them.

The fine grained molecular architecture of the trophoblast is further complicated by its ability to produce and incorporate into its plasma membrane a variety of steroid and protein hormones. Heterologous antisera to intact HCG is not cytotoxic to cultured trophoblast but causes the release of chromium from HCG secreting Bewo cells (Paul and Talwar, 16.2.09). It is postulated that the trophoblastic epithelium is indeed a treadmill releasing or shedding antigen (HCG) or antigen–antibody complexes too rapidly for cytotoxic reactions to occur. Lang (16.2.06) reported poor immunogenicity of the C-terminal portion of the beta subunit of HCG. This molecule as an immunogen appears committed to inducing a suppressor T cell response that blocks helper cells from participating in the expression of the immune response.

Nebel (16.2.07) showed that HCG could block the efforts of cytotoxic sensitized lymphocytes highlighting further the immunomodulatory activities of HCG.

It is obvious that we have nearly exhausted our *in vitro* tricks to force the trophoblast to reveal itself antigenically. Perhaps techniques of perfusion and organ culture described for the renal nephron adapted for the placenta villus blocked of certain of its well defined *in vivo* functions will assist us in understanding the potential vulnerability of its plasma membrane when confronted with immunological effectors. Work of this nature is being conducted by Gagnon and Beer.

Differentiation antigens in embryonic development

Differentiation involves the proliferation of cells and the emergence of cells different from either parent. These organize into different cell types and into discrete functional units. Cell surface displays of molecules allow differentiating cells to interact among themselves and with their environments. Workshop evidence was presented here that HY antigens can be detected on embryonic cells and that the molecules identified with monoclonal antibodies are involved in sexual differentiation. Studies by Danon *et al.* (16.3.04) on a neural cell surface antigen shed light that embryonic antigen identification may show tumour cell types prone to metastasize and predict the malignant potential of the cell.

Although the use of monoclonal antibodies to study differentiation antigens has yielded much information the fact that differentiation antigens are stage-specific and often of limited life span makes it difficult not only to produce the proper antibody but also to select the proper one for the questions being asked. In summary the study of differentiation antigens will prove of particular interest in elucidating the relationship between differentiation and the process of malignant transformation.

Definition of these "neogens" has alerted workers in maternal/foetal immunology that their view of syngeneic pregnancies based on the MHC coded antigens is simplistic and incomplete for in these pregnancies immuno confrontation of the mother is afforded by a multitude of "neogens".

Immunological approaches to fertility regulation

Immunological approaches to fertility regulation is not a new concept since similar approaches have been employed effectively in the prevention and control of viral and bacterial diseases on a mass scale. Specific antigenic components studied as targets are associated with spermatozoa, ova and components of the placenta.

New information in four areas has surfaced:

(a) definition of autoantigens of the zona pellucida and autoantibodies produced to these;

(b) affinity and effectiveness of antibodies to HCG;

(c) *In vivo* effects of antibodies to prolacti(PRL) in females; and

(d) immunosuppressive molecules from human seminal plasma.

Das (16.6.02) and Mori (16.6.09) reported the isolation and partial characterization of porcine and human zona pellucida extracts. Heteroantibodies to both extracts showed tissue specificity with immunofluorescence testing. These antibodies were capable of blocking human fertilization *in vitro*. Contrary to earlier evidence it now appears that primate and ungulate zonae exhibit partial species specificity and there may be allo-specificity in the pig.

Confusion persists regarding the incidence and significance of naturally occurring antizona antibodies in infertile women, when compared with appropriate control patients.

Extensive absorption of test sera with both human and porcine erythrocytes reduces but does not eliminate positive reactions in fertile women and men. The immunological significance of these reactions as tested by immunofluorescence or immunoprecipitation on porcine zonae remains uncertain. The present status of HCG as a trophoblastic target antigen was discussed.

Thanavala (16.6.12) characterized antibodies developed in baboons immunized with the C-terminal Peptide (C-TP) of βhCG. Antibody concentration and affinity correlated with the antifertility effects in immunized animals. Tissue localization of baboon antihuman C-TP antibodies using IF showed a strong reaction with human syncytiotrophoblast and a weaker reaction with baboon trophoblast conferring partial immunologic identity. No cross-reactivity with baboon or human pituitary was seen. No cross-reactivity with HLH was shown by radiobinding assays.

Natural immune regulatory mechanisms in reproduction are relevant to immunological fertility control. Marcus (16.6.08) presented data of a high mol. wt glycoprotein fraction of human seminal plasma with *in vitro* suppressive effects on T cell function. Studies to date show no clear correlation of this immunosuppressive activity of seminal plasma with either fertility status or naturally occurring immunity to sperm in females or males.

In the quest for immunological control of fertility regulation we are faced with the toughest battery of antigens placed on cell surfaces. When asked if he thought fertility control could ever be achieved by immune mechanisms Professor Billingham commented "You all have faith in what you are doing and faith has moved mountains". We have a long way to go before a suitable antifertility vaccine becomes a reality. The effectiveness of an antigen(s) and the attendant immune responses to it to prevent pregnancy has not as yet been demonstrated in humans. I predict that when we understand the immunological contributions to the immunologically privileged status of the trophoblast in full we will surely create a vaccine that is ultimately safe and sure.

Immune reactivity of the mother towards the conceptus

Having discussed trophoblast behaviour as an immunologically privileged tissue, we must ask the following questions:

(1) *Is the conceptus immunogenic?*

(a) as early as the first cleavage stages murine embryos express non H-2 alloantigens.
(b) H-2 alloantigens are expressed on mouse blastocysts.
(c) loss of antigen or case of antigen detection occurs as implantation approaches.
(d) HLA antigens are not detected in human placentae by immunofluorescence.
(e) H-2 antigens are detected on 12–15 day murine placentae.
(f) H-2 antigens can be detected on 14–16 day murine trophoblast using a 3-step radioautographic technique.

Other evidence suggests the presence of alloantigens on trophoblast:

(a) hydatidiform molar pregnancies lacking foetal blood cellular elements and of probable androgenic origin evoke high titres of anti-HLA antibodies;
(b) both murine and human trophoblast are capable of adsorbing IgG alloantibodies to paternal antigens with greater efficiency than IgG alloantibodies directed against third party antigens;
(c) immunoglobulins eluted from semiallogeneic placentae enhance the growth of paternal tumour test allografts.

(2) *Is there an antipaternal alloantibody response?*

Bell (16.5.04) utilizing a modified haemadsorption assay showed that H-2b mice pregnant by H-2k males produced IgG, antipaternal antibodies during their second pregnancy but not during their first.

Antczak (16.5.01) reported that pregnant mares consistently produce cytotoxic antibodies to paternal lymphocytes. These findings are similar to those of Minami and Shreffler who studied the role of *I* region gene products in primary and secondary MLR against $K + D$ region products. Similarly trophoblast may express $K + D$ determinants and lack *Ia* region determinants.

(3) *Is there maternal T cell sensitization during pregnancy?*

Contributions by Stern (16.5.32), Jondor (16.5.33), Burton (16.5.08), MacCullagh (16.5.20) addressed this question. Stern showed that maternal antipaternal MLC reaction is suppressed during pregnancy but recovers in the postpartum period. Cytotoxicity to paternal strain antigens is detected by mid pregnancy; and that suppression is specific for the paternal haplotype. Smith found that alloantigen regulatory cells displaying both helper and suppressor activities could be recovered from the nodes draining the uterus during pregnancy. Burton demonstrated the emergence of cytotoxic cells by day 10–15 of pregnancy, an increase in natural killing, and a priming but lack of expression in cytotoxic responses in allogeneically mated mice. Clark reported that lymphocytes from para-aortic nodes of allogeneically pregnant females were less efficient in inducing GVH disease in appropriate target neonates than those from females gestating syngeneic foetuses.

(4) *What are the immunoregulatory mechanisms and what do they accomplish?*

Papers by Chaouat (16.5.9), Smith (16.5.24), Clark (16.5.10), Blank (16.5.6), Morton (16.5.23), Rolfe (16.5.28) and Granberg (16.5.14) addressed this question.

These workers showed that regulation occurs at the level of induction of immunity as well as at the level of its expression. The immunoregulatory processes have been identified. They include: 1. Blocking antibodies; 2. Subsets of T cells that influence MLR; 3. Placental molecular products that lead to suppressor T cell emergence; 4. Suppressed cytotoxic precursor cells; 5. Immunosuppressive molecules of foetal origin, EFP, AFP and other ovum factor soluble suppressive factors.

We are presented with a surfeit of immunoregulatory phenomena. Although some may be epiphenomena most appear tailored to assist in immunodetente between mother and the foetoplacental unit.

Cellular and molecular traffic between one mother and the conception during gestation and lactation

Cellular and molecular exchange between mother and conceptus can occur at various times during pregnancy and the postpartum period.

One of the earliest events following successful mating is the appearance of the immunosuppressive protein EPF (early pregnancy factor) in maternal serum shortly after fertilization and prior to implantation. The ovum releases a low mol. wt factor (1500 daltons) which triggers production of EPF by the mother (Cavanagh *et al.*; Giddley-Baird *et al.*, 16.4.05; 16.4.09). The mechanism of production of OF is still a mystery, and the possible role of EPF in survival of the "foetal allograft" requires further study.

Several papers dealt directly with the issue of placental transport of maternal IgG. Ibanez and Uriel (16.4.10) immunized female rats with horseradish peroxidase (HRP) and then in a subsequent pregnancy examined the localization of anti-HRP antibodies in the placenta. Maternal antibodies were seen only on the maternal side of the yolk sac epithelium whereas other molecules such as α-foetoprotein were seen on both sides. These observations suggested that little maternal IgG is transported to the foetus in the rat. Laliberte *et al.* (16.4.12) studied transport of anti-HRP antibodies in the rat placenta by electron microscopy. Transport via microvesicles was reported to occur in yolk sac but not trophoblast. Antibodies deprived of the Fc piece did not appear to be transported. No information concerning the possible presence of maternal anti-HRP antibodies in the foetal blood was forthcoming to quantify the magnitude of any transport that might be occurring. Wegmann (16.5.17) described the localization of monoclonal antibodies to H-2 and Ia antigens injected into pregnant mice. In syngeneic matings anti-H-2 alloantibodies appeared in the foetal circulation and did not localize in the placenta. In allopregnant mice bearing H-2 (K,D) and Ia antigens in the foetus capable of reacting with the antibodies, a different result occurred. The anti-H-2 did not appear in the foetus but bound to the placenta to a "Hofbauer"-like cell on the foetal side of Reichert's membrane in the lateral region of the placenta near the yolk sac. Anti-Ia did not bind, however. These data suggested that IgG transport to the foetus occurs via the placenta in the mouse, and that antibodies reactive with foetal H-2 (K,D) transplantation antigens are "filtered out" by a macrophage-like cell in placenta. No binding of antibody to trophoblast was seen, suggesting that little if any H-2 (IC, D) antigen is expressed at the maternal-foetal interface in the central part of the placenta. We were reminded that autoantibodies present in mothers with certain autoimmune diseases can cross the human placenta and cause transient autoimmune disease in the foetus.

Several laboratories reported experiments in which maternal immunity was transmitted to the foetus. Some attempts were made to discern whether mistransmission was occurring via the placenta (prenatally) or via the breast milk (postnatally). Appleby and Catty (16.4.01) studied transfer of anti-Ig-1^b allotype IgG molecules from BALB/c mothers to BALB/c × SJL/JF_1 foetuses. Antiallotype antibody appeared in the circulation of the neonate by the 5th day after birth, suggesting transfer had occurred via breast milk. Bratanov and Hristova-Koleva (16.4.04) reported that human breast milk contains, in addition to IgA, concentrations of IgE and IgD which exceed that found in maternal serum. The audience noted that presence of IgE might explain a toxic diarrhoea associated with vasoactive amine release that occurs when certain breast milks are ingested by human neonates. Smithyman *et al.* (16.4.14) studied transfer of immunity to Sendai virus to the mouse foetus. A single injection of vaccine into the mother one week before parturition followed by oral administration of the vaccine to the mother appeared to provide maximal protection against an intranasal challenge with live virus. The degree of protection did not correlate with serum antibody found in some other studies of secretory immunity at mucosal surfaces. Weisz-Carrington *et al.* (16.4.19) described selective uptake of IgA by mammary glands in pregnant mice which appears to facilitate excretion of IgA in colostrum, and some of the workshop participants suggested his localization may be prolactin-dependent.

Stern *et al.* (16.4.11) reported that immunization of pregnant mice can result in suppression of the immune responsiveness of the neonate. Reduction of the response to DNP was most frequently seen when DNP-coated SRBC were given to the mothers shortly after mating. When protein carriers such as BCG were used, and when immunization was carried out later in pregnancy, the responsiveness of the neonate was enhanced. Cross-foster nursing experiments showed pre- and postnatal transmission of the effect. These types of experiments illustrated the problem of determining whether the effects on the foetus were mediated by transfer of antigen or maternal antibody, and whether the transfer occurred pre- or postnatally. A further complication was demonstrated by Toms (16.4.16) who reported that breast feeding of the human neonate was associated with a reduced risk of hospitalization at 2–6 months of age from respiratory syncytial virus (RSV). The mothers were primigravida who lacked IgA reactive with RSV in their milk which could proliferate in response to RSV antigen. The long duration of protection of the neonate suggested that transfer of the cellular elements of breast milk to the foetus might be important.

With respect to possible pathogenic effects of maternal T cells in colostrum following transfer to the semiallogeneic neonate, Parmely and Williams (16.4.13) reported that while colostral T cells responded to paternal allogeneic stimulators in a MLC reaction, no cytotoxic T cells were generated. The colostral cells could also respond to the antigens of various pathogens. Failure to generate cytotoxic T cells was not caused by a T suppressor cell. Weiler *et al.* (16.4.18) presented evidence that colostral cell could prolong the lifespan of colostral antibody that entered the circulation of the neonate. Further studies are needed to determine the immunologic role and mechanism by which colostral cells play in the immunologic status of the neonate.

With respect to transport of intact maternal lymphoid cells to the foetus prenatally, new information was provided: it is thought that virus-infected maternal cells (as with CMV and rubella) may play a role in infecting the foetus.

Many questions remain to be answered and new data are anticipated by the time of the next congress. However, during this Congress we have learned much of immunoregulatory mechanisms operating during all places of reproductive processes.

To date we have no singular immunological explanation for the establishment of immunological coexistence between sexual partners and between the mother and her foetus during gestation. We have heard the results of well designed studies using sophisticated immunological tools that have documented unequivocally immunoregulatory processes and of factors initiated during germ cell formation-maturation, conception, gestation, and lactation. Maternal responses to MHC antigens of the foetus do occur and are not inimicable to their survival. In fact there is cogent evidence that alloreactivity may be beneficial to the foetoplacental unit. This normal reactivity of the female to alloantigens of the foetoplacental unit has not been shown to bring about cytotoxic destruction of the "trophoblastic dialysis membrane" *in vivo* or *in vitro*.

I conclude that, based on studies presented, alterations in immunoreactivity coupled with the production of unique protein and steroid hormones and other molecules by the trophoblast result in an effective block of the efferent limit of the immunological reflex arc and allows the trophoblastic epithelium to experience an immunologically privileged status as a tissue. Nature has developed her own reproductive immunological telephone system to facilitate appropriate cell to cell communication or to interrupt or short circuit communications.

This system appears foolproof without major cost to the mother and certainly of benefit to the foetoplacental unit preserving the individuality of both. A forward leap in infertility, fertility control, transplantation and developmental biology will certainly derive from our ability to more fully comprehend and utilize similar methods and processes.

Theme 17

Manipulation of the Immune System

Presidents:
I. M. ROITT
P. GALANAUD

Symposium chairman:
S. KOTANI

60

Manipulation of the Immune Response by Anti-idiotype

CHARLES A. JANEWAY

Department of Pathology, Yale University School of Medicine, New Haven, Connecticut, USA

Introduction

One of the primary practical goals of modern immunology is to manipulate the immune system such that a greater or lesser response is obtained. Drugs, hormones and ionizing radiation have all been used with varying degrees of success. Their signal disadvantage is their lack of immunological specificity. More precise manipulation of the immune system may derive from the use of monoclonal antibodies directed at individual functional sets of lymphocytes. These can serve both as agonists and as antagonists. However, frequently the goal is to affect only the response to a particular antigen, without influencing the response to other antigens. To achieve this selectivity, two approaches have been attempted. One is to use the antigen itself. However, in the particular case of inducing tolerance to tissue grafts, which is one of the major goals of such research, the results obtained using antigen have been disappointing. Furthermore, large amounts of antigen are difficult to obtain. A second approach has therefore been attempted. This is to manipulate the immune response using antibodies directed at unique antigenic determinants in T or B cell receptors, of a particular specificity (idiotypes) or by immunizing actively with the idiotype itself. In this paper, I will briefly review the results obtained in attempts to manipulate the immune response by means of anti-idiotype immunity. I will also set these observations in the framework of our current understanding of idiotype–anti-idiotype interactions and their influence on the immune response in general. From this analysis, it becomes clear that a great deal of detailed analysis of the effects of anti-idiotype antibody on individual components of the immune apparatus still needs to be done before one can reliably predict the outcome of injection of idiotype or anti-idiotype on an immune response.

Manipulation of the immune response with anti-idiotype

Idiotypes or individually specific antigenic determinants found on antibody of a particular specificity, were initially described in rabbits (Oudin and Michel, 1963) and in human myeloma proteins (Kunkel *et al.*, 1963). These early studies suggested that each individual made a unique set of idiotypes upon immunization with a particular antigen. However, studies in inbred mice subsequently revealed that certain idiotypes appeared reliably in every individual of a particular strain immunized with that antigen (Weigert and Riblet, 1978). Furthermore, these studies demonstrated that the inheritance of the ability to produce a particular idiotype was largely determined by genes encoding the variable regions of the heavy and light chains of immunoglobulin.

The availability of anti-idiotype antibody directed at these inherited or so-called germ line idiotypes led to experiments aimed at either suppressing or enhancing immune responses by injecting such antibody into animals. The results of such experiments can be divided into those in which anti-idiotype served as an agonist, leading to activation of idiotype production, and those in which anti-idiotype served as an antagonist, leading to the suppression of idiotype production.

Lymphocyte activation by anti-idiotypic antibody

It has been possible in some instances to demonstrate an increase in the number and/or activity of idiotype-bearing B and T lymphocytes following injection of anti-idiotypic antibody. The system that has been studied in most detail is that of Eichmann (1978). In these experiments, antibody raised in guinea-pigs to an idiotype found on about 30% of the antibody of strain A/J mice directed at streptococcal group A carbohydrate (A-CHO) is divided into the IgG1 and IgG2 subclasses. IgG1 anti-idiotype antibody injection leads to priming of idiotypic B and T lymphocytes bearing the common idiotype, yet no anti-A-CHO antibody can be detected in these animals. Actual activation of lymphocytes to secrete antibody using anti-idiotype as the inducing signal has thus far been achieved *in vitro* by Trenkner and Riblet (1975) and *in vivo* by Frischknecht *et al.* (1978). Thus, anti-idiotype antibody appears to be far less effective at activating the immune system to secrete antibody than is antigen.

On the other hand, activation of T cells by injection of anti-idiotype antibody is a frequently observed occurrence. It has been shown that anti-idiotype antibody can activate helper T cells (Eichmann and Rajewsky, 1975; Cosenza *et al.*, 1977). Further experiments have shown activation of both idiotypic and anti-idiotypic T cells by anti-idiotype (Hetzelberger and Eichmann, 1978). Anti-idiotype antibody raised against T cell blasts activated to alloantigens has also been used to activate cytolytic effector T cells specific for that alloantigen *in vitro* (Frishknecht *et al.*, 1978). In some of these instances, it has been shown that anti-idiotype is more effective than antigen in activating T cell responses (Binz *et al.*, 1979). Suppressor T cells have also been activated by the injection of anti-idiotypic antibody (Eichmann and Rajewsky, 1975; Nisonoff *et al.*, 1977). In this instance, Eichmann and Rajewsky (1975) find that it is the IgG2 fraction of guinea-pig anti-idiotype that induces suppressor T cell activity in their system. The dose-response characteristics and requirement for antigenic stimulation in the maintenance of these suppressor T cells demonstrate the complexity of these systems. Therefore, anti-idiotype antibody can be shown to activate T cells and B cells. Amongst T cells, it can activate idiotypic and anti-idiotypic T cell sets, and these can be helper, suppressor or cytotoxic sets of T cells.

Suppression of immune responses by anti-idiotypic antibody

Most studies have focused on the suppression of the immune response by anti-idiotype antibody. The most dramatic of these findings is the long-term suppression of antiphosphorylcholine (PC) antibody production by neonatal injection of anti-idiotype antibody directed at the BALB/c PC-binding myeloma TEPC 15 (T15) (Cosenza *et al.*, 1977). In such mice, B cell responses are absent over prolonged periods; upon recovery of the ability to make anti-PC antibody, little T15 idiotype is produced. These effects seem to be primarily on B cells; suppressor cells have not been shown in this system. Similar findings in other idiotypic systems have largely demonstrated suppression of idiotype production but *not* suppression of antibody production (Nisonoff *et al.*, 1977; Eichmann, 1978). Thus, while anti-idiotype antibody clearly can suppress production of idiotype, its usefulness in the regulation of immune responsiveness in antibody responses may be limited by production of antibody bearing alternate idiotypic determinants.

Numerous studies suggest that anti-idiotype antibody has more profound effects on the regulatory T cell apparatus. Thus, anti-idiotype antibody clearly can lead to activation of suppressor T cells (Eichmann, 1974; Nisonoff *et al.*, 1977; Bottomly *et al.*, 1978) and in some cases a concomitant decrease in helper T cells needed for idiotype production (Ward *et al.*, 1977). Furthermore, extensive experiments by Binz, Wigzell and co-workers (Andersson *et al.*, 1977; Auget *et al.*, 1978; and Binz and Wigzell, 1978) have demonstrated the potential for regulation of T cell responses to MHC by means of anti-idiotype antibody either actively induced or passively administered.

Anti-idiotype and the immunoregulatory network

Taken together, these and many other similar studies clearly demonstrate that anti-idiotype antibody can profoundly influence specific immune responsiveness. On the other hand, they represent an important first step on a long journey, in which hopefully similar experiments will also be the last step. That is, they very clearly point to a role for anti-idiotype in the modulation of an immune response to a particular antigenic determinant. However, in general such studies have not been informative as to the mechanism of action of the anti-idiotype in the animal. This, in turn, reflects our relative ignorance about various aspects of immunoregulation and the organization of the immune system. It has become clear that the immune system is made up of a complex set of interacting lymphocytes which can be discriminated from one another on the basis of function, cell surface antigenic determinants, specificity, and state of activation. Furthermore, these lymphocytes interact with one another, such that the outcome of an immune response is a complex function of the interactions of antigen with this "network" (Jerne, 1974) of cells. The idiotypic and/or anti-idiotypic nature of cellular receptors, of secreted immunoregulatory products, including antibody, and indeed the precise chemical nature of idiotypy itself are all in the process of being further defined. Thus, it is not surprising that injection of anti-idiotype should produce such a multiplicity of effects. Before such manipulation of the immune system can be placed on a purely rational basis, it will be necessary to have a complete picture of the following:

(a) The individual cellular components of the immunoregulatory apparatus.

(b) The receptors used by these components, particularly those that determine their interactions with other cells in the apparatus (restrictions).

(c) The nature of idiotype at the genetic and molecular level.

(d) The role of non-binding site components (e.g. isotype) of the anti-idiotype antibody in their biological activity.

This discussion will focus on the first two of these points, as little can be said at present about the latter two, other than that answers in these areas will be highly complex (see Kelsoe *et al.*, 1980; Eichmann, 1978).

The structures of the immunoregulatory apparatus

Apart from the major distinction of lymphocytes into T cell and B cells, many different populations of lymphocytes have now been defined. These can be distinguished on the basis of function and, in general, associated cell surface antigenic determinants, or differentiation antigens. In particular, the Lyt antigens have been useful in dissecting these cells. This complexity makes experiments in which anti-idiotype is injected into an intact animal leading to alterations in that animal's immune response difficult to attribute to a particular agonist or antagonist effect of the antibody on a particular cell. That is to say, increases in immune responses induced by anti-idiotype could be due to activation of B cells or helper T cells, or to inactivation of suppressor T cells, and vice versa for decreased responses. In this section, we will describe some of these lymphocyte types and then attempt to portray their interactions that lead to a normal immune response.

Idiotypic receptors on lymphocytes

One of the implications of injecting animals with anti-idiotype antibody is that a lymphocyte can be affected by the action of the anti-idiotype antibody on that cell's receptors. This has been clearly shown for both T cells and B cells. However, whether this is the total explanation for the effects of anti-idiotype antibody is not clear, since interaction of anti-idiotype with idiotypic T or B cell products could also affect the response.

B cells have been shown to be inactivated by exposure to anti-idiotype antibody (Cosenza *et al.*, 1977). Only those B cells bearing the idiotype were known to have been affected. The same is true of B cell priming with anti-idiotypic antibody (Eichmann, 1978). In many cases, suppression of idiotypic B cells by anti-idiotype does not affect the overall B cell response to the antigen; the early work with anti-T15 antibody on the anti-PC response appears to be the exception rather than the rule. From this, it has become clear that B cells do bear idiotypic receptors, and that these cells can become activated or inactivated by anti-idiotype acting upon those receptors. However, it is also clear that in most instances this does not abolish the entire response to the antigen.

T cells have been shown to be activated (Eichmann, 1978; Cosenza *et al.*, 1977; Frishknecht *et al.*, 1978) as well as inactivated (Binz *et al.*, 1979) by anti-idiotype. Here, the story appears to be somewhat different from the results obtained with B cells. That is, T cells specific for a particular antigenic determinant appear to all bear the same idiotype. While this definition of idiotype is subject to change based on an emerging picture of far greater complexity of idiotypic antibody as the analysis becomes more precise, the message is still clear. T cell receptor idiotypes are clearly less heterogeneous than B cell receptor idiotypes (Binz and Wigzell, 1977; Eichmann, 1978; Nisonoff *et al.*, 1977; Krawinkel *et al.*, 1978; Mozes and Haimovich, 1979).

In fact, there are so many examples of this rule, that it is difficult to find an exception. Thus, two lessons emerge. T cells are more idiotypically homogeneous than are B cells, where the two have been compared. It follows that anti-idiotype manipulation of the immune response should focus on manipulation of T cells by anti-idiotype. Thus, it is on T cells that this article will primarily focus.

T lymphocyte subpopulations

As stated above, T lymphocyte receptors both for conventional antigen and for major histocompatibility complex (MHC) antigen appear to bear commonly occurring or germ line idiotypes (Janeway *et al.*, 1976). Recently, it has become obvious that T cells can also be anti-idiotypic, and that idiotypic and anti-idiotypic T and/or B lymphocytes can interact in various ways to influence the immune response. T lymphocytes can also be subdivided by physiologic function and by the cell surface antigens that they bear. Here, I will focus on two broad classes of lymphocytes, and I will term these TMHC, for those T cells that bear receptors specific for self MHC determinants, and TIg, for those T cells that bear receptors for self immunoglobulin (Ig) determinants (Bottomly and Mosier, 1980). Within each of these classes of lymphocytes, both helper and suppressor T cells have been described. It seems likely that some T cells will also exist which have no receptor for self specificities, but act directly upon antigen.

TMHC. These T cells would appear to bear two receptor sites. One is specific for MHC determinants, recognizing self MHC determinants with low affinity, and allogenic MHC determinants with a high affinity. This receptor plays a critical physiological role in directing T cells to recognize antigen in the context of self MHC determinants only. The second receptor is specific for the nominal or foreign antigen. Either (or both) receptors will be marked by idiotypic determinants (Janeway *et al.*, 1976, 1980). In particular, helper T cells will bear receptors for self *I*-region encoded determinants, which direct them to interact with B cells and/or macrophages bearing the nominal antigen for which they are also specific. Helper cells of this type have been clearly defined in numerous studies, most clearly where they were removed by binding to antigen-coated macrophages (Swierkosz *et al.*, 1978). Suppressor cells that are clearly MHC restricted have not been satisfactorily demonstrated. However, Yamauchi *et al.* (pers. comm.) have described a suppressor-effector factor that is MHC restricted in its action on the Ly-1 helper T cells it affects.

TIg. This more recently described set of cells appears to bear receptor sites for self Ig determinants and for antigen, although unlike TMHC, recognition of each determinant appears to be independent. Thus far, clear evidence for TIg exists only in a limited number of idiotypic systems, most clearly the anti-PC response (Bottomly *et al.*, 1978, 1979, 1980), the anti-Ars response (Nisonoff *et al.*, 1977; Ward *et al.*, 1977), and the anti-A-CHO response (Hetzelberger and Eichmann, 1978). These cells are restricted in their interactions with other cells by anti-idiotype receptors. Recently, Bottomly and

Maurer (1980) and Bottomly and Janeway (1980) have produced evidence suggesting that such cells are not MHC recognizing. Thus, these anti-idiotypic T cells form a separable set of T cells from TMHC, based on their anti-self receptor sites. Their ontogenic development can be shown to depend on the presence of idiotype as circulating Ig in the mouse (Bottomly and Mosier, 1979; and Bottomly *et al.*, 1980). Thus far, such cells have been examined for their influence on B cells only; whether they affect idiotypic T cells is not presently clear. However, this seems likely to be so.

These TIg cells probably need to be distinguished from a seemingly similar set of T cells that is also anti-idiotypic. Thus, many investigators have shown that injection of idiotype in adjuvant will activate anti-idiotypic T cells (Janeway *et al.*, 1975; Eichmann *et al.*, 1978; Binz and Wigzell, 1978). The cells generated in this manner will probably belong to the TMHC family, and use their *anti-nominal antigen receptor* in recognizing idiotypic determinants. This matter could be clarified by further examining MHC restriction or its absence in various classes of anti-idiotypic T lymphocytes. It is also clear that, while such anti-idiotypic T cells may not play a major role in the physiological regulation of an antibody response, they may be useful in attempts to manipulate immunity with idiotype or anti-idiotype, and should be studied and understood accordingly.

Networks and interactions

Given that there are B cells, helper T cells and suppressor T cells, all of which can be idiotypic or anti-idiotypic, and can produce products bearing idiotypic or anti-idiotypic determinants, how do all of these components interact in the generation of an immune response? And how might they be best manipulated by anti-idiotype to alter that response?

Clearly, such questions can not be completely answered at the present time. In part, this is because the complexity of the immune system is even greater than that briefly outlined above. For instance, it has been shown that a T cell which has helper characteristics (Ly-1^+2^-) also serves to activate a suppressor T cell, and does so via immunoglobulin variable region (e.g. idiotypic) structures, presumably via idiotype-anti-idiotype interactions (Eardley *et al.*, 1979). However, the effect is not directly upon the actual suppressor T cell, but rather acts indirectly through a transducing cellular apparatus, which may convert the signal from one type of interaction (idiotype–anti-idiotype) to another (idiotype–antigen), since the effector cell in this system *is* MHC restricted (Yamauchi *et al.*, pers. comm.). Another problem is that much of our detailed knowledge of immunoregulation comes from short term *in vitro* or *in vivo* experiments. Such experiments give precise answers about individual components and their initial interactions, but tell us little about long-term modulation of the immune response. The role of idiotype–anti-idiotype interactions in antibody feedback systems has yet to be fully clarified. In longer term *in vivo* experiments, it is common to find the endogenous production of anti-idiotypic antibody (Cosenza *et al.*, 1977; Brown and Rodkey, 1979). Furthermore, it is clear that idiotypes can vary very widely in the course of an antibody response (Dzierzak *et al.*, 1980), whereas many studies have measured but a single time point, thus perhaps arriving at only partially correct answers to questions.

The need for information about idiotypic regulation

On the more positive side, the explosion in technology in the study of immunology allows us optimism that many answers will be obtained to these questions before the next international congress. Thus, there are certain clear needs that should soon be met.

Further development of idiotypic systems

Much of our knowledge of idiotypes and anti-idiotypes depends on either the random occurrence of antigen-binding myelomas or on induced antibody as a source of idiotype, and use of heterologous or isologous anti-idiotype antibody. Such studies suggested relative homogeneity in responses to several antigens, such as PC, Ars, NP, etc. The development of monoclonal antibodies has allowed access to numerous examples of induced idiotype for serological and structural analysis. This has begun to reveal a startling complexity to idiotypic systems previously assumed to be quite homogeneous (Reth *et al.*, 1979; Marshak-Rothstein *et al.*, 1980; Berek-Jack *et al.*, 1980). This analysis has been pursued to some extent at the B cell level. Current understanding of T cell idiotypes is even less complete. However, access to monoclonal idiotype and anti-idiotype antibodies should greatly refine our analysis of idiotypic regulation.

The effect of anti-idiotype on isolated T cell populations

Amongst B cells, it appears that anti-idiotype can activate or prevent the activation of a subpopulation of antigen-specific B cells, but will probably not alter an entire response, since alternate idiotypes specific for the same antigen exist on B cells. However, anti-idiotype treatment of T cells, which besides being more homogeneous idiotypically are also capable of helping or suppressing entire responses in an *antigen-specific* fashion after activation by anti-idiotype (Eichmann, 1978), may play an important role in the future of anti-idiotypic manipulation of the immune response. Therefore, it is to be hoped that isolated T cell subsets and/or T cell clones bearing idiotypes will be treated in isolation with anti-idiotype antibody to determine the effect of anti-idiotype directly upon that cell type. Such cells, once activated or inactivated by anti-idiotype, could then be added to intact immune systems to determine their effect on an immune response. From this, it should be possible to determine the effect of anti-idiotype directly on T cells. A related experiment, equally important, involves determining the effect of anti-idiotype antibody given to intact animals in activating or inactivating subsequently isolated T and B cell sets. Both approaches are essential to our understanding of how anti-idiotype may be used to regulate the immune response.

The role of nonidiotype binding regions of anti-idiotype antibody

Different classes of antibody to antigen or to idiotype have differential effects on antibody and T cell responses to antigen (Henry and Jerne, 1968; Eichmann and Rajewsky, 1975; Murgita and Vas, 1972). It is clear that the reasons for this can now be obtained precisely using monoclonal anti-idiotypic antibody, which is homogeneous as to class. Antibody class and species of origin may play a critical role in the effect of anti-idiotype on different classes of cells, and in turn, on the immune response. Such work could clearly point to the type of anti-idiotype to use in trying to activate or suppress the immune response of an intact organism.

Summary

It is clear from the few examples cited that an animal's immune response can be affected by anti-idiotypic antibody administered to it. Often strikingly small amounts are needed for these effects. Likewise, active immunization with idiotype to produce anti-idiotype endogeneously can greatly influence an animal's immune response. However, it has not been possible up to the present time to answer the following question: What is the precise mechanism by which the anti-idiotype produces its effect, and particularly, which cell type(s) are activated or inactivated by injection of anti-idiotype? Secondly, anti-idiotype often prevents idiotype formation without affecting other components of the immune response to the same antigen. Third, it is not yet clear in previously untested systems what effect anti-idiotype antibody will have on a particular immune response. Until this can be reliably predicted, use of anti-idiotypic manipulation of the immune response in clinical settings must be viewed with extreme caution. However, the rapid progress in defining the immunoregulatory apparatus, and the advent of monoclonal antibody technology, should allow the resolution of many of these questions in the near future, so that this means of manipulating the immune response will become an increasingly valuable component of the immunologic armamentarium.

References

Andersson, L. C., Auget, M., Wright, E., Andersson, R., Binz, H. and Wigzell, H. (1977). *J. Exp. Med.* **146**, 1124.

Auget, M., Andersson, L. C., Andersson, R., Wright, E., Binz, H. and Wigzell, H. (1977). *J. Exp. Med.* **147**, 50.

Berek-Jack, C., Schreier, M. H., Sidman, J. L., Jaton, J. C., Kocher, H. P. and Cosenza, H. (1980). *Eur. J. Immunol.* **10**, 287.

Binz, H. and Wigzell, H. (1977). *Contemp. Top. Immunobiol.* **7**, 113.

Binz, H. and Wigzell, H. (1978). *J. Exp. Med.* **147**, 63.

Binz, H., Frischknecht, H. and Wigzell, H. (1979). *Ann. Immunol. (Inst. Pasteur)* **130**, 273.

Bottomly, K. and Mosier, D. E. (1979). *J. Exp. Med.* **150**, 1399.

Bottomly, K. and Mosier, D. E. (1980). *In* "Strategies in Immune Regulation" (E. Sercarz and A. Cunningham, eds) Academic Press, New York (in press).

Bottomly, K. and Maurer, P. H. (1980). Submitted for publication.

Bottomly, K. and Janeway, C. A., Jr (1980). Submitted for publication.

Bottomly, K., Mathieson, B. J. and Mosier, D. E. (1978). *J. Exp. Med.* **148**, 1216.

Bottomly, K., Mathieson, B. J., Cosenza, H. and Mosier, D. E. (1979). *In* "B Lymphocytes in the Immune Response" (M. Cooper, D. Mosier, I. Scher, E. Vitetta, eds) p. 323. Elsevier-North Holland, New York.

Bottomly, K., Janeway, C. A., Jr, Mathieson, B. J. and Mosier, D. E. (1980). *Eur. J. Immunol.* **10**, 159.

Brown, J. C. and Rodkey, L. S. (1979) *J. Exp. Med.* **150**, 67.

Cosenza, H., Julius, M. H. and Augustin, A. A. (1977). *Immunol. Rev.* **150**, 67.

Dzierzak, E. A., Janeway, C. A., Jr, Rosenstein, R. W. and Gottlieb, P. D. (1980). *J. Exp. Med.* (in press).

Eardley, D. D., Shen, F.-W., Cantor, H., and Gershon, R. K. (1979). *J. Exp. Med.* **150**, 44.

Eichmann, K. (1974). *Eur. J. Immunol.* **4**, 296.

Eichmann, K. (1978). *Adv. Immunol.* **26**, 195.

Eichmann, K., Falk, I. and Rajewsky, K. (1978). *Eur. J. Immunol.* **8**, 853.

Eichmann, K. and Rajewsky, K. (1975). *Eur. J. Immunol.* **5**, 661.

Frischknecht, H., Binz, H. and Wigzell, H. (1978). *J. Exp. Med.* **147**, 500.

Henry, C. and Jerne, N. K. (1968). *J. Exp. Med.* **128**, 113.

Hertzelberger, D. and Eichmann, K. (1978). *Eur. J. Immunol.* **8**, 846.

Janeway, C. A., Jr, Jones, B., Binz, H., Frischknecht, H. and Wigzell, H. (1980). *Scand. J. Immunol.* (in press).

Janeway, C. A., Jr, Sakato, N. and Eisen, H. N. (1975). *Proc Natn. Acad. Sci. U.S.A.* **72**, 2357.

Janeway, C. A., Jr, Wigzell, H. and Binz, H. (1976). *Scand. J. Immunol.* **9**, 993.

Jerne, N. K. (1974). *Ann. Immunol. (Inst. Pasteur)* **125C**, 373.

Kelsoe, G., Reth, M. and Rajewsky, K. (1980). *Immunol. Rev.* **52** (in press).

Krawinkel, U., Cramer, M., Melchers, I., Imanishi-Kari, T. and Rajewsky, K. (1978). *J. Exp. Med.* **147**, 1341.

Kunkel, H. G., Mannik, M., and Williams, R. C. (1963). *Science* **140**, 1218.

Marshak-Rathstein, A., Siekevitz, M., Mudgett-Hunter, M., Margolies, M. N., and Gefter, M. L. (1980). *Proc. Natn. Acad. Sci. U.S.A.* **77**, 1120.

Mozes, E. and Haimovich, J. (1979). *Nature (Lond.)* **278**, 56.

Murgita, R. A. and Vas, S. I. (1972). *Immunology* **22**, 319.

Nisonoff, A., Ju, S.-T. and Owen, F. L. (1977). *Immunol. Rev.* **34**, 89.

Oudin, J. and Michel, M. (1963). *C. R. Acad. Sci. (Paris)* **257**, 805.
Owen, F. L., Ju, S.-T. and Nisonoff, A. (1977). *J. Exp. Med.* **145**, 1559.
Reth, M., Imanishi-Kari, T. and Rajewsky, K. (1979). *Eur. J. Immunol.* **9**, 1004.
Swierkosz, J. E., Rock, K., Marrack, P. and Kappler, J. W. (1978). *J. Exp. Med.* **147**, 554.
Trenkner, F. and Riblet, R. (1975). *J. Exp. Med.* **142**, 1121.
Ward, K., Cantor, H. and Boyse, E. A. (1977). *In* "The Immune System: Genetics and Regulation" (E. Sercarz, L. Herzenberg and C. F. Fox, eds) p. 397. Academic Press, New York.
Weigert, M. and Riblet, R. (1978). *Springer Symp. Immunopathol.* **1**, 133.

61

Nonspecific and Specific Immunosuppression by Total Lymphoid Irradiation (TLI)

S. SLAVIN, S. YATZIV, I. ZAN BAR* Z. FUKS, H. S. KAPLAN and S. STROBER****

Immunobiology Research Laboratory, Hadassah University Hospital, Jerusalem, Israel
*and **Stanford University School of Medicine, Stanford, California*

Abbreviations
TLI: total lymphoid irradiation; BM: bone marrow; GVHD: graft versus host disease; HVG: host versus graft; MLR: mixed lymphocyte reaction; WBI: whole body irradiation; T cells: thymus-derived lymphocytes; B cells: immunoglobulin-bearing lymphocytes; PHA: phytohaemagglutinin; Con A: concanavalin A; NZB/NZW: New Zealand Black × New Zealand White F_1 hybrid mice; CFA: complete Freund's adjuvants; BSA: bovine serum albumin; BGG: bovine γ globulin.

*Present address: Department of Cell Biology, the Weizmann Institute of Science, Rehovot, Israel.

This work was supported by grants from the National Institutes of Health—grant Nos AI-15387 and AI-11313, from the United States—Israel Binational Science Foundation—grant No. 1786/79, and from the Howard Hughes Medical Institute.
The authors wish to thank Dr Lola Weiss, Ms S. Morecki, Ms P. Abeliuk, Ms G. Garrelts, and Ms C. Doss for their fine technical assistance.

Total lymphoid irradiation (TLI)—general background

Total lymphoid irradiation (TLI) was originally introduced as a technique of supravoltage radiotherapy used for the treatment of Hodgkin's disease and nonHodgkin lymphoma and has become a standard programme for treatment all over the world. This treatment technique has been designed to permit high radiation doses to all of the major lymphoid structures of the body, while shielding adjacent vital organs and tissues (Kaplan, 1972). More recently, it has been demonstrated that TLI is also an effective mode of immunosuppression in strains of rodents (Slavin *et al.*, 1976, 1977a, b, 1978a, b, 1979a; Strober *et al.*, 1979; Zan Bar *et al.*, 1979), dogs (Slavin *et al.*, 1979b, c; Strober *et al.*, 1979), primates (Bieber *et al.*, 1979), as well as in man (Fuks *et al.*, 1976; Najarian *et al.*, 1980 in prep.).

Based on the use of TLI as the basic conditioning regimen, we developed a method for the induction of permanent tolerance to soluble protein antigens (Zan Bar *et al.*, 1979) and transplantation antigens which allows for the permanent survival of bone marrow and organ allografts in both inbred and outbred adult animals which differ at the major histocompatibility complex (Slavin *et al.*, 1976, 1977a, 1978a, b, 1979b, c; Strober *et al.*, 1979). TLI has few severe side effects, and a negligible mortality rate (Kaplan, 1972). We review here the essential features of our experimental findings with stress on possible applicability of TLI conditioning for experimental and, hopefully, clinical bone marrow and organ transplantation.

The TLI procedure is based on two general principles: a) selective irradiation of lymphoid organs including the thymus and the spleen with proper shielding of nonlymphoid organs as well as bone marrow-containing bones. Irradiation ports used for different animal models and man were previously described in detail (Slavin *et al.*, 1976, 1977b, 1978a, 1979b; Kaplan, 1972). b) Daily fractionation of the irradiation to well tolerated doses of 100–200 rads.

If the radiation is selectively restricted to lymphoid tissues and the total dose is fractionated, high cumulative doses of irradiation (3000–4400 rads) can be administered without the severe side effects of WBI.

Nonspecific immunosuppressive effects of TLI

Effects of TLI on the lymphoid organs and lymphocyte subpopulations

TLI is accompanied by severe leukopenia with total elimination of circulating lymphocytes but the total white blood cell count increases upon completion of irradiation (Slavin *et al.*, 1976, 1977b). The total number of peripheral white blood cells in rodents returns to the normal range within a few weeks, however, differential counts reveal an inversion of the lymphocyte/polymorphonuclear ratio with absolute lymphocytopenia. The lymphocyte/polymorphonuclear ratio increases steadily, and reaches normal levels at 3 months. The total number of leukocytes is maintained in the normal range (Slavin *et al.*, 1977b). T lymphocytes are usually undetectable in the peripheral blood for the first 4 weeks following TLI. A steep rise in the absolute number of T lymphocytes is usually observed in the second month. A slow increase in T cell count continues thereafter but T lymphocytopenia persists for more than 250 days in mice (Slavin *et al.*, 1977b) and for more than 10 years in man (Fuks *et al.*, 1976). Absolute B lymphocytosis persists following TLI in both rodents and man (Slavin *et al.*, 1977b; Fuks *et al.*, 1976). The size and cellularity of lymphoid compartments in all lymphatic organs decrease following TLI but the lymphoid follicles as well as T and B lymphocyte domains appear otherwise normal (unpublished observations).

T dependent immune responses following TLI

In the immediate post-TLI period PBL are unable to respond in the one-way MLR and to mitogens (PHA, ConA) (Slavin *et al.*, 1977b). TLI-treated mice show no primary responses (IgM) to sheep red blood cells (T dependent) for more than one month. The IgG response returns approximately 200 days after TLI, but returns within 28 days after single dose whole body irradiation (Zan Bar *et al.*, 1979). Mice primed prior to TLI are able to mount vigorous IgG responses, indicating that memory cells can survive this irradiation regimen. First set organ allograft survival is markedly prolonged following TLI. In mice the survival of skin allografts across major histocompatibility differences is prolonged 5-fold (Slavin *et al.*, 1977b). Heterotopic heart allograft survival is prolonged 9-fold in rats (Slavin *et al.*, 1978a). Kinetic studies on the recovery of MLR reactivity in mice show a good correlation with the ability to reject skin allografts (Slavin *et al.*, 1977b). Similar potent immunosuppressive effects are also observed in patients with Hodgkin's disease undergoing TLI. After radiotherapy, the PHA response of patients with Hodgkin's disease falls significantly below that of the pretreatment level. Reduced PHA responsiveness persists for at least 10 years after radiotherapy without disease recurrence. Similarly, the MLR is virtually eliminated for about 20 months following radiotherapy. Thereafter, a slow recovery is observed such that normal responses were uniformly observed 5 or more years after treatment (Fuks *et al.*, 1976).

The pattern of regeneration of murine lymphocyte subpopulations following the severe depletion caused by radiotherapy is unique. Thus, in addition to the persistent T lymphocytopenia with a concomitant B lymphocytosis, TLI results in enrichment of TL positive cells in the spleen and lymph nodes (Strober *et al.*, 1979), depletion of PHA-responsive T cells, enrichment of Con-A responsive T cells (Slavin *et al.*, 1977b), and enrichment of nonspecific suppressor T cells (Zan Bar *et al.*, 1978) as well as non-B non-T suppressor cells (Slavin, unpublished observations). The unique recovery pattern following TLI suggests that the process of T cell maturation may be altered due to changes in the thymus, impairment of the normal matrix of the lymphatic tissues, and/or an imbalanced cellular proliferation due to different radiosensitivities of different lymphocyte subsets.

Immunosuppression of autoimmune diseases by TLI

Female F_1 hybrid New Zealand Black/New Zealand White (NZB/NZW) mice provide an ideal animal model for the study of systemic lupus erythematosus (SLE). The immunosuppressive effects of TLI were tested on the autoimmune manifestations of the NZB/NZW model of autoimmune disease, based on the previously reported responsiveness of both NZB/NZW disease and SLE to immunosuppressive regimens. A marked beneficial effect of fractionated lymphoid irradiation on the autoimmune disease of NZB/NZW mice was demonstrated in two reports (Slavin, 1979; Kotzin and Strober, 1979). Disease activity seemed to be controlled by TLI as could be demonstrated by kinetic studies of the proteinuria, anti-DNA activity and the survival following TLI. Significant prolongation of survival was also recently demonstrated in both MRL/lpr and MRL/n animal models of autoimmune disorders (Moscovitch and Slavin, in prep.).

A marked remission of adjuvant induced "autoimmune" polyarthritis in Lewis rats as indicated by direct objective evaluation of the synovitis in the affected joints as well as by improved roentgenological signs of joint involvement was also demonstrated (Schurman *et al.*, 1978).

The potential of TLI for the treatment of autoimmune disorders in man is also suggested by the encouraging preliminary results obtained from a pilot study in a small group of patients with intractable rheumatoid arthritis (Strober *et al.*, 1980, in prep.).

The efficacy of TLI in induction of immunosuppression and remission of some of the autoimmune manifestations in the animal models and in the few patients tested so far suggests that TLI should be further investigated as a new clinical therapeutic approach for the treatment of selected cases of autoimmune disorders refractory to conservative therapeutic modalities.

Induction of specific unresponsiveness following conditioning with TLI

Tolerance to protein antigens

Injection of nondeaggregated BSA in saline following TLI treatment of BALB/c mice results in specific unresponsiveness following a challenge with DNP_{15}-BSA in CFA up to 120 days following TLI. A similar challenge given to TLI-treated BALB/c mice not injected with tolerogen results in a normal response. Tolerance to BSA can be induced even when BSA in saline is injected 100 days following completion of TLI treatment. BSA injected mice generate normal antibody responses following a challenge with DNP_{15}-BGG in CFA, indicating antigen-specific unresponsiveness (Zan Bar *et al.*, 1978).

BM transplantation and allograft tolerance in rodents

Infusion of allogeneic BM cells (about 10^9 nucleated cells/kg body weight) within 24 h following TLI (200 rads × 17, total 3400 rads) results in permanent chimaerism in rodents. Thus, infusion of 30 × 10^6 BM cells following TLI results in permanent (> 360 days) chimaerism in each of the following combinations of strongly incompatible donor-recipient strains: C57BL/Ka (H-2^b) → BALB/c (H-2^d); A/J (H-2^a) → (BALB/c × C57BL/6) F_1 (H-$2^{d/b}$); BALB/c (H-2^d) → C3H/HeJ (H-2^k), and C3H/HeJ (H-2^k) → BALB/c (H-2^d) (Slavin *et al.*, 1977b; 1978b; Slavin *et al.*, submitted for publication). Similarly, Lewis (Ag-B^1) rats treated with TLI accept permanently ACI (Ag-B^4), Brown–Norway (Ag-B^3) or Wistar–Furth (Ag-B^2) BM (Slavin *et al.*, 1978a). None of the BM recipients developed lethal GVHD which was uniformly observed when similar recipients were conditioned with WBI instead of TLI (Slavin *et al.*, 1978b). Chimaerism can be best documented by the presence of donor-type cells in the blood, lymph nodes, spleen, and BM of the recipients.

Chimaeras maintain permanent and specific tolerance to donor-type alloantigens, thus donor's skin or heart allografts are permanently accepted (> 360 days), whereas third-party skin grafts are promptly rejected. Specific unresponsiveness can also be documented *in vitro* by MLR assays. Lymph node or spleen lymphocytes of chimaeras lose their ability to respond against either parental lymphocytes in a one-way MLR, whereas a positive response can be documented against third-party lymphocytes (Slavin *et al.*, 1978b; Slavin and Strober, 1979).

BM and organ transplantation in dogs

Successful marrow transplantation can also be documented in large outbred animals after TLI. Stable chimaerism was documented in 2 out of 5 unrelated mismatched mongrels conditioned with heavy doses of TLI to separate chest and abdominal fields administered over long periods of time (Slavin *et al.*, 1979b). Continuing work at Stanford University (Gottlieb *et al.*, 1980) demonstrated success in establishing stable BM chimeras in 12 out of 12 unrelated, randomly matched mongrels following conditioning with 18 daily fractions of 100 rads each to chest and abdominal fields in continuity. Chimaerism was confirmed by both karotype analysis and typing of donor's-type red blood cell antigens in recipients following BM transplantation (Gottlieb *et al.*, 1980). In a series of as yet unpublished independent studies, work at Hadassah University Hospital failed to induce consistent chimaerism in mongrels conditioned with TLI using daily fractions of 100–200 rads up to a total of 3000 rads (Slavin *et al.*, in prep.). The reason for the discrepancy in results at the two centres is currently being investigated.

Application of TLI conditioning for successful perfused organ allotransplantation was also recently attempted in unmatched beagles. Untreated dogs uniformly rejected a kidney allograft within a median of 5 days. Long term (>18 months) kidney allograft survival was demonstrated in 2 out of 4 dogs conditioned with TLI (total dose 2400 rads) and infused with a low dose of donor BM cells ($0{\cdot}5 \times 10^8$ cells/kg) (Slavin *et al.*, 1979c; Howard *et al.*, submitted for publication). No further immunosuppressive treatment was applied. The dogs showed no evidence of GVHD in the post-operative recovery period, although no definite chimaerism was demonstrable.

More recently, TLI with and without additional BM cell administration was successfully applied as an adjunct to low dose conventional immunosuppressive treatment (imuran and prednisone) for conditioning of human recipients for transplantation of totally mismatched allografts in poor risk patients who have previously rejected one or more kidney allografts within the first 12 months following transplantation (Najarian *et al.*, submitted for publication). Longer observation periods are necessary to fully assess the advantages and possible long-term side effects of TLI conditioning in clinical organ transplants.

The use of TLI and BM transplantation for correction of metabolic disorders

There has been little progress in finding a practical mode of treatment for the many metabolic diseases in man, including enzyme deficiency disorders. Enzyme-producing allogeneic cells or whole organs may provide a potential intrinsic physiological source of deficient enzymes. Whole organs (kidney, liver, pancreas) and cellular (fibroblasts and bone marrow) transplantations have already been attempted experimentally for the treatment of enzymatic and metabolic disorders (Desnick *et al.*, 1972; Matas *et al.*, 1976; Sutherland *et al.*, 1978; Hong *et al.*, 1979). Unsolved problems in overcoming the rejection phenomenon stand in the way of further clinical trials of whole organ allografts for the treatment of enzyme deficiency disorders. The major obstacles in further application of allogeneic BM transplantation for reconstitution of enzyme-deficient recipients are the HVG and GVHD. The feasibility of enzyme reconstitution in deficient mice was recently explored by evaluating the effectiveness of continuous enzyme supply by allogeneic BM cells.

We report here a new approach for enzyme replacement therapy by allogeneic BM allografts obtained from normal enzyme-producing donors using TLI conditioning of enzyme-deficient recipients to ensure engraftment and prevent GVHD. Inbred β-glucuronidase-deficient C3H/HeJ (H-2^k) mice were used as a model system of enzyme-deficient recipients. Normal enzyme producing BALB/c (H-2^d) mice were used as donors. Enzyme-deficient C3H/HeJ underwent TLI (200 rads $\times$ 17) and 30 $\times$ 10^6 nucleated BALB/c BM cells were administered intravenously one day following radiotherapy. Fresh plasma and liver tissue samples were obtained from experimental mice and intact age and sex matched BALB/c and C3H/HeJ controls at different time intervals following BM inoculation. β-glucuronidase activity was measured in each sample. Chimaerism was detected by measuring the percentage of donor-type (BALB/c) cells in the peripheral blood of BM recipients. C3H/HeJ recipients were fully reconstituted with BALB/c cells ($>90\%$ in the blood) following BM transplantation (Slavin *et al.*, 1980a). Chimaerism persisted throughout an observation period of 7 months but no GVHD was noted. Enzyme activity increased significantly ($P < 0{\cdot}001$) to normal BALB/c levels in all chimaeras tested. The mean specific enzyme activity increased approximately 9-fold in the liver and 2-fold in the plasma. The increase of enzyme activity was attributable to marrow repopulation since no increased activity was noted in mice that underwent radiotherapy without marrow reconstitution (Slavin *et al.*, 1980a). Our data indicate that TLI can be used for establishment of stable GVHD-free, BM chimaeras, using histoincompatible marrow cells as a continuous source of enzyme replacement in enzyme-deficient recipients, providing enzyme activity extracellularly in the cell-free plasma and in the liver tissue.

Mechanisms of tolerance in TLI treated mice

Active suppression of cell-mediated immune responses by different subsets of suppressor cells seems to play an important role in the mechanism of tolerance and in the induction and/or maintenance of the state of tolerance following TLI conditioning. No evidence could be generated so far in support of any major role of humoral blocking factors (Slavin *et al.*, 1980b). Nevertheless, the final basis of the HVG and GVH bilateral transplantation tolerance seen in BM chimaeras prepared with TLI remains to be elucidated.

The cellular basis for tolerance to soluble protein antigens

Antigen specific suppressor T cells in tolerant mice

The active role of specific suppressor T cells in the induction of the state of tolerance to BSA can be documented by experiments involving adoptive transfer of spleen cells obtained from BSA-tolerant mice. Transfer of 1×10^6 BSA-primed T cells and 5×10^6 DNP-BSA primed B cells obtained from spleens of primed mice concomitantly with 5×10^6 spleen cells from TLI-induced BSA-tolerant BALB/c mice results in relative unresponsiveness to a challenge of $DNP_{15}BSA$ in CFA ($\log_{10}$ anti-DNP titre of $0{\cdot}8 \pm 0{\cdot}1$ compared to $1{\cdot}9 \pm 0{\cdot}1$ obtained without coinjection of suppressor spleen cell). The suppressive effect of spleen cells from tolerant mice can be completely abolished ($\log_{10}$ anti-DNP titre of $1{\cdot}9 \pm 0{\cdot}1$) by treating spleen cells with anti-Thy-1·2 and complement prior to transfer, indicating that the suppressor cells are T lymphocytes. The suppressive effects of the spleen cells are specific, since 5×10^6 BSA-tolerized spleen cells fail to suppress the anti-DNP response of mice adoptively transferred with 1×10^6 BGG primed T cells and 5×10^6 DNP-BGG primed B cells following $DNP_{15}BGG$ in CFA challenge (Zan Bar *et al.*, 1978).

Tolerance to soluble protein antigens at the level of B cells

The generation of tolerance on the level of B cells was recently documented by adoptive transfer of spleen B cells obtained from mice rendered tolerant to BSA following conditioning with TLI and injection of nondeaggregated BSA in saline. Control mice were injected with spleen B cells obtained from normal mice or from animals given WBI. Normal T cells were injected into both groups and all irradiated recipients were challenged with BSA in CFA within 24 h of cell transfer. Determination of serum antibody responses 3 weeks later indicated that tolerance was induced only in recipients of B cells from TLI-treated mice (Zan Bar and Slavin, manuscript in prep.).

Suppressor cells of MLR

The suppressive activity of cells obtained from TLI treated (BALB/c × C57BL/6) F_1 mice and from C57BL/Ka → BALB/c chimeras can best be demonstrated by coculturing spleen cells in one-way MLR system, assaying the proliferative capacity (H^3-TDR uptake) of responding cells in the presence of assayed spleen cells as compared to normal (C57BL/Ka × BALB/c) F_1 or inactivated C57BL/Ka spleen cells (in both cases the added spleen cells are unresponsive against either the responding or the stimulating lymphocytes, thus the response remains one-way despite the presence of cells from different sources). The suppressive effects of TLI-treated spleen cells and chimeric spleen cells are relatively radioresistant (1500–3000 rads) and cell-dose dependent. The suppression of MLR by spleen cells obtained from TLI treated mice is maintained for 4–6 weeks, whereas spleen cells obtained from stable chimaeras are able to maintain suppressive capacity for many months with predominantly responder-specific specificity (Slavin and Strober, 1979; 1979f; Slavin *et al.*, 1980d; Zan Bar *et al.*, 1978; Slavin *et al.*, manuscript in prep.). Figure 1 represents an example of MLR suppression by increased proportions of spleen cells obtained from chimaeras in an MLR system in which the relative proportion of suppressor to responder ratio is increased.

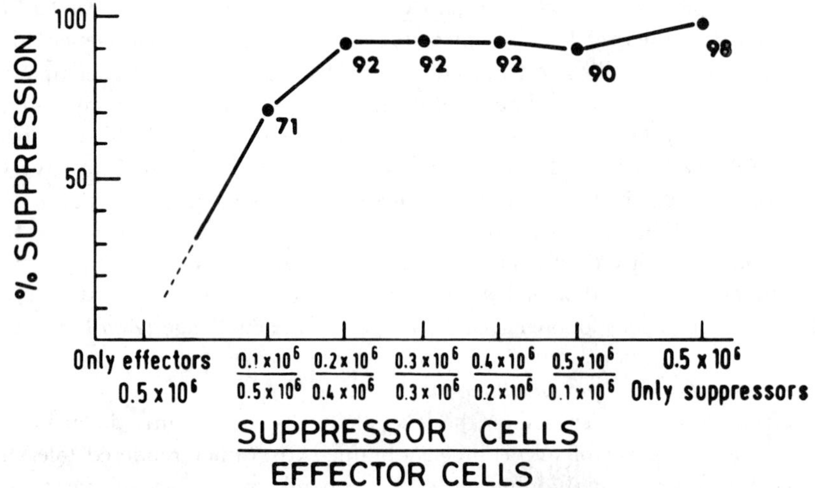

FIG. 1. *Suppression of MLR by increased proportions of spleen cells obtained from 70-day-old C57BL/Ka→BALB/c chimaera. The suppressive effects of different suppressor/responder ratios were measured by comparing H^3-TDr uptake of one-way MLR with cocultured chimaeric and normal (C57BL/Ka × BALB/c)F_1 spleen cells. Responding BALB/c lymph node cell number varied between 0·5 × 10^6 to 0·1 × 10^6, cocultured spleen cell numbers varied between 0·1 × 10^6 to 0·5 × 10^6, and the stimulating C57Bl/Ka lymph node cell number was kept constant (1 × 10^6). The total number of cells per well remained constant (1·6 × 10^6), such as only the ratio of suppressors to responders was altered, increasing from 1/5 to 5/1. Control responses of responders without suppressors, and suppressors without responders was also determined. The data represent the calculated per cent of relative suppression of MLR by chimaeric as compared to normal (C57BL/Ka × BALB/c) F_1 cells as determined by the ratio of the mean H^3-TDR uptake, respectively.*

Adoptive transfer of tolerance to alloantigens

Specific transplantation tolerance can be transferred to sublethally irradiated recipients by the intravenous injection of chimaeric spleen cells. Adoptive BALB/c recipients of 25 × 10^6 C57BL/Ka → BALB/c spleen cells maintain C57BL/Ka skin grafts for more than 250 days, but reject third-party skin grafts within 2–3 weeks. Although normal C57BL/Ka spleen cells injected intravenously into sublethally irradiated BALB/c mice produce vigorous GVHD, the injection of similar numbers of C57BL/Ka cells present in chimaeric spleens produce no clinically evident GVHD. The adoptively transferred allogeneic spleen cells are not rejected as documented by typing donor-type cells in the recipient (Slavin and Strober, 1980, 1979f).

The findings indicate that the C57BL/Ka cells obtained from the chimaeras are unable to respond to the BALB/c alloantigens, since they cannot inititate fatal GVHD in an *in vivo* transfer system. This is consistent with the lack of GVHD in chimaeric donors. It is unclear whether functional or actual clonal deletion, active suppression or both operate in these experiments.

Conclusions and future directions

TLI produces a unique and potent immunomanipulative effect on both arms of the immune system. Nonspecific immunosuppression is extremely potent in the immediate postradiotherapy period. The nonspecific immunosuppressive effects of TLI can be utilized for the treatment of various autoimmune disorders and as a powerful tool in organ transplantation. In addition, TLI conditioning can be used for successful induction of tolerance to soluble protein antigens as well as BM and organ allografts in adult animals. The potential application of TLI for BM and organ transplantation across major genetic barriers merits further study since it may have important clinical implications.

References

Bieber, C. P., Jamieson, S. J., Raney, A., Burton, N., Bogarty, S., Hoppe, R., Kaplan, H. S., Strober, S. and Stinson, E. B. (1979). *Transplantation* **28**, 347.

Desnick, R. J., Allen, K. Y., Simmons, R. L., Woods, J. E., Anderson, C. F., Najarian, J. S. and Krivit, W. (1972). *Surgery* **72**, 203.

Fuks, Z., Strober, S., Bobrove, A. M., Sasazuki, T., McMichael, A. and Kaplan, H. S. (1976). *J. Clin. Invest.* **58**, 803.

Gottlieb, M., Strober, S., Hoppe, R., Grimet, C. and Kaplan, H. S. (1980). *Transplantation* (in press).

Hong, C., Sutherland, D. E. R., Matas, A. J. and Najarian, J. S. (1979). *Transplant. Proc.* **11**, 498.

Howard, R. J., Sutherland, D. E. R., Lum, C. T., Lewis, W. I., Kim, T. H., Slavin, S. and Najarian, J. S. (Submitted for publication.)

Kaplan, H. S. (1972). *In* "Hodgkin's Disease" (H. S. Kaplan, ed.) pp. 216–279. Harvard University Press, Cambridge.

Kotzin, B. L. and Strober, S. (1979). *J. Exp. Med.* **150**, 371.

Matas, A. J., Sutherland, D. E. R., Steffes, M. W., Mauer, S. M., Lowe, A., Simmons, R. L. and Najarian, J. S. (1976). *Science* **192**, 892.

Schurman, D., Hirschman, P., Slavin, S., Singer, M., Moser, K. and Strober, S. (1978). *Trans. Orth. Res. Soc.* **3**, 38.

Slavin, S. (1979). *Proc. Nat. Acad. Sci.* **76**, 5274.

Slavin, S., Strober, S. (1979). *J. Immunol.* **123**, 942.

Slavin, S. and Strober, S. (1980). *In* "Immunobiology of Bone Marrow Transplantation" (S. Thierfelder, H. Rodt and H. J. Kolb eds.) pp. 323–331. Springer-Verlag, New York.

Slavin, S., Strober, S., Fuks, Z. and Kaplan, H. S. (1976). *Science* **193**, 1252.

Slavin, S., Strober, S., Fuks, Z. and Kaplan, H. S. (1977a). *Transplant. Proc.* **9**, 1001.

Slavin, S., Strober, S., Fuks, Z. and Kaplan, H. S. (1977b). *J. Exp. Med.* **146**, 34.

Slavin, S., Reitz, B., Bieber, C. P., Kaplan, H. S. and Strober, S. (1978a). *J. Exp. Med.* **147**, 700.

Slavin, S., Fuks, Z., Kaplan, H. S. and Strober, S. (1978b). *J. Exp. Med.* **147**, 963.

Slavin, S., Fuks, Z., Bieber, C. P., Hoppe, R. T., Kaplan, H. S. and Strober, S. (1979a). *In* "Cell Biology and Immunology of Leukocyte Function". (M. R. Quastel, ed.) pp. 917–924. Academic Press, New York.

Slavin, S., Gottlieb, M., Bieber, C., Hoppe, R., Kaplan, H. S., Strober, S. and Grumet, C. (1979b). *Transplantation* **27**, 139.

Slavin, S., Fuks, Z., Strober, S., Kaplan, H. S., Howard, R. and Sutherland, D. E. R. (1979c). *Transplantation* **28**, 359.

Slavin, S., Zan-Bar, I. and Strober, S. (1979d). *Transplant. Proc.* **11**, 891.

Slavin, S., Fuks, Z., Weiss, L. and Morecki, S. (1980a). *In* "Biology of Bone Marrow Transplantation". ICN-UCLA Symposia on Molecular and Cellular Biology, Vol. XVII (R. Gale and C. Fred Fox, eds.) (in press). Academic Press, New York.

Slavin, S., Yatziv, S., Weiss, L., Morecki, S., Abeliuk, P. and Fuks, Z. (1980b). *Transplant. Proc.* (in press).

Strober, S., Slavin, S., Gottlieb, M., Zan-Bar, I., King, D., Hoppe, R. T., Fuks, Z., Grumet, F. C. and Kaplan, H. S. (1979). *Immunol. Rev.* **46**, 87.

Sutherland, D. E. R., Matas, A. J. and Najarian, J. S. (1978). *Surg. Clin. North Am.* **58**, 365.

Sutherland, D. E. R., Gifford, R. M., Lum, C. T., Lewis, W. I., Howard, R. J., Ferguson, R. M., Kersey, J., Simmons, R. L., Slavin, S., Kim, T. H., Levitt, S. H. and Najarian, J. S. (1980). (Submitted for publication.)

Zan-Bar, I., Slavin, S. and Strober, S. (1978). *J. Immunol.* **121**, 1400.

Zan-Bar, I., Slavin, S. and Strober, S. (1979). *Cell Immunol.* **45**, 167.

62

The Use of Regulatory Biological Products to Manipulate Immune Responses

JEAN-FRANÇOIS BACH

Hôpital Necker, Paris, France

Introduction

The treatment of immunological diseases has been based over the last 20 years on the use of chemical or biological agents that alter immunocompetent cells nonspecifically.

Immunosuppressive agents include antimetabolites (6-mercaptopurine, azathioprine, amethopterin), agents or methods acting directly on nucleic acids (alkylating agents or irradiation, eventually limited to the lymphoid system) and drugs selected by chance screening (the best example being Cyclosporin A) or xenogeneic antisera produced against lymphocytes. Immunostimulating agents include nonphysiologic products such as bacterial extracts, eventually available in a well-defined chemical form like the muramyl dipeptide (MDP) or chemicals (levamisole, bestatin, synthetic polyribonucleotides, isoprinosine, etc).

Recent progress in basic cellular immunology makes it now possible to think of new approaches based on the use of the very numerous and diverse regulatory materials produced by the immune system itself, which are often physiologically active on immunocompetent cells. Some of these products are now well defined and are available in synthetic form. Others, less well defined, can be used in sufficient amounts to permit clinical application. As conventional immunosuppressive or immunostimulating agents, these regulatory biological products are not antigen-specific, with the possible exception of transfer factor. At variance with these products, however, they have the advantage of acting in a physiological way on the regulatory mechanisms whose abnormal function probably explains most immunological diseases. Their natural origin is associated with a lower toxicity and hence an easier clinical use. Their main drawback remains their general lack of availability and their imprecise mode of action.

This is a very wide topic if one thinks of all the mediators released by T cells or macrophages that affect *in vitro* immune responses, as well as the pharmacologically active biological substances, such as prostaglandins or cyclic nucleotides, which also alter lymphocyte functions. Since this theme is devoted to immunomanipulation, I shall restrict myself to those products released by immunocompetent cells that regulate immune responses and have been evaluated *in vivo* in experimental models and, eventually, in man (Table I).

TABLE I

Regulatory biological products used to manipulate immune responses

	Origin	*Main products*
Thymic hormones	Thymic epithelial cells	Thymosins Thymopoietin Thymic humoral factor Serum thymic factor (FTS)
Lymphokines	Activated T cells	TCGF (IL-2) SIRS Immune interferon
Monokines	Macrophages and monocytes	LAF (Il-1)
Leukocyte extracts	Peripheral leukocytes	Transfer factor Immune RNA

Thymic hormones

As soon as the central function of the thymus in immunity was discovered, the hypothesis of a secretion of endocrine factors was postulated. However, it was not until the 1970s that convincing data were produced which demonstrated the stimulation of immunocompetence of thymectomized mice by injections of thymic extracts. Since then, major progress has been achieved concerning both the chemical nature and the biological significance of thymic factors. It has permitted us to envisage the therapeutical application of these factors (or hormones) in various clinical conditions associated with T cell deficiencies.

Two approaches have been used to isolate and characterize thymic hormones. Goldstein extracted from the thymus gland a crude fraction called "thymosin Fraction 5". This preparation, which contains many substances (more than 30 polypeptides including probably many, if not all, the other available thymic factors), is biologically active in various assay systems, both in animals and in man. Starting from this global preparation, Goldstein engaged in a systematic screening of the peptides present in Fraction 5. Other workers started from calf thymus extracts or serum, basing the characterization of their factors on well-defined bioassays: enhancement of an *in vitro* graft v. host reaction for THF (Trainin *et al.*, 1975), depression of neuromuscular conduction for thymopoietin (Goldstein, 1974), increase in θ antigen expression for FTS (Bach *et al.*, 1971). These approaches each led to the isolation of a single but apparently different product. Before discussing the potential relationships between the various products, I shall give a brief review of their main characteristics.

Thymosins

Thymosin Fraction 5 is composed of a group of polypeptides with mol. wts ranging from 1000 to 15 000. They are heat-stable up to 80°C. Goldstein and his associates have undertaken the isolation and characterization of each polypeptide component in thymosin Fraction 5 and a detailed study of their individual biological functions.

To facilitate the identification and comparison of all the thymic peptides from one laboratory to another, they have proposed a nomenclature based on the isoelectric pattern of thymosin Fraction 5 in the pH ranges 3·5–9·5. Peptides are divided into 3 regions: the α region consists of peptides with pI below 5·0, the β region between 5·0 and 7·0, and the γ region above 7·0. The subscripts (1,2 ...) are used to identify the peptides from that region as they are isolated.

With the combination of ion exchange chromatography and gel filtration, 16 polypeptide components have been isolated from Fraction 5 for further characterization: 10 from the α region (a_1–α_{10}) and 6 from the β region (β_1–β_6). Thymosins α_1, β_1 and β_4 have been sequenced, thymosin α_7 and β_3 have been totally purified. α_1 Thymosin has been synthesized and shown to have several of the biological activities of Fraction 5 (Low *et al.*, 1979).

Thymosin Fraction 5 can also induce certain functional changes in lymphocytes, such as the production of macrophage migration inhibitory factor (MIF) and increased production of antibody-forming cells (Low and Goldstein, 1978; Thurman *et al.*, 1978). Thymosin Fraction 5 has been found to be active in an MLR assay measuring the differentiation of murine thymocytes in an allogeneic mixed leukocyte culture, a human E rosette assay (Wara *et al.*, 1975) and mouse mitogen assays *in vitro* (Thurman *et al.*, 1978). Thymosin Fraction 5 can act in lieu of the thymus gland to reconstitute certain immune functions in thymus-deprived and/or immunodeprived individuals. Thus it has been found to induce T cell differentiation and enhance immunological functions in genetically athymic mice, in adult Tx mice, in NZB mice with severe autoimmune reactions, in tumour-bearing mice, and in mice with casein-induced amyloidosis.

Thymosin has also been shown to increase alloantigenic markers in lymphocyte populations (Goldstein *et al.*, 1972; Scheid *et al.*, 1973). Thymosin Fraction 5 can also induce terminal deoxynucleotidyl transferase (TdT), an enzyme found almost exclusively in cortical thymocytes *in vivo* and *in vitro* in the less dense layers of bone marrow cells of nude mice and adult Tx mice (Pazmino *et al.*, 1978).

Thymopoietin

Thymopoietin, a polypeptide hormone of the thymus, was isolated by its neuromuscular effects rather than by its action on the immune system. The development of experimental models of myasthenia gravis led to the detection of a thymic hormone influence on neuromuscular transmission, and electromyographic assays were used to monitor the fractionation of thymus extracts (Goldstein, 1974). By this means, thymopoietin was isolated and the biochemically homogeneous polypeptide was shown to have appropriate potency (4 ng/mouse) in the neuromuscular assay. Thymopoietin was also shown to be capable of inducing various T cell specific alloantigens *in vitro* in the Komuro and Boyse (1973) assay (Goldstein, 1977).

Thymopoietin is a 49 amino acid polypeptide isolated to chemical homogeneity from thymus extracts. The complete amino acid sequence of thymopoietin has been determined (Goldstein, 1977). Two forms, termed thymopoietin I and II, differ by only 2 amino acid substitutions. A synthetic pentapeptide has the complete activity of thymopoietin, being selective for T cell differentiation *in vitro*. Recently, thymopoietin or its pentapeptide fragment (TP-5) have been shown to enhance several T cell functions *in vivo* (rejection of carcinoma, prevention of autoimmunity in mice, generation of cytotoxic T cells) (Goldstein, 1977; Lau and Goldstein, 1980a, b).

Thymic humoral factor

Using an *in vitro* graft versus host assay, Trainin and colleagues have characterized a small mol. wt peptide called "thymic humoral factor" (THF). Using a crude thymic extract dialysate as a source of THF, Trainin showed that THF was capable of restoring the ability of lymphoid cells from neonatally Tx mice to participate in mixed lymphocyte reaction (Umiel and Trainin, 1975), to kill tumour cells (Carnaud *et al.*, 1973) and to react to T lectins (Rotter and Trainin, 1974). The administration of THF to humans suffering either from primary or from secondary immunodeficiencies results in the restoration of cellular immunocompetence, while progressive clinical improvement of these patients was observed (Zaizov *et al.*, 1979). Immune maturation of thymus-deprived lymphoid cells after *in vitro* or *in vivo* exposure to THF occurs via an obligatory rise in cellular cAMP levels (Kook and Trainin, 1974; Yakir *et al.*, 1978). THF was isolated by a procedure which consisted of a stepwise gel filtration through Sephadex columns. When tested in terms of the acquisition of competence by spleen cells from neonatally Tx mice in an *in vitro* assay of GVh reactivity, it appeared that the pure material of THF is a polypeptide of 3000 mol. wt (Yakir *et al.*, 1978)

Serum thymic factor (FTS)

Using the rosette θ and/or azathioprine conversion assay, we have characterized a serum factor capable of inducing T cell markers in T cell precursors. This serum factor (Facteur Thymique Sérique) (FTS) is absent in the serum of nude or Tx mice and reappears after thymus grafting. Chemical analysis (Dardenne *et al.*, 1977) showed that it is a peptide of mol. wt close to 900, with the following sequence: <Glu-Ala-Lys-Ser-Gln-Gly-Gly-Ser-Asn (Bach *et al.*, 1976; Pleau *et al.*, 1977).

Synthesis of this factor was accomplished by several laboratories, notably that of Bricas. Recently, the latter synthesized a series of analogues which made it possible to identify the biologically active site and the antigenic site of the molecule (Bricas *et al.*, 1977; Bach *et al.*, 1978).

We have compared synthetic FTS and natural FTS (extracted from pig serum) in many biological and biochemical tests, without being able to detect the least difference between the two products.

The presence of FTS in the thymus has been demonstrated by different approaches (Bach *et al.*, 1978). Firstly, fractionation of a thymic extract on Sephadex G-25 gel reveals the presence of molecules with a mol. wt close to that of FTS that are fully biologically active in the rosette assay. The relationship between such molecules and FTS is detected by the identical amino acid composition and the binding of such molecules to an antibody raised in rabbits against synthetic FTS (Dardenne *et al.*, 1980). We cannot exclude the possibility that the material thus extracted from the thymus is, or also exists as, a slightly larger molecule than FTS, and might be, for example, a precursor. In any case, this material is closely related to FTS since, in addition to having a very similar mol. wt, it shares the same antigenicity and biological activity. Lastly, the anti-FTS antibody has been shown to bind specifically to mouse thymic epithelium (Monier *et al.*, 1980).

Discussion of the multiplicity of thymic factors

The multiplicity of thymic factors is puzzling, and the relationships of the various thymic factors discussed above are still a matter of some confusion. The list of available peptides is already long. It should be made clear that the various factors (apparently all peptides) that have been charcterized in the thymus or in the serum, have not all been sequenced and thus direct comparison is not possible. In addition, it is likely that not all of these factors are involved in T cell differentiation. In fact, one may classify them into 3 categories:

(1) factors involved in T cell differentiation physiologically *in vivo*;

(2) factors, pharmacologically active on lymphocytes, able to induce T cell markers and eventually to modulate some T cell functions, but not capable of inducing long-term T cell differentiation in Tx mice;

(3) factors that show no activity whatsoever on lymphocytes.

It is likely that some of thymosin Fraction 5 peptides should be included in the third category. Whether a given factor belongs to the first or the second category is a difficult question which has not been adequately resolved for most of these peptides. The bioassays generally used do not always discriminate between true, long-term differentiation and "marker" induction. It is, however, a crucial question since, in the absence of a strict definition, ubiquitin (Goldstein, 1977) or cyclic AMP (Scheid *et al.*, 1973; Kook and Trainin, 1974; Bach *et al.*, 1975) would be considered to possess the full activity of thymic hormones. It is reassuring to see that some well-defined factors, such as FTS of THF show a large variety of properties, some of which are directly related to T cell differentiation.

Finally, can we deduce any significant relationship between the various available factors that we have cited: in other words, are all "biologically relevant" thymus factors independent ones, as if the use of different methodology had led each investigator to the discovery of different molecules, or did these differences in chemical and biological approaches provide, in some instances, products which are chemically different, but which are related in some way (precursors, carriers ...)?

Chemical relationships

Several types of chemical relationship may be considered. The precursor hypothesis is the most attractive one. It does not apply to thymopoietin, thymosin α_1 or β_4 nor FTS, that do not present any homology in their amino acid sequence. It could, however, operate for thymosins other than α_1, or β_4, THF with regard to smaller factors, such as FTS. In fact, we have found FTS or a related product to be present in Fraction 5 (Dardenne *et al.*, 1980), and it could be that one of the Fraction 5 peptides is a FTS precursor.

Another type of chemical relationship between peptides relates to the cleavage of large molecules into smaller fragments. Thus, renin induces the appearance of angiotensin in the circulation, and growth hormone that of the somatomedins that mediate many of its biological effects. FTS could be, for example, a sort of "thymomedin" generated in the thymus and perhaps also in the periphery under the effect of another substance that could be any of the other thymic peptides.

Target cells of thymic hormones

Thymic factors do not act identically on various lymphocyte subsets. The analysis and the discussion of the functions that are the most readily affected by the various available thymic factors should prove useful for the understanding of the role of thymic factors in T cell differentiation.

Indirect evidence, essentially based on Stutman's work (1978), indicates that thymic factors probably act at the level of a so-called "post-thymic precursor cell", as found in neonatal spleen. Such a post-thymic cell has already encountered the thymic influence, probably by direct contact with the epithelium, where, in addition to receiving the nonantigen-specific maturation signal, it has gained its anti-H-2 (or Ia) receptors that will be needed for the various T cell cognitive functions.

Data obtained with purified or synthetic thymic factors are generally compatible with this hypothesis. There are some reports according to which thymic factors might act in nude mice or totally T cell deprived mice (thymectomized, irradiated, reconstituted with antitheta serum-treated bone marrow cells), but these publications either concern cell markers (Bach *et al.*, 1975; Scheid *et al.*, 1975) and do not provide direct information on functional T cell differentiation, or do not relate to T cell functions (Ikhehara *et al.*, 1975), but have not been confirmed. Most data, whether obtained *in vitro* or *in vivo*, derive from studies in normal adult Tx, partially T cell deprived, NZB or aged mice, which may show some degree of T cell deficiency, but which share the property of possessing post-thymic cells.

Marker studies indicate that the various types of T cell differentiation antigens may be induced in precursor cells which are devoid of such markers. This was initially shown for the θ antigen, using various thymic extracts (Bach *et al.*, 1971), and has now been confirmed and extended for Lyt-1,2 and 3 antigens, TL antigens and xenogeneic antigens (Scheid *et al.*, 1975). Most available thymic factors appear to induce such differentiation antigens. In particular, FTS induces the θ and Ly antigens in the mouse, and xenogeneic T cell antigens in the human (Bach *et al.*, 1978; Incefy *et al.*, 1980).

Other T cell markers are induced by thymic factors. In particular, terminal deoxynucleotidyl transferase (TdT) expression is modified by incubation of immature lymphoid cells with thymic factors. Interestingly, the effects differ according to the cell type considered. TdT is increased by thymosin in nude mouse spleen cells (Pazmino *et al.*, 1978) and decreased in normal bone marrow cells by synthetic FTS in BSA gradient-separated human bone marrow cells (Incefy *et al.*, 1980). Human E rosettes are seemingly increased *in vitro* and *in vivo* by all available factors (Wara *et al.*, 1975; Zaizov *et al.*, 1979; Incefy *et al.*, 1980; Incefy *et al.*, 1975).

Most T cell functions have been reported to be induced or enhanced by thymic factors (provided the adequate recipient is selected, as discussed above).

Thymic hormones enhance T cell mediated cytotoxicity in Tx mice. This effect is particularly clear in adult Tx mice using the Brunner assay (Bach, 1977). Similarly, FTS also acts on T cells involved in delayed-type hypersensitivity induced by DNFB (Erard *et al.*, 1979). It restores a normal response in adult Tx mice. The effect of thymic hormones on helper T cells as studied on anti-SRBC antibody production is much less clear, perhaps due to a simultaneous action on suppressor T cells.

In fact, thymic hormones have recently proved to be remarkably active on suppressor T cells in various *in vitro* and *in vivo* systems (Bach *et al.*, 1978; Erard *et al.*, 1979). Given *in vivo* to normal mice, FTS suppresses the generation of alloantigen reactive T cells or DNFB-sensitive T cells. Given at 10–100 ng, it may prolong skin allograft survival. Lastly, *in vitro*, FTS and thymosin Fraction 5 (Horowitz, 1977) reconstitute, in a very significant fashion, the depressed capacity of most lupus patients to generate suppressor T cells after con A activation, assessed on PWM-driven immunoglobulin synthesis.

This new effect of thymic factors complicates the interpretation of the biological data observed in various functions, but widens the potential therapeutic applications. It appears, as far as FTS is concerned, that the suppressor effect is essentially observed at high "pharmacological" FTS doses, while other effects are seen at lower, presumably physiological, doses. Whether this difference in dose is related to a difference in the cellular receptors of suppressor T cells compared to helper T cells or other T cells, is not known. Whether it is related to a pharmacological stimulation of mature suppressor cells or to an induction or maturation of suppressor T cell precursors is similarly not determined. Note, however, that a nonspecific inhibitory effect on immune responses is made unlikely by the prevention of the effect by pretreatment of recipient mice by low doses of cyclophosphamide, known to inhibit suppressor T cells selectively in various systems.

It is interesting to note that this effect of FTS on suppressor cells probably explains most of its preventive effects observed in NZB autoimmune mice (decrease in anti-PVP antibody production, prevention of Sjögren syndrome (Bach *et al.*, 1978). A simultaneous effect on helper T cells probably explains the accelerated production of IgG anti-DNA antibodies also observed in these mice.

Mode of action at the cellular level

The cellular mode of action of thymic hormones may be studied at two levels: cellular receptors and cAMP. We have recently demonstrated the presence of specific FTS receptors on T cell lines derived from patients with acute lymphoblastic leukaemia (Pleau *et al.*, 1980). FTS was labelled by tritium, using sodium borohydride. Cultured lymphocytes were incubated with labelled FTS for 90 min; 12–15% FTS bound to the cell lines and the specificity of the binding was assessed by the strong inhibition of the binding obtained by addition of unlabelled FTS (10^{-8} M). In fact, it was even possible to displace labelled FTS by secondary addition of unlabelled FTS after 90 min incubation. The fact that some T cell lines did not bind FTS indicates that T cells do not express FTS receptors at all stages of T cell differentiation.

Finally, receptors with a high binding affinity for FTS ($K_D = 10^{-9}$) appear to exist on T cells. That these receptors are associated with the biological effects of FTS is likely but remains to be demonstrated.

The effect of thymic hormones on cAMP and GMP remains a matter of controversy and speculation. In brief, cAMP and products increasing its intracellular level mimic the induction of markers achieved by thymic factors (Scheid *et al.*, 1973; Kook and Trainin, 1974; Bach and Bach, 1972, 1973). However, with the exception of THF, thymic factors do not stimulate cAMP synthesis as evaluated directly at the total lymphocyte level (Low and Goldstein, 1978; Hadden, 1978; Bach, 1977). Thymopoietin and thymosin Fraction 5 have been reported to increase cGMP level (Naylor *et al.*, 1976; Sunshine *et al.*, 1978), but this effect has not been found with other thymic extracts. The paradox between indirect evidence suggesting cAMP involvement and difficulties in showing a direct cAMP increase could relate (1) to the dilution of thymic hormone target cells among other lymphoid cells, rendering impossible the evaluation of a modest increase in cAMP level in such a minority of cells, and (2) to an effect restricted to a cytoplasmic or nuclear cAMP pool. Studies in progress using the T cell line mentioned above should provide an interesting and new approach to this problem, since the cultured T cells in question represent an homogeneous source of FTS-responsive cells. The description by Astaldi *et al.* (1976) of a thymus-dependent serum factor that stimulates cAMP synthesis in mouse thymocytes should be recalled here.

Clinical applications

The diversity of the biological effects of thymic factors and, more generally, the central role of the thymus in the regulation of immune responses indicate that thymic hormones could have major therapeutical applications.

Thymic extracts have been injected into patients with various types of immunodeficiency or malignancy. Crude extracts have exclusively been used so far—thymosin Fraction 5 (Wara *et al.*, 1975; Wara and Amman, 1978;

Schafer *et al.*, 1976a, b; Aleksandrowicz *et al.*, 1975; Ishizawa *et al.*, 1978), thymus dialysate (Zaizov *et al.*, 1979). Clinical cases included congenital immunodeficiencies (Wara *et al.*, 1975; Schafer *et al.*, 1976a; Aleksandrowicz *et al.*, 1975), malignancies (Schafer *et al.* 1976a; Chretien *et al.*, 1979), viral infections complicating leukaemia (Zaizov *et al.*, 1977) and thermal burns (Ishizawa *et al.*, 1978).

Clinical results are difficult to evaluate, except in some series where randomized trials have been performed. No obvious signs of toxicity were observed and no clear accident of hypersensitivity has been noted, even in fairly long-term treatments, as used in some cases of congenital immunodeficiency (Wara and Amman, 1978). An overall favourable effect on T cell markers has been observed in most series, in particular normalization of T cell numbers, assessed by the E rosette test, an effect apparently predictable *in vitro* in individual cases by the restoration of normal E rosette numbers by pre-incubation of the lymphocytes with the thymic extract (Wara *et al.*, 1979). Effect on mitogen responsiveness and on delayed hypersensitivity reactions has been observed in some cases and favourable clinical effects have been suggested in many cases. However, the only convincing results are those obtained in a randomized trial of lung cancer (Chretien *et al.*, 1979). In brief, patients with small cell carcinoma of the lung receiving intensive chemotherapy were randomized to receive thymosin Fraction 5 at a dose of 60 mg/m^2, thymosin at a dose of 20 mg/m^2, or placebo twice weekly. Increased survival occurred in patients receiving the thymosin dose of 60 mg/m^2. The increase in survival was greater in patients with low pretreatment T cell and HS-glycoprotein levels. Note, however, that the mechanism of action of thymosin on lung cancer is not easy to understand, since the existence and role of T cell deficiency in such malignancy are still ill-defined. Particularly promising results have also been obtained with THF in postleukaemia-varicella (Zaizov *et al.*, 1979). One must hope that in the coming months more randomized trials will be performed and that synthetic thymic factors will be used instead of crude thymic extracts. Three synthetic factors are already available (α-1 thymosin, thymopoietin or its shorter analogues, and FTS) and the large-scale use of thymic extracts is hardly conceivable.

In addition to the indications mentioned above, other clinical conditions might benefit from thymic hormone therapy. Acute viral infections, such as measles, zoster and herpes, occurring on immunodeficient background and/or complicated by severe brain or lung localizations should represent important future indications, particularly when associated with patent signs of T cell deficiency, as assessed by marker studies. A particular case should be made for ageing patients who are likely to present with T cell deficiency secondary to thymic involution and are known to lack circulating thymic hormone. Lepromatous leprosy, cutaneomucous candidiasis are also apparently associated with some type of T cell deficiency and could be favourably influenced by thymic hormones.

The problem of autoimmune diseases is more complex. On the one hand, data have accumulated to show that most experimental and clinical autoimmune diseases are associated with a defect in suppressor T cells. Such a defect is also suspected in multiple sclerosis and atopic asthma. On the other hand, it is not proven that such a deficiency is a primary event in the disease and, in particular, one cannot exclude the risk of stimulating simultaneously suppressor and helper T cells. In fact, when treating NZB and B/W mice with synthetic FTS, we have observed improvement or prevention of the Sjögren syndrome and haemolytic anaemia, simultaneously with an enhancement of the production of anti-DNA antibodies (Bach *et al.*, 1978). It is likely that Sjögren syndrome and haemolytic anaemia are exclusively under suppressor T cell control, whereas the production of anti-DNA antibodies is regulated by both helper and suppressor T cells, and that, in the protocol used, helper T cells have been operationally more stimulated than suppressor cells. This observation, similar to others recently reported in the literature, does not deny there is a future for the thymic hormone treatment of lupus and other autoimmune diseases (with a better choice of doses or association with agents selectively inhibiting helper T cells), but it does urge for caution in the use of thymic hormones or any other T cell stimulating agent in autoimmune diseases.

Finally, the potential scope of the clinical action of thymic hormones is very large. Much uncertainty persists, however, at the level of the mode of action of the available factors on the different T cell subsets, and on the cellular abnormalities involved in immunological diseases. These limitations should not prevent the development of future clinical trials, but call for particular caution in the follow-up of patients and in the interpretation of immunological and clinical data.

Lymphokines

Activated T cells produce a wide array of soluble mediators. Some of them are antigen specific and are possibly related to the antigen recognition T cell receptors. They include both helper and suppressor factors. Although such antigen-specific factors have been used *in vivo* (Taussig, 1974), their clinical use still appears a very remote possibility.

In addition to such factors, activated T cells produce a number of non-antigen-specific factors with very diverse biological properties, involving multiple targets. Many of these mediators, for which the general term "lymphokines" has been coined, modify the level or the quality of immune responses and may be considered as physiological regulatory molecules. A limited number of attempts to evaluate the *in vivo* effects of lymphokines have been reported. Cohen and Yoshida (1979) have shown that the injection of MIF-containing preparations induced a monocytopenia and transiently suppressed delayed hypersensitivity reactions in the guinea-pig. Some of them have been used in *in vivo* experiments such as the skin reactive factor(s) and could be used in the future in clinical conditions. I will discuss in more detail 3 of these products with particularly promising activities in the context of immunomanipulation: (1) T cell growth factor (TCGF); (2) soluble immune response suppressor (SIRS); (3) interferon.

T cell growth factor (TCGF)

Alloantigen or mitogen-induced stimulation of T cells leads to the production of nonantigen-specific soluble mediators that may enhance immune responses in *in vitro* assays, e.g. antibody production against thymus-dependent antigens, the mixed lymphocyte reaction, and the generation of cytotoxic T cells (Altman and Cohen, 1975; Möller, 1980). In addition, supernatants of mitogen or alloantigen activated T cells are capable of supporting the long-term growth of antigen-activated functional T cells (Gillis and Smith, 1977; Morgan *et al.*, 1976). Numerous authors have reported factors with similar activity with mol. wts ranging between 15 000 and 50 000. Such factors include the thymocyte stimulating factor, the costimulator and TGCF (Möller, 1980). These factors which are, as yet, undistinguishable, have been grouped under the name of interleukin 2 (IL-2) (Möller, 1980), by contrast to the macrophage-produced lymphocyte activating factor (LAF) called interleukin 1 (IL-1). IL-2 is produced by T cells, but converging arguments indicate that adherent cells are also necessary for its production. More precisely, the hypothesis has been put forward that the macrophage product LAF IL-1, which has no direct IL-2 activity, induces the production of IL-2. Small numbers of adherent cells are required for optimal IL-2 production. LAF (IL-1) totally replaces the requirement for adherent cells. LAF has no proliferative effect on nude mouse spleen cells.

IL-2 has so far essentially been used in *in vitro* experiments. It could also eventually be used *in vivo* and is likely to produce strong immunostimulating effects. In fact, in his initial experiments on the allogeneic effect Katz showed that allogeneic reaction products could substitute for helper T cells in antibody production and eventually in T cell-mediated immunity (Katz *et al.*, 1971, 1972). Retrospectively, it is likely that the allogeneic effect is mediated by IL-2 or a related molecule expressing Ia antigens at variance with IL-2.

More recently, Wagner *et al.* (1980) have shown that when IL-2 is injected locally into lymph nodes, the local generation of TNP specific cytotoxic T cells may be increased dramatically. However, the same authors also reported on the existence of an IL-2 serum inhibitor which blocks IL-2 effects in a dose-related fashion. Such an inhibitor could play an important role physiologically in the regulation of IL-2 effects. Therapeutically, it could pose a difficult pharmacological problem.

IL-2 has been shown to stimulate various aspects of T cell functions in immature T cells, particularly in nude mouse spleen cells (Gillis *et al.*, 1979 and in cortical thymocytes (Wagner *et al.*, 1980). These effects are reminiscent of those previously discussed for thymic hormones (Table II). One may

TABLE II
Comparison of thymic hormones and of interleukin 2

	Thymic hormones	*Interleukin 2 (TCGF)*
Site of production	Thymic epithelium	Lyt-1 T^+ cells
Mol. wt	1000–5000	15 000–40 000
Sensitivity to serum inhibitor	+ (FTS)	+
Functions		
T cell markers	+ +	+
Mitogen responses		
Nude mouse	+	+ +
Neonatally Tx mouse	+	
Adult Tx mouse	+ +	
Thymocytes	+ (?)	
Allogeneic responses		
MLR nude	–	+ +
thymocytes	+	
CTL nude	–	+ +
adult Tx mouse	+ (*in vivo*)	
Regulatory T cells		
helper	+	+
suppressor	+	?

hypothesize that IL-2 acts as an amplification circuit for T cell differentiation, once Lyt-1 T cells have been produced in sufficient amounts under the control of the thymic epithelium and thymic hormones. In any case, the recent demonstration of the *in vivo* immunoenhancing effects of IL-2 in nude mice (Gillis *et al.*, 1979) and in neonatally thymectomized mice (Stutman, pers. comm.) indicates that IL-2 could also be used in immunodeficiency syndromes.

Finally, IL-2 appears as one of the most potent lymphokines. Its potential clinical use can be foreseen. One should recall, however, that IL-2 is still not well defined (chemically it is not certain whether one or several molecular entities are involved). It is to be hoped that the recent report of IL-2 producing tumours will help to obtain sufficient amounts of material for chemical characterization.

Suppressor factors (SIRS)

Supernatants from con A-activated T cells contain a mediator, named soluble immune response suppressor (SIRS), which suppresses nonspecifically *in vitro* antibody formation against several thymus-dependent and thymus-independent antigens (Pierce and Kapp, 1976; Pierce and Tadakuma, 1978; Kapp *et al.*, 1978). SIRS is produced by T cells (namely the Lyt-23+ subset) and macrophages are required for its production. The action of SIRS is not due to transferred con A. It is fairly selective of antibody responses and there is no action on cytotoxic or proliferative activities of T cells (Pierce and Kapp, 1976; Kapp *et al.*, 1978). Physicochemical studies have revealed that SIRS is a glycoprotein with a mol. wt of the order of 50 000. No difference has been detected biochemically so far with MIF and it is suggested that SIRS and MIF represent different biological functions of the same molecule. Conversely, SIRS should be distinguished from a mediator described by Rich and Rich (1976; Rich *et al.*, 1979) which is present in the supernatant of the mixed lymphocyte reaction. This factor bears MHC determinants and nonspecifically suppresses mixed lymphocyte reactions and cytotoxic responses of T cells syngeneic at the I-C subregion with the cells producing the factor. The target cell of SIRS is the macrophage, as shown by separate exposure of purified macrophages and spleen lymphocytes to SIRS for 2 h, followed by washing and recombination (Pierce and Kapp, 1976). The suppression exerted by SIRS-treated macrophages is an active process mediated by soluble factors released by the macrophages, which will in turn inhibit B cell proliferation and differentiation.

SIRS has been used *in vivo* in an attempt to suppress autoimmune responses. Spontaneously autoimmune (NZB × NZW)F_1 mice prematurely lose their capacity to produce SIRS after exposure of their spleen cells to con A, but keep their sensitivity to SIRS-induced suppression (Krakauer *et al.*, 1976). Long-term treatment of (NZB × NZW)F_1 mice has been shown to prevent very significantly the onset of antinuclear autoantibodies and of immune complex glomerulonephritis (Krakauer *et al.*, 1977). Note, however, that when injected too late in the life of autoimmune mice, SIRS no longer shows its protective effect and may, conversely, accelerate the disease (Steinberg *et al.*, 1978). This adverse effect is possibly due to the presence of factors other than SIRS in the supernatant of con A-activated T cells, such as helper factors of the IL-2 type.

Interferons

Interferon has been known for 20 years as an antiviral molecule produced by virus-infected cells. Two lines of findings have indicated in recent years that interferon may have tight relationships with the immune system.

An interferon-like molecule is produced by lymphoid cells activated by an antigen, an alloantigen, or by a polyclonal T cell activator such as phytohaemagglutinin or con A (Younger and Salvin, 1973). This "immune interferon" (Type II) is biochemically similar to, but distinct from, the classical virus-induced leukocyte or fibroblast interferon (Type I) (Younger and Salvin, 1973). It has analogous biological effects, including the antiviral activity which defines it. It should be noted, however, that in many experiments using immune interferon, partially purified material is used and proof that the immunomodulatory effect is due to interferon (and not to another lymphokine) has not been established.

In addition to their direct antiviral effects, interferons (Type I or Type II) have modulatory effects on the immune system. It is these effects which will be reviewed here in view of their potential clinical applications.

It has been known for several years that Type I interferon inhibits the proliferative response of mouse lymphocytes to mitogens or allogeneic cells (Sonnefeld and Merigan, 1979). It has also been shown that interferons alter antibody production both *in vitro* (Gisler *et al.*, 1974) and *in vivo* (Brodeur and Merigan, 1975). In fact, the effect of interferon on the humoral immune response is time-dependent. Given between 4 and 48 h before antigenic stimulation, interferons are immunosuppressive, but given between 48 and 72 h before, immunostimulation is observed (Sonnefeld *et al.*, 1977; Virelizier *et al.*, 1977).

Interferons can also modulate cell-mediated immune responses. They inhibit the development of delayed-type hypersensitivity reactions in the mouse (De Maeyer *et al.*, 1975a, b), suppress graft v. host reactions (Hirsch *et al.*, 1973), and may prolong skin allograft survival (Hirsch *et al.*, 1974).

The effect of interferon on cytotoxic cells has recently been the matter of extensive investigation. Cytotoxic T cells, cytotoxic macrophages and natural killer (NK) cells all show increased activity after *in vivo* or *in vitro* treatment with Type I interferon (Trinchieri *et al.*, 1978). The effect on NK cells is a very striking one, whether interferon is used directly or whether interferon-inducing agents such as polyriboinosinic-polyribocytidylic acid are administered. It is not known whether interferon activates existing NK cells, as with the activation of macrophages by lymphokines, or triggers the differentiation of a precursor to the NK cells into an effector cell (Bloom, 1980). One should note that, paradoxically, the enhancement of cytotoxic T cell activity is associated with a depression of mixed lymphocyte reaction (Heron *et al.*, 1976).

In addition to these effects on immune responses, interferons have been shown to alter the expression of the antigens present on lymphocyte membranes. In particular, the H-2D and H-2K molecules show increased expression on the surface of thymocytes or fibroblasts after *in vivo* or *in vitro* exposure to interferons (Lindahl *et al.*, 1976; Vignaux and Gresser, 1977). This action could contribute to the enhancement of T cell cytotoxicity against virus-infected cells, since such cytotoxicity involves the simultaneous recognition of H-2 and virus-induced membrane antigens. More recently it has been shown that Type I interferon can cause an increase in the expression of antigen-binding receptors on T cell receptors (Lonai and Steinman, 1977). Type I and Type II interferons show similar immunomodulatory activities. Several reports would tend to suggest that for identical antiviral activity, immune interferon is a much more potent immunomodulator than leukocyte interferon. In fact, one may wonder whether immune interferon does not represent the major "suppressive" lymphokine. Its chemical relationship with SIRS would be important to determine. Its interrelations with thymic hormones should also be studied, since thymic factors possess analogous immunomodulatory effects and recent reports have shown that they induce interferon production

(Eshel *et al.*, 1980) and increase NK cell activity (Bardos *et al.*, 1980).

Interferon (Type I) has been used clinically in several conditions where an antiviral effect was desired. More recently, interferon has been given to patients showing a decreased production of interferon, either as part of a complex immune disorder or as a selective defect (Virelizier and Griscelli, 1980).

Lymphocyte activating factor (LAF)

Macrophages and monocytes synthesize several substances that are known to regulate immune responses such as prostaglandins, free radicals and proteins. Such proteins, to which the general name of monokines has been given, have the property of replacing macrophages in a number of macrophage-dependent *in vitro* lymphocyte activation processes, such as mitogen and antigen-induced proliferation, generation of cytotoxic T cells, and enhancement of antibody responses to thymus-dependent antigens.

The lymphocyte activating factor (LAF) also named recently interleukin 1 (IL-1) was initially described as a macrophage produced mediator with thymocyte mitogenic activity. Its production is enhanced by lipopolysaccharides and allogeneic reactions. LAF size is of the order of 10 000–20 000. Recently, its production by a macrophage cell line has been reported (Mizel, 1979). The initial LAF target cell is a matter of controversy. Some authors favour the antibody forming cell precursor (B cell), as the primary target (Wood *et al.*, 1976; Hoffmann, 1979).

Others (Farrar *et al.*, 1979) favour a primary action on T cells which then participate in secondary T–T or T–B interactions. This latter hypothesis is strengthened by the demonstration of LAF effect on the generation of cytotoxic T cells. Recent data would suggest that LAF and TCGF are sequentially linked (Smith *et al.*, 1980; Wagner *et al.*, 1980). LAF has not yet been thoroughly evaluated *in vivo*. One may think however, that when it is purified and chemically characterized LAF could represent an important therapeutic tool.

Transfer factor

It is now more than 25 years since Lawrence (1949) reported transfer, in humans, of delayed skin sensitivity to streptococcal M substance and tuberculin with disrupted leukocytes. It was soon noted that, at variance with what is observed in guinea-pigs, the passively, acquired sensitive state persisted for many months. It was then possible to obtain the transfer by using dialysable extract. Transfer factor (TF) was then defined as a dialysable component of leukocyte extracts having the property of transferring antigen-specific immunological reactivity from a sensitive donor to a naïve recipient. Major efforts have been devoted since first discoveries to resolve the following 4 major issues: 1) true antigen specificity of transfer; 2) chemical nature of active molecule(s); 3) *in vitro* assay to evaluate active preparations; 4) clinical efficacy. It is fair to recognize that in spite of the multitude of published reports on these 4 points, no consensus has emerged.

Antigen specificity

The problem of the antigen specificity of TF should be approached in precise terms. Four nontotally mutually exclusive main hypotheses may theoretically be distinguished:

(1) TF may transfer true antigen-specific (and antigen free) chemical information, as in Lawrence's original hypothesis;

(2) TF contains antigen, with or without adjuvant factor;

(3) TF is essentially acting by enhancing pre-existing subliminal immunity;

(4) TF stimulates *de novo* the immune system nonspecifically.

These four hypotheses have already been the matter of extensive discussion that we shall not reiterate here. We shall discuss later the possibility that some of the peptides known to be present in TF preparations are responsible for the nonantigen-specific TF effects and are in fact thymic hormones that are bound to the lymphocytes from which TF is extracted.

The antigen specificity of the transfer has been demonstrated in several settings in a very conclusive way, using *de novo* sensitization by well defined antigens. Thus, TF prepared in KLH-sensitized subjects confers sensitivity to KLH, whereas TF prepared in the same subjects before KLH sensitization does not (Burger *et al.*, 1977).

The problem, thus, is not to question the antigen specificity but to evaluate the contribution of concomitant, nonantigen-specific stimulation of the immune system which might obscure the specificity and the clinical effects of TF. There is, indeed, compelling evidence for nonantigen-specific effects that we shall review below. In the very domain of DTH itself, it has been shown that DTH could be induced to antigens against which the donor was anergic (Kirkpatrick, 1978) and more generally, it is striking to note how efficacious TF preparations from normal (nonhyperimmune) subjects are in different clinical conditions. The erratic results observed in the specificity of immune reactivity induced by TF could be explained in individual cases by the non-specific enhancement of host subliminal immunity or by a specific transfer of a DTH state that was not expressed in the donor.

Transfer factor has been shown to possess a number of nonantigen-specific immunological activities such as:

enhancement of E rosette formation, notably after *in vitro* trypsin treatment (Valdimarsson *et al.*, 1974) or heat treatment (Mendes *et al.*, 1975);

increase of PHA responses (Arala-Chaves *et al.*, 1974; Hamblin *et al.*, 1976);

increase of antigen driven DNA synthesis (Burger *et al.*, 1976) in a non antigen specific manner;
induction of LAF release by macrophages (Togawa *et al.*, 1980);
increase in the synthesis of cyclic GMP by monocytes (Sandler *et al.*, 1975) and of cAMP by both monocytes and lymphocytes (Kirkpatrick and Smith, 1976);
chemotactic activity for granulocytes and monocytes (Gallin and Kirkpatrick, 1974).

It is interesting to note that many of these actions are also produced by the thymic hormones mentioned above. It is possible that the peptides found in TF preparations which could explain these effects are related to thymic hormones or even represent circulating thymic hormone contaminating leukocytes.

This hypothesis of TF contamination by thymic factors could be tested in several ways: comparison of TF obtained in normal or thymectomized (or aged) donors who lack thymic hormone, direct demonstration of the presence of thymic factor in TF by use of a radioimmunoassay, removal of some of the TF biological activities by passage on an anti-FTS immunoadsorbent or study of the binding of TF to FTS receptors.

Search for an *in vitro* assay

Only few and sometimes controversial data are available on the *in vivo* effects of transfer factor in other species than man, even if some progress has been made recently in guinea-pigs, subhuman primates, dogs and especially in mice for which 3 laboratories have independently reported successful transfer of delayed type hypersensitivity with leukocyte extracts.

This limitation has represented a severe handicap for the chemical characterization and the clinical application of TF. It has led numerous investigators to set up an *in vitro* assay that would detect the antigen-specific activity of TF. Some authors used the various *in vitro* assays of lymphokines. Paque *et al.* (1969) reported that when lymphoid cells were exposed to whole leukocyte lysates, they responded to *in vitro* stimulation in a fashion apparently specific for the antigens to which the lysate donor was reactive. Unfortunately, these experiments have not been convincingly reproduced with leukocyte dialysates, i.e. TF, although isolated positive reports have appeared in the literature. In any case, there is an obvious disparity between the relative ease in obtaining lymphokine production by lymphocytes from persons who have received TF *in vivo* and the results obtained when lymphocytes are treated with TF *in vitro*.

Still more elusive data have been obtained with lymphocyte transformation where most enhancing effects appear to be nonantigen-specific.

Characterization

The lack of suitable *in vitro* assay has seriously hampered the biochemical characterization of TF. Most authors who fractionated TF preparations had to follow up the biological activity by injecting the fractions into humans and studying the skin test conversion; such a methodology represents a major limitation due to its difficulty to perform on a large scale and to its internal pitfalls. Consequently, one must accept published chemical data with circumspection. We shall only mention the main results published in the recent years:

Baram and co-workers (1966) have found TF activity associated with a polynucleotide;

Arala-Chaves *et al.* (1967) found no evidence for nucleic acids in his preparation but detected proteins;

Gottlieb *et al.* (1973) proposed that TF is composed of a polypeptide chain joined to 3–4 residue ribonucleic acids.

Enzymatic studies have provided complex results from which one may isolate the sensitivity to several proteolytic enzymes, which corroborates the Arala-Chaves's data mentioned above, which indicate the presence of polypeptides.

The knowledge of the chemical nature of TF active principle is essential for understanding its mode of action. The antigen-independent activities could be explained by several mechanisms, including contaminating thymic hormones (as discussed above), other immunoactive peptides, ribonucleic acid fragments, or other adjuvant or rather immunostimulant-like molecule. The antigen-specific activities are more difficult to explain, at least if one assumes that true *de novo* antigen-specific immunity without concomitant antigen transfer, can be transferred to a naïve individual. It will be crucial to determine whether putative antigen specificity bears on polypeptides, or polynucleotide moieties and how to reconcile their expression of multiple specificities with the present knowledge on the generation of antibody diversity. A structural model for TF has been proposed by Burger *et al.* (1979) containing inosine or IMP, ribose, a phosphodiester group and a polypeptide chain. Recently, Borkowsky and Lawrence (1980) have reported that TF preparations bind specifically the antigen, hence the hypothesis that the TF antigen specific moiety could be a T cell receptor fragment.

Hypotheses involving immune RNA have also been put forward. RNA-rich extracts (of larger mol. wt than TF) have been obtained from tissues of animals immunized with various antigens and have been shown to transfer specific immune responsiveness either to nonimmune recipients *in vivo* or *in vitro* (Friedman, 1979). However, it is difficult to exclude, as stated in some of these studies, that such immune RNA are in fact RNA-antigen complexes in which the RNA serves as a potent nonspecific immunostimulator.

In conclusion, transfer factor (TF) is still an ill-defined biological preparation. The reality of specific transfer is well established. It is often obscured, however, by the presence in the dialysate of nonantigen-specific potent enhancers of immune responses. TF has already been used in numerous clinical conditions with variable results (Petersen and Kirkpatrick, 1979). Its potential use is, however, limited by the lack of an *in vitro* assay (and consequently an insufficient standardization of batches used in patients) and the poor chemical definition of biologically active moieties.

Conclusions

One of the main technological recent progress of immunology is without question the possibility now available to maintain in very long-term culture all types of immunocompetent cells. The feasibility of culturing cloned cells provides a remarkable source for all the regulatory products discussed in this review. In some cases of tumour, lines producing the factors are known, as in the case of interleukin 2.

One may predict that this major breakthrough will permit us to obtain large quantities of pure mediators and consequently learn their structure, and start synthesizing them, eventually under the form of smaller analogues.

In parallel to these efforts, the subtle interactions between lymphocyte and macrophage subsets in immune and autoimmune responses will be better understood and agents or protocols selective for a given subset will probably be discovered. Then, and only then, immunomanipulation by regulatory products will have reached the scientific status of modern pharmacology. One may thus hope that it will not be long before immunologists will provide the clinicians with a set of new chemicals that will substitute for the nonantigen-specific and especially nonselective drugs or methods presently used.

References

Aleksandrowicz, J., Blicharski, J., Czyzewskawazewska, M., Janicki, K., Lisiewicz, J., Skotnicki, A. B., Sliwzynska, B., Torowski, G. and Szmigiel, Z. (1975). *In* "The Biological Activity of Thymic Hormones" (D. W. Van Bekkum, ed.) p. 37. Kooyker Scientific Publications. Rotterdam.

Altman, A. and Cohen, I. R. (1975). *Eur. J. Immunol.* **5**, 437.

Arala-Chaves, M. P., Lebacq, E. G. and Heremans, J. F. (1967). *Int. Arch. All.* **31**, 353.

Arala-Chaves, M. P., Proenca, R. and De Sousa, M. (1974). *Cell. Immunol.* **10**, 371.

Astaldi, A., Astaldi, G. C. B., Schellekens, P. Th. A. and Eijsvoogel, V. P. (1976). *Nature* **260**, 713.

Bach, J. F., Bach, M. A., Blanot, D., Bricas, E., Charreire, J., Dardenne, M., Fournier, C. and Pleau, J. M. (1978). *Bull. Inst. Past.* **76**, 325.

Bach, J. F., Dardenne, M., Goldstein, A. L., Guha, A. and White, A. (1971). *Proc. Natn. Acad. Sci. U.S.A.* **68**, 2734.

Bach, J. F., Dardenne, M., Pleau, J. M. and Rosa, J. (1976). *C. R. Acad. Sci.* **283**, 1606.

Bach, M. A. (1977). *J. Immunol.* **119**, 641.

Bach, M. A. and Bach, J. F. (1972). *C. R. Acad. Sci. (Paris)* **275**, 2783.

Bach, M. A. and Bach, J. F. (1973). *Eur. J. Immunol.* **3**, 778.

Bach, M. A., Dardenne, M. and Droz, D. (1978). *In* "Pharmacology of immunoregulation" (G. H. Werner and F. Floc'h, eds) p. 201. Academic Press. New York and London.

Bach, M. A., Fournier, C. and Bach, J. F. (1975). *Ann. N. Y. Acad. Sci.* **249**, 316.

Baram, P., Yuan, L. and Mosko, M. M. (1966). *J. Immunol.* **97**, 407.

Bardos, P., Carnaud, C. and Bach, J. F. (1980). *C. R. Acad. Sci.* **289**, 1251.

Bloom, B. R. (1980). *Nature* **284**, 593.

Borkowsky, W. and Lawrence, H. S. (1980). *In* "Abstracts 4th International Congress of Immunology", (19.8.02) Paris.

Brandriss, M. W. (1968). *J. Clin. Invest.* **47**, 2152.

Bricas, E., Martinez, T., Blanot, D., Auger, G., Dardenne, M., Pleau, J. M. and Bach, J. F. (1977). *In* "Proc. 5th Intern. Peptide Symposium" (M. Goodman and J. Meienhofer, eds) p. 564. J. Wiley, New York.

Brodeur, B. R. and Merigan, T. C. (1975). *Proc. Natn. Acad. Sci. U.S.A.* **190**, 574.

Burger, D. R., Vandenbark, A. A., Finke, P., Nolte, J. E. and Vetto, R. M. (1976). *J. Immunol.* **117**, 782.

Burger, D. R., Vandenbark, A. A., Finke, P. and Vetto, R. M. (1977). *Cell Immunol.* **29**, 410.

Burger, D. R., Wamplen, P. A., Vandenbark, A. A. and Regan, D. H. (1979). *Ann. N. Y. Acad. Sci.* **332**, 236.

Carnaud, C., Ilfeld, D., Brook, I. and Trainin, N. (1973). *J. Exp. Med.* **138**, 1521.

Chester, T. J., Paucker, K. and Merigan, T. C. (1973). *Nature* **246**, 92.

Chretien, P. B., Lipson, S. D., Makuch, R., Kenady, D. E. and Cohen, M. H. (1979). *Ann. N. Y. Acad. Sci.* **332**, 135.

Cohen, S. and Yoshida, T. (1979). *Ann. N. Y. Acad. Sci.* **332**, 356.

Dardenne, M., Pleau, J. M., Man, N. K. and Bach, J. F. (1977). *J. Biol. Chem.* **252**, 8040.

Dardenne, M., Pleau, J. M., Blouquit, J. Y. and Bach, J. F. (1980). *Clin. Exp. Immunol.* (in press).

Degre, M., and Rollag, J. (1979). *J. Ret. End. Soc.* **25**, 489.

De Maeyer, E. J., De Maeyer-Guignard, J. and Vandeputte, M. (1975a). *Proc. Natn. Acad. Sci. U.S.A.* **190**, 574.

De Maeyer, E., De Maeyer-Guignard, J., and Vandeputte, M. (1975b). *Proc. Natn. Acad. Sci. U.S.A.* **72**, 1733.

Erard, D., Charreire, J., Auffredou, M. T. and Galanaud, P. (1979). *J. Immunol.* **123**, 1573.

Eshel, J., Shoham, J., Aboud, M. and Salzberg, S. (1980). *In* "Abstracts 4th Int. Cong. Immunology" (17.2.11), Paris.

Farrar, J. J., Simon, P. L., Farrar, W. L., Koopman, W. J. and Fuller-Bonar, J. (1979). *Ann. N. Y. Acad. Sci.* **332**, 303.

Friedman, H. (1979). *Ann. N. Y. Acad. Sci.* **332**, 236.

Gallin, J. I. and Kirkpatrick, C. H. (1974). *Proc. Natn. Acad. Sci. U.S.A.* **71**, 498.

Gidlund, M., Orn, A., Wigzell, H., Senik, A. and Gresser, I. (1978). *Nature* **273**, 759.

Gillis, S. and Smith, K. A. (1977). *Nature* **268**, 154.

Gillis, S., Urrion, N. A., Baker, P. E. and Smith, K. A. (1979). *J. Exp. Med.* **149**, 1460.

Gisler, R. H., Lindahl, P. and Gresser, I. (1974). *J. Immunol.* **113**, 438.

Goldstein, A. L., Guha, A., Zatz, M. M., Hardy, A. and White, A. (1972). *Proc. Natn. Acad. Sci. U.S.A.* **69**, 1800.

Goldstein, G. (1974). *Nature* **247**, 11.

Goldstein, G. (1977). *In* "Progress in Immunology" Vol. III (T. E. Mandel, C. Cheers, C. S. Hosking, I. F. C. McKenzie and G. J. V. Nossal, eds) p. 390. North Holland, Amsterdam.

Goldstein, G., Scheid, M. P., Boyse, E. A., Schlesinger, D. H. and Van Wauve, J. (1979). *Science* **204**, 1309.

Gottlieb, A. A., Foster, L. G., Waldman, S. R. and Lopez, M. (1973). *Lancet* **2**, 822.

Hadden, J. (1978). *In* "Pharmacology of Immunoregulation" (G. H. Werner and F. Floc'h, eds) p. 380. Academic Press, New York and London.

Hamblin, A. S., Dumonde, D. C. and Maini, R. N. (1976). *Clin. Exp. Immunol.* **23**, 303.
Heron, I., Berg, K. and Cantell, K. (1976). *J. Immunol.* **117**, 1370.
Hirsch, M. S., Ellis, D. A., Proffitt, M. R., Black, P. H. and Chirigos, M. A. (1973). *Nature New Biol.* **244**, 102.
Hirsch, M. S., Ellis, D. A., Black, P. H., Monaco, A. P. and Wood, M. L. (1974). *Transplantation* **17**, 234.
Hoffmann, M. K. (1979). *Ann. N. Y. Acad. Sci.* **332**, 557.
Horowitz, S., Borcheling, W., Moorthy, A. V., Chesney, R., Shulte-Wissermann, H. and Hong, R. (1977). *Science* **197**, 999.
Ikhehara, S., Hamashima, Y. and Masuda, T. (1975). *Nature* **258**, 335.
Incefy, G. S., Mertelsmann, R., Dardenne, M., Bach, J. F. and Good, R. A. (1980). *Clin. Exp. Immunol.* **40**, 396.
Incefy, G. S., Boumsell, L., Kagan, W., Goldstein, G., De Sousa, M., Smithwick, E., O'Reilly, R. and Good, R. A. (1975). *Trans. Assoc. Am. Phys.* **88**, 135.
Ishizawa, S., Sakai, H., Sarles, H. E., Larson, D. L. and Daniels, J. C. (1978). *J. Trauma* **18**, 48.
Kapp, J. A., Pierce, C. W., Theze, J. and Benacerraf, B. (1978). *Fed. Proc.* **37**, 2361.
Katz, D. H., Davie, J. M., Paul, W. E. and Benacerraf, B. (1971). *J. Exp. Med.* **134**, 201.
Katz, D. H., Ellmann, L., Paul, W. E., Green, I. and Benacerraf, B. (1972). *Cancer Res.* **32**, 133.
Kirkpatrick, C. H. (1978). *Cell Immunol.* **41**, 62.
Kirkpatrick, C. H. and Smith, T. K. (1976). *J. Invest. Derm.* **67**, 425.
Komuro, K. and Boyse, E. A. (1973). *Lancet* **i**, 740.
Kook, A. I. and Trainin, N. (1974). *J. Exp. Med.* **139**, 193.
Krakauer, R. S., Waldmann, T. A. and Strober, W., (1976). *J. Exp. Med.* **144**, 662.
Krakauer, R. S., Strober, W., Rippeon, D. L. and Waldmann, T. A. (1977). *Science* **196**, 56.
Lau, C. and Goldstein, G. (1980a). *J. Immunol.* **124**, 1861.
Lau, C. and Goldstein, G. (1980b). *In* "Abstracts 4th International Congress of Immunology" (19.8.02), Paris.
Lawrence, H. S. (1949). *Proc. Soc. Exp. Biol. Med.* **71**, 516.
Lindahl, P., Leary, P. and Gresser, I. (1972). *Proc. Natn. Acad. Sci. U.S.A.* **69**, 721.
Lindahl, P., Gresser, I., Leavy, P. and Rovey, M. (1976). *Proc. Natn. Acad. Sci. U.S.A.* **73**, 1284.
Lindahl-Magnusson, P., Leary, P. and Gresser, I. (1972). *Nature New Biology* **237**, 120.
Lonai, P. and Steinman, I. (1977). *Proc. Natn. Acad. Sci. U.S.A.* **74**, 5662.
Low, T. L. K., and Goldstein, A. L. (1978). *In* "The Year in Hematology" (R. Silber, J. Lobue and A. S. Gordon, eds) p. 281, Plenum Press, New York.
Low, T. L. K., Thurman, G. B., Chincarini, C., McClure, J. E., Marshall, G. D., Hus, K. and Goldstein, A. L. (1979). *Ann. N. Y. Acad. Sci.* **332**, 33.
Mendes, N. F., Saraiva, P. S. and Santos, O. B. O., (1975). *Cell. Immunol.* **17**, 560.
Mizel, S. B. (1979). *Ann. N. Y. Acad. Sci.* **332**, 539.
Moller, G. (1980). *Immunol. Rev.* **51**.
Monier, J. C., Dardenne, M., Pleau, J. M., Schmitt, D., Descheaux, P. and Bach, J. F. (1980). *Clin. Exp. Immunol.* (in press).
Morgan, D. A., Ruscetti, F. W. and Gallo, R. (1976). *Science* **193**, 1007.
Naylor, P. H., Sheppard, H., Thurman, G. B. and Goldstein, A. L. (1976). *Biochem. Biophys. Res. Commun.* **73**, 843.
Paque, R. E., Kniskern, P. J., Dray, S. and Baram, P. (1969). *J. Immunol.* **103**, 1014.
Pazmino, N. H., Ihle, J. M. and Goldstein, A. L. (1978). *J. Exp. Med.* **147**, 708.
Petersen, E. A. and Kirkpatrick, C. H. (1979). *Ann. N. Y. Acad. Sci.* **332**, 216.
Pierce, C. W. and Kapp, J. A. (1976). *Cont. Topics Immunobiol.* **5**, 91.
Pierce, C. W. and Tadakuma, T. (1978). *Prog. Immunol.* **3**, 405.

Pleau, J. M., Dardenne, M., Blouquit, Y. and Bach, J. F. (1977). *J. Biol. Chem.* **252**, 8045.

Pleau, J. M., Fuentes, V., Morgat, J. L. and Bach, J. F. (1980). *Proc. Natn. Acad. Sci. U.S.A.* **77**, 2861.

Rich, S. S. and Rich, R. R. (1976). *J. Exp. Med.* **144n**, 1214.

Rich, S. S., David, C. S. and Rich, R. R. (1979). *J. Exp. Med.* **149**, 114.

Rotter, V. and Trainin, N. (1974). *Cell Immunol.* **16**, 413.

Sandler, J. A., Smith, T. K., Manganiello, V. C. and Kirkpatrick, C. H. (1975). *J. Clin. Invest.* **56**, 1271.

Schafer, L. A., Goldstein, A. L., Gutterman, J. U. and Hersh, E. M. (1976a). *Ann. N. Y. Acad. Sci.* **277**, 609.

Schafer, L. A., Gutterman, J. U., Hersh, E. M., Mavligit, G. M., Dandridge, K., Cohen, G. H. and Goldstein, A. L. (1976b). *Cancer Immunol. Immunotherap.* **1**, 259.

Scheid, M. P., Hoffmann, N. K., Komuro, K., Hammerling, V., Abbott, J., Boyse, E. A. Cohen, G. H. Hooper, J. A., Schulof, R. S. and Goldstein, A. L. (1973). *J. Exp. Med.* **138**, 1027.

Scheid, M. P., Goldstein, G. and Boyse, E. A. (1975). *Science* **190**, 1211.

Smith, K. A., Lachman, L. B., Oppenheim, J. J. and Favata M. F. (1980). *J. Exp. Med.* **151**, 1551.

Sonnefeld, G. and Merigan, T. C. (1979). *Ann. N. Y. Acad. Sci.* **332**, 345.

Sonnefeld, G., Mandel, A. D. and Merigan, T. C. (1977). *Cell. Immunol.* **34**, 193.

Steinberg, A. D., Krakauer, R., Reinertsen, J. L., Klassen, L. W., Ilfeld, D., Reeves, J. P. and Williams, G. W. (1978). *Arth. Rheum.* **21**, 204.

Stewart, W. E. (1979). *In* "The Interferon System" p. 305. Springer Verlag.

Stutman, O. (1978). *Immunol. Rev.* **42**, 138.

Sunshine, G. S., Bash, R. S., Coffey, R. G., Cohen, K. W., Goldstein, G. and Hadden, J. W. (1978). *J. Immunol.* **120**, 1594.

Taussig, M. J. (1974). *Nature* **248**, 234.

Thurman, G. B., Rossio, J. L. and Goldstein, A. L. (1978). *In* "Regulatory Mechanisms in Lymphocytes Activation" (D. O. Lucas, ed.) p. 629. Academic Press, New York and London.

Togawa, A., Oppenheim, J. J. and Kirkpatrick, C. H. (1980). *Cell. Immunol.* (in press).

Trainin, N., Small, M., Zipori, D., Umiel, T., Kook, A. I. and Rotter, V. (1975). *In* "The Biological Activity of Thymic Hormones" (D. W. Van Bekkum, ed.) p. 117. Kooyker Scientific Pub., Rotterdam.

Trinchieri, G., Santoli, D. and Koprowski, H. (1978). *J. Immunol.* **120**, 1849.

Umiel, T. and Trainin, N. (1975). *Eur. J. Immunol.* **5**, 85.

Valdimarsson, H., Hambleton, G., Henry, K. and McConnell, I. (1974). *Clin. Exp. Immunol.* **16**, 141.

Vignaux, F. and Gresser, I. (1977). *J. Immunol.* **118**, 721.

Virelizier, J. L., Chan, E. L. and Allison, A. L. (1977). *Clin. Exp. Immunol.* **30**, 299.

Virelizier, J. L. and Griscelli, C. (1980). *In* "Primary immunodeficiencies" (M. Seligmann, ed.). Elsevier, Amsterdam (in press).

Wagner, H., Hardt, C., Heeg, K., Pfizenmaier, K., Solbach, W., Bartlett, R., Stockinger, H. and Rollinghof, M. (1980). *Immunol. Rev.* **51**, 215.

Wara, D. and Ammann, A. J. (1978). *Transpl. Proc.* **10**, 203.

Wara, D. W., Goldstein, A. L., Doyle, W. and Amman, A. J. (1975). *New Engl. J. Med.* **292**, 70.

Wood, D. D., Cameron, P. M., Poe, M. T. and Morris, C. A. (1976). *Cell. Immunol.* **21**, 88.

Yakir, Y., Kook, A. I. and Trainin, N. (1978). *J. Exp. Med.* **148**, 71.

Youngner, J. S. and Salvin, S. B. (1973). *J. Immunol.* **11**, 1914.

Zaizov, R. R., Vogel, I., Wolack, B., Cohen, I. J., Varsano, I., Shohat, B., Handzel, Z., Rotter, V., Yakir, Y. and Trainin, N., (1979). *Ann. N. Y. Acad. Sci.* **332**, 172.

63

Immunostimulation: Recent Progress in the Study of Natural and Synthetic Immunomodulators Derived from the Bacterial Cell Wall

EDGAR LEDERER

Institut de Biochimie, Université de Paris-Sud, Centre d'Orsay
Laboratoire de Biochimie, C.N.R.S., Gif-sur-Yvette, France

The many imperfections of this text are due to the fact that I was asked only 48 h before the beginning of the Congress to replace the scheduled speaker, Dr P. Dukor, who was unfortunately unable to attend the Congress. Due to this special circumstance, this review covers only a small part of the field of immunostimulation. I am greatly indebted to Drs J. F. Petit and P. Lefrancier for their critical reading of the manuscript and useful suggestions for its improvement.

The work of the author was supported by CNRS and, in part, by grants from DGRST, INSERM, Fondation de la Recherche Médicale, Ligue Nationale Française contre le Cancer, the Cancer Research Institute, New York, and a contract with Laboratoires Choay and Institut Pasteur.

The last decade has witnessed the discovery of an ever increasing number of natural compounds which have interesting immunostimulant properties. They belong to a large variety of chemical structures: peptides, such as tuftsin, the thymic hormones, the protease inhibitor bestatine, liposoluble vitamins and their derivatives, such as retinoic acid, the ubiquinones, etc. Amongst synthetic compounds derived from natural substances, we find polynucleotides, lysolecithin analogues, etc. Some purely synthetic compounds, such as levamisole and tilorone are also widely studied. Some of these are known to be inducers of interferon (see the excellent revue of Dukor *et al.*, 1979).

We shall restrict our review, however, to two classes of immunomodulators, which have been at the centre of our interest for some time (Petit and Lederer, 1978), both of which are derived from the mycobacterial cell wall: trehalose diesters (natural cord factor and synthetic derivatives) (for reviews see Asselineau and Asselineau, 1978; Lederer, 1979) and MDP (muramyl-dipeptide and derivatives) (for reviews see Chedid *et al.*, 1978; Dukor *et al.*, 1979; Parant, 1979). The perspectives of both categories of compounds have been recently reviewed by the author (Lederer, 1980). The chemistry of MDP and its derivatives is reviewed by Lefrancier and Lederer (1981).

Trehalose 6,6′-diesters (cord factor and synthetic analogues)

Known since 1950 as "toxic lipid" extracted from whole mycobacteria (Bloch, 1950), cord factor was shown to be a 6,6′-dimycolate of trehalose (Noll *et al.*, 1956) (Formula **1**). It took 20 years until its interesting immunological properties were discovered, by Bekierkunst *et al.* (1969, 1971a, b, 1974) who showed that i. v. injections of 10 μg cord factor into mice in the presence of 1% mineral oil, produce granulomas in the lung and local immunity against airborne infection by tubercle bacilli; when injected into the footpad of mice it increases the antibody response to SRBC.

Three main activities of natural and synthetic trehalose diesters have been studied recently *in vivo*: anti-infectious, antiparasitic and antitumour.

Anti-infectious activity

I.p. injection of cord factor (TDM)* in oil emulsion protects mice against an i.p. challenge from *Salmonella typhi* and *S. typhimurium* (Yarkoni and Bekierkunst, 1976); aqueous suspensions of TDM are active in mice against *Klebsiella pneumoniae* and *Listeria monocytogenes* (Parant *et al.*, 1977). A synthetic lower homologue of TDM, called C76 (an isomer of the trehalose dicorynomycolate produced by corynebacteria) (Formula **2**) was shown to be just as active as TDM (Parant *et al.*, 1978b). These synthetic analogues have the great advan-

* The terms cord factor, P_3, TDM (for trehalose dimycolate) are synonymes for the mixture of trehalose 6,6′-dimycolates produced by mycobacteria.

Total carbon number	Structure of $R-\overset{O}{\overset{\|\|}{C}}-OH$
$\sim C_{180}$ (cord factor = TDM = P_3)	Mycobacterial mycolic acids, i.e.: $CH_3(CH_2)_{19}\underset{\diagdown\;CH_2\;\diagup}{CH-CH}(CH_2)_{14}\underset{\diagdown\;CH_2\;\diagup}{CH-CH}-(CH_2)_{17}\overset{OH}{CH}-\underset{C_{24}H_{49}}{CH}-CO_2H$
1	$C_{84}H_{164}O_3$
C_{76}	Synthetic racemic $CH_3(CH_2)_{14}\overset{OH}{\underset{H}{C}}-\underset{C_{14}H_{29}}{CH}-CO_2H$
2	$C_{32}H_{64}O_3$

TABLE I
Toxicity of emulsified TDM and its synthetic analogues

Material injected[a]	No. of deaths/no. treated Exp. 1	Exp. 2
TDM	10/10	10/10
$C_{76\alpha}$	0/10	1/10
$C_{76\beta}$	0/10	1/10
Emulsion	0/10	1/10

[a] Oil (9%)/water emulsions of TDM, its synthetic analogues (0·1 mg/0·2 ml/mouse) or emulsion alone were prepared by ginding and aminístered in volumes of 0·2 ml i.v. (from Yarkoni *et al.*, 1978).

tage of being nontoxic (Table I) and much less granulomagenic than TDM (Yarkoni *et al.*, 1978).

Antiparasitic activity

TDM in aqueous suspension injected 3–7 weeks before infection protects mice against the protozoan parasite *Babesia microti* (Clark, 1979) (Fig. 1); similarly,

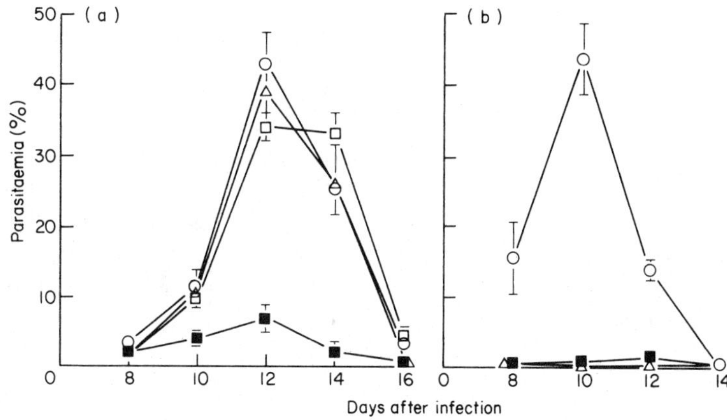

FIG. 1. *(a) Minimum effective dose of cord factor when given 3 weeks before* B. microti*:* □ *10 μg;* △ *50 μg;* ■ *200 μg;* ○ *control; 2 s.e. range indicated. (b) Different intervals between 200 μg cord factor with* B. microti. *Cord factor given* ■ *5 weeks or* △ *7 weeks before parasite,* ○ *controls; 2 s.e. range indicated (Clark, 1979).*

mice can be partially protected against infection by *Schistosoma mansoni* by TDM, or even by trehalose dipalmitate, in suspension in paraffin oil (Olds *et al.*, 1980). A significiant prolongation of survival time of mice infected by *Toxoplasma gondii* was obtained by vaccination with protoplasm of disrupted *T. gondii* in an oil-in-water emulsion containing TDM (Masihi *et al.*, 1979).

Antitumour activity

I.p. injection of TDM in Bayol F, or in an emulsion of saline and peanut oil protects mice against L 1210 leukaemia cells (Leclerc *et al.*, 1976). TDM and the synthetic C_{76} analogue, injected intralesionally into a methylcholanthrene-induced fibrosarcoma inoculated to mice, cause up to 100% regression of the established tumour, in the presence of 9% paraffin oil. Most of the cured mice were resistant to growth of tumour cells of a challenge inoculum (Yarkoni *et al.*, 1978) (Table II). The growth of an ascitic rat hepatoma is suppressed by i.p. injection of TDM or, to a lesser extent, by some synthetic analogues when emulsified in peanut oil; paraffin oil gives better results (Pimm *et al.*, 1979), squalene is better still (Pimm *et al.*, 1980).

Most of the biological effects of natural and synthetic trehalose diesters can be explained by the interaction of these glycolipids with cell membranes and mitochondrial membranes (Kato *et al.*, 1978). Structural modifications, or simplifications of the trehalose diester model have mostly led to less active molecules (Yarkoni *et al.*, 1979).

TABLE II

Regression of a murine fibrosarcoma by intralesional administration of emulsified TDM or synthetic analogues

Exp. no.	*Material injected*[a]	*Dose (mg)*	*No. tumour-free animals/no. animals treated (60 days)*	*Percentage regression*	*P*
1	Emulsion	—	1/12	8	—
	TDM	0·15	11/12	92	<0·001
	C76 (β)	0·15	10/12	83	<0·001
2	No treatment	—	0/12	0	—
	Emulsion	—	0/12	0	
	C76 ($\alpha + \beta$)	0·05	12/12	100	<0·001
	TDP	0·15	3/12	25	NS[b]
	TDB	0·15	4/12	33	NS
3	No treatment	—	0/12	0	—
	TDM	0·1	11/12	92	<0·001
	TDP	0·15	3/10	30	NS
	TDB	0·15	4/10	40	NS

[a] Emulsions (9% oil) were injected into 5- to 6-day-old tumours (3–5 mm in diameter).
[b] NS, number of tumour-free animals not significantly different from controls (from Yarkoni *et al.*, 1978). TDP = trehalose dipalmitate; TDB = trehalose dibehenate.

MDP (muramyl-dipeptide and derivatives)

In 1974 it was shown that *N*-acetyl-muramyl-L-alanyl-D-isoglutamine (Formula **3**) (MDP, for muramyl-dipeptide) is the simplest structural unit of bacterial peptidoglycans capable of replacing whole killed mycobacteria in Freund's adjuvant, for increasing antibody titres and for establishing delayed hypersensitivity (Ellouz *et al.*, 1974; Merser *et al.*, 1975; Adam *et al.*, 1975; Kotani *et al.*, 1975) Chedid *et al.* (1977) then showed that synthetic MDP also increases resistance to bacterial infections and is also active in saline (Audibert *et al.*, 1976) and even by the oral route (Chedid, *et al.*, 1976). It

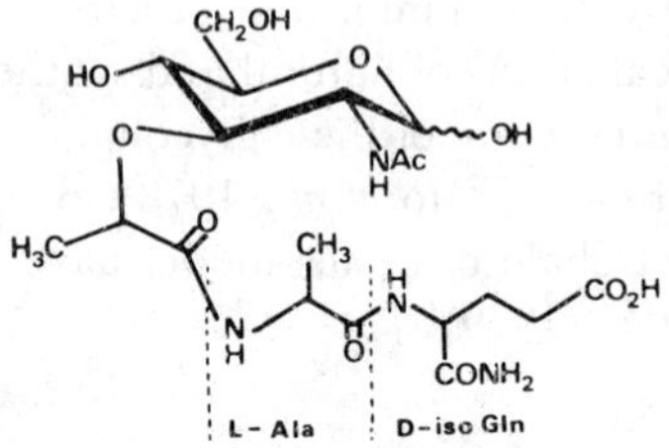

3

MDP

is adjuvant-active even in neonatal mice, where endotoxin (LPS) is inactive (Parant *et al.*, 1978a) (for reviews on MDP see Chedid *et al.*, 1978; Dukor *et al.*, 1979; Parant, 1979; Lederer, 1980).

MDP has, however, several unexpected untoward effects, such as pyrogenicity (Kotani *et al.*, 1976; Dinarello *et al.*, 1978) thrombocytolysis (Rotta *et al.*, 1979), production of a transitory leukopenia (Kotani *et al.*, 1976) etc. Fortunately, the molecule of MDP is an exquisite model for the inventive chemist, allowing a large number of variations of each of the three principal parts of the molecule. Indeed, several hundred derivatives of MDP have already been described and even more mentioned in the patent literature. Some of these new compounds open interesting perspectives for clinical applications.

In the restricted space available, we can only mention a few structural types and the resulting changes in activity.

Structural variations

The *carbohydrate* moiety has been simplified, giving nor-MDP (in which the methyl group of the lactyl side-chain of muramic acid is replaced by an H atom) (Adam *et al.*, 1976), which is, in some tests, less active, but is also less toxic (Dukor *et al.*, 1979). MDP has been coupled to *N*-acetyl-glucosamine, giving disaccharide dipeptides, which seem more active than MDP (Tsujimoto *et al.*, 1979; Durette *et al.*, 1979), but are certainly more difficult to prepare. Larger peptidoglycan fragments, for instance tetra- to hexasaccharides of di- to pentapeptides, have greater activity for inducing arthritogenicity (Koga *et al.*, 1979) and for inhibiting plasminogen activator secretion from macrophages (Drapier *et al.*, 1979).

The *peptide moiety* is essential for the immunological activities of MDP; L-Ala can be replaced by other L-amino-acids (the L-seryl and L-valyl derivatives for instance, are more active than MDP) (Dukor *et al.*, 1979; McLaughlin *et al.*, 1980)), but the replacement of L-Ala by D-Ala gives an immunosuppressor (Chedid *et al.*, 1976). The replacement of the D-glutamic acid residue by D-Asp, or by L-Glu, gives inactive compounds, whereas the α and γ substituents can be varied in different ways (Dukor *et al.*, 1979; Parant, 1979).

Pyrogenicity can be strongly diminished, or nearly abolished, by some simple modifications, such as the *N*-methylation of L-Ala, or the esterification of the α-carboxyl of D-glutamine by *n*-butanol (F. Audibert, M. Parant, L. Chedid, di Choay and P. Lefrancier, unpub. experiments).

Lipophilic derivatives

Lipophilic derivatives have attracted great interest. It was known that adjuvant-active chloroform-soluble wax D fractions of mycobacteria contain a peptidoglycan moiety linked to an arabinogalactan esterified by mycolic acids (White *et al.*, 1958). For a long time it was even thought that a mycobacterial adjuvant had to be liposoluble, until the discovery of the first water-soluble adjuvant (WSA) (Adam *et al.*, 1972) proved the contrary. Now the pendulum has swung back and Japanese authors (Azuma *et al.*, 1978; Kusumoto *et al.*, 1978; Shiba *et al.*, 1978; Uemiya *et al.*, 1979) were the first to prepare 6-*O*-acyl esters of MDP; they showed, that indeed, 6-*O*-mycolyl-MDP, 6-*O*-nocardomycolyl-MDP, and 6-*O*-corynomycolyl-MDP have interesting antitumour properties and are less pyrogenic than MDP. Lipophilic MDP derivatives bearing a mycolyl group at the end of the peptide chain, such as MurNAc-L-Ala-D-isoGln-L-Ala-glycerol-mycolate (Lefrancier *et al.*, 1979) stimulate strongly adjuvant activity and nonspecific antibacterial resistance (Parant *et al.*, 1980). When the corresponding "desmuramyl" compound, i.e. L-Ala-D-isoGln-L-Ala-glycerol-mycolate was tested, it came as a great surprise

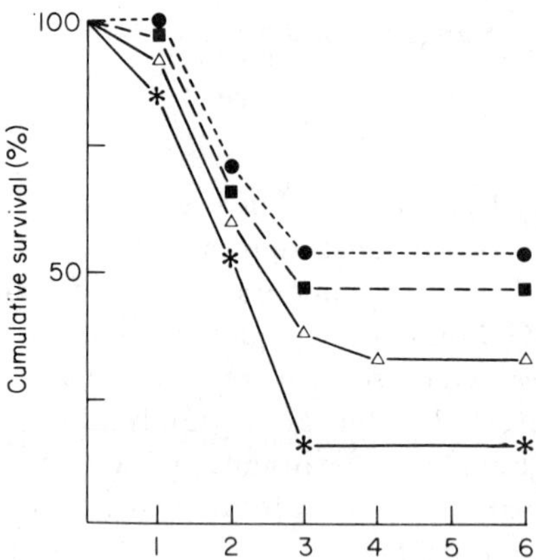

FIG. 2. *Protective activity of lipophilic MDP derivatives in adult mice infected intramuscularly with 4* × *10*^{6} P. aeruginosa. *Mice were given 300 μg intravenously of each compound 7 days before being infected.* ●, *L-alanyl-D-isoglutaminyl-L-alanyl-glycerol-mycolate (17/32,* P < *0·01);* ■, N-*acetyl-muramyl-L-alanyl-D-isoglutaminyl-D-alanyl-glycerol-mycolate (15/32,* P < *0,05);* △, *MDP (16/48); *, controls (5/32) (Parant* et al., *1980).*

that it was as active as the MurNAc derivative in stimulating antibacterial resistance, but entirely inactive for increasing humoral antibodies (Parant *et al.*, 1980) (Fig. 2). This shows the important role played by the MurNAc moiety in the latter activity.

Another interesting peptidoglycan derivative has been prepared by Migliore *et al.* (1979) by *N*-laurylation of an inactive cell wall tetrapeptide of a *Streptomyces* strain. A synthetic lauryl-tetrapeptide analogue (N^2-[*N*-(*N*-lauryl-L-alanyl)-γ-D-glutamyl]-N^6-glycyl-DD-LL-diamino-2,6-pimelamic acid) is adjuvant-active and protects mice against *Listeria monocytogenes.*

A very lipophilic nonapeptide L-Ala-D-isoGln-L-Lys(Ac)-D-Ala-$(Gly)_5$-OMe has also been reported to produce delayed hypersensitivity when injected in FIA with an antigen. All these compounds contain the sequence L-Ala-D-Glu which thus seems to be specifically recognized by the target cell, most probably the macrophage.

Oligomers, polymers, carriers

MDP is not antigenic, it does not react with antipeptidoglycan antibodies (Audibert *et al.*, 1978) and does not sensitize to tuberculin (Ellouz *et al.*, 1974; Kotani *et al.*, 1975). It is, however, very rapidly excreted unchanged in the urine. In mice, more than 50% are found after 30 min, and more than 90% after 2 h (Parant *et al.*, 1979). It is thus obvious that larger molecules carrying the MDP unit could have longer lifetimes in the body. For studying this problem, a *p*-aminophenyl-glycoside of MDP was cross-linked with glutaraldehyde (Parant *et al.*, 1978c); the resulting polymer of about 6000 daltons had an increased activity for stimulating antibacterial resistance, but difficulty in preparing a well defined compound in sufficient quantity hindered further experimentation.

Following the pioneer work of Sela and colleagues (Sela and Mozes, 1979), MDP was coupled to a synthetic multi (poly(DL-alanyl)-poly(L-lysine) carrier. The resulting conjugate had a 100-fold increased anti-infectious activity, but also a very strong pyrogenicity. It came as a great surprise, however, that the analogous conjugate with the inactive (or even immunosuppressive) MDP-DD was also strongly anti-infectious, but nonpyrogenic; it does not sensitize, nor induce an immune response to the glycopeptide moiety (Chedid *et al.*, 1979). These experiments open the way for the realization of the "dream" of Sela and Mozes (1979) of synthetic adjuvants coupled through a synthetic carrier to a synthetic antigen.

MDP in vaccines

MDP increases the efficacy of influenza vaccines in mice, either with an inactivated viral vaccine, or with a purified subunit (Audibert *et al.*, 1977; Webster *et al.*, 1977).

Immunization of monkeys against malaria has been shown to be possible with MDP or some of its derivatives. Protective immunity was produced in *Aotus* monkeys and in macaques, using MDP, or nor-MDP and merozoites of *Plasmodium falciparum* or *P. knowlesi* in FIA as antigens (Reese *et al.*, 1978; Mitchell *et al.*, 1978) (Fig. 3). Siddiqui *et al.* (1978) used liposomes containing 6-*O*-stearoyl-MDP and obtained full protection of *Aotus* monkeys, using a *P. falciparum* antigen. This work showed for the first time the advantage of using lipophilic MDP derivatives in liposomes.

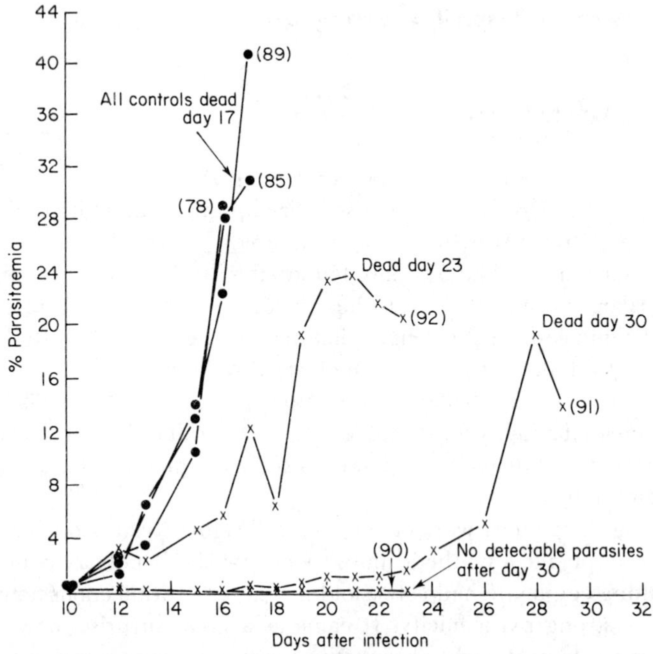

FIG. 3. *Protective immunity induced in* Aotus *monkeys immunized with an antigen/muramyl dipeptide mixture emulsified in oil. Monkeys 78, 85, and 89 were injected with the muramyl dipeptide/oil emulsion* (⊙)*; all were dead by day 17. Monkeys 90, 91 and 92 were injected with a merozoite-rich fraction of* P. falciparum *obtained from organisms cultivated* in vitro *emulsified in the same adjuvant* (*x*)*. Monkey 90 had no detectable parasites after day 30; monkey 91 was dead by day 30; monkey 92 was dead by day 23. All animals had been challenged with* 5×10^5 *parasitized monkey erythrocytes* (*Reese* et al. *1978*).

MDP for stimulation of nonspecific resistance

A partial protection of mice against *Trypanosoma cruzi* was obtained by Kierszenbaum and Ferraresi (1979) by applying MDP in an Alzet minipump (which releases 1 μl/h over several days) or by repeated doses of MDP (Fig. 4). In the case of *Schistosoma mansoni*, it was found that MDP diminishes the degree of infection in rats when used either with or without an antigen; it is clear that here too the effect is principally due to nonspecific stimulation of resistance (Tribouley *et al.*, 1979). MDP also restores nonspecific immunity in immunosuppressed mice; such animals, pretreated with cyclophosphamide, have a greatly increased susceptibility to various infections and much larger doses of antibiotics are necessary to overcome the infection. Nor-MDP has been shown to counteract the effect of immunosuppression "indicating a potential clinical usefulness of immunostimulation in immunocompromised and infected human patients" (Sackmann and Dietrich, 1980).

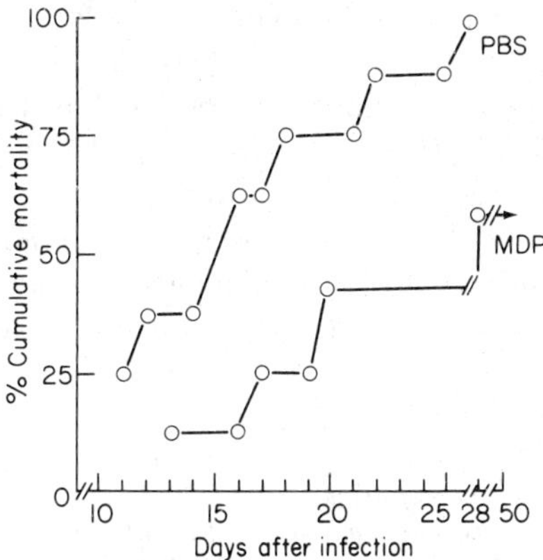

FIG. 4. *Effect of continuous administration of MDP on the mortality rate of mice infected with* T. cruzi. *MDP (4 mg) was contained in an osmotic minipump inserted s.c. 2 days before infection:* P < *0·27; PBS = phosphate buffered saline.* (*From Kierszenbaum and Ferraresi, 1979.*)

Mechanism of action of MDP

The primary action of MDP seems to be on the macrophage, leading to the liberation of monokines activating B cells and T cells (Février *et al.*, 1978; Taniyama and Holden, 1979; Pabst and Johnson (1980). MDP *in vitro* causes secretion of prostaglandins, of a collagenase and a fibroblast proliferation factor, all known to be produced by activated macrophages (Wahl *et al.*, 1979). It also inhibits migration of macrophages (Adam *et al.*, 1978; Nagao *et al.*, 1979). For more details on cellular immunology of MDP the reader is referred to the reviews of Chedid *et al.* (1978), Dukor *et al.* (1979) and Parant (1979).

Like other adjuvants, MDP can also be *immunosuppressive*, depending on the timing in relation to the administration of antigen and also on the dosage (Leclerc *et al.*, 1979; Souvannavong and Adam, 1980). A selective suppression of an IgE response has been obtained with antigen-conjugated muramyl-peptides and seems to be due to the induction of allergen-specific suppressor cells (Kishimoto *et al.*, 1979); this work indicates new posibilities for the treatment of allergies.

Combined immunostimulation with trehalose esters and MDP

The lipopolysaccharides (endotoxins) of Gram-negative bacteria are well known immunostimulations (Louis and Lambert, 1979). A special endotoxin preparation (ET) from an O antigen-deficient (Re) mutant of *Salmonella typhimurium* has been used by Meyer *et al.* (1974) and Ribi *et al.* (1976), in emulsion with TDM and paraffin oil, for intralesional injection into an established line 10 hepatocarcinoma growing intradermally in line 2 guinea-pigs. Up to 100% regression was obtained. Then, some synthetic analogues of TDM were shown to be able to replace TDM and, later, the combined injection of a purified ET preparation called B_4 (50 μg) + MDP (ser) (the serine analogue of MDP) (150 μg) + TDM (50 μg) were shown to produce complete regression (Ribi *et al.*, 1979). Quite recently, however, McLaughlin *et al.* (1980) have obtained nearly 100% cures, using only two compounds—150 μg of an MDP derivative + 150 μg TDM, in emulsion with 0·75% paraffin oil (Table III). They showed

TABLE III

Tumour regression after treatment. Values are numbers of guinea-pigs cured of dermal and metastatic tumours over numbers of animals treated. Data shown are pooled from two separate experiments. No cures were observed in animals treated with any muramyl dipeptide in the absence of trehalose dimycolate (from McLaughlin et al., *1980)*

Synthetic muramyl dipeptide (150 μg) tested with trehalose dimycolate (150 μg)	*Observed tumour regression*
N-Acetylmuramyl-L-alanyl-D-isoglutamine	1/17
N-Acetylmuramyl-D-alanyl-D-isoglutamine	0/9
N-Acetyl-4,6-di-*O*-octanoylmuramyl-L-alanyl-D-isoglutamine	1/9
N-Acetyldesmethylmuramyl-L-alanyl-D-isoglutamine[a]	2/19
N-Acetylmuramyl-L-threonyl-D-isoglutamine	3/9
N-Acetylmuramyl-L-seryl-D-isoglutamine	10/17[b]
N-Acetyldesmethylmuramyl-L-valyl-D-isoglutamine[a]	10/17[b]
N-Glycolyldesmethylmuramyl-L-alanyl-D-isoglutamine	7/9[b]
N-Acetyl-4,6-di-*O*-octanoylmuramyl-L-valyl-D-isoglutamine	16/18[b]
N-Acetyldesmethylmuramyl-L-α-aminobutyryl-D-isoglutamine	17/18[b]
Trehalose dimycolate alone (control)	0/17
Emulsion of oil, Tween 80 and phosphate-buffered saline (control)	0/14

[a] These are trivial names for 2-acetamido-2-deoxy-D-gluco-3-*O*-yl-acetyl dipeptides.
[b] Significantly different from the value for trehalose dimycolate-treated controls.

that it is necessary to emulsify both compounds together, because the joint injection of emulsions prepared separately, each with only one type of compound, gives no cures. "A tertiary complex of muramyl-dipeptide, trehalose dimycolate and oil droplets is required" (McLaughlin *et al.*, 1980).

Parallel experiments with the same line 10 hepatocarcinoma in line 2 guinea-pigs of Yarkoni *et al.* (1978) had shown that the ET preparation of Ribi *et al.*, (1976) combined with TDM was fully active and that the synthetic C_{76} analogue can replace TDM. More recently, Yarkoni *et al.* (1980) have obtained 100% cures using MDP and TDM in 10% paraffin oil. After a detailed study of the optimum percentage and nature of oil (Yarkoni and Rapp, 1980), it was shown that 2% squalene with 0·2% Tween gave the best results. Squalene or hexadecane are much less effective. Table IV shows that the synthetic C_{76} analogue can replace TDM with MDP, and Table V shows a dose-response study using MDP and TDM emulsified in 2% squalane + 0·2% Tween.

TABLE IV

Tumour regression induced in guinea-pigs by intralesional injection of emulsified mixtures of MDP and TDM, or of MDP and C_{76} (from Yarkoni et al., *1980).*

Material injected[a] *(mg)*			*Emulsification method*	*No. of cured animals*[b]*/no. of animals tested (90 days)*
MDP	*TDM*	C_{76}		
0·3	1	—	Grinding	7/7
0·3	1	—	Sonication	7/7
0·3	—	1	Grinding	6/7
0·3	—	1	Sonication	5/7
—	—	—	Sonication	0/8

[a] A chloroform solution of TDM (or C_{76}) was added to a polypropylene tube containing MDP. The chloroform was evaporated. The mixture was ultrasonically dispersed in 10% squalene and then emulsified in saline containing 0·2% Tween. The emulsified preparations were injected intralesionally in 0·4 ml volumes. [b] Complete disappearance of the dermal tumour, no clinical evidence of metastatic disease, and rejection of contralateral challenge (10^6 tumour cells) 2 months after the inoculation of the tumour transplant.

TABLE V

Tumour regression induced in guinea-pigs by intralesional injection of emulsified mixtures of MDP and TDM: Dose response (from Yarkoni et al., *1980).*

Material injected[a] *(mg)*		*No. of cured animals*[b]*/no. of animals tested (90 days)*
MDP	*TDM*	
0·25	—	0/7
0·25	1·0	8/8
0·25	0·2	8/8
0·25	0·04	6/8
0·05	0·2	7/8
0·05	0·04	7/8
0·01	1·0	7/8
0·01	0·2	7/8
0·01	0·2	7/8
0·01	0·04	6/7
—	1·0	0/7

[a] Emulsions were prepared by ultrasonication and contained 2% squalane and 0·2% Tween. [b] Complete disappearance of the dermal tumour, no clinical evidence of metastatic disease, and rejection of contralateral challenge (10^6 tumour cells) 2 months after the inoculation of the tumour transplant.

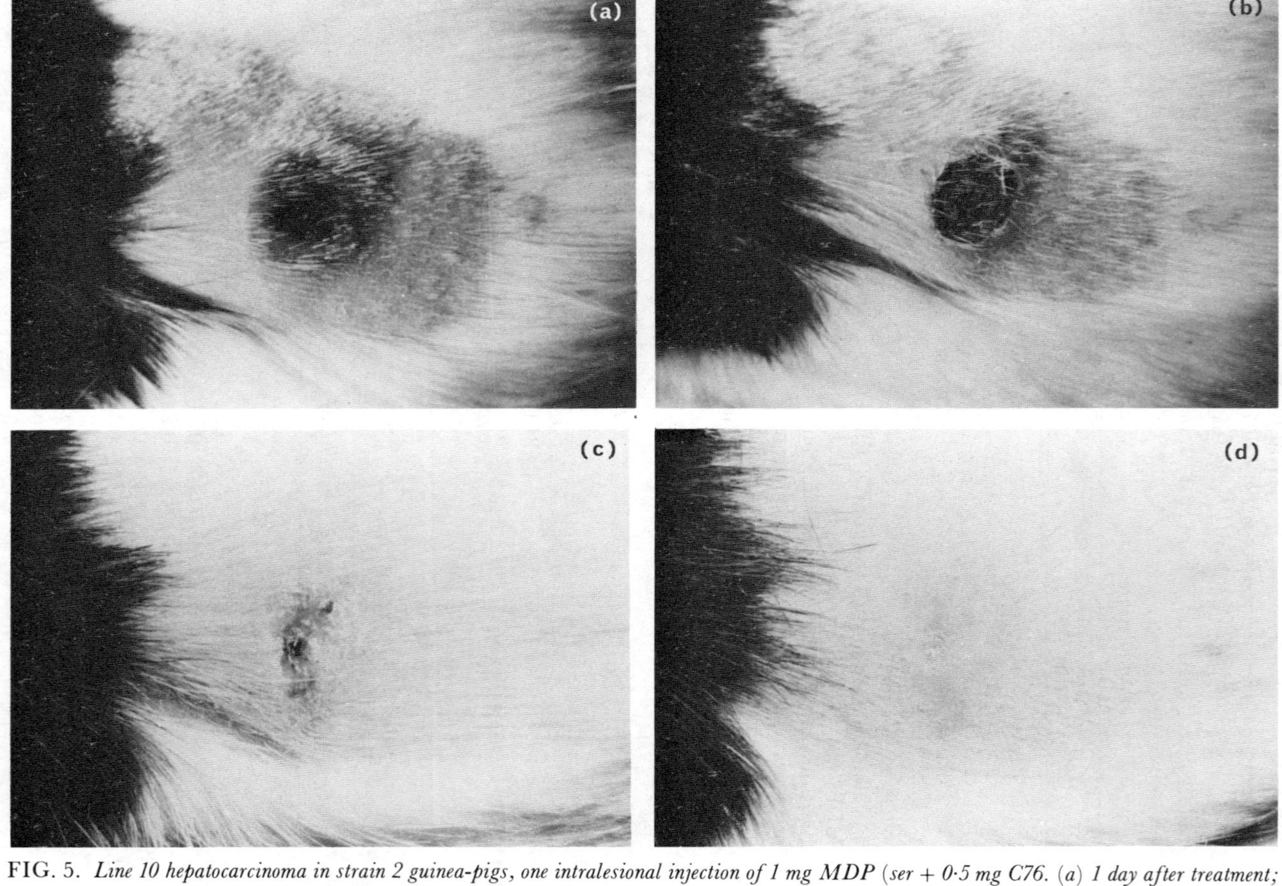

FIG. 5. *Line 10 hepatocarcinoma in strain 2 guinea-pigs, one intralesional injection of 1 mg MDP (ser + 0·5 mg C76. (a) 1 day after treatment; (b) 5 days after treatment; (c) 11 days after treatment; (d) 20 days after treatment. (Photo. E. Yarkoni.)*

Here again it was confirmed that both immunostimulants should be emulsified together to cause regression. In all cured animals there was a complete disappearance of the dermal tumour (Fig. 5) and no evidence of metastases; all animals rejected a contralateral challenge 2 months after the inoculation of the tumour transplant

Table III shows a striking discrepancy with Tables IV and V. In Table III MDP itself is inactive, other MDP derivatives being very active, whereas in Tables IV and V MDP itself is fully active. This discrepancy can be explained by experimental differences, in particular the lower oil content used by McLaughlin *et al.* (1980).

TABLE VI

Thymocyte mitogenic protein secretion in supernatants of trehalose dimycolate elicited mouse peritoneal macrophages (from Tenu et al., *1980).*

Macrophage stimulation in vivo	in vitro	^{3}H-*TdR incorporation in thymocytes*	*Relative effect*	*No. of experiments*
None	None	489 ± 93	1	6
(resident	MDP 10 μg/ml	490 ± 83	1	6
macrophages)	LPS 50 μg/ml	4868 ± 632	10	6
Trehalose	None	1767 ± 245	3·6	12
dimycolate	MDP 10 μg/ml	5769 ± 749	11·7	12
elicited on day 7	MPP 50 μg/ml	3555 ± 462	7·3	5
(50 μg in	LPS 50 μg/ml	5921 ± 767	3·4	11
saline, i.p.)				

TMP is assayed at dilution 1/2 on thymocytes of C_3H/He J mice (8–9 weeks old). Results (mean ct/min ± s.e. from triplicate cultures) correspond to the average incorporation of ^{3}H-TdR obtained in the number of experiments indicated. Relative effect: ratio of the average value for each assay to the average value for unstimulated resident macrophages. MPP = muramyl pentapeptide.

In an attempt to reach an understanding of the cellular mechanism of these *in vivo* experiments, Tenu *et al.* (1980) have studied the activation of macrophages in mice by TDM and MDP. The criteria for activation were secretion of a monokine, the thymocyte mitogenic protein (TMP, also called LAF, or lymphocyte activating factor) and cytostaticity to a mastocytoma *in vitro*. Adherent cells from the peritoneal cavity of untreated mice do not secrete significant amounts of TMP and are poorly cytostatic. In contrast, adherent peritoneal cells from mice, to which at day-7 50 μg of TDM in saline emulsion had been injected intraperitoneally, secrete significant amounts of TMP (Table VI) and are strongly cytostatic for P 815 cells. The addition of 10 μg of MDP *in vitro* to such "activated" macrophages increases TMP production (Table VI) and compensates for the decline of activity observed during culture of the macrophages *in vitro*. Trehalose dimycolate is also active when added *in vitro*: (a) it enhances the cytostatic action of thioglycollate-elicited macrophages; (b) alone, or in sequence with MDP, it induces an appreciable cytostatic activity in resident macrophages (Table VII); (c) it limits the decline of the cytostatic activity of TDM-elicited macrophages occurring during *in vitro* cultivation. Here again, the synthetic C_{76} can replace TDM in obtaining cytostatic macrophages (Petit, Tenu and Drapier, unpub. experiments).

TABLE VII

Cytostatic activity of resident macrophages: sequential stimulation in vitro *by TDM and MDP, as measured by tritiated thymidine incorporation into syngeneic mastocytoma P 815 cells (from Tenu* et al., *1980)*

	In vitro *stimulation with*						
	12h (μg/ml)	*5% FCS*	*36h (μg/ml)*	*5% FCS*	*^{3}H-TdR incorporation culture*	*Growth inhibition (%)*	*No. of experiments*
P815 alone	—	—	—	—	35 358 ± 3394		14
P815	—	—	—	—	31 695 ± 3042		3
+	—	+	—	+	26 702 ± 3050	0	4
Resident							
macrophages	MDP 10	—	MDP 10	—	17 553 ± 877	34	3
	TDM 10	+	—	+	15 698 ± 941	41	5
	TDM 10	+	MDP 10	+	11 397 ± 3500	57	6
	TDM 10	+	MPP 50	+	14 199 ± 1800	47	3

FCS = foetal calf serum. MPP = muramyl pentapeptide.

These *in vivo* and *in vitro* studies show that mouse macrophages are highly susceptible to the action of TDM and MDP and that they can be the primary target of these immuno-modulators. The *in vivo* effects of TDM could be related to its chemotactic activity. The synergistic action of TDM and MDP might be explained by a modification of the macrophage membrane conformation by TDM, which then allows the approach of MDP to more or less specific surface receptors.

Some successful clinical experiments with injection of mycobacterial cell walls and TDM in melanoma lesions have been described (Vosika *et al.*, 1979), and a few cases of skin tumours have been treated with an ointment containing killed BCG + TDM (Cohen and Bekierkunst, 1979). In both instances, however, only a few cases have been treated and the beneficial effect of the adjunction of TDM has not been proven.

Conclusions

We have seen that natural and synthetic trehalose diesters, as well as muramylpeptides (MDP and derivatives) are potent adjuvants for stimulating antibody production and are also capable of increasing nonspecific resistance, as shown in various animal models by their antibacterial, antiparasitic and antitumour activities. We have also learnt that combined immunostimulation with emulsions containing trehalose diesters and muramylpeptides offers new possibilities for regression of tumours in animal models and we might suggest that such emulsions should also be tried as adjuvants for vaccines. Both categories of immunostimulants should find useful applications in immunodepressed animals or human beings.

The near future will tell whether these compounds will become widely used, relatively harmless drugs in veterinary and clinical medicine, or whether they will be superseded by one or several of the many new, natural and synthetic immunostimulants described in the recent literature. In that case TDM and MDP and their derivatives will still remain useful reagents for fundamental experiments in immunology.

References

Adam, A., Ciorbaru, R., Petit, J. F. and Lederer, E. (1972). *Proc. Natn. Acad. Sci. U.S.A.* **69**, 851.

Adam, A., Ellouz, F., Ciorbaru, R., Petit, J. F. and Lederer, E. (1975). *Z. Immun. Forsch.* **149**, 341.

Adam, A., Devys, M., Souvannavong, V., Lefrancier, P., Choay, J. and Lederer, E. (1976). *Biochem. Biophys. Res. Comm.* **72**, 339–346.

Adam, A., Souvannavong, V. and Lederer, E. (1978). *Biochem. Biophys. Res. Comm.* **85**, 684–690.

Asselineau, C. and Asselineau, J. (1978). *Prog. Chem. Fats Other Lipids* **16**, 59.

Audibert, F., Chedid, L. and Hannoun, C. (1977). *C. R. Hebd. Séanc. Acad. Sci. Ser. D.* **285**, 467.

Audibert, F., Heymer, B., Gros, C., Schleifer, K. H., Seidl, P. H. and Chedid, L. (1978). *J. Immunol.* **121**, 1219.

Azuma, I., Sugimura, K., Yamawaki, M., Uemiya, M., Kusumoto, S., Okada, S., Shiba, T. and Yamamura, Y. (1978). *Tetrahedron Lett.* **49**, 4899.

Bekierkunst, A., Levij, I. S., Yarkoni, E., Vilkas, E., Adam, A. and Lederer, E. (1969). *J. Bacteriol.* **100**, 95.

Bekierkunst, A., Levij, I. S., Yarkoni, E., Vilkas, E. and Lederer, E. (1971a). *Science* **174**, 1240.

Bekierkunst, A., Levij, E., Yarkoni, E., Flechner, J., Morecki, S., Vilkas, E. and Lederer, E. (1971b). *Infect. Immun.* **4**, 256.

Bekierkunst, A., Wang, L., Toubiana, R. and Lederer, E. (1974). *Infect. Immun.* **10**, 1044–1050.

Bloch, H. (1950). *J. Exp. Med.* **91**, 197.

Chedid, L., Audibert, F., Lefrancier, P., Choay, J. and Lederer, E. (1976). *Proc. Natn. Acad. Sci. U.S.A.* **73**, 2472–2475.

Chedid, L., Parant, M., Parant, F., Lefrancier, P., Choay, J. and Lederer, E. (1977). *Proc. Natn. Acad. Sci. U.S.A.* **74**, 2089–2093.

Chedid, L., Audibert, F. and Johnson, A. G. (1978). *Progr. Allergy* **25**, 63–105.

Chedid, L., Parant, M., Parant, F., Audibert, F., Lefrancier, P., Choay, J. and Sela, M. (1979). *Proc. Natn. Acad. Sci. U.S.A.* **76**, 6557.

Clark, I. A. (1979). *Parasite Immunol.* **1**, 179.

Cohen, H. A. and Bekierkunst, A. (1979). *Dermatologia* **158**, 117–125.
Dinarello, C. A., Elin, R. J., Chedid, L. and Wolff, S. M. (1978). *J. Infect. Dis.* **138**, 760–767.
Drapier, J. C., Lemaire, G., Tenu, J. P. and Petit, J. F. (1979). *In* "The Molecular Basis of Immune Cell Function" (J. G. Kaplan, ed.), p. 458. Elsevier, Amsterdam.
Dukor, P., Tarcsay, L. and Baschang, G. (1979). *Ann. Rep. Med. Chem.* **14**, 146–166.
Durette, P. L., Meitzner, E. P. and Shen, T. Y. (1979). *Carbohydr. Res.* **77**, C1.
Ellouz, F., Adam, A., Ciorbaru, R. and Lederer, E. (1974). *Biochem. Biophys. Res. Comm.* **59**, 1317–1325.
Février, M., Birrien, J. L., Leclerc, C., Chedid, L. and Liacopoulos, P. (1978). *Eur. J. Immunol.* **8**, 558.
Kato, J., Tamura, T. Siove, G. and Asselineau, J. (1978). *Eur. J. Biochem.* **87**, 497.
Kierszenbaum, F. and Ferraresi, R. W. (1979), *Infect. Immunol.* **25**, 273.
Kishimoto, T., Hirai, Y., Nakanishi, K., Azuma, I., Nagamatsu, A. and Yamamura, Y. (1979). *J. Immunol.* **123**, 2709.
Koga, T., Maeda, K., Onoue, K., Kato, K. and Kotani, S. (1979). *Mol. Immunol.* **16**, 153.
Kotani, S., Watanabe, Y., Kinoshita, F., Shimono, T., Morisaki, I., Shiba, T., Kusumoto, S., Tarumi, Y. and Ikenaka, K. (1975). *Biken J.* **18**, 105.
Kotani, S., Watanabe, Y., Shimono, T., Harada, K., Shiba, T., Kusumoto, S., Yokogawa, K. and Taniguchi, M. (1976). *Biken.* **19**, 9–13.
Kusumoto. S., Inage, M., Shiba, T., Azuma, I. and Yamamura, Y. (1978). *Tetrahedron Lett.* **49**, 4899.
Leclerc, C., Lamensans, A., Chedid, L., Drapier, J. C., Petit, J. F., Wietzerbin, J. and Lederer, E. (1976). *Cancer Immunol. Immunother.* **1**, 227–232.
Leclerc, C., Juy, D., Bourgeois, E. and Chedid, L. (1979). *Cell. Immunol.* **45**, 199.
Lederer, E. (1979). *Springer Sem. Immunopathol.* **2**, 133–148.
Lederer, E. (1980). *J. Med. Chem.* **23**, 819.
Lefrancier, P. L. and Lederer, E. (1980). *Prog. Chem. Org. Natn. Prod.* **40** (in press).
Lefrancier, P., Petitou, M., Level, M., Derrien, M., Choay, J. and Lederer, E. (1979). *Int. J. Pept. Protein Res.* **14**, 437.
Louis, J. A. and Lambert, P. H. (1979). *Springer Sem. Immunopathol.* **2**, 215.
Masihi, K. N., Brehmer, H. and Werner, H. (1979). *Zbl. Bakt. Hyg. I. Abt. Orig. A.* **245**, 377.
McLaughlin, C. A., Schwartzman, S. M., Horner, E. L., Jones, G. H., Moffat, G. J., Nestor, J. J. Jr and Tegg, D. (1980). *Science* **208**, 415–416.
Merser, C., Sinaÿ, P. and Adam, A. (1975). *Biochem. Biophys. Res. Comm.* **66**, 1316.
Meyer, T. J., Ribi, E. E., Azuma, I. and Zbar, B. (1974). *J. Natn. Cancer Inst.* **52**, 103–111.
Mitchell, G. H., Richards, W. H. G., Voller, A., Dietrich, F. M. and Dukor, P. (1979). *In* "Proceedings of NMRI/USAID/WHO. Workshop on the Immunology of Malaria", p. 189. Bethesda, Maryland, USA.
Nagao, S., Tanaka, A., Yamamoto, Y., Koga, T., Onoue, K., Shiba, T., Kusumoto, K. and Kotani, S. (1979). *Infect. Immun.* **24**, 308–312.
Noll, F., Bloch, H., Asselineau, J. and Lederer, E. (1956). *Biochem. Biophys. Acta* **20**, 299.
Olds, G. R., Chedid, L., Lederer, E. and Mahmoud, A. F. (1980). *J. Infect. Dis.* **141**, 473–478.
Pabst, M. J. and Johnston, R. B. (1980). *J. Exp. Med.* **151**, 101.
Parant, M. (1979). *Springer Sem. Immunopathol.* **2**, 101–118.
Parant, M., Parant, F., Chedid, L., Drapier, J. C., Petit, J. F., Wietzerbin, J. and Lederer, E. (1977). *J. Infect. Dis.* **135**, 771–777.
Parant, M., Parant, F. and Chedid, L. (1978a). *Proc. Natn. Acad. Sci. U.S.A.* **75**, 3395.
Parant, M., Audibert, F., Parant, F., Chedid, L., Soler, J., Polonsky, J. and Lederer, E. (1978b). *Infect. Immun.* **20**, 12–19.

Parant, M., Damais, C., Audibert, F., Parant, F., Chedid, L., Sache E., Lefrancier, P. and Lederer, E. (1978c). *J. Infect. Dis.* **138**, 378–386.

Parant, M., Parant, F., Chedid, L., Yapo, A., Petit, J. F. and Lederer, E. (1979). *Int. J. Immunopharmac.* **1**, 35–41.

Parant, M. A., Audibert, F. M., Chedid, L. A., Level, M. R., Lefrancier, P. L., Choay, J. P. and Lederer, E. (1980). *Infect. Immun.* **27**, 826–831.

Petit, J. F. and Lederer, E. (1978). *Symp. Soc. Gen. Microbiol.* **XXVIII**, 177–199.

Pimm, M. V., Baldwin, R. W., Polonsky, J. and Lederer, E. (1979). *Int. J. Cancer* **24**, 780–785.

Pimm, M. V., Baldwin, R. W. and Lederer, E. (1980). *Eur. J. Cancer* (in press).

Reese, R. T., Trager, W., Jensen, J. B., Miller, D. A. and Tantravahi, R. (1978). *Proc. Natn. Acad. Sci. U.S.A.* **75**, 5665.

Ribi, E. E., Takayama, K., Milner, K., Gray, G. R., Goren, M. B., Parker, R., McLaughlin, C. and Kelly, M. (1976). *Cancer Immunol. Immunother.* **1**, 265–270.

Ribi, E. E., Parker, R., Strain, S. M., Mizuno, Y., Notwotny, A., von Eschen, K. B., Cantrell, J. L., McLaughlin, C. A., Hwang, K. W. and Goren, M. B. (1979). *Cancer Immunol. Immunother.* **7**, 43.

Rotta, J., Rye, M., Mašek, K. and Zaoral, M. (1979). *Exp. Cell Biol.* **47**, 258.

Sackmann, W. and Dietrich, F. M. (1980). Abstract, Int. Symp. Infect. in Immunocompromised Host. June 1980. Veldhoven, The Netherlands.

Sela, S. and Mozes, E. (1979). *Springer Sem. Immunopathol.* **2**, 119.

Shiba, T., Okada, S., Kusumoto, S., Azuma, I. and Yamamura, Y. (1978). *Bull. Chem. Soc. (Jpn)* **51**, 3307.

Siddiqui, W. A., Taylor, D. W., Kan, S. Ch., Kramer, K., Richmond- rum, S. M., Kotani, S., Shiba, T. and Kusumoto, S. (1978). *Science* **201**, 1237.

Souvannavong, V. and Adam, A. (1980). *Eur. J. Immunol.* **10**, 645.

Taniyama, T. and Holden, H. T. (1979). *Cell. Immunol.* **48**, 369.

Tenu, J. P., Lederer, E. and Petit, J. F. (1980). *Eur. J. Immunol.* **10**, 647.

Tribouley, J., Tribouley-Duret, J. and Appriou, M. (1979). *C. R. Soc. Biol.* **173**, 1046.

Tsujimoto, M., Kinoshita, F., Okunaga, T., Kotani, S., Kusumoto, S., Yamamoto, K. and Shiba, T. (1979). *Microbiol. Immunol.* **23**, 933.

Uemiya, M., Sugimura, K., Kusama, T., Saiki, I., Yamawaki, M., Azuma, I. and Yamamura, Y. (1979). *Infect. Immun.* **24**, 83.

Vosika, G. S., Schmidtke, J. R., Goldman, A., Ribi, E., Parker, R. and Gray, G. R. (1979). *Cancer* **44**, 495–503.

Vosika, G. S., Schmidtke, J. R., Goldman, A., Parker, R., Ribi, E. and Gray, G. R. (1980). *Cancer Immunol. Immunother.* **4**, 221–224.

Wahl, S. M., Wahl, L. M., McCarthy, J. B., Chedid, L. and Mergenhagen, S. E. (1979). *J. Immunol.* **122**, 2226–2231.

Webster, R. G., Glezen, W. P., Hannoun, C. and Laver, W. G. (1977). *J. Immunol.* **119**, 2073.

White, R. G., Bernstock, L., Johns, R. G. and Lederer, E. (1958). *Immunol.* **1**, 54.

Yarkoni, E. and Bekierkunst, A. (1976). *Infect. Immun.* **14**, 1125.

Yarkoni, E., Rapp, H. J., Polonsky, J. and Lederer, E. (1978). *Int. J. Cancer* **22**, 564–569.

Yarkoni, E., Rapp, H. J., Polonsky, J., Varenne, J. and Lederer, E. (1979). *Infect. Immun.* **26**, 462–466.

Yarkoni, E. and Rapp, H. J. (1980). *Infect. Immun.* **28**, 881–886.

Yarkoni, E., Lederer, E. and Rapp, H. J. (1980). Abstracts. Fourth International Congress of Immunology, Paris, 1980.

Theme 17: Summary
Manipulation of the Immune System

ERNA MÖLLER

Department of Immunology, Karolinska Institut Medical School, Stockholm, Sweden

This theme included many diverse subjects, ranging from drug effects on immune responses (17.1,3,7), to thymic hormones, lymphokines and monokines (17.2), to specific manipulation of immune responses by antigenic determinants (17.4,8) and specific manipulation of immune responses by anti-idiotypic immunizations, tolerance and enhancement (17.6).

It has been said that it is easy to perform immunological experiments, since you can simply inject something into a mouse and obtain an antibody. Then you can characterize it. If there is no response, it might be even more interesting. Certainly, manipulations of immune response offers even more advanced possibilities, since responses in conjunction with various drugs offer unique possibilities of variability, and evidently, all results are true whether they are relevant or not.

One of the lessons I have learnt during this conference, is that all immunosuppressive drugs are also immunostimulatory and vice versa depending upon dose, kinetics, type of immunocompetent subpopulation affected, or, not least, whether you test effects of drugs *in vitro* or *in vivo*. For instance, the best adjuvants which are often and conveniently bacterial products, which increase B cell activity, are also excellent inducers of T suppressor cells (17.3). All this is of course understandable, if, and as Niels Jerne foresaw, the immune system is a network of specific effector molecules. However, we have also learnt during this week that nonspecific mediator molecules interact in similar feedback systems and that many different kinds of molecules interact in immune responses (17.2).

It is extremely difficult to conclude anything about effects of drugs on immune responses as a whole, before we know the physiological process of immune reactions. Other difficulties include the fact that different investigators use highly divergent test systems, and in most cases it is not known how a particular *in vitro* system reflects the status of the individual as a whole. Even more difficult are studies in man, where the only source of cells for *in vitro* experiments are blood lymphocytes, where many different variables can affect traffic and localization of immunocompetent cells.

Immune responses can be modulated using different antigenic determinants (17.4). Some structures or ways of presentation of antigen are believed to selectively facilitate induction of suppression over help etc. Various experimental protocols have revealed that different antigenic determinants induce T and B cell proliferation (17.4:14,16,17). This possibly reflects on different repertoires of specific receptors in these two cell populations, but that does not surprise me. Other experiments hinted at different requirements and antigenic determinants for activation of help versus suppression in T cells (17.4.03,04,09). However, the molecular structure of these determinants are not yet known, and I personally believe that studies on "self" molecules recognized by various T cell subsets could give more information than studies on more or less conventional "nonself" antigens. If T_s and T_H represent distinct subpopulations of T cells, different antigen binding receptor repertoires can be expected, but if they represent functional subsets of one single differentiation line of T cells, direct receptor specificity differences become harder to explain.

The ultimate goal for manipulations of immune responses is the specific interference with clonal reactions. Anti-idiotypic reactions induced after immunization with alloantibodies or with MLC activated blasts, according to the model by Leif Andersson *et al.* (*Nature, Lond.* **264**, 778, 1976) using cells enriched for idiotypic determinants, has been advocated as useful means for specific immunosuppression of alloimmune responses. However, as yet, no experimental models have been devised which will ensure specific loss of alloreactivity. Anti-idiotypic antibodies can sometimes be induced after blast immunization, which block *in vitro* reactions, such as MLC responses, but *in vivo* reactions have not indicated lack of reactivity (17.6.06,07).

This raised the issue of the type of cell to be used for immunizations, as well as the possibility of too narrow a specificity of the anti-idiotypic response. However, various studies even using the original experimental protocols have failed to reproduce good results. Hans Binz recently stated that graft prolongation only occurred in 30% of his animals. In this congress, Capel (17.6.06) demonstrated that alloreactive H-2L anti-idiotypic antibodies could indeed be raised by blast immunization, without effect on graft survival. However, the serum was effective *in vitro*, and separation into the IgG1 and IgG2a classes demonstrated graft prolongation with the IgG2a, but not with the IgG1 antibodies, which in fact had the reverse effect. These effects of different anti-idiotypic isotypes have clear and interesting correlates in other experimental systems and warrant further documentation. The implication that binding of the idiotype by effector cells or antibodies is not enough for effects is important enough.

Tolerance has usually been considered to result from specific clonal deletion. However, the issue has been raised as to whether this phenomenon could be mediated by suppressor cells. Clear examples of active suppression have been demonstrated even in neonatally tolerant animals, and an important contribution by Dorsch and Roser (17.6.10) revealed T suppressor cells of donor phenotype present in the thoracic duct, but not in bone marrow of recipients in neonatally tolerant animals.

Other tolerance-inducing regimens also clearly indicated suppressor mechanisms, like the intriguing finding of Brent and his colleagues (17.6.04), that injection of minute but not high amounts of blood (1 μl), to mice given conventional immunosuppressive drugs can ensure a high rate of alloskingraft tolerance. The similarities to and the implications of these findings for the human allotransplant situation is obvious, and might explain the hitherto unclear blood transfusion effects in transplant patients.

Of course, the initial concept of clonal deletion in tolerance is still very much valid. However, it might be pointed out here that in B cell tolerance to thymus-independent antigens, unresponsiveness never involves clonal deletion, but only affects that part of the clone which carries activation receptors for the tolerogen. Specific clonal reactivity can be achieved with the tolerated determinant present on another activation ligand (C. Fernandez and G. Möller, *J. Immunol.* **7**, 137, 1978). Maybe we should think of T cell subpopulations in the same way, and try to analyse situations where only one of several cell populations are tolerized. It might even be conceivable that a straightforward primary immune response is only obtained in situations where suppressor cells are tolerized, or where clones of anti-idiotypically reactive cells are specifically eliminated within that subset. It is hard for me to understand how secondary responses can ever occur in the presence of the now well documented regulatory networks of extreme complexity. One can also ask, as did Czitrom, and also Gruchalla and Streilein (17.6.08,27), if H-2 I-J molecules always induce suppressive phenomena? They found it did, and I think, if true, this might indicate that I-J molecules are in fact the physiological activating ligands for suppressor T cells.

Much debate was initiated by the presentation by Gorszynski (17.6.13) that neonatal tolerance can be transferred from tolerant males to their offspring both in the first and second generation, and also by the revival of the demonstration that immune RNA can confer specific immune reactivity (17.6.24,25). As the chairman, Dr Brent, pointed out, we should not forget that in his early experiments, tolerant males mated to tolerant females had normally reactive offspring. This, I believe, is very important. Not only need new conclusions and experiments be repeated in other experimental situations and by other scientists, but the new discoveries should be discussed in terms of older data on the same subject, which might not be easily reconciled with a new phenomenon. I personally believe that this is one of the most important aspects of immunology today. If your data do not fit with earlier findings, you are obliged to explain why they do not.

Specific immunosuppression can also be achieved by TLI (Total Lymphoid Irradiation) in rodents as pioneered by Strober and Slavin (17.1.19,46). Fractionated doses of irradiation according to Kaplan's scheme for treatment of patients with Hodgkin's disease are given during a couple of weeks, followed by bone marrow injection. Injection of allogenic bone marrow leads to chimaerism, and eventually to specific graft acceptance.

Experiments were shown which indicate that TLI treatment in mice leads to the formation of suppressor cells, at first acting nonspecifically, and to the appearance in the peripheral lymphoid organs of more immature lymphoid cells, as evidenced by different IgM/IgG and IgM/IgD ratios in B cells, and peripheral T cells carrying the TL marker. According to Ellen Vitetta, cells from TLI mice can be readily tolerized *in vitro*. Possibly, such phenomena are the reasons for induction of allograft acceptance in these animals, and establishment of chimaerism. This very appealing way of immunosuppression has not yet been successful in other species, such as dogs and humans (17.1.29,36). The reasons for these discrepancies are not yet known, but warrant caution for the immediate use of TLI as the tool for human allograft acceptance.

In the area of thymic hormones substantial progress has been made recently (17.2). Many different thymic peptide hormones have been described, some of which have now been completely sequenced. To these belong thymosin a_1, b_3, b_4, the Tp-5 peptide of thymopoietin and of course the nonapeptide, FTS. These peptides can now be synthesized chemically, and new techniques of recombinant DNA cloning have introduced the gene for *N*-a-desacetyl-thymosin a_1 into *E. coli* (A. Goldstein, pers. comm.). These peptides interestingly show little sequence homology, which fits well with their action at different stages of maturation of the T cell lineage. Some factors have also been found to have immune restorating properties *in vitro* and *in vivo*, but interpretation is difficult because of multiple influences of these agents on various immune responses.

Lymphokines are becoming ever more central in immunology. Not only do we need TCGF for continuous growth of T cell lines, but we need to understand the interacting systems of monokines and lymphokines in immune responses. Cell lines producing TCGF will of course aid in these studies (17.2.13, R. T. Smith, pers. comm.). TCGF can restore thymus-dependent responsiveness in nude mice, and in neonatally thymectomized mice, and clinical experiments using both hormones and lymphokines are underway. Let us hope that we shall soon learn that immunomodulating drugs interfere with specific hormones and "kines" at specific stages of differentiation and immune reactions, so that their use will be understood in the light of the ever increasing knowledge of physiological modulating molecules.

The last lesson for now concerns immunostimulatory and immunosuppressive drugs. As already mentioned, effects can vary, and the best adjuvants for humoral responses, such as various bacterial products, seem to be powerful for the induction of suppressor T cells and enhancement of cell-mediated immunity.

As one example of new information in the workshop on Immunopharmacology, I cite the chairman's summary: "The new drug Isoprinosin, made its pharmacological debut in this workshop. Several abstracts dealt with the effects of this new drug". In spite of the scientific debut, everyone of you was supplied with a folder in your congress bag from a company selling this drug, which according to them, I quote, "safely and effectively restores impaired cell-mediated immunity" and advocated the drug for the treatment of influenza, Herpes infections and infectious hepatitis.

Clinical studies are said to be underway, and we can only hope that they will be critically reviewed and presented in scientific journals before they make their way to the newspaper front pages, and patients demand treatment with the drug. Dr White, the chairman of one of these workshops stated: "Attention should be alerted to the potential hazards of immunopotentiation in man including induction of auto-immune disease, enhancement of tumor growth, arthritis and other immune complex disorders and amyloid disease".

I would like to end this summary with a beautiful example of how the use of these new drugs can elucidate basic functions of the immune response. Cyclosporin, a fungus derivative, in clinical use already, with efficient immunosuppressive effects, but unfortunately, a high lymphoma incidence in patients, was shown by Graham Bird to completely block T cell dependent polycolonal activation of immunoglobulin synthesis in human lymphocytes, without any demonstrable effect of thymus-indpendent activation by EB-virus. However, he found that the presence of this drug in *in vitro* cultures will allow the formation of cell lines from all individuals, whether seropositive for EBV or not; thus probably interfering with regulatory T cell mechanisms. However, the implication of this finding for the high incidence on lymphoma tumours in cyclosporin treated patients is enormous, since activation of dormant EB-virus has been implicated as the agent responsible for at least some of the lymphomas in transplanted patients. This is one way, in which work with special drugs and characterization of their effect, can have important clinical implications.

Theme 18

Human and Experimental Immunopathology

Presidents:
F. ROSEN
M. SELIGMANN

Symposium chairman:
J. HUMPHREY

64

The Amyloid Diseases

EDWARD C. FRANKLIN and PETER D. GOREVIC

Department of Medicine, Irvington House Institute, New York Medical Center, and Division of Allergy, Rheumatology and Clinical Immunology, State University of New York, New York, USA

Introduction and clinical features

Almost since the discovery of amyloidosis by Virchow in 1854, it has been suspected that amyloidosis is not a single entity but rather a group of diseases, all characterized by the deposition of a homogenous infiltrate with very typical staining properties. If they progress, these deposits ultimately cause destruction of the involved organs and if the liver, heart or kidney are involved, they lead to death. The initial suspicion of heterogeneity among the amyloid diseases was based on the variability of the clinical features. The characteristic patterns of organ involvement together with the nature of the associated diseases and in some instances a typical familial distribution have given rise to a variety of classifications (Dahlin, 1950), one of which is listed in Table I. In recent years, the concept that amyloid is a generic term encompassing a variety of different diseases has been borne out as a result of the demonstration by biochemical and immunologic techniques that there are striking differences in the nature of the major components of several of these clinically distinguishable types of amyloid deposits, even though all of them appear identical by light and electron microscopy (Franklin and Zucker-Franklin, 1972; Glenner *et al.*, 1973; Glenner and Page, 1976; Rosenthal and Franklin, 1977). So far these approaches have been applied successfully only to the most common

Supported by USPHS Research Grant Nos AM 01431, AM 02594, and The Michael and Helen Schaffer Fund.

TABLE I
Clinical and biochemical classification of the amyloid diseases

Type–clinical	*Associated diseases*	*Protein subunit*[a]
Primary and myeloma associated	Myeloma, macroglobulinaemia, monoclonal gammopathy and related plasma cellular neoplasma	AL (λ or κ) with λ predominant
Secondary	Chronic infections, inflammatory conditions, Hodgkin's, etc.	AA
Hereditary—many types		
FMF	—	AA
Portuguese	—	AF_P (prealbumin)
Localized		
Endocrine organs	Medullary carcinoma of the thyroid	AE_E (Thyrocalcitonin)
	Diabetes	AE(? glucagon)
		AE(? glucagon)
	Others	AE(? other hormones)
Senile		
Cardiac		AS_c (6000–14 000 mol. wt)
Brain, etc.		$AS_?$
Cutaneous	Localized amyloid	$AD_?$
Others		?

A stands for amyloid; the second letter identifies the type of deposit, and the subscript defines the deposit more precisely when known.
[a] Nomenclature as suggested at a meeting in Portugal in 1979. Glenner, G. G., Coste, P. P. and Freitas, F. (eds). *In* "Amyloid and Amyloidosis". *Excerpta Medica* (in press).

and widespread forms of the disease. However, it seems likely that in the next few years some of the blanks in Table I will be filled in by analysis of the rarer and more localized forms of amyloidosis and that a more precise biochemical classification will replace the current clinical one (Glenner, 1980).

In this discussion, we will attempt to summarize some of the recent advances in our understanding of the two major types of amyloid diseases, i.e. the primary or light chain related type and the secondary or AA related type, and point out some of the approaches currently employed in trying to understand the pathogenesis of some of these disorders. We will also attempt to predict some of the advances we are likely to encounter in the next few years. The approach we will use to examine their pathogenesis is somewhat mechanistic and is based on currently available information related to the nature of the amyloid substances and the discovery of larger circulating precursors whose synthesis is increased in certain pathologic states and which appear to be processed by proteolysis in the two most common types. This escapes the need to go deeply into the role of disordered B cell or T cell function, an area replete with contradictory information that is often difficult to evaluate critically. This confusion is in large part due to the existence of a plethora of animal models of amyloidosis, in many of which the disease appears to be induced and influenced by a variety of different and often contradictory factors, whose complexity makes it difficult to delineate clearly the aetiologic mechanisms underlying the disease. Consequently, no effort will be made to cover exhaustively the complex and often confusing immunologic phenomena that have been described in several experimental models of amyloidosis other than to emphasize the fact that all seem to involve components of the immune system.

Before discussing the nature of the amyloid substances, a few words dealing with the clinical features of the L chain (primary) and AA protein (secondary) types of amyloid seem warranted since they will place the inciting agents in proper perspective. With the decrease in chronic infectious and inflammatory diseases and the widespread clinical use of serum and urine electrophoresis and immunoelectrophoresis, the primary or perhaps better referred to as the L chain type of amyloidosis associated either with a full blown neoplasm of plasma cells or lymphocytes, or at times with a very localized or latent form of such a neoplastic process which is difficult or even impossible to document, has become the most common type of amyloidosis in the Western World. This type of amyloidosis has been estimated to occur in 6–15% of patients with otherwise typical multiple myeloma (Cohen, 1967), often in association with marked Bence Jones proteinuria most frequently of the λ type. In about half the patients with this type of amyloid disease, a plasma cell neoplasm is obvious, whereas in the other half its existence can only be suspected. Regardless of this, in all instances the disorder appears to be a result of the overproduction by plasma cells or lymphocytes of light chains which may or may not be detectable in serum or urine.

In the past, and in many parts of the world where parasitic and bacterial infections continue to be prevalent, secondary or AA protein amyloidosis is the most common type of this disease. The incidence of the "secondary form" of amyloidosis in the Western World is on the decline owing to the virtual eradication of chronic suppurative conditions such as osteomyelitis, tuberculosis, bronchiectasis, and syphilis, which used to be largely reponsible for the development of this disease (Cohen, 1967; Brandt *et al.*, 1968). This type of amyloidosis is now more often encountered in chronic illnesses, such as paraplegia and other neurologic diseases, chronic pyelonephritis, Hodgkin's disease, renal cell carcinoma, leprosy, regional ileitis, rheumatoid arthritis, and other types of inflammatory arthritis, and in drug addicts with chronic suppurative diseases. In general, the feature common to all these underlying diseases is the prolonged and persistent stimulation of the RES.

It is important to emphasize that virtually all types of amyloidosis in experimental animals, regardless of the inciting regimen, correspond to the AA type of amyloidosis. Consequently all experimental models provide information related only to this form of amyloidosis and offer no insights into the light chain related forms.

Just for the sake of completeness—though they will not be discussed in detail—it seems appropriate to mention the amyloid deposits of the brain and aorta, pancreas, testes and heart, that accompany ageing, several localized forms of amyloid deposits of endocrine organs including the pancreas and thyroid, a host of familial forms differing in organ involvement in different regions of the world, and some other types localized to skin, lung, and other organs. The limited information about these forms of the disease and the nature of their major protein constituents are summarized in Table I.

Nature of the amyloid deposits

All amyloid appears as a homogeneous eosinophilic extracellular deposit that destroys the surrounding cells by compression. This material is metachromatic with several dyes like toluidine blue and crystal violet, binds Congo red avidly, and gives a characteristic green birefringence when viewed by polarizing

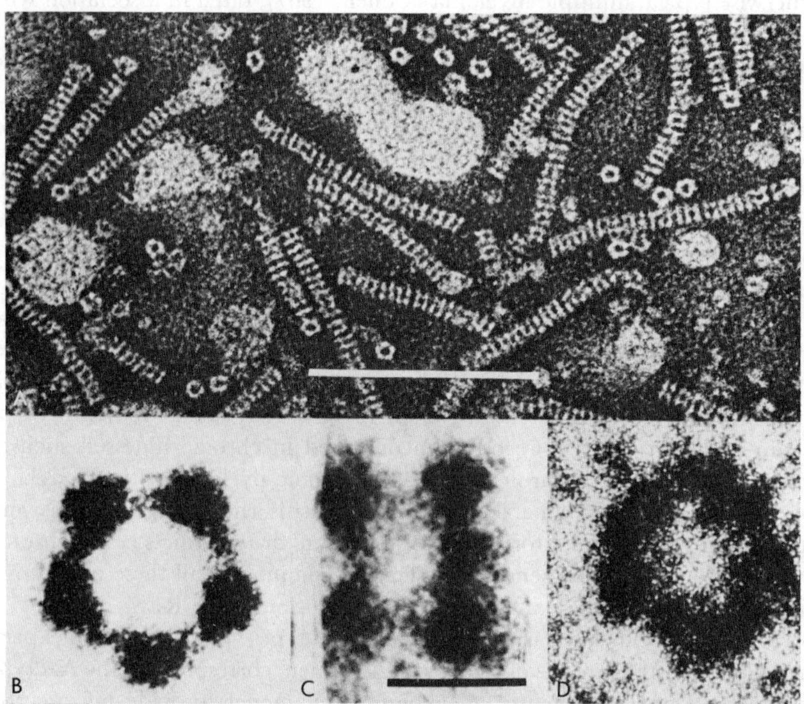

FIG. 1. *Amyloid fibrils negatively stained with 1% phosphotunstic acid* (× *60 000*). (*Courtesy of Dr D. Zucker-Franklin, NYU Medical Center.*)

microscopy (Glenner and Page, 1976; Rosenthal and Franklin, 1977). Nevertheless, when viewed in the electron microscope, amyloid was found to consist of long fibrils with a diameter of 10–15 nm and made up of two longitudinal 4 to 6 filaments separated by a clear space of 2·5–5·0 nm. The fibrils are long and twisting and tend to polymerize (Fig. 1). The possible existence of additional subunits of the fibrils that can be resolved morphologically has been raised by some (Shirahama and Cohen, 1967; Pras *et al.*, 1968, 1969) but still remains in doubt. In spite of this morphologic uniformity and striking similarity of all types of amyloid even on X-ray diffraction analysis, recent biochemical studies have provided convincing evidence for the uniqueness of different amyloid substances. This progress is a direct result of our ability to isolate the fibrils in a state of purity by a variety of techniques, the simplest of which takes advantage of the fact that the fibrils are insoluble in the presence of salt and can be extracted as a colloidal suspension in distilled water after repeated extractions of contaminating proteins with physiological saline (Pras *et al.*, 1968).

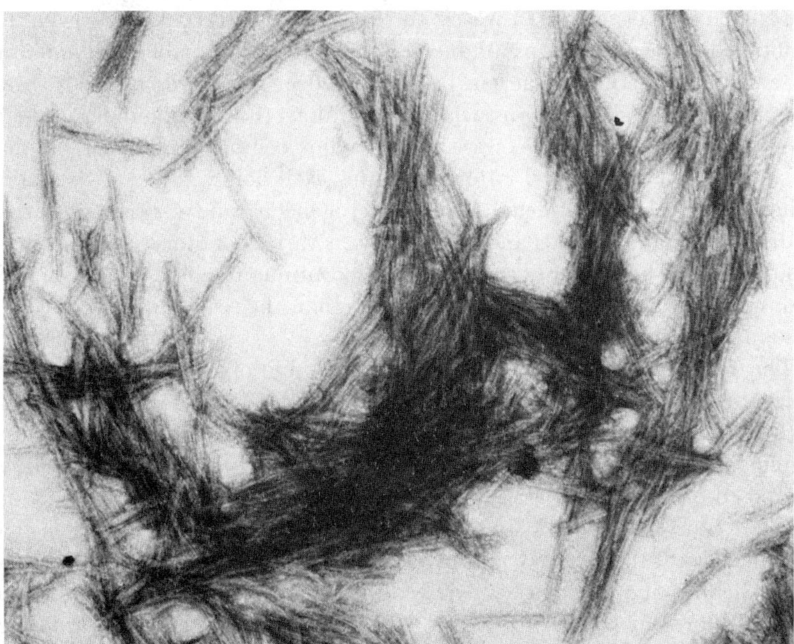

FIG. 2. *Electronmicrograph of SAP in 1 mM EDTA, negatively stained with silicotungstate. The micrograph shows: (top) pentagonal macromolecules and rod-like supramolecular assemblies. The marker is equal to 1000 Å; (B) a photographic integration of the pentagon prepared by superimposing a number of selected negative images; (C) a similar technique was used to produce an integrated image of the side view of the macromolecule prepared from the rods; (D) in some fields decagons are evident as shown in the integrated image. (From Pinteric and Painter, 1972.)*

The saline supernatant in all forms of amyloid contains another substance with a unique ultrastructural appearance known as the P component (Bladen *et al.*, 1966; Skinner *et al.*, 1974). In the EM, this protein has the appearance of a doughnut with 5 subunits that tend to stack in the form of long filaments (Fig. 2). The P component, although it makes up less than 10% of all amyloid deposits, is undoubtedly important because it is present in all types of naturally occurring and experimental amyloid and is of interest because of its striking homology with C-reactive protein (Osmand *et al.*, 1977; Levo *et al.*, 1977). The P component in amyloid has a molecular weight of 180 000 to 200 000, is composed of 10 identical noncovalently linked subunits, and is antigenetically related to an α_1 serum glycoprotein (Skinner *et al.*, 1974). Like CRP, it interacts with a variety of cells and proteins in the presence of calcium. However, its precise biologic function remains to be elucidated since it appears to behave only to a limited extent as an acute phase reactant, especially in situations or species where C reactive protein is lacking. It seems likely that together with CRP it serves an as yet undefined function in the response of the host to his environment.

After removal of these saline extractable components, the amyloid fibrils are recovered in a state of purity in the distilled water fraction which has the appearance of serum. In water, the fibrils tend to precipitate slowly and spontaneously, but do so instantaneously after the addition of small amounts of salt. The material which can be released from the fibrils prepared from all types of amyloid under dissociative conditions (using guanidine, urea, or alkali) has been shown to consist of two major components. One, common to all amyloid substances, is found in the exclusion volume of Sephadex columns. It remains ill-defined and heterogeneous and consists of carbohydrates, free amino acids and presumably a variety of other substances. Its molecular weight and antigenic properties continue to elude analysis and it seems possible that it represents little more than the scaffolding upon which the amyloid substance is deposited.

The second component, usually a protein subunit of low molecular weight, differs depending on the type of amyloid from which it is derived. Only two of these will be discussed in detail since they appear to be related to the immune system in their origin. All types of amyloid fibrils, however, seem to be composed of molecules with a β pleated sheet structure.

The first of the amyloid subunits to be characterized in detail was that associated with the primary and myeloma associated form of the disease. In 1971 Glenner and coworkers (reviewed in Glenner and Page, 1974) showed that the fibrils are composed of the amino terminal fragments of immunoglobulin light chains; to date, no heavy chain fragments have been found, although one heavy chain disease protein has been converted into amyloid-like fibrils by proteolysis *in vitro* (Pruzanski *et al.*, 1974). This heterogeneous group of proteins is now called AL (amyloid L chain) protein and is usually, but not always, associated with a similar or related L chain containing immunoglobulin in the serum. The AL proteins range in size from 5000–25 000 and generally begin at the amino terminal end of the variable region (Glenner *et al.*, 1971b). They usually include the variable region in addition to part of the constant region and may sometimes even consist of the entire L chains, in which case they appear to be absolutely identical to the related urine or serum protein (Terry *et al.*, 1973). Their relation to light chains of immunoglobulins was shown by 3 types of studies. The first and most clearcut evidence was the demonstration that the amino acid sequence of the amino terminal region of the amyloid proteins was homologous or identical to that of κ or λ light chain variable regions (Glenner *et al.*, 1971b). A byproduct of such studies has been the discovery of new $V\lambda$ ($V\lambda6$) subclass, which has been found in 6 amyloid-related λ chain proteins (Sletten *et al.*, 1974; Solomon and Franklin, 1980). Additional support for this conclusion was provided when fibrils with the appearance of amyloid fibrils were produced *in vitro* by proteolytic digestion of some, but not all Bence Jones proteins, especially those belonging to the $V\lambda_1$ subclass (Glenner *et al.*, 1971a; Linke *et al.*, 1973a), and by the finding that antisera to amyloid subunits cross-reacted with κ or λ light chains (Isersky *et al.*, 1972). There can be little doubt that these immunoglobulin-related proteins or their precursors are synthesized by plasma cells or lymphoid cells. Some are deposited intact, while others appear to result from the degradation of an L chain, either as a consequence of some inherent structural property of some light chain proteins or as a result of some unusual features of the degradative mechanisms by which the individual metabolized his light chains. The former possibility is supported by the demonstration that certain Bence Jones proteins, especially of the $V\lambda_1$ subclass, assume the appearance of amyloid fibrils when degraded by several proteolytic enzymes, including those from renal lysosomes (Epstein *et al.*, 1974), and that so far all $V\lambda6$ proteins have been found in patients with amyloidosis, while the role of degradative processes is suggested by the fact that amyloid fibrils can be prepared *in vitro* from proteins from patients without amyloidosis (Linke *et al.*, 1973b). For reasons that are not yet clear, the frequency of λ-related proteins in amyloid fibrils and in the sera of patients with amyloidosis is much higher than that of proteins of the κ chain class which constitute the predominant L chain class in all immunoglobulins and myeloma proteins (Isobe and Osserman, 1974). It is of interest that one rare subclass of λ chains appears only in association with amyloidosis (Sletten *et al.*, 1974).

The origin of this type of amyloid subunit in plasma cells and lymphocytes is abolutely certain. The processing to the fibril can, on occasion, occur within or in direct proximity to the plasma cell producing it since at times intracellular amyloid fibrils have been observed. However, more commonly processing seems to occur at distant sites. The exact nature of the cell responsible for processing and factors responsible for the typical tissues distribution remain uncertain. However, it seems likely that proteolytic processing of the L chain subunit is essential for fibril formation to occur.

Amyloid fibrils from patients with the secondary type of amyloidosis and certain familial forms such as Familial Mediterranean Fever, as well as those isolated from all experimentally induced and naturally occurring amyloid deposits in all species examined so far (Glenner and Page, 1976; Rosenthal and Franklin, 1977), consist primarily of a protein known as the amyloid A (AA) protein. It is unrelated to any immunoglobulin and has no relationship to any hitherto described protein (Benditt and Eriksen, 1971a, b; Levin *et al.*, 1972). This protein generally has a mol. wt of 8500, although a fragment half this size was isolated from the fibrils of one patient with rheumatoid arthritis and several intermediate fragments have been found in the tissues of other patients. The amino acid sequence of proteins from man, baboons, ducks, guinea-pigs, mice, and mink have demonstrated significant homologies among different species (Eriksen *et al.*, 1976). The several human proteins that have been sequenced have been shown to be virtually identical in the amino terminal half but to have some differences in the carboxy terminal half (Sletten *et al.*, 1974).

In considering its possible origin, it is of interest that the human protein is often heterogeneous at the amino terminus and that several additional residues precede the first in duck and guinea-pig amyloid. These findings suggest that, like the L chain-related amyloid, AA amyloid is derived by proteolysis from a larger precursor. Support for this mechanism was provided by the discovery in serum of a larger antigenically related component known as SAA, which is an α_1 globulin with a mol. wt of 12 000 to 14 000 and which exists in the serum complexed to other proteins such as high density lipoproteins (Anders *et al.*, 1975; Benditt and Eriksen, 1977) or albumin (Rosenthal *et al.*, 1976; Rosenthal and Franklin, 1977). Amino acid sequence studies of SAA have demonstrated sequence identity for the entire 76 residues and have documented the existence of multiple polymorphic species of SAA within a single individual (Franklin, 1980). Only a partial sequence is available for the additional 30 residue carboxyterminal extension which is presumably cleaved by proteolysis in the process of AA deposition. Recent studies of SAA and AA in a number of inbred strains of mice subjected to different inducing regimens have demonstrated the existence of several closely related species of SAA, only some of which appear to be deposited in the tissue amyloid deposits (Gorevic *et al.*, 1978; Franklin, 1980).

Studies of the biologic behaviour of this serum component have shown a number of features that may have some bearing on pathogenetic mechanisms in this type of amyloidosis (Husby and Natvig, 1974; Rosenthal and Franklin, 1975; Gorevic *et al.*, 1976). Its concentration is very low (less than 200 μg/ml) during the first 5 decades of life and has been found by several observers to increase significantly in older age, often to a level 10 or more times as great in the eighth and ninth decades. This finding of an age-related increase has not been confirmed by another group (Hijmans and Sipe, 1979). In addition, its concentration increases markedly in many chronic diseases, including all types of amyloidosis, cancer, infections, rheumatoid arthritis, multiple myeloma, macroglobulinaemia, lymphomas, and a variety of other disorders, and also in pregnancy. In acute infections, and in acute exacerbations of chronic diseases, the protein often behaves like an acute phase reactant, quickly returning to normal levels as the disease is brought under control. The prolonged liberation of this protein during many chronic diseases may well exceed the body's degradative capacity for this protein and may explain the deposition of this type of amyloidosis in association with many chronic diseases. Whether this is due simply to overproduction or perhaps also to faulty degradation is currently under study. In any case, the acute phase reactant properties of SAA preclude its use as a simple tool for the diagnosis of AA related amyloidosis.

The site of synthesis of SAA has been difficult to establish, but early studies have implicated fibroblasts (Linder *et al.*, 1976), blood mononuclear cells (Zucker-Franklin, 1977), and polymorphonuclear leukocytes (Rosenthal, 1977). Recently the hepatocyte has been shown to be the major site of synthesis (Sipe *et al.*, 1979; Benson and Kleiner, 1979) and it seems possible that each of these tissues may play a role. Processing to the AA fibril appears to occur at sites far removed from the site of synthesis. Of interest is the SAA response and the ability to induce amyloidosis in the endotoxin resistant C3H/Hej mouse. Endotoxin is one of the best agents to induce an SAA response and amyloid deposits in mice. In this particular strain, however, endotoxin is ineffective, other agents like casein are equally as effective as they are in all other strains of mice. In addition, it is possible to circumvent the defect by administering a serum fraction obtained from other strains of endotoxin-treated mice, thus clearly proving that this resistant strain can develop amyloidosis provided that proper stimulus is used (Lavie *et al.*, 1980; Sipe *et al.*, 1979). There appear to be, however, variations, in the susceptibility of different strains of mice with the A/J strain the most resistant.

The biological functions of SAA or AA have not been elucidated. However, there are two reports which suggest that perhaps they have an immunosuppressive function or that they can interact and perhaps modify certain subsets of lymphocytes (Benson *et al.*, 1975; Rosenthal, 1977). Since the SAA protein is a significant serum component that has been conserved during evolution, an elucidation of its function is urgent.

It is now clear that amyloid is a generic term that encompasses a number of different diseases and chemical subunits. In addition to the two major types already described, systemic amyloidosis developing in association with certain malignancies appears to be AA protein and may reflect striking SAA elevations noted in neoplastic states. Localized amyloid occurring with medullary thyroid carcinoma appears to originate from prohormone forms of thyrocalcitonin (Sletten *et al.*, 1976) and so may some of the localized deposits in the pancreas, which may be derived from insulin and glucagon, since these hormones can be converted to fibrils appearing like amyloid by treatment with acid and other procedures (Linke *et al.*, 1976). Preliminary evidence indicates senile cardiac amyloid to be unique and composed of low mol. wt subunits that are structurally and antigenically unrelated to other forms of amyloid examined to date (Westermark *et al.*, 1977). Nothing is known about the chemical nature of other localized forms of any of the familial types with the exception of FMF, which consists of the AA protein (Levin *et al.*, 1972), and the Portuguese type, which is related to prealbumin (Costa *et al.*, 1978). A feature common to all amyloid-related proteins appears to be a β-pleated sheet structure. Perhaps this is related to the propensity of these proteins to form fibrils (Glenner and Page, 1976).

A great deal of contradictory information pointing to dysfunction of B and T cells in the aetiology of amyloidosis is difficult to interpret. Perhaps the application of newly described reagents to measure surface markers characteristic of different subsets of B and T cells in the near future may illuminate this important aspect of the problem. In the meantime, some information can be obtained from studies of the amyloid substances and possible factors involved in their production and degradation. Viewed in its simplest form, amyloid deposits of the two major types tend to occur in association with exposure to a large antigenic load (casein administration, hyperimmunized horses, and chronic infection in man), or with depression and in some instances with neoplastic proliferation of certain components of the immune system. In most instances, there appears to be the conversion of a soluble precursor to the insoluble fibril by proteolysis. In addition, it is recognized that amyloid fibrils are inert once deposited and that they resist removal by phagocytosis and proteolysis. Hence, the possibility remains that amyloid occurs because of overproduction of the precursor in hosts who are, genetically or for other reasons, defective in processing the precursor or fibril. This type of dual mechanism is suggested by the fact that SAA production in resistant and susceptible mice given endotoxin appears to be identical (Benson *et al.*, 1977; McAdam and Sipe, 1976), and by recent studies suggesting a defect in the processing of SAA and AA by macrophages of patients with amyloidosis and about 40% of normal subjects who are perhaps genetically more susceptible to developing the disease under appropriate stimuli (Lavie *et al.*, 1978). Studies of peripheral blood monocytes in man and peritoneal macrophages in mice have identified a group of membrane-associated serine proteases, which appear to cleave SAA either completely to dialysable peptides or to a transient or persistent AA-like intermediate. Studies are currently in progress to determine if one or more of these enzymes is absent or defective in cells from individuals with the disease and in about one-third of normal individuals who process SAA and AA in a manner similar to the patients with the disease. Preliminary studies suggest that the pattern of processing may be an inherited trait (Mornaghi *et al.*, 1980).

One last point is worthy of mention in discussing the course of the disease. Once deposited, it is difficult to remove amyloid. This is probably due to the fact that amyloid fibrils are poorly immunogenic and resistant to both phagocytosis and to proteolysis (Franklin and Pras, 1969; Zucker-Franklin and Franklin, 1970).

In conclusion, though much is known about the structure of several of the amyloid substances, we are still far removed from a clear understanding of the pathogenesis of the secondary AA type of the disease which seems to be associated with hyperactivity of the RES. It is hoped that work in the next few years will provide insights into this provocative problem.

References

Anders, R. E., Natvig, J. B., Michaelsen, T. E. and Husby, G. (1975). *Scand. J. Immunol.* **4**, 397.

Benditt, E. P. and Eriksen, N. (1971a). *Am. J. Pathol.* **65**, 231.

Benditt, E. P. and Eriksen, L. H. (1971b). *FEBS Lett.* **19**, 169.

Benditt, E. P. and Eriksen, N. (1977). *Proc. Natn. Acad. Sci. U.S.A.* **74**, 4025–4028.

Benson, M. D., Aldo-Benson, M. A., Shirahama, T., Borel, I. and Cohen, A. S. (1975). *J. Exp. Med.* **142**, 236.

Benson, M. D. and Kleiner, E. (1979). *Clin. Res.* **27**, 321.

Benson, M. D., Scheinberg, M. A., Shirahama, T., Cathcart, E. S. and Skinner, M. (1977). *J. Clin. Invest.* **59**, 412.

Bladen, H. A., Nylen, M. U. and Glenner, G. G. (1966). *J. Ultrastruct. Res.* **14**, 449–459.

Brandt, K., Cathcart, E. S. and Cohen, A. S. (1968). *Am. J. Med.* **44**, 955.

Cohen, A. S. (1967). *N. Engl. J. Med.* **277**, 522.

Costa, P. P., Figueira, A. S. and Bravo, F. R. (1978). *Proc. Natn. Acad. Sci. U.S.A.* **75**, 4499.

Dahlin, D. C. (1950). *Med. Clin. North Am.* **34**, 1107.

Epstein, W. V., Tan, M. and Wood, I. S. (1974). *J. Lab. Clin. Med.* **84**, 107.

Eriksen, N., Ericsson, L. H., Pearsall, N., Lagunoff, D. and Benditt, E. P. (1976). *Proc. Natn. Acad. Sci. U.S.A.* **73**, 964.

Franklin, E. C. (1980). Unpublished observation.

Franklin, E. C. and Pras, M. (1969). *J. Exp. Med.* **130**, 797.

Franklin, E. C. and Zucker-Franklin, D. (1972). *Adv. Immunol.* **15**, 249.

Glenner, G. G. (1980). *In* "Third International Symposium on Amyloidosis". Elsevier/North-Holland, Amsterdam (in press).

Glenner, G. G., Ein, D., Eanes, E. D., Bladen, H. A., Terry, W. and Page, D. L. (1971b). *Science* **174**, 712.

Glenner, G. G. and Page, D. L. (1976). *Int. Rev. Exp. Pathol.* **15**,1.

Glenner, G. G., Terry, W., Harada, M., Isersky, C. and Page, D. (1971a). *Science* **171**, 1150.

Glenner, G. G., Terry, W. D. and Isersky, C. (1973). *Semin Hematol.* **10**, 65.

Gorevic, P. D., Rosenthal, C. J. and Franklin, E. C. (1976). *Clin. Immunol. Immunopathol.* **6**, 83.

Gorevic, P. D., Levo, Y., Frangione, B. and Franklin, E. C. (1978). *J. Immunol.* **121**, 138.

Hijmans, W. and Sipe, J. P. (1979). *Clin. Exp. Immunol.* **35**, 96.

Husby, G. and Natvig, J. B. (1974). *J. Clin. Invest.* **53**, 1054.

Isersky, C., Ein, D., Page, D. L., Harada, M. and Glenner, G. G. (1972). *J. Immunol.* **108**, 486.

Isobe, T. and Osserman, E. F. (1974). *N. Engl. J. Med.* **290**, 473.

Lavie, G., Zucker-Franklin, D. and Franklin, E. C. (1978). *J. Exp. Med.* **148**, 1020.

Lavie, G., Flechner, E., Gallo, G. and Frangione, B. (1980). *In* "Amyloidosis" (G. Glenner, ed.). In press.

Levin, M., Franklin, E. C., Frangione, B. and Pras, M. (1972). *J. Clin. Invest.* **51**, 2773.

Levo, Y., Frangione, B. and Franklin, E. C. (1977). *Nature* **268**, 56.

Linder, E., Anders, R. F. and Natvig, J. B. (1976). *J. Exp. Med.* **144**, 1336–1346.

Linke, R. P., Zucker-Franklin, D. and Franklin, E. C. (1973a). *J. Immunol.* **111**, 10.

Linke, R. P., Tischendorf, F. W., Zucker-Franklin, D. and Franklin, E. C. (1973b). *J. Immunol.* **111**, 24.

Linke, R. P., Eanes, E. D., Termine, J. D., Bladen, H. A. and Glenner, G. G. (1976). *In* "Amyloidosis" (O. Wigelius and A. Pasternak, eds) pp. 371–374. Academic Press, New York.

McAdam, K. P. W. J. and Sipe, J. D. (1976). *J. Exp. Med.* **144**, 1121.

Mornaghi, R., Rubenstein, P. and Franklin, E. C. (1980). Unpublished observation.

Osmand, A. P., Friedenson, B., Gewurz, H., Painter, R. H., Hofmann, T. and Shelton, E. (1977). *Proc. Natn. Acad. Sci. U.S.A.* **74**, 739.

Pinteric, L. and Painter, R. H. (1972). *Can. J. Biochem.* **57**, 729.

Pras, M., Schubert, M., Zucker-Franklin, D., Rimon, A. and Franklin, E. C. (1968). *J. Clin. Invest.* **47**, 924.

Pras, M., Zucker-Franklin, D., Rimon, A. and Franklin, E. C. (1969). *J. Exp. Med.* **130**, 777.

Pruzanski, W., Katz, A., Nyburg, S. C. and Freedman, M. H. (1974). *Immunol. Comm.* **3**, 469.

Rosenthal, C. J. (1977). *Clin. Res.* **25**, 366.

Rosenthal, C. J. and Franklin, E. C. (1975). *J. Clin. Invest.* **55**, 746.

Rosenthal, C. J. and Franklin, E. C. (1977). *J. Immunol.* **119**, 630.

Rosenthal, C. J., Franklin, E. C., Frangione, B. and Greenspan, J. (1976). *J. Immunol.* **116**, 1415.

Shirahama, T. and Cohen, A. S. (1967). *J. Cell Biol.* **33**, 679.

Sipe, J. D., Vogel, S. N., Ryan, J. L., McAdam, K. P. W. J. and Rosenstreich, D. L. (1979). *J. Exp. Med.* **150**, 597.

Skinner, M., Cohen, A. S., Shirahama, T. and Cathcart, E. S. (1974). *J. Lab. Clin. Med.* **84**, 604.

Sletten, K., Husby, G. and Natvig, J. B. (1974). *Scand. J. Immunol.* **3**, 833.

Sletten, K., Westermark, P. and Natvig, J. B. (1976). *J. Exp. Med.* **143**, 993.

Solomon, A. and Franklin, E. C. (1980). Unpublished observation.

Terry, W. D., Page, D. L., Kumura, S., Isobe, I., Osserman, E. F. and Glenner, G. G. (1973). *J. Clin. Invest.* **52**, 1276.

Westermark, P., Natvig, J. and Johansson, B. (1977). *J. Exp. Med.* **140**, 631.

Zucker-Franklin, D. (1977). *In* "Amyloidosis" (O. Wigelius and A. Pasternak, eds). Academic Press, New York.

Zucker-Franklin, D. and Franklin, E. C. (1970). *Am. J. Pathol.* **59**, 23.

65

Immunological Aspects of Leprosy

M. HARBOE and O. CLOSS

University of Oslo, Institute for Experimental Medical Research, Ullevaal Hospital, Oslo, Norway

Leprosy may to a great extent be considered as an immunological disease. The causative organism, *Mycobacterium leprae*, is virtually nontoxic and may occur in great numbers in the skin with almost no clinical symptoms. Most symptoms of the disease are due to immune reactions against the bacilli. Complications such as nerve damage which is responsible for the deformities so often associated with the disease, are directly due to immune reactions. The case is the same for erythema nodosum leprosum (ENL) which is a classical example of an immune complex disease in man (Wemambu *et al.*, 1969). It has become increasingly apparent that leprosy offers unique opportunities for studies of the relationship between host and parasite during a chronic infection, particularly development of clinical symptoms due to immune reactions against antigenic substances liberated from micro-

Abbreviations

CMI: cell mediated immunity; CIE: crossed immunoelectrophoresis; DTH: delayed-type hypersensitivity; ENL: erythema nodosum leprosum; LTT: lymphocyte transformation test; MLM: *Myobacterium leprae*; RIA: radioimmunoassay.

organisms. Leprosy is thus developing as a "model disease" which provides essential information on the importance of immune reactions in several chronic infectious diseases.

In this position paper, we present our view on the current state of knowledge on essential immunological features of leprosy. We have deliberately focused attention on areas where current concepts may need to be challenged and where the available information is incomplete, thus pointing to areas in need of further work.

A portrait of the infection

The early events occurring after infection with *M. leprae* are incompletely known. The main current view is that most individuals do not develop symptoms after infection, as indicated in Fig. 1. We know little about the mechanisms of resistance in these cases. It may be due to an efficient immune response, or it may be an example of innate immunity largely depending on nonimmunological factors. If resistance is inadequate, the bacilli multiply with development of clinical disease which shows a highly variable course, forming a spectrum between two polar groups: tuberculoid leprosy (TT) with few lesions containing few bacilli, and lepromatous leprosy (LL) with multiple lesions where the bacilli grow without inhibition due to defective cell mediated immunity (Ridley and Jopling, 1966). The area between the polar groups is denoted "borderline leprosy" and is subdivided into various groups as indicated in the figure. The intention of this classification is "an ordering of the clinical, histological, and bacteriological spectrum of the disease in such a way that it expresses the immunity of the patient, since it is the immune response that determines both the spectrum and the prognosis of the patient" (Ridley, 1977). The histological classification depends on several criteria: the type of granuloma cell divides the spectrum in half, with epithelioid cells from TT to BB, and macrophages in BL and LL. The density of bacilli in the granuloma varies directly with the position in the spectrum between BT and BL. Infiltration of the subepidermal zone is almost invariable in TT, inconstant in BT, and this zone is clear in BB, BL and LL. Nerve involvement and

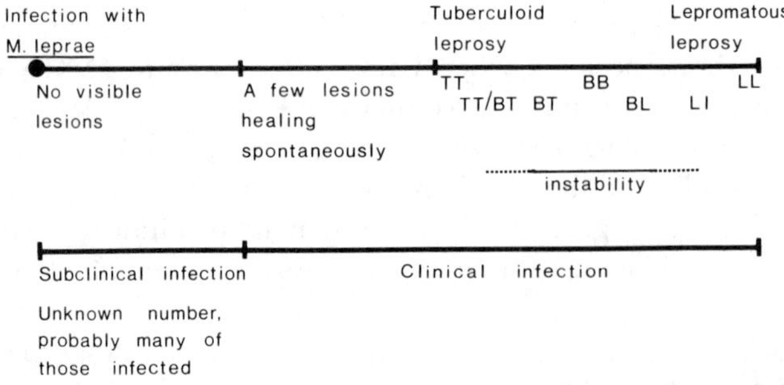

FIG. 1. *The course after infection with* M. leprae.

degree of lymphocyte infiltration are also important features. The lymphocyte number shows striking variation, being variable in TT and BT, few in BB, most numerous in BL and most scanty in LL. The polar groups are stable. Elsewhere in the spectrum evolution of the disease may be associated with changes in immune reactions and classification. Untreated patients tend to move towards the lepromatous end.

Mycobacterium leprae is an obligate intracellular parasite residing mainly in macrophages and Schwann cells. The localization in Schwann cells is of particular importance for development of "reactions" resulting in nerve damage, and often permanent loss of nerve function. These episodes of reactions are associated with increased cell mediated immune reactivity against *M. leprae* (Godal *et al.*, 1973; Barnetson *et al.*, 1975; Bjune *et al.*, 1976), and this hypersensitivity reaction against antigens of *M. leprae* is considered to be directly responsible for induction of nerve damage.

ENL is another form of reaction in leprosy. It occurs frequently in patients towards the lepromatous end of the spectrum (Waters *et al.*, 1967) and leads to development of small tender subcutaneous nodules which persist for a few days, and new lesions may develop constantly. Some patients have marked generalized symptoms of malaise, fever and signs of arthritis and iridocyclitis. Histologically, the lesions are characterized by local vasculitis with infiltration of neutrophilic granulocytes. The lesions have been demonstrated to contain immune complexes (Wemambu *et al.*, 1969). Bjorvatn *et al.* (1976) have demonstrated characteristic changes in the complement system during ENL with increased concentration of the complement split product C3d in serum in patients with active ENL. As there was no apparent correlation between amount of circulating immune complexes and occurrence of ENL, this indicated that the immune complex formation leading to ENL mainly occurs extravascularly.

Properties of *Mycobacterium leprae*

Mycrobacterium leprae cannot be grown *in vitro*, and until recently very little information was available on the antigenic structure of the leprosy bacillus. The availability of larger amounts of *M. leprae* due to the fact that it can grow and establish a systemic mycobacterial infection in the armadillo (Kirchheimer and Storrs, 1971) has made studies of the antigenic constitution of *M. leprae* possible.

Immunological techniques are particularly valuable for taxonomic studies of *M. leprae* since it cannot be grown *in vitro*. By double diffusion tests in gel Stanford *et al.* (1975) found 4 antigens "specific to the leprosy bacillus" and claimed that immunodiffusion studies and skin testing indicated an especially close relationship with *M. vaccae*.

By crossed immunoelectrophoresis (CIE) with rabbit antisera against *M. leprae*, 7 different antigenic components of *M. leprae* were initially identified and numbered (Harboe *et al.*, 1977b). By the use of concentrated antigenic preparations for immunization and testing and concentrated rabbit anti-*M. leprae* immunoglobulins, more than 20 distinct antigenic components have been demonstrated in *M. leprae* by CIE (Closs *et al.*, 1979). CIE with lepromatous leprosy serum as antibody reagent has provided additional information on the antigenic structure of *M. leprae*. Studies of antigen 21 of *M. smegmatis* which cross-reacts with antigen 4 of *M. leprae* led to the demonstration of antigenic determinants that are specific for the leprosy bacillus on the latter component (Kronvall *et al.*, 1976, 1977).

Demonstration and isolation of "*M. leprae* specific antigens" would be important and has been given high priority in attempts to develop new diagnostic reagents and techniques in leprosy. Claims for demonstration of *M. leprae* specific antigens have been made by several authors including Abe *et al.* (1972), Stanford *et al.* (1975), Reich (1978) and Caldwell *et al.* (1979).

Strict criteria should be established and met to accept an antigen as *M. leprae* specific.

Firstly, it should be documented that the antigen is of mycobacterial origin. To prove that this is the case and to establish suitable controls may be difficult. Since *M. leprae* does not grow *in vitro* whereas the mycobacteria used for control are obtained by *in vitro* culture, antigens of host origin induced by the disease process may easily be mistaken as microbial constituents.

Secondly, it should be established whether the reaction is due to an *M. leprae* specific component or *M. leprae* specific determinants on a cross-reacting component. We see it as essential that the nomenclature should distinguish clearly between these two alternatives and are of the opinion that the term "*M. leprae* specific antigen" should be reserved for the first type. An *M. leprae* specific antigen should then react with anti-*M. leprae* antibodies produced experimentally or obtained from leprosy patients, whereas it should not react with antisera against other mycobacteria. Antisera against the antigen should react with *M. leprae* but not with other mycobacteria. Selection of test system is essential since antigens which appear to be specific in precipitation assays may prove to be cross-reactive in other assays, e.g. immunofluorescence.

Using such criteria, we have so far not been able to demonstrate any *M. leprae* specific antigen. Neither has the *M. leprae* specific nature of the antigens described so far been sufficiently documented according to these criteria.

The taxonomic position of *M. leprae* has not been established. Our data indicate that *M. leprae* is more closely related to *M. tuberculosis*, *M. avium* and *M. lepraemurium* than to *M. nonchromogenicum*, *M. phlei* and *M. smegmatis*.

Immune reactions in relation to the clinical spectrum of leprosy

Myrvang *et al.* (1973) studied the response in the lymphocyte transformation test (LTT) in patients throughout the clinical spectrum of leprosy. Patients with tuberculoid leprosy usually reacted strongly to *M. leprae* in culture. The mean response of groups of patients was recorded clinically and histologically classified according to the extended Ridley and Jopling scale and found that the mean response showed a continuous decrease towards the lepromatous end of the spectrum where the lymphocytes did not respond to stimulation with *M. leprae in vitro*. At least for a decade the main view has been that cell mediated immune reactions and antibody formation are inversely related throughout the leprosy spectrum, antibody concentration being low in tuberculoid leprosy and increasing towards the lepromatous end (cf. Fig. 1 in Bullock, 1978).

Various observations indicate that our immunological concepts of the clinical spectrum of leprosy should be carefully reconsidered and may need considerable revision.

Bjune *et al.* (1976) found that the variation in LTT response in patients with tuberculoid leprosy earlier observed by Myrvang *et al.* (1973) was related to clinical symptoms. Patients with BT leprosy with silent skin lesions frequently had fairly low LTT responses, whereas BT leprosy patients with lesions showing signs of inflammation usually had strong LTT responses. Similar observations were made in the borderline lepromatous group where patients with lesions showing signs of inflammation had fairly strong LTT responses, and these might even be stronger than the responses in BT patients with lesions showing no signs of inflammatory reactivity. From clinical observations it is apparent that resistance to infection is lower in the BL group than in the BT group. These observations indicate strongly that the LTT response is more related to hypersensitivity than to resistance to infection in the individual patient. Development of hypersensitivity to tuberculin in guinea-pigs after infection with *M. tuberculosis* was described by Robert Koch (1891) shortly after his discovery of the tubercle bacillus. The relationship between tuberculin hypersensitivity and resistance to infection with *M. tuberculosis* has been discussed since then, and it is not yet clear how these phenomena are related to each other. The same problem is of great significance in leprosy.

According to several current descriptions, the leprosy spectrum is "continuous", e.g. as expressed by Godal (1978): "The gradual shift in changes observed with all parameters would suggest that the spectrum is, in fact, continuous and that each point merely represents an arbitrary point along this spectrum".

Various observations indicate that some parameters do not change gradually, e.g. the number of lymphocytes in the granulomas as described above. The original observations of Myrvang *et al.* (1973) showed that patients with similar clinical classification, e.g. the BT/TT group, showed wide variation in response in the lymphocyte transformation test. A similar variation in amount of antibody against *M. leprae* antigen 7 (and the cross-reacting BCG antigen 60) in patients with the same clinical classification has been demonstrated by Harboe *et al.* (1977a) and by Yoder *et al.* (1979). Even though the median anti-*M. leprae* 7 antibody concentration determined by radioimmunoassay decreases from lepromatous to tuberculoid leprosy, the variation within each group is almost as great as throughout the spectrum.

Recently, Ridley (1976) has pointed out that important features of the spectrum need clarification: "Turning to classification, the foregoing results with the LTT raise a number of questions. Does the Ridley–Jopling scale reflect any sort of useful immunity or only a destructive hypersensitivity? Can the two in practice be separated in leprosy? And if so does the disease really present two spectra instead of one?"

Careful clinical, histopathological, and immunological investigations on the same patients are needed to establish how the different clinical groups in the spectrum are related to differences in hypersensitivity and resistance. Further information is also needed on the factors that determine the patient's position in the spectrum, changes in classification and progression of the disease.

Immunodeficiency in lepromatous leprosy

It is widely recognized that patients with lepromatous leprosy are unable to mount an efficient cell mediated immune (CMI) response to *M. leprae*. Evidence for this view has been obtained *in vivo*, e.g. through the consistent finding of a negative lepromin test (Rees, 1964) and *in vitro* through the lack of response to stimulation by *M. leprae* in the LTT (Godal *et al.*, 1971, 1972; Myrvang *et al.*, 1973). The uninhibited growth of *M. leprae* is generally considered to be due to this defect. The current view is that patients with lepromatous leprosy have both a generalized depression of CMI and a specific deficiency of CMI reactivity against *M. leprae*. The latter deficiency is more pronounced and irreversible upon treatment of the disease (Rees, 1964; Godal *et al.*, 1972). Godal *et al.* (1971) demonstrated that patients with lepromatous leprosy lacked circulating lymphocytes with ability to respond to *M. leprae* in the LTT and later Godal *et al.* (1972) provided additional evidence that the mechanism of immunological tolerance ("central failure") is responsible for the lack of host resistance in lepromatous leprosy. Other hypotheses under current consideration are abnormal macrophage function with defective presentation of *M. leprae* antigens to the immune system (Hirschberg, 1978; Convit *et al.*, 1980) and depression of CMI by suppressor cells (Mehra *et al.*, 1979). The mechanism of this deficiency is still an open question of essential importance to the understanding of the immunological features of leprosy. Stoner *et al.* (1978) studied patients with lepromatous leprosy and their siblings. They found that HLA-D identical siblings of patients with lepromatous leprosy showed equally strong LTT responses to *M. leprae* as HLA-D nonidentical siblings of the same patients. This indicates that the deficient CMI in lepromatous leprosy is not due to genetic factors closely linked with the HLA complex. The use of cells from leprosy patients and their HLA-D identical normal siblings makes it possible to perform experiments on mixtures of lymphocytes and macrophages from the sick and the healthy individual to localize the deficiency in specific cell types. Detailed understanding of this basic immunodeficiency in lepromatous leprosy may provide new means for immunotherapy directed against correction of the defect, which would be of utmost importance for prevention of relapse. Increased knowledge of the nature of the defect is also essential for development of techniques for prevention of lepromatous leprosy, e.g. by vaccination.

Antibody formation in leprosy

Antibodies have been demonstrated in sera from leprosy patients by a variety of methods, the general view being that antibodies occur in greatest amounts and in a high proportion of patients with lepromatous leprosy, whereas the frequency is lower and the amount smaller towards the tuberculoid end of the spectrum. Recent experiments based on crossed immunoelectrophoresis (CIE) with patient serum in the intermediate gel have provided additional information on the specificity of the antibodies. In lepromatous leprosy, the specificity varies in individual patients, the most frequently occurring antibodies being directed against *M. leprae* antigens 2, 5 and 7 (Harboe *et al.*, 1977b). The antibody response in armadillos, who develop systemic mycobacterial infection after inoculation with *M. leprae*, has similar specificity (Harboe *et al.*, 1978b). Antibodies against 7 components of *M. leprae* were detected by incorporation of concentrated immunoglobulins from a lepromatous serum pool in the intermediate gel of a CIE plate showing more than 20 antigenic components in *M. leprae* (Closs *et al.*, 1979). In view of the large antigenic load in lepromatous leprosy patients, the restriction in antibody specificity is as striking as the frequently described increased amount. This observation should be extended and explained. The influence of absorption *in vivo* is unknown. One explanation is limited production, i.e. only a few components of the bacillus being able to induce a humoral immune response. Instead of an inverse relationship between cell mediated and humoral immunity in lepromatous leprosy, there may be a dual lack of response to most components of *M. leprae*.

A radioimmunoassay (RIA) has been developed for demonstration and quantification of antibodies against *M. leprae* antigen 7 (Melsom *et al.*, 1978). The median concentration of anti-*M. leprae* 7 antibodies decreases from the lepromatous to the tuberculoid end of the spectrum, but there is a marked variation in antibody concentration in individual sera from patients with similar clinical classification, e.g. in BT leprosy (Yoder *et al.*, 1979). During dapsone treatment of lepromatous leprosy, there is a gradual, slow decline in antibody concentration (Rees *et al.*, 1965; Melsom *et al.*, 1978). In tuberculoid leprosy, anti-*M. leprae* 7 antibody concentration in groups of patients decreased during DDS treatment, suspected and proven relapse being associated with renewed synthesis and increased concentration of antibody (Yoder *et al.*, 1979).

Kronvall *et al.* (1976) showed that antibodies in lepromatous sera are particularly useful as antibody reagents to demonstrate antigenic determinants that are highly specific for *M. leprae* on components which also contain determinants cross-reacting with many species of mycobacteria, and various assays have been developed to demonstrate antibodies reacting with these determinants after absorption with other mycobacteria. Published tests of this kind are the leprosy fluorescent antibody absorption test (Abe *et al.*, 1976, 1980) and a radioimmunoassay (Harboe *et al.*, 1978a). Further work in this area is currently pursued in our laboratory, based on RIA and the ELISA technique. Production of monoclonal anti-*M. leprae* antibodies by the hybridoma technique is also expected to provide valuable information on the antigenic structure of *M. leprae*, for development of immunological reagents and techniques for identification of *M. leprae* in tissues, and related to further development of antibody assays in man.

In development of diagnostic procedures, antibodies will probably be particularly valuable for demonstration of individuals in the incubation stage of lepromatous leprosy and with diffuse lepromatous leprosy, a highly infectious form of the disease with only moderate clinical symptoms. Patients with highly bacilliferous disease are particularly important from the prophylactic point of view and are usually characterized by negative tests for CMI. There is thus a great need for an antibody assay of moderate sensitivity, where antibody concentration is correlated to bacterial load, and with high specificity for *M. leprae*.

Principles and possibilities for prophylaxis

The lesions of patients with lepromatous leprosy often contain vast amounts of bacilli. If untreated, the patients may shed large numbers of viable bacilli, particularly through nasal discharge (Davey, 1978). These patients are therefore particularly important for dissemination of the disease, and the major effort should be concentrated on making them less infectious or noninfectious to break the chain of infection. Despite decades of continuous drug treatment, there is a high risk of relapse, and their characteristic immunodeficiency persists (Rees, 1964; Godal *et al.*, 1972). Development of techniques for reversal and prevention of this immunodeficiency would therefore be of utmost importance in leprosy. Prevention of tuberculoid leprosy is also of obvious importance, but probably more from the point of view of prevention of nerve damage and chronic deformities.

Development of a leprosy vaccine has been given major priority in the WHO immunology of leprosy (IMMLEP) programme, and many laboratories are involved in the initial, preparative stage of this work. The principles on which a leprosy vaccine may be developed have been extensively discussed by Godal *et al.* (1974), Stanford (1976) and Convit *et al.* (1980). From a theoretical point of view, there are three main ways by which a potential leprosy vaccine could be developed: (1) by the use of a selected, living, nonpathogenic mycobacterium with high cross-reactivity to *M. leprae*; (2) by the use of killed *M. leprae* in an appropriate adjuvant; (3) by the use of a living vaccine containing an attenuated nonpathogenic strain of *M. leprae*.

The third alternative is not practical today since *M. leprae* cannot be grown in sufficient quantity *in vitro*. Selection of an attenuated strain and the proof that it is nonpathogenic would be extremely difficult in view of the long incubation time of leprosy in man and the uncertainty of extrapolation from tests of pathogenicity in other species to conditions in man. Selection between the two first alternatives is also difficult on the basis of current knowledge. If an adjuvant should be used, living BCG bacilli is probably the main candidate today. This will however impose difficulties in testing of efficiency. BCG vaccination has previously been tested for its efficiency in protection against leprosy. The degree of protection varied considerably, ranging from 80% in Uganda (Brown *et al.*, 1968) to insignificant in Burma (Bechelli *et al.*, 1973). The main reason for this difference has been discussed extensively but still remains unknown. To establish that a new leprosy vaccine works better than BCG, it would require, however, that the new vaccine should be compared with the use of BCG alone in simultaneous testing in the same population.

For selection between different vaccination procedures and for evaluation of their potential effect, it would be of tremendous value, if not a requirement, to have an immunological assay for efficiency, *in vitro* or *in vivo*. The assay should have a high correlation to induction of protective immunity. Conversion of immunological reactivity demonstrated by currently available lymphocyte transformation tests or skin tests is related to hypersensitivity but not necessarily to protective immunity.

Genetic aspects and experimental models

Evidence from twin-, family- and population studies indicate that genetic factors of the host play an important role in determining susceptibility and type of response after infection with *M. leprae*, and thus for development and type of clinical disease in man (cf. Harboe, 1980). Recent population studies have demonstrated an association between leprosy and HLA antigens (Thorsby *et al.*, 1973; Kreisler *et al.*, 1974; Dasgupta *et al.*, 1975; Smith *et al.*, 1975). In various populations, the association has been with different HLA types, which indicates that susceptibility to leprosy is due to genes linked with, but not included in the HLA complex. Family studies (de Vries *et al.*, 1976, 1979) indicate that there is a strong genetic predisposition for development of tuberculoid leprosy, the responsible gene(s) being linked to HLA-DRw2. The observations with regard to lepromatous leprosy are so far too few to permit definite conclusions. Several hypotheses are compatible with the observations made. Several gene loci may be involved partly determining susceptibility to develop leprosy after infection, and another linked with the

HLA complex determining the tendency for development of the tuberculoid type of leprosy.

In experimental models based on the use of another slow growing mycobacterium, *M. lepraemurium* (MLM), it has been shown that different inbred strains have completely different levels of natural resistance to MLM infection (Closs, 1975a). After footpad inoculation of about 1×10^6 acid-fast bacilli in C3H/Tif mice, the mice have no ability to resist the infection. The bacilli grow continuously, disseminate in the body, and the mice eventually die in a cachectic state. Similar inoculation of C57BL mice results in local growth of the bacilli for about four weeks until a local reaction with footpad swelling occurs, and there is no further increase in number of acid-fast bacilli. The histological pattern of the lesions differs markedly in the two strains (Closs and Haugen, 1975), the granulomas being surrounded by a dense infiltration of mononuclear cells in the C57BL mice, whereas the mycobacteria-loaded macrophages in the C3H/Tif mice occur in completely naked granulomas without any surrounding infiltration of mononuclear cells.

These strains offer unique opportunities to study the genetic factors involved and the mechanisms of resistance to a leprosy-like infection.

In the susceptible strain, delayed-type hypersensitivity (DTH) against a total ultrasonicate of MLM can be induced without any apparent effect on the resistance to the infection. A local DTH reaction against an MLM sonicate may be induced repeatedly in the footpad of C3H/Tif mice inoculated at the same site with living MLM bacilli, and the multiplication of the bacilli is not affected by this simultaneous cell mediated immune reaction (Løvik and Closs, 1980). In the resistant strain, increased ability to resist the infection can be induced by prior inoculation with a small amount of living MLM bacilli (Closs, 1975b). In C57BL mice it has further been shown that immunization with an MLM sonicate induces a strong DTH response against the sonicate. This in itself induces no resistance but accelerates the process in the C57BL mice which provides increased resistance upon inoculation with living MLM bacilli (Closs and Løvik, 1980). These findings indicate that DTH is a poor parameter of induction of true protective immunity, i.e. increased ability to prevent bacterial multiplication in MLM infection.

In experimental models in mice, resistance to various infections has been shown to be determined by genes in the H-2 locus and on several other chromosomes. This shows that genes are essential at different points in the host response which determines susceptibility to the particular infection. Detailed demonstration of the genetic basis of resistance, or lack of resistance to a particular infection thus provides new, and very potent means for studies of mechanisms of protective immunity and lack of resistance. The value of this approach has been illustrated in murine typhoid. Two genes were originally identified that determine the susceptibility of inbred mice to infection with *Salmonella typhimurium*, an autosomal gene on chromosome 1 (Plant and Glynn, 1979) and an X-linked gene (O'Brien *et al.*, 1979). Subsequently, O'Brien *et al.* (1980) studied C3H/HeJ mice who are highly susceptible to *S.*

typhimurium and defective in their response to bacterial lipopolysaccharide (LPS) due to a mutation at the Lps locus on chromosome 4. Their data indicate strongly that susceptibility of C3H/HeJ mice to *S. typhimurium* is due either to the Lps^d allele or to a closely linked gene. The former is a particularly attractive view, showing how genetic techniques may provide information pointing directly to the mechanism of susceptibility to infection. This approach should be intensively explored in mycobacterial infection studying MLM infection in selected congenic strains of mice. Cell mediated immune reactions are of main importance for development of resistance (WHO, 1973), but the mechanisms of protective immunity in mycobacterial disease are very incompletely known (Lagrange and Closs, 1979). We do not know the role of individual antigens for development of protective immunity. Many data indicate that living mycobacteria are needed to induce efficient protective immunity (Youmans and Youmans, 1969), and it is therefore still largely unknown how these antigens should be demonstrated and defined. The T cell subpopulation of main importance for development of protective immunity and its relation to the subpopulation responsible for development of hypersensitivity reactions have still not been defined. Additional knowledge of these essential immunological mechanisms is needed to obtain an equally good understanding of the immunological basis of resistance, lack of resistance, and development of complications in leprosy and other mycobacterial diseases as in other important infectious diseases in man.

References

Abe, M., Minagawa, F., Yoshino, Y. and Okamura, K. (1972). *Int. J. Lepr.* **40**, 107.

Abe, M., Izumi, S., Saito, T. and Mathur, S. K. (1976). *Lepr. India* **48**, 272.

Abe, M., Yoshino, Y., Saikawa, K. and Saito, T. (1980). *Int. J. Lepr.* (in press).

Barnetson, R. StC., Bjune, G., Pearson, J. M. H. and Kronvall, G. (1975). *Brit. Med. J.* **4**, 435.

Bechelli, L. M., Carbajosa, P. G., Gyi, M. M., Uemura, K., Sundaresan, T., Dominguez, V. M., Matejka, M., Tamondon, C., Quagliato, R., Engler, V. and Altmann, M. (1973). *Bull. Wld Hlth Org.* **48**, 323.

Bjorvatn, B., Barnetson, R. S., Kronvall, G., Zubler, R. H. and Lambert, P. H. (1976). *Clin. Exp. Immunol.* **26**, 388.

Bjune, G., Barnetson, R. StC., Ridley, D. S. and Kronvall, G. (1976). *Clin. Exp. Immunol.* **25**, 85.

Brown, J. A. K., Stone, M. M. and Sutherland, I. (1968). *Brit. Med. J.* **1**, 24.

Bullock, W. E. (1978). *J. Infect. Dis.* **137**, 341.

Caldwell, H. D., Kirchheimer, W. F. and Buchanan, T. M. (1979). *Int. J. Lepr.* **47**, 477.

Closs, O. (1975a). *Infect. Immun.* **12**, 480.

Closs, O. (1975b). *Infect. Immun.* **12**, 706.

Closs, O. and Haugen, O. A. (1975). *Acta Path. Microbiol. Scand.* **83**, Sect. A, 59.

Closs, O. and Løvik, M. (1980). *Infect. Immun.* (in press).

Closs, O., Mshana, R. N. and Harboe, M. (1979). *Scand. J. Immunol.* **9**, 297.

Convit, J., Ulrich, M. and Aranzazu, N. (1980). *Int. J. Lepr.* **48**, 62.

Dasgupta, A., Mehra, N. K., Ghei, S. K. and Vaidya, M. C. (1975). *Tissue Antigens* **5**, 85.

Davey, T. F. (1978). *Lepr. Rev.* **49**, 269.
Godal, T. (1978). *Prog. Allergy* **25**, 211.
Godal, T., Myklestad, B., Samuel, D. R. and Myrvang, B. (1971). *Clin. Exp. Immunol.* **9**, 821.
Godal, T., Myrvang, B., Frøland, S. S., Shao, J. and Melaku, G. (1972). *Scand. J. Immunol.* **1**, 311.
Godal, T., Myrvang, B., Samuel, D. R., Ross, W. F. and Løfgren, M. (1973). *Acta Path. Microbiol. Scand.* Sect. A Suppl. **236**, 45.
Godal, T., Myrvang, B., Stanford, J.-L. and Samuel, D. R. (1974). *Bull. Inst. Pasteur* **72**, 273.
Harboe, M. (1980). *In* "Symposium on Modern Genetic Concepts and Techniques in the Study of Parasites". WHO, Geneva.
Harboe, M., Closs, O., Bjorvatn, B. and Bjune, G. (1977a). *Brit. Med. J.* **2**, 430.
Harboe, M., Closs, O., Bjorvatn, B., Kronvall, G. and Axelsen, N. H. (1977b). *Infect. Immun.* **18**, 792.
Harboe, M., Closs, O., Bjune, G., Kronvall, G. and Axelsen, N. H. (1978a). *Scand. J. Immunol.* **7**, 111.
Harboe, M., Closs, O., Rees, R. J. W. and Walsh, G. P. (1978b). *J. Med. Microbiol.* **11**, 525.
Hirschberg, H. (1978). *Clin. Exp. Immunol.* **34**, 46.
Kirchheimer, W. F. and Storrs, E. E. (1971). *Int. J. Lepr.* **39**, 693.
Koch, R. (1891). *D. Med. Wschr.* **17**, 101.
Kreisler, M., Arnaiz, A., Perez, B., Cruz, E. F. and Bootello, A. (1974). *Tissue Antigens* **4**, 197.
Kronvall, G., Stanford, J. L. and Walsh, G. P. (1976). *Infect. Immun.* **13**, 1132.
Kronvall, G., Closs, O. and Bjune, G. (1977). *Infect. Immun.* **16**, 542.
Lagrange, P. H. and Closs, O. (1979). *Scand. J. Immunol.* **10**, 285.
Løvik, M. and Closs, O. (1980). *Scand. J. Infect. Dis.* (in press).
Mehra, V., Mason, L. H., Fields, J. and Bloom, B. R. (1979). *J. Immunol.* **123**, 1813.
Melsom, R., Naafs, B., Harboe, M. and Closs, O. (1978). *Lepr. Rev.* **49**, 17.
Myrvang, B., Godal, T., Ridley, D. S., Frøland, S. S. and Song, Y. K. (1973). *Clin. Exp. Immunol.* **14**, 541.
O'Brien, A. D., Scher, I., Campbell, G. H., MacDermott, R. P. and Formal, S. B. (1979). *J. Immunol.* **123**, 720.
O'Brien, A. D., Rosenstreich, D. L., Scher, I., Campbell, G. H., MacDermott, R. P. and Formal, S. B. (1980). *J. Immunol.* **124**, 20.
Plant, J. and Glynn, A. A. (1979). *Clin. Exp. Immunol.* **37**, 1.
Rees, R. J. W. (1964). *Prog. Allergy* **8**, 224.
Rees, R. J. W., Chatterjee, K. R., Pepys, J. and Tee, R. R. (1965). *Amer. Rev. Resp. Dis.* **92**, Suppl., 139.
Reich, C. V. (1978). *In* "Proc. XIth Int. Leprosy Congress, Mexico D.F. 1978" Excerpta Medica, Amsterdam, 1980.
Ridley, D. S. (1976). *Lepr. Rev.* **47**, 171.
Ridley, D. S. (1977). *In* "Skin Biopsy in Leprosy", pp. 37–45. Documenta Geigy.
Ridley, D. S. and Jopling, W. H. (1966). *Int. J. Lepr.* **34**, 255.
Smith, G. S., Walford, R. L., Shepard, C. C., Payne, R. and Prochazka, G. J. (1975). *Vox Sang.* **28**, 42.
Stanford, J. L. (1976). *Lepr. Rev.* **47**, 87.
Stanford, J. L., Rook, G. A. W., Convit, J., Godal, T., Kronvall, G., Rees, R. J. W. and Walsh, G. P. (1975). *Brit. J. Exp. Path.* **56**, 579.
Stoner, G. L., Touw, J., Belehu, A. and Naafs, B. (1978). *Lancet* **ii**, 543.
Thorsby, E., Godal, T. and Myrvang, B. (1973). *Tissue Antigens* **3**, 373.
de Vries, R. R. P., Lai A. Fat, R. F. M., Nijenhuis, L. E. and Rood, J. J. van (1976). *Lancet* **ii**, 1328.

de Vries, R. R. P., Rood, J. J. van, Lai A Fat, R. F. M., Mehra, N. K. and Vaidya, M. C. (1979). *In* "Immune Mechanisms and Disease" (D. B. Amos, R. S. Schwarz and B. W. Janicki, eds), pp. 283–296. Academic Press, New York.

Waters, M. F. R., Rees, R. J. W. and Sutherland, J. (1967). *Int. J. Lepr.* **35**, 311.

Wemambu, S. N. C., Turk, J. L., Waters, M. F. R. and Rees, R. J. W. (1969). *Lancet* **ii**, 933.

World Health Organization (1973). *Wld Hlth Org. Techn. Rep. Ser.* **No. 519**.

Yoder, L., Naafs, B., Harboe, M. and Bjune, G. (1979). *Lepr. Rev.* **50**, 113.

Youmans, G. P. and Youmans, A. S. (1969). *J. Bact.* **97**, 107.

66

Genetics of Complement and Complement Deficiencies

DONALD RAUM, VIRGINIA H. DONALDSON,* CHESTER A. ALPER and FRED S. ROSEN**

** Children's Hospital, Cincinnati, Ohio, USA and **Children's Hospital Medical Center, Boston, Massachusetts, USA*

Introduction

Inherited deficiencies of complement proteins and their associated clinical syndromes have provided knowledge of the biologic activities and physiology of individual components and their cleavage fragments. Extensive genetic polymorphism of the complement proteins has made them useful as tools for genetic mapping of the human genome. Remarkably, the genetic loci for some of these components have been shown both in families with inherited deficiency and with inherited structural variation to be closely linked to suspected immune response genes. This picture has been pieced together from study of man and animals, *in vitro* and *in vivo*, and has also yielded knowledge of the molecular nature of complement defects and the mechanism of the synthesis of the complement proteins. These studies have revealed the multiple contributions of the complement system to immune function.

Polymorphism of C4

Polymorphism of C4 in humans has been described. Two dimensional immunoelectrophoresis of EDTA plasma against anti-C4 serum gave patterns demonstrating differences in individuals which were constant for any single person over long periods of time, suggesting genetic polymorphism. C4 patterns differed in paired maternal and foetal sera, suggesting foetal synthesis of C4 and failure of C4 to cross the placenta. Various attempts to resolve these patterns consistent with Mendelian inheritance of alleles at a single locus have failed. A significant advance was made with the recognition that Chido and Rodgers blood groups are distinct antigenic components of human C4. O'Neill and coworkers, using agarose gel electrophoresis followed by immunofixation with anti-C4, were able to demonstrate a common polymorphism in which all individuals had 4 fast, 4 slow, or all 8 bands. Calling these individuals F, S or FS, they noted that the distribution of phenotypes was not consistent with a single locus model, but required a 2 locus model. O'Neill and coworkers proposed 2 closely linked loci for C4, one marked by Chido and the other by Rodgers reactivity. One determines the presence or absence of 4 fast bands, C4F or $C4F^0$, and the other the presence or absence of 4 slow bands, C4S or $C4s^0$. Individuals who lacked slow bands (s^0/s^0) were always Chido negative [*Ch*(*a* −)] while individuals homozygous for f^0 (lacking the four anodal bands) were always Rodgers negative [Rg(a −)]. In addition, Ch(a +) and Rg(a +) antigens from an individual with C4 type FS were removed after passing the serum over an affinity chromatography column in which anti-C4 was covalently bound. C4 isolated from pooled sera was able to inhibit either anti-Ch^a or anti-Rg^a. In O'Neill's system it was not possible to detect $C4f^0$ and $C4s^0$ in heterozygotes. By desialation prior to electrophoresis and subsequent crossed immunoelectrophoresis it has been possible to type all individuals in a manner predicted by the 2 locus model of O'Neill. Since the frequency of homozygous C4 deficiency appears to ber very low, it is proposed that the alleles at these loci are in linkage disequilibrium so that there are few haplotypes of the type s^0f^0. Recently, Awdeh and Alper have extended these studies and have detected 6 common or relatively common structural variants at the Rodgers (*C4A*) locus and two common variants at the Chido (*C4B*) locus. Nine C4*A*-*B* haplotypes, of 21 predicted possible, have been identified in initial studies. In this system, C4f^0 is designated as *C4A*Q0* and C4s^0 as *C4B*Q0*.

Polymorphism of C2

Genetic polymorphism in human C2 was first described by isoelectric focusing of human sera followed by overlay consisting of sensitized sheep erythrocytes and C2 deficient serum. Like the other components discussed, C2 in homozygous individuals is heterogeneous, showing many bands, though one

TABLE I

Frequencies of common variants of complement components in the major races

	Race				
C3					
Whites	N. America	S 0·77	F 0·22		
	Norway	S 0·80	F 0·19		
	Germany	S 0·78	F 0·19		
Orientals	N. America	S 0·99			
Blacks	N. America	S 0·93	F 0·06		
BF					
Whites	N. America	S 0·8055	F 0·1755	F1 0·0095	S1 0·0095
Orientals		S 0·890	F 0·110		
Blacks		S 0·437	F 0·512	F1 0·051	
Whites	W. German	S 0·808	F 0·174	F1 0·008	S1 0·009
C6					
Whites		A 6·01	B 0·37	R 0·015	
Orientals		A 0·59	B 0·35	R 0·05	
Blacks		A 0·56	B 0·38	R 0·06	
C8					
Blacks	N. America	A 0·700	B 0·246	A1 0·054	
	Brazil	A 0·662	B 0·309	A1 0·029	
Whites		A 0·649	B 0·348	A1 0·003	
Orientals		A 0·655	B 0·345		
C2					
Whites		C 0·95	B 0·04	A 0·01	
C7					
Whites		C 0·989	R 0·011		

R, all rare alleles; S, slow; F, fast; A, acidic; B, basic; C, common.

prominent band can be identified for the type C2 C (for common). Variations described are termed C2 B (for basic), in which there is a duplication of the C2 C pattern closer to the cathode, and C2 A (for acidic), in which there is a duplication of the C2 C bands closer to the anode. In the observations made by Hobart and Lachmann and Meo and colleagues, C2 C is designated C2-1 and C2 B is C2-2. Several rare variants have also been seen with a total frequency less than 1%. The frequency of these variants is presented in Table I for the major races. The inheritance of C2 types is regulated by autosomal codominant alleles. Human variants of C2 have been examined for haemolytic activity and no difference has been detected between homozygous C2 C and C2 B.

Polymorphism of B

Factor B had earlier been termed glycine-rich β-glycoprotein or GBG, C3 proactivator or C3PA. On electrophoresis at pH 8·6, heterogeneous patterns given by homozygous individuals consist of 5 bands of varying intensity and

TABLE IA

Frequency of C4 haplocytes in healthy caucasians

C4	AQ0	B1	0·123
	AQ0	B2	0·038
	A1	BQ0	0·004
	A1	B1	0·004
	A2	B1	0·035
	A2	BQ0	0·004
	A2	B2	0·019
	A2	B3	0·004
	A3	BQ0	0·088
	A3	B1	0·546
	A3	B2	0·015
	A3	B3	0·004
	A4	B2	0·065
	A6	B1	0·050
	A3	B4	Rare
	A5	B1	Rare
	A7	B?	Rare

are designated BF (for factor B). The difference between BF F (for fast) and BF S (for slow) consists of displacement of all the bands by 1 electrophoretic position. BF types are inherited as autosomal codominant traits in family studies. The distribution of progeny was close to the predicted Mendelian ratios and the distribution of phenotypes was close to the predictions of the Hardy-Weinberg law. Gene frequencies in the major races are given in Table I.

B has also been visualized by isoelectric focusing or agarose gel electrophoresis followed by an overlay consisting of guinea-pig erythrocytes and human serum heated to 50°C for 15 min in 10 mM EGTA, 7 mM $MgCl_2$ in normal saline.

No functional differences between the BF variants have been detected. During activation, B undergoes cleavage to yield the major products Bb and Ba. The determinants of the common variants BF F and BF S are on the Ba fragment, while those for the rarer variants, F1 and S1, are located on the Bb fragment. The determinants for several other rare BF types have also been shown to be located on the Bb fragment.

Chromosomal positions of C2 and BF

The structural locus for *BF* is closely linked to *HLA* in man. In the initial family studies, no cross-overs were observed, though subsequent studies have identified *HLA-BF* cross-overs. The structural locus for *C2* is also known to be linked to the *HLA* region and *C2 deficiency* is known to be *HLA*-linked. No cross-over has yet been observed between *C2 deficiency* and *BF* or *C2* and *BF*, and these 2 loci, *C2* and *BF*, are therefore thought to be products of a tandem gene duplication. This view is also supported by family studies and partial amino acid sequence analysis of these proteins. Purified C2 has an amino acid composition very similar to that of BF.

Conflicting evidence has been presented concerning the order of genes of the *HLA* complex and *BF-C2*. Several authors have suggested that the *BF* locus is between *HLAB* and *HLAD* loci on the sixth human chromosome and others that the order is *HLAB,D* (*BF,C2*). In family studies of the C2 structural polymorphism, an observed recombination fraction of 0·02 between *C2* and *HLAB* was in accord with the recombination rate observed in the same population between *C2*Q0* and *HLAB* (0·03) and *BF* and *HLAB* (0·04), which is considerably greater than the observed recombination rate between *HLAB* and *HLAD*.

Two other family studies of C2 deficiency suggested that *C2*Q0* is located outside the *HLA* region. Other recombination fractions for *BF* and *HLAB* include 0·021 and 0·0166. One group has reported a substantially lower fraction.

Several specific cross-overs in the literature are worth special notice. The family Krist, described by Lamm and colleagues, has 5 offspring. Each parent has but one HLAD typing response identified by available D cells and an individual offspring with an apparent *HLAB,BF* cross-over from her mother showed low stimulation in mixed lymphocyte culture with a sibling who inherited the same paternal haplotype, but the mother's other *HLA* haplotype. In this case, it was concluded that the cross-over occurred between *HLAB* and *D* and the *BF* allele followed *HLAB*, not *HLAD*. From the pedigree Mu-0111 described by Rittner it was concluded from mixed lymphocyte culture data that a cross-over occurred in the father between *BF* and *HLAD* loci. In this family the *BF* allele in the recombinant travelled with the *HLAB* locus.

In the family Bon, presented by Hauptmann, the conclusion that BF was between *HLAB* and *HLAD* rested upon mixed lymphocyte culture data suggesting a paternal recombination of *HLAD*, but not of *BF*. There has been considerable suggestive evidence that *C4* is also coded in the same region as *C2* and *BF*. In the family Bru, presented by Bijnen and colleagues, an apparent maternal recombination between *HLAB* and *HLAD* did not result in a recombination for Rodgers antigen negativity. These data would place the Rodgers antigen (a C4 antigen) between the *HLAB* and *HLAD* loci. It should be noted that the father was not typed and that it was not possible to detect Rodgers negative heterozygotes. It seems likely that recent advances in HLAD, DR, and C4 typing should resolve some of the differences in the literature, as will repeat attempts to determine whether there were previous errors in ascertainment of HLAA, HLAB phenotypes or inferences about genotypes, or BF and C2 types. In a study of the association of HLAA, HLAB, and BF types, *HLAB*18* was shown to be in linkage disequilibrium with *BF*F1*. In a similar study, a correlation was found between *HLAB*7* and *BF*S*, though less than between *HLAB*7* and *HLAD*2*, which was not expected if *BF* is between *HLAB* and *HLAD*. This may be the result of the size of the sample or of undefined HLAD specificities.

Arnason and colleagues have pointed out that the frequency of laboratory and other errors in ascertaining recombinants may be greater than the recombination frequency and have attempted to infer the order of these genes from frequencies of specific haplotypes with the *HLAB* allele, *B8*, in several populations with a common ancestor. They concluded that *BF* is very close to *HLAB* because among 100 haplotypes there was an apparent absence of the *HLAB*8-BF*F* haplotype, suggesting no recombinant events between *HLAB* and *BF* in the past 1000 years. Nevertheless, Bender and colleagues reported 4 of 69 haplotypes to be *HLAB*8-BF*F* and 1 to be *HLAB*8-BF*S1*, suggesting at least some recombinant events between *HLAB* and *BF* in the past. In a gene marker study of a partial 6p trisomic child resulting from a balanced maternal translocation, it was concluded that *BF* is localized between *HLAB* and *HLAD*. It was surmised that the break occurred through the *HLAD* region; however, the mother of the proposita with the balanced translocation had only one *HLADR* specificity.

One other remarkable fact has emerged from these studies. C2 deficiency *C2*Q0* shows a remarkable linkage disequilibrium with *HLAA*10*, *B*18*, *D*2* and *BF*S* and *C2*B* with *HLAB*15* and *BF*S*. This has been interpreted to mean that *C2*Q0* and *C2*B* are recent mutations in the population which have not yet reached equilibrium, though the possibility of selective pressure for maintenance of linkage of these alleles has not been ruled out. In addition, *BF*S* appears to be in linkage disequilibrium with *HLAB*27*.

Linkage of C4

The linkage of the C4 structural locus to HLA has been inferred from the study of two reported C4 deficient families. Both showed linkage of C4 to HLA, though the conclusion rests on the ascertainment of heterozygous C4 deficient individuals within these families. The definition of heterozygotes is susceptible to several errors because of the wide range of normal for C4 (25–175% nl) and the frequency of partially deficient haplotypes. The allotypes of C4 described by Teisberg and colleagues and Mauff are said to show close linkage to HLAB.

Disease association of BF and C4 allotypes

Twenty-four of 106 white patients in Boston with insulin-dependent diabetes melitus (IDDM) were found to carry the *BF*F1* allele even though *BF*F1* is rare in the general population. Previous studies had shown the association of IDDM with several HLAB and HLAD types. Disease associations with HLA or complement loci in this region are taken as evidence for genetic linkage of susceptibility genes for these diseases. Therefore, it has been postulated that there is a diabetogenic gene (Dm) closely linked to *BF* and *HLADR* and in linkage disequilibrium with *BF*F1* and *HLADR*W3* and *W4*. In this population, most patients developed clinical diabetes before 20 years of age.

The association of *BF*F1* with IDDM has been confirmed in several other populations. Among those examined by Bertrams and colleagues, 151 were HLAA,B,C typed and increased frequencies of *HLAB*18*, *B*15* and *C*W3* were noted. *BF*F1* is known to be in linkage disequilibrium with *HLAB*18*.

The frequency of *BF*F1* is highly age-dependent. Among a French population (not included in Table I) of 531 IDDM patients there also was an excess of BF F1 types. Reviews of these data suggest that differences in *BF*F1* frequency between studied populations is due to age of onset of IDDM.

Polymorphism of C3

C3 is a major serum protein and its polymorphism can be detected by zonal electrophoresis of whole serum in agarose gel with direct staining of protein. Prolonged electrophoresis in agarose gell or high voltage starch gel electrophoresis allowed the detection of extensive common genetic polymorphism in human C3.

In a buffer without calcium, human C3 has a mobility similar to transferrin, but when the buffer contains calcium ions, migration of C3 is slower than that of the other major β globulins, transferrin and β lipoprotein, using a standardized electrophoretic procedure. At pH 8·6 and ionic strength 0·05 and with 0·0018 M calcium 2+, over 20 variants of C3 have been detected. Each consists of a single major band and 2 anodal minor bands. The most frequent type in Caucasians is called C3 S (for slow) and another frequent variant is designated C3 F. Variants are named according to their relative migration distance towards the cathode or anode from C3 S. The distance from C3 S to C3 F1·0 is arbitrarily assigned unity and other mobilities are expressed as a decimal with respect to this distance. No functional differences in serum concentrations of C3 are found between individuals who are C3 F and C3 S.

C3 variants are inherited as autosomal codominant traits. Gene frequencies for C3 types are given in Table I. No significant differences in specific activity have been found between a number of C3 variants tested for haemolytic complement activity. It has been claimed but not confirmed that C3 F is better at producing rosettes with macrophages than is C3 S.

In studies of the relationship of C3 types to various diseases, suggestive but inconclusive associations have been reported for rheumatoid arthritis and hepatitis and atherosclerotic disease.

An unusual C3 variant with the electrophoretic mobility of C3 F has been found in a man, his mother, and his son. The decreased quantity of this variant, called C3f or C3 FQD, was shown to be the result of decreased synthesis. It has been found in other families. C3 polymorphism has also been reported in other mammals.

Polymorphism of C6

Like C3 and BF, C6 exhibits genetic polymorphism. Typing can be performed by prolonged agarose gel electrophoresis and immunofixation with specific antiserum. However, the method of choice is isoelectric focusing followed by overlay consisting of sensitized sheep red cells and C6 deficient serum. C6 is heterogeneous in all individuals, forming at least 7 bands of varying intensity in persons homozygous for any given allotype. The patterns from individuals homozygous for the acidic form (A) differ from those homozygous for the basic form (B), in that the latter are shifted 1 electrophoretic position towards the cathode. The AB pattern consists of the 2 patterns superimposed and can be reproduced by mixing equal parts of A and B sera. In family studies, these and several rare variants were shown to be inherited as simple autosomal codominant alleles.

The gene frequencies for the major races are given in Table I with the rarer genes collectively designated as $C6^R$. The frequencies of phenotypes observed correspond to the prediction of the Hardy–Weinberg equilibrium.

Polymorphism of C7

C7 can be typed, like C2 and C6, by C7 deficient serum and sensitized sheep erythrocytes as an overlay of samples after isoelectric focusing, and C7 1, C7 2, and C7 3 variant proteins are demonstrable. Most of the later complement components except C7 increase in acute phase sera. Therefore, activation of the alternative pathway in acute phase sera produces a reagent deficient in C3 and C7. Using a euglobulin fraction (which is rich in C3) from such a serum with sensitized guinea-pig erythrocytes to produce an overlay for C7 after isoelectric focusing, serum from 1215 of 1228 unrelated individuals gave the same pattern, C7 1. Two rare phenotypes were detected, C7 2,1 in 4 individuals and C7 3,1 in 9 individuals. The inheritance was shown to be consistent with three codominant autosomal alleles.

Polymorphism of C8

The availability of C8 deficient serum from 1 individual has made it possible to examine C8 polymorphism. After serum samples have been subjected to isoelectric focusing on polyacrylamide, the plate is overlaid with a gel consisting of agarose, sensitized sheep erythrocytes, and C8 deficient serum. C8 is found to produce multiple lysis zones in the pH range 6·2–6·8. The alleles are named *C8*A* (for acidic) and *C8*B* (for basic). A pattern identical to C8 AB can be produced by a mixture of equal proportions of C8 A and C8 B sera. The variants are inherited as codominant autosomal alleles at a single locus. In addition, another frequent allele, termed C8 A1, producing zones of lysis anodal to C8 A is found in blacks (and in a single case in a white). The frequency of phenotypes in family studies corresponds to the prediction of Mendelian genetics and the distribution of types among random individuals closely fits the predictions of the Hardy–Weinberg Law. Table I gives the distribution of alleles in the major races. Examination of 18 structural genetic markers, including HLA, failed to show any linkage.

Clinical syndromes associated with complement deficiency

Three syndromes are associated with complement deficiency: oedema due to changes in vascular permeability, immune complex diseases, and increased susceptibility to infection. These are summarized in Table II.

Hereditary angioneurotic oedema

$C\bar{1}$ inhibitor deficiency

Hereditary angioneurotic oedema is associated with an inherited deficiency

TABLE II
Clinical disorders associated with hereditary complement deficiency

Deficient component	*Clinical disorder*
C1q	Renal disease and lupus-like syndrome (2 of 2)
C1r	Systemic lupus erythematosus (SLE) or glomerulonephritis (4 of 7)
C2	None (about 33% of 38 known cases)
	Immune complex disease (23 of 38)
	Propensity to infection (7 of 38)
C3	Severe immunodeficiency (4 of 5 cases)
C4	Lupus or lupus-like syndrome (4 of 4)
C5	SLE (1), *Neisseria* infections (6 of 8)
C6	*Neisseria* infections (7 of 8)
C7	*Neisseria* infections (5 of 13), glomerulonephritis (6), Raynaud's (1), rheumatoid arthritis (1)
C6 and C7	Healthy (1 case)
C8	*Neisseria* infections (4 of 9), xeroderma pigmentosus (3), SLE (1), lupus-like syndrome (2)
C9	No disease (2 of 2)
C3b inactivator	Severe immunodeficiency (3)
$C\bar{1}$ inhibitor	Many cases of HANE and immune complex disease

of the function of the serum inhibitor of the activated first component of complement ($C\bar{1}$). Its distinctive clinical features include recurrent bouts of noninflammatory submucosal oedema which can cause severe colicky abdominal pain when the gastrointestinal tract is involved. When the respiratory tract swells, there may be sudden death from suffocation. These signs and symptoms of internal swellings are typical of this disorder and are important diagnostic clues to be sought in obtaining historical support for this diagnosis.

The symptoms of hereditary angioneurotic oedema appear to be due in part to a polypeptide kinin which can enhance vascular permeability. This polypeptide may be released by plasmin from a fragment cleaved from C2 by $C\bar{1}$

Deficiency of $C\bar{1}$ inhibitor

Although both the symptoms and the biochemical defect associated with hereditary angioneurotic oedema are transmitted within a given kindred as autosomal dominant traits, the inheritance of the biochemical defect is more complicated. A majority of patients with this disorder are deficient for the antigenic and the functional properties of serum $C\bar{1}$ inhibitor, as if the protein were synthesized at a lower rate than normal. The remainder of patients (15–30%), however, have a normal or greater than normal serum concentration of a protein with the antigenic properties of the normal $C\bar{1}$ inhibitor, demonstrable by quantitative immunological assays, but the proteins upon which these antigenic determinants reside do not function. In addition, the nonfunctional forms of the inhibitor are heterogeneous. Some are able to block the digestion of synthetic amino acid esters by $C\bar{1}$, but not the destruction of C4 by $C\bar{1}$. Some bind to $C\bar{1}s$, others do not. A few kindred have nonfunctional proteins in their serum of normal electrophoretic mobility, some of slightly faster electrophoretic mobility, and some of very fast electrophoretic mobility. Another group has serum inhibitor demonstrable with immunoelectrophoretic assay as a 2 component protein, one of which represents the binding of the nonfunctional inhibitor to albumin. These individuals have a very high concentration (400% of the normal) of nonfunctional protein and no normal protein.

The deficiency of $C\bar{1}$ inhibitor in hereditary angioneurotic oedema is due to defects in biosynthesis of the protein. When radiolabelled purified normal serum inhibitor has been administered to persons with hereditary angioneurotic oedema in remission, the time for clearance of the protein from their plasma was not significantly different from the time for clearance of the protein from a normal individual's plasma. Therefore, the deficiency did not reflect an increased rate of catabolism or excretion. In addition, examination of hepatic cells, known to synthesize $C\bar{1}$ inhibitor in normal individuals, by immunofluorescent techniques revealed that the hepatic parenchymal cells of individuals with the decreased antigen variety of hereditary angioneurotic oedema failed to fluoresce significantly in sharp contrast to the fluorescence found in sections of normal livers. This observation provided support for the view that the deficiency of $C\bar{1}$ inhibitor is due to a failure of its synthesis. To date, there is no evidence of linkage of the genetic regulation of synthesis of serum $C\bar{1}$ inhibitor to that of other plasma proteins.

The therapy of hereditary angioneurotic oedema has recently provided added insights into the mechanism of the genetic regulation of synthesis of $C\bar{1}$ inhibitor. It has been known since 1961 that the administration of androgenic steroids could prevent the occurrence of the symptoms of hereditary angioneurotic oedema. It was our experience that treatment of patients with methyl testosterone accomplished this frequently, but not always, but did not significantly change the level of $C\bar{1}$ inhibitor in the serum of these patients in whom remission had been induced by this means. More recently, Gelfand and his colleagues used a nonmasculinizing anabolic steroid (danazol) which had been synthesized for use in the treatment of endometriosis. This induces the synthesis or release of normal $C\bar{1}$ inhibitor into the plasma of affected individuals. Coincident with the rise towards normal of the inhibitor, the symptoms of the disease remitted, and prolonged remission have been obtained. The secondary defects in C4 and C2, as well as the deficiency of $C\bar{1}$ inhibitor, were also corrected by this therapy. Once significant levels of inhibitor appear in the serum of these individuals, the action of $C\bar{1}$ is blocked, and C4 and C2 are no longer destroyed. More recently, Gadek and his associates have demonstrated that danazol can induce biosynthesis of normal serum inhibitor in patients with nonfunctional $C\bar{1}$ inhibitor in their blood in crossed immunoelectrophoretic studies. The nonfunctional inhibitor protein of abnormal electrophoretic mobility remains demonstrable during successful therapy, but a new peak of normal serum inhibitor appears in the serum of the patient. Thus, the therapy appears to allow the effective function of the normal gene which designates synthesis of a normal inhibitor. Since all individuals with hereditary angioneurotic oedema presently known are heterozygous for this defect, it has been difficult to explain the failure to find half normal levels of serum inhibitor antigens or of functional serum inhibitor in these persons (which is the dilemma in explaining many autosomal dominant traits). Since therapy with danazol apparently causes the appearance of normal serum inhibitor in significant concentrations in serum of these individuals, one might postulate that it in some way 'de-represses'' a genetic mechanism which is blocked from functioning in heterozygous individuals with hereditary angioneurotic oedema, but there is no proof for such a mechanism.

C1 subcomponent deficiency states

Three families with an inherited deficiency of C1r have been found. One was associated with chronic glomerulonephritis and depressed C1s levels. In a second case, the propositus was a 16-year-old boy with a lupus-like syndrome with malar rash, subacute focal membranous glomerulitis, arthralgia, and negative LE test. A female sibling also had recurrent fever and malar rash and was C1r deficient. While 5 other siblings are alive and well, 3 had died in childhood of overwhelming infections or lupus-like disease. In the propositus and his sister, C1s was also depressed. Functional and immunochemical studies of this family have shown the propositus and affected sister to be deficient in C1r, while parents and unaffected siblings have half normal or normal levels of C14. The establishment of heterozygous deficient individuals is not unambiguous because of the wide range of C1r concentration in normal sera. In a third case, the propositus was a 20-year-old male who presented with severe discoid lupus erythematosus involving the upper body, recurrent fevers and polyarthritis. A sister was similarly affected and also both C1r and C1s-deficient. Both siblings had a positive latex fixation test; the proposita's ANA test was negative while her brother's was positive. Two other affected siblings were well, as were 5 unaffected siblings. Three untested siblings died in childhood. In the 4 affected siblings, C1s was nearly absent also. A patient with a lupus-like disorder and deficiency of C1q has been reported, but this may be an acquired abnormality. In man, C1r deficiency segregates independently of HLA.

A 4-year-old Asian boy who presented with a lupus-like syndrome and glomerulonephritis was found to have absent serum haemolytic complement function even during remission. The serum complement activity was restored by purified C1q. A C1q-like protein was present in the serum, but was antigenically deficient and appeared to differ from normal in charge, mol. wt, chain structure and amino acid composition. This protein bound immune complexes, but did not activate C1r and C1s. This abnormal molecule was also found in several other family members, all of whom were well. Another propositus, a 10-year-old male, with recurrent skin lesions and chronic infections was found to have selective C1q deficiency. Though the C1q titres were normal in 8 of 9 family members, the propositus' maternal great grandmother and paternal grandmother, in whom C1q was reduced, were sisters. This child had antismooth muscle antibodies, circulating immune complexes and anti-HBsAg antibody and died of sepsis. *Post mortem* examination demonstrated mesangioproliferative glomerulonephritis.

C4 deficiency

An 18-year-old girl presenting with a lupus-like syndrome with malar rash, arthralgia and negative LE test, was found to be deficient in C4. The patient's mother had approximately half normal levels of C4. A 5-year-old male with fever, arthritis, and diffuse proliferative glomerulonephritis was C4 deficient by both functional and immunochemical assays. However, the identification of heterozygous deficient individuals is made difficult by the wide range of normal C4 levels. In this family, the obligate heterozygous deficient parents of the propositus had normal levels of C4.

This C4 deficient child showed diminished antibody formation after immunization with bacteriophage ΦX174 antigen and the secondary response showed neither the amplification nor the transition from IgM to IgG seen in normal controls. This patient also showed persistent lymphopaenia and T cell depletion as evidenced by a decreased percentage of erythrocyte rosette forming cells. In addition, the chemotactic index of the patient's granulocytes was low. This child also had SLE and was treated with cytotoxic drugs, making interpretation of these findings somewhat difficult. When the C4 deficient serum was incubated with zymosan or endotoxin to activate the alternative pathway, little chemotactic activity was generated. Restitution of this activity with purified C4 did not occur in Mg EGTA, suggesting that this patient was also deficient in an alternative pathway activity.

C2 deficiency

C2 deficiency (*C2*Q0*) is perhaps the most common complement deficiency. Its incidence in the population approaches 1 homozygous deficient individual/10 000 blood donors. In another study, 1·2% of random individuals were found to be heterozygous C2 deficient. First discovered in healthy individuals, homozygous C2 deficiency was next described in association with systemic lupus erythematosus, Henoch-Schönlein's purpura and polymyositis.

The normal range of serum levels of C2 is narrow enough that half normal levels lie outside the normal range. This has made possible the detection of heterozygous C2 deficient individuals. C2 deficiency is due to a silent allele at the C2 structural locus.

C3 deficiency

The existence of homozygous *C3*Q0* deficient individuals was predicted from the observation that individuals with half normal levels of C3 carried a silent allele of the C3 structural locus, *C3*Q0*. These heterozygous *C3*Q0* deficient individuals were healthy, but some had minor reductions in total haemolytic complement levels and there was suboptimal enhancement of phagocytosis of antibody-sensitized pneumococci by their sera. Later a 15-year-old female proposita with numerous episodes of pyogenic infections was discovered to have little or no detectable serum C3, but all other components of complement were present in normal concentrations. In this family, the parents of the proposita had half normal levels of C3. In the same Afrikaner population, another unrelated heterozygous C3 deficient and an unrelated homozygous C3 deficient individual were found. This suggests a high frequency of the *C3*Q0* allele in this population, possibly secondary to a "founder effect". In the first individual there was no leukocytosis in the face of sepsis. Nevertheless, skin lesions contained perivascular neutrophils. Several other C3-deficient individuals have been described. One had several episodes of pneumonia and has 1–2% normal concentration of C3 as a young child, but by the age of 5 her C3 level was that of other C3 deficient subjects, around 20 ng/ml (normal = 1–2 mg/ml). This child showed blunted leukocytosis. Two other partially C3 deficient children have had abnormalities of total haemolytic complement and phagocytic functions, but developed appropriate leukocytosis with bacterial infection.

In order to study the biochemical basis of C3 deficiency, the ability of monocytes from C3 deficient and normal individuals to synthesize C3 was compared. Monocytes from 2 C3-deficient individuals produced radiolabelled C3 protein at a rate of 20–30% of normal counterparts.

C3b inactivator (I) deficiency

Four individuals with inherited deficiency of I have been investigated. The first patient reported, who is now in his mid-30s, also has Klinefelter's syndrome. He has a lifelong history of severe infections with such organisms as *Diplococcus pneumoniae*, *Haemophilus influenzae*, and β-haemolytic streptococci. These infections have included septicaemia, pneumonia on several occasions, meningitis, sinusitis, and otitis media. Another patient is an 11-year-old girl who has had several episodes of meningitis, but no other serious infections. In a third family, 2 preteenage female siblings have I deficiency. One has had severe repeated meningococcal infections, while the other is entirely well. In individuals with absence of this inhibitor there is continuous activation of the alternative pathway *in vivo* and consumption of B and C3. Thus, native

C3 is markedly reduced and there is no detectable native B; C3b, Ba and Bb are found in fresh plasma. C5 and P levels are only minimally affected. The first patient's serum is deficient in haemolytic complement activity, bactericidal activity for smooth Gram negative organisms, opsonic activity for antibody sensitized pneumococci and endotoxin particles, and chemotaxis and the sera of the other patients show the same abnormalities.

That the I deficiency was the patient's primary defect and that the other protein deficiencies were secondary to their consumption was supported when the concentration of I declined exponentially after plasma infusion, whereas C3, B and C5 gradually rose. This was later confirmed when all the effects of whole plasma were mimicked by an infusion of purified I. P concentration, which was initially slightly low, also rose following the infusion of either plasma or I, but a metabolic study with labelled P failed to show increased catabolism in the patient's resting state. The concentration of I in the serum of his mother, 3 of his 6 siblings, and 2 nephews was approximately 40–50% the normal concentration. The father's serum could not be tested.

Dysfunctional BF

In a family reported for the occurrence of a rare BF allotype F0.55, functional haemolytic detection of BF bands on isoelectric focusing revealed the inability of the variant in serum from 5 heterozygotes to lyse guinea-pig red blood cells via the alternative pathway when C3 and D were supplied.

C5 deficiency

Three families with isolated deficiency of the fifth component of complement have been found. In the first, the proband, a black female, developed SLE at age 11 years with positive LE preparation and ANA test, hyper-γ-globulinaemia and renal biopsy showing focal nephritis. Later she developed cutaneous vasculitis and a second renal biopsy showed diffuse membranous glomerulonephritis. She also had prolonged localized herpes zoster, multiple skin infections and a single episode of enterococcal meningitis at age 18 years. A second C5 deficient half sibling (with 1–2% normal level of C5) had frequent infections in childhood, but was otherwise healthy. Family studies showed this defect to be inherited as an autosomal codominant trait. Total haemolytic complement in the serum of the apparent (obligate) heterozygotes was normal or elevated, indicating that heterozygous C5 deficiency would not be detected by this screening test. Obligate heterozygotes displayed haemolytic C5 levels 34–65% of the normal mean.

The proband mounted a marked peripheral blood leukocytosis on several occasions. Studies of the sera of both C5 deficient members of this family showed that they were unable to generate optimal chemotactic activity on incubation with aggregated γ globulin or *E. coli* endotoxin. This function was restored by addition of highly purified human C5 to normal serum concentrations.

Sera from 8 family members who were apparently heterozygous for C5 deficiency gave normal chemotactic scores and C5 homozygous deficient serum opsonized Baker's yeast, *Candida albicans*, or *Staphylococcus aureus* for ingestion and killing by neutrophils normally. The proband's serum failed to lyse erythrocytes from a patient with paroxysmal nocturnal haemoglobinuria and lacked bactericidal activity against sensitized and unsensitized *Salmonella typhi*, though serum from the C5 deficient half sister had some bactericidal activity (i.e., lysed *S. typhi*).

A second proband with C5 deficiency and her homozygous deficient twin sister both had disseminated gonococcaemia and recurrent fever and they had less than 2% of the normal serum level of C5. Neither had manifestations of collagen vascular disease. The mother, a brother, and his son had half normal levels of C5. Chemotactic activity for polymorphonuclear luekocytes could not be generated in the C5 deficient sera.

In a study of 2 families with known C5 deficiency, C6 polymorphism was informative in 17 meioses with at least 6 recombinations, excluding close linkage between C5 and C6. C5 deficiency in three families has not shown HLA linkage.

C6 deficiency

Hereditary deficiency of the sixth component of complement in man was first described in an 18-year-old black woman with Raynaud's phenomenon and recurrent gonococcal infection. Only C6 was absent and both parents and 5 of 6 siblings had approximately half normal levels of C6, suggesting Mendelian autosomal inheritance. The C6 deficient serum of the proband lacked whole haemolytic complement and bactericidal activity against *S. typhi* and *H. influenzae* and lacked ability to mediate lysis of red cells from patients with paroxysmal nocturnal haemoglobinuria in acidified serum or the sugar water test. These deficiencies were corrected by addition of purified human C6 to the serum. The serum exhibited normal capacity to generate chemotactic activity on incubation with bacterial endotoxin or aggregated IgG. The proposita had normal coagulation functions.

The second patient with inherited deficiency of C6 was a 6-year-old black male with meningococcal meningitis and a third black patient with recurrent meningococcal meningitis has been found. In a fourth family, the C6 deficient proband, a black female, presented with recurrent *Neisserial* infections. However, heterozygous C6 deficiency defined by half normal serum level of C6 transmitted in a family and confirmed by anomalous inheritance of C6 allotypes (similar to C3 deficiency and C2 deficiency) has been observed in whites, as well as blacks, and demonstrated deficiency of C6 to be allelic with the C6 structural locus.

C7 deficiency

Deficiency of C7 is also inherited as an autosomal trait. In a Caucasian woman with severe Raynaud's phenomenon, sclerodactyly and telangiectasia, C7 was around 10% of normal. About half normal levels were found in the serum of the patient's parents and children. This patient did not have increased susceptibility to infection, but was among a large number of patients with immunologic diseases who were screened for complement abnormalities.

In another report, a 13-year-old male lacked detectable C7 in his serum. His parents were first cousins. He was well and had been admitted to donate bone marrow for his sister with acquired a-γ-globulinaemia and lymphocytopaenia. Both parents and one sister had half normal serum levels of C7 and a C7-inactivating principle was found. Apparently C7 deficient serum is normal with respect to opsonizing activity, immune adherence, and the ability to generate chemotactic activity, but bactericidal and haemolytic activity are absent.

The third report of C7 deficiency was of a 44-year-old Caucasian woman with HLAB 27 positive ankylosing spondylitis who was deficient in C7, determined by both haemolytic and immunochemical methods. In this case, no C7 inhibitor was detected and opsonic and coagulation studies were normal. Numerous relatives were found with half normal levels of C7 and two well siblings were also homozygous C7 deficient. None of the 3 showed an unusual susceptibility to infection. Some members of the family also had an inherited partial deficiency of C2.

A fourth case of C7 deficiency in a 46-year-old black female with renal disease and recurrent urinary infection has been described. A C7 inactivator was detected, but appeared to be $C\overline{56}$.

In other reports there was an association between C7 deficiency and recurrent *Neisseria* infection, an association between C7 deficiency and SLE, and one case associated with recurrent meningococcal meningitis.

Finally, a single case has been reported of a healthy propositus with low, but detectable levels of both C6 (1%) and C7 (8%). Family study demonstrated both deficiencies to be inherited together. This combined defect may have important genetic implications in that there may be a common gene regulating biosynthesis of these 2 proteins produced by closely linked genes. Other possible mechanisms by which this combined defect originated include unequal crossing over with loss of part of both genes and the normal production of C6 and C7 by a single "supergene" with postsynthetic processing of a single polypeptide chain product into the 2 serum complement components. C7 polymorphism and deficiency do not appear to be HLA linked.

C8 deficiency

Several reports of C8 deficiency have appeared. A black woman with disseminated gonococcal infection was discovered to lack normal ability to promote haemolysis of sensitized sheep erythrocytes. No inhibitor of C8 was detected. Her fresh serum lacked bacterial activity against *Neisseria gonorrhoeae*, but purified C8 restored this activity. This serum was normal with regard to opsonization of yeast particles and staphylococci and ability to generate chemotactic activity. Blood coagulation was normal. Inheritance of the defect in this family was consistent with an autosomal trait and heterozygous deficient family members were identified by half normal levels of C8. However, subsequent analysis of C8 allotypes in this family showed misidentification both of normal and deficient family members, suggesting that half normal levels are not sufficient criteria for identification of heterozygous C8 deficient individuals, because of the wide range of serum C8 concentrations in normals.

In a second instance the proposita had xeroderma pigmentosum. Both parents had normal C8 serum concentration, but she had 2 siblings who were also C8 deficient. Subsequent analysis of C8 allotypes in this family confirmed the impression that C8 deficient heterozygous individuals may have C8 levels within 2 standard deviations of the normal mean, making their ascertainment difficult. This deficient subject had no unusual infection.

The third case of C8 deficiency was associated with SLE. A 56-year-old black woman presented with malar rash, polyarthritis, and nephronic syndrome and her serum had characteristics like that of the first described patient.

Two further brief reports of C8 deficiency have appeared, one in a patient with thalassaemia, and another of a 27-year-old male with a history of gonococcal endocarditis and staphylococcal sepsis who had C8 less than 1%, as did his healthy mother. All siblings and half siblings had serum C8 levels between 62% and 92% of normal.

A family with antigenically detectable, though functionally inactive, C8 had also been observed. A second patient has been described with recurrent meningococcal infection and his serum also contained abnormal C8 which lacked some of the antigenic determinants of normal C8.

C9 deficiency

A 76-year-old white male was found to have low total haemolytic activity in serum and plasma. All the components of complement were normal or elevated by functional haemolytic assay except C9. C9 antigen was undetectable. The patient had no unusual propensity to infection. A family study demonstrated autosomal inheritance and lack of linkage to HLA. C9 deficient serum mediated lysis of sensitized sheep cells more slowly than normal sera. Bactericidal activity was likewise slower, but approached normal with longer incubation times. A second unrelated asymptomatic elderly person with complete deficiency of C9 has been identified by the same group of investigators.

Immunologic disease associations

Numerous observations have been made of the association of inherited complement component deficiency states and immunologic diseases. Whether this association is causative or fortuitous is not clear. Large numbers of patients with rheumatic diseases have been screened for complement abnormalities, in part because acquired abnormalities of complement are used to diagnose and monitor some of these disease states. While patients with homozygous deficiency states are rare, those with heterozygous states are necessarily much more common. For C2 deficiency, the predicted incidence from homozygous deficiency and from screening random blood donors for heterozygous deficiency is about 1 in 50 to 1 in 100 of the population. If this is so, then systemic lupus erythematosus (SLE) occurs 2–3 times more frequently among heterozygous C2 deficient individuals than in the normal population. In 38 reported homozygous C2 deficient individuals, 23 had autoimmune diseases, of which 14 had SLE or discoid lupus. Whether this predisposition to lupus in C2 deficient individuals is secondary to an abnormal function of the complement system is not clear. Of note, homozygous C2 deficient relatives of propositi have a lower incidence of autoimmune disease than the propositi, suggesting bias in ascertainment. Alternatively, this predisposition may be due to linkage disequilibrium of the C2 deficiency genes to postulated immune response genes in the MHC. This possibility is also supported by data suggesting viral infection as aetiologic in lupus. Several patients with $C\bar{1}$ inhibitor deficiency have also been reported with systemic or discoid lupus erythematosus.

Though patients with homozygous deficiency of C5 and C8 have been reported with immune complex diseases, no adequate theory to explain this association has been advanced. On the other hand, the association of homozygous defects of the early complement components, C1r, $C\bar{1}$ inhibitor, C4, C2 and C3, with possible immune complex disease may be due to the defect in itself, since complement is necessary for the solubilization of immune complexes. In addition, antibody-independent lysis of oncornaviruses does not occur in C2 or C4 deficient sera, though it does in normal sera.

Theme 18: Summary

Human and Experimental Immunopathology

R. J. WINCHESTER

The Rockefeller University, New York, USA

The diverse subjects of Theme 18 had as their unifying principle the mechanism of diseases with immune features and diseases of the immune system itself.

One group of disorders that were discussed share the fact that their susceptibility is influenced by alleles of the major histocompatibility complex, but that there is no clearly defined environmental cause.

Systemic lupus erythematosus (SLE)

In the instance of SLE and the related family of diseases, the antibody aspect of both the human and murine lupus-like disease has provided the most clearly etched findings.

The application of hybridoma methodology to the analysis of naturally occurring autoantibodies in strains of mice with "lupus-like" disorders has been initiated in a number of laboratories. This approach affords an important opportunity to examine the immune response of these animals from a clonal point of view with emphasis on both precise specificities and avidities of the combining sites as well as on the *V* and *J* gene repertoire from which the autoantibodies are constructed. The extraordinary leap in resolution that was evident in the Scatchard and competitive inhibition plots of anti-DNA antibodies made for the confidence that this aspect of the field was poised on the threshold of a most exciting era.

In human SLE the nature of the various antigens to which the antinuclear antibodies are directed was also the subject of very considerable interest. This was particularly the case with antibodies directed to nuclear antigens other than those of the classic DNA type. For example, certain sera contain antibodies with specificities for components of the centromere: one variety reacts with the special 4-6S DNA found only in the centromere and another specificity reacts with protein subunits found within the centromere. Another example is that antinuclear antibodies with specificity for ribonucleoprotein appear to be directed to gene splicing enzymes. In the same vein, evidence was presented that antibodies to the SM antigen are directed to topoisomerases responsible for the uncoiling of the DNA superhelix.

The meaning of the development of antibodies for these enzymes remains the subject of intriguing speculation, particularly since similar enzymes are found in certain viruses.

Multiple sclerosis (MS)

In the area of multiple sclerosis research it has proved difficult to advance evidence for an immune mechanism. A number of laboratories confirmed the tantalizing finding of elevated levels in blood and CSF (cerebrospinal fluid) of T lymphocytes with the suppressor phenotype. These fall sharply during acute exacerbation of the disease only to rise again. However, the significance of this characteristic remains undeciphered.

An elevation CSF IgG is a diagnostic feature of multiple sclerosis. An intriguing feature of this elevation is that it is oligoclonal in character, a fact demonstrated particularly well by isoelectric focusing. The idiotypes of the bands have not been demonstrated to share specificities. Thus far, the only antibody activity demonstrable in them was to components of a normal brain. Nonetheless, it is difficult to abandon the hope that the bands hold a real clue for determining if there is a viral agent underlying MS.

From the approach of laboratory models of multiple sclerosis a new direction in the field of experimental allergic encephalitis involved the development of a chronic remitting, severely demyelinating encephalitis model. The immunogen found in whole brain was shown to be unrelated to myelin basic protein and to be of a highly labile nature. The development of the disease was dependent on host age and genetic factors. Its characteristics suggest that it may provide an improved model for the demyelinating diseases.

Antireceptor antibodies

One of the areas which evoked far ranging discussion was the topic of antireceptor antibodies. These antibodies have been found in a wide variety of diseases in which altered immunity is evident and at least in some they may play an important role. For example, in patients with myasthenia gravis or occasional patients with insulin resistant diabetes mellitus, antibodies to the acetyl choline or insulin receptor are associated with marked functional inhibition of the target cell. This leads to muscle paralysis or failure of insulin secretion. Reciprocally, the antireceptor antibodies under other circumstances result in stimulation of the target organ. Here, perhaps the best example is in thyrotoxicosis where antibodies directed to components of the thyroid stimulating hormone (TSH) receptor, evoke thyroid enlargement as well as endocrine overactivity. These precisely mimic the actions of TSH, a fact that favours the parallel between these antibodies and anti-idiotypes. Furthermore, another important thyroid antigen previously thought to be restricted to the microsomal fraction has been identified on the cell surface making a pathogenetic role far easier to comprehend.

One common characteristic of many of the antireceptor antibodies is that they have restricted light and heavy chain specificities. This raises the possibility of searching for cross-reactive idiotypes and could lead to further insights into their mechanisms of production. Susceptibility to the major diseases with antireceptor antibodies is known to be associated with particular alleles of the major histocompatibility complex. This raises the question of whether the basis of the disease stems from the recognition of a particular receptor antigen in the context of Ia allotypes expressed on the macrophage.

Tropical and parasitic diseases

The vast group of tropical and parasitic diseases stand in complete contrast to the previous conditions because of the unambiguous presence of an inciting organism. And by definition, the immune response is ineffective and often protracted.

Immunoreactants abound, including circulating and organism-associated immune complexes, as well as autoantibodies. The autoantibodies have specifities for antinuclear and various cell membrane determinants. However, these autoantibodies remain as yet unincriminated as proximate causes of tissue injury. In contrast to diseases like multiple sclerosis and diabetes mellitus, where one struggles to identify immune phenomena that would be relevant to pathogenesis, here the cornucopia is filled with phenomena as well as the presence of an inciting organism.

A number of studies were centred on the purification of antigens from the inciting organisms. These antigens are being used to dissect the elements of the complex host immune responses to the parasite. Particular success is being met with in studies on leprosy. This chemical reductionist approach should soon allow the posing of appropriate questions regarding the role of the immune system in determining susceptibility resistance and mediating some of the complications of parasitic and tropical diseases.

Intestinal immune system

The martial aspect of the immune response as mediator of disease and defender against hostile micro-organisms assumed a more gentle and conservative role in the sessions on the role of the intestinal immune system. Here one sees it is a homeostatic suppression in the sense of Claude Bernard. IgA antibodies to food antigens received emphasis as a physiological means of clearing the circulation of normally absorbed macromolecular food components such as β-lactoglobulin. The complexes of IgA and food antigens circulated briefly. In contrast, in states of food allergy, the offending antigens circulate complexed to IgG as well as IgA antibodies.

The "Chase phenomenon" or systemic hyporesponsiveness to antigens originally presented by an oral route, was shown not to depend on serum factors involving IgA complexes, as was thought previously. Rather the phenomenon has been related to the generation of large numbers of suppressor T cells that seed to the nongut associated lymphoid system. This finding fits well with the previous observations on the physiological role of IgA and provided a mechanism for its occurrence.

Several diseases were known to be characterized by the deposition of IgA on the kidney glomerulus and certain of these are known to be MHC linked. These include Berger's disease, Henoch-Schoenlein purpura, and the nephropathy of alcoholic cirrhosis. This IgA was characterized as being primarily of the IgA2 class and polymeric, a finding that suggests the IgA could originate from the gastrointestinal tract, possibly representing an immune complex involving a mucosal or enteric antigen.

Immunoproliferative diseases

The interrelationships of clinical and basic immunology have nowhere been as great as in the realm of immunoproliferative diseases, first with multiple myeloma and now with the leukaemias and lymphomas. The concept of leukaemia as a malignant transformation of a cell that freezes it at a particular point in its lineage is well established. In particular, the acute leukaemia have served to permit studies of precursor cells that would otherwise be extremely difficult because of their low frequency.

For example, studies of the acute lymphatic leukaemic cell led to the concept of a pre-B cell expression an H-chain gene produced intracellularly in the absence of L chains. This finding has been confirmed and its genetic basis delineated by recombinant DNA technology. Using these leukaemias, it was demonstrated that the H chain genes are selectively rearranged into functional units while the L chain genes are arrested in the extended germ line configuration.

Of course, the concept of the distinct nature of T and B lineages is well established even getting the support of recombinant DNA technology with which it has been demonstrated that the *Ig* genes of T cell chronic lymphatic leukaemias are still in the germ line configuration. However, the irrevocable nature of this commitment to T or B lineage has been questioned by perplexing reports on "hairy" cell leukaemia. Here the hairy cells which expressed surface Ig, typically IgD, were induced to express T cell markers and lose their Ig.

What is a leukaemia or a lymphoma? The phenomenologic criteria of recent years have included tissue invasion and death of the untreated patient. This question was the subject of an interesting discussion in which the use of the more sophisticated definitions of an monoclonal nature of the proliferation and the presence of chromosomal abnormalities were advocated as primary markers of malignancy. This point was in turn questioned as being only a late selective consequence of the malignant proliferations that reflect the preponderant growth of the most anaplasic clone.

Evidence was brought forward that in the early stages of immunoangioblastic lymphoma or progressive infectious mononucleosis disease the earliest recognizable stage could be characterized as being polyclonal or more properly oligoclonal, due to the presence of κ and λ type cells. The issue was not resolved but precedent for an oligoclonal origin exists in studies of *in vitro* transformation of lymphocytes by EB virus as well as in the classic Potter studies of the induction of myelomas in BALB/c mice.

Conclusion

In summary, the process of physicochemical reduction of disease phenomena is progressing surely, if also slowly, like the inexorable advance of pawns. Yet somehow it is not quite enough. Perhaps what we need is a series of intellectual knight's moves—bold and far-reaching. There is no doubt that in these diseases we have the answers to some of the most fascinating questions of immunology ... If only we could discuss what was the exact question that was being asked.

The assistance of the Workshop chairmen, and Drs Seligmann, Ballet, Clot and Hurez in the preparation of this report is gratefully acknowledged.

Subject Index

D

E

R

S

U